# Clinical Anatomy and Physiology for Veterinary Technicians

# Clinical Anatomy and Physiology for Veterinary Technicians

## Third Edition

**Thomas Colville, DVM, MSc**
Attending Veterinarian
Red River Zoo
Fargo, North Dakota

**Joanna M. Bassert, VMD**
Program Director and Professor
Program of Veterinary Technology
Manor College
Jenkintown, Pennsylvania

ELSEVIER

# ELSEVIER

3251 Riverport Lane
St. Louis, Missouri 63043

---

**Notices**

Knowledge and best practice in this field are constantly changing. As new research and experience broaden
our understanding, changes in research methods, professional practices, or medical treatment may become
necessary.

Practitioners and researchers must always rely on their own experience and knowledge in evaluating and
using any information, methods, compounds, or experiments described herein. In using such information
or methods they should be mindful of their own safety and the safety of others, including parties for
whom they have a professional responsibility.

With respect to any drug or pharmaceutical products identified, readers are advised to check the most
current information provided (i) on procedures featured or (ii) by the manufacturer of each product to be
administered, to verify the recommended dose or formula, the method and duration of administration,
and contraindications. It is the responsibility of practitioners, relying on their own experience and
knowledge of their patients, to make diagnoses, to determine dosages and the best treatment for each
individual patient, and to take all appropriate safety precautions.

To the fullest extent of the law, neither the Publisher nor the authors, contributors, or editors, assume
any liability for any injury and/or damage to persons or property as a matter of products liability,
negligence or otherwise, or from any use or operation of any methods, products, instructions, or ideas
contained in the material herein.

---

**Previous editions copyright © 2008, 2002.**
**Library of Congress Cataloging-in-Publication Data**

Colville, Thomas P., author.
    Clinical anatomy and physiology for veterinary technicians / Thomas Colville, Joanna M. Bassert.—Third edition.
      p. ; cm.
    Includes bibliographical references and index.
    ISBN 978-0-323-22793-3 (pbk. : alk. paper)    1. Veterinary anatomy.    2. Veterinary physiology.    I. Bassert,
Joanna M., author.    II. Title.
    [DNLM:    1. Animals, Domestic—anatomy & histology.    2. Animal Technicians.    3. Animals,
Domestic—physiology.  SF 761]
    SF761.C65 2016
    636.089'1—dc23
                                                                              2015002278

*Content Strategist:* Shelly Stringer
*Content Development Manager:* Ellen Wurm-Cutter
*Senior Content Development Specialist:* Maria Broeker
*Publishing Services Manager:* Catherine Jackson
*Senior Project Manager:* Rachel E. McMullen
*Designer:* Ashley Miner

Printed in Canada

Last digit is the print number:    9    8    7    6    5    4    3    2    1

Working together
to grow libraries in
developing countries

www.elsevier.com • www.bookaid.org

*To Amy Ellwein, Amy Jordahl, Carolyn Colville,*
*Erick Lamun, Erin Teravskis, Gary Stende, Janelle Meyer,*
*Jennifer Jacobsen, Jeff Colville, Jeremiah Gard, Joanie Knab,*
*Kelsey Hoium-Johnson, Linda Goos, Linda Wilm, Lisa Tate,*
*Marcy Thompson, Nathan Schlagel, Nicole Lee, Peggy Gaynor,*
*Rachel Fritz, Raina Fritz, Sally Jacobson, Samantha Bruers—family, friends,*
*and colleagues who inspire me.*

**Tom Colville**

*To my students and colleagues at Manor College who inspire me.*

**Joanna M. Bassert**

# Contributors

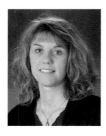

**Lori R. Arent, MS**
Clinic Manager
The Raptor Center,
College of Veterinary Medicine
University of Minnesota
St. Paul, Minnesota

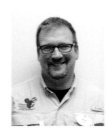

**Ryan DeVoe, DVM, MSpVM, Dipl ACZM-Avian**
Senior Veterinarian
North Carolina Zoological Park
Asheboro, North Carolina

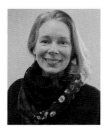

**Joanna M. Bassert, VMD**
Program Director and Professor
Program of Veterinary Technology
Manor College
Jenkintown, Pennsylvania

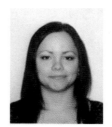

**Christina Jeffries, AAS, BVSc**
Veterinary Technology Instructor
Pima Medical Institute
Certified Veterinary Technician
Valley Animal Hospital
Tucson, Arizona

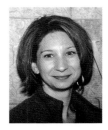

**Angela Beal, DVM**
Program Director
Vet Tech Institute at Bradford School
Columbus, Ohio

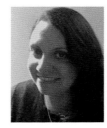

**Jennifer A. Maniet, BS, DVM**
Instructor, Program of Veterinary Technology
Manor College
Jenkintown, Pennsylvania

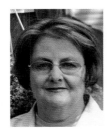

**Joann Colville, DVM**
North Dakota State University
Veterinary Technology Program
(Retired)
Fargo, North Dakota

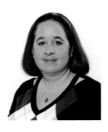

**Morgan Rodgers, CVT**
Veterinary Technology Instructor
Pima Medical Institute
Tucson, Arizona

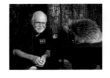

**Thomas Colville, DVM, MSc**
Attending Veterinarian
Red River Zoo
Fargo, North Dakota

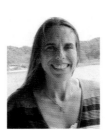

**Sabrina Maria Timperman, DVM**
Assistant Professor
Veterinary Technology
Mercy College
Dobbs Ferry, New York

# Preface

Textbooks are, by their nature, works in progress. Each published edition is an updated snapshot of that ongoing process. To make this edition of the book relevant and useful to students and instructors, we had to address some difficult questions such as: what material from the preceding edition should be retained, and what should be left out? What new knowledge and terminology should replace older information? What new features would make the book more useful? How has clinical veterinary technology changed since the last edition?

This third edition continues the logical progression from the first edition to the second edition. Popular features, such as "Test Yourself" boxes, a complete glossary of anatomy and physiology terms, "Clinical Application" boxes, and much of the original content have been retained. The accompanying Laboratory Manual has been revised for this edition and now includes critical thinking activities. The Laboratory Manual is filled with interactive exercises, step-by-step guidelines, and full-color photos and illustrations. It is designed to enhance understanding of A&P in in the clinical setting and allows for the application of knowledge in the laboratory setting.

New features and expanded content in this edition include:

- The sequence of the chapters has been reordered.
- All chapters were revised and updated, and many illustrations were added.
- The Amazing Cell chapter from the second edition has been divided into two separate chapters: Anatomical Structure of the Cell and Physiology of the Cell.
- The Blood, Lymph, and Immunity chapter from the second edition has been divided into two separate chapters: Blood, Lymph, and Lymph Nodes and Immunity and Defense.
- "Vocabulary Fundamentals," a listing of key terms with phonetic pronunciations, has been added to each chapter. This pronunciation system is an easy-to-learn approach for mastering the sounds of veterinary language. It is not overloaded with linguistic marks and variables. The following rules apply:
  1. Hyphens are used to separate syllables.
  2. Stressed syllables are noted in bold type, as in **class**-room.

3. Any vowel that has a dash above it represents the long sound:

| ā | as in | sāy |
| ē | as in | wē |
| ī | as in | pīe |
| ō | as in | gō |
| ū | as in | ūniform |

4. Any vowel that is followed by the letter "h" represents the short sound:

| ah | as in | about |
| eh | as in | pet |
| ih | as in | pit |
| oh | as in | hot |
| uh | as in | mutt |

5. Unique vowel combinations are as follows:

| aw | as in | caught |
| eər | as in | care |
| eer | as in | here |
| ər | as in | butter |
| oo | as in | loot |
| ou | as in | out |
| oy | as in | boy |

- Evolve Resources
  - Instructor resources include a 1000 question test bank in ExamView format with rationales. Two image collections are included; one with all figures from the textbook and the second with all figures from the Laboratory Manual. A PowerPoint collection is arranged chapter-by-chapter with the textbook. The answers to the Laboratory Manual are available. Instructors also have access to all student resources.
  - Student resources include Chapter Summaries, Test Yourself Answers, and Crosswords that correspond to each chapter of the Laboratory Manual.

Our goal for this third edition continues what we have undertaken from the start: to provide a practical, interesting, clinically relevant source of veterinary anatomy and physiology information to you, the reader. We hope it will foster an appreciation for the elegant organization, intricate relationships, and functional beauty of the wonderful living machine that is the animal body.

# Acknowledgments

This book was a continuation of the team effort that produced the first two editions, and we would like to acknowledge the contributions of new and returning people who helped make it possible. Dr. Bassert's students Amanda Arduino, Krista Gabarro, Amanda Hadley, Melena Petit, Bernadette Rogers, and Samantha McWilliams offered invaluable suggestions and assembled several of the chapter outlines for the Evolve site. Dr. Joann Colville returned to revise and edit several chapters. Lori Arent, MS and Dr. Ryan DeVoe returned to enhance their chapters from previous editions. We also welcomed new contributors Dr. Angela Beal, Christina Jeffries, CVT, Dr. Jennifer Maniet, Morgan Rodgers, CVT, and Dr. Sabrina Timperman. We thank Sharon Oien for preparing phonetic pronunciations for the Vocabulary Fundamentals section of each chapter. Before her retirement, Teri Merchant, our editor at Elsevier for the first two editions of this book, started this edition taxiing toward the runway. Shelly Stringer, Maria Broeker, and Rachel McMullen ably took over the controls and, through persistence, good humor, and more than a little cajoling, got the project off the ground. To each of these individuals, and others who aided the book's progress, we express our sincere gratitude and appreciation for a job well done!

Finally, we would like to once again thank our families for tolerating the many hours we spent working on this book. Their encouragement and understanding helped make the book possible.

# Vet Tech Threads

With this revision of *Clinical Anatomy and Physiology for Veterinary Technicians,* we continue using features and design elements that are shared with other vet tech titles on the Mosby and Saunders lists. The purpose of the "Vet Tech Threads" is to make it easier for students and instructors to incorporate multiple books into the fast-paced and demanding vet tech curriculum.

The shared features in *Clinical Anatomy and Physiology for Veterinary Technicians,* Third Edition, include the following:

- Cover and internal **design similarities:** the colorful, student-friendly design encourages reading and learning of the core content

- A **Chapter Outline** and list of **Objectives** begins each chapter
- **Clinical Application** boxes demonstrate clinical relevance of anatomy and physiology principles
- An extensive **Glossary** of the key terms at the end of the text

# Contents

# 1 Introduction to Anatomy and Physiology

*Thomas Colville*

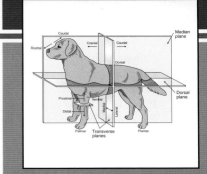

## OUTLINE

## LEARNING OBJECTIVES

*When you have completed this chapter, you will be able to:*

1. Define the terms *anatomy* and *physiology*.
2. Differentiate between microscopic and macroscopic anatomy.
3. Differentiate between the study of regional anatomy and the study of systemic anatomy.
4. Describe the four anatomic planes of reference.
5. List and describe the anatomic terms of direction.
6. List and describe common regional terms for the body.
7. List the components of the dorsal body cavity.
8. List the components of the ventral body cavity.
9. List the four basic types of body tissue.
10. Define *homeostasis*.

## VOCABULARY FUNDAMENTALS

*Adipose* **ahd**-ih-pōs
*Anatomy* ah-**naht**-ah-mē
*Anterior* ahn-**teer**-ē-ər
*Barrel* **beər**-uhl
*Bilateral symmetry* bī-**laht**-ər-ahl **sihm**-ih-trē
*Brisket* **brihs**-kiht
*Cannon* **kahn**-nuhn
*Cardiac muscle* **kahr**-dē-ahck **muhs**-uhl
*Carpus* **kahr**-puhs
*Caudal* **kaw**-dahl
*Connective tissue* kuh-**nehck**-tihv **tihsh**-yoo
*Cranial* **krā**-nē-ahl
*Cranium* **krā**-nē-uhm
*Deep* dēp
*Digestive system* dih-**jehs**-tihv **sihs**-tehm
*Distal* **dihs**-tahl
*Dorsal* **dohr**-sahl
*Dorsal body cavity* **dohr**-sahl **boh**-dē **kahv**-ih-tē
*Dorsal plane* **dohr**-sahl plān
*Epithelial tissue* ehp-ih-**thē**-lē-ahl **tihsh**-yoo
*Equilibrium* ē-kwuh-**lihb**-rē-uhm
*External* ehcks-**tər**-nahl

*Fetlock* **feht**-lohck
*Fight or flight system* fīt *or* flīt **sihs**-tehm
*Flank* flahngk
*Gastrointestinal (GI) tract* gahs-trō-ihn-**tehs**-tih-nahl trahkt
*Gross anatomy* grōs ah-**naht**-ah-mē
*Health* hehlth
*Hock* hohck
*Homeostasis* **hō**-mē-ō-**stā**-sihs
*Inferior* ihn-**feer**-ē-ər
*Inflammation* ihn-fluh-**mā**-shuhn
*Internal* ihn-**tər**-nahl
*Knee—carpus of hoofed animals* nē—**kahr**-puhs *of* hooft **ahn**-uh-muhlz
*Lateral* **laht**-ər-ahl
*Macroscopic anatomy* mah-krō-**skohp**-ihck ah-**naht**-ah-mē
*Medial* **mē**-dē-ahl
*Medial plane* **mē**-dē-ahl plān
*Microscopic anatomy* mī-krō-**skohp**-ihk ah-**naht**-ah-mē
*Muscle tissue* **muhs**-uhl **tihsh**-yoo
*Organ* **ohr**-gahn

*Palmar* **pahl**-mər
*Parietal layer* pah-**rī**-eh-tahl **lā**-ər
*Pastern* **pahs**-tərn
*Physiology* fihz-ē-**ohl**-uh-jē
*Plane of reference* plān *of* **rehf**-ər-uhnz
*Plantar* **plahn**-tahr
*Pleura* **ploor**-ah
*Poll* pōl
*Posterior* pō-**steer**-ē-ər
*Proximal* **prohck**-sih-mahl
*Regional anatomy* **rē**-juhn-ahl ah-**naht**-ah-mē
*Rostral* **rohs**-trahl
*Sagittal plane* **sahj**-ih-tahl plān
*Skeletal muscle* **skehl**-ih-tahl **muhs**-uhl
*Smooth muscle* smooth **muhs**-uhl
*Spinal canal* **spī**-nahl kuh-**nahl**
*Stifle* **stī**-fuhl

*Superficial* soo-pər-**fihsh**-ahl
*Superior* suh-**peer**-ē-ər
*System* **sihs**-tehm
*Systematic anatomy* sihs-tuh-**maht**-ihck ah-**naht**-ah-mē
*Tailhead* **tā**-uhl-hehd
*Tarsus* **tahr**-suhs
*Thorax* **thohr**-ahx
*Tissue* **tihsh**-yoo
*Transverse plane* trahnz-**vərs** plān
*Ventral* **vehn**-trahl
*Ventral body cavity* **vehn**-trahl **boh**-dē **kahv**-ih-tē
*Viscera* vih-**sər**-ah
*Visceral layer* **vih**-sər-ahl **lā**-ər
*Withers* **wihth**-ərz
*Xiphoid process* **zī**-foyd **proh**-sehs

## INTRODUCTION

Life is a tricky proposition. It is difficult, messy, fragile, and a lot of work. The bodies of living animals have to be organized just right and maintained within very narrow limits to allow the hectic choreography of life to unfold throughout their lives.

We don't usually think of animals as living mechanisms, but the study of anatomy and physiology is really the study of the animal machine, what makes it up, and how the whole thing works. The language of anatomy and physiology uses terms like *cells, tissues, organs,* and *systems,* but we're really talking about the component parts of this living machine. These living parts are amazingly intricate and their functions delicately interrelated. As veterinary health care professionals, we must understand how animals are put together and how their bodies work. Fortunately, the animal body is fascinating to study in and of itself, but even more so when we appreciate how important normal anatomy and physiology are to animal health.

The various parts of the body must work together in near-perfect harmony to maintain the life and well-being of an animal. The interesting part of this truth is that the apparently simple and automatic states of life and health are not as they seem. Life is not simple, and health is not automatic. Life is extraordinarily complicated, and health is the result of numerous things going just right. At first glance it seems as though health is the normal state of affairs, and disease and death result from some awful *outside* influences attacking the body. However, outside influences alone usually play smaller roles than we might think. Disease and death often result from the *absence of normal body structure and functioning.* Normal anatomy and physiology are critical to an animal's health and survival, and our knowledge of them is critical to our ability to *influence* the animal's health and survival in cases of disease or injury.

## ANATOMY AND PHYSIOLOGY

Anatomy and physiology describe two complementary but different ways to look at the animal body. **Anatomy** deals with the *form and structure* of the body and its parts—what things look like and where they are located. **Physiology** deals with the *functions* of the body and its parts—how things work and what they do. They can be studied as separate subjects, but such an approach makes it difficult to gain a complete picture of how the amazing animal machine works. This book examines anatomy *and* physiology together as we go along.

We can approach the study of anatomy in different ways, for example *microscopic anatomy* versus *macroscopic anatomy.* **Microscopic anatomy** deals with structures so small we need a microscope to see them clearly, such as cells and tissues.

**Macroscopic anatomy**, also called **gross anatomy**, deals with body parts large enough to be seen with the unaided eye, such as organs, muscles, and bones. Both aspects are presented in this book as we examine the animal body in detail. We also delve into the submicroscopic level occasionally to explain things occurring at the microscopic and macroscopic levels. Discussions at the submicroscopic level include the components that make up cells and the chemical molecules and ions that serve important roles in the body.

Another way to approach anatomy is to study individual *regions* of the body (**regional anatomy**) versus individual *systems* of the body (**systemic anatomy**). In the regional approach, all the components of each region of the body are examined; for example, the anatomy of the neck (*cervical*) region would include all the cells, tissues, blood vessels,

| TABLE 1-1 | Main Body Systems |
| --- | --- |
| **SYSTEM** | **MAIN COMPONENTS** |
| Skeletal | Bones and joints |
| Integumentary | Skin, hair, nails, and hooves |
| Nervous | Central nervous system and peripheral nerves |
| Cardiovascular | Heart and blood vessels |
| Respiratory | Lungs and air passageways |
| Digestive | Gastrointestinal tube and accessory digestive organs |
| Muscular | Skeletal, cardiac, and smooth muscle |
| Sensory | Organs of general and special sense |
| Endocrine | Endocrine glands and hormones |
| Urinary | Kidneys, ureters, urinary bladder, and urethra |
| Reproductive | Male and female reproductive structures |

nerves, muscles, organs, and bones present in the neck. The problem is that the body is not always easy to subdivide this way, and there is often overlap between adjacent regions; that is, where does the neck region end and the shoulder region begin? It's not always clear.

The systematic approach to anatomy, however, deals with the systems of the body, such as the nervous system and the skeletal system, as separate topics. The many interrelationships between the body systems can be described as the systems are examined. This approach lets us look at the whole body by breaking it down into clear, logical components. The main systems of the body are listed in Table 1-1. We will take a systematic approach to anatomy and physiology in this book, and in addition to these systems, we examine cells, epithelial and connective tissues, and blood, lymph, and immunity.

---

✓ **TEST YOURSELF 1-1**

1. How does the anatomy of a muscle or bone differ from its physiology? Which describes appearance and location and which describes function?
2. How might abnormalities in an animal's anatomy or physiology have a negative impact on its health and well-being?

---

## TERMINOLOGY

To be clear and accurate with descriptions of body parts, we have to use terms that leave no doubt about their meanings. Terms such as *up, down, above, below,* and *beside* are not very useful because they depend on the orientation of the animal (upright, on its side, on its back, and so on). If an animal is lying on its left side, is its right lung *above* its left lung or *beside* it? If the animal stands up, what is the relationship between the lungs then? Even the position of the observer can make a difference in terms such as *left* and *right.* If a structure in an animal is located "to the right" of another structure, does the meaning change if

the observer is facing the animal head-on or facing the same direction as the animal? Anatomic terms must have the same meaning regardless of the orientation of the animal or the position of the observer. Basic anatomic terminology is based on imaginary slices, called *planes,* through the animal body that can be used as points or areas of reference and on sets of directional terms that have opposite meanings from each other.

## ANATOMIC PLANES OF REFERENCE

There are four anatomic **planes of reference,** two of which are variations of each other. Each plane is an imaginary slice through the body that is oriented at right angles to the other two. The four reference planes (Figure 1-1) are as follows:

**Sagittal plane:** A plane that runs the length of the body and divides it into left and right parts that are not necessarily equal halves.

**Median plane:** A special kind of sagittal plane that runs down the center of the body lengthwise and divides it into *equal* left and right halves. It could also be called a *midsagittal plane,* but that term is not commonly used.

**Transverse plane:** A plane across the body that divides it into cranial (head-end) and caudal (tail-end) parts that are not necessarily equal.

**Dorsal plane:** A plane at right angles to the sagittal and transverse planes. It divides the body into *dorsal* (toward the animal's back) and *ventral* (toward the belly) parts that are not necessarily equal. If an animal stands in water with its body partially submerged, the surface of the water describes a dorsal plane. In humans this plane is called the **frontal plane** (Figure 1-2).

 **CLINICAL APPLICATION**

### Radiography Positioning Terminology

Radiographs, commonly called *x-rays,* are two-dimensional images of what is inside an animal. Radiographs are described according to the path the x-ray beam takes through the body using anatomic directional terms. For example, imagine a dog lying on an x-ray table on its back. The x-ray tube is above it, and the x-ray film is beneath it in a light-tight case called a *cassette.* During the exposure, the x-rays will enter the animal's ventral surface, pass through the abdomen, and exit the animal's dorsal surface before striking the film. We call this a *ventro-dorsal (VD) view* of the abdomen, because the x-rays enter the ventral surface and exit the dorsal surface of the body. A *dorso-palmar (DP) view* of a horse's front fetlock joint, which is the joint between the large metacarpal bone and the proximal phalanx, will have the x-ray machine positioned in front of the leg and the x-ray cassette behind the joint. The x-rays will enter the dorsal surface of the leg and exit the palmar surface. Lateral radiographic views are taken by passing the x-ray beam through the area of study from side to side. They are named according to which side of the animal is closest to the film. If the animal's right side is closest to the film for an abdominal radiograph, the view is called a *right lateral view* of the abdomen.

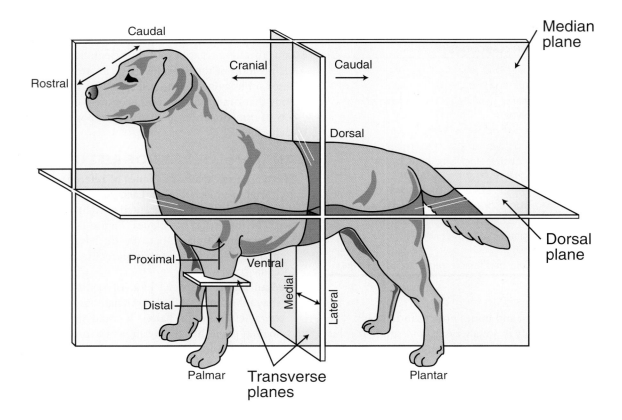

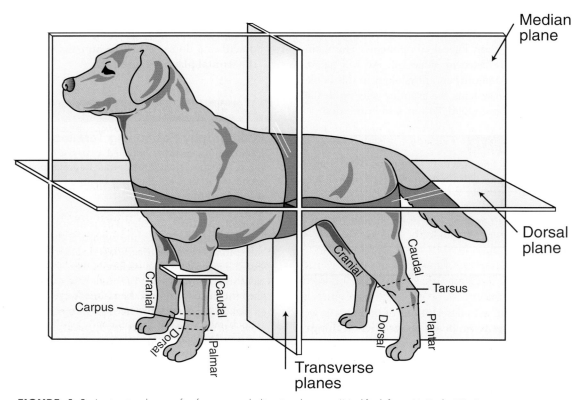

**FIGURE 1-1** Anatomic planes of reference and directional terms. (Modified from McBride DF: Learning veterinary terminology, ed 2, St Louis, 2002, Mosby.)

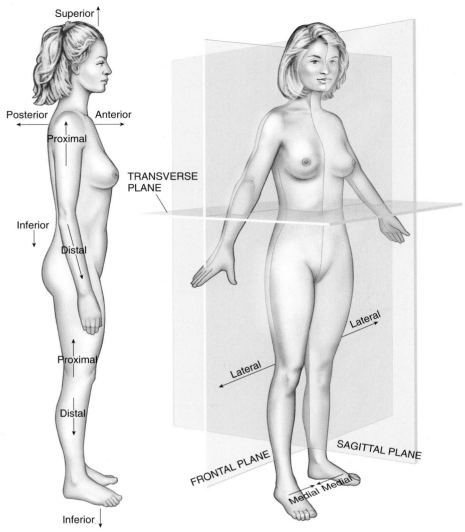

**FIGURE 1-2** Directions and planes of the human body. (From Thibodeau GA, Patton KT: Anatomy and physiology, ed 8, St Louis, 2013, Mosby.)

## DIRECTIONAL TERMS

Directional terms in anatomy provide a common language for accurately and clearly describing body structures regardless of the position of the animal's body. These terms generally occur in pairs that have opposite meanings and are used chiefly to describe relative positions of body parts. Since humans walk upright, there are a few differences between human directional terms and those of nonhuman animals (Table 1-2).

*Left* and *right* always refer to the *animal's* left and right sides. The spleen, an organ with several important functions, is located on the left side of a cow's abdomen. The duodenum, the first short portion of the small intestine, exits the stomach on the right side of a dog's abdomen.

*Cranial* and *caudal* refer to the ends of the animal as it stands on four legs. **Cranial** means toward the head *(cranium),* and **caudal** means toward the tail *(cauda).* A horse's shoulder is located cranial to its hip. The caudal end of the sternum (breastbone) is called the **xiphoid process.**

In humans **superior** is used in place of *cranial,* and **inferior** is used in place of *caudal.*

*Rostral* is a special term used only to describe positions or directions on the head. The term *cranial* loses its meaning on the head because the cranium is part of the head. *Caudal* retains its normal meaning on the head because it still means toward the tail end of the animal. **Rostral** means toward the tip of the nose *(rostrum).* An animal's eyes are located rostral to its ears. In humans the term *nasal* means toward the nose.

*Dorsal* and *ventral* refer to "up and down" directions or positions with the animal in a standing position. **Dorsal** means toward the back (top surface) of a standing animal, and **ventral** means toward the belly (bottom surface) of a standing animal. Dorsal and ventral are easiest to visualize in a standing animal, but they retain their meanings regardless of the animal's position. When one prepares to ride a horse, the saddle is placed on the animal's dorsal surface, and the cinch goes around the horse's ventral surface. In humans **posterior** takes the place of *dorsal,* and **anterior** takes the place of *ventral.*

| TABLE 1-2 | Directional Terms: Domestic Animals versus Humans | |
|---|---|---|
| **DIRECTION** | **DOMESTIC ANIMAL** | **HUMAN** |
| Individual's left | Left | Left |
| Individual's right | Right | Right |
| Toward the head end of the body | Cranial | Superior |
| Toward the tip of the nose (head only) | Rostral | Nasal |
| Toward the tail end of the body | Caudal | Inferior |
| Toward the back | Dorsal | Posterior |
| Toward the belly | Ventral | Anterior |
| Toward the median plane | Medial | Medial |
| Away from the median plane | Lateral | Lateral |
| Toward the center (whole body or part) | Deep (internal) | Deep (internal) |
| Toward the surface (whole body or part) | Superficial (external) | Superficial (external) |
| Toward the body (extremity) | Proximal | Proximal |
| Away from the body (extremity) | Distal | Distal |
| "Back" of forelimb from carpus distally | Palmar | Palmar |
| "Back" of hindlimb from tarsus distally | Plantar | Plantar |
| "Front" of forelimb and hindlimb from carpus and tarsus distally | Dorsal | Anterior |

| TABLE 1-3 | Common Regional Terms |
|---|---|
| **TERM** | **REGION** |
| Barrel | Trunk of the body—formed by the rib cage and the abdomen |
| Brisket | Area at the base of the neck between the front legs that covers the cranial end of the sternum |
| Cannon | Large metacarpal or metatarsal bone of hoofed animals |
| Fetlock | Joint between cannon bone (large metacarpal/metatarsal) and the proximal phalanx of hoofed animals |
| Flank | Lateral surface of the abdomen between the last rib and the hind legs |
| Hock | Tarsus |
| Knee | Carpus of hoofed animals |
| Muzzle | Rostral part of the face formed mainly by the maxillary and nasal bones |
| Pastern | Area of the proximal phalanx of hoofed animals |
| Poll | Top of the head between the bases of the ears |
| Stifle | Femorotibial/femoropatellar joint—equivalent to human knee |
| Tailhead | Dorsal part of the base of the tail |
| Withers | Area dorsal to scapulas |

*Medial* and *lateral* refer to positions relative to the median plane. **Medial** means toward the median plane (toward the center line of the body), and **lateral** means away from the median plane. The medial surface of an animal's leg is the one closest to its body. The lateral surface of the leg is the outer surface.

*Deep (internal)* and *superficial* (external) refer to the position of something relative to the center or surface of the body or a body part. **Deep** means toward the center of the body or a body part. (**Internal** is sometimes used in place of deep.) **Superficial** means toward the surface of the body or a body part. (**External** is sometimes used in place of superficial.) The deep digital flexor muscle is located closer to the center of the leg than the superficial digital flexor muscle, which is located nearer to the surface of the leg.

*Proximal* and *distal* are used to describe positions only on extremities, such as legs, ears, and tail, relative to the body. **Proximal** means toward the body, and **distal** means away from the body. The proximal end of the tail attaches it to the body. The toes are located on the distal end of the leg.

When it comes to describing the front and back surfaces of the legs, things get just a little more complicated. There are different terms depending on whether we are referring to the distal or proximal parts of the legs. The

proximal–distal dividing line for the front leg is the proximal end of the **carpus** (equivalent to our wrist), and the dividing line for the rear leg is the proximal end of the **tarsus** (equivalent to our ankle). The back surface of the front leg from the carpus distally is called the **palmar** surface—like the palm of our hand—and proximal to the carpus it is the caudal surface. The back of the hind leg from the tarsus distally is called the **plantar** surface—like the plantar or *ground* surface of our foot—and proximal to the tarsus it is called the caudal surface, just like the front leg. The "front" surface of both the front and hind legs is termed *dorsal* from the carpus and tarsus distally and *cranial* proximal to them.

## COMMON REGIONAL TERMS

Common regional terms (Figure 1-3) give us a shorthand way of recording anatomic locations in veterinary records. It is easier to refer to the "fetlock" of a horse than to have to write "the joint between the large metacarpal or metatarsal bone and the proximal phalanx." Table 1-3 gives the meanings of commonly used regional terms, including some that are unique to the horse and other hoofed animals.

## GENERAL PLAN OF THE ANIMAL BODY

Before studying the individual parts of the animal body, let's take a look at the overall arrangement of the body. Our focus is on the principle of bilateral symmetry, the two main cavities (spaces) in the body, and the levels of organization that make up the body.

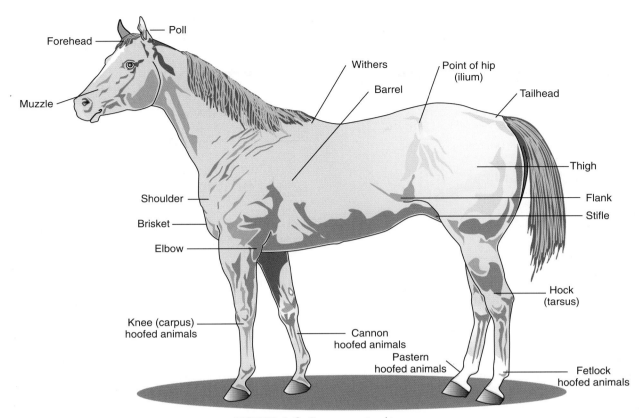

**FIGURE 1-3** Common regional terms.

✓ *TEST YOURSELF 1-2*

1. How does each of the anatomic planes of reference (sagittal, median, transverse, and dorsal) divide a cow's body?
2. If you are facing a cat head-on, is its left ear on your left or right side?
3. Why must the term *rostral* be used instead of *cranial* to describe structures on a hedgehog's head, but the term *caudal* works just fine?
4. If your left hand is on a goat's belly and your right hand is on its back, which hand is on the animal's dorsal surface and which is on its ventral surface?
5. The next time you see a dog, differentiate between the medial and lateral surfaces of one of its elbows and the proximal and distal ends of one of its legs.
6. If you insert a hypodermic needle into a horse's muscle to give it an injection, which end of the needle—the tip or the hub—is located deep in the muscle, and which end is located superficially?
7. What surface of a hamster's front leg is in contact with the ground when it is walking normally? What surface of the hind leg?

## BILATERAL SYMMETRY

**Bilateral symmetry** means that the left and right halves of an animal's body are essentially mirror images of each other. Although not absolute, the principle of bilateral symmetry accurately reflects the basic inner and outer structure of the body. Paired structures, such as the kidneys, lungs, and legs, are approximately mirror images. For example, in looking at your hands, you see that they are not identical—the thumb of one of your hands is where the little finger is on the other hand—but they are mirror images of each other. Paired internal organs are similar.

Single structures in the body are generally found near the center of the body, near the median plane. This is true of structures such as the brain, the heart, and the **gastrointestinal (GI) tract**. At first glance the GI tract does not seem to obey this rule. After all, it is extensively folded and more or less fills the abdominal cavity. Actually the GI tract *is* located near the median plane, but it is so long that it has to be intricately folded so it fits in the abdomen. If we were to stretch it out, it would form one long tube. Even with all its twists, turns, and convolutions, the GI tract does not wander far from the median plane.

## BODY CAVITIES

The animal body has two main cavities (spaces)—a small dorsal cavity and a much larger ventral cavity (Figure 1-4).

### DORSAL BODY CAVITY

The **dorsal body cavity** contains the brain and spinal cord, that is, the central nervous system. It consists of two parts: a somewhat spherical *cranial cavity* in the skull and a long, narrow *spinal cavity* running down the spine. The cranial cavity is also known as the **cranium**. It is formed from several

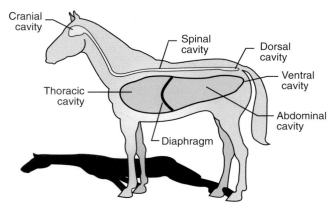

**FIGURE 1-4** Body cavities.

bones of the skull, and it houses and protects the brain. The spinal cavity is also known as the **spinal canal**. It is formed from the vertebrae of the spine, and it houses and protects the spinal cord.

## VENTRAL BODY CAVITY

The **ventral body cavity** is much larger than the dorsal one. It contains most of the soft organs (**viscera**) of the body. It is divided by the thin diaphragm muscle into the cranial thoracic cavity, also known as the **thorax** or *chest,* and the *caudal abdominal cavity,* also known as the *abdomen.*

Major structures in the thoracic cavity include the heart, lungs, esophagus, and many major blood vessels coming to and going from the heart. All of the organs in the thoracic cavity are covered by a thin membrane called the **pleura**. Even the cavity itself is lined by pleura. The layer that covers the organs is called the **visceral layer** of pleura because it lies right on the viscera (the organs). The layer that lines the whole thoracic cavity is called the **parietal layer** of pleura. The potential space between the two layers is filled with a small amount of lubricating fluid. The smooth pleural surfaces are lubricated by the pleural fluid to ensure that the two surfaces slide over each other easily during breathing. If the pleural surfaces become thickened and roughened by **inflammation**, a condition called *pleuritis* or *pleurisy,* the surfaces scrape over each other with each breath, making breathing very painful.

The abdomen contains the digestive, urinary, and reproductive organs. It is lined by a thin membrane called the *peritoneum,* which also covers its contents. The visceral layer of peritoneum covers the abdominal organs, and the parietal layer lines the abdominal cavity. As in the thorax, a potential space filled with peritoneal fluid separates the two layers. Inflammation of the peritoneum *(peritonitis)* is very painful and most commonly results either from a wound that penetrates into the abdomen from the outside or from a rupture or perforation of the GI tract. When performing surgery on the digestive tract, we must take care to suture it securely closed to prevent leakage, which could lead to peritonitis.

## LEVELS OF ORGANIZATION

### CELLS

Cells are the basic functional units of animal life—the smallest subdivisions of the body that are capable of life. A simple, single-celled animal like an ameba has to carry out all the life functions necessary to support itself within its one cell. It must do things such as: grow; respond to positive and negative stimuli; seek out, engulf, and absorb food; eliminate wastes; and reproduce. It has no ability to influence its environment and has to take things as they come. If environmental conditions are favorable, the amoeba survives. If not, it dies.

In the complex animals we discuss in this book, the body's cells must divide the work. The sheer size of a dog or horse results in most of the animal's cells being far removed from the outside environment. The animal's body must create and support an internal environment that allows all of its cells to live and function. To accomplish this, cells must specialize in some functions and eliminate others. For example, some cells specialize in absorbing nutrients (intestinal lining cells), others in carrying oxygen (red blood cells), and still others in organizing and controlling body functions (nerve cells). A particular cell in the body depends on the rest of the body's cells all doing their jobs to ensure its survival. At the same time, all the other cells in the body rely on that cell doing its job to contribute to their survival.

### TISSUES

When specialized cells group together, they form **tissues**. The entire animal body is made up of only four basic tissues: *epithelial* tissue, *connective* tissue, *muscle* tissue, and *nervous* tissue. The basic characteristics and functions of the four body tissues are summarized in Table 1-4.

**Epithelial tissue** is composed entirely of cells, and its main jobs are to *cover* body surfaces, *secrete* materials, and *absorb* materials. The surface of the skin is covered by epithelium, as are the linings of the mouth, intestine, and urinary bladder. Epithelial tissue also forms glands, which are structures that secrete useful substances and excrete wastes. The secreting units of sweat glands, salivary glands, and mammary glands are all composed of specialized epithelial tissues. The epithelium that lines the GI tract is specialized to absorb nutrients from the lumen of the tube.

**Connective tissue** holds the body together (connects its cells) and gives it support. Cells are very soft and cannot support themselves without outside help. Connective tissues

| TABLE 1-4 | Body Tissues | |
|---|---|---|
| **TISSUE** | **CHARACTERISTICS** | **FUNCTIONS** |
| Epithelial | Composed only of cells | Covers and protects (surfaces) |
| | | Secretes (glands) |
| | | Absorbs (intestinal lining) |
| Connective | Composed of living cells and non-living intercellular substances | Binds cells and structures together and supports the body |
| Muscle | Skeletal (voluntary) | Movements |
| | Cardiac (heart) | |
| | Smooth (involuntary) | |
| Nervous | Composed of nerve cells (neurons) and supporting cells | Transmits information around body; Coordinates and controls activities |

range from very soft, such as **adipose** tissue (commonly called *fat*) to very firm, such as cartilage and bone. Connective tissues are composed of cells and a variety of nonliving intercellular substances, such as fibers, that add strength.

**Muscle tissue** moves the body inside and out. It exists as three types: *skeletal* muscle, *cardiac* muscle, and *smooth* muscle. **Skeletal muscle** moves the bones of the skeleton and is under conscious nervous system control. **Cardiac muscle** makes up the heart and works "automatically" (no conscious effort is required). **Smooth muscle** is found in internal organs such as the digestive tract and urinary bladder. It also works pretty much automatically.

**Nervous tissue** transmits information around the body and controls body functions. It transmits sensory information from the body to the brain, processes the information, and sends instructions out to tell the body how to react to changing conditions.

Epithelial and connective tissues are discussed in more detail in Chapter 5. Muscle and nervous tissues are more complicated, so each has its own chapter.

## ORGANS

The next level up from tissues is *organs*. **Organs** are made up of groups of tissues that work together for common purposes. For example, the kidney is an organ composed of various tissues that function together to eliminate wastes from the body. Some organs, such as the eyes, lungs, and kidneys, occur in pairs. Others, such as the brain, heart, and uterus, are single structures.

## SYSTEMS

**Systems** are the most complex level of body organization. Systems are groups of organs that are involved in a common set of activities. For example, the **digestive system** is concerned with obtaining, digesting, and absorbing nutrients to fuel the rest of the body. It is composed of the organs that make up the digestive tube, such as the esophagus, stomach,

and intestine, as well as accessory digestive organs, such as the salivary glands, pancreas, and liver. Table 1-1 lists all the major systems of the body.

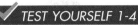

**TEST YOURSELF 1-4**

1. What is the difference between a cell, a tissue, an organ, and a system in an animal's body?
2. What are the four basic tissues that make up an animal's body?

## HEALTH

The term **health** has a lot of meanings. Probably the simplest way to think of health is as a state of normal anatomy and physiology. When the structures or functions of the body become abnormal, disease results. Maintaining health is a complicated process. In terms of the levels of organization of the body, the health of the body as a whole depends on the health and proper functioning of each of its systems, organs, tissues, and cells. On the other hand, each of the body's cells depends on the health and proper functioning of all the tissues, organs, systems, and the body as a whole. All structures and functions in the body are interrelated; nothing takes place in isolation. We can represent these interrelationships with the following diagram:

Body health ⟷ System health ⟷ Organ health ⟷ Tissue health ⟷ Cell health

## HOMEOSTASIS

Imagine that you are driving a car. To reach your destination, you cannot just put the car in gear and then sit back, relax, and expect it automatically to take you there. You have to be actively involved in the process. You must accelerate to the proper speed, monitor and avoid other traffic, steer as the road twists and turns, accelerate up hills, brake while going down hills, stop when necessary, and generally oversee conditions and make adjustments throughout the journey. This description is an analogy for homeostasis in the body. The road is life, the car is the animal's body, and homeostasis is all the little inputs and corrections necessary to keep the body (car) alive (on the road).

**Homeostasis** is the maintenance of a dynamic equilibrium in the body. The word *dynamic* implies activity, energy, and work, and **equilibrium** refers to balance. Together they summarize all the physiological processes that actively maintain balance in the various structures, functions, and properties of the body. Consider this: An animal's body temperature cannot vary more than a few degrees from either side of the normal range without starting to interfere with other body functions. Or consider how acid–base balance, fluid balance, hormone levels, nutrient levels, and oxygen levels cannot vary by much if the body is to operate normally; they must be kept within fairly narrow operational ranges. The processes that monitor and adjust all the various essential parameters of the body are summarized by the term *homeostasis*.

Is some particular part of the body responsible for homeostasis? The answer is no. The *whole body* is responsible for homeostasis. All the body systems are involved in the many mechanisms of homeostasis, which require a lot of energy and work. Like all the little inputs and corrections that keep a car safely traveling down the road, the various homeostatic mechanisms in the body keep it functioning amid the twists and turns of life. To put it more mechanistically, the processes of homeostasis help maintain a fairly constant internal environment in the body as conditions inside and outside the animal change. Along with normal functioning of the body's cells, tissues, organs, and systems, the processes of homeostasis make life possible.

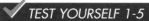

**TEST YOURSELF 1-5**

1. How does the normal anatomy and physiology of cells in an animal's body impact the health of the animal as a whole? How does the normal anatomy and physiology of the animal's body as a whole impact the health of each of its cells?
2. How do homeostatic mechanisms influence the health of an animal?

If you are beginning to view the concepts of life and health as a little less ordinary and more unique, you are starting to appreciate the amazing complexity of the animal body. Only by understanding what is normal in the body can we hope to help sick or injured animals. With this in mind, we can proceed with our examination of the fascinating machine that is the animal body.

    **CLINICAL APPLICATION**

### Homeostasis and Congestive Heart Failure

The processes in the body that try to maintain the functioning of a failing heart offer some excellent illustrations of how important homeostasis is as it attempts to maintain the health and life of an animal. *Congestive heart failure* is a clinical term used to describe a heart that is not pumping adequate amounts of blood. This results in blood "backing up" in the body, which produces *congestion*, or abnormal fluid accumulation, upstream from the failing heart. There are many causes and forms of congestive heart failure, but the overall homeostatic mechanisms that attempt to maintain normal blood circulation in the body are basically the same.

The first indication that the heart is starting to fail is a drop in the cardiac output, that is, the amount of blood the heart pumps out per minute. The decreased blood flow and blood pressure are picked up by receptors in the vascular system and relayed to the central nervous system. Signals then go out to activate the sympathetic portion of the nervous system. This system, also called the **fight-or-flight system**, helps prepare the body for intense physical activity. Its effect on the cardiovascular system is to increase blood flow and blood pressure by stimulating the heart to beat harder and faster and by constricting blood vessels. In the short term, these mechanisms help bring blood flow and blood pressure back up to normal levels.

Unfortunately, these compensatory mechanisms cause the weak heart to work harder, which is kind of like whipping an exhausted horse to get it to move faster or pull harder. The result is a further weakening of the heart and further decreases in cardiac output. This causes more sympathetic nervous system stimulation. The cycle continues to repeat until either the heart gives up completely or we intervene with medical therapy. Homeostatic mechanisms cannot change the basic defects that are causing the heart to fail, but they help the damaged heart maintain vital blood flow to the rest of the body for as long as possible. By adding good medical care to the body's natural homeostatic mechanisms, we can often extend the length and quality of life of an animal in congestive heart failure.

# 2 Chemical Basis for Life*

Joanna M. Bassert

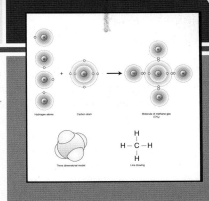

## OUTLINE

## LEARNING OBJECTIVES

**When you have completed this chapter, you will be able to:**

1. List the characteristics of each of the subatomic particles.
2. Differentiate between a molecule and a compound.
3. List and describe the types of chemical bonds that may form between elements.
4. Give the general equations for synthesis, decomposition, and exchange reactions.
5. Differentiate between organic and inorganic compounds.
6. Differentiate between hydrophobic and hydrophilic molecules.
7. List the unique properties of the water molecule.
8. Differentiate between acids and bases.
9. Describe the actions of a buffer system.
10. List the components of carbohydrates, lipids, proteins, and nucleic acids.
11. List the functions of body proteins.
12. Describe the actions of enzymes.

## VOCABULARY FUNDAMENTALS

*Acid* **ah**-sihd
*Activation energy* ahck-tuh-**vā**-shuhn **ehn**-ər-jē
*Adenosine diphosphate* ah-**dehn**-ō-sēn dī-**fohs**-fāt
*Adenosine triphosphate* ah-**dehn**-ō-sēn trī-**fohs**-fāt
*Amino acid* ah-**mē**-nō **ah**-sihd
*Anion* **ahn**-ī-uhn
*Atom* **aht**-uhm
*Atomic number* ah-**tohm**-ihck **nuhm**-bər
*Atomic weight* ah-**tohm**-ihck wāt
*Base* bās
*Carbohydrate* kahr-bō-**hī**-drāt
*Catalyst* **kaht**-ah-lihst

*Cation* **kaht**-ī-ohn
*Cellular respiration* **sehl**-ū-lər res-puh-**rā**-shuhn
*Chemical element* **kehm**-ih-kuhl **ehl**-uh-mehnt
*Chemical equation* **kehm**-ih-kuhl ē-**kwey**-shuhn
*Chemical reaction* **kehm**-ih-kuhl rē-**ahck**-shuhn
*Chemical symbol* **kehm**-ih-kuhl **sihm**-buhl
*Chromosome* **krō**-mō-sōm
*Colloid* **kohl**-oyd (or emulsion ē-**muhl**-shuhn)
   *is a heterogeneous* heht-ər-**rohj**-uh-nuhs
   ***mixture*** **mihcks**-chər *that contains a much*
      *larger sized*
   ***solute*** **sohl**-yoot *than those found in a*

---

*The author and the publisher wish to acknowledge Dr. Mary Ann Seagren for her previous contributions to this chapter.*

*solution* suh-**loo**-shuhn
*Compound* **kohm**-pohwnd
*Covalent bond* kō-vā-lehnt bohnd
*Decomposition reaction* dē-kohmp-ō-**zihsh**-uhn
    rē-**ahck**-shuhn
*Dehydration synthesis* dē-hī-**drā**-shuhn **sihn**-thuh-sihs
*Deoxyribonucleic acid (DNA)* dē-**ohck**-sē-rī-bō-noo-**klā**-
    ihck **ah**-sihd
*Disaccharide* dī-**sahck**-uh-rīd
*Eicosanoid* ī-**kō**-seh-noyd
*Electron* ē-**lehck**-trohn
*Electron shell* ē-**lehck**-trohn shehl
*Electrostatic attraction* ē-lehck-trō-**staht**-ihck
    ah-**trahck**-shuhn
*Element* **ehl**-eh-mehnt
*Enzyme* **ehn**-zīm
*Exchange reaction* ehcks-**chānj** rē-**ahck**-shuhn
*Fatty acid* **faht**-ē **ah**-sihd
*Functional group* **fuhngk**-shuh-nuhl groop
*Functional protein* **fuhngk**-shuh-nuhl **prō**-tēn
*Glycerol* **glihs**-ər-ahl
*Glycoprotein* glī-kō-**prō**-tēn
*Hydrolysis* hī-**drohl**-uh-sihs
*Hydrophilic* hī-drō-**fihl**-ihck
*Hydrophobic* hī-drō-**fō**-bihck
*Inorganic compound* ihn-ohr-**gahn**-ihck **kohm**-pohwnd
*Ion* ī-ohn
*Ionic bond* ī-**ohn**-ihck bohnd
*Isotope* ī-sō-tōp
*Lipid* **lihp**-ihd
*Lipoprotein* lī-pō-**prō**-tēn
*Macromolecule* **mah**-krō-**mohl**-uhl-kyool
*Matter* **maht**-ər
*Mixture* **mihcks**-chər

*Molecule* **mohl**-uhl-kyool
*Monosaccharide* mohn-ō-**sahck**-ah-rīd
*Neutral fat* **noo**-truhl faht
*Neutralize* **noo**-truhl-īz
*Neutron* **noo**-trohn
*Nucleotide* **noo**-klē-ō-tīd
*Organic compound* ohr-**gahn**-ihck **kohm**-pohwnd
*Peptide bond* **pehp**-tīd bohnd
*Periodic Table of the Elements* peer-ē-**ohd**-ihck **tā**-buhl
    *of the* **ehl**-eh-mehntz
*Phospholipid* fohs-fō-**lihp**-ihd
*Polypeptide* pohl-ē-**pehp**-tīd
*Primary structure* **prī**-meər-ē **struhckt**-shər
*Product* **prohd**-uhckt
*Protein* **prō**-tēn
*Proton* **prō**-tohn
*Radioactive isotope* **rād**-ē-ō-ahck-tihv
    ī-**sō**-tōp
*Reactant* rē-**ahck**-tuhnt
*Ribonucleic acid (RNA)* rī-bō-noo-**klā**-ihck
    **ah**-sihd
*Salt* sahlt
*Saturated fatty acid* **sahch**-ər-ā-tihd **faht**-ē ahs-ihd
*Solute* **sohl**-yoot
*Solution* suh-**loo**-shuhn
*Solvent* **sohl**-vuhnt
*Steroid* **steər**-oyd
*Structural protein* **struhck**-shər-uhl prō-tēn
*Substrate* **suhb**-strāt
*Suspension* suh-**spehn**-shuhn
*Synthesis reaction* **sihn**-thuh-sihs rē-**ahck**-shuhn
*Triglyceride* trī-**glihs**-ər-rīd
*Unsaturated fatty acid* uhn-**sahch**-ər-ā-tihd
    **faht**-ē **ah**-sihd

## INTRODUCTION

When our universe was less than 1 second old, astronomers tell us, waves of hydrogen and energy streamed across an ever-expanding space. Gravity swirled these small atoms closer and closer until they were crushed against one another, igniting the nuclear reactions that formed the stars. The products of the nuclear reactions were new elements that were blown into the cosmos when stars exploded into supernova. Oxygen, nitrogen, iron, silicone, and other elements were forged in these nuclear furnaces. Carbon was blown off of slowly aging, medium-sized stars and condensed into minute dust particles. Four and a half billion years ago the debris from these stellar explosions coalesced by the force of gravity to form celestial bodies that circled our sun. Earth was created literally from stardust (Figure 2-1).

The atmosphere of the primordial earth contained methane gas ($CH_4$), water ($H_2O$), and ammonia ($NH_4$) but little free oxygen. These molecules contain the

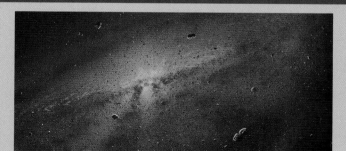

**FIGURE 2-1** Illustration of the early cosmos. A painting of early events in the universe (NASA/JPL). (From Weissman P, McFadden L, Johnson T: Encyclopedia of the solar system, Burlington, Mass, 1999, Academic Press.)

elements—hydrogen, oxygen, carbon, and nitrogen—that make up 96% of living organisms. Scientists believe that the combined activity of lightning, ultraviolet (UV) light, meteorite strikes, and thermo-reactions in the earth's crust and core provided the energy needed to convert $CH_4$,

$H_2O$, and $NH_4$ into life-generating organic molecules such as amino acids and nucleic acids. The most successful molecules were self-replicating. From these self-replicating molecules, scientists believe early cells evolved. These early cells were tiny, bacteria-like units without a **nucleus**, and they had the new ability to use energy from the environment to make their own chemical energy.

*Archaebacteria* are ancient bacteria that survived the harsh, oxygen-free environment of young earth. Some forms still exist today in the extreme environments of hot springs, salt flats, and the intestines of mammals. Early bacteria had various ways of creating the chemical energy needed to maintain themselves and to reproduce. Some developed enzymes that created oxygen gas as a waste product and, later, cells evolved that used oxygen to produce their own molecular energy. As oxygen concentrations in the earth's atmosphere climbed, expansion of the number and size of living organisms became possible (Figure 2-2).

Life on earth comes in a multitude of forms, but the biochemistry that defines living things is remarkably consistent. All living entities are formed from inorganic chemicals, such as water and salts, as well as from organic chemicals, such as proteins, lipids, carbohydrates, and nucleic acids. The same physical forces that caused the formation of the stars, planets, and elements also governed biochemical reactions and interactions in living organisms.

The body of an animal is composed of thousands of chemicals, interacting with one another at rapid speed. Their dynamic collisions with and separations from one

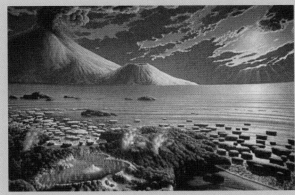

**FIGURE 2-2** The Precambrian sea. The earliest evidence of life is shown by calcified algal structures called *stromatolites* that existed during the Precambrian period. Scientists believe that the energy from asteroid strikes, lightning strikes, and the reactions in the earth's melted crust and core supplied the energy for common molecules, such as ammonia and methane, to be converted into organic molecules such as proteins and nucleic acids. (Courtesy the National Museum of Natural History, Smithsonian Institution.)

another underlie the physiological processes of life: respiration, digestion, reproduction, movement ... they are all the result of chemical interaction. Each organic and inorganic molecule found in living systems is composed of atoms, the elemental units of matter. It is fitting, therefore, to begin our discussion of anatomy and physiology with an introduction to biochemistry, the chemistry of life.

## MATTER

Matter is defined as anything that occupies space and has mass (Figure 2-3). We can often identify matter with our senses by feeling, seeing, tasting, and smelling. Though matter has mass and takes up space, keep in mind that mass is not the same as weight. The mass of an animal is based on how much matter it contains, whereas an animal's weight is determined by the pull of gravity on the matter. On earth, for example, a unit of matter would weigh more than the same unit of matter on the moon, because the acceleration of gravity on the moon is far less than that on earth. However, the mass is the same on both the earth and the moon.

## STATES OF MATTER

Matter can exist in one of three states, as a gas, liquid, or solid. The bodies of animals contain examples of each state. The air that is inhaled and the carbon dioxide that is exhaled

are examples of gases in the living system. Blood, which is primarily composed of water, is a vital liquid that helps transport critical nutrients to hungry tissues. Finally, the musculoskeletal system composed of bones, tendons, ligaments and muscles are examples of solid features that give the body shape and strength.

## COMPOSITION OF MATTER: ELEMENTS AND ATOMS

### ELEMENTS

All matter is made of one or more elements. Each element is a single pure substance consisting of only one type of atom. All of the 118 elements known today are listed in the Periodic Table of Elements where they are divided into three general categories: metals, metalloids, and nonmetals (Figure 2-4). Only 92 of the elements occur in nature; the rest are made artificially or are theoretical and not known to exist.

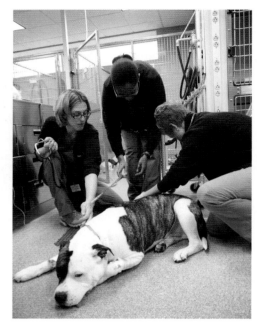

**FIGURE 2-3** Matter. Everything you see in this picture is made of matter. Matter is anything that takes up space and has mass. The page it is printed on is also matter. (Courtesy Dr. Joanna Bassert.)

Each known element has its own unique properties, but it can be joined in various combinations with other elements to form all of the matter that exists on earth. Some common examples of elements are aluminum, gold and carbon as pictured in Figure 2-5. Others include oxygen, chlorine, and helium. At room temperature, gold is a solid metal, whereas oxygen and chlorine are gases. Pure carbon can exist as coal or, with enough time and pressure, can be compressed into diamonds.

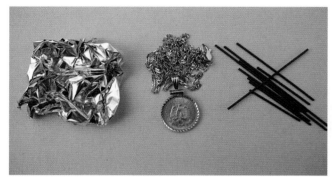

**FIGURE 2-5** Examples of elements. Aluminum foil is 98.5% aluminum. Twenty-four carat gold is 99.9% gold. Graphite is 100% carbon.

# Periodic Table

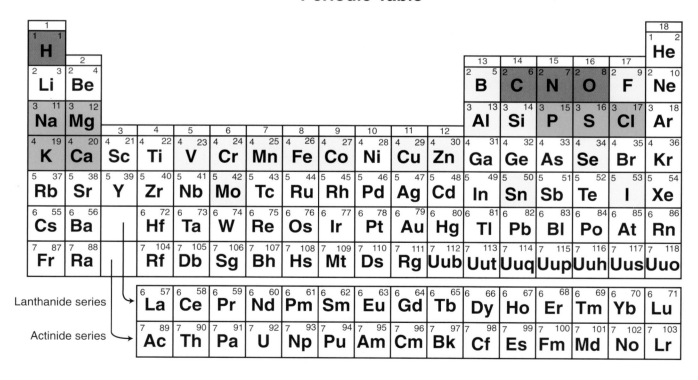

Lanthanide series

Actinide series

Key:

■ = Major elements     ■ = Minor elements     □ = Trace elements

**FIGURE 2-4** Periodic Table of the Elements. The Periodic Table of the Elements gives us important information about each element: the chemical symbol, atomic number, and atomic weight. The table groups elements with similar properties. The metallic elements are on the left and the inert gases are in the right-hand column. The elements shaded in red are the major elements that make up 96% of the matter in the animal body. The elements shaded in blue are the minor elements, and those shaded in yellow are trace elements.

Surprisingly, living organisms are made up of only a few of the 118 known elements. Only four elements, nitrogen, oxygen, hydrogen, and carbon, make up 96% of the matter found in all living organisms. Several other elements are found in relatively small quantities. Table 2-1 shows the most common elements found in living organisms and their function in the body. These are divided into major and minor categories.

Each element is referenced using a **chemical symbol**, which is derived from its name in English, Latin, or Greek. The chemical symbol for oxygen, for example, is O from the English word "oxygen," whereas the chemical symbol

for gold is Au from the Latin word *aurum*, meaning gold (Figure 2-4).

## ATOMS

An **atom** is the smallest unit of an element that retains the unique properties of the element (Figure 2-6). Atoms themselves are made of smaller, subatomic particles called **protons**, **neutrons**, and **electrons**, but these particles do not retain the physical and chemical properties of the element when they are isolated. The protons and neutrons are the heaviest particles—each has an atomic mass of one—and these are grouped together in the center of the atom and collectively

| TABLE 2-1 | Elements in the Animal Body | | | |
|-----------|------------------------------|---|---|---|
| | The Percentage of Each Element Found in an Animal's Body is Listed. Note That the First Few Elements Make Up the Vast Majority of Matter in the Animal Body | | | |
| **ELEMENT** | **CHEMICAL SYMBOL** | **ATOMIC NUMBER** | **BODY MASS (%)** | **FUNCTION IN THE ANIMAL BODY** |
| **Major Elements** | | | | |
| Oxygen | O | 8 | 65.0 | Necessary for cellular respiration; component of water |
| Carbon | C | 6 | 18.5 | Primary component of organic molecules |
| Hydrogen | H | 1 | 9.5 | Component of water and organic molecules; necessary for energy transfer and respiration; ion influences pH of fluids |
| Nitrogen | N | 7 | 3.3 | Component of all proteins and nucleic acids |
| Calcium | Ca | 20 | 1.5 | Component of bones and teeth; required for muscle contraction, nerve impulse transmission, and blood clotting |
| Phosphorus | P | 15 | 1.0 | Principal component in backbone of nucleic acids; important in energy transfer (part of ATP); component of bones |
| Potassium | K | 19 | 0.4 | Principal positive ion within cells; important in nerve function |
| Sulfur | S | 16 | 0.3 | Component of most proteins |
| Sodium | Na | 11 | 0.2 | Important positive ion in extracellular fluid; important in nerve function |
| Chlorine | Cl | 17 | 0.2 | Ion is most abundant negative ion in extracellular fluids |
| Magnesium | Mg | 12 | 0.1 | Component of many energy-transferring enzymes |
| **Trace Elements** | | | | |
| Silicone | Si | 14 | 0.1 | Component of some enzymes |
| Aluminum | Al | 13 | 0.1 | Component of some enzymes |
| Iron | Fe | 26 | 0.1 | Critical component of hemoglobin |
| Manganese | Mn | 25 | 0.1 | Needed for fatty acid synthesis |
| Fluorine | F | 9 | 0.1 | Component of bones and teeth |
| Vanadium | V | 23 | 0.1 | Component of some enzymes |
| Chromium | Cr | 24 | 0.1 | Needed for proper glucose metabolism |
| Copper | Cu | 29 | 0.1 | Needed for hemoglobin and myelin |
| Boron | B | 5 | 0.1 | Component of some enzymes |
| Cobalt | Co | 27 | 0.1 | Needed for maturation of red blood cells |
| Zinc | Zn | 30 | 0.1 | Important component of many enzymes and proteins |
| Selenium | Se | 34 | 0.1 | Antioxidant |
| Molybdenum | Mo | 42 | 0.1 | Key component of many enzymes |
| Tin | Sn | 50 | 0.1 | Component of some enzymes |
| Iodine | I | 53 | 0.1 | Component of thyroid hormones |

From Patton KT, Thibodeau GA: Anatomy and physiology, ed 8, St Louis, 2013, Mosby, p 35.

## CLINICAL APPLICATION

### Iron Deficiency Anemia

There are trace amounts of some elements in the body that are essential for life. Iron is an example of an essential element. As a percentage of the mass of the body, iron exists in extremely small amounts. Healthy animals have only 9 to 22 mg of iron in their bodies, most of which is found in the globular protein, hemoglobin, in red blood cells. Iron is used to bind oxygen and carry it to tissues where it is needed in the mitochondria to generate adenosine triphosphate (ATP). Without iron, the level of oxygen that can be carried by the blood is reduced, leading to fatigue and exercise intolerance. Chronic blood loss reduces the level of iron stored in the body. Without adequate levels of iron, the body is not able to make hemoglobin and adequate numbers of red blood cells. In this way, ongoing blood loss results in a condition called *iron deficiency anemia*. A puppy or kitten with a severe flea infestation, for example, can lose 100 ml of blood a day. When the stores of iron in the body are depleted, hemoglobin can no longer be manufactured and the red blood cell count decreases. Clinical signs include pale mucous membranes, fatigue, bounding pulses, and galloping heart rhythm. Microscopic examination of the blood shows small (microcytic) pale (hypochromic) red blood cells with large central areas. The oxygen carrying capacity of blood affected by iron deficiency is greatly reduced and the animal becomes weak. If the animal is stressed and the demand for oxygen increases, such as during a physical examination at the vet's office, the puppy or kitten can die suddenly from heart failure. Iron deficiency anemia is treated by stabilizing the patient with blood transfusions, giving oral and injectable iron supplements, and eliminating the cause of the blood loss.

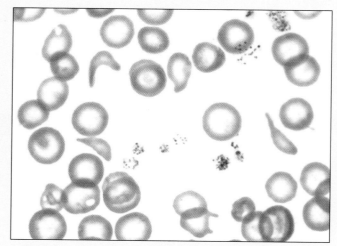

From Harvey JW: Veterinary hematology: a diagnostic guide and color atlas, St Louis, 2012, Elsevier Saunders.

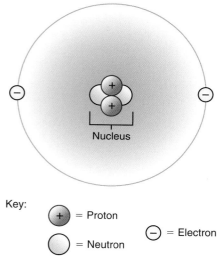

Key:
+ = Proton
− = Electron
= Neutron

**FIGURE 2-6** Diagram of a helium atom (planetary model). The neutrons and protons group together in the center of the atom, which is called the nucleus. Electrons move around the outside of the nucleus in an orbit. The charges of the particles are shown. Note that there are equal numbers of protons and electrons, giving the atom no net electrical charge.

are called the **atomic nucleus.** The neutrons and protons together determine the **atomic weight** of the atom. Electrons are tiny "wavicles" that possess the properties of both waves and particles. They can collide with other electrons and can be diffracted like light. Electrons exist in a state of constant motion moving continuously around the nucleus and

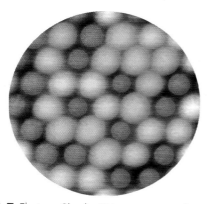

**FIGURE 2-7** Electron Clouds. Using an atomic force microscope (AFM), the outer surfaces of electron clouds are visible in atoms clustered together along the flat surface of a crystal. The different colors represent different types of atoms. (From Sugimoto Y, Pou P, Abe M, et al: Chemical identification of individual surface atoms by atomic force microscopy, Nature 466:64-67, 2007.)

generate regions where they are statistically most likely to be found called electron clouds (Figure 2-7). Electrons are so tiny that their mass does not contribute to the atomic weight of the atom as a whole. Protons have a positive electrical charge, electrons have a negative electrical charge, and neutrons have no electrical charge and are therefore neutral. The net electrical charge of many atoms is neutral, because the atom contains equal numbers of protons and electrons, so the positive and negative charges of these particles cancel each other out.

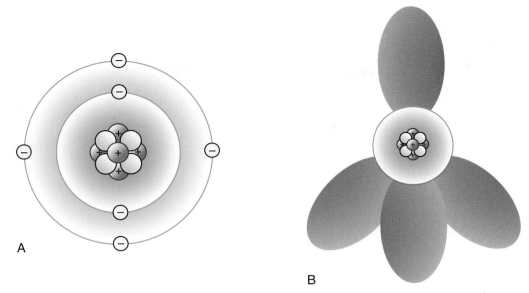

**FIGURE 2-8** Atomic models. **A**, The planetary model of an atom of carbon. Carbon has six protons, six electrons, and six neutrons. (Note: Not all the nuclear particles are shown.) **B**, An orbital model of carbon. The neutrons and protons are grouped together in the nucleus. The shaded shapes show the most likely positions of the various electrons that surround the nucleus.

There are two common models used to represent atoms graphically. The planetary model shows the protons and neutrons of the nucleus encircled by electrons, which orbit like planets around a sun. This is not physically accurate, but it makes the atom easy to understand and allows us to explain interactions between two atoms in a clearer fashion. A more accurate representation is the orbital model, which shows a three-dimensional view of the most likely location of the electrons at any given time. Figure 2-8 shows the difference between a planetary model and an orbital model of a carbon atom. Keep this model in mind while studying the interaction of atoms and molecules. Electrons exist in a cloud around the nucleus, and can move closer to one side of the nucleus than another. Each atom of an element has the same number of protons as other atoms of that element. For example, every oxygen atom has eight protons, and every carbon atom has six protons. If the number of protons is changed—which can only be done with extraordinary means, like nuclear reactions—then the element is changed to another element. In each atom, the number of electrons is the same as the number of protons. The **atomic number** of the element is equal to the number of protons found in the nucleus. Sometimes an atom can lose or gain an electron, giving it a positive or negative charge: This charged atom is called an **ion**. Each element has a naturally occurring, specific number of neutrons. Figure 2-8 shows examples of common elements that make up the animal body.

Sometimes atoms exist that contain a different number of neutrons. These atoms are called **isotopes** of the element. For example, carbon normally has six protons, six electrons, and six neutrons, so the atomic weight of carbon is normally 12. There are some isotopes of carbon, however, that have *eight* neutrons, giving them the atomic weight of 14. This

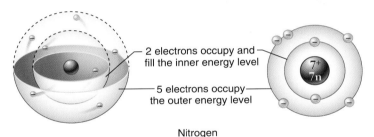

- 2 electrons occupy and fill the inner energy level
- 5 electrons occupy the outer energy level

Nitrogen

**FIGURE 2-9** The principal quantum numbers or energy levels of the electron shells of a nitrogen atom are depicted in three dimensions *(left)* and using a planetary model *(right)*. (From Patton KT, Thibodeau GA: *Anatomy and physiology*, ed 8, St Louis, 2013, Mosby, p 37, Figure 2-5.)

form of carbon is a **radioactive isotope** called *carbon-14*. A radioactive isotope spontaneously emits particles of energy at a constant rate and thereby changes into a stable, nonradioactive element. The rate at which this happens is called the *rate of decay*. Carbon-14's rate of decay can be measured in rock and is used to date fossils.

The area around the nucleus where the electrons have their most likely position is called the **electron shell**. An electron's energy level determines which electron shell it will inhabit. An atom has one or more electron shells surrounding the nucleus, depending on the number of electrons and their energy. Lower energy electrons exist in the first electron shell, which is found closest to the nucleus. Higher energy electrons are in the second electron shell (Figure 2-9).

We will use the planetary model to describe the electron shell (Figure 2-10). The first electron shell can only hold two electrons. Hydrogen has only one electron, so it has only one electron shell. Helium has two electrons, so its first and only

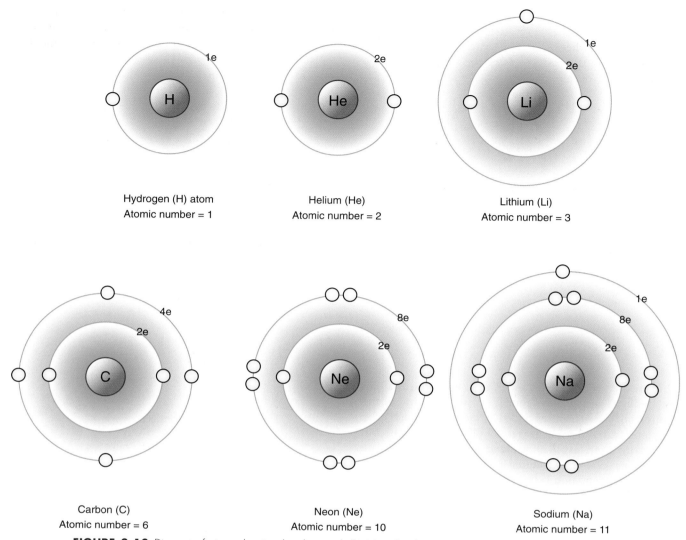

**FIGURE 2-10** Diagram of atoms showing the electron shells. Note that the outer shells of hydrogen, lithium, carbon, and sodium are incomplete, but the outer shells of helium and neon are complete. This renders the atoms of helium and neon less chemically active; indeed, they are referred to as *inert gases.*

electron shell is full. The next element in the Periodic Table is lithium, which has three electrons; so the first electron shell is full, and the second electron shell contains one electron. The second electron shell can hold up to eight electrons. Carbon has six electrons, so its first shell is full, and its second shell contains four electrons. Neon has 10 electrons, so its first and second shells are completely filled. It is important to understand whether the electron shell of a particular atom is full or incomplete. Atoms are most stable when their electron shells are full. Helium and neon have full electron shells and are therefore chemically inactive or *inert.* Atoms like hydrogen, carbon, and oxygen are more chemically active, because their electron shells are incomplete. These atoms are constantly trying to find electrons to complete their outer shell (Table 2-2). The forces that drive the activities of electrons account for the formation of bonds between atoms.

| TABLE 2-2 | Capacity of Electron Shells Electron Capacity = $2n^2$, Where n Equals the Principal Quantum Number or Energy Level | | |
|---|---|---|---|
| **SHELL NUMBER = ENERGY LEVEL (PRINCIPAL QUANTUM NUMBER)** | | **SHELL LETTER** | **ELECTRON CAPACITY** |
| 1 | | K | 2 |
| 2 | | L | 8 |
| 3 | | M | 18 |
| 4 | | N | 32 |
| 5 | | O | 50 |
| 6 | | P | 72 |

## MOLECULES AND COMPOUNDS

A molecule forms when atoms are joined together by chemical bonds. If two or more atoms of the *same* element are joined together, we call the result a *molecule of the element*. For example, oxygen does not usually exist as a single atom. Oxygen gas exists as a molecule of two oxygen atoms joined together, and this is expressed by the symbol $O_2$ (Figure 2-11). The subscript 2 denotes the number of atoms in the molecule.

Atoms of *different* elements may also join together to form a molecule. For example, carbon dioxide is formed from one atom of carbon and two atoms of oxygen. The chemical symbol for carbon dioxide is $CO_2$ (Figure 2-12). A molecule of table salt is called *sodium chloride* and has the chemical symbol NaCl. A molecule of this **compound**

consists of one atom of sodium bonded to one atom of chlorine (Figure 2-13). A **molecule** is the smallest unit of a compound that retains the properties of that compound. This is important because often the properties of the compound are much different than the properties of the elements from which it is made. Table salt is very different from sodium (a metal) and chlorine (a poisonous gas).

## MIXTURES

Most matter is combined into mixtures of two or more substances. There are three types of mixture: solutions, colloids, and suspensions (Figure 2-14).

Solutions are homogeneous mixtures of various substances. The components can be gases, liquids, and/or solids. A component that is present in the greatest amount is called the solvent, while the substances present in smaller amounts

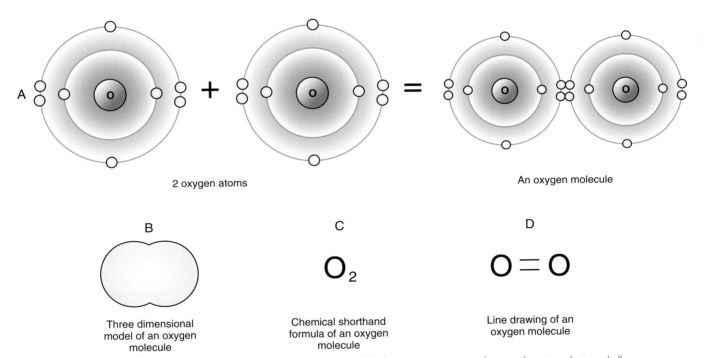

2 oxygen atoms

An oxygen molecule

B
Three dimensional model of an oxygen molecule

C
$O_2$
Chemical shorthand formula of an oxygen molecule

D
$O = O$
Line drawing of an oxygen molecule

**FIGURE 2-11** A molecule of oxygen. **A,** A planetary model of two oxygen atoms, showing the outer electron shells touching so that the electrons can be shared by both atoms. **B,** A three-dimensional representation of the molecule. **C,** Chemical formula for oxygen. **D,** Line drawing. Because the oxygen atoms are sharing two electrons, a double covalent bond exists. This is represented by two lines between the atoms.

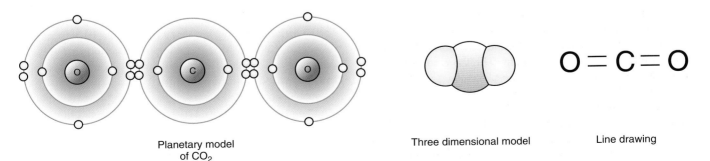

Planetary model of $CO_2$

Three dimensional model

Line drawing
$O = C = O$

**FIGURE 2-12** A molecule of carbon dioxide. Methods of representing a molecule of carbon dioxide ($CO_2$) are shown. The carbon atom is sharing two electrons with each of the oxygen atoms to form double covalent bonds.

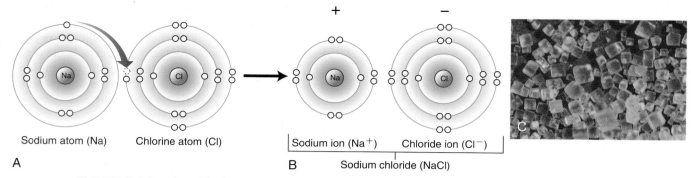

**FIGURE 2-13** Sodium chloride (NaCl) is formed from ionic bonding. **A,** Within the aqueous environment of the body, ionic bonds are frequently formed as electrons are transferred from sodium ions to chloride ions. This gives both atoms an electrical charge. **B,** Table salt takes on cube-shaped crystals. **C,** A photomicrograph captures crystals of sodium chloride after the water has been removed. (**C,** Courtesy Michael Godomski/Tom Stack & Associates.)

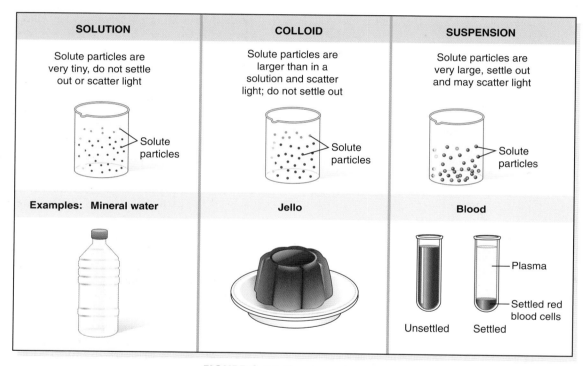

**FIGURE 2-14** Three types of mixture.

are called solutes. Water is the most important solvent in animal bodies. Solutes in solutions are very tiny, consisting of molecules, such as glucose and sodium chloride, or of individual atoms. Because the solutes are minute, they are found evenly distributed throughout the solvent, do not settle out and do not refract light. Therefore solutions are usually clear.

Colloids (or emulsions) are heterogeneous mixtures that contain much larger sized solutes than those found in solutions. Despite their increased size, solutes do not precipitate out of colloids but they often reflect light. Colloids appear translucent or milky. Among the many interesting properties of colloids is their ability to transform from a fluid to a solid and

back again. This ability is called the sol–gel transformation. Jello is an excellent example of a colloid and is well known for changing from a fluid to a gel when chilled in the refrigerator. Later, when heated on a hot day, it may change back from a gel to a fluid. Cytosol, the fluid component found inside living cells, is also a colloid. The cytosol's ability to undergo sol–gel transformations is important during cell division.

Suspensions are heterogeneous mixtures containing large solutes that readily separate from the solution when there is no movement of the suspension. Blood is an example of a suspension in living systems. When left to sit in a glass tube without any movement, the cellular components of blood settle to the bottom of the liquid portion, which is known as plasma. Shaking the blood tube will resuspend the cells.

## DISTINGUISHING COMPOUNDS FROM MIXTURES

Mixtures and compounds differ from one another in the following ways:

1. The components of mixtures are physically mixed, not chemically bonded to one another. Each component is physically unchanged when they are combined in a mixture.
2. The components of a compound are chemically bonded to one another and can only be separated by breaking the chemical bonds. In contrast, the components of mixtures can be separated in a variety of ways, including filtration, straining, evaporation, and centrifugation.
3. All compounds are homogeneous, whereas some mixtures are homogeneous and others are heterogeneous.

---

### ✓ TEST YOURSELF 2-1

1. What is an element?
2. What is a chemical symbol?
3. Name the three subatomic particles.
4. What is the electrical charge of each particle?
5. Which particles are in the nucleus of an atom?
6. How many electron shells would an atom have if it had four electrons?
7. What is a mixture?
8. List three types of mixture. How is each type similar to or different from the others?
9. How are compounds and mixtures different from one another?

---

## CHEMICAL BONDS

The way that atoms join together to form molecules is through a process called *chemical bonding*. A **chemical bond** between two atoms means that the atoms are sharing or transferring electrons between them. Think back to the concept of the electron shell, and remember that atoms are most stable when their outer electron shells are full. If they have an incomplete electron shell, they will either try to fill the shell by gaining more electrons or lose the shell entirely by giving up the extra electrons. If there is a possibility of the atom becoming more stable by transferring or sharing electrons, then the atoms will naturally do so. There are three types of chemical bond: *covalent* bonds, *ionic* bonds, and *hydrogen* bonds.

## COVALENT BONDS

A **covalent bond** is a strong chemical bond formed when atoms share electrons: The electron spends part of the time in the outer electron shell of one atom and the rest in the outer electron shell of the other. The previous examples of the molecules $O_2$ and $CO_2$ are examples of covalent bonding. Note that an oxygen atom has eight electrons, two in the first shell and six in the second electron shell. The oxygen atom would be more stable with eight electrons in the outer shell, so it would be inclined to gain two electrons. If another oxygen atom is available, the two atoms can bond together by sharing two electrons, and each will have a complete set of eight in its electron shell (see Figure 2-11). In the case of the carbon dioxide molecule, the outer shell of the carbon atom has four electrons so carbon would be more stable by gaining four more electrons. This stability is gained when a carbon atom shares two electrons from each of two oxygen atoms. This completes the electron shell of the carbon atom, as well as that of each oxygen atom (see Figure 2-12).

Another example of covalent bonding is found in a molecule of methane gas ($CH_4$). Each hydrogen atom shares its one electron with a carbon atom, thereby completing carbon's outer electron shell. At the same time, two electrons borrowed from the carbon atom fill the first, and only, electron shell of hydrogen. A *single covalent bond* is formed when one electron is shared. When two electrons are shared the bond is called a *double covalent bond*. A *triple covalent bond* is formed when three electrons are shared (Figure 2-15).

The shared electrons in a covalently bonded molecule spend part of their time in the electron shell of each of the atoms. Sometimes the electrons spend more time in one atom than in the other. For example, the water molecule $H_2O$ is made of two hydrogen atoms and one oxygen atom. The shared electrons spend more time near the oxygen atom because oxygen is a good electron acceptor and hydrogen is a good electron donor (Figure 2-16). Because of this distribution of electrons and the three-dimensional arrangement of the molecule, there will be a slight positive charge on the hydrogen side of the molecule and a slight negative charge on the oxygen side. The position of the covalent bonds in water arranges the hydrogen atoms toward the same side of the oxygen molecule. This makes the molecule a **polar molecule**, meaning it has oppositely charged ends. This special electromagnetic property of water will be important in the interactions of many molecules in the body. We will explore this further when we discuss the properties of water.

## IONIC BONDS

An **ionic bond** is formed when electrons are transferred from one atom to another. Ionic bonds are most often formed between two types of atom: those with fewer than two electrons in their outer shell and those with nearly full outer shells. An atom with one electron in its outer shell will be inclined to give up that electron so its "new" outer shell will be stable. Similarly, an atom that needs only one electron readily accepts electrons that will make its outer shell full and stable. For example, the sodium atom (Na) has 11 electrons: two in the first shell, eight in the second shell, and one in the

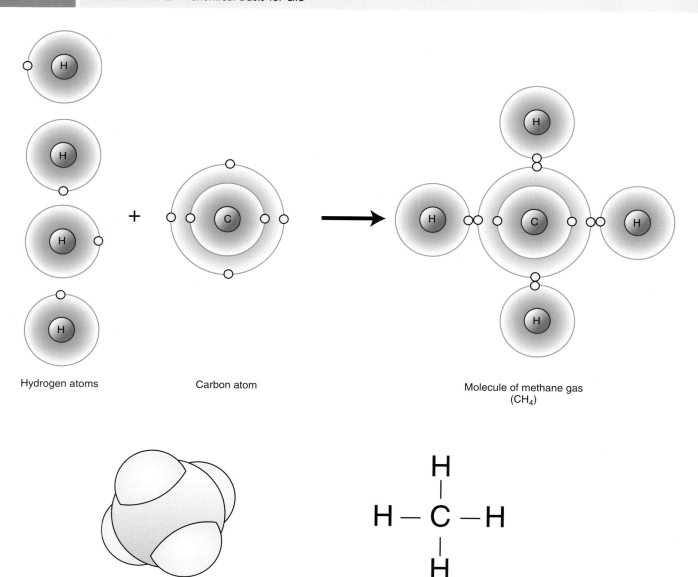

Hydrogen atoms                 Carbon atom                              Molecule of methane gas
(CH₄)

Three dimensional model                                      Line drawing

**FIGURE 2-15** Formation of single covalent bonds. Planetary model, three-dimensional model, and line drawing of a methane molecule (CH₄). Since each hydrogen atom is sharing only one electron with the carbon atom, a single covalent bond is formed, represented by a single line.

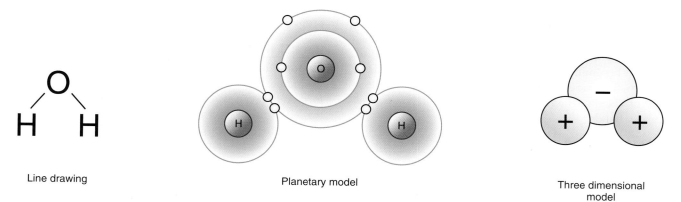

Line drawing                         Planetary model                          Three dimensional
model

**FIGURE 2-16** The polar water molecule. Bonded electrons spend more time near the oxygen atom, giving that aspect of the molecule a slightly negative charge. The hydrogen side of the molecule carries a slightly positive charge.

third shell. It would be more stable without the 11th electron. Suppose a handy atom like chlorine is nearby, with 17 electrons: two in the first shell, eight in the second shell, and seven in the third shell. It badly needs one more electron to make its third shell stable (see Figure 2-13). As the atoms approach each other, sodium's outer electron is strongly attracted to the third shell of the chlorine atom. This does a few things: When the sodium atom loses its electron, it develops a positive charge, because it has more protons than electrons. When the chlorine atom gains the extra electron, it gains an overall negative charge, because now it has more electrons than protons. Thus, these two atoms are drawn to each other by their respective electrical charges, which is an **electrostatic attraction**. This is an ionic bond, and the resulting compound is a molecule of sodium chloride, or table salt (NaCl) (Figure 2-17). Sodium and chloride are **ions** because they have an electrical charge. Sodium is a **cation** because its electrical charge is positive. All cations have positive charges. You can remember this if you think of the "T" in "cation" as a "+" sign. For those of you who really like cats, you will not find it difficult to remember that **cat**ions are positively charged ions. Chloride has a negative charge and is called an **anion**. **All anions have a negative charge**. All ions (cations and anions) are involved in essential functions in the animal body including, for example, contraction of muscle fibers, transmission of nerve impulses, and maintenance of water balance.

## HYDROGEN BONDS

A **hydrogen bond** is more of an electrostatic *attraction* than a true bond because electrons are neither shared nor transferred. It is far weaker than either a true ionic bond or a covalent bond, and is formed when a hydrogen atom (that is already covalently bonded to an atom) is electrostatically attracted to another hydrogen atom that is covalently bonded to a separate atom on a separate portion of the same molecule or on a separate molecule altogether. When hydrogen is covalently bonded in a molecule, it usually has a slight positive charge. As we have already discussed, hydrogen is a willing electron donor, so the shared electron spends more time away from the hydrogen atom, giving it a relative positive charge. A good example of hydrogen bonding occurs in water ($H_2O$). In this molecule, the hydrogen atoms' electrons are electrostatically attracted toward the oxygen atom. This gives the hydrogen side of the molecule a slight positive charge, so the hydrogen side is subsequently attracted by electrostatic forces to the negatively charged portion (the oxygen side) of other water molecules (Figure 2-18). Hydrogen bonds are formed mostly *between molecules*— such as between water molecules—and act to stabilize the solution. Hydrogen bonding is key to water's unique properties as a universal solvent and medium for life processes. Hydrogen bonds also can form *between parts of the same molecule*, which helps to stabilize the molecule. The shape of large complex molecules, such as proteins and DNA, is maintained by hydrogen bonding within the macromolecule (Figure 2-19).

> **TEST YOURSELF 2-2**
> 1. What is a molecule?
> 2. How does an ionic bond differ from a covalent bond?
> 3. In what circumstance does a hydrogen bond commonly occur?
> 4. What important function do hydrogen bonds perform in organic and inorganic chemicals?

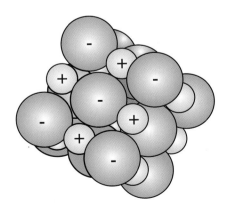
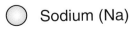 Sodium (Na)
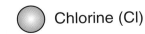 Chlorine (Cl)

A

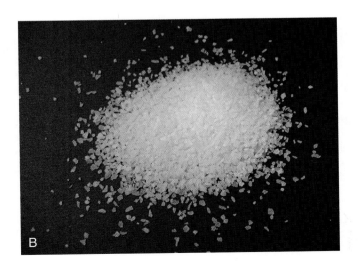

**FIGURE 2-17** Ionic bonding. **A,** The positive charge of the sodium ion and the negative charge of the chloride ion hold the molecule together by electrostatic attraction, forming ionic bonds. **B,** The molecules of sodium chloride are also held together by electrostatic attraction, creating the solid form of sodium chloride called table salt.

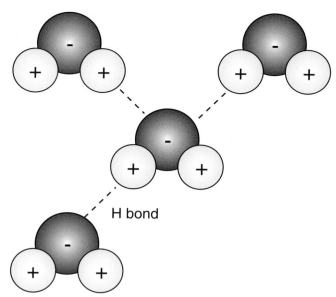

**FIGURE 2-18** Hydrogen bonding between water molecules. In this diagram of water molecules, note that the positively charged hydrogen atom of one water molecule is attracted to the negatively charged oxygen atom of another water molecule.

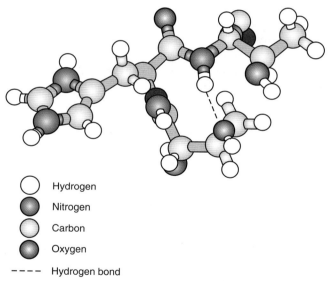

- ○ Hydrogen
- ● Nitrogen
- ○ Carbon
- ● Oxygen
- ---- Hydrogen bond

**FIGURE 2-19** Hydrogen bonding within protein molecules. In this protein molecule, note the attraction between the hydrogen atom in one part of the molecule and the negatively charged oxygen atom in another portion of the same molecule. Hydrogen bonds hold the protein molecule in its specific shape.

## CHEMICAL REACTIONS

A **chemical reaction** involves the formation and breaking of chemical bonds. A **chemical equation** is the way in which the reaction is described in writing; it shows the molecular formula of the **reactants** (X and Y), the **products** (Z) and the direction of the reaction (shown by an arrow).

$$X + Y \rightarrow Z$$

Surprisingly, there are only three types of chemical reaction: *synthesis*, *decomposition*, and *exchange* reactions (Figure 2-20).

During a **synthesis reaction** a new and more complex chemical is made by combining multiple smaller molecules or elements together. Bonds are formed in all synthesis reactions.

$$X + Y \rightarrow XY$$

For example, the formation of the oxygen molecule ($O_2$) can be written:

$$O + O \rightarrow O_2$$

Synthesis reactions occur in the body when simple molecules such as amino acids are assembled to form larger peptide chains, which in turn can be assembled to form proteins needed by the body. Synthesis reactions underlie all **anabolic** (constructive) processes and are particularly evident during growth and the repair of tissues.

In a **decomposition reaction** a single chemical is broken down into multiple, smaller, chemical units.

$$XY \rightarrow X + Y$$

An example is the breakdown of water into hydrogen and oxygen gas.

$$2H_2O \rightarrow 2H_2 + O_2$$

Notice that the number used as a subscript to an element denotes the number of atoms of the element in the molecule (e.g., $H_2$). The number used as a prefix to a molecule denotes the number of molecules of reactant used or of product created (e.g., $2H_2O$).

Decomposition reactions are the reverse of synthesis reactions and involve the breakdown of chemical bonds. Decomposition reactions are the foundation of **catabolic** (degradative) reactions. Proteins for example are degraded into smaller peptide chains or even further into individual amino acids. Decomposition reactions are particularly conspicuous during digestion.

In an **exchange reaction** certain atoms are exchanged between molecules. It is a combination of a synthesis and decomposition reaction. Bonds are both broken and made. In an exchange reaction, new molecules are produced when chemical partners are exchanged.

$$WX + YZ \rightarrow WY + XZ$$

An example is the reaction of sodium bicarbonate, often given for relief of indigestion, with hydrochloric acid in the stomach:

$$NaHCO_3 + HCl \rightarrow NaCl + H_2O + CO_2$$

Note that the number of atoms of each element is the same on both sides of all chemical equations.

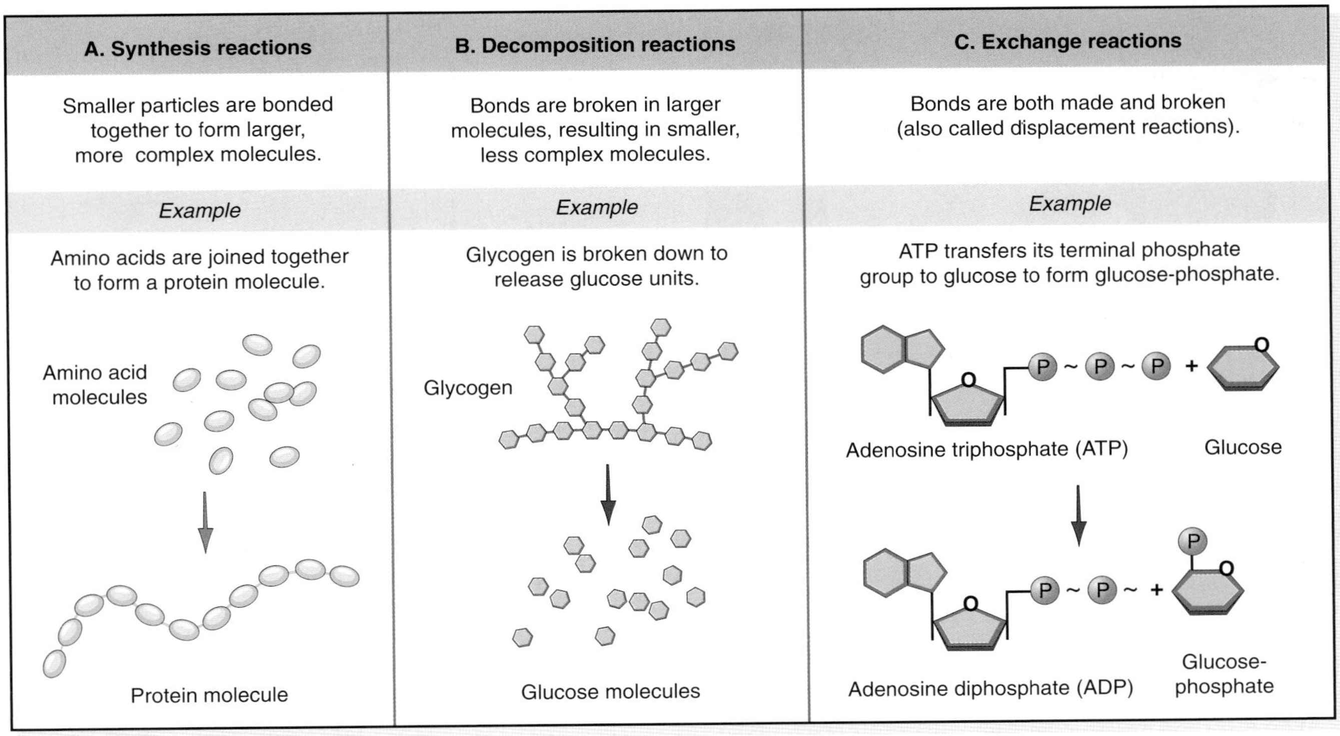
A. Synthesis reactions
Smaller particles are bonded together to form larger, more complex molecules.
Example
Amino acids are joined together to form a protein molecule.
Amino acid molecules
Protein molecule
B. Decomposition reactions
Bonds are broken in larger molecules, resulting in smaller, less complex molecules.
Example
Glycogen is broken down to release glucose units.
Glycogen
Glucose molecules
C. Exchange reactions
Bonds are both made and broken (also called displacement reactions).
Example
ATP transfers its terminal phosphate group to glucose to form glucose-phosphate.
Adenosine triphosphate (ATP)
Glucose
Adenosine diphosphate (ADP)
Glucose-phosphate

**FIGURE 2-20** Three types of chemical reaction: **A**, synthesis, **B**, decomposition and **C**, exchange.

Chemical reactions either require the input of energy or they release energy. In synthesis reactions new bonds are formed, so energy is required. After the bonds are formed, potential energy is stored in the chemical bonds between the atoms. In decomposition reactions energy is released from the breaking of the chemical bonds (i.e., the potential energy stored in the bonds is released). Exchange reactions have no net energy requirement. The energy released from breaking bonds is used to create the new bonds. This concept will be explored in more detail in Chapter 17, Nutrients and Metabolism.

Several factors can influence the rate of reaction. One is the availability of the reactants, referred to as the *concentration of reactants*. The more reactants that are available, the more likely they will come in contact and be able to react with one another. The temperature of the environment influences the rate of reaction. When the temperature increases, the speed of molecular movement increases, and the chance of molecules meeting improves. Temperature also increases the velocity at which reactants meet, and the velocity provides the energy for the reaction. **Activation energy** is the energy required for the reaction to happen. Some reactions have a higher activation energy and require the input of more energy for the reaction to occur; these reactions will occur at a slower pace. Certain reactions require the presence of a **catalyst**. In living organisms, catalysts are usually special proteins that hold the reactants together so they may interact. The catalyst protein is not destroyed or used up by the reaction, and the reaction speed is increased when there are more catalyst proteins present. These special catalyst proteins are called **enzymes**.

### TEST YOURSELF 2-3

1. What is a chemical reaction?
2. What are the three types of chemical reaction?
3. The digestion of food uses which type of chemical reaction?
4. What factors influence the rate of chemical reactions?

## CHEMICAL COMPONENTS OF LIVING ORGANISMS

With the myriad of **chemical elements** available on earth and the millions of combinations of those elements, it is amazing that all living organisms are composed of only a few elements. The compounds that make up living organisms such as a cow, for example, are divided into two categories: *organic* and *inorganic* (Figure 2-21). **Organic compounds** tend to be large, complex molecules that contain carbon–carbon (C–C) covalent bonds or carbon–hydrogen (C–H) covalent bonds. Examples of organic molecules include proteins, carbohydrates, triglycerides, and nucleic acids. **Inorganic molecules**, such as water, salts, acids, and bases, rarely contain carbon and do not contain C–C or C–H bonds. They tend to be small molecules and often have ionic bonding. Both organic and

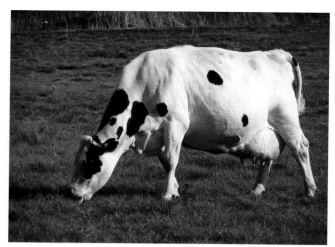

**FIGURE 2-21** Organic versus inorganic matter. The molecules that make up a living organism, such as this Holstein cow and the grass she is eating, are primarily organic compounds. Nonliving structures, such as rocks and metal fencing, contain mostly inorganic compounds.

inorganic molecules are essential components of all living organisms.

Why is carbon an essential component of organic molecules? Carbon is small in size and is electrically neutral so it never gains or loses electrons. Instead, it shares electrons with other atoms. Because it has four valence shell electrons, carbon is able to form four covalent bonds with other elements, including other carbon atoms. In this way, carbon enables the formation of long hydrocarbon chains, which can form a linear shape or a ring shape. Collections of atoms called **functional groups** may be attached to the carbon chains (or rings) and determine the functionality of the molecule as a whole (Figure 2-22). The functional group, though small relative to the entire molecule, is the reactive part of the molecule and determines the molecule's chemical activity.

> ✓ **TEST YOURSELF 2-4**
> 1. What is the difference between organic and inorganic compounds?
> 2. Are only organic compounds necessary for life?
> 3. List four types of inorganic molecule that are important for life.
> 4. List four types of organic molecule that are important for life.
> 5. What features does carbon possess that makes it particularly well suited for creating the chemistry of living creatures.
> 6. Define the term "functional group."

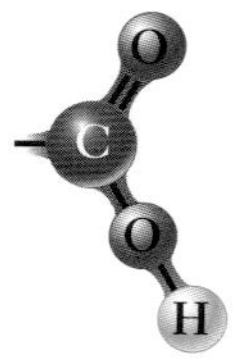

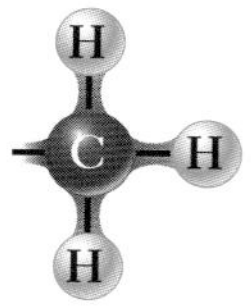

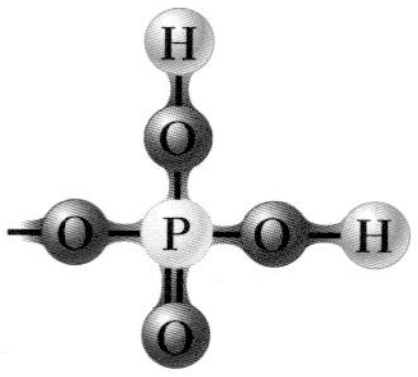

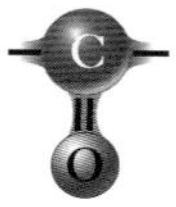

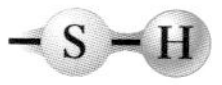

## INORGANIC COMPOUNDS

### WATER

Water is a very simple molecule that has unique properties. As mentioned, the water molecule is composed of one

| Functional Group | Structural Formula | Models |
|---|---|---|
| Hydroxyl | $-OH$ | |
| Carbonyl | $-\overset{\|\|}{\underset{O}{C}}-$ | |
| Carboxyl | $-C\overset{O}{\underset{OH}{\nwarrow}}$ | |
| Methyl | $-\overset{H}{\underset{H}{C}}-H$ | |
| Amino | $-N\overset{H}{\underset{H}{\diagdown}}$ | |
| Sulfhydryl | $-SH$ | |
| Phosphate | $-O-\overset{OH}{\underset{O}{P}}-OH$ | |
| Acetyl | $-\overset{O}{\overset{\|\|}{C}}-\overset{H}{\underset{H}{C}}-H$ | |

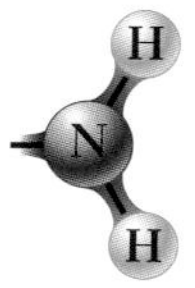

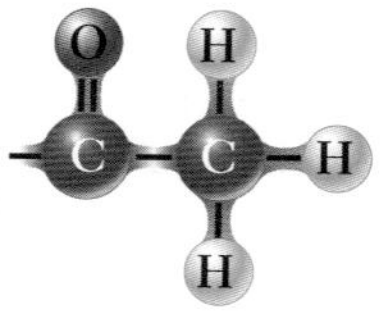

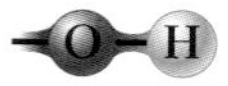

**FIGURE 2-22** Common functional groups. Functional groups are attached to the carbon backbone of organic molecules and represent the metabolically active portion of the molecule that determines its biochemical activity.

oxygen atom covalently bonded to two hydrogen atoms. It is a polar molecule that has a slight positive charge in the area of the hydrogen atoms and a slight negative charge in the area of the oxygen atom. This polarity allows water molecules to form hydrogen bonds with each other and with other polar molecules. The polarity of the water molecule allows it to fulfill the following important roles within the living organism.

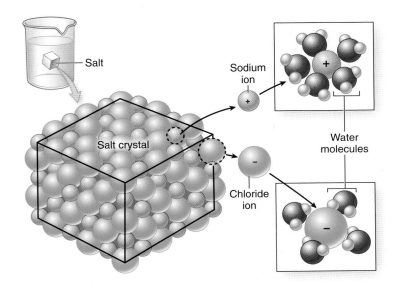

**FIGURE 2-23** Water as the universal solvent. A crystal of sodium chloride (NaCl) dissociates in water forming sodium (Na⁺) and Chloride (Cl⁻) ions. During this process, water molecules surround each ion. The positively charged ends of the water molecule (hydrogen) are attracted to the negative chloride ions (Cl⁻), forming hydrogen bonds. Similarly, the negatively charged end of the water molecule (oxygen) is attracted to the positive Na⁺ ions. In this way, water serves as a universal solvent.

*Water is the universal solvent.* Chemicals added to water are called **solutes**, and the combination of the chemicals plus the water is called a **solution**. More chemicals can be dissolved in water than any other known **solvent**. Water molecules surround molecules of solute; the negatively charged ends of water surround positively charged molecules, forming a layer of water around each molecule (Figure 2-23). Or, conversely, the positive ends of the water molecule surround or *blanket* negatively charged molecules. Chemicals that dissolve or mix well in water are called **hydrophilic** (literally *water loving*) and are usually polar molecules or ions. Molecules that do not mix well with water are called **hydrophobic** (*water hating*). They are usually electrically neutral, nonpolar molecules such as lipids. Hydrophobic molecules gather together into a droplet when they are added to water, and a layer of water molecules then surrounds the droplets. There are no bonds between the water molecules and the hydrophobic molecules (Figure 2-24).

*Water is an ideal transport medium.* The blanketing property of water allows molecules in the water to move around freely and to be cushioned from each other. Because many molecules dissolve readily in water, they can be carried easily to locations in the body or a cell via blood, lymph, and intracellular and extracellular fluid. Blood is a suspension of cells and chemicals in water and is used to carry cells and chemicals around the body. Urine is a solution of waste products in water and is used to eliminate such waste products from the body.

*Water has a high heat capacity and a high heat of vaporization.* As the chemicals in solution react, they often give off

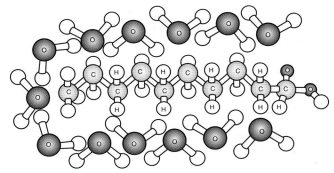

**FIGURE 2-24** Water and hydrophobic molecules. Water molecules surround a fatty acid molecule (hydrocarbon chain), which is hydrophobic. No bonds form between hydrophobic molecules and water.

energy as heat. Water is able to absorb heat from biochemical reactions so that the overall temperature of the solution does not rise too rapidly. This stabilization of heat is necessary to keep living organisms in a stable temperature range so that the reactions of life's processes can occur at a steady rate without interruption. The *high heat of vaporization* means that water needs a fairly high temperature to change from a liquid to a gas; therefore, water will remain in a liquid state through a wide range of temperatures.

*Water is used for lubrication.* The ability of water to surround molecules allows it to be a lubricant for moving parts in the body. Examples abound in the animal body: the fluid in the pericardial sac allows the heart to move freely within the sac and synovial fluid in the joints allows bones to rub without pain when a limb is moved.

## SALTS

**Salts** are mineral compounds that have ionic bonds, and they are the principal form of minerals that enter and are stored in the body. An example of a salt is sodium chloride (NaCl), which is present in large amounts in blood and other tissues. Another example is calcium phosphate $Ca^3(PO_4)^2$, which is the substance that gives bones their rigidity. When salts are added to water they immediately *ionize*, or divide into separate ions. Salts in their ionic form are known as **electrolytes**, substances that have the ability to transmit an electrical charge. The transmission of nerve impulses, for example, requires sodium ions ($Na^+$) and potassium ions ($K^+$). In addition, the contraction of muscle requires sodium, potassium, and calcium ions ($Ca^{2+}$).

## ACIDS AND BASES

**Acids** are ionically bonded substances that, when added to water, freely release hydrogen ions ($H^+$). In other words, acids ionize in water and one of their ions is $H^+$. Acids are therefore called *$H^+$ donors* or *proton donors*, since $H^+$ is a proton with

no electron. **Bases**, which are alkaline compounds that are ionically bonded, also ionize in water but release a hydroxyl ion ($OH^-$), not hydrogen ions, therefore bases are known as *proton acceptors*. Hydroxyl ions are attracted to $H^+$ ions to form water.

Acids and bases are also electrolytes because, when they ionize in water, they can transmit electricity. An example of an acid is hydrochloric acid (HCl). When added to water, the $H^+$ and $Cl^-$ ions disassociate and are free to join with other substances. If hydrochloric acid is added to water containing a base such as sodium hydroxide (NaOH), the acid and base **neutralize** each other. The protons from the acid join with hydroxyl groups from the base and the resulting solution has a neutral pH.

$$HCl + NaOH \rightarrow H^+ + Cl^- + Na^+ + OH^- \rightarrow H_2O + NaCl$$

## THE pH SCALE

Acidity and alkalinity are measured on a pH scale. The scale ranges from 1 (the most acidic) to 14 (the most alkaline or basic). A pH of 7 is the middle of the scale and is neutral. For example, lemon juice is very acidic and has a pH of 2.3, and ammonia is very basic and has a pH of 11.6. To function properly the tissues and blood in the animal body must maintain a pH of around 7.4, which is slightly basic (Figure 2-25).

## BUFFERS

Weak acids and bases are those that do not completely ionize in water. They are important in the physiology of living systems because they act to **buffer** the solution where chemical reactions take place. *Buffering the solution* means keeping the pH in the neutral range. As metabolic chemical reactions

---

**CLINICAL APPLICATION**

### Kidney Failure: Low Potassium

A 16-year-old cat has kidney failure. One of the findings on the serum chemistry test is a low serum potassium concentration. Potassium (K) is an electrolyte that is important for muscle contraction and nerve function. The low level of potassium is caused by the cat's lack of appetite over the last few weeks: kidney disease makes the cat feel nauseated, so she has a reduced intake of potassium-containing foods and loss of potassium through the damaged kidneys. The lack of potassium makes her feel weak, and it can slow her gastrointestinal contractions and cause constipation. More dangerously, because potassium plays an important role in muscle contraction, the low potassium makes it difficult for the heart muscle to contract. This reduces blood flow to the tissues and can also cause irregular heartbeat; these arrhythmias can be life threatening. We treat this condition by supplementing her intravenous fluids with potassium or by giving her oral potassium supplements.

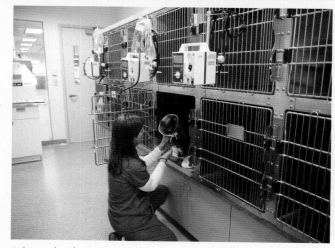

A hospitalized cat in renal failure is examined at regular intervals by veterinary technicians. Fluid therapy is a critical part of treatment. Therefore, an Elizabethan collar is applied to prevent the patient from removing the intravenous catheter. (Courtesy Dr. Joanna Bassert.)

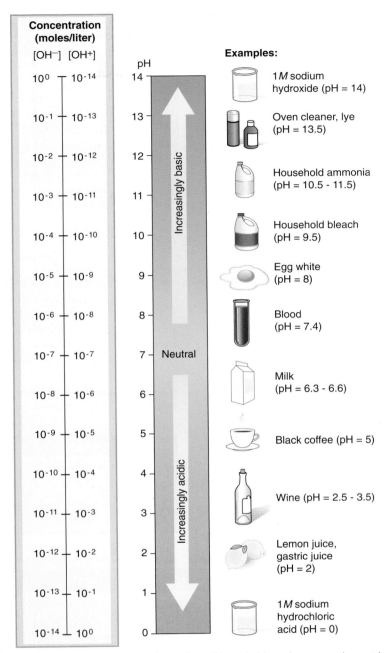

**FIGURE 2-25** The pH scale. Many common chemicals and household products are either acidic or basic. As the concentration of H⁺ increases, the solution becomes more acidic and the pH value decreases. As the OH⁻ concentration increases, the solution becomes more basic or alkaline, and the pH value increases.

take place in the body, strong acids such as lactic acid and strong bases such as ammonia are produced as waste products. If these substances were allowed to accumulate, the pH of the cell or tissue would quickly become too high or too low for chemical reactions to continue. When placed in water, a weak acid will not ionize completely. The product of ionization is a weak base; in other words, a weak acid will initially ionize into free H⁺ ions, a weak base product, and weak acid molecules (Figure 2-26). The pH of the solution is not changed greatly because some of the chemical remains in acid form and some remains a weak base. If a strong base

is added to the solution, the hydrogen ion will attach to the base and neutralize it, and the remaining weak acid will ionize Further.

Buffers help the cell maintain a neutral pH by not allowing excessive hydrogen or hydroxyl ions to accumulate. An example of the most common buffer system is carbonic acid and bicarbonate. Carbonic acid ($H_2CO_3$) ionizes, when placed in water, to free hydrogen ions and the weak base, bicarbonate ($HCO_3^-$).

$$H_2CO_3 \rightarrow H^+ + HCO_3^-$$

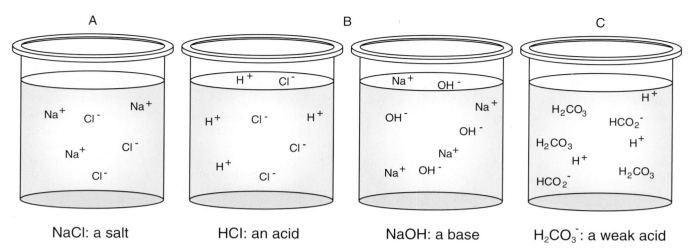

**FIGURE 2-26** Salts, acids, and bases. **A,** When placed in water, salt (NaCl) ionizes completely. **B,** Hydrochloric acid (HCl) is a strong acid, and sodium hydroxide (NaOH) is a strong base; they ionize completely in water. **C,** Carbonic acid ($H_2CO_3$) is a weak acid and ionizes incompletely to hydrogen ions ($H^+$) and a weak base, bicarbonate ($HCO_3^-$).

Bicarbonate ($HCO_3^-$) can further ionize by losing a proton, resulting in carbonate ($CO_3^{2-}$).

$$HCO_3^- \rightarrow H^+ + CO_3^{2-}$$

This means bicarbonate can act as both a weak acid, by losing a proton, and a weak base, by gaining one; this is what makes it such an effective buffer. The complete reaction is written as:

$$H_2CO_3 \leftrightarrow H^+ + HCO_3^- \leftrightarrow 2H^+ + CO_3^{2-}$$

Notice that this equation can run in either direction. What happens when a stronger acid, say lactic acid, is added to the solution? The strong acid disassociates, and the extra $H^+$ ions increase the speed of the reaction, so more carbonic acid is produced. This is eventually excreted as $CO_2$ via the **respiratory system**.

$$H_2CO_3 + C_3H_5O_3^- \text{ (lactate)} \rightarrow HCO_3^- + C_3H_6O_3 \text{ (lactic acid)}$$

If a base is added to the blood, the bicarbonate will donate its hydrogen ion and more carbonate will be formed.

---

### ✓ TEST YOURSELF 2-7

1. Which type of compound is known as a proton donor: acid or base?
2. What does pH measure?
3. Is a solution with a pH of 8.5 acidic or basic?
4. How does a weak acid act as a buffer?

---

 **CLINICAL APPLICATION**

## Metabolic Acidosis

Sometimes so much acid accumulates in the animal body that the buffering system is overwhelmed, and the pH of the blood is lowered. This condition is called *metabolic acidosis*. Two common causes are fatty acid accumulation in diabetes mellitus, due to the excessive breakdown of lipids for energy, and the accumulation of hydrogen ions in kidney disease caused by the kidney's inability to excrete them. In these conditions the blood and tissue have a high level of acid: weak acids from the buffering system and strong acids caused by the underlying condition. Metabolic acidosis can cause several uncomfortable and dangerous symptoms including anorexia, vomiting, lethargy, and muscle wasting. Severe metabolic acidosis can decrease cardiac output, reducing blood flow to the tissues, which further damages the kidneys and other organs. Life-threatening cardiac arrhythmias can also develop. Administering balanced electrolyte solutions treats metabolic acidosis since these fluids contain the buffers needed by the body to decrease the acid concentration in the blood.

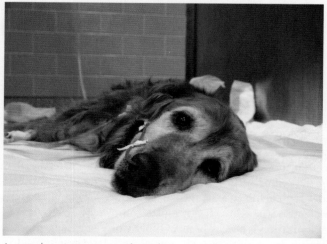

A critical canine patient with acidosis receives intravenous fluids with buffers and electrolytes. Humidified nasal oxygen via a nebulizer is also provided to assist with respiration. (Courtesy Dr. Joanna Bassert.)

# ORGANIC COMPOUNDS

Organic compounds are composed of large molecules containing carbon. The molecules are divided into four groups: carbohydrates, lipids, proteins, and nucleic acids. What is it about the element carbon that makes it so omnipresent in organic chemistry? Carbon has four electrons in its outer electron shell, so it is moved to share these electrons with other atoms to complete its outer shell. For this reason, carbon is most stable when it has four covalent bonds with other atoms. This allows molecules containing carbon to exist in many forms including chains, rings, and branches. This flexibility allows for various structures to be built using a small selection of atoms. Many of the organic molecules used in the body are **macromolecules**—long, complex molecules, often with repeating units. Table 2-3 lists the important organic molecules and macromolecules used by the animal body.

## CARBOHYDRATES

**Carbohydrate** molecules are used for energy, storage of energy, and cellular structures; table sugar, starch, and cellulose are all examples. Carbohydrates are composed of atoms of carbon, hydrogen, and oxygen, with hydrogen and oxygen in the same ratio as in water—two to one. You can think of carbohydrates as *hydrated carbon* or *water-containing carbon*.

The simplest form of a carbohydrate is called a *simple sugar* or **monosaccharide**. Monosaccharides contain three to seven carbon atoms in a chain or ring. An example is glucose, with the chemical formula $C_6H_{12}O_6$ (Figure 2-27); this molecule is the primary fuel of the body. Since glucose contains six carbon atoms, it is known as a **hexose sugar**. A sugar with five carbons is a **pentose sugar**. Another example of a hexose sugar is fructose. It also has the molecular formula $C_6H_{12}O_6$, but the arrangement of the atoms is different. This molecule is consumed as the primary sugar in fruit and then converted to glucose in the body. Figure 2-28 shows diagrams of these important monosaccharides.

When two monosaccharides are joined together the reaction is a synthesis reaction, and a **disaccharide** is formed. Because water is created during the reaction—it is extracted from the saccharides—the reaction is called **dehydration synthesis**. An example is the combination of glucose and fructose to make sucrose, which is table sugar. Cells use synthesis reactions to build molecules needed for cellular functioning. This process is called *anabolism*. The opposite reaction is when sucrose is decomposed into its monosaccharide components, glucose and fructose. Since water is used in the reaction to break down sucrose this type of reaction is called **hydrolysis** (Figure 2-29). Cells use decomposition reactions to release energy held in bonds between atoms and to generate the simple molecular building blocks needed by the cell. The decomposition of nutrients is a process called

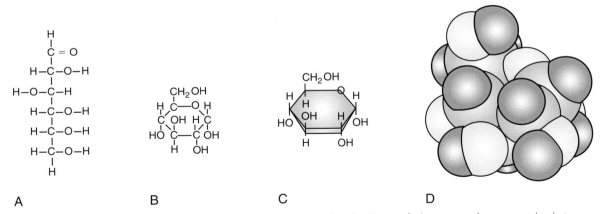

**FIGURE 2-27** Structure of carbohydrate molecule. **A,** The carbon backbone of glucose may form a straight chain. **B,** A more stable carbon ring structure. **C,** Shorthand for the glucose molecule, omitting the carbon atoms at the angles of the carbohydrate ring. **D,** The three-dimensional view of the glucose molecule.

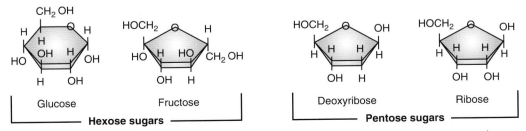

**FIGURE 2-28** Monosaccharides. Glucose and fructose are example of hexose sugars. They contain six carbons each. Deoxyribose and ribose are examples of five-carbon pentose sugars.

| TABLE 2-3 | Organic Molecules in the Body | |
|---|---|---|
| **MOLECULAR CLASSIFICATION** | **CONSTITUENTS AND MOLECULAR STRUCTURE** | **EXAMPLES AND NOTATIONS** |
| **Carbohydrates** | | |
| Simple carbohydrates | Monosaccharide: most stable as a single pentose ring | Glucose, fructose, ribose, deoxyribose |
| | Disaccharide: two pentose rings | Sucrose |
| Complex carbohydrates | Polysaccharide | Starches; glycogen: stores energy in liver; cellulose: derived from plants and provides insoluble fiber in diet |
| **Proteins** | | |
| | Amino acids link to form peptide and polypeptide chains; proteins form primary, secondary, tertiary and quarternary structures | <u>Contractile structural proteins</u> that make up muscle (e.g. actin and myosin) <br> <u>Other structural proteins</u> that make up cartilage and tendons (collagen), and hair and skin (keratin) <br> <u>Globular functional proteins</u> such as enzymes, antibodies, hemoglobin and many integral and peripheral proteins in the cell membrane |
| **Lipids** | | |
| Neutral fats | Triglycerides: one glycerol molecule (backbone) and three fatty acid chains; fatty acid chains that lack double bonds are "saturated" while those with double bonds are "unsaturated" | Saturated fatty acids are solid (fats) at room temperature and unsaturated fatty acids are liquid (oils) at room temperature; both are concentrated sources of energy |
| Phospholipids | Phosphate head, glycerol backbone and two fatty acid chains | Key component of the bilayer of the cell membrane |
| Steroids | Four flat interlocking rings | Cholesterol, cortisol, testosterone, estrogen |
| **Other Lipid Substances** | | |
| Fat-soluble vitamins | Variable molecular structure depending upon the specific vitamin; stored in liver and fat | Vitamins A, D, E, and K: stored in body fat; can be toxic if given in excess |
| Eicosanoids | Derived from arachidonic acid, a 20-carbon fatty acid | Regulatory molecules that enhance the immune system and elicit inflammatory responses (e.g., prostaglandins, mediate inflammation; leukotrienes, mediate bronchoconstriction; thromboxanes, mediate platelet function) |
| **Nucleic Acids** | | |
| Deoxyribonucleic acid (DNA) | Two parallel strands of nucleotides connected via hydrogen bonds; each nucleotide is composed of: a phosphate group, a **2-deoxyribose** sugar, and a nitrogenous base (e.g., cytosine, guanine, alanine, or **thymine**) | Found in the nucleus where it condenses with histone proteins to form chromosomes; also found in mitochondria, providing the molecular instructions for making the enzymes needed for cellular respiration |
| Ribonucleic acid (RNA) | A **single strand** of nucleotides; each nucleotide is composed of: a phosphate group, a **ribose** sugar, and one nitrogenous base (e.g., cytosine, guanine, alanine, or **uracil**) | Three types of RNA: ribosomal RNA (rRNA), forms ribosomes and found in the nucleolus; transfer RNA (tRNA), carries amino acids to docking stations on mRNA; messenger RNA (mRNA), carries the genetic code from the nucleus to the cytosol |
| Adenosine triphosphate (ATP) | An ATP molecule is composed of: adenine, a ribose sugar, and three phosphate groups | ATP is used by the cell to carry out all active metabolic processes; when the terminal phosphate group is removed, energy is released and the molecule becomes adenosine diphosphate (ADP). ADP is transported back to the mitochondria where it is converted back to ATP |

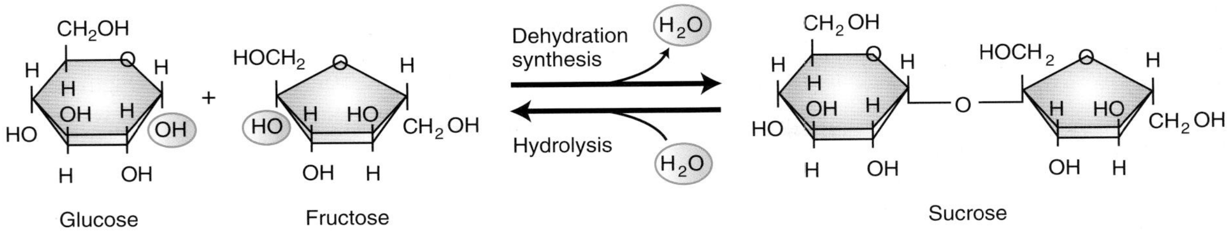

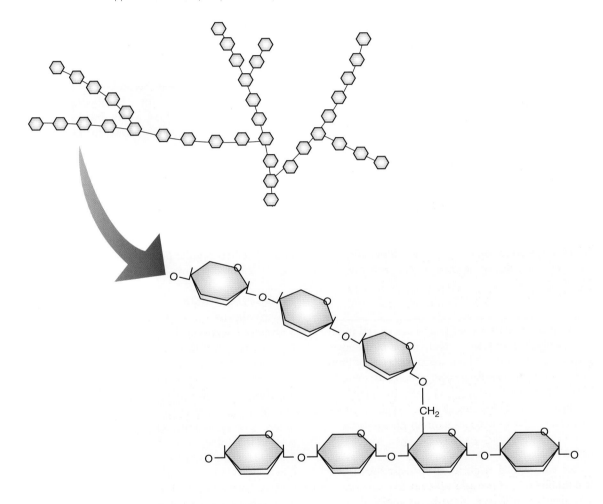

**FIGURE 2-29** Disaccharide. Glucose and fructose are joined in dehydration synthesis to make sucrose, a disaccharide, and water. The opposite reaction, hydrolysis, decomposes sucrose into glucose and fructose.

**FIGURE 2-30** Polysaccharide. A simplified model of a molecule of glycogen. Glycogen is a polysaccharide made of the multiple glucose molecules bonded in a branching chain. Glucose is stored in the liver in form of glycogen. The branching of the molecules creates many ends that allow for reactions at each end to break glucose molecules off very rapidly when the animal needs energy.

*catabolism*, and this process, along with anabolism, will be explored in more detail in Chapter 17.

**Polysaccharides** are combinations of many monosaccharides, all joined by dehydration synthesis. Polysaccharides can have a structural or a fuel storage function. Glycogen (Figure 2-30) is an important polysaccharide that stores fuel

in body tissues, and starch is a polysaccharide that has a similar function in plant tissues. Cellulose is the most abundant organic molecule in the biosphere; it is a polysaccharide that provides structural strength to plants. Herbivores can digest cellulose and use the component monosaccharides as fuel.

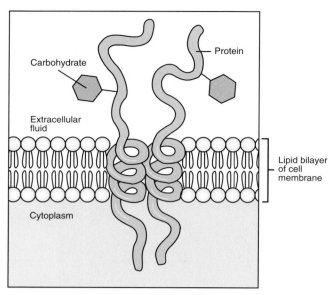

**FIGURE 2-31** Glycoprotein. Glycoproteins, macromolecules made of amino acid and carbohydrate units, are found in cell membranes. The carbohydrate recognizes molecules that are to be transported into the cell by the protein channel.

Carbohydrates can also be joined to other molecules, such as proteins or lipids, to create macromolecules important to life. For example, a **glycoprotein** is a macromolecule composed of a carbohydrate attached to a protein. The carbohydrate component of a cell membrane glycoprotein has important roles in the adhesion of the cell to other cells and in recognition of molecules to be transported into the cell (Figure 2-31).

## LIPIDS

**Lipids** are used in the body for energy and are stored in fat for future energy needs. Lipids serve as chemical messengers in the form of some hormones. There are four classes of lipid that are important for life: *neutral fats, phospholipids, steroids,* and *eicosanoids.* Like carbohydrates, lipids are made of carbon, hydrogen, and oxygen, though their oxygen content is much lower. They also sometimes contain phosphorus.

## NEUTRAL FATS

**Neutral fats** are also called *triglycerides* or, simply, *fats.* A **triglyceride** contains three fatty acids (hence the "tri" in the name) and a glycerol molecule. A **glycerol** molecule is a modified, three-carbon simple sugar. It has the formula $C_3H_8O_3$. A **fatty acid** is a chain of carbon atoms with one or two hydrogen atoms attached to each carbon by single or double bonds. A fatty acid is called a **saturated fatty acid** when all the bonds in the hydrocarbon chain are single bonds and as many hydrogen atoms as possible are attached to the carbon. Saturated fatty acids are mainly found in animal fats such as butter and lard. A fatty acid is called an **unsaturated fatty acid** when there are some double bonds between the carbon and hydrogen atoms. Unsaturated fatty acids are mainly of plant origin, such as corn oil and olive oil. The glycerol molecule and the three fatty acid molecules connect together in the shape of an "E" with the glycerol molecule making the backbone of the E (Figure 2-32). They are joined by dehydration synthesis: three water molecules are produced by joining the hydrogen from the fatty acids to the hydroxyl (OH) groups of the glycerol.

---

✓ **TEST YOURSELF 2-8**
1. What three elements are found in all carbohydrates?
2. What is the name of a simple sugar?
3. What process joins multiple simple sugars?
4. What is another name for a complex, multiunit carbohydrate?

---

When triglycerides are decomposed, the reaction is called hydrolysis, and water molecules are consumed. These reactions should be familiar because they are similar to the reactions that occur with carbohydrate synthesis and decomposition. Neutral fats are mainly used for energy; the body gets energy by breaking down the bonds in the neutral fats and stores energy by transporting the excess neutral fats to adipose tissue. The fat-filled cells act to pad vital organs from trauma and act as insulation to help maintain body temperature. Neutral fats are hydrophobic and do not mix in water.

A **lipoprotein** is a macromolecule composed of proteins and lipids. Lipoproteins are used to transport fats within the body. The hydrophilic proteins allow the fats to be shielded from the blood plasma and to be transported.

### PHOSPHOLIPIDS

**Phospholipids** are similar to triglycerides in that they have a glycerol backbone. They have two fatty acids attached to the glycerol extending in one direction. In place of the third fatty acid, they have a phosphate group ($PO_4$) attached to a nitrogen-containing compound extending in the other direction. The phosphate group side, or head end of the phospholipid, is water soluble, meaning it is hydrophilic and polar, whereas the fatty acid side, or tail end of the molecule, is water insoluble, that is, hydrophobic and nonpolar (Figure 2-33). This unique property is what makes phospholipids line up in two layers, called a *lipid bilayer,* when placed in a polar substance such as water. The hydrophilic heads form hydrogen bonds with the water and the tails are repelled from the water and are most stable when abutting another tail. Phospholipids are the main component of cellular membranes. They also form the myelin sheath of nerve cells.

### STEROIDS

**Steroids** are lipids that take the form of four interlocking hydrocarbon rings. They are hydrophobic, nonpolar substances with very little oxygen. Different types of steroid are formed by attaching unique functional groups to the four-ring structure of the molecule (Figure 2-34). The basic cholesterol ring structure is synthesized from acetyl CoA (see

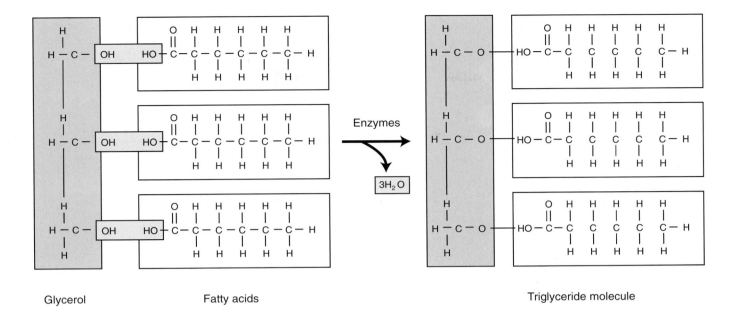

Glycerol                          Fatty acids                                                    Triglyceride molecule

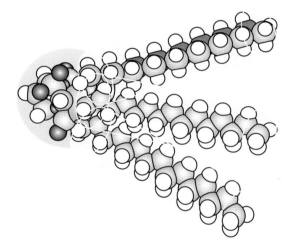

**FIGURE 2-32** Triglyceride. A triglyceride molecule is formed by dehydration synthesis and is composed of three fatty acids and one glycerol molecule. A three-dimensional view is also shown.

Chapter 17). Cholesterol is used in the formation of bile salts, which aid in fat digestion. Cholesterol is also used by the adrenal glands, testes, and ovaries for creation of steroid hormones including cortisone, estrogen, progesterone, and testosterone.

### EICOSANOIDS

**Eicosanoids** are lipids formed from a 20-carbon fatty acid and a ring structure (Figure 2-35). The prefix *eicosa* derives from the Greek word for *twenty*. Eicosanoids are important substances for the mediation of complex chemical processes in the body and include: **prostaglandins (PGs)**, which mediate inflammation; **thromboxane**, which mediates platelet function; and **leukotrienes**, which mediate bronchoconstriction and increased mucus production.

### PROTEINS

**Proteins** are the most abundant organic molecules in the body. They also have the widest variety of functions (Table 2-4). Proteins are used for cell structures and structural body tissues, for controlling chemical reactions, for regulating growth, and for defending the body from invaders. Proteins **catalyze** or speed up all reactions occurring in the body, and

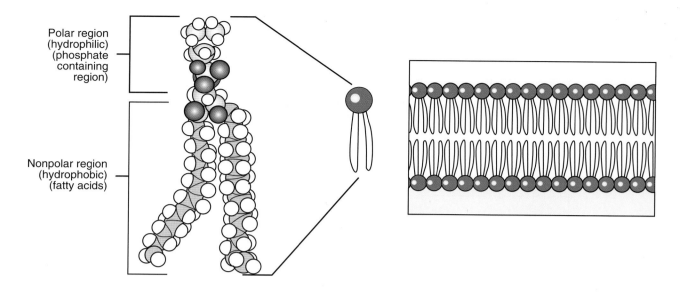

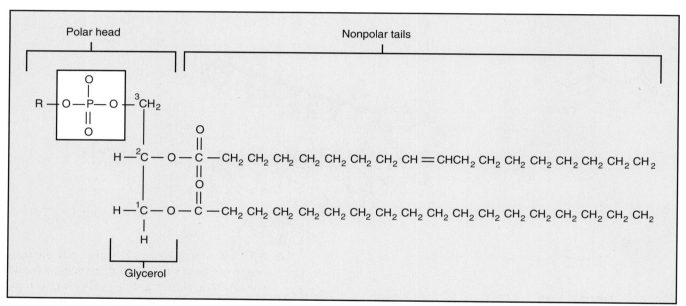

**FIGURE 2-33** Anatomy of a phospholipid. Example of hydrophilic and hydrophobic regions of a phospholipid molecule. In the diagram of the cell membrane, note that the phospholipids form a lipid bilayer with the polar part of the phospholipid molecules hydrogen-bonded to and facing the water molecules.

| TABLE 2-4 | Functions of Proteins | |
|---|---|---|
| **PROTEIN STRUCTURE** | **FUNCTION** | **EXAMPLE** |
| Functional (globular) | Chemical reactions | Protein enzymes: essential to almost every biochemical reaction in the body |
| | Transport of molecules | Hemoglobin transports oxygen in the blood |
| | Regulation of metabolism | Peptide hormones: regulate metabolic activity, growth, and development (e.g., thyroid hormone regulates metabolic rate and insulin regulates blood sugar levels) |
| | Immune system | Antibodies (immunoglobulins) are proteins created by immune cells that recognize foreign substances such as viruses |
| Structural (fibrous) | Structural framework | Collagen: gives strength to bones, tendons, ligaments<br>Keratin: hair, nails, waterproofing of skin |
| | Physical movement | Actin and myosin: contractile proteins found in muscle; actin also used for intracellular transport |

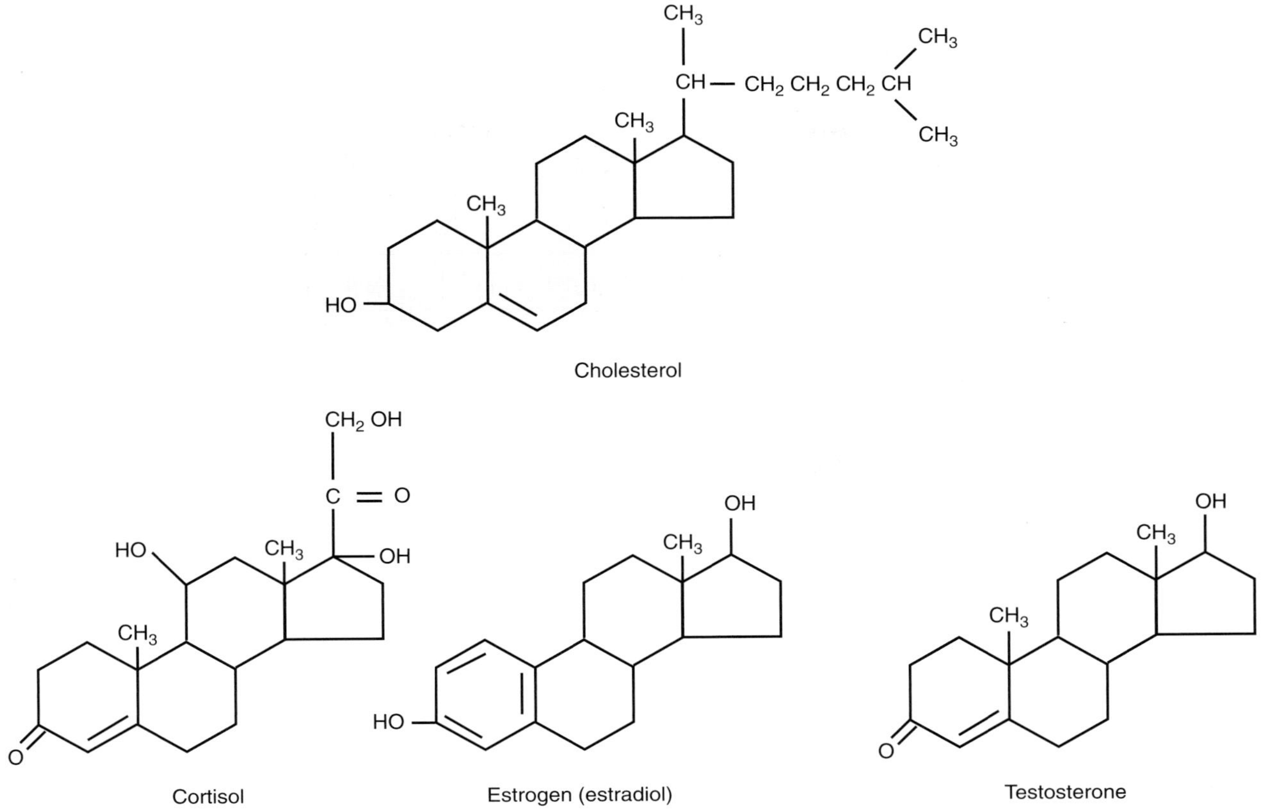

CH₃
CH — CH₂ CH₂ CH₂ CH
CH₃          CH₃
CH₃              CH₃

CH₃

CH₃

HO

Cholesterol

CH₂ OH

C = O

HO          CH₃          OH

CH₃

O

Cortisol

OH

CH₃          OH

HO

Estrogen (estradiol)

OH

CH₃          OH

CH₃

O

Testosterone

**FIGURE 2-34** The steroid nucleus. The steroid nucleus (highlighted) found in cholesterol is a four-ring structure. Attaching a different functional group to the basic four-ring structure forms a different steroid compound. You can see how easy it is for any steroid to be converted into another type of steroid. The clinical significance of this is exemplified by the high cholesterol seen in horses and dogs with Cushing's syndrome (high cortisol is converted to cholesterol). This also plays an important role in women with breast cancer. Hormones in meats, dairy products, and some therapeutic drugs consumed by women, as well as xenoestrogens found in insecticides and other environmental pollutants, can be converted to estrogens and other tumor-enhancing steroid hormones (progesterone).

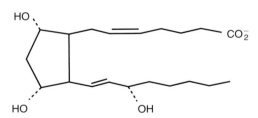

HO

HO          OH          $CO_2^-$

**FIGURE 2-35** Eicosanoid. This is a diagram of prostaglandin F2alpha, which is used to lyse the corpus luteum to alter the reproductive cycle in female cattle. The 20-carbon fatty acid is in the classic *hairpin* formation of all eicosanoids.

they transport ions and other molecules into and out of the cell and around the body. You can think of proteins as the worker molecules of the body that organize and facilitate all metabolic processes. Proteins are organic molecules made chiefly of carbon, oxygen, hydrogen, and nitrogen, though some proteins also contain sulfur, iron, or phosphorus. The building blocks of proteins are amino acids, linked together like the cars of a long train. The sequence of the amino acids is what makes each protein unique and defines the function of the protein.

## AMINO ACIDS

There are 20 different amino acids used by the body, but they all share the same basic structure. The **amino acid** molecule contains a central carbon atom attached to a hydrogen atom, an *amino group* ($NH_2$), a *carboxyl group* (COOH), and a unique group of atoms called a *side chain* designated by the letter *R* (Figure 2-36). The *R* group defines each amino acid. Amino acids can be linked together in an infinite variety of combinations to form proteins. The specific combination of amino acids is ordered by the cell's DNA, and this is what determines the nature and function of the resultant protein. Two amino acids are linked together by a dehydration synthesis reaction. The carboxyl group of one amino acid links with the amino group of another amino acid via a **peptide bond**. A short chain of two amino acids is called a **dipeptide** (Figure 2-37). A **tripeptide** is a chain of three amino acids linked together, and a **polypeptide** is a chain of 10 or more amino acids linked together. When the chain exceeds 100 amino acids it is called a *protein*.

## STRUCTURE OF PROTEINS

The shape of a protein molecule directly determines its function. For example, fibrous proteins such as collagen are

A

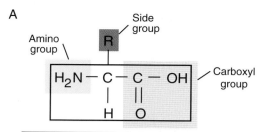

B

| Nonpolar | | Polar (but uncharged at pH 7) | | Acidic (negatively charged at pH 7) | |
|---|---|---|---|---|---|

**FIGURE 2-36** Structure of amino acids. **A,** Every amino acid is composed of an amino group, carboxyl group, and side chain (R). The side group can be simple or complex, depending on the amino acid. **B,** The 20 standard amino acids required for animal life to exist. Alanine is an example of an amino acid with a simple side group. Tryptophan has a more complex side group.

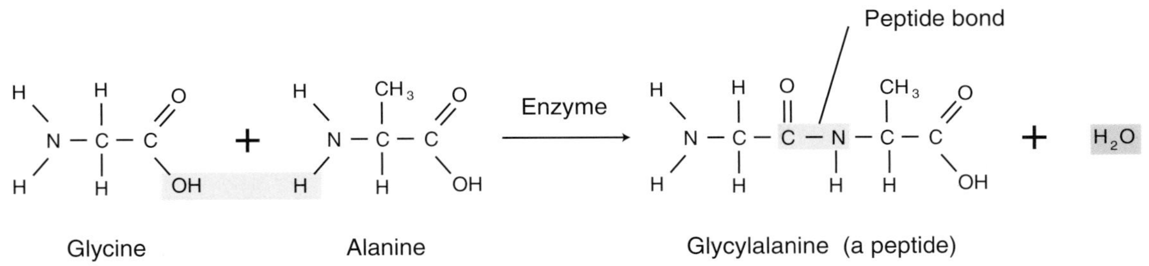

**FIGURE 2-37** Formation of a dipeptide. A dipeptide is formed when two amino acids combine by dehydration synthesis. The carboxyl group of one amino acid is bonded with the amino group of another amino acid by a peptide bond, releasing a molecule of water.

long and firm, which allows them to be used to add strength to tissues, for example the connective tissue in ligaments and tendons. Globular proteins such as immunoglobulins, also known as *antibodies,* have a specific shape, so they may join like a puzzle piece with a specific foreign protein that invades the body. The structure of proteins is often described in four levels. The **primary structure** is the sequence and number of amino acids that link together to form the peptide chain. The secondary structure is the natural bend of parts of the peptide chain as it is formed in three dimensions. The bends are stabilized when the atoms of the protein molecule form weak hydrogen bonds with each other (Figure 2-38).

The most common shapes that chains of amino acids assume are the alpha helix and the beta-pleated sheet. The alpha helix occurs when the chain of peptides winds into a spring shape, like a "Slinky" toy or a curl of hair. A beta-pleated sheet occurs when the peptide chain folds into a shape like an accordion. These shapes can both occur within the same protein at different places in the peptide chain. The tertiary structure is the overall shape of a single protein molecule. A protein molecule further folds in on itself, often shielding the inner, hydrophobic amino acids from the watery environment of the cell or blood. The outer, hydrophilic amino acids allow the protein to be water soluble. The folds are held in place by more hydrogen bonds and also some covalent bonds, such as the **disulfide bond**, which is a sulfur atom in one part of the protein covalently bonded to a sulfur atom in another part of the protein. The quaternary structure is when two or more protein chains join to form a complex macromolecule. Again hydrogen and covalent bonds between atoms of the proteins stabilize the shape of the macromolecule.

## STRUCTURAL PROTEINS

**Structural proteins** are stable, rigid, water-insoluble proteins that are used for adding strength to tissues or cells. Because they often have a long, stringy shape they are called *fibrous proteins.* Examples include: collagen, which is the main protein in connective tissues such as ligaments, cartilage, bone, and tendons; fibrin, which is the fibrous connective tissue in blood clots; and keratin, which

is the main protein in hair, hooves, horns, and the outer layer of skin.

## FUNCTIONAL PROTEINS

**Functional proteins** are generally water soluble and have a flexible, three-dimensional shape, which can change under different circumstances. Because they have a convoluted, changeable shape they are called *globular proteins.* Globular proteins are highly chemically active molecules. Examples include hemoglobin, antibodies, protein-based hormones, and **enzymes,** which are proteins that catalyze or speed up chemical reactions (Figure 2-39).

*HOW ENZYMES WORK.* Enzymes are essential to the body in their role of catalyzing chemical reactions; without them, most chemical reactions in the body would occur too slowly to produce the chemicals needed. Enzymes speed up a chemical reaction without being destroyed or altered, and they are specific to the reaction that they catalyze and to their **substrates,** which are the substances they act upon. This specificity is determined by the shape, charge, and hydrophilic/hydrophobic properties of the enzyme and its substrates. This specificity is often referred to as the *lock and key* property of enzymes, because an enzyme fits its substrates exactly and is itself unaltered at the end of the reaction. Enzymatic reactions often take place in a series of reactions with the products of one reaction acting as the substrate for the next reaction. Often these reactions occur along lipid membranes with the enzymes existing as proteins within the membrane aligned in order of the reaction. An example of this is seen in the description of the Krebs cycle and the **electron transport system** for the production of ATP molecules (see Chapter 17).

✓ *TEST YOURSELF 2-10*
1. What element is found in all proteins that is not found in carbohydrates or lipids?
2. What is the building block for proteins?
3. What is the name of the bond holding two amino acids together?
4. What is a peptide?
5. How does an enzyme work?

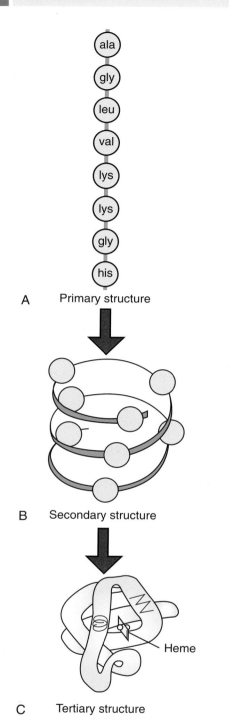

A  Primary structure

B  Secondary structure

C  Tertiary structure

Heme

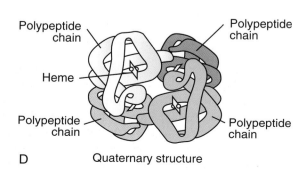

Polypeptide chain

Polypeptide chain

Heme

Polypeptide chain

Polypeptide chain

D  Quaternary structure

**FIGURE 2-38** Levels of organization of proteins. **A,** The primary structure of proteins consists of a sequence of amino acids. Amino acids are linked to one another like beads in a necklace. **B,** The secondary structure can be either helical or pleated and is held by hydrogen bonds between nearby amino and carboxyl groups. **C,** The tertiary structure consists of either folded alpha helixes or beta pleats. **D,** The quaternary structure refers to the combination of more than one polypeptide chain; such chains unite to form the complete protein molecule.

### CLINICAL APPLICATION

### Hyperthermia and Protein Denaturation
*Hyperthermia* is the scientific name for elevated body temperature, and it can have many causes such as a fever, heatstroke, or prolonged seizures. When the body temperature becomes too elevated for too long, the chemical bonds between and within molecules start to break. The hydrogen bonds holding proteins in their tertiary and quaternary structures are especially sensitive to this stress. When these bonds break, proteins are released from their complex structures and stretch into a straight chain of amino acids. Because they no longer have their unique shape these proteins lose their function. This is called the *denaturation of proteins*. Once this happens on a large scale it is irreversible, and the tissues of the body are irreversibly damaged. Some body proteins denature at 40°C (104°F), and death will usually occur around 41.7°C (107°F) if that temperature is maintained for 30 minutes.

## NUCLEIC ACIDS

**Nucleic acids** are the largest molecules in the body and are composed of carbon, oxygen, hydrogen, nitrogen, and phosphorus. There are only two classes of nucleic acids: DNA and RNA. **DNA** or *deoxyribonucleic acid* exists mainly in the nucleus but also in mitochondria; it is the molecule that contains all the instructions needed by the cell to build proteins. These instructions determine the shape and function of every tissue in the body and therefore the shape and function of the living organism (Figure 2-40). The instructions are coded in segments of the DNA called *genes*. **RNA** or *ribonucleic acid* transfers the instructions out of the nucleus and into the cytoplasm of the cell and builds the proteins. You can think of DNA as the blueprint for the cell and the RNA as the scanner/fax/printer that brings the instructions to where they are needed. The proteins created then catalyze all the reactions performed in the cell, creating and breaking down all the substances needed by the body.

## NUCLEOTIDES

The molecular building blocks of nucleic acids are the **nucleotides**. There are five different nucleotides but they all have the same basic structure. They are composed of a nitrogenous base, plus a five-carbon (*pentose*) sugar, plus a phosphate group (Figure 2-41). The sugar in DNA is

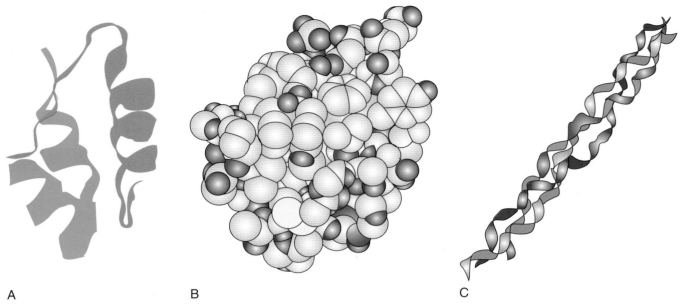

A                                B                                C

**FIGURE 2-39** Examples of proteins. **A,** Proteins are commonly depicted in a ribbon-like form to show the complex secondary and tertiary structure of the chain of amino acids. Here is a model of the insulin molecule showing the helical and straight chains of amino acids. **B,** A three-dimensional view of the atoms of a functional (globular) protein (insulin) shows the true space-filling, solid shape of proteins. The solid shape is essential to the specific function of the protein because the shape determines which substrates will react with the protein. **C,** Interwoven strands of amino acid chains are used to create structural (fibrous) proteins. The protein collagen has three strands of amino acids woven in a coil.

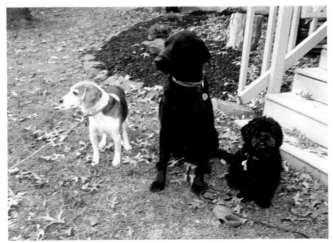

**FIGURE 2-40** Differences in living organisms. DNA is the nucleic acid that forms genes. Genes determine the shape and function of all living tissues and therefore the shape and function of living organisms. Even in animals with almost completely identical genes, such as within the same species, there are vast differences in how the animals look and how they behave.

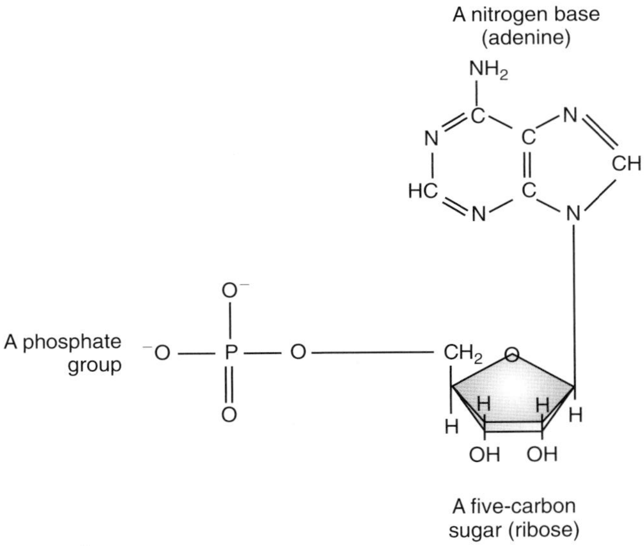

A nitrogen base
(adenine)

A phosphate group

A five-carbon
sugar (ribose)

**FIGURE 2-41** Nucleotide. Nucleotides are the building blocks of nucleic acids. Each nucleotide contains a phosphate group, a five-carbon sugar, and a nitrogenous base.

deoyxribose and the sugar in RNA is ribose, thus giving DNA and RNA their respective names. The five nucleotides are named for their nitrogenous base: adenine, guanine, cytosine, uracil, and thymine. Three nucleotides, adenine (A), guanine (G), and cytosine (C), occur in both DNA and RNA. Uracil (U) occurs only in RNA and thymine (T) occurs only in DNA.

The nucleic acid is formed by the sugar and phosphate groups joined in a long chain with the nitrogenous base open and available for metabolic activity (Figure 2-42). The information needed to produce proteins is determined by the order of the nucleotides; a grouping of three nucleotides is the code for a specific amino acid. For example, C-G-T is the code for the amino acid alanine. A gene is a sequence of

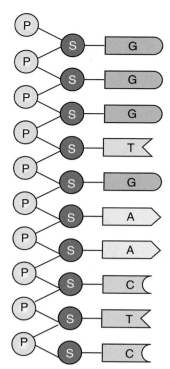

**FIGURE 2-42** Segment of a nucleic acid molecule, DNA. The phosphate of one nucleotide bonds with the sugar group of another nucleotide. These phosphate–sugar bonds make up the "backbone" of the nucleic acid molecule. A nitrogenous base sequence is formed, which provides the cell with coded information. The exposed nitrogenous base is available to bond to a nitrogenous base that is part of a complementary chain.

nucleotides that carries the information to make one peptide chain. Long chains of genes are combined with protein to form **chromosomes**. Chromosomes replicate during cell division so that all daughter cells inherit an identical copy of the chromosomes from the parent cell.

## DNA

Deoxyyribonucleic acid molecules consist of two parallel strands of the nucleotides adenine, guanine, cytosine, and thymine. The strands are connected by hydrogen bonds between the nitrogenous bases. Each nitrogenous base can only bond with one other, specific nitrogenous base: adenine can bond only with thymine and guanine can bond only with cytosine. The two strands of bonded nucleic acid twist around each other in a spiral called a *double helix* (Figure 2-43). The order of the nucleotides is unique to each individual and is carried in every cell of the individual.

## RNA

RNA consists of only one strand of the nucleotides adenine, guanine, cytosine, and uracil. There are three types of RNA that have unique roles in protein synthesis: *transfer, messenger,* and *ribosomal* RNA. Transfer RNA copies the information in the DNA molecule, messenger

**TEST YOURSELF 2-11**
1. How does a nucleotide differ from an amino acid?
2. What three parts compose a nucleotide?
3. How many nitrogenous bases are there?
4. Explain the structure of DNA.
5. Why is DNA important to life?

### CLINICAL APPLICATION

#### Genetic Disease: Be Careful What You Breed For

Genetic disease is caused by inheritable mutations of DNA. Any change to DNA, such as insertion, deletion, or mixing of the nitrogenous base pairs, leads to a nonsense sequence in the DNA. This defect can manifest as a disease in an organ system. Genetic diseases exist that affect the eyes, skeleton, skin, kidney, immune system, and enzymatic pathways. The defect may result in an incidental finding, such as microcytosis in Akitas, or the defect may cause life-threatening organ failure, such as copper-storage disease in Bedlington Terriers.

Owing to the frequency of inbreeding in small animals, the most common type of disease that is seen is caused by inheritance of recessive traits. To inherit a recessive trait the animal must receive an affected chromosome from both parents. Obviously, affected animals are not bred, but a *carrier* animal may be inadvertently used in the breeding program. A carrier animal appears unaffected because it has an unaffected chromosome that is dominant over the recessive, affected chromosome. If two carrier animals are bred, each of the offspring has a 25% chance of being affected, inheriting the affected chromosome from each parent. They have a 50% chance of being a carrier by inheriting an affected chromosome from only one parent. When choosing which animals to breed, the ethical breeder will not breed relatives of any affected animals. If a relative of an affected animal must be used for breeding, there are tests available for some genetic diseases that will confirm whether or not the animal is a carrier. Some tests measure the production of abnormal proteins generated because of the DNA mutation. Carriers usually produce a small amount of the abnormal proteins. DNA tests can also detect the mutant genes for some diseases directly.

RNA carries the information out of the nucleus, and ribosomal RNA uses the information to create the proteins needed by the body.

## ATP

When a cow eats its meal of grain and grasses, the food is broken down into nutrients such as glucose and proteins. Glucose that is derived from food is converted into energy by the cells. As glucose is broken down into monosaccharides, the energy created is stored in a molecule called **adenosine triphosphate (ATP)**. You can think of

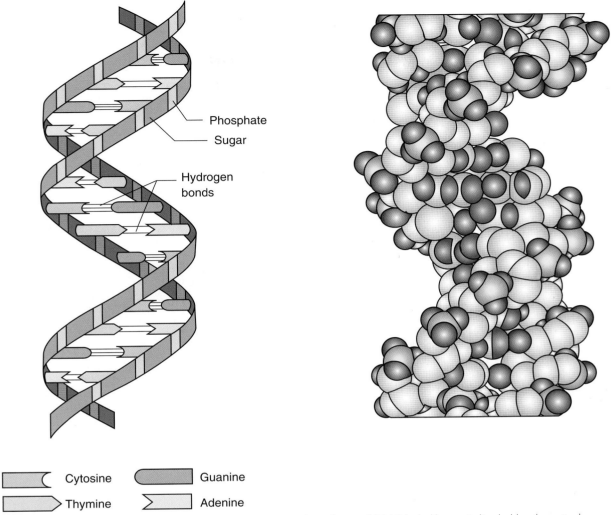

| | Cytosine | | Guanine |
| | Thymine | | Adenine |

**FIGURE 2-43** Structure of the DNA double helix. Deoxyribonucleic acid (DNA) looks like a spiraling ladder, the vertical portion of which is composed of alternating phosphate and sugar groups; the "rungs" of the ladder are composed of nitrogenous bases. A three-dimensional model is also shown.

ATP as the *energy currency* of cells. The cells need ATP to fuel any work that they do. Just as wood is added to a fire, and the fire burns the wood to create heat, nutrients are added to the body, and the cells use up the nutrients in a process called **cellular respiration** to create ATP (see Chapter 17).

The energy needed by the body is stored in the phosphate bonds of the ATP molecule. ATP is an RNA nucleotide containing the nitrogen base adenine with two additional phosphate groups attached (Figure 2-44). The bonds between the phosphate groups are called **high-energy bonds**. It is when these bonds are broken that energy is released from the ATP molecule. To use the energy stored in ATP, enzymes must move the terminal phosphate group to another molecule. The receiving molecule is then termed *phosphorylated* and temporarily has energy to do some work. During this process

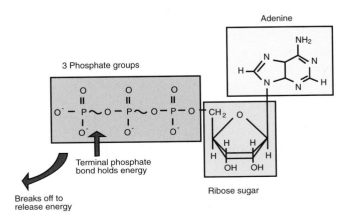

**FIGURE 2-44** Structure of ATP. ATP is formed from a ribose sugar, the nitrogenous base adenine, and three phosphate groups. Bonds between the phosphate groups hold energy.

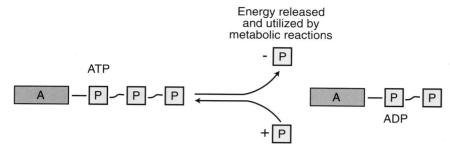

**FIGURE 2-45** Conversion of ATP to ADP. Energy is released and available for cellular work when a phosphate group breaks off from the ATP molecule. The resultant molecule, with two phosphate groups, is ADP. A phosphate group can be added back to the ADP, creating ATP through the process of cellular respiration.

the ATP molecule loses a phosphate group and becomes **adenosine diphosphate (ADP)** (Figure 2-45).

Another phosphate group can be used, resulting in the creation of a molecule of **adenosine monophosphate (AMP)**. As more glucose and other nutrients are metabolized, phosphate groups are joined to AMP, creating a renewed source of ATP. Without ATP, muscle cells could not contract, enzymatic reactions could not take place, and molecules could not be actively transported across cell membranes.

# 3 Anatomy of the Cell

*Joanna M. Bassert*

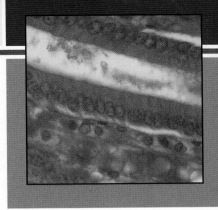

## CHAPTER OUTLINE

## LEARNING OBJECTIVES

*When you have completed this chapter, you will be able to:*

1. Explain how scientists believe the earliest cells may have formed on earth.
2. Differentiate between prokaryotic and eukaryotic cells.
3. List the early discoveries of the 17th, 18th, and 19th centuries that led to our modern understanding of cells.
4. List the physiologic factors that limit cell size.
5. Describe the molecular structure of the cell membrane.
6. Explain the importance of cilia and flagella.
7. List and describe the components of cytoplasm.
8. Describe the structure and functions of the cytoskeleton.
9. Describe the consistency and molecular components of cytosol.
10. Describe the structure and functions of each of the cellular organelles, inclusions, and vesicles.
11. List the parts that make up the nucleus; for each part, explain its structure and function.
12. Compare and contrast the molecular structure of DNA and RNA.
13. Define the term "chromatin" and explain the relationship between chromatin and chromosomes.

## VOCABULARY FUNDAMENTALS

*Adenine* **ahd**-eh-nīn
*Autolysis* aw-**tohl**-uh-sihs
*Basal body* **bās**-sahl **boh**-dē
*Catalyze* **kaht**-ih-līz
*Caveolae* kā-vē-eh-lē
*Cell* sehl
*Cell adhesion molecule* sehl ahd-**hē**-shuhn **mohl**-uhl-kyool
*Cell-mediated immune response* sehl **mē**-dē-ā-tehd ih-**myoon** reh-**spohns**
*Cell membrane* sehl **mehm**-brān
*Centriole* **sehn**-trē-ōl
*Chemical signaling* **kehm**-ih-kuhl **sihg**-nahl-ihng
*Chromatin* **krō**-mah-tihn
*Chromosome* **krō**-mō-sōm
*Cilia* **sihl**-ē-ah
*Cristae* **krih**-stē
*Cytoplasm* **sī**-tō-plahz-uhm
*Cytosine* **sī**-tō-sēn
*Cytoskeleton* sī-tō-**skehl**-ih-tuhn
*Cytosol* **sī**-tuh-sahl

*Deoxyribonucleic acid (DNA)* dē-**ohck**-sē-rī-bō-noo-**klā**-ihck **ah**-sihd
*Electron microscopy* ē-**lehck**-trohn mī-**kraw**-skō-pē
*Endoplasmic reticulum* ehn-dō-**plahz**-mihck reh-**tihck**-ū-luhm
*Enzyme* **ehn**-zīm
*Eukaryote* yoo-**keər**-ē-ōt
*Flagella* flah-**jehl**-ah
*Fluid mosaic* **floo**-ihd mō-**zā**-ihck
*Genetic material* jeh-**neht**-ihck mah-**teer**-ē-ahl
*Globular protein* **glohb**-yoo-lər **prō**-tēn
*Glycolipid* glī-kō-**lihp**-ihd
*Glycoprotein* glī-kō-**prō**-tēn
*Golgi apparatus* **gōl**-jē ahp-uh-**raht**-uhs
*Guanine* **gwah**-nēn
*Histone* **hihs**-tōn
*Immunization* ihm-ū-nī-**zā**-shuhn
*Inclusion* ihn-**kloo**-shuhn
*Integral protein* **ihn**-teh-grahl **prō**-tēn
*Intermediary fiber* ihn-tər-**mē**-dē-eər-ē **fī**-bər
*Keratin fiber* **keər**-ah-tihn **fī**-bər
*Ligand* **lī**-gahnd

*Light microscopy* līt mī-**kraw**-skō-pē
*Lipid bilayer* **lihp**-ihd **bī**-lā-ər
*Lysosome* **lī**-sō-sōm
*Mathias Scheiden* mah-**thī**-uhs **shī**-dehn
*Matrix* **mā**-trihks
*Membrane receptor* **mehm**-brān reh-**sehpt**-ər
*Microfilament* mī-krō-**fihl**-ah-mehnt
*Microtrabeculae* mī-krō-truh-**behck**-ū-lā
*Microtubule* mī-krō-**too**-būl
*Mitochondria* mī-tō-**kohn**-drē-ah
*Multicellular organism* muhl-tī-**sehl**-ū-lər
    **ohr**-gah-nihz-uhm
*Myofibril* mī-ō-**fī**-brihl
*Neurofilament* nər-ō-**fihl**-ah-mehnt
*Nuclear envelope* **noo**-klē-ər **ehn**-veh-lōp
*Nucleoli* noo-**klē**-ō-lī
*Nucleoplasm* **noo**-klē-ō-plahzm
*Nucleosome* **noo**-klē-ō-sōm
*Nucleus* **noo**-klē-uhs
*Organelle* ohr-gah-**nehl**
*Organism* **ohr**-gah-nihz-uhm
*Osteocyte* **ohs**-tē-ō-sīt
*Peripheral protein* puh-**rihf**-ər-ahl **prō**-tēn
*Peroxisome* pər-**ohcks**-ih-sōm

*Plasma membrane* **plahz**-mah **mehm**-brān
*Plasmalemma* plahz-mah-**lehm**-ah
*Prion* **prī**-ohn
*Prokaryote* prō-**keər**-ē-ōt
*Proteasome* prō-**tē**-ah-sōm
*Protoplasm* **prō**-tō-plahz-uhm
*Raft* rahft
*RNA: Ribonucleic acid* rī-bō-noo-**klā**-ihck
    **ah**-sihd
*Robert Hooke* **rohb**-ərt hook
*Scanning electron microscopy* **skah**-nihng eh-**lehck**-trohn
    mī-**kraw**-skō-pē
*Scrapie* **skrā**-pē
*Specialization* spehsh-uh-lah-**zā**-shuhn
*Spindle apparatus* **spihn**-duhl ahp-uh-**raht**-uhs
*Spindle fiber* **spihn**-duhl **fī**-bər
*Theodor Schwann* **thē**-uh-dohr shwahn
*Thymine* **thī**-mihn
*Tonofilament* toh-nō-**fihl**-ah-mehnt
*Transmission electron microscopy* trahnz-**mihsh**-uhn
    eh-**lehck**-trohn mī-**kraw**-skō-pē
*Uracil* **yər**-ah-sihl
*Vault* vahlt
*Virus* **vī**-ruhs

## INTRODUCTION

The **cell** is the remarkable basic unit of living things. It can exist alone as a single, free-living plant or animal, or it can combine with other cells to form elaborate complex **organisms**, such as trees, horses, and people. The cell is dynamic and performs all of the functions by which life is defined. It has a metabolism, can grow, develop, reproduce, adapt, respire, become influenced by outside stimuli, maintain a stable internal environment, and convert food into usable energy. Each cell carries vital **genetic material** that governs its own development, metabolism, and **specialization**. A great diversity is seen in the appearance of cells. They can be small, biconcave red blood cells; long, thin **myofibrils**; or octopus-like **osteocytes**. Each form reflects its own specialized function (Figure 3-1). In a **multicellular** organism, such as a dog, cells have differentiated and become grouped into specialized tissues that work collaboratively to sustain life for the animal as a whole. These tissues, as well as the systems they form, are the focus of anatomy and physiology, but it is important to remember that their functional unit is the cell. It is in the cell that molecular messages are transmitted and received, electrical impulses generated, oxygen absorbed, and energy manufactured. Thus we must first learn about cells before we can understand the anatomy and physiology of the tissues and systems they compose.

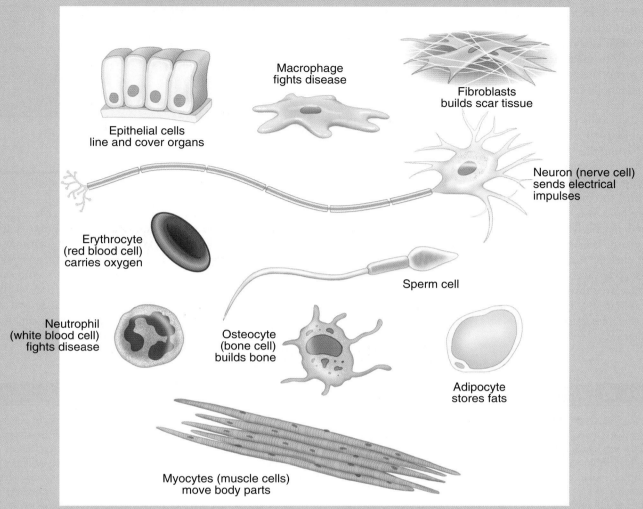

**FIGURE 3-1** Examples of cell types. Differentiation and specialization of cells in the multicellular organism has led to a diverse array of cell types. The shape and size of the cell are related to its function.

## OUR EARLY UNDERSTANDING OF CELLS

### EVOLUTION OF CELLS

The first cells are thought to have evolved in the massive oceans of our primitive earth about 3 billion years ago. Jolted by the fierce electrical energy from frequent lightning storms and by the intense, unabated radiation from the sun, the three molecules that made up the primitive atmosphere—methane gas ($CH_4$), water ($H_2O$), and ammonia ($NH_3$)—were forced to collide and split apart. The first organic molecules, similar to amino acids, were thought to have formed in this tempestuous environment. Clustering into heavy droplets, these molecules are thought to have been washed from the atmosphere by driving rains into the warm, shallow seas below. There, proteins, lipids, and carbohydrates evolved, which in turn arranged themselves over time into sophisticated, organized structures to become the first cells.

These primitive cells resembled present-day bacteria and contained a single strand of deoxyribonucleic acid (DNA), which floated freely in gelatinous **protoplasm**. The cells did not possess a nucleus and were therefore called **prokaryotes**, which means *before nucleus*. For 1.5 billion years prokaryotes were the only forms of life on this planet. **Eukaryotes**, meaning *true nucleus*, developed later and are found in all multicellular organisms today. Eukaryotic cells are characterized by a distinct nucleus, in which the DNA has combined with protein to form chromosomes. These, in turn, are surrounded by a protective **nuclear envelope**, which, like a guard station, monitors the flow of molecules in and out of the nucleus.

### SIZE LIMITATIONS

The size of most animal cells is restricted to a range of 10 to 30 μm in diameter because of the relationship between the surface area and the volume of a cell. Small cells have smaller nutritional requirements than large cells but have a proportionately large surface through which they can absorb the substances they need. Thus a small cell with a proportionately large surface area will be able to complete its metabolic functions more rapidly and efficiently than a large cell with a relatively small surface area. In other words, if cells were the size of basketballs, they would not be able to take in nutrients fast enough to feed themselves and would die.

A second factor limiting cell size is related to the governing capability of the nucleus. A single nucleus can control the metabolic activity of a small cell better than a large one. Also, the more active a cell is, the greater are its metabolic needs. Therefore it is not surprising that some very large cells or cells that are very active, such as cardiac and skeletal muscle cells, have two or more nuclei. Also, these cells are long and thin, thereby creating a larger surface area through which nutrients can be absorbed. The combination of increased nuclei and expanded surface area enables muscle cells to function at a very high metabolic rate.

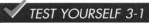

### TEST YOURSELF 3-1

1. What are the basic cellular functions that define life?
2. Describe the series of events that scientists believe led to the formation of the first cells on earth.
3. What is the difference between a prokaryote and a eukaryote?
4. Why are cells not the size of watermelons?

## LOOKING INSIDE THE CELL
### MAMMALIAN CELL ANATOMY

Today with the aid of sophisticated microscopes, scientists have been able to look inside cells and focus on their minute, fantastic internal world (Box 3-1). For over 3 billion years, cells have evolved into diverse shapes and have taken on a wide range of specialized functions within multicellular organisms. Despite these changes and the **morphological** diversity that evolved among them, there are three essential structures found in all mammalian cells

---

### BOX 3-1 | An Introduction to Microscopy

In the 1600s, a Dutch scientist named Anton van Leeuwenhoek found microscopic creatures in pond water. He was able to make this exciting discovery using a single-lens microscope that he had fabricated himself. The Englishman Robert Hooke also made his own microscope, which allowed him to observe the tiny units that make up cork. These early, homemade tools were the first light microscopes and marked the beginning of three and a half centuries of impressive exploration in the frontiers of microspace.

#### Light Microscopy

Light microscopy works by using visible light to see tiny structures. Tissues and other items being examined are sliced or spread out into thin layers, affixed to glass slides, and stained. When placed on the *stage* of the microscope, as shown in the drawings below, the tissues can be examined through the ocular lens. Light comes from underneath the slide and is concentrated on the tissue by the condenser. The effect of this backlighting is dramatic and colorful. Pictures taken of microscopic objects using a light microscope are called *light micrographs* and are found throughout this and other anatomy texts. Use of stains, including fluorescent stains, has markedly improved the visibility of microscopic structures using light microscopy.

#### Electron Microscopy

As its name implies, electron microscopy uses electrons rather than light to create an image. An electron beam generated by an electron gun is directed with precision toward the specimen by magnets. Some of the electrons pass through the specimen, but some of them bounce off and are deflected to the sides. Electron

beams are not visible to humans, and the generation of images in electron microscopes is therefore dependent upon an electron *detector*, which translates the pattern of incoming electrons into a readable image. The electron microscope is so powerful that it can make extraordinarily minute intracellular structures visible, including the organic molecules that compose cells. Interestingly, there is no color at this level of magnification, because the structures being examined are as small as, or smaller than, the wavelength of the colors we humans can see. However, computer enhanced coloration is used to augment the black and white world, creating images with greater clarity and definition.

There are two types of electron microscope: *transmission electron microscopes (TEM)*, which generate two-dimensional images; and *scanning electron microscopes (SEM)*, which generate three-dimensional images. Transmission electron microscopy works by sending a beam of electrons *through* a specimen in the same way that light microscopy sends a beam of light through a specimen. Thus the specimen used in TEM, like light microscopy, must be very thin so that the electron beam can pass through it. Once the electrons pass through the specimen, they strike phosphorescent particles on a viewing screen, which release photons (visible light). In this way, the screen literally glows with the microscopic image.

Specimens in scanning electron microscopy are first "sputtered" or covered with tiny particles of gold before they are examined. Inside the microscope, an electron beam is generated and is scanned back and forth over the specimen, hence the term *scanning* electron microscope. The electrons from the beam are deflected at the surface and secondary electrons are displaced from the surface as well. These primary and secondary electrons are detected by a sensor that relays the

BOX 3-1   An Introduction to Microscopy—cont'd

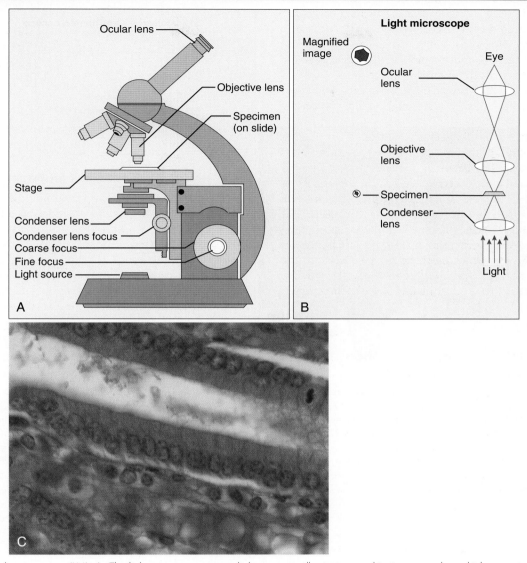

Light microscopy (LM). **A,** The light microscope uses a light source to illuminate very thin tissue samples, which are put on glass slides and placed on the microscope's stage. The objective lens and ocular lens together create the magnification needed to enlarge the image. **B,** Specimens under examination are backlit by visible light, which is focused on the stage by the condenser. **C,** The simple **columnar epithelial cells** that cover the folded lining of the abomasum (stomach) in a steer come to life with LM. Stain is absorbed by the nuclei, making them appear purple. Cytoplasm and the cell membranes are various shades of pink. (**A, B,** From Thibodeau GA, Patton KT: Anatomy & physiology, ed 6, St Louis, 2007, Mosby; **C,** courtesy Joanna Bassert.)

signal to an amplifier. The magnified image is subsequently displayed on a monitor.

### Atomic Force Microscopy

An atomic force microscope (AFM) generates a three-dimensional image of incredibly small structures using a minute sharp-tipped probe attached to a delicate cantilever (arm). The tiny probe meticulously scans the surface of specimens, allowing the forces between the tip and the sample surface to deflect the cantilever. This deflection is recorded by a computer, which generates a digital image. Some of the forces that can cause deflection include capillary forces, chemical bonding,

*Continued*

## BOX 3-1    An Introduction to Microscopy—cont'd

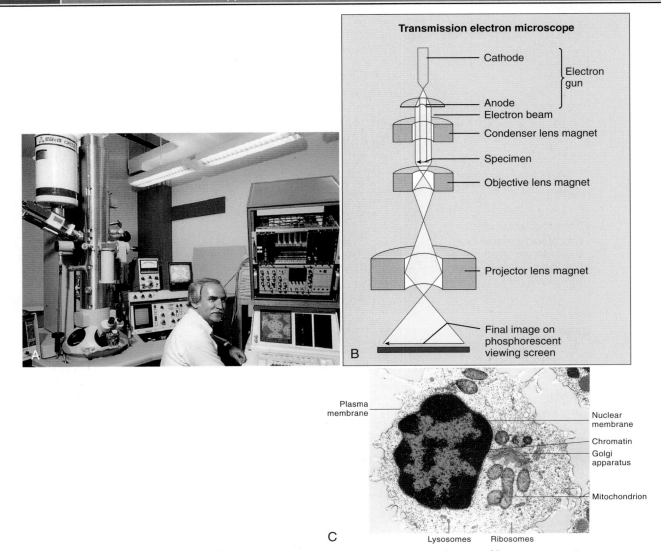

**Transmission electron microscope**

Cathode
Electron gun
Anode
Electron beam
Condenser lens magnet
Specimen
Objective lens magnet
Projector lens magnet
Final image on phosphorescent viewing screen

A

B

C

Plasma membrane
Nuclear membrane
Chromatin
Golgi apparatus
Mitochondrion
Lysosomes    Ribosomes

Transmission electron microscopy (TEM). **A,** An electron microscope and the associated monitors fill an entire room. During examination of specimens, it is helpful if the room is dark. **B,** An electron beam is generated by the electron gun. The direction of the beam is focused on a specimen by condenser magnets. Electrons that pass through the specimen bombard phosphorescent particles on the viewing screen, where the image is seen. **C,** A transmission electron micrograph of a mammalian cell. Far greater levels of magnification are possible with electron microscopy than light microscopy. (From Thibodeau GA, Patton KT: Anatomy & physiology, ed 6, St Louis, 2007, Mosby.)

electrostatic and magnetic forces, as well as mechanical contact forces. In most AFMs, a feedback mechanism is employed by the computer to adjust the tip-to-sample distance so that a constant force is maintained between the tip and the sample. In this way, the tip and sample are prevented from banging into one other causing damage to either the sample or the tip. The tip of the probe is often covered with an array of special coatings depending upon what forces are being investigated. For example, a gold coating is used to trace covalent bonding in organic molecules, diamond coatings are used to increase the wear resistance of the probe and magnetic coatings are used to evaluate magnetism on the surface of a

**BOX 3-1** | An Introduction to Microscopy—cont'd

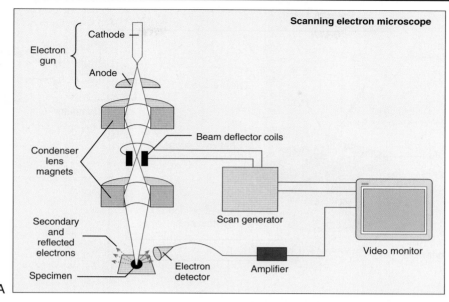

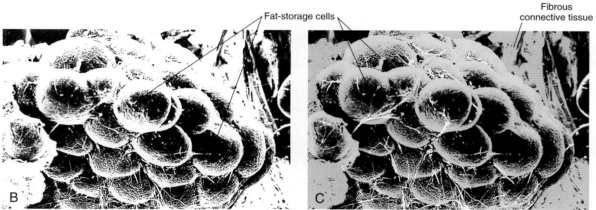

Scanning electron microscopy (SEM). **A,** An electron beam is scanned back and forth over a specimen. The electrons that bounce off the specimen, and secondary electrons that come from the surface of the specimen, are detected, amplified, and transcribed into an image, which is visible on a video monitor. **B** and **C,** SEM brings adipose tissue to life in three-dimensional images. Electron micrographs can be enhanced with color by computers to add a greater level of detail and clarity. Notice that the pink added to the background helps to delineate the fibrous connective tissue from the fat cells. (From Thibodeau GA, Patton KT: Anatomy & physiology, ed 6, St Louis, 2007, Mosby.)

specimen. The probe can scan the surface of specimens in a static (or contact mode), or via a dynamic (noncontact) mode in which the probe is vibrated. The results are magnificent three-dimensional images on a scale far smaller than previously thought possible. The use of AFM technology has enabled scientists to look more deeply inside cells and to visualize the minute anatomical structures that are necessary for life. Thus, AFM has led to a greater understanding of the cause of some diseases that have devastated both humans and animals.

*Continued*

**BOX 3-1** | An Introduction to Microscopy—cont'd

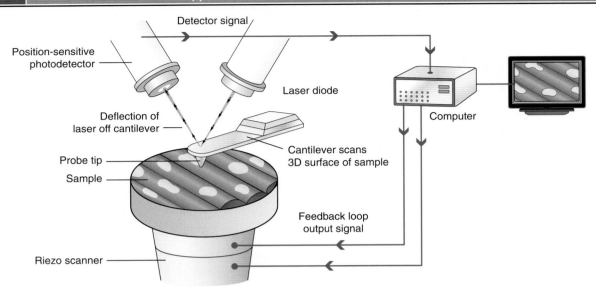

**Atomic Force Microscopy (AFM)**

Atomic force microscopy (AFM) uses a minute probe and cantilever system to scan the surfaces of specimens. A laser and a position-sensitive photodetector translate the minute movements of the probe into data that are subsequently used to generate a three-dimensional image on a computer screen.

regardless of their shape, size and function. These structures are:

- The **cell membrane** (plasmalemma)
- The cytoplasm:
  - Cytosol
  - Cytoskeleton
  - Organelles
- The nucleus

All cells are separated from their environment by a cell membrane, which is also known as a **plasma membrane** or **plasmalemma** (plaz-ma-LEM-a; *lema* meaning *husk*). Everything inside the cell membrane, other than the nucleus and genetic material, is known as the *cytoplasm* (*cyto* means "*cell*"). **Cytoplasm** includes: *cytosol*, a **colloidal**, jamlike protoplasm that is highly structured and composed of proteins, electrolytes, and **metabolites**; a flexible *cytoskeleton*; and complex structures called *organelles*. **Organelles**, like the organs in our own bodies, work collaboratively to carry out necessary metabolic functions (Table 3-1). As already mentioned, all mammalian cells are eukaryotic and therefore possess a nucleus, which contains vital genetic material in the form of chromosomes. Figure 3-2 is an illustration of a composite cell that includes many of the important structures students are asked to learn and study. Keep in mind that, in reality, no single cell includes all of these features and cells have a diverse array of shapes and sizes depending upon their function within the body. Also, be aware that nuclei have many shapes also and that many of them are not positioned in the center of the cell.

## CELL MEMBRANE

The cell membrane acts as a flexible, elastic barrier between the inner cytoplasm and the outside environment (Figure 3-3). It includes many infoldings and outpouchings that provide extra surface area, and it is continually removing and recycling different segments of itself, updating surface receptors and renewing its sticky outer coating. Like our own skin, the cell membrane is capable of self-repair, but if it is damaged to the extent that intracellular contents are released, the cell quickly dies. The cell membrane governs the movement of atoms and molecules in and out of the cell. Although the actual consistency and complexity of the cell membrane are based largely on the function of the cell, cell membranes usually consist primarily of protein (55%) and phospholipids (25%) but also include quantities of cholesterol (13%), miscellaneous lipids (4%), and carbohydrates (3%).

## MEMBRANE STRUCTURE

Because of its surprising thinness (about 60 to 100 angstroms), the cell membrane is not visible using light microscopy. Under the transmission **electron microscope**, however, the cell membrane appears as two thin, dark layers with a seemingly empty space between them. At the molecular level, the cell membrane is composed of two layers of phospholipid molecules arranged so that the hydrophilic heads are on the outside and the hydrophobic, fatty acid tails are on the inside. This is called a **lipid bilayer**. Proteins that are suspended in this bilayer can move easily throughout the membrane to create a constantly changing mosaic pattern

| TABLE 3-1 | Anatomical Parts of the Cell | | |
|---|---|---|---|
| **MORPHOLOGY** | **PART** | **DESCRIPTION** | **FUNCTION** |
| **Cell Membrane** | | | |
| | Cell membrane | Phospholipid bilayer with integral and peripheral proteins; a fluid mosaic with discrete areas of stiff "rafts," covered in a sugary glycocalyx | Boundary between extracellular and intracellular compartments; controls passage of substances into and out of cell; maintains membrane receptors for attachment of ligands |
| | Cilia | Many fine hairlike structures on luminal surface of cells that beat rhythmically in unison | Fast phase of rhythmic beat propels mucus and fluid across luminal surface of cell in one direction |
| | Flagellum | Single long hairlike structure found in sperm, cells and some pathogens | Thrashing movement of flagellum propels cell forward |
| **Nucleus** | | | |
| | Nucleus | Wide variety of shapes, sizes and number of nuclei within each cell type; contains nucleoplasm, DNA, rRNA, and ribosomal subunits | Site of transcription; (transfer of genetic code from DNA to mRNA) and production of ribosomal subunits |
| | Nuclear envelope | Double-layered membrane punctated by countless nuclear pore complexes; outer membrane is continuous with endoplasmic reticulum | Separates nucleus from surrounding cytosol; restricts movement of molecules into and out of nucleus |
| | Chromatin | Located in nucleoplasm. Composed of nucleosomes (DNA wrapped around 8 histone proteins) connected by sections of linker DNA; normally arranged in loose strands | DNA portion contains sequence code for making proteins and enzymes that control molecular interactions; supercoils to form X-shaped chromosomes during cell division |
| | Nucleolus | Dense cluster of ribosomal RNA and protein; nucleoli are not membrane bound | Location of synthesis of ribosomal subunits |

*Continued*

| TABLE 3-1 | Anatomical Parts of the Cell—cont'd | | | |
| --- | --- | --- | --- | --- |
| MORPHOLOGY | PART | DESCRIPTION | FUNCTION | |

**Cytoplasm (Includes Organelles)**

| MORPHOLOGY | PART | DESCRIPTION | FUNCTION |
| --- | --- | --- | --- |
| | Cytosol | Protoplasm containing water, dissolved enzymes, electrolytes, nutrients, and protein | Medium for transport of intracellular molecules and organelles; supports cell membrane |
| | Inclusions | Vesicles, vacuoles, and lipid droplets suspended in cytosol | Storage and transportation vesicles of intracellular substances |
| | Cytoskeleton | Structural complex within cytosol composed of: microtubules intermediary filaments and microfilaments | Provides, strength, structure, and support; maintains cell shape, and affects cell division, and movement of organelles and the cell membrane |
| | Centrioles | Found in the center of the centrosome near the nucleus. Composed of microtubules arranged in a pin-wheel. Asters radiate away from the centrioles. | Duplicate prior to cell division. Mother and daughter centrioles. Help anchor spindle fibers. Two pairs of centrioles move apart as the spindle fibers lengthen. |

**Organelles**

| MORPHOLOGY | PART | DESCRIPTION | FUNCTION |
| --- | --- | --- | --- |
| | Mitochondria | Double-membrane bound organelle, internal membrane folds inward forming cristae; increased internal surface area maximizes metabolic processes | Site of cellular respiration, which produces ATP |
| | Endoplasmic reticulum (ER) | A system of collapsed sacs extending from the outer layer of the nuclear envelope; has two forms: RER with ribosomes, and SER without ribosomes. | RER produces, modifies and packages secretory proteins; SER produces, modifies and packages lipids and carbohydrates |
| | Ribosomes | Composed of two subunits: one large and one small. These fit together like cupped hands. Each subunit is made of RNA and protein. Fixed ribosomes are found on RER; free ribosomes float in cytosol. | Site of protein synthesis. Protein manufactured on fixed ribosomes (RER) is intended for export; protein manufactured on free ribosomes is intended for intracellular use. Ribosomal subunits are manufactured in nucleoli. |

| TABLE 3-1 | Anatomical Parts of the Cell—cont'd | | |
|---|---|---|---|
| **MORPHOLOGY** | **PART** | **DESCRIPTION** | **FUNCTION** |
| | Proteasome | Hollow cylinder composed of protein subunits and caps on each end. It is about half the size of a ribosome. | Responsible for breaking down individual misfolded or abnormal protein molecules. Like ribosomes, is found throughout the cytosol. |
| | Golgi apparatus | Network of connected flattened tubes stacked on top of one another. | Refines and alters molecules intended for both secretion and internal use. Produces lysosomes. |
| This figure shows both entries Golgi apparatus and lysosome | Lysosome | Vesicle filled with hydrolytic enzymes; formed by golgi apparatus. | Digestion of absorbed material and internally produced waste; rupture causes cellular autolysis |
| | Peroxisomes | Membrane-bound vesicle containing enzymes: produced by fission | Detoxify various molecules such as alcohol and formaldehyde; remove free radicals |
| | Vault | Tiny barrel-shaped capsule composed of RNA (vRNA) and protein. Thought to be very numerous in cells. | Perhaps able to fit into nuclear pore complexes where one end opens to pick up or drop off molecules entering or exiting the nucleus. |

known as the **fluid mosaic**. Most lipid-soluble materials, such as oxygen and carbon dioxide molecules, pass through the membrane with ease, whereas ionized and water-soluble molecules, such as amino acids, sugars, and proteins, which are not lipid soluble, do not readily pass through.

The membrane also contains cholesterol molecules that wedge themselves between phospholipids and help to stabilize the membrane. In this way cholesterol not only prevents the lipids from aggregating, which helps to keep the membrane fluid, but it also adds to the oily nature of the internal layer, which increases the membrane's impermeability to water-soluble molecules.

The cell membrane is composed of a wide variety of important structural and **globular proteins**, which are responsible for the membrane's special functions. Compact globular proteins may occur either on the cell surface or inside the lipid bilayer. Those that occur within the bilayer are called **integral proteins**. These molecules span the entire width of the membrane and may create channels through which other molecules can pass. Some integral proteins form selective passageways that permit only particular substances to enter or exit the cell, whereas others create **pores**, such channels within the protein molecule that allow substances

such as water to pass through with no resistance. Pores are scattered over the surface of the cell and make up approximately 0.2% of the cell's surface area.

Other globular proteins form **peripheral proteins**, which are bound to the inside or outside surfaces of the cell membrane. The internal peripheral proteins are more restricted in their movement than integral proteins, because they are often attached to portions of the internal cytoskeleton or to the exposed parts of some integral proteins. Peripheral proteins sometimes act as **enzymes** to **catalyze** specific chemical reactions and may be involved in the mechanics of changing the cell's shape, an event that is quite dramatically seen, for example, during the contraction of a muscle cell.

The inner and outer layers of the cell membrane are different from one another. Proteins that reside on the inner surface of the membrane, for example, may be bound to components of the cytoskeleton, **keratin fibers**, or peripheral proteins, whereas proteins and lipids on the outer layer are attached to sugar groups. These **glycoprotein** (sugar and protein) and **glycolipid** (sugar and phospholipid) molecules are the principal components of the "sugar coating" that covers the surface of cells. This coating is called the **glycocalyx**. Like the pattern of stripes on a zebra or the fingerprints

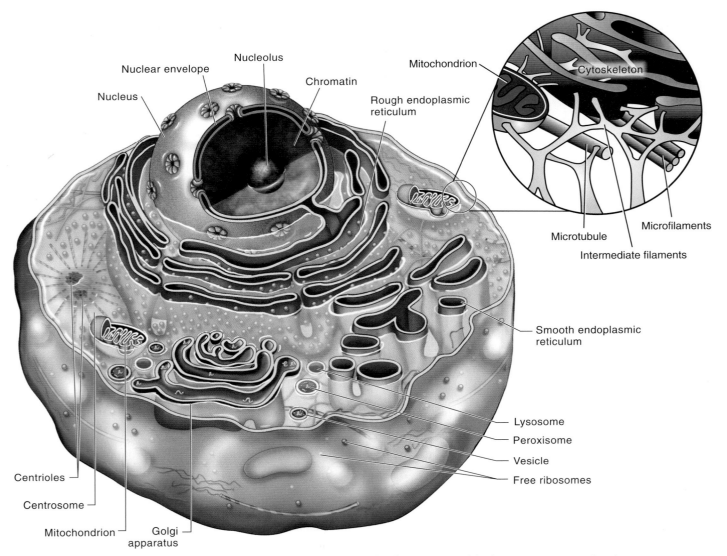

**FIGURE 3-2** Composite example of a mammalian cell. (Modified from Patton KT, Thibodeau GA: *Anatomy & physiology,* ed 8, St Louis, 2013, Mosby.)

on a human hand, the glycocalyx is unique. It provides improved cell-to-cell adhesion and represents an important biological marker for intercellular recognition and for the interactions between the cell and antibodies or the cell and viruses. The interaction between the glycocalyx and extracellular molecules may bring about changes in the membrane and possibly in the activity of the cell as a whole.

The glycocalyx is composed of two families of molecules: *cell adhesion molecules* and *membrane receptors.* **Cell adhesion molecules (CAMs)** are sticky glycoproteins that cover the surfaces of almost all of the cells in mammals; they allow the cells to bond to extracellular molecules and to each other. These molecules are also important in helping cells move past one another and in signaling circulating cells, such as white blood cells, to areas of inflammation or infection.

**Membrane receptors** are integral proteins and glycoproteins that act as binding sites on the cell surface. Some of

them play a vital role in cell-to-cell recognition, a process called *contact signaling.* This is particularly important during the **cell-mediated immune response** and assists bacteria and viruses in finding preferred target cells. Membrane receptors are also involved in a process called **chemical signaling.** Hormones, neurotransmitters, and other chemical messengers called **ligands** bind to specific binding sites on cell surfaces Once bound to the cell membrane, ligands can bring about a change in the cell's activity. Some ligands act as enzymes to activate or inactivate a particular cellular activity.

Molecules that make up the fluid mosaic are not evenly distributed across the cell membrane. Some areas, for example, are stiffer and more rigid than others. As molecules react with one another within the fluid mosaic, rigid areas of densely packed phospholipids, cholesterol, and protein form plaquelike structures called **rafts** within the cell membrane. They appear to move on the surface of the cell much

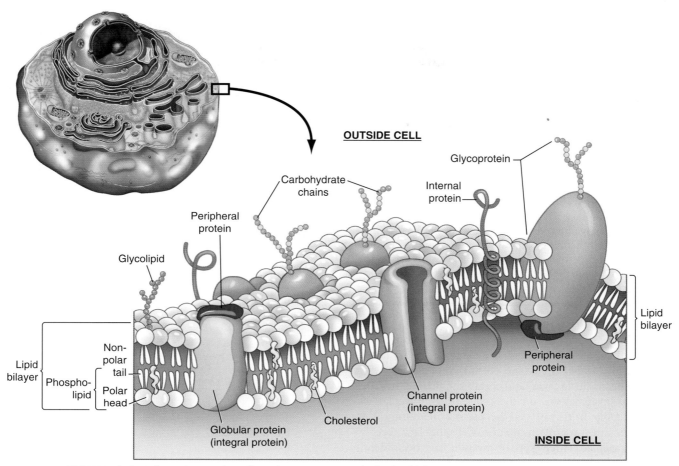

**FIGURE 3-3** Cell membrane. The cell membrane is composed of a lipid bilayer. Proteins help govern the movement of atoms and molecules in and out of the cell. (*Top left*, Modified from Patton KT, Thibodeau GA: *Anatomy & physiology*, ed 8, St Louis, 2013, Mosby.)

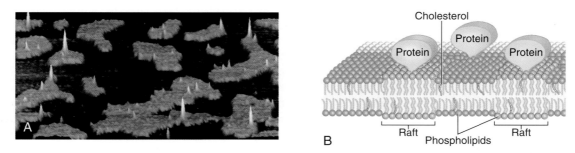

**FIGURE 3-4 A,** An image generated by an atomic force microscope shows rigid orange-colored rafts surrounded by darkly colored phospholipids on the surface of a cell. Proteins are visible reaching upwards into the spaces above the rafts. **B,** An illustration of the molecular structure of a fluid mosaic membrane containing rigid rafts. Notice that the rafts are rich with cholesterol molecules and protein. These molecules cling to one another, forming a single unit that moves through the phospholipid bilayer, much like a raft on water. Rafts are important in membrane-bound organelles as well as in the cell membrane, where they facilitate molecular interactions and functions. (**A,** Used with permission: Henderson R et al: Lipid rafts: feeling is believing, *Physiology* 19(2):39-43, © 2004 Int Union Physiol Sci/Am Physiol Soc.)

like a log floating on water. Rafts are important in helping to organize functional areas on the cell surface, in initiating cytokinesis during cell division, and in forming depressions on the cell surface that may lead to involution and vesicle formation. With use of atomic force microscopy, rafts are visible as discrete plaques in a sea of phospholipids on the cell membrane (Figure 3-4).

**CAVEOLAE.** Caveolae are small (50 nm) invaginations of the plasma membrane. Often the caveolae pinch off and

Insulin is an important ligand that binds to specific receptors on the surface of cells, particularly liver, fat, and cardiac and skeletal muscle cells. Insulin stimulates glucose uptake by triggering the movement of glucose transporter protein 4 (GLUT4) from an intracellular storage compartment to the plasma membrane. Once inside the cell, glucose is used to manufacture adenosine triphosphate (ATP), a vital energy source that fuels metabolic functions. Without adequate amounts of ATP the cell may not be able to function properly, can weaken and may even die. In many patients with type 2 diabetes (also known as diabetes mellitus), the number of insulin receptors on the cell surface is decreased. This is a physiologic response to excessive fat stores in the animal and is one form of insulin resistance. With fewer insulin docking sites in the cell membrane, diminished amounts of glucose are brought inside the cell. Paradoxically, the cell begins to starve even though the level of glucose outside the cell is very high (too high).

migrate inside the cell to form tiny vesicles. Depending upon the type of cell, caveolae can form single vesicles or clusters of them, like grapes on a vine or tiny rosettes. The word caveolae means "little caves" and pertains to their appearance as minute invaginations on the cell surface. Caveolae are produced only from rafts in the plasma membrane that contain the integral protein caveolin. Cells that lack caveolin also lack caveolae. Three types of caveolin have been identified thus far (caveolin-1, caveolin-2, and caveolin-3). All of them possess a similar loop structure that looks as though it was inserted into the cell membrane like a hairpin. Caveolin-1 and caveolin-2 have been found in the cell membranes of endothelial, fibrous, and adipose cells, while caveolin-3 has been found in striated and smooth muscle cells.

Many cellular functions have been associated with caveolae including endocytosis, transcytosis, and contact signaling. Caveolae with specialized receptors can capture extracellular material and bring it into the cell. In endothelial cells, for example, caveolae are known to shuttle substances such as low density lipoprotein (LDL—the infamous "bad" cholesterol) from the luminal side of the cell to the basal side (Figure 3-5). As the caveolae discharge their LDL cargo, the space behind the endothelium fills with cholesterol, forming a plaque that over time will thicken and narrow the lumen of the vessel. These atherosclerotic plaques can obstruct blood flow and lead to heart disease and stroke.

### FLAGELLA AND CILIA

Flagella and cilia are extensions of the plasma membrane that extend into the extracellular space. They are energetic, motile "hairs" that are structurally identical but function differently from one another. Cilia and flagella are composed of nine pairs of microtubules that encircle a central pair of microtubules. Both cilia and flagella originate from a pair of **centrioles**, called **basal bodies**, which are located at the periphery of the cell, just under the plasma membrane.

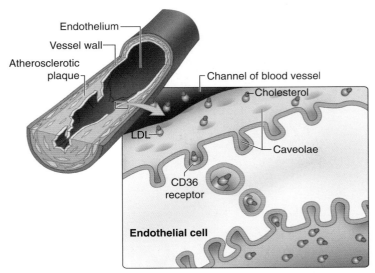

**FIGURE 3-5** Caveolae. The endothelial lining of blood vessels is rich with caveolae. The caveolae fitted with CD36 receptors will attract low density lipoproteins (LDL), also known as the "bad" cholesterol. The caveolae involute and pinch off from the plasma membrane, forming transport vesicles that carry the cholesterol to the other side of the endothelial cell. Here the LDL is discharged into the space behind the endothelium. Over time, a plaque forms in the wall of the vessel, narrowing the lumen and increasing the likelihood of a blockage. If the vessel blocks completely, the tissues that it normally supplies with nutrients and oxygen will die. Tissue death due to hypoxia is called an *infarct*. If an infarct occurs in the heart, it is called a *myocardial infarct*, which is a common cause of a *heart attack*. (From Patton KT, Thibodeau GA: Anatomy & physiology, ed 8, St Louis, 2013, Mosby.)

During their formation, cilia and flagella grow outward from the basal bodies and exert pressure on the plasma membrane.

**Cilia** occur in large numbers on the exposed surface of some cells (Figure 3-6). They are shorter than flagella and measure only about 10 μm long. They move synchronously, one after the other, creating waves of motion that propel fluid, mucus, and debris across the cellular surface. Cilia are best known for their important functions: (1) in the upper respiratory tract, where they propel bacteria and mucus away from the lungs; and (2) in the oviduct, where their beating motion pulls the expelled egg away from the ovary and into the opening of the oviduct.

**Flagella** generally occur singly and are significantly longer than cilia. They are typically attached to individual cells and propel the cell forward by undulating. Flagella move cells through fluid, whereas cilia move fluid across cell surfaces. The tail of a sperm cell is an example of a **flagellum**. A sperm is the only mammalian cell that is propelled by a single flagellum, although many disease-causing organisms are propelled in this manner.

### CYTOPLASM

The **cytoplasm** is the inner substance of the cell, excluding the nucleus. Initially, seen under light microscopy, it appears as a nondescript bag of gel with a few opaque speckles. Now, with the increased use of electron microscopy, **cytologists**

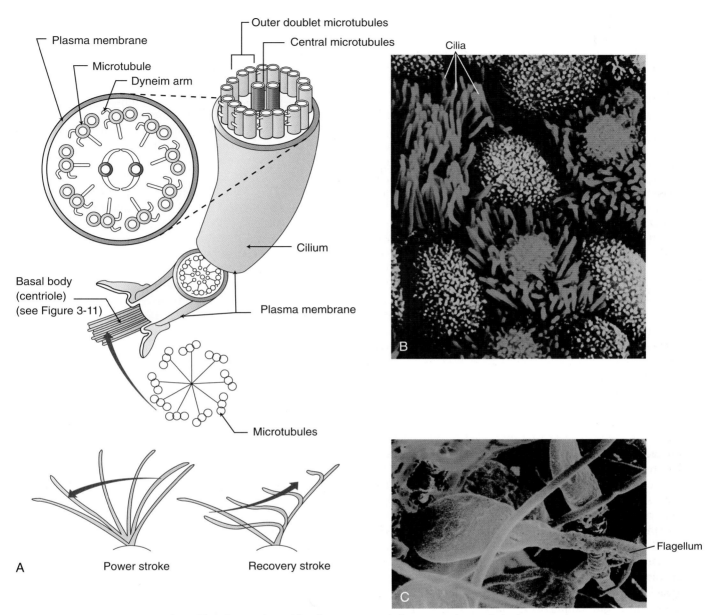

**FIGURE 3-6** Cilia and flagella. **A,** Cilia and flagella are composed of nine pairs of microtubules that surround a central pair. Cilia have a fast, powerful, and synchronized stroke in one direction. In the trachea, this helps to propel particles away from the lungs toward the mouth where they can be coughed up and swallowed. Unlike cilia, which are numerous on the surface of some cells, flagella occur singly. **B,** A scanning electron micrograph of cilia on the apical surface of epithelial cells in the lung airways. **C,** A scanning electron micrograph of sperm. The single elongated flagellum enables the sperm cell to move rapidly through the female reproductive tract. (**B,** Courtesy Charles Flickinger, University of Virginia. **C,** From Thibodeau GA, Patton KT: Anatomy & & physiology, ed 8, St Louis, 2013, Mosby.)

✓ *TEST YOURSELF 3-2*
1. Name three structures that all mammalian cells possess.
2. Draw a picture of the lipid bilayer. Which part is hydrophobic and which part is hydrophilic?
3. What types of protein are found in the cell membrane?
4. Where are these proteins located and what are their functions? Add them to your drawing.
5. What are the molecular components of rafts and what role do rafts play in the life of a cell?
6. What is the glycocalyx and what important role does it play in cellular interaction?
7. What are CAMs and what do they do?
8. What are membrane receptors and ligands, and what role to they play in the health of the cell? How does obesity affect cell membrane receptors for insulin?
9. What are caveolae and what role do they play in the cell membrane?
10. How are cilia and flagella different?
11. Which are found more commonly in mammalian cells: cilia or flagella?

have the ability to visualize minute internal structures that define the complex internal workings of the cell. The principal components of cytoplasm are the cytosol, cytoskeleton, organelles, and inclusions.

## CYTOSOL

The fluid of the cell is called **cytosol**. It is a viscous, semi-transparent liquid composed of dissolved electrolytes, amino acids, and simple sugars. Proteins are also suspended in the cytosol and give it its thick, jellylike consistency. These proteins are mostly enzymes that are important in the metabolic activities of the cell.

## CYTOSKELETON

Like the skeleton in our bodies, the **cytoskeleton** is a three-dimensional frame for the cell; but unlike our bones, it is neither rigid nor permanent (Figure 3-7, *A* and *C*). It is a flexible, fibrous structure that changes in accordance with the activities of the cell. It gives support and shape to the cell, enables it to move, provides direction for metabolic activity, and anchors the organelles. Three different types of fiber comprise the cytoskeleton, all of which are made of protein. They are *microtubules*, *intermediate fibers*, and *microfilaments* (Figure 3-7, *B*). These fibers are not enclosed in a membrane.

The thickest fibers are the **microtubules**, which are long, hollow tubes that grow out from the cell center near the nucleus. They form secure "cables" to which mitochondria, lysosomes, and **secretory granules** attach. Proteins that act as motors move the attached organelles along the microtubule from one location in the cell to another. Because microtubules act as the railroad tracks for organelle travel, they can be easily disassembled and then reassembled to form new paths or to take on new direction. They appear, for example, in greater numbers during cell division to assist in the separation of chromosomes and organelles. Microtubules are composed of a pair of spherical molecules called **tubulins**, which are linked together into a spiral chain. The spiral shape provides strength and flexibility to cilia and flagella, as well as to the cell as a whole.

**Intermediate fibers** are woven, ropelike fibers that possess high tensile strength and are able to resist forces pulling on the cell by acting as internal guy wires. These fibers are the toughest and most permanent element of the cytoskeleton. They are composed of different proteins, depending on the function of the cell, and often take on different names depending on the type of cell in which they are found. In epithelial cells, for example, intermediate fibers are composed primarily of keratin and are known as **tonofilaments** or *keratin filaments*, whereas in nerve cells they are known as **neurofilaments**.

**Microfilaments** are located near the cell surface on the cytoplasmic side of the plasma membrane and are arranged in bundles and meshworks. They are composed of the contractile protein **actin** and, together with the motor protein **myosin**, play a key role in the cell's ability to change shape, break apart during cell division, and form outpouchings and involutions. In most cells, microfilaments are assembled where and when they are needed. Their position and quantity within the cell vary depending on the cell's activity. In muscle cells, however, the microfilaments are permanent, highly developed myofibrils, which shorten to cause muscle contraction.

Some cytologists believe that minute **microtrabeculae** exist as a fourth component of the cytoskeleton. These fibers are thought to form a lattice that interconnects larger cytoskeletal elements, suspends free ribosomes, and gives cytosol its jamlike consistency.

***CENTROSOME.*** A important region of the cytoskeleton, located near the nuclear envelope, is called the *centrosome*. The centrosome is responsible for the coordination of building and breaking down microtubules in the cell and is composed of several parts: centrioles, pericentriolar material, and asters (Figure 3-8). The centrosome helps manufacture microtubules, the thickest and strongest fibers in the cell. Microtubules are not only important parts of the cytoskeleton but also key elements in cell division and the formation and function of cellular extensions such as cilia and flagella. In these ways, the centrosome is vital to cellular life.

A pair of small cylinders, called **centrioles**, is found in the central portion of the centrosome. Each centriole is composed of nine triplets of microtubules arranged like a pinwheel around a hollow core. Long rods of microtubules, called *asters*, radiate away from the centrioles, forming anchors to the larger centrosome. In the center of this region, a concentrated amorphous collection of proteins forms the *pericentriolar material (PCM)*, where formation of microtubules is initiated.

In preparation for cell division, centrioles must first duplicate themselves; each one forms a "daughter" centriole that is oriented perpendicular to the "mother" centriole. Mother and daughter centrioles are linked to one another by a thin interconnecting fiber. The mother centriole is equipped with an array of molecular appendages that help anchor the newly formed microtubules that emerge from the PCM. As the fibers lengthen, the two centriole teams move slowly apart from one another, holding fast to the fibrous ends of the elaborate construction that ultimately becomes the **spindle apparatus**.

The centrosome plays an important role in the formation of microvilli, cilia, and flagella. Refer to the section in this chapter on the cell membrane for more information about these microtubular cell extensions.

## ORGANELLES

Organelles, or "little organs," are membrane-bound structures within the cytoplasm that possess specialized cellular functions. The membranes of the organelles are similar in composition to those in the plasma membrane but do not have glycocalyx coatings. In this way, each organelle is separated from the surrounding cytosol and is able to maintain its own internal environment. This compartmentalization is crucial for effective metabolic processes, because it enables the cell to separate and control various molecular

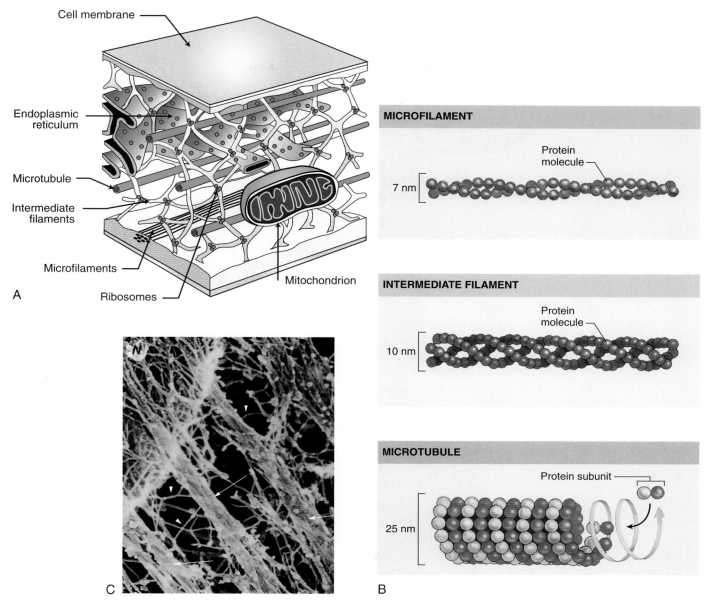

**FIGURE 3-7** Cytoskeleton. **A,** The cytoskeleton is an important structural frame for the cell. It is strong but flexible and can be dismantled in some regions and rearranged as needed. **B,** Left: Cytoskeleton is composed of three different types of fiber: *microtubules, intermediate fibers,* and *microfilaments*. Middle: Electron micrographs of each type of fiber. Right: Light microscopy reveals parts of the cytoskeleton using fluorescent stains to illuminate specific molecules. **C,** Color-enhanced scanning electron micrograph showing cytoskeleton. Note that the microtubules *(arrows)* are thicker than the minute intermediate filaments *(arrowheads)*. (**B,** *Top,* Courtesy I. Herman, Tufts University; *middle,* Courtesy E. Smith and E. Fuchs, University of Chicago; *bottom,* courtesy G. Borisy, University of Wisconsin, Madison.)

interactions, which are the basis for food absorption, energy production, and excretion.

***MITOCHONDRIA.*** Among the largest of the organelles is the **mitochondrion** (plural, *mitochondria*). This is known as the *powerhouse* of the cell because it produces 95% of the energy that fuels the cell. In the mitochondria, large nutrient molecules, such as glucose, are processed and broken down into smaller ones, which can be used intracellularly to fuel most metabolic processes (Figure 3-9). It is also where

respiration takes place: oxygen is consumed, and carbon dioxide is excreted. Numerous biochemical reactions occur in the mitochondria, such as amino acid and fatty acid catabolism, respiratory electron transport, oxidative phosphorylation, and the oxidative reactions of the citric acid cycle. (See Chapter 17 for more detailed descriptions of these metabolic processes.)

Active cells, which have high energy demands, have greater numbers of mitochondria within their cytoplasm than inactive cells. Heart muscle cells, for example, have far

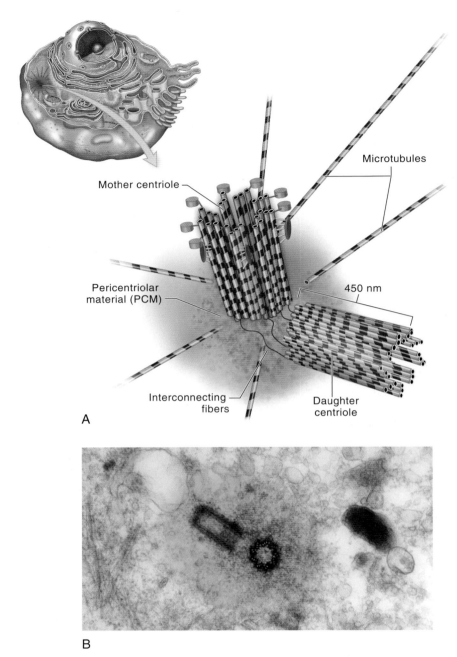

**FIGURE 3-8** Centrosome. **A,** A mother and daughter pair of centrioles form the focus of the centrosome. Each centriole is composed of nine triplets of microtubules arranged around a central axis, much like a pinwheel. Minute fibers connect the centrioles to one another while microtubules called asters radiate outward from the pericentriolar material. **B,** A transmission electron micrograph (TEM) of a centrosome. (**B,** Photograph by Dr. Conly L. Rieder, East Greenbush, NY.)

more mitochondria than relatively inactive endothelial cells. When cellular requirements for energy increase, the mitochondrion divides by pinching itself in half via a process called **fission**. Both halves subsequently grow to normal size. In addition, mitochondria tend to congregate in areas of the cell where greater amounts of energy are required, such as at the base of a flagellum.

Mitochondria contain the DNA, RNA, and enzymes necessary to make protein, but they provide themselves with only 13 of the proteins required for their metabolic functions; the nucleus provides the remaining 50. Thus most of the protein needed by the mitochondria is produced elsewhere in the cell and is later taken up by the mitochondria.

Mitochondria may take on a variety of shapes but tend to be elliptical or round. They can move throughout the cell and can elongate or change shape with ease. Mitochondria are enclosed by two membranes: the outer one is smooth and featureless, and the inner one involutes dramatically, forming

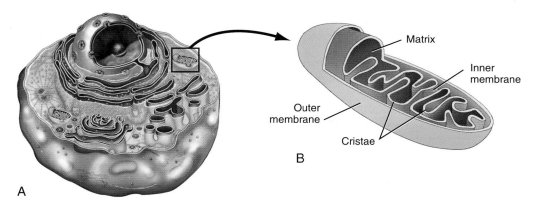

**FIGURE 3-9** Mitochondrion. **A,** The mitochondrion is the powerhouse of the cell. Using oxygen, it produces 95% of the energy that fuels the cell. **B,** Transmission electron micrograph of a mitochondrion. Note the convolutions of the inner membrane, which create increased workspace for the manufacturing of adenosine triphosphate (ATP). (Modified from Thibodeau GA, Patton KT: Anatomy & physiology, ed 6, St Louis, 2007, Mosby.)

shelflike folds called **cristae**. These folds increase the internal working area and allow greater contact between the cristae and the enzyme-rich liquid, called the **matrix**, which fills the spaces between the cristae. In addition to containing vital enzymes, the matrix is composed of calcium ions and the substrates required for metabolic reactions. Additional enzymes are available in the form of small particles that are found attached to some of the cristae. Because the cristae are the site of ATP production, it is not surprising that active mitochondria possess more cristae than inactive ones.

The DNA and RNA found in mitochondria are similar to those found in bacteria but are quite different from those found in the nucleus and cytoplasm. Mitochondria are thought to have originated as independent, bacteria-like organisms billions of years ago that later moved into the bodies of unicellular plants and animals, developing a symbiotic relationship with them.

**RIBOSOMES.** The most common and smallest organelle in the cell is the dark-staining **ribosome** (Figure 3-10). It is composed of two globular subunits, which fit together like cupped hands. These subunits contain protein and a specific type of RNA, known as *ribosomal RNA (rRNA)*. Although only 25 μm in diameter, the ribosome is an important site for protein synthesis. Soluble protein intended for intracellular use is manufactured on ribosomes that are evenly distributed freely throughout the cytoskeleton. Protein intended for use in the plasma membrane or meant for cellular export, on the other hand, is synthesized on ribosomes attached to the endoplasmic reticulum. Ribosomes are flexible in their abilities to attach and detach from membranes and to move freely within the cell. Thus they can move back and forth between the cytoskeleton and endoplasmic reticulum, depending on the type of protein they are making. When manufacturing protein, the ribosomes assemble the amino acids into long chains using specific instructions that are determined by the cell's genetic material. In this way, a wide range of proteins, such as cellular enzymes, hormones,

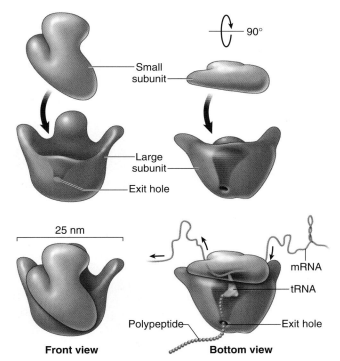

**FIGURE 3-10** Ribosome. Each ribosome is composed of one large and one small subunit. When joined together, these two subunits form one ribosome. The small subunit attaches to a strand of messenger RNA (mRNA). Amino acids are carried to the ribosome by transfer RNA (tRNA). The amino acids are assembled in order according to the recipe in the genetic code. As a chain of amino acids forms and lengthens, it leaves the ribosome via an exit hole in the bottom of the large subunit. When the polypeptide is fully formed, it will be released from the ribosome. (From Patton KT, Thibodeau GA: *Anatomy & physiology*, ed 8, St Louis, 2013, Mosby.)

collagen, and mucus, may be created, based on the needs of the cell and of the organism as a whole.

**ENDOPLASMIC RETICULUM.** The **endoplasmic reticulum (ER)** is a series of flattened tubes stacked on one another and bent into a crescent shape. Its surface area is enormous and may be 30 times larger than that of the plasma membrane. The walls of the ER are composed of a single lipid bilayer and are continuous with the membranes of the nucleus.

The two types of ER are *rough*, which has ribosomes on its surface, and *smooth*, which lacks ribosomes. **Rough ER** is involved in the production of protein, which is assembled by the ribosomes. These newly manufactured protein molecules are moved inside the ER into passageways known as *cisternae* (sis-TUR-ne; a reservoir of water). Here the proteins are modified before being moved on to the Golgi apparatus for further modification and packaging. **Smooth ER**, which is connected to rough ER, is active in the synthesis and storage of lipids, particularly phospholipids and steroids, and is

therefore seen in large quantities in gland cells. In liver cells, it may also function to eliminate drugs and break down glycogen into glucose. The proportion of smooth to rough ER varies depending on the synthetic activities of the cell.

***GOLGI APPARATUS.*** The **Golgi apparatus**, like the ER, is composed of stacks of flattened, crescent-shaped cisternae (Figure 3-11). Small, spherical transfer sacs from the ER containing newly manufactured proteins are received by the Golgi apparatus. These sacs fuse with the membrane at the ends of the Golgi apparatus and dislodge their contents into the Golgi cisternae. The protein molecules are then moved from stack to stack through the Golgi body, where they are modified. For

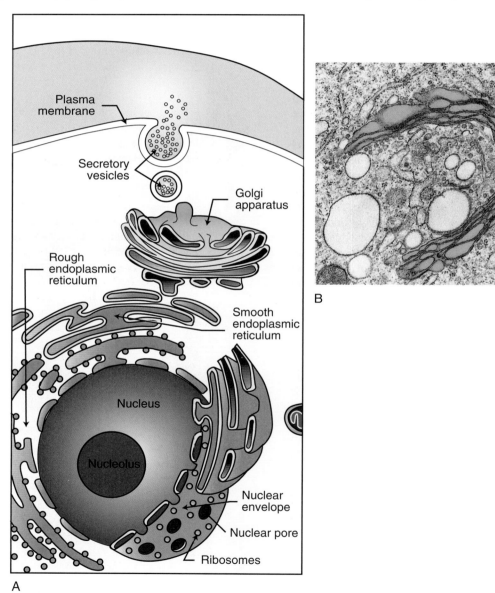

Plasma membrane

Secretory vesicles

Golgi apparatus

Rough endoplasmic reticulum

Smooth endoplasmic reticulum

Nucleus

Nucleolus

Nuclear envelope

Nuclear pore

Ribosomes

A

B

**FIGURE 3-11** Golgi apparatus and endoplasmic reticulum. **A,** Endoplasmic reticulum (ER) is continuous with the nuclear envelope and is divided into two types: *rough ER,* which is covered by ribosomes, and smooth *ER,* which does not have ribosomes. Molecules produced by ER are transported to the Golgi apparatus, where they are modified and packaged into vesicles. Vesicles transport molecules to other regions of the cell. **B,** A transmission electron micrograph of the Golgi apparatus. (**A,** Courtesy Charles Flickinger, University of Virginia. **B,** From Thibodeau GA, Patton KT: Anatomy & physiology, ed 8, St Louis, 2013, Mosby.)

example, sugar groups, which the Golgi apparatus manufactures, may be added to the proteins to form glycoproteins. When the modified proteins reach the outermost layer of the Golgi's flattened tubes, they are packaged into small spherical *vesicles*. The vesicles are formed as they pull away from the cisternae and venture out into the cytosol, where they travel to other parts of the cell, particularly the cell membrane. Thus the Golgi body acts as a modification, packaging, and distribution center for molecules destined either for secretion or for intracellular use. It also functions in polysaccharide synthesis and in the coupling of polysaccharides to proteins to create glycoproteins found on the cell surface.

**LYSOSOMES.** The **lysosome** is a specialized vesicle formed by the Golgi apparatus (Figure 3-12). It contains powerful enzymes enclosed in a single, protective membrane, which fuses with other vesicles carrying nutrients, microbes or aged cellular parts. Both the ER and the Golgi apparatus are skilled in policing the cytosol for unused and damaged protein, organelles, and cellular debris. Their membranes reach out into the cytosol and envelope this unwanted material. Subsequently, the vesicles fuse with lysosomes, which dump their digestive enzymes into the vesicles to break down the contents. A small residual body is all that is left behind, carrying amino acids and other molecular subunits that can be recycled to form new molecules or neatly expelled from the cell if not needed. It is not surprising, therefore, that the lysosome is considered the "stomach" or "garbage disposal" vessel of the cell. Its

principal responsibilities are to break down nutrient molecules, aged organelles, and cellular debris and to destroy phagocytosed microinvaders. Lysosomes also remove accumulations of protein that might otherwise obstruct normal cellular processes.

When cells die, the lysosomes within them are triggered to burst open and release their caustic enzymes into the cytosol; these enzymes immediately begin to dismantle and digest the various organelles and nuclear components of the cell. The process of self-digestion is called **autolysis**. The organism as a whole recycles the used parts of the dead cell to create new cells or to help maintain existing ones. Not surprisingly, as cells age, the number of lysosomes within them increases.

Lysosomes may also release their enzymes outside the cell to assist with the breakdown of extracellular material. During the process of bone remodeling, for example, osteocytes use lysosomes to help break down and remove unnecessary bone. This process is seen radiographically (in an x-ray film) as bone resorption, with a decrease in opacity of the affected area. In addition, lysosomal digestion is responsible for decreasing the size of body tissues, for example after parturition, with shrinkage of the uterus, and in the atrophy of muscles in paralyzed animals.

**PROTEASOMES.** The proteasome is a small cylindrical structure composed of multiple protein subunits. Like the lysosome, it assists with the breakdown and removal of misfolded and unwanted protein in the cell. Unlike the lysosome, however, which can digest large amounts of cellular debris, the proteasome can only break down one protein at a time.

The proteasome is barrel-shaped and composed of a stack of flattened protein subunits with a hollow core that extends down its center (Figure 3-13). Regulatory molecules form

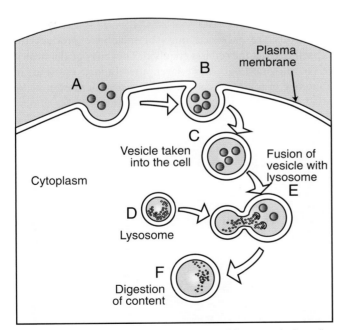

**FIGURE 3-12** Lysosomal action. **A,** Material from outside the cell is drawn into a forming vesicle. **B,** The plasma membrane surrounds the material and pinches off to form a vesicle. **C,** The vesicle transports material to internal regions of the cell. **D,** A lysosome approaches the vesicle. **E,** The lysosome fuses with the vesicle and dumps digestive enzymes into it; these break down the material. **F,** The contents of vesicle are digested and transported to other regions of the cell.

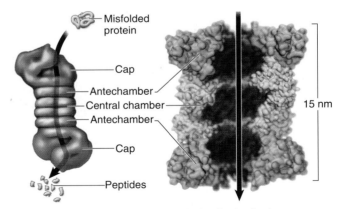

**FIGURE 3-13** Proteasome. Vital to the health of cells, the proteasome disposes of damaged, old or unwanted protein in cytoplasm that otherwise might build up and obstruct normal metabolic activity. The tiny organelle is a little more than half the size of a ribosome and is made of protein subunits with caps at each end. Following the route indicated by the arrows, a misfolded protein enters the hollow core of the proteasome where it is broken down into short peptide chains. The peptide chains exit the proteasome at the opposite end, and are further broken down into amino acids, which are used to make new proteins.

caplike structures at each end of the proteasome. These molecules control the entry and release of the proteins that it processes.

Before a protein can enter the proteasome, a short-chained protein called *ubiquitin* is attached to the misfolded protein. The ubiquitin then "pulls" the protein into the central core of the proteasome. As the protein passes through the cap, the protein is unfolded to prepare it for processing in the central chamber where it is broken into short peptide chains 4 to 25 amino acids in length. These short peptides are subsequently expelled from the distal cap into the cytosol where they are further broken down into amino acids that are recycled to make new proteins.

Scientists have learned that normal functioning of proteasomes is essential for healthy cells. In diseases such as Parkinson's disease in humans, for example, accumulations of misfolded proteins kill cells in the brain that regulate muscle function, because the proteasome system is not functioning properly.

**PEROXISOMES.**  Like lysosomes, **peroxisomes** are membranous sacs containing enzymes that are found throughout the cell. But unlike lysosomes, which are formed by the Golgi apparatus, peroxisomes are formed by vesicles pinching in half via fission or by pinching off from the ER. They commonly occur in liver and kidney cells and are important in the detoxification of various molecules. Peroxisomes contain enzymes that use oxygen to detoxify a number of harmful substances, including alcohol and formaldehyde. They also assist in the removal of *free radicals*, which are normal products of cellular metabolism but can be harmful to the cell in large quantities because they interfere with the structure of proteins, lipids, and nucleic acids. Peroxisomes carry two major types of enzyme: **peroxidases**, which assist in the conversion of free radicals to hydrogen peroxide, and **catalases**, which reduce hydrogen peroxide to water.

**VAULTS.**  A new tiny organelle has recently been discovered, called a vault (Figure 3-14). Its minute barrel-shaped structure with tapered ends is reminiscent of a straight "crescent" dinner roll, but unlike dinner rolls, vaults are hollow inside. Vaults are thought to be extremely numerous throughout the cell and may play a role in transporting molecules to and from the nucleus. They appear to be attached to microtubules in the cytoskeleton and are thought to act as transportation pods, sliding rapidly from one end of the cell to another. Their tiny size enables them to dock in nuclear pore complexes where they can open into a rosette shape that echoes that of the nuclear pore complex. In this way, they can open one end to pick up or drop off ribosomal subunits or large molecules. They are made of protein and a small amount of RNA. This RNA is called vault RNA (vRNA or vtRNA for short).

> ✓ **TEST YOURSELF 3-3**
> 1. What are the principal components of cytoplasm?
> 2. What is cytosol and what kind of molecules are found in it?
> 3. What is the centrosome and what important roles does it play in the life of the cell?
> 4. What is the cytoskeleton and what is its function?
> 5. How many types of fiber make up the cytoskeleton? Can you name them? How do they function differently?
> 6. Draw a picture of each of the eight organelles described earlier.
> 7. How does each of these organelles function within the cell?

## INCLUSIONS

**Inclusions** are packaged units of metabolic products or substances that the cell has engulfed. They may be delineated by a surrounding, single-layer membrane, as seen in secretory granules, vacuoles, and vesicles, or they may be

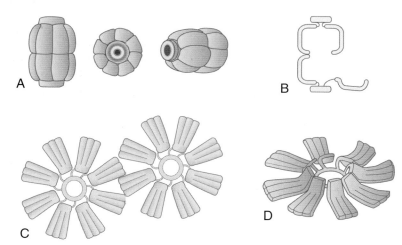

**FIGURE 3-14** Vaults. Vaults are recently discovered organelles. They resemble tiny hollow pods and are thought to transport small structures to and from the nucleus. They can attach themselves to microtubules and rapidly zip from one part of the cell to another. The ends of each vault open to allow it to pick up or drop off loads.

non-membrane bound inclusions, such as lipid droplets and fat globules. **Vacuoles** are larger than vesicles but are otherwise identical in structure. They are often filled with water and solutes that are transported to and from the cell surface. Some vesicles act simply as storage units, holding substances within the cell until the contents can be used.

## NUCLEUS

The nucleus is the largest organelle in the cell and is considered the control center, the central processing unit, the CEO of operations, or the "brain" of the cell. It is a dominating, dark-staining, ovoid, spherical, flattened, or multisegmented body. The primary functions of the nucleus are to maintain the hereditary information of the species and to control cellular activities through protein synthesis. Thus the nucleus contains the hereditary information (DNA) that enables the cell to divide and produce an identical daughter cell and, on a larger scale, determines whether an animal will develop into a dog, cat, or horse. It also contains all of the instructions, blueprints, and information required to make over 2000 proteins that are needed for normal cell activity.

Although most cells have at least one nucleus, extremely large cells, such as muscle cells, may have many nuclei and are therefore called **multinucleated**. Mature mammalian red blood cells, on the other hand, have no nuclei, because the nuclei are removed from the cells during their development in the bone marrow. These cells are therefore called **anucleate**. Without a nucleus, they cannot divide, make protein or enzymes, or repair themselves as they start to age. For this reason, the supply of vital molecules in mammalian red blood cells allows them to survive in circulation for only 3 or 4 months. The red blood cells found in birds and reptiles, on the other hand, are nucleated and therefore are able to produce the proteins and other molecules needed by the cells to survive for longer periods.

The anatomy of the nucleus is divided into the following four parts:
- Nuclear envelope or membrane
- Nucleoplasm
- Chromatin
- Nucleoli

### NUCLEAR ENVELOPE AND NUCLEOPLASM

The nucleus is separated from the cytosol by a nuclear envelope composed of a lipid bilayer. The outer layer is continuous with the ER and is studded with ribosomes. Over 10% of the nuclear surface consists of **nuclear pore complexes**—places where the two layers of the nuclear envelope have fused to form a channel that spans its entire thickness (Figure 3-15). With improved microscopy techniques, the structure of nuclear pore complexes has become better understood, and they are relatively large (120 nanometers in diameter). Typically, protein molecules are moved into the nucleus from the cytoplasm, and mRNA and rRNA molecules are exported. The nuclear pore complexes represent the principal channels of communication between the cytoplasm and the nucleus. Between the bilayers of the nuclear envelope is a space called

the **perinuclear cisterna**. The nucleus is filled with a gel-like substance called **nucleoplasm** that resembles cytosol and which contains chromatin.

## DNA, RNA, AND CHROMATIN

The structure of genetic material, which was known to exist within the nucleus, was a mystery until the early 1950s, when research on heredity was to take a great leap forward. Rosalind Franklin (Box 3-2), a British physical chemist working at Kings College in London, used x-ray crystallography techniques to examine the structure of DNA. In 1953, she discovered that there are two forms of DNA, which she called *A* and *B*. It was her photograph 51 of the *B* form of DNA that showed the helical and double coaxial structure of the molecule, better known as the **double helix**. This critical discovery became the basis for the model that was subsequently developed by James Watson and Francis Crick (Figure 3-16) for which they won the Nobel Prize for Medicine and Physiology in 1962. Today, with the aid of advanced technology, cell biologists have an even better understanding of nucleic acids—DNA and RNA—and of the proteins that are central to the continuation of life.

DNA and RNA are made up of chains of **nucleotides**. Nucleotides are composed of three subunits: a *nitrogenous base*, a *five-carbon sugar*, and a *phosphate group*. In DNA the sugar is deoxyribose and in RNA the sugar is ribose. DNA and RNA nucleotides are linked in such a way as to form a "backbone" of alternating sugar and phosphate groups. The nitrogenous bases project out of this backbone and in DNA they are weakly bonded to nitrogenous bases on an opposing strand. In this way, DNA forms a double-stranded molecule, the basic structure of which is analogous to a twisted ladder in which the vertical poles are composed of alternating sugar and phosphate groups and the horizontal rungs are paired nitrogenous bases. DNA's molecular structure is therefore called the **double helix** (see Figure 3-16). RNA, however, is a single-stranded molecule that has no opposing strand. The single strand of RNA is similar in structure to each of the strands found in DNA.

Four kinds of nitrogen base are found in DNA and RNA nucleotides (Figure 3-17). The three that are found in *both* RNA and DNA are **adenine (A)**, **cytosine (C)**, and **guanine (G)**. However, only DNA contains **thymine (T)**, and only RNA contains **uracil (U)**. In addition, the structure of each nitrogenous base permits the bonding of only certain pairs of nucleotides. For example, thymine can only bond to adenine, and cytosine can only bond to guanine. Uracil, the RNA base, can only bond to the DNA base adenine. These nitrogenous bases and their corresponding bonding parameters are the foundation for the storage of genetic information.

**Chromatin** appears as light or dark fibers in the nucleoplasm of the nucleus and is made up of DNA and globular proteins called **histones**. A single strand of DNA winds around eight histone molecules, forming a granule called a **nucleosome**. The nucleosomes are held together by short

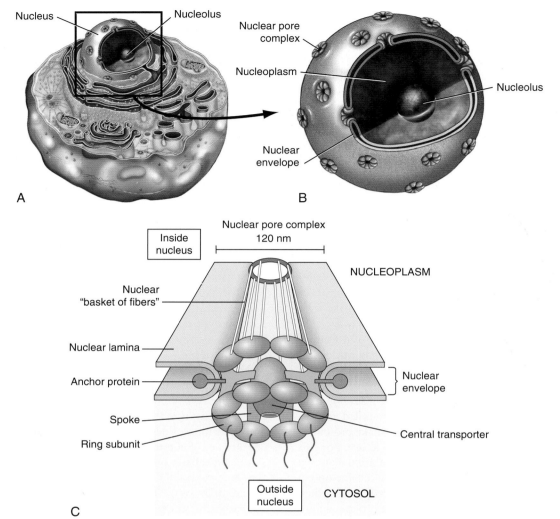

**FIGURE 3-15** Nucleus. **A,** The nucleus contains a nonmembrane bound region containing rRNA, called the nucleolus, and colloidal nucleoplasm that contains chromatin. The entire nucleus is surrounded by a nuclear envelope that is perforated by thousands of nuclear pore complexes (NPC). The NPCs have a rosette appearance comprising eight "petals" arranged around a central transporter "pore." The NPC permits selective passage of substances in and out of the nucleus. **B,** A computer-enhanced transmission electron micrograph shows a nuclear pore and the details of the two lipid bilayer membranes that make up the nuclear envelope. Keep in mind that the outer lipid bilayer is continuous with the endoplasmic reticulum. Nucleoplasm *(gray)* inside the nucleus and cytoplasm *(yellow)* outside the nucleus are also visible. **C,** A nuclear pore complex is composed of many parts. (**A,** Modified from Patton KT, Thibodeau GA: *Anatomy & physiology,* ed 8, St Louis, 2013, Mosby. **B,** From Thibodeau GA, Patton KT: *Anatomy & physiology,* ed 5, St Louis, 2003, Mosby.)

---

| BOX 3-2 | Rosalind Elsie Franklin |

In the early 1950s, when research on heredity was moving forward rapidly, Dr. Rosalind Franklin, at King's College in Cambridge University, used crystal chromatography to study the structure of DNA. She made meticulous preparations and produced several excellent photographs. One in particular, photograph 51, showed the helical structure of the molecule. Without her permission, Maurice Wilkins, who worked with Franklin in the same laboratory, showed her data and photograph 51 to James Watson and Francis Crick. Immediately, Watson and Crick began work on a new 3-dimensional model that included two helical strands, discarding their previous 3-helix model. On March 17th, 1953, Franklin wrote a draft

paper based on her own research describing the structure of DNA and detailed the placement of the sugars, phosphates and nitrogenous bases. However, before her paper was published, James Watson and Francis Crick's paper appeared on April 25, 1953 in *Nature.*

By the time Watson and Crick's paper was published, Franklin had left King's College for a new appointment at Birkbeck College, where she was given charge of a new research group working on the tobacco mosaic virus. At Birkbeck, Franklin found a collaborative working environment in which she became highly productive. She enthusiastically initiated work on the structure and assembly of the tobacco mosaic

**BOX 3-2** | Rosalind Elsie Franklin—cont'd

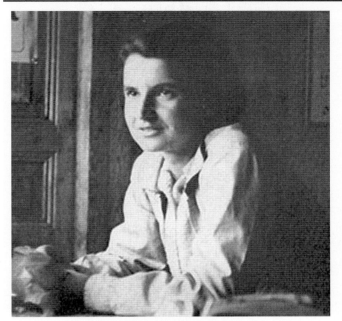

Rosalind Elsie Franklin. (From Piper A: Light on a dark lady. Trends Biochem Sci 23:151-154, 1998.)

virus and, during the four and a half years she spent at Birkbeck, published 17 papers. This was an impressive feat in the best of circumstances, but was particularly so for Franklin, because in 1956 she was diagnosed with ovarian cancer, which may have been caused by her lengthy exposures to x-ray radiation. Despite her illness, she maintained an arduous schedule and continued working in the laboratory until shortly before her death two years later. She died in London on April 16th, 1958 at the age of 37. After her death, her colleague Aaron Klug, who had been working with Franklin since 1954, took over the directorship of the laboratory at Birkbeck. He continued the research that Franklin had started on the tobacco mosaic virus and completed new research on the polio virus. Klug was subsequently awarded the Nobel Prize for this work.

In 1962, four years after Rosalind Franklin's death, the Nobel Prize for Medicine or Physiology was awarded to Francis Crick, James Watson, and Maurice Wilkins for determining the structure of DNA. Regrettably, the Nobel Prize is only awarded to the living. Nominations cannot be made posthumously. The premature death of Rosalind Franklin arguably robbed her of two chances to win the Nobel Prize herself. Nevertheless, it is widely felt that her contribution to the discovery of the structure of DNA is comparable to those who did receive the prize, and that she is indeed among the most brilliant scientists of our time.

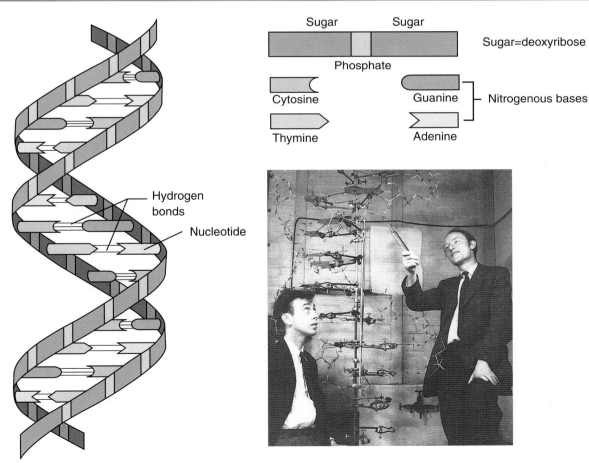

**FIGURE 3-16** DNA. With the aid of data collected by Rosalind Franklin, of Britain, James Watson, of the United States, and Francis Crick, of Britain (photo, right), developed the double-helix model of deoxyribonucleic acid (DNA). Like a spiraling ladder, the vertical portion is composed of alternating molecules of sugar and phosphate, while the "rungs" are paired nitrogenous bases. Watson, Crick, and Maurice Wilkins were awarded the Nobel Prize in 1962 for this famous work. (Photo from Cold Spring Harbor Laboratory.)

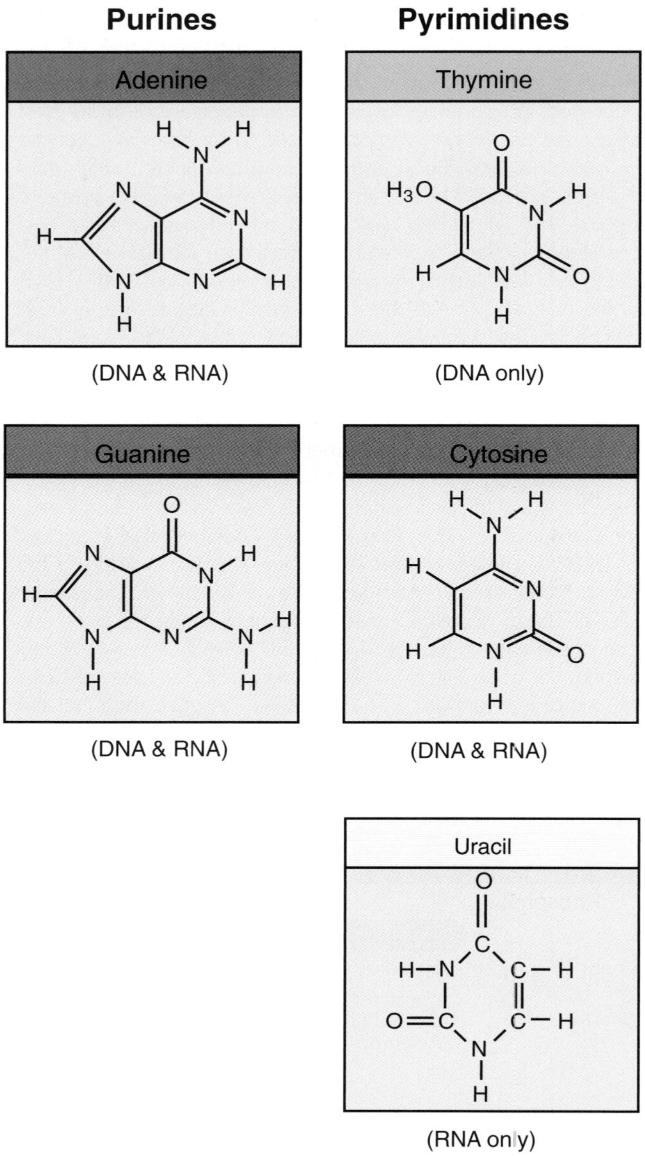

## Purines

### Adenine

(DNA & RNA)

### Guanine

(DNA & RNA)

## Pyrimidines

### Thymine

(DNA only)

### Cytosine

(DNA & RNA)

### Uracil

(RNA only)

**FIGURE 3-17** Nitrogenous bases. DNA and RNA are composed of two types of nitrogenous base: *purines* and *pyrimidines*. Purine molecules each have two rings and are found in both DNA and RNA. Pyrimidines, in contrast, are single-ringed molecules. Cytosine is the only pyrimidine that occurs in both RNA and DNA. Thymine occurs only in DNA, and uracil occurs only in RNA.

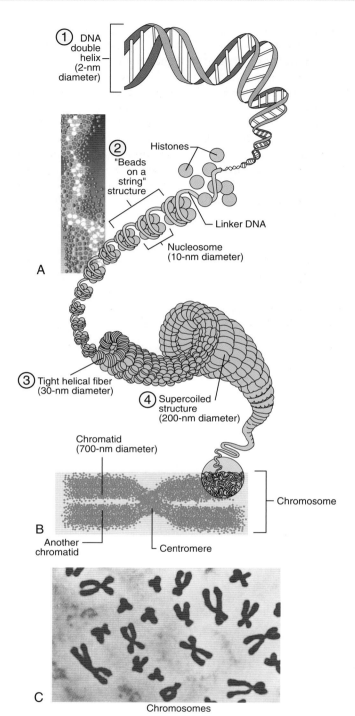

**FIGURE 3-18** Chromatin (DNA and protein) comprises chromosomes. **A,** The double helix of DNA (1) wraps twice around eight histone proteins, forming a nucleosome. The nucleosomes are joined together by linker-DNA strands (2). Nucleosomes compress into a fiber, which coils tightly (3). The coiled fiber is then supercoiled and compressed into chromosomes (4). **B,** During cell division, the chromosome becomes shaped like an X, representing two chromatids held together at the centromere. **C,** Light micrograph of chromosomes in a cell preparing to divide. (**C,** From Thibodeau GA, Patton KT: Anatomy & physiology, ed 5, St Louis, 2003, Mosby.)

strands of DNA called *linker DNA*. Not only do the histone proteins help keep the DNA strand organized and untangled, they also expose small sections of the DNA to the outside nucleoplasm. These sections of DNA are called **genes**. By changing shape, the histones can expose different genes at different times. The exposed genes determine what proteins will be made by the cell. In this way, histones play an important role in the control of gene expression. We call this process **gene regulation**.

The DNA contains all of the important instructions required for the synthesis of thousands of different proteins, but not all of them are made: only a small percentage are actually manufactured. The histones help to determine which segments of the DNA will be expressed and therefore which proteins will be made. When not being used to make protein, chromatin coils into tight helical fibers, which appear as dark strands in the nucleoplasm. This arrangement protects the delicate strands of DNA when they are not being used and saves space within the nucleoplasm. Strands of chromatin that are actively engaged in protein synthesis are uncoiled and called *extended chromatin*. The extended chromatin is lighter and is usually not visible under light microscopy. During cell division the chromatin condenses into supercoiled, X-shaped structures called **chromosomes** (Figure 3-18).

## NUCLEOLI

Nuclei usually contain one or more small, dark-staining spherical patches known as **nucleoli**. The nucleoli are not membrane bound but are the places in the nucleus where ribosomal subunits are made. These subunits are exported separately from the nucleus and are assembled in the cytoplasm to form functional ribosomes. In addition, nucleoli contain the DNA that governs the synthesis of ribosomal RNA (rRNA).

---

### ✓ TEST YOURSELF 3-4

1. Why do inclusions vary in appearance? What function do they perform?
2. What role does the centriole play in the formation of cilia and flagella?
3. How are centrioles structurally similar to cilia and flagella?
4. Why is the nucleus considered the "CEO of operations"?
5. Can a cell that does not contain a nucleus live as long as a cell that does contain one? Why or why not?
6. Describe the nuclear envelope. How is it different from the cell membrane?
7. How do histones play a role in gene regulation?
8. What is the significance of the nucleolus? What happens in that region of the nucleus?

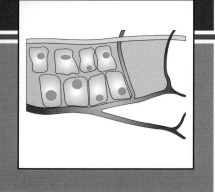

# Cell Physiology 4

*Joanna M. Bassert*

## OUTLINE

## LEARNING OBJECTIVES

*When you have completed this chapter you will be able to:*

1. Differentiate between active and passive transport processes.
2. Describe the factors that determine whether a molecule can pass through a plasma membrane by passive diffusion.
3. Differentiate between diffusion and facilitated diffusion.
4. Describe the process of osmosis.

5. Describe the process of active transport.
6. Describe the processes of endocytosis and exocytosis.
7. Describe the role of ions in maintaining a cell's resting membrane potential.
8. List the phases of mitosis and describe the events that occur in each phase.
9. List the steps in replication of DNA.
10. List the steps in the synthesis of proteins.

## VOCABULARY FUNDAMENTALS

*Absorption* ahb-**sohrp**-shuhn
*Active membrane process* **ahck**-tihv **mehm**-brān
 **proh**-sehs
*Active transport* **ahck**-tihv **trahnz**-pohrt
*Alkaline* **ahl**-kah-līn
*Anaphase* **ahn**-uh-fāz
*Anion* **ahn**-ī-uhn
*Anticodon* ahn-tē-**kō**-dōn
*Antiport system* **ahn**-tē-pohrt **sihs**-tehm
*Ascites* ah-**sī**-tēz
*Carrier protein* **keər**-ē-ər **prō**-tēn
*Cation* **kaht**-ī-ohn
*Coated pit* **kō**-tihd piht
*Codon* **kō**-dohn
*Concentration gradient* kohn-sehn-**trā**-shuhn
 **grā**-dē-ehnt

*Contact inhibition* **kohn**-tahckt ihn-ih-**bihsh**-ihn
*Cytokinesis* sī-tō-**kihn**-ē-sihs
*Cytosis* sī-**tō**-sihs
*Diffusion* dihf-**fyoo**-shuhn
*Electrolyte* ē-**lehck**-trō-līt
*Endocytosis* ehn-dō-sī-**tō**-sihs
*Equilibrium* ē-kwuh-**lihb**-rē-uhm
*Excretion* ehck-**skrē**-shuhn
*Exocytosis* ehcks-ō-sī-**tō**-sihs
*Exon* **ehck**-sohn
*Extracellular fluid* ehcks-trah-**sehl**-ū-lahr
 **floo**-ihd
*Facilitated diffusion* fah-**sihl**-ih-tā-tehd
 dihf-**fyoo**-shuhn
*Filtration* fihl-**trā**-shuhn
*Gene* jēn

*Genetic code* jeh-**neht**-ihck kōd
*Growth one phase* grōth wuhn fāz
*Growth two phase* grōth too fāz
*Hydrostatic pressure* hī-drō-**staht**-ihck **prehsh**-ər
*Hypertonic* hī-pər-**tohn**-ihck
*Hypotonic* hī-pō-**tohn**-ihck
*Interphase* **ihn**-tər-fāz
*Interstitial fluid* ihn-tər-**stihsh**-ahl **floo**-ihd
*Intracellular fluid* ihn-trah-**sehl**-ū-lər **floo**-ihd
*Intron* **ihn**-trohn
*Ion* **ī**-ohn
*Isotonic* ī-sō-**tohn**-ihck
*Messenger RNA (mRNA)* **mehs**-ehn-jər RNA
*Metaphase* **meht**-ah-fāz
*Metaphase plate* **meht**-ah-fāz plāt
*Mitosis* mī-**tō**-sihs
*Mitotic phase* mī-**toh**-tihck fāz
*Mutagen* **myoo**-ta-jehn
*Mutation* **myoo**-tā-shuhn
*Oncotic pressure* ohn-**kaw**-tihck **prehsh**-ər
*Osmosis* ohs-**mō**-sihs
*Osmotic pressure* ohs-**moh**-tihck **prehsh**-ər
*Passive membrane process* **pah**-sihv **mehm**-brān **proh**-sehs

*Phagocytize* fahg-ō-**sih**-tīz
*Phagocytosis* fahg-ō-sī-**tō**-sihs
*Phagosome* **fahg**-ō-sōm
*Pinocytosis* pih-nō-sī-**tō**-sihs
*Polymerase* **pohl**-ē-mər-āz
*Prophase* **prō**-fāz
*Pseudopodia* soo-dō-**pōd**-ē-ah
*Receptor-mediated endocytosis* reh-**sehpt**-ər **mē**-dē-ā-tehd ehn-dō-sī-**tō**-sihs
*Resting membrane potential* **rehs**-tihng **mehm**-brān puh-**tehn**-shahl
*Ribosomal RNA (RNA)* rī-boh-**sōm**-ahl RNA
*Secretion* seh-**krē**-shuhn
*Selectively permeable* seh-**lehck**-tihv-lē pər-mē-ah-buhl
*Simple diffusion* **sihmp**-ehl dih-**fyoo**-shuhn
*Symport system* **sihm**-pohrt **sihs**-tehm
*Synthetic phase* sihn-**theht**-ihck fāz
*Telophase* **tehl**-ō-fāz
*Transcription* trahnz-**skrihp**-shuhn
*Transfer RNA (tRNA)* **trahnz**-fər RNA
*Translation* trahnz-**lā**-shuhn

## INTRODUCTION

The survival of a cell depends upon its ability to manufacture and transport molecules and to moderate their intricate and vital interactions with one another. Survival also depends upon the cell's selective control over what will and what will not cross the cell membrane that delineates the intracellular and extracellular spaces. The building, modification, placement and subsequent destruction of molecules are the foundational activities that underlie all of the events by which life is defined. Cellular respiration, growth, development, repair, adaptation, reproduction, and the ability to maintain an internal homeostasis are all based upon molecular activities within the cell. This chapter focuses on some of the most important physiologic events in the cell and, where relevant, correlates them to the clinical work of veterinary technicians.

## BODY FLUIDS

### BODY FLUIDS AND FLUID COMPARTMENTS

Water is essential for life. Roughly 60% of an animal's body is composed of water (Figure 4-1). Water is found in all cells, tissues and organs, as well as in blood and lymph. Healthy animals maintain normal hydration by consuming the same amount of water as they lose. Animals take in water from eating moist or wet foods and by drinking fluids. In addition, a small amount of water is produced as the by-product of cellular metabolism. This water is called **water of oxidation** or **metabolic water**. Conversely, animals lose water in a wide variety of ways. It is vaporized away from the body during respiration and diffuses passively away from skin. This water loss is called **insensible water loss**. However, greater quantities of water are lost overtly via sweating, vocalizing, urinating and defecating. In sick animals, it is lost more rapidly as a result of vomiting, diarrhea, excessive sweating, hemorrhage, and elevated body temperatures.

Despite the remarkable ability of the kidney to conserve water by concentrating urine, some fluid is inevitably lost from the production of urine regardless of how concentrated it may be. In addition, insensible water loss from respiration and evaporation on skin cannot be prevented. Therefore, all animals—including the inactive couch potatoes that may live with us—must consume water or they

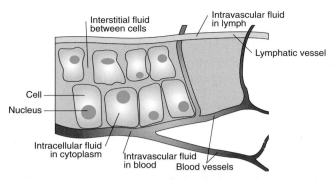

**FIGURE 4-1** Fluid spaces. Most fluid in the body is found inside the cell and is therefore called *intracellular fluid*. *Extracellular fluid* is found outside the cell and includes *intravascular fluid*, found in blood and lymphatic vessels, and *interstitial fluid*, found in the tissue-spaces surrounding cells. Arterial blood delivers oxygen, nutrients and ions to needy cells while venous blood carries away $CO_2$ and waste products.

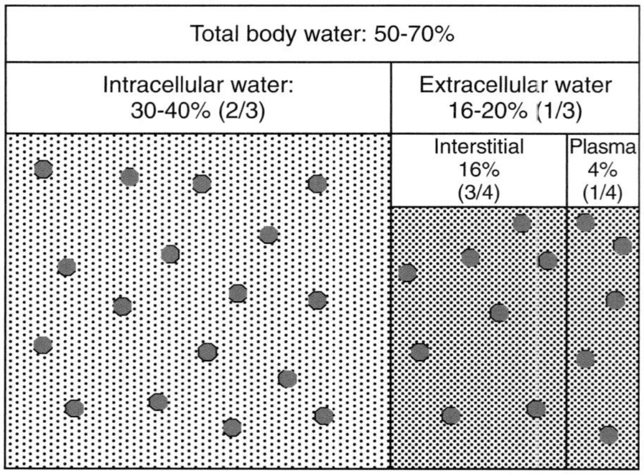

| Total body water: 50-70% | | |
|---|---|---|
| Intracellular water:<br>30-40% (2/3) | Extracellular water<br>16-20% (1/3) | |
| | Interstitial<br>16%<br>(3/4) | Plasma<br>4%<br>(1/4) |

**FIGURE 4-2** Roughly 60% of a mammal's body is composed of water. Two thirds of this water is found inside the cell while one third is found outside the cell. (From Bassert JM, Thomas JA: McCurnin's clinical textbook for veterinary technicians, ed 8, St Louis, 2014, Elsevier.)

will die in a relatively short period of time. Dogs, for example, die within 2 to 4 days, while cattle die within 6 to 8 days. Small animals, particularly neonates, with rapid metabolisms may die within several hours without water. Extraordinarily, some types of camels have been known to survive for 1 to 2 months in the winter desert, and 6 to 10 days in the summer desert, without drinking. Regardless of the species, evaluating the initial and changing hydration status of veterinary patients and carrying out and maintaining fluid therapy orders are important responsibilities for veterinary technicians.

Two thirds, the vast majority, of total body water (TBW) is found inside cells and is called **intracellular fluid**. Fluid outside the cell is called **extracellular fluid** and makes up the other third of TBW. Extracellular fluid found in lymphatic and blood vessels is called **intravascular fluid**, while the extracellular fluid found outside vessels and surrounding cells is called **interstitial fluid** (Figure 4-2). Keep in mind that the epithelia that comprise vascular walls separate intra-vascular and interstitial fluid, while the cell membrane delineates intracellular from interstitial fluid.

## SOLUTES AND OSMOLALITY

Body fluids are filled with many different kinds of particles called **solutes**. The solutes range in size, level of abundance, and whether or not they have an electrical charge. Charged particles, called **ions**, are the most abundant type of solute found in body fluid. Ions may be either positively or negatively charged. Salt is an excellent example of an ionic compound because it is composed of oppositely charged ions that separate from one another (i.e., it ionizes) when mixed in water. The salt sodium sulfate ($Na_2SO_4^{2-}$), for example, separates into two sodium ions ($Na^+$) and one sulfate ion ($SO_4^{2-}$). Positively charged ions, such as $Na^+$, are called **cations** (pronounced "cat-ions"), and negatively charged ions, such as $SO_4^{2-}$, are called **anions** (unfortunately, they are not called *dogions*, which would seem logical in the veterinary world). A salt, by definition, is made up of anions other than the hydroxyl ion ($OH^-$) and cations other than the hydrogen ion ($H^+$). Because anions and cations are capable of conducting an electrical current in solution, they are called **electrolytes**. All ions are electrolytes.

The concentration of electrolytes in body fluids is usually expressed in milliequivalents per liter (mEq/L), which is a measure of the number of electrical charges in 1 liter of solution. Figure 4-3 illustrates relative quantities of the most commonly found electrolytes in the body. Notice that the electrolytes are generally distributed unevenly between the intracellular and extracellular fluid compartments. Remember, intracellular fluid is only found inside cells, whereas extracellular fluid is found outside cells ... in tissues (interstitial fluid) and in lymphatic and blood vessels (intravascular fluid). Notice that sodium, bicarbonate, and chloride have the highest concentrations outside the cell, while the concentrations of potassium, magnesium, hydrogen phosphate, and sulfate are highest inside the cell.

Acids and bases are also electrolytes, because they dissociate in water and can conduct an electrical impulse. However, unlike salt, acids release hydrogen ions ($H^+$) and bases release hydroxyl ions ($OH^-$) when in solution. Because the nucleus of a hydrogen atom contains one proton, a hydrogen ion is therefore simply a proton. For this reason, acids are molecules that release protons and are called *proton donors*. Conversely, bases are *proton receivers* because they release hydroxyl ions, which readily bind to free hydrogen ions (protons). When a hydroxyl anion and a hydrogen cation unite, two things happen: water is formed, and the acidity of the solution is reduced.

The more free protons or hydrogen ions ($H^+$) in a solution, the greater is its acidity. In contrast, the greater the concentration of hydroxyl ions, the more basic or **alkaline** the solution becomes. Body fluids are rich in hydrogen and hydroxyl ($OH^-$) ions, and their relative proportion

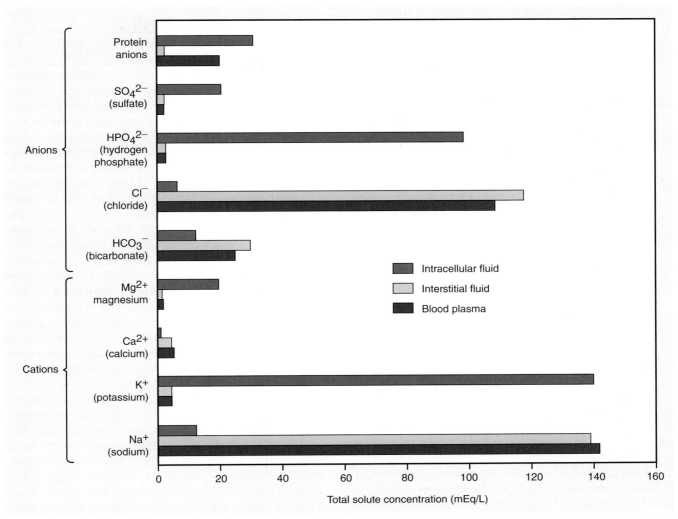

**FIGURE 4-3** Distribution of electrolytes in fluid compartments. Notice that electrolytes sodium, bicarbonate, and chloride are abundant in the *extracellular* space, while potassium, magnesium, hydrogen phosphate, and sulfate are abundant in the *intracellular* space.

determines the acidity or alkalinity of the fluid. The concentration of hydrogen ions in fluid is measured *inversely* by pH units on a scale from 0 to 14. Pure water, for example, has a neutral pH of 7, while blood is slightly alkaline with a pH of around 7.4. Gastric juices, on the other hand, are acidic, which means a lot of $H^+$ ions are present in them. Therefore they have a pH *below* 7. In contrast, an alkaline substance, such as bleach, has a pH *above* 7 because it contains a low concentration of hydrogen ions and a high concentration of hydroxyl ions, as shown below:

| 0 (Acidic) | 7 (Neutral) | 14 (Alkaline) |
| --- | --- | --- |
| Many $H^+$ ions | Equal concentration | Few $H^+$ ions |
| Few $OH^-$ ions | of $H^+$ and $OH^-$ ions | Many $OH^-$ ions |

In sick or injured animals, the electrolyte concentrations and pH of intracellular and extracellular fluid can become

abnormally high or low. Normal body functions, such as the transmission of nervous impulses, muscle contraction, and respiration, can be adversely affected by changes in electrolyte concentration and pH. For this reason, intravenous fluids can be used to help balance the pH of body fluids. There are a number of different types of intravenous fluids, which used selectively can help correct imbalances and abnormalities in pH.

## OSMOLALITY OF BODY FLUIDS

Osmolality is a measurement of the solute concentration in fluid. Fluids that have a high concentration of solutes have a high osmolality. Ranges of serum osmolality in mammals are roughly between 278 and 300 milliosmoles per kilogram (mOsml/kg), but this varies among species. Mammals are able to maintain the osmolality of body fluids within a very narrow range. This is carried out by a hormonal feedback loop. An increase in the osmolality of blood, for example, triggers the desire to drink and also simulates the release of antidiuretic hormone (ADH) from stores in the pituitary (in the brain). Once released, ADH travels through the circulatory system to the kidney where it stimulates the resorption of water from proto-urine, resulting in the production and excretion of concentrated urine. Conversely, a decrease of osmolality in body fluids inhibits the desire to drink and inhibits the release of ADH. Water subsequently is NOT resorbed from proto-urine in the kidney and dilute urine is produced and excreted that helps to rid the body of its excess fluid. (Refer to Chapter 18 for more information about the role of ADH in controlling osmolality in the body.)

Veterinarians sometimes request serum osmolality tests to better understand what is happening physiologically in sick patients. For example, a serum osmolality test might be performed when the following are **suspected** in a patient:

- Problems with the hydration status, either dehydration (high osmolality) or overhydration (low osmolality).
- The presence of hyperglycemia caused by diabetes (high osmolality).
- Problems with the functioning of the hypothalamus in the brain, which produces ADH (low osmolality with trauma to the head).
- Poisoning by ethylene glycol (high osmolality) or excessive use of steroids (low osmolality).

There is a variety of fluid products used to treat osmolality disorders. Products with an osmolality comparable to that of normal blood, such as 0.9% NaCl (normal saline), are called **isotonic**. Fluids with an osmolality greater than that of blood are called **hypertonic** and those with an osmolality less than that of blood are called **hypotonic**. It is important to select a fluid product that appropriately compensates for osmolar anomalies so that the cells within the patient are not damaged from excessive expansion or shrinkage due to tonicity imbalances. (Refer to Clinical Application: The Importance of Fluid Therapy.) Evaluating the initial and changing hydration statuses of patients, communicating this information to the veterinary health care team and carrying out and maintaining fluid therapy as ordered are the responsibilities of veterinary technicians.

## MOVEMENT OF BODY FLUIDS

Water moves freely between intracellular, interstitial, and intravascular fluid compartments in the body, based on changes in the osmolality of the fluid in each compartment. Because electrolytes, though small, are the most abundant solutes in the body, changes in their concentration have the greatest ability to cause fluid shifts between compartments. However, large organic molecules, such as soluble proteins, phospholipids, cholesterol, and triglycerides, though not as numerous as electrolytes, constitute the *bulk* (mass) of the solutes. These large solutes are unequally distributed among the fluid compartments because of variations in their size, electrical charge, and dependence on transport proteins. When there are changes in the concentrations of any solute, including these larger molecules as well as tiny electrolytes, there is movement of water from one compartment to another. Keep in mind that the movement of water between interstitial and intracellular compartments crosses the **cell membrane**. The movement of water between intravascular fluid and interstitial fluid crosses **capillary walls**. Thus, any change in the osmolality between compartments, for any reason, results in the movement of water from one compartment to another (see Figure 4-1).

**Edema** is a common sign of an abnormal movement of fluid from the vascular space into the interstitial space. Albumin, which is made in the liver, together with other soluble proteins and electrolytes, establish the osmolality needed to keep fluid within blood and lymphatic vessels. Abnormally low levels of these large solutes decrease the oncotic "pull" that holds fluid inside vessels. The fluid subsequently leaks out across the vessel wall and enters the delicate structures of extravascular tissues. If fluid leaks from vessels into the surrounding lung tissue, the condition is called **pulmonary edema.** If fluid leaks into skin, it is called **cutaneous edema**. **Pitting cutaneaous edema** is identified if an indentation remains in the skin after pressure, such as pushing with ones thumb, is removed.

---

 **CLINICAL APPLICATION**

### The Importance of Fluid Therapy

Fluid therapy is used to maintain hydration, to treat dehydration and to address ongoing fluid losses. It is also commonly used to maintain venous access during surgical procedures and in patients receiving intravenous medications. During emergencies, fluid therapy is used to increase oncotic pressure during hypovolemia and shock. It is used to improve urine production and output, and also to correct acid–base and electrolyte imbalances.

### Types of Fluid

There are two general types of fluid administered: cystalloids and colloids.

- Crystalloid fluids are composed of water that is rich in many different types of electrolytes. The solution can be either hypotonic (such as 5% dextrose in water, 0.45% sodium chloride, Normasol M, and Plasmalyte 56), or isotonic (such as Plasmalyte 148, Normasol R, and lactated Ringers solution). Because the solutes in crystalloids are small, allowing them to cross the vascular wall, crystalloids are particularly good for rehydrating extravascular spaces. They are also useful in correcting acid–base imbalances.
- Colloid fluids are solutions containing large, heavy molecules suspended in an isotonic crystalloid. Because the large solutes are too big to cross the vascular wall, they

remain in blood vessels and improve blood pressure by "holding" fluid in the intravascular space. Colloids may contain natural proteins such as albumin or synthetic molecules such as hetastarch. Therefore, they work well in patients with low plasma protein levels and in patients that are in cardiovascular shock.

## Administration of Fluids

Fluid therapy is administered in three phases:
1. Resuscitation.
2. Replacement.
3. Maintenance.

### Resuscitation

The goal of fluid therapy during resuscitation is to increase the volume of fluid in the intravascular space and to raise blood pressure quickly. Patients in hypovolemic shock have lost about 30% of their blood volume. Shock doses for the colloid hetastarch are 20 to 30 ml/kg in dogs and 10 to 15 ml/kg in cats. The shock doses of an isotonic crystalloid are 80 to 90 ml/kg for dogs and horses and 40 to 60 ml/kg for cats. Using a mixture of both a colloid and a crystalloid during resuscitation has the benefit of an expansion effect with reduced side effects and a reduction in the total fluid dose.

### Replacement

Replacement fluid therapy is administered to correct dehydration, replace fluid losses, and to provide for maintenance fluid requirements. Isotonic crystalloids are typically used during the replacement phase.

Replacement fluid = losses from dehydration + ongoing losses + maintenance fluid needs

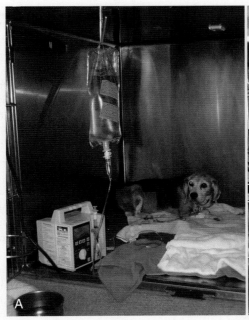
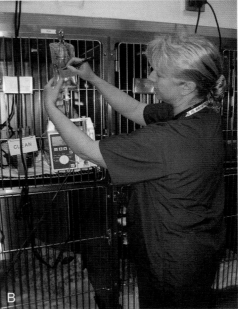

**A,** Intravenous (IV) fluids can be administered to patients using infusion pumps, such as the one shown above. The infusion pump ensures that the animal will not receive more than the desired amount and that fluid will be administered at a constant rate. An alarm mechanism in the pump alerts veterinary technicians of any interruption in the infusion. When the prescribed dose is administered, the pump automatically stops. **B,** Veterinary technicians often put additives, such as potassium chloride (KCl) and complex B vitamins, in IV fluids to help stabilize the patient. It is important that the fluid bag be carefully labelled, as shown, with the names and amounts of the additives.

*Continued*

## CLINICAL APPLICATION—cont'd

### Estimating Percent of Dehydration Based on Physical Examination in Dogs

| CLINICAL SIGNS | PERCENTAGE OF DEHYDRATION |
|---|---|
| No clinical signs of dehydration detected. Mentation is normal<br>Mucous membranes (MM) wet or moist, capillary refill time (CRT) <2 s<br>Skin turgor: strong snap <1 s return | <5% |
| Patient may be quiet.<br>MM tacky, CRT 2.5-3 s<br>Skin turgor: delayed slightly, 1-2 s return | 5%-7% |
| Patient is subdued and likely to be either sitting or recumbent<br>MM dry, tongue is tacky, CRT 3-4 s<br>Skin turgor: delayed return (3-4 s) | 8%-9% |
| Patient is depressed and recumbent, but conscious with rapid, weak pulses. Eyes are slightly shrunken and recessed in orbits<br>MM dry, tongue is dry, CRT 4-5 s<br>Skin turgor severely delayed: 5-8 s | 10%-12% |
| Animal is recumbent, unconscious and in cardiovascular shock with very rapid, thready pulses. Eyes are severely shrunken and recessed in orbits. Death is imminent<br>MM very dry and contracted, tongue is dry and contracted, CRT 5-8 s<br>Skin remains tented with no skin turgor | 12%-15% |

### Estimating Dehydration (see Table)

As animals become dehydrated, they manifest a set of clinical signs that worsen as the percentage of dehydration in the patient increases. Each patient demonstrates these signs differently. However, the chart below offers specific clinical guidelines for estimating the percentage of dehydration in dogs.

### Estimating Fluid Deficit from Dehydration

An estimate of the amount of fluid lost from dehydration (in liters) can be calculated by multiplying the percentage of dehydration by the weight of the animal in kilograms. For example:

$$\text{Body weight (kg)} \times \% \text{ Dehydration} = \text{Fluid deficit (L) from dehydration}$$

$$\text{Body weight (kg)} \times \% \text{ Dehydration} \times 1000 = \text{Fluid deficit (ml) from dehydration}$$

### Estimating Ongoing Fluid Losses

Sick animals lose fluid at a faster rate than healthy animals because of vomiting, blood loss, diarrhea, and elevated body temperature. Ongoing fluid losses can be quantified in hospitalized patients by collecting lost fluid. Urine, for example, can be collected in bags via urethral catheters and measured. Other body fluids can be collected from drains or in absorbable pads and subsequently weighed. The weight of the pad is subtracted to obtain the weight of the fluid alone. Assuming that a milliliter of lost fluid weighs one gram, an estimate of fluid loss can be calculated. For outpatients, getting a thorough history and knowing the frequency of incidents of vomition, urination, and diarrhea, as well as the volume of each incident, is helpful in estimating ongoing losses. However, this approach often underestimates the true fluid loss, so it is recommended that estimates be doubled to obtain a more accurate value. In general, replacement fluids should be administered over the same period of time as that in which they were lost. Fluids lost slowly, for example, should be replaced slowly and vice versa.

### Maintenance

Isotonic crystalloids are typically used at a maintenance fluid rate in patients that are not drinking but have no level of dehydration and no ongoing fluid losses.

### Estimating Maintenance Fluid Needs

Maintenance fluids are administered to replace the fluids lost from normal physiologic activities such as sweating, breathing, urination, and defecation. The hourly maintenance rate in ml/hour is calculated using the formulae $132 \times \text{body weight (kg)}^{(0.75)}$ for dogs and $80 \times \text{body weight (kg)}^{(0.75)}$ for cats. In horses, 40 to 60 ml/kg/day is used to calculate the daily maintenance rate in adult horses, and 90 ml/kg/day is used for young foals.

### Case Scenario

Leonard is a 2-year-old male castrated Yorkshire Terrier that has vomited six times in the past 36 hours. The owner says that Leonard has been sleeping more than usual and did not want to go for a walk as he normally does. After examining the patient, the veterinarian recommends that Leonard be hospitalized, given fluid therapy, and have further testing performed. The physical examination findings include the following information: Leonard weighs 10 lb (or 4.5 kg). His skin has lost some of its turgor and his gums are tacky. You

## CLINICAL APPLICATION—cont'd

estimate the percentage of dehydration to be about 8%. As you prepare to administer intravenous fluids, you make the following calculation:

1. Fluid losses from dehydration: $4.5 \text{ kg} \times 0.08 \times 1000 = 360$ ml.
2. Ongoing fluid losses from vomiting: $40 \text{ ml} \times 6 = 240 \text{ ml} \times 2 = 480$ ml.
3. Maintenance fluid needs: $132 \times (4.5\text{kg})^{(0.75)} = 408$ ml.

4. Total replacement fluids: $360 + 480 + 408 = 1248 \text{ ml} = 1.25$ L.
5. Hourly rate = 1248 ml/36 hours = 35 ml/hour.

After 36 hours, Leonard is rehydrated, and the rate per hour is decreased. Maintenance fluids and ongoing fluid losses are combined to estimate the lower rate.

$$408 \text{ ml} + 480 \text{ ml} = 888 \text{ ml/day} = 37 \text{ ml/hour}$$

## MEMBRANE PROCESSES: EXCRETION, SECRETION AND ABSORPTION

In addition to containing electrolytes, tissue fluids are loaded with fatty acids, vitamins, amino acids, regulatory hormones, and dissolved gases. For the cell to maintain homeostasis, it must select what it needs from the extracellular fluid and bring it into the intracellular environment. Similarly, it must excrete waste products or transport resources needed in other parts of the body to the extracellular compartment.

The function of the plasma membrane is complex, and therefore it may work differently at various times and locations on the cell surface (Table 4-1). For example, the absorption of nutrients or excretion of waste may occur with or without the expenditure of energy (adenosine triphosphate; ATP) from the cell. Absorptive or excretory processes that require energy are considered active, whereas those that do not require energy are passive. In addition, the cell membrane may be **impermeable** to some substances and freely **permeable** to others. Thus the cell membrane is generally considered to be **selectively permeable** because it allows some molecules to pass through, but not others. It is important to keep in mind that water ($H_2O$) is a small molecule and can pass freely though the lipid bilayer of the cell membrane.

## PASSIVE MEMBRANE PROCESSES
### DIFFUSION

Whether in liquid or in gas, molecules are constantly moving, gyrating, and, at times, bouncing into one another. This activity, called *kinetic energy*, can be increased in warmer temperatures and slowed in cooler ones. Concentrated molecules gyrate away from one another until they are evenly distributed within the space that confines them. The spectrum between the most concentrated region and the area that is least filled with molecules is called the **concentration gradient**. As the molecules move from an area of high

| TABLE 4-1 | Summary of Membrane Processes | | | |
|---|---|---|---|---|
| **TYPE OF PROCESS** | **DESCRIPTION** | **SUBSTANCES TRANSPORTED** | | **EXAMPLE** |
| | | **PASSIVE PROCESSES (DO NOT REQUIRE ATP)** | | |
| 1. Diffusion | Kinetic movement of molecules from higher to lower concentration | 1. Small molecules diffuse through membrane  2. Lipid-soluble gases pass through lipid bilayer  3. Charged ions move through specialized channel proteins | | 1. Water  2. Oxygen and carbon dioxide  3. Chloride and urea |
| 2. Facilitated diffusion | Selective carrier proteins assist in movement of molecules from higher to lower concentration; speed of diffusion is limited by saturation of carrier molecules | Some large molecules and non–lipid-soluble molecules | | Movement of glucose into muscle and fat cells |

*Continued*

| TABLE 4-1 | Summary of Membrane Processes—cont'd | | | |
|---|---|---|---|---|
| **TYPE OF PROCESS** | **DESCRIPTION** | **SUBSTANCES TRANSPORTED** | | **EXAMPLE** |
| **PASSIVE PROCESSES (DO NOT REQUIRE ATP)** | | | | |
| 3. Osmosis | Passive movement of water through a semipermeable membrane from dilute solution to more concentrated one | Water | | Water moves from stomach into bloodstream |
| 4. Filtration | Hydrostatic pressure (caused by the beating heart) forces liquid and small molecules through a membrane | Water and small molecular solutes but not large molecules such as protein; separates molecules by size | | Filtration of blood in kidney enables small solutes and liquid to pass through it but not blood cells, proteins, and other large molecules |
| **ACTIVE PROCESSES (USE ATP)** | | | | |
| 1. Active transport | Active movement of molecules by specific carrier protein; molecules may move against concentration gradient | Molecules too large to pass through channels or unable to penetrate lipid bilayer because of polarity; may be on wrong side of concentration gradient | | Ions such as $K^+$, $Na^+$, and $Ca^{2+}$ |
| 2. Endocytosis a. Phagocytosis | Cell engulfs solid substances | Microinvaders and foreign debris | | White blood cell or macrophage engulfs bacteria |
| b. Pinocytosis | Cell engulfs liquid substances | Water and other solutes | | Absorptive cells in small intestine take water into intracellular vesicles |
| c. Receptor mediated | Specialized protein receptors bind to ligands specific to receptors | Hormones, iron, and cholesterol | | Insulin, produced by pancreas, only binds to cells with insulin receptors |
| 3. Exocytosis | Excretion of waste products and secretion of manufactured substances; these substances are packaged in secretory vesicles, which fuse with cell membrane; contents are ejected to the extracellular space | Waste products, secretory proteins, hormones, and lipids | | Digestive enzymes produced in pancreas and released into ducts connected to small intestine |

Illustrations from Thibodeau GA, Patton KT: Anatomy & physiology, ed 5, St Louis, 2003, Mosby.

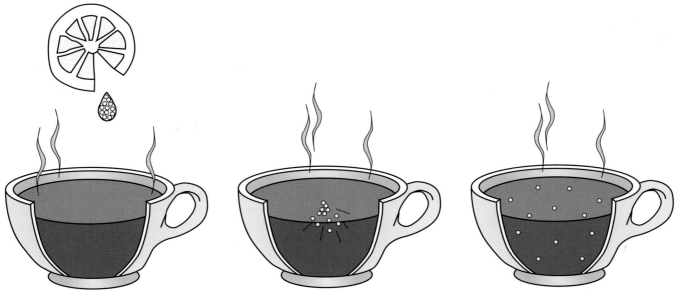

**FIGURE 4-4** Diffusion. Molecules in solution are active and collide into one another. The hotter the solution, the more active the collisions. With time, molecules become evenly distributed throughout the liquid, having moved from the highest concentration to the lowest. This process, called *diffusion*, occurs more rapidly in hot liquids than in cold ones.

concentration to a region of low concentration, they are said to be moving *down* the concentration gradient; therefore **diffusion** can be defined as the process of moving down the concentration gradient. Examples of diffusion are everywhere. When you place a drop of lemon in your tea, the drop slowly spreads out until it is uniformly mixed within the liquid (Figure 4-4). The rate of diffusion depends upon the temperature of the tea: it occurs faster in hot tea than in iced tea.

When a dog expresses its anal sacs in the waiting room of a veterinary office because it is nervous, it may not be noticeable at first to the people waiting on the other side of the room; however with time, diffusion of anal sac molecules released into the air will make everyone aware of a foul odor.

The plasma membrane forms an obstacle to the diffusion of some molecules into or out of the cell. Molecules such as water, oxygen, and carbon dioxide pass through the membrane easily, whereas others, such as sodium, may not. The following three principal factors determine whether a molecule may pass through the cell membrane by passive diffusion:

1. *Molecular size:* Very small molecules, such as water ($H_2O$), may pass through cellular membrane pores, which are approximately 0.8 μm in diameter; larger molecules, such as glucose, cannot pass through.
2. *Lipid solubility:* Lipid-soluble molecules, such as alcohol and steroids, and dissolved gases, such as oxygen ($O_2$) and carbon dioxide ($CO_2$), can pass through the lipid bilayer with ease, whereas other molecules may not.
3. *Molecular charge:* Ions are small in size, but their charge prevents easy passage through the membrane pores. Specialized pores called *channels* selectively allow certain ions to pass through, but not others. For example, chloride channels permit only chloride ions through, and urea channels permit only urea.

## FACILITATED DIFFUSION

Some large molecules and non–lipid-soluble molecules can pass through the cell membrane with the assistance of an integral protein or carrier protein that is located in the bilayer. The molecule outside the cell binds to a particular binding site on the carrier protein. This causes the carrier protein to change its shape in such a way that the molecule is able to pass through the membrane and enter the cell. Once exposed to the cytoplasm, the molecule is released intracellularly. This process is known as **facilitated diffusion** and requires no energy from the cell.

An example of facilitated diffusion in animals is the movement of glucose into the cell (Figure 4-5). Glucose is normally of a higher concentration outside the cell, but it is too large to fit through the tiny membrane pores and therefore cannot rely on **simple diffusion** to enter the cell. However, glucose is able to pass with the assistance of a carrier protein. Each carrier protein in the cell membrane is selective about the molecules that it transports. As the level of glucose in the bloodstream rises, more carrier molecules specific for glucose are employed. Eventually, if the blood sugar level becomes high enough, all of the carrier molecules become engaged and glucose is unable to enter the cell at a faster rate. Thus facilitated diffusion is different from ordinary diffusion in that the process is limited by the number of available **carrier proteins**. Increasing the amount of glucose given to an animal under these circumstances is not going to increase the rate at which glucose is taken into the cell. Hormones such as insulin, however, play an important role in controlling the activity of the glucose-specific carrier proteins and can act on them to speed up their rate of transport.

## OSMOSIS

**Osmosis** is the passive movement of water through a semipermeable membrane into a solution in which the water concentration is lower. In other words, when two solutions of different concentrations are separated by a semipermeable membrane, water molecules move from the dilute

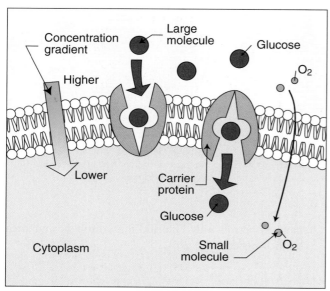

**FIGURE 4-5** Simple and facilitated diffusion. Large lipid-soluble molecules, such as glucose, are transported into the cell by binding to a transmembrane carrier protein. Small lipid-soluble molecules, on the other hand, can pass through the cell membrane via simple diffusion.

solution, across the membrane, to the concentrated solution (Figure 4-6). In osmosis, the movement of water occurs to achieve the same concentration of solution on both sides of a semipermeable membrane. This state is called a *concentration balance* or **equilibrium**. The greater the difference in solute concentration, the greater the osmotic flow. The force of water moving from one side of the membrane to the other is called the **osmotic pressure**. Note that osmosis occurs in the opposite direction to diffusion and that in osmosis the water, not the solute, is moving. In addition, osmosis requires a selective membrane, whereas diffusion does not.

Water can move rapidly into and out of cells through the pores in integral proteins, but large molecules and lipophobic substances cannot pass through. Normally the extracellular fluid has the same concentration of dissolved solutes as the intracellular fluid and is therefore called **isotonic**. In isotonic environments, the cell does not change size and water moves freely in and out of the cell. If the extracellular fluid is **hypotonic**, however, the inside of the cell is more concentrated than the outside. In this scenario, water flows into the cell and causes it to swell and possibly burst. If the extracellular fluid is **hypertonic** and more concentrated than the cytoplasm, water is excreted into the extracellular space, causing the cell to shrink and become shriveled (Figure 4-7).

Osmosis is an important aspect of passive membrane physiology. It illustrates the importance of the extracellular environment and the necessity for stable concentration gradients. In regions of the body where isotonic environments cannot always be maintained, such as the kidney, the body has developed protective mechanisms. The endothelial cells, for example, that line the ducts of the urinary system are coated with thick mucus to separate them from urine, which would

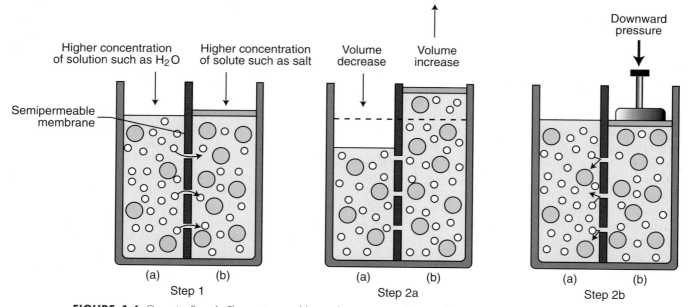

**FIGURE 4-6** Osmosis. Step 1: The semipermeable membrane prevents larger solute molecules on side *b* from passing into side *a*. However, smaller solution molecules can pass readily from side *a* to side *b*. Step 2a: As solution moves from side *a* to side *b*, the volume of side *b* increases until the concentration of solute is the same on both sides. Step 2b: Osmosis can be reversed via filtration when hydraulic pressure is added to side *b*. This forces solution back through the semipermeable membrane to side *a*.

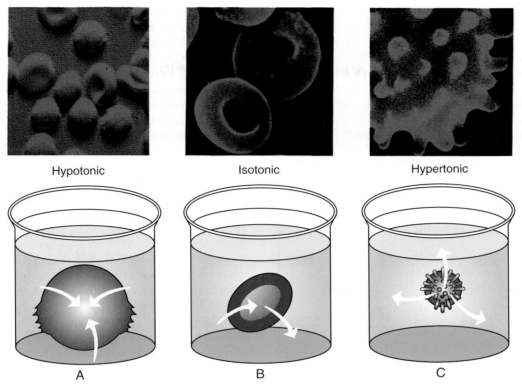

Hypotonic          Isotonic          Hypertonic

A          B          C

**FIGURE 4-7** Effects of osmosis on red blood cells. **A,** In hypotonic solutions, red blood cells swell and can burst as a result of movement of water into the cell. Notice, in the scanning electron micrograph, the spherical appearance of the normally biconcave cells. **B,** In isotonic solutions, cells maintain the same size and internal pressure because movement of water into the cell is equal to movement of water out of the cell. **C,** In hypertonic solutions, the cell loses fluid and deflates as water moves out of the cell by osmosis. Projections from the cytoskeleton become visible and look like spikes on the cell's surface. (Photomicrographs from Thibodeau GA, Patton KT: Anatomy & physiology, ed 8, St Louis, 2013, Mosby.)

otherwise be caustic to the cells. Urine can be hypertonic, isotonic, and hypotonic at various times. These large swings in concentration would be fatal to unprotected cells.

The difference between the osmotic pressure of blood and the osmotic pressure of interstitial fluid or lymph is called the **oncotic pressure**. This is an important force in maintaining fluid balance between the blood and lymph in vessels and the fluid in surrounding tissues. In some disorders the balance of fluid between these two spaces is disrupted, particularly if there is a decrease in the number of protein molecules in blood plasma. Starvation, liver failure, and intestinal disorders, for example, can cause the levels of plasma proteins to decrease. If the levels become low enough, fluid can move via osmosis across the vessel wall into surrounding tissue or into open body cavities. When fluid leaks into the tissue under the skin, it is called *subcutaneous edema*. When it leaks into the abdomen, it is called **ascites**.

## FILTRATION

Unlike the processes of diffusion and osmosis, which rely on concentration gradients to drive the activity of molecules, **filtration** is based on a *pressure gradient*. Liquids may be pushed through a membrane if the pressure on one side of the membrane is greater than that on the other side. The force that pushes a liquid is called **hydrostatic pressure**.

In animals, hydrostatic pressure is blood pressure and is generated by the pumping heart. Blood, as it circulates in the body, is forced through vessels and minute capillaries. Small molecules and cells may be pushed through, but large cells may not. One of the best examples of filtration in animals is evident in the kidney, where blood is filtered through specialized capillaries in the process of making urine.

## ACTIVE MEMBRANE PROCESSES

The movement of molecules and substances across the cell membrane is considered active when the cell is required to use energy. Some molecules are unable to enter the cell via the passive routes, perhaps because (1) they are not lipid soluble and therefore cannot penetrate the lipid bilayer, (2) they are too large to pass through a membrane pore, or (3) they are on the wrong side of the concentration gradient.

Regardless of the reason, these substances must rely on an active cellular process to enter the cell. Substances can be actively moved into or out of the cell by two processes: *active transport* and *cytosis*.

### ACTIVE TRANSPORT

Some amino acids and ions must enter and exit cells without the assistance of a concentration gradient. They cannot move through the plasma membrane passively and must rely on energy, in the form of ATP, to assist in their transport across the cell membrane. Like facilitated diffusion, the **active transport** of a substance relies on a carrier protein with a specific binding site, but unlike facilitated diffusion, it does not require a concentration gradient. All cells

demonstrate the active transport of electrolytes, specifically, sodium ($Na^+$), potassium ($K^+$), calcium ($Ca^{2+}$), and magnesium ($Mg^{2+}$). In addition, specialized cells can transport iodide ($I^-$), chloride ($Cl^-$), and iron ($Fe^{2+}$). Many active transport systems move more than one substance at a time. If all of the substances are moved in the same direction, the system is called a **symport system**. However, if some substances are moved in one direction and others moved in the opposite direction, the system is called an **antiport system**.

One of the best understood examples of active transport is the antiport sodium–potassium pump. $Na^+$ and $K^+$ are the most common cations in the cell, and active transport sites for them can be found speckled throughout the plasma membrane. Normally, the concentration of potassium in the cell is 10 to 20 times higher than it is outside the cell. Conversely, sodium is 10 to 20 times higher outside the cell than it is inside. Because of this concentration gradient, potassium tends to diffuse out of the cell and sodium diffuses in. To maintain appropriate levels of intracellular potassium and extracellular sodium, the cell must pump potassium in and move sodium out. Because diffusion is ongoing, the active transport system must work continuously. The rate of transport depends on the concentration of sodium ions in the cell.

When an ion is transported, it binds to a specific carrier protein in the cell membrane that triggers the release and use of cellular energy. This response, in turn, causes the orientation of the carrier protein to be altered, renders the ion lipid soluble, and allows the carrier protein to move the ion through the cell membrane. ATP is provided by cellular respiration and, with the assistance of the enzyme ATPase, is broken down on the inner surface of the cell membrane to release energy. The pump can cycle several times using one molecule of ATP, so that for every molecule of ATP, two $K^+$ ions are moved intracellularly and three $Na^+$ ions are moved extracellularly (Figure 4-8).

Differences in ionic concentrations are critical for maintaining proper fluid balance in all cells and tissue types. In

---

### ✓ TEST YOURSELF 4-1

1. List three fluid compartments in the body.
2. What is an electrolyte?
3. Give specific examples of both cations and anions.
4. Which electrolytes are normally more concentrated outside the cell and which ones are more concentrated inside the cell?
5. What is the relationship between solutes and osmolality?
6. Give specific examples of solutes in the body.
7. Why do changes in osmolality cause fluid to move from one compartment to another?
8. Give two examples of conditions that result from fluid shifts.
9. How do changes in the osmolality of body fluids affect an animal's desire to drink and its ability to concentrate or dilute urine?
10. What is diffusion? Is it an active or a passive membrane process?
11. What molecules are more likely to diffuse into a cell? What three principles are involved?
12. How is facilitated diffusion different from simple diffusion? What is the limiting factor in the rate of facilitated diffusion?
13. What effect does a hypotonic solution have on a cell? What passive membrane process causes this effect?
14. What is the relationship between hydrostatic pressure and filtration?
15. What is another name for hydrostatic pressure in the body?
16. What defines a passive membrane process?

---

## CLINICAL APPLICATION

### Dialysis

Dialysis is a type of diffusion used most commonly in animals with acute kidney failure, though animals with chronic renal failure may also be dialyzed as well *(A)*. Common causes of acute renal failure may include infections, such as leptospirosis in dogs, pyelonephritis in cats, or toxins from the consumption of nonsteroidal anti-inflammatory drugs and ethylene glycol. Hypovolemic shock, which causes profound hypotension, may also cause an acute renal crisis. Hemodialysis can be performed in some veterinary hospitals to remove toxic substances that accumulate with renal failure, such as urea, uric acid, and creatinine. At abnormally high levels, these uremic toxins make animals feel nauseated, so they stop eating, lose weight, and become lethargic. Clinically, nausea in dogs often causes them to lick their lips excessively and often causes cats to drool.

To remove these toxic substances, the animal's blood is circulated through a machine that includes a filtering

apparatus called a *dialyzer* or *artificial kidney (B and C)*. The dialyzer consists of a plastic cylinder filled with hundreds if not thousands of hollow, semipermeable filaments. Small molecules such as creatinine pass through the semipermeable membranes, but larger molecules, such as the protein albumin, cannot. Blood from the animal is pumped into the dialyzer (from the top, in this case) and flows within the thin fibers. A special electrolyte solution called *dialysate* is driven through the dialyzer filter in the opposite direction to the blood (from the bottom). This enables small solutes such as creatinine and blood urea nitrogen (BUN) to move out of the blood in the filaments and into the dialysate solution (i.e., to move from a higher concentration to a lower one).

Dialysis is an excellent example of the use of basic scientific principles to help resolve a clinical problem. This deductive ingenuity has saved countless animal and human lives.

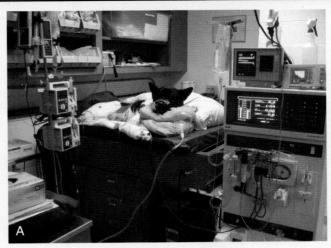

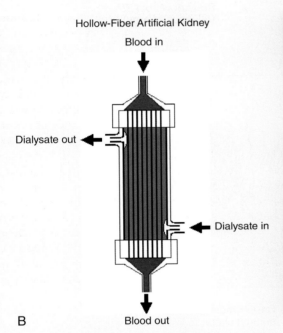

Hollow-Fiber Artificial Kidney

Blood in

Dialysate out

Dialysate in

Blood out

B

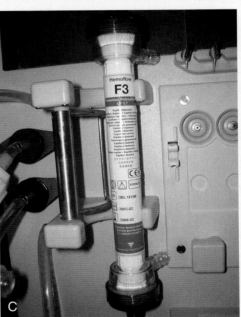

C

**A,** Maggie, a 2-year-old Akita, is undergoing dialysis to prepare her for a kidney transplant operation. **B,** Blood from the animal enters the dialyzer from the top and flows through thin, threadlike, hollow fibers within the cylinder. Dialysate solution, which surrounds the fibers, enters from the bottom and moves up the filaments in the opposite direction to the blood flow. The surface area and number of pores of each filament promote the movement of toxins from the blood into the dialysate. This cleansed blood exits the dialyzer at the bottom and is returned to the patient. The patient's blood is commonly circulated through the dialyzer several times before the desired blood values are achieved. **C,** Dialyzers come in different sizes to accommodate different blood volumes (differently sized animals). (**C,** Courtesy Joanna Bassert.)

addition, differences in ionic concentrations are of particular importance in the normal functioning of so-called *irritable cells*, such as myofibrils and neurons, where up to 40% of the energy produced from cellular respiration is used to fuel active transport.

## CYTOSIS

**Cytosis** is another mechanism for bringing nutrients into the cell and ejecting waste. Like active transport, cytosis requires ATP and is therefore considered an active process. The two types of cytosis are **endocytosis**, which means *going into the cell*, and **exocytosis**, which means *going out of the cell.*

***ENDOCYTOSIS.*** **Endocytosis** enables large particles, liquid substances, and even entire cells to be taken into a cell by engulfing them (Figure 4-9). In this case, the plasma membrane involutes, engulfs the particle or liquid, and

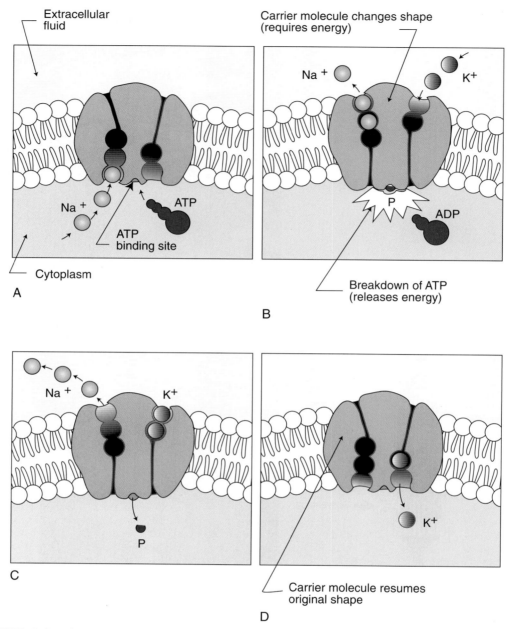

**FIGURE 4-8** Sodium–potassium pump (an antiport system). Sodium and potassium ions are transported in and out of cells against their concentration gradients; therefore the pump is called an *antiport system*. **A,** A carrier molecule located in the plasma membrane accommodates three sodium (Na⁺) ions. **B,** Energy in the form of adenosine triphosphate (ATP) binds to the carrier molecule and releases energy by breaking off one phosphate; adenosine diphosphate (ADP) remains. **C,** For each molecule of ATP, one carrier protein can transport three sodium ions and two potassium (K⁺) ions. **D,** The carrier protein returns to its original shape when transport of molecules is complete. It is once again prepared to accept Na⁺ ions.

forms a vesicle by closing the cell membrane around it. If the cell engulfs solid material, the process is called **phagocytosis,** which means *cell eating*. The vesicle formed from phagocytosis is called a **phagosome.** If the cell engulfs liquid, the process is called **pinocytosis,** which means *cell drinking*.

In mammals the macrophage, a giant cell found in many tissues throughout the body, is notorious for its ability to gobble up debris, dead cells, and outside invaders with ease. The phagosomes of macrophages often fuse with lysosomes,

which empty their digestive enzymes into the vesicles and digest their contents. The small molecules formed from this digestion can diffuse through the phagosome's membrane into the surrounding cytoplasm. Some white blood cells also can **phagocytize** material. They police tissues and keep them free of foreign invaders, such as bacteria and viruses. Many macrophages and white blood cells have very dynamic and motile cell membranes that allow them to move via **amoeboid motion.** Their steaming cytoplasm can branch out into

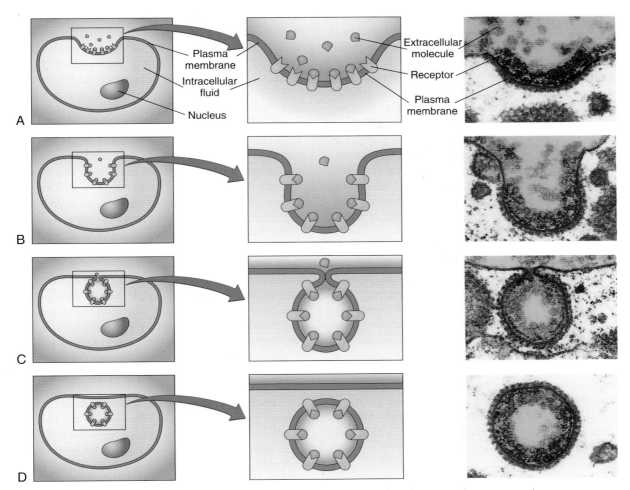

**FIGURE 4-9** Receptor-mediated endocytosis. An artist's interpretation *(left and center)* and transmission electron micrographs *(right)* show the basic steps of receptor-mediated endocytosis. **A,** Membrane receptors bind to specific molecules in the extracellular fluid. **B,** A portion of the plasma membrane is pulled inward by the cytoskeleton and forms a small pocket around the material to be moved into the cell. **C,** The edges of the pocket eventually fuse and form a vesicle. **D,** The vesicle is then pulled inward—away from the plasma membrane—by the cytoskeleton. In this example, only the receptor-bound molecules enter the cell. In some cases, some free molecules or even entire cells may also be trapped within the vesicle and transported inward. (Electron micrographs: Courtesy M.M. Perry and A.B. Gilbert, Edinburgh Research Center.)

armlike projections called **pseudopodia** or *false feet*, which enable these cells to move throughout tissue.

Unlike phagocytosis, pinocytosis involves only a minute infolding of the plasma membrane. Tiny droplets of liquid and the particles dissolved in them are taken into pinocytotic vesicles, which pinch off from the plasma membrane. Eventually the membrane surrounding the vesicle breaks down, and the liquid contents spill into the surrounding cytoplasm. Pinocytosis is particularly important in cells that have absorptive responsibilities, such as the cells lining the small intestine and the cells that line the renal tubules in kidneys.

Unlike the processes of phagocytosis and pinocytosis, which are primarily nonspecific ingestion processes, **receptor-mediated endocytosis** is very specific, occurring in cells that have specific proteins in their plasma membrane. These proteins act as specialized receptor sites for ligands such as hormones, iron, and cholesterol, which are found in

the extracellular fluid. Insulin, for example, is a ligand that, once secreted from the pancreas, will only bind to those cells in the body that display the specialized protein receptor for insulin.

When a ligand successfully binds to a cell, it is taken into the cell with a small amount of involuted cell membrane and forms a vesicle called a **coated pit**. Like other endocytotic vesicles, receptor-mediated coated pits fuse with lysosomes so that the ligands they contain can be broken down into smaller units and used by the cell.

***EXOCYTOSIS.*** Cells may export substances from the intracellular environment into the extracellular space by **exocytosis**. Exocytosis of waste products is called **excretion**, and the exocytosis of manufactured molecules is known as **secretion**. Substances to be exported are packaged in vesicles by the endoplasmic reticulum (ER) and Golgi body. The vesicles move through the cytoplasm to the cell surface, fuse with the plasma membrane, and release their contents into the extracellular fluid. A neuron, for example, stores packages of acetylcholine, a neurotransmitter, in the synaptic region of the axon. When the proper electrical stimulus is initiated, these packages are released into the extracellular space, where they quickly affect the postsynaptic neuron. Other examples of exocytosis are seen in the secretion of mucus by the endothelial cells lining the trachea and in the secretion of hormones by the adrenal and pituitary glands. One of the most dramatic examples of exocytosis, however, is evident during an allergic reaction, in which thousands of granules containing histamine are released from mast cells. (Some of us are all too aware of the clinical signs of histamine secretion during ragweed season.)

## RESTING MEMBRANE POTENTIAL

Charged particles (ions) exist within the intracellular and extracellular environments of all tissues. The amount, type, and distribution of these ions are important in maintaining cellular homeostasis. The plasma membrane, as you now know, is more permeable to some of these molecules than to others. This difference in permeability leads to changes in the distribution of the charged particles on either side of the cell membrane, which, in turn, forms a **membrane potential** or **voltage** (Figure 4-10). A *voltage* is potential electrical energy created by the separation of opposite charges. All cells possess and maintain a membrane potential, which can

range from −20 to −200 millivolts (mV), depending on the type of cell. The minus sign indicates that the cell is negative along the inner layer of the cell membrane relative to the outer cell surface. Cytoplasm and extracellular fluid generally have no net charge, although they are both rich in ions.

How does the cell control the distribution and flow of the ions that create the membrane potential? Although many ions are contained within the intracellular and extracellular fluids, the principal ions involved in maintaining membrane potential are $K^+$ and $Na^+$. As mentioned earlier, there are normally more potassium ions inside the cell than outside, and therefore potassium moves out of the cell via diffusion. Sodium, on the other hand, is more concentrated outside the cell than inside but, unlike potassium, it cannot enter the cell easily. The influx of sodium is lower than the outflow of potassium. In addition, for every cycle of active transport, three sodium molecules exit the cell for every two potassium molecules that are retrieved. Thus both active and passive membrane processes help to place more positively charged ions on the outside of the cell than on the inside. Cytoplasmic proteins, which are too large to leave the cell, tend to be negatively charged and further add to the voltage potential.

Cells are acutely aware of changes in the membrane potential. Changes in environmental tonicity, osmotic pressures, temperature, and contact with neighboring cells may alter **resting membrane potentials**, which, in turn, alter the flow of metabolites and the behavior of some structural and enzymatic proteins. Some specialized cells, such as muscle cells, owe their ability to contract to changes in membrane potential. Later chapters (Chapters 7, 8, and 13) further address the role of membrane potential in the normal functioning of cardiac muscle and neuronal tissue, respectively.

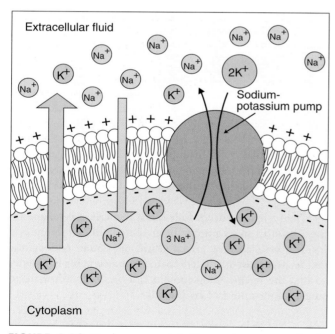

**FIGURE 4-10** Membrane potentials. The *membrane potential* is the voltage or electrical potential caused by the separation of oppositely charged particles. Typically, the outside of the cell is slightly more positive than the inside of the cell as a result of the sodium–potassium pump and because sodium ($Na^+$) diffuses into the cell more slowly than potassium ($K^+$) diffuses out.

---

✓ **TEST YOURSELF 4-2**

1. When is a membrane process considered *active*?
2. How do electrolytes enter the cell?
3. What is the difference between a symport and an antiport system?
4. Describe how sodium and potassium enter and exit the cell.
5. Describe the three types of endocytosis.
6. What is the difference between excretion and secretion? These are both examples of what?
7. What are the principal ions involved in maintaining a cell's resting membrane potential?
8. Is there normally a higher concentration of sodium inside or outside the cell? Where is there a higher concentration of potassium?

## LIFE CYCLE OF THE CELL

In multicellular animals, cells are divided into two broad categories based on the way in which they divide. **Reproductive cells**, which are found in ovaries and testicles and give rise to eggs and sperm, divide via a process known as **meiosis**. (Meiosis is discussed later, in Chapter 19, Reproduc-

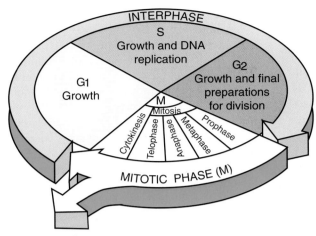

Another cell is formed

**FIGURE 4-11** Life cycle of somatic cells. During its life, the cell spends most of its time in interphase, which is an important time for metabolic activity and growth. Interphase is divided into three stages: growth one (G1), synthesis, and growth two (G2). The cell divides during the mitotic phase, which is relatively brief in most cells. The metabolic phase is composed of four stages: prophase, metaphase, anaphase, and telophase.

System.) Reproductive cells may also be referred to as "sex cells" or "germ cells." **Somatic cells**, on the other hand, constitute all of the cells in the body except the reproductive cells. These cells divide via **mitosis.**

## MITOSIS

An animal's ability to grow and repair tissue is based on the division of somatic cells. In mitosis a cell divides by separating into two roughly equal parts. The cytoplasm, organelles, and genetic material separate to form two daughter cells, each of which grows and performs countless biochemical reactions before becoming ready to divide again. The life cycle of the cell has been divided into two major periods: *interphase*, when the cell is growing, maturing, and differentiating, and the *mitotic phase*, when the cell is actively dividing (Figure 4-11).

## INTERPHASE

**Interphase** is the period between cell divisions. Early cytologists were not aware of the complex metabolic activities of the cell and therefore erroneously considered interphase to be the *resting* phase. However, the cell is carrying out its normal life-sustaining activities during this time and therefore it might be more accurately called the *metabolic* phase. During this time, the nucleus and nucleoli are visible, and the chromatin is arranged loosely throughout the nucleus. In addition, the centrioles can be seen in various stages of replication. Interphase has been divided into three subphases: *growth one, synthetic,* and *growth two*; and cell growth occurs throughout all of them.

The first part of interphase is called the **growth one (G1) phase.** This stage can last for variable periods, from a few

minutes in rapidly dividing cells to several weeks or even years in slowly dividing cells. The G1 phase is defined by intensive metabolic activity and cellular growth. During this time, the cell doubles in size and the number of organelles also doubles. In addition, centrioles begin to replicate in preparation for cell division.

The last two phases of interphase progress more rapidly. The **synthetic (S) phase** is marked by DNA replication. New histones are formed and are assembled into chromatin, forming new identical replicas of the genetic material. The **growth two (G2) phase** is very brief and includes the synthesis of enzymes and proteins necessary for cell division and continued growth of the cell. The centrioles complete their replication by the end of the G2 phase. Although interphase is divided into distinct stages, these phases flow as a smooth, continuous process.

> ✓ *TEST YOURSELF 4-3*
>
> 1. What are the two major periods that comprise the life cycle of the cell?
> 2. Is interphase a time when the cell is resting? Why or why not?
> 3. What are the four stages of the mitotic phase?
> 4. What happens in each of these stages?
> 5. Why is it important for chromatin to coil and form discrete chromosomes before cell division?
> 6. What three factors play a role in the control of cell division?
> 7. What is the genetic basis of cellular differentiation?

## DNA REPLICATION

The bodies of animals are composed of cells that are continually replicating to maintain body tissues, to heal wounds, or to enable growth. However, before each cell can divide, a perfect copy of the DNA must be created to pass on to the daughter cells. This replication occurs during the interphase period of the cell's life cycle. There is a great deal that is still unknown about how DNA replicates, but most scientists agree that the process includes the following steps (Figure 4-12):

1. In the nucleoplasm of a cell, chromosomes uncoil from their superhelical and helical formations to form loose strands of chromatin (DNA and histone proteins).
2. The portion of DNA to be copied unwraps and separates from the histone proteins.
3. A special protein, called a *helicase enzyme*, initiates the untwisting of the DNA helix and separates portions of the DNA into two nucleotide chains. Each region along the long strand where the DNA has separated is called a *replication bubble*. The spot at which the bubble begins and ends is called a *replication fork*.
4. Free DNA nucleotides, which are dissolved in the surrounding nucleoplasm, are attracted to the exposed complementary nucleotides. These molecules pair to one another in complements. Remember that the purines, adenine and guanine, always bond to the

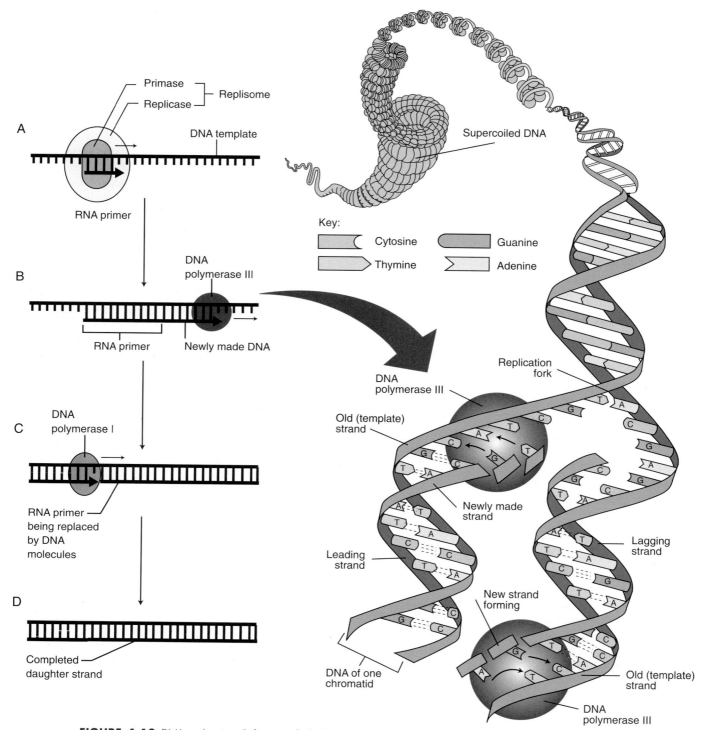

**FIGURE 4-12** DNA replication. Before a cell divides, it makes an identical copy of its genetic material. To do this, DNA uncoils and the hydrogen bonds between the base pairs are broken, causing the double helix to separate. **A,** A molecular "machine" called a *replisome* generates a short strand of RNA called the *RNA primer.* The RNA primer is the *start here* sign for DNA replication. **B,** The RNA primer signals DNA polymerase III to begin DNA synthesis by pairing free nucleotides with the exposed bases on the template strand. Note that there is an obligatory pattern of base pairing; for example, adenine (A) pairs with thymine (T), and cytosine (C) pairs with guanine (G). **C,** After the strands of DNA have been replicated, DNA polymerase I replaces the RNA primer with DNA nucleotides. **D,** In this way, an identical copy of the genetic material is created, which can be passed on to the daughter cell when the cell divides.

| TABLE 4-2 | Examples of Codons in the Genetic Code | |
|---|---|---|
| **AMINO ACID** | **DNA SEQUENCE** | **RNA SEQUENCE** |
| Alanine | CGT | GCA |
| Aspartic acid | CTA | GAU |
| Cysteine | ACA | UGU |
| Glutamine | GTT | CAA |
| Histidine | GTA | CAU |
| Isoleucine | TAG | AUC |
| Phenylalanine | AAA | UUU |
| Tryptophan | ACC | UGG |
| Valine | CAA | GUU |

A, Adenine; C, cytosine; G, guanine; T, thymine; U, uracil.

pyrimidines, thymine and cytosine, respectively (refer to Chapter 2 and to Table 4-2 for more details). Thus, the original DNA strand is a template for the formation of a complementary new strand. If the original strand reads "GATTAG," the complementary new strand will read "CTAATC."

5. DNA replication is carried out by a kind of molecular "machine" called a *replisome*. The replisome is composed of a collection of proteins including two types of enzymes called *primases* and *replicases*.

6. Interestingly, the replication process begins when the primases attach a short chain of RNA to the DNA template strand. These *RNA primers* are about 10 bases long.

7. Once the RNA primer is in place, DNA replication can begin in earnest. An enzyme called *DNA polymerase III* places complementary nucleotides along the template strand and covalently links them together. In this way, polymerase III is responsible for assembling the majority of the new nucleotide strand.

8. DNA polymerase III moves only in one direction, so the first strand, the *lead strand*, is made continuously while the second strand, the *lagging strand*, is made in segments and subsequently joined together by an enzyme called *DNA ligase*. When DNA polymerase III has finished building a new strand, *DNA polymerase I* moves in and replaces the RNA primer with DNA nucleotides.

9. Finishing touches are added. Telomeres, nucleoprotein caps, are placed on the ends of each DNA strand to protect the ends from damage. In addition, histone proteins are imported into the nucleus from the cytoplasm, and DNA is wrapped around them, forming chains of nucleosomes.

10. The identical DNA strands become chromatids, joined together at a central point called the **centromere**. Each chromatid is an exact replica of the other, each containing one strand of the original DNA molecule and one strand of the new complement.

## MITOTIC PHASE, CELL DIVISION

The mitotic (M) phase is the time when the cell is actively dividing. From a single cell, two daughter cells are produced,

each with the identical genetic material of the mother cell and each with the potential to divide and, once again, to pass on an identical copy of its DNA. Mitosis is separated into four stages—*prophase, metaphase, anaphase,* and *telophase*—and concludes with the division of the cytoplasm, which is called **cytokinesis** (Figure 4-13).

A clue that a cell is about to divide is evident in the nucleus. During prophase, the chromatin, which is normally invisible and spread thinly throughout the nucleoplasm, condenses, coils, supercoils and forms discrete X-shapes. The DNA and histone proteins within the X are so densely packed together that they become visible under a light microscope. It is as though the chromosomes magically emerge from the nucleoplasm to dominate the nucleus. The formation of duplicate chromosomes is essential for life and enables the cell to divide its genetic material equitably for a new generation, without tangling or breaking the long, delicate chains of genetic code. The X-shaped chromosomes are composed of two identical **chromatids** linked together at a constriction in their middle, known as the *centromere* or **kinetochore**. The cytoplasm becomes more viscous as microtubules from the cytoskeleton are disassembled and the cell becomes round. Two pairs of centrioles form anchors on which new microtubules are constructed, and as the microtubules lengthen, they push the centrioles farther and farther apart. In this way a mitotic spindle is formed that provides the structure and machinery necessary to separate the chromosomes. Because transcription and protein synthesis cannot occur while the DNA is tightly coiled, the appearance of chromosomes marks the cessation of normal synthetic processes. Prophase is thought to conclude with the disintegration of the nuclear envelope.

**Metaphase** is distinguished by the lining up of chromosomes in the exact center of the spindle, known as the equator. The chromosomes are evenly spread apart and form what is called the **metaphase plate** midway between the poles of the cell. The centromere of each chromosome is attached to a single spindle fiber.

In **anaphase**, the centromere of each chromosome splits in half and each single strand becomes its own, independent chromosome. As each spindle fiber shortens, the spindle as a whole separates, and the single-stranded chromosomes are pulled away from their mate toward opposite poles. During this time, each strand takes on a V-shape as they are dragged limply by their midpoint toward the centrioles at opposite ends of the cell. The cell elongates dramatically, changing the shape of the cell. The cytoplasm constricts along the plane of the metaphase plate as though forming a waist. Although anaphase is the shortest phase of mitosis and usually lasts only a few minutes, its importance is clear in light of the devastating consequences of any error during chromosomal separation. In anaphase the advantage of separating compact chromosomes, rather than long thin threads of delicate chromatin, is particularly obvious.

**Telophase** is the final stage of mitosis and is said to begin when chromosomal movement stops. The chromosomes, having reached the poles, begin to unravel, elongate, and

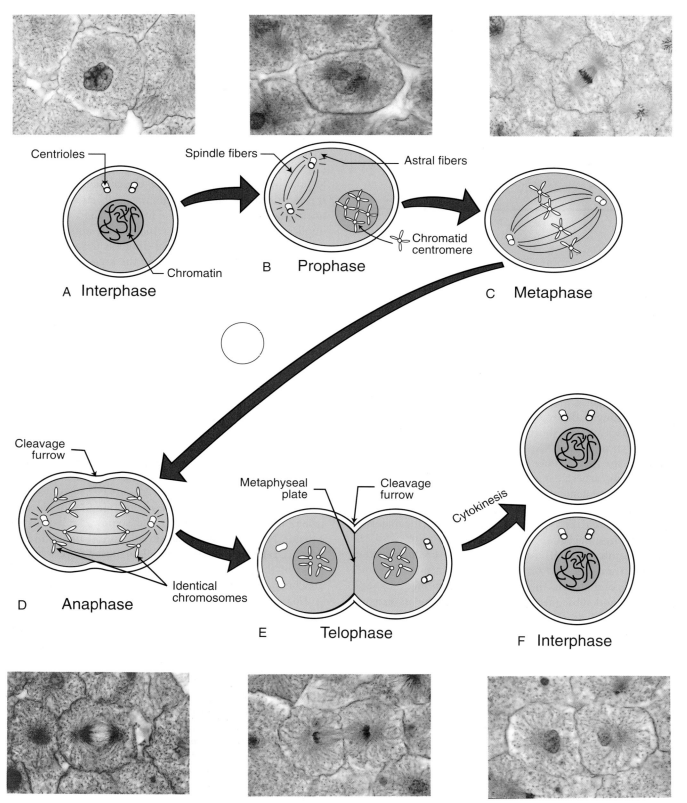

**FIGURE 4-13** Stages of mitosis. **A,** Interphase: Before a cell can divide, it must first make a copy of its DNA and another pair of centromeres. **B,** Prophase: Chromatin strands coil and condense to form chromosomes, which are linked at a central kinetochore. A spindle apparatus takes form while the nuclear envelope disintegrates. **C,** Metaphase: Chromosomes line up in the center of the spindle. The centromere of each chromosome is attached to a spindle fiber. **D,** Anaphase: Chromatids are pulled apart by spindle fibers to form a duplicate set of chromosomes. The cytoplasm constricts at the metaphyseal plate. **E,** Telophase: Chromatin begins to unravel at the poles of the cell, and a nuclear envelope appears. Cytokinesis marks the end of telophase. **F,** Interphase: The cycle of growth is repeated. (From Dennis Strete.)

return to the diffuse, threadlike form characteristic of *chromatin*. A nuclear envelope appears around each new set of chromosomes. RNA, protein, and ribosomal subunits combine into discrete regions within the new nucleus, reestablishing nucleoli. The microtubules that made up the spindle in the earlier phases of mitosis disassemble, and a ring of peripheral microfilaments begins to squeeze the cell into two parts. Ultimately, the cell pinches itself in half, dividing the cytoplasm and forming two completely separate daughter cells. Cytokinesis is the dramatic process of cytoplasmic division and marks the end of cell division. After cytokinesis, the daughter cells immediately enter interphase, and begin intense metabolic activity and growth so that ultimately they too can divide and produce daughter cells.

## CONTROL OF CELL DIVISION

Cell division is important in the growth of an animal, but once adult size is reached, cell division becomes primarily a function of tissue repair and cellular replacement. Some cells, such as skin cells, must divide continuously to replace outer layers that have sloughed off. Nerve cells and fat cells, however, do not divide readily and are held in check. Why do some cell types divide rapidly whereas others do not divide at all? The control of cell division is poorly understood, but some important observations have been made.

First, normal cells stop dividing when they come into contact with surrounding cells. This phenomenon is called **contact inhibition**. Second, growth-inhibiting substances are released from cells when their numbers reach a certain point. Third, a number of checkpoints are reached during cell division, when the cell reassesses the division process. These checkpoints occur during the G1 and G2 phases of interphase. For example, when the proper level of maturation promoting factor (MPF) is acquired at the end of the G2 phase, the cell is stimulated to begin the mitotic phase of the cell cycle. So far, there have been two proteins isolated that allow the cell to enter mitosis: **cyclins** and **cyclin-dependent kinases (CDKs)**. Cyclins are regulatory proteins whose levels increase and decrease throughout each cell life cycle. CDKs, on the other hand, are present at constant levels in the cell and are activated when they bind to cyclin proteins. When the CDKs are activated, they trigger a cascade of enzymatic activity, which enables cell division. When the mitotic phase is completed, the cyclins are destroyed.

## PROTEIN SYNTHESIS

Cell division and most metabolic activities are possible because of the intricate interactions of proteins and enzymes (specialized proteins). All cell function would come to an abrupt halt and life would end without continued protein synthesis. Protein synthesis begins in the nucleus, where the instructions for building proteins are contained within DNA.

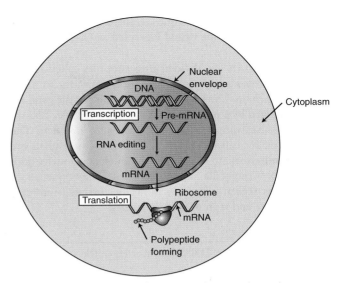

**FIGURE 4-14** Summary of protein synthesis. In the nucleus, a pre-mRNA molecule is made via transcription. Fine tuning and small adjustments are made to the pre-mRNA molecule to produce mRNA, which is exported from the nucleus into the cytoplasm. Ribosomes in the cytoplasm attach to the mRNA strand, and act like landing pads for circulating tRNA molecules with attached amino acids. Through the process of translation, polypeptide chains are assembled, which are further combined to make protein.

Although amino acids are assembled in the cytoplasm, DNA does not leave the nucleus. Instead, the valuable instructions for protein synthesis are transferred to a messenger molecule that carries the information out of the nucleus and into the cytoplasm.

The messenger is a special type of RNA called **messenger RNA (mRNA)**. The process of making mRNA is called **transcription**. Carrying the transcribed genetic code, the mRNA molecule leaves the nucleus and moves into the cytoplasm, where it connects with ribosomes. Another type of RNA, called **transfer RNA (tRNA)**, carries amino acids. Each molecule of tRNA carries one amino acid, which it brings to the ribosome and pairs with the complementary base on the mRNA molecule. The amino acids are linked together in the prescribed order to form chains of peptides and, subsequently, protein. The latter process, of making protein from mRNA templates, is called **translation** (Figure 4-14).

A single cell contains the information to make over 100,000 different types of protein. However, only a few hundred kinds of protein are actually made by any one cell. The type of proteins made is determined by the *function* of the cell. Note that *all* of the somatic cells in an animal contain the same genetic information, that is, the same DNA; however, a single cell cannot and does not make use of all of it.

The sequence of nitrogenous bases along the length of the DNA strand can be translated into the sequence of amino acids that make up a protein. Three nitrogenous bases represent one amino acid. This sequence is called the **genetic code**. The triplet CGT, for example, codes for the amino acid alanine, and the triplet GTA codes for the amino acid histidine. When the genetic code is transferred to the mRNA, these same amino acids would be coded as GCA and CAU, respectively.

DNA molecules are divided into subunits called **genes**. Each gene carries all of the information necessary to make one peptide chain. The beginning and ending of the gene are each delineated by a nucleotide triplet. For example, TAC on DNA codes for *start here,* and ATT codes for *stop here.* The start signals are called **promoters**, and the stop signals are called **terminators**. In this way, the sequence of nucleotides on the DNA molecule not only defines the sequence of amino acids within a protein molecule but also indicates where to start and stop protein synthesis.

## TRANSCRIPTION

As mentioned earlier, DNA does not leave the nucleus, but the genetic information it contains is copied onto a carrier molecule, mRNA, and transported out of the nucleus to the cytoplasm, where it is used to make protein. The formation of mRNA in the nucleus is called **transcription** (Figure 4-15).

The mRNA is assembled one nucleotide at a time. Normally, RNA nucleotides drift freely in the nucleoplasm, but during transcription a special enzyme called **RNA polymerase** binds to a DNA molecule and coordinates bonding between DNA nitrogenous bases and circulating RNA nucleotides. When RNA polymerase bonds to the DNA molecule, it initiates separation of the double helix and causes the nitrogenous bases of a particular gene to be exposed. Transcription begins at the promoter: the first segment of the gene.

As RNA polymerase moves along the exposed strand of DNA, a molecule of mRNA forms, as the enzyme systematically pairs each DNA nucleotide with its corresponding RNA nucleotide. For example, U is bonded to A, and C is bonded to G. So a DNA code that reads T, C, A, A, T, C, C, A is transcribed as A, G, U, U, A, G, G, U in the developing mRNA molecule. Each group of three RNA nucleotides, such as AGU, for example, is called a **codon**. Each codon represents a different amino acid; therefore the order of the codons will translate into the order of the amino acids in the protein (see Table 4-2).

When RNA polymerase reaches the terminator, the transcription is finished and the new strand of mRNA is complete. At this time, RNA polymerase detaches from the DNA molecule, and the two complementary strands of DNA reconnect to form a double helix once again.

DNA has noninformational or "nonsense" triplets called **introns** that separate informational triplets called **exons**. The first strand of mRNA that is manufactured from transcription therefore contains noninformational codons that must be removed from the mRNA molecule before it can be used for protein synthesis. Special RNA–protein complexes found in the nucleus form assembly lines called **spliceosomes** to remove the nonsense portions of the mRNA molecule. The complexes, called **small ribonucleoproteins**, cut out the introns and splice together the exons in the order in

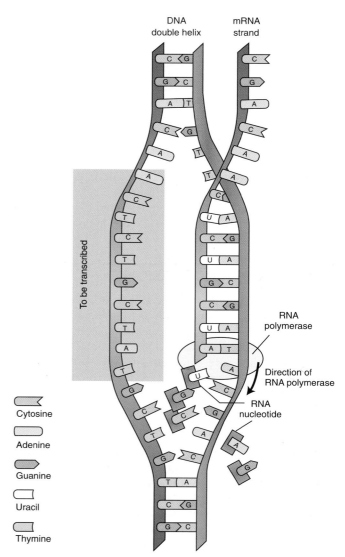

**FIGURE 4-15** Transcription (formation of RNA). In the nucleus, the enzyme RNA polymerase initiates separation of the double helix so that a single strand of DNA is exposed. It then coordinates pairing and bonding of circulating RNA nucleotides to corresponding DNA nucleotides. In this way, mRNA is assembled one nucleotide at a time. When transcription is complete, the two strands of DNA reunite and the newly formed mRNA molecule leaves the nucleus to convey its important genetic message to the cytoplasm.

which they occurred in the DNA gene (Figure 4-16). After this editing process is complete, the mRNA molecule leaves the nucleus and enters the cytoplasm by passing through a nuclear pore.

## TRANSLATION

The process of building a new protein using the information on the mRNA molecule is known as *translation* because information is translated from one language (nucleotides) into another (amino acids). After leaving the nucleus, mRNA enters the cytoplasm, where one or more ribosomes bond to the mRNA strand. The ribosomes act as "translation

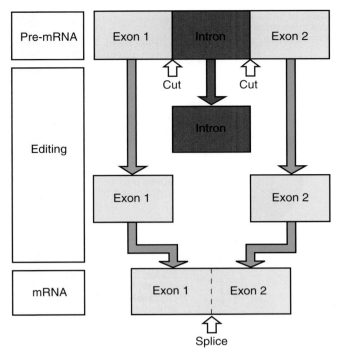

| Pre-mRNA | Exon 1 | Intron | Exon 2 |
| --- | --- | --- | --- |

**FIGURE 4-16** *Fine tuning after transcription. In the last stage of mRNA production, final "edits" in the genetic code are completed. Here an intron is cleaved from between two exons and discarded. Exons are subsequently bonded together.*

stations." Carrier molecules bring amino acids to the ribosome, where the amino acids are linked together to form a peptide chain using the sequence mapped out on the mRNA molecule (Figure 4-17). Several ribosomes can bond to one mRNA molecule at once, and translation can occur simultaneously at different sites along the strand to form multiple copies of the same polypeptides and protein (Figure 4-18).

Ribosomes are composed of protein and a second type of RNA called **ribosomal RNA (rRNA)**. The protein and rRNA molecules are interwoven to form two, unequally sized, globular units. Protein synthesis begins when the two ribosomal units interlock around the initial codon of an mRNA strand. The larger ribosomal unit contains an **active site** that serves as a docking site for the third type of RNA, transfer RNA (tRNA). The active site has room for only two tRNA molecules at a time.

The tRNA is a small, cloverleaf-shaped molecule and consists of approximately 80 nucleotides. There are at least 20 different kinds of tRNA in a cell, one for each type of amino acid. Each tRNA binds to a specific amino acid found in the cytoplasm and subsequently transports the amino acid to the active site of a ribosome bound to mRNA. At this time, a trio of nitrogenous bases on tRNA, called the **anticodon**, binds to the mRNA codon. Bonds between mRNA and tRNA molecules occur only if the nitrogenous bases in the codon and anticodon are complementary. In this way, transfer RNA provides the link between the forming protein and the mRNA molecule, because part of it binds to an amino

**Nucleus**
*Transcription*
1. RNA polymerase binds to a DNA molecule and initiates separation of the double helix. A specific section of DNA, called a *gene*, is exposed.
2. RNA polymerase moves along the DNA strand and coordinates the pairing of RNA nucleotides to corresponding DNA nucleotides. The RNA nucleotides are linked to one another to form a strand of mRNA.
3. When RNA polymerase reaches the end of the gene, the newly formed mRNA molecule is released and travels through the nuclear envelope to the cytoplasm.
4. The separated strands of DNA are reunited to form a double helix once again.

**Cytoplasm**
*Translation*
1. A ribosome binds to the beginning of the mRNA strand.
2. Transfer RNA molecules move into the vicinity of the ribosome. The tRNA anticodon is paired with the appropriate codon on the mRNA molecule.
3. The amino acid carried by the tRNA molecule is released and linked to the neighboring amino acid.
4. The ribosome continues to move along the mRNA molecule until all of the codons have been paired.
5. As the developing chain of amino acids lengthens, it coils and folds into the structure of a functional protein.
6. When translation is complete, the new protein is released and later modified. The mRNA, tRNA, and ribosome are free to repeat the process and form more of the same type of protein.

acid and another part binds to a particular codon on the mRNA.

After tRNA binds to the active site, enzymes on the ribosome break the link between the tRNA molecule and the amino acid it is carrying. A peptide bond is then created to link the amino acid to its new neighbor on the active site. The tRNA molecule, now free of its amino acid, disembarks from the active site on the ribosome and ventures into the cytoplasm, where it may collect another amino acid. Subsequently, the ribosome moves to the next codon on the mRNA strand and receives another amino acid-carrying tRNA molecule. A peptide chain is created from the successive additions of amino acids to a chain of increasing length. The order of the amino acids is determined by the sequence of nucleotides in the mRNA (Figure 4-19). (See Box 4-1 for a summary of protein synthesis.)

## GENETIC MUTATIONS

The body of a large dog is composed of trillions of cells, and each cell is derived from the division of the parent cell. The number of cell divisions made within the lifetime of a dog

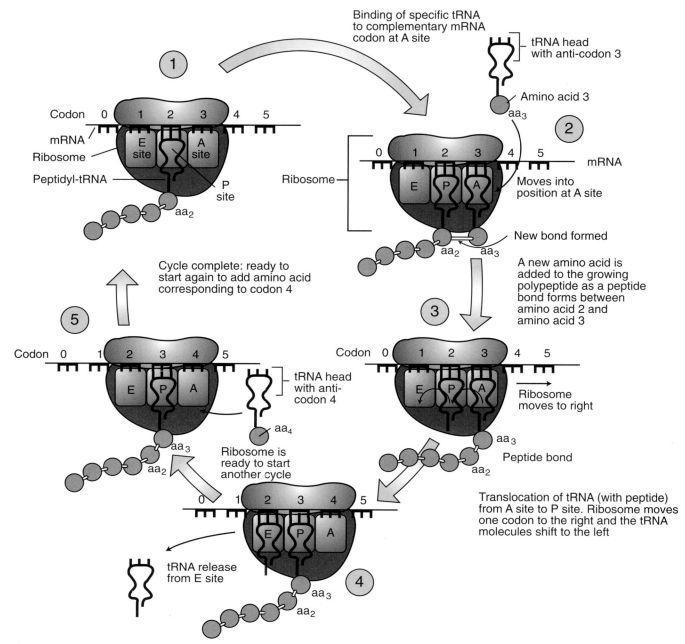

**FIGURE 4-17** Translation: Protein synthesis (up close). In the cytoplasm, ribosomal subunits attach to the mRNA strand and begin the process of translation. Transfer RNA (tRNA) molecules transport specific amino acids to the mRNA molecule as prescribed by codon sequence on the mRNA. A codon of mRNA is paired with the corresponding anticodon of tRNA. As tRNA molecules line up next to one another along the mRNA strand, they bring attached amino acids into close proximity to one another. This allows peptide bonds to form between the amino acids so that a long chain of amino acids (a polypeptide) is subsequently formed. Some proteins are composed of several polypeptide chains bonded together.

is, therefore, staggering. The process of DNA replication must not only be efficiently orchestrated, but it must be highly accurate as well. Given the enormous amount of information held within a single chromosome, it is not surprising that mistakes in the genetic code occasionally occur during the countless replications of DNA. These errors lead to alterations in chromosomes, and if the cell is able to survive such an error, it will be passed on to future generations of cells. A genetic error is called a **mutation**. Mutations

found in the mitochondrial DNA have been particularly helpful in genetically mapping the origins of species. It is the basis of some genetic testing in laboratories today.

Mutations can be caused by a wide variety of factors. Some of them seem to arise spontaneously, but others have been associated with some kinds of virus, ionizing radiation, and certain chemicals. These factors are called **mutagens**.

Mutagens can affect genetic material in several ways. For example, sections of DNA may be left out during the

## Translation
### (other view)

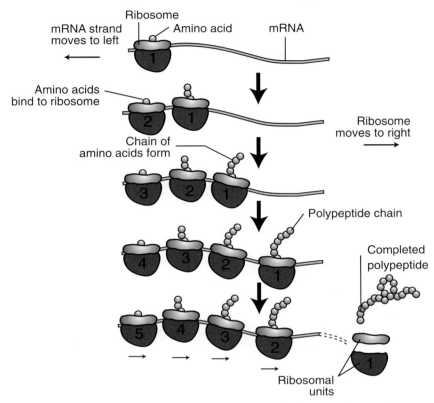

mRNA strand
moves to left

Ribosome
Amino acid

mRNA

Amino acids
bind to ribosome

Ribosome
moves to right

Chain of
amino acids form

Polypeptide chain

Completed
polypeptide

Ribosomal
units

**FIGURE 4-18** Polyribosomes. A polyribosome consists of a single strand of mRNA with many ribosomes attached to it. With electron microscopy, polyribosomes look like a string of pearls. This process allows hundreds of copies of the same polypeptide to be generated in a short period of time.

replication process, a gene may be spliced into the wrong position, or the wrong nucleotide may be paired to a nitrogenous base. Ionizing radiation, such as x-rays and ultraviolet light, is most likely to cause adjacent nucleotides to bond to one another or to cause a single strand of DNA to break apart. Chemical mutagens tend to cause bases to be left out, as well as causing the abnormal formation of linkages between strands. There are many ways in which an error can be made, but no matter how the mutation occurs, the consequence is the same: an alteration in genetic information.

Some mutations are so severe that the cell is not able to survive. For example, if the gene that codes for the production of RNA synthetase is left out of the DNA, the cell will die. But mutations can also have relatively little effect. For example, if a cell is unable to manufacture an enzyme that is relatively unimportant, the cell can continue to function normally. The mutations that cause the greatest harm are those that fall in between these two extremes. These mutations do not kill the cell or preclude cellular reproduction, but they affect the normal function of the cell in ways that

can be harmful. In time, the increasing numbers of mutant cells may cause structural and functional abnormalities in the tissues and organs they make up.

It is important to recognize that the effect of mutation is more severe in young animals than it is in adults. A mutation in a growing embryo, for example, will produce large numbers of abnormal cells that may occur in multiple tissue systems. In addition, a mutation that occurs in a fertilized egg would affect every cell in the animal's body and would, therefore, have the most extreme consequences. A mutant cell in an adult, on the other hand, is surrounded by normal cells and may go undetected.

Fortunately, cells are equipped with special repair enzymes that can detect certain kinds of errors in the newly forming DNA strands. These enzymes are able to detach defective nucleotides and replace them with the correct complement to those nucleotides on the opposite strand. Unfortunately, the repair enzymes are unlikely to correct errors in a mutation that involves both strands of the DNA at the same region. If the cell survives, this type of mutation is likely to be passed on to future generations of cells.

## Summary of transcription and translation

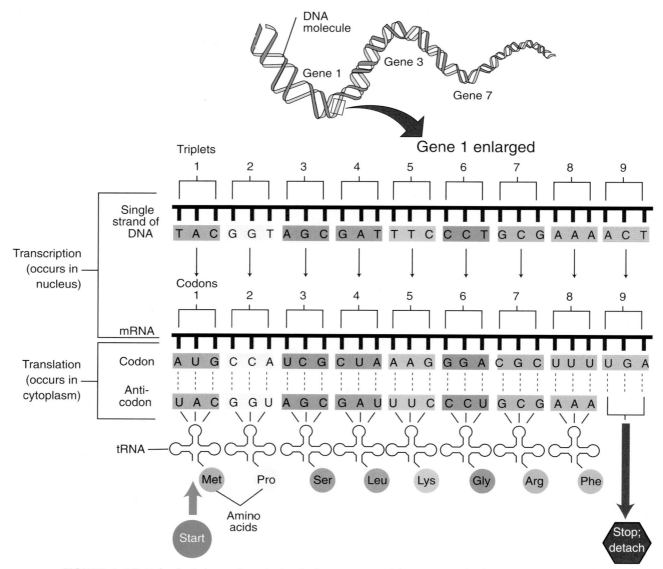

**FIGURE 4-19** Molecular "whisper down the lane": Communication of the genetic code. The genetic code is communicated as clusters of three (triplet) nucleotide bases. Each triplet represents a specific amino acid. In the nucleus, DNA triplets are transcribed into the language of mRNA (triplets called *codons*). The codons are subsequently translated into the language of tRNA. These triplets are called *anticodons*. The anticodon on each tRNA molecule indicates the type of amino acid that it carries. The order of the triplets, codons, and anticodons communicates the order in which the amino acids will be lined up in the polypeptide chain. This sequence is critical, because it determines the shape and activity of the protein.

## CELL DIFFERENTIATION AND DEVELOPMENT

The **development** of a complex, multicellular animal from a single fertilized egg is a miraculously choreographed event. It incorporates that which we understand biologically and that which is incomprehensible, for all living, breathing, thinking animals begin life as a single cell: the fertilized egg. The egg divides to form two cells, which in turn divide to form four cells, then eight, then sixteen, and so on. Each generation of new cells gives rise to greater specialization. Ultimately the cells assume the diverse shapes and functions of the various tissues and organs with which we are familiar: heart, lung, kidney, liver, and so on. But if all of the cells in an individual contain the same genetic material, how can they take on diverse forms, shapes, and functions if they are all given the same set of instructions?

The answer lies in the position of genes in chromosomes. Some genes may be located on a region of the chromosome that is available for transcription, whereas other genes may be located inside the molecule and cannot be reached by transcription molecules. We say that one gene is *turned on* while the other gene is *turned off*. Genes can be turned off permanently or temporarily. Chromosomes are dynamic in their ability to twist so that a gene that was once inaccessible on the inside can be moved to the outside of the molecule for use.

Some genes, like the ones that code for protein synthesis, are active in all cells; but the genes that govern the production of hormones and neurotransmitters are only turned on in some cells. The DNA that codes for the production of acetylcholine, for example, is turned off in a muscle cell because it is not needed; but the same gene in a nerve cell is turned on. Thus **differentiation** involves the temporary or permanent inhibition of genes that may be active in other cells.

Differentiation is important, because no one cell can contain all of the metabolic and structural machinery needed to perform the secretion, absorption, contraction, conduction, storage, and elimination processes that are required for homeostasis in the body. The genetic material therefore tells the cell what types of protein to make and, consequently, what functions to perform. The proteins may be enzymes or catalysts for specific metabolic reactions. Thus the types of proteins that a cell makes are key to its specialization.

The specialization of cells also leads to a morphologic or structural variation and influences the types and quantities of organelles contained within the various cell types. Some cells, such as striated muscle cells, are long and thin because the contractile proteins that they contain are long and thin. On the other hand, other cells, such as lymphocytes, are small and spherical, enabling them to pass through tiny blood vessels. In addition, cells such as macrophages, which are important phagocytic cells, are rich with lysosomes, whereas red blood cells contain no lysosomes, because they do not need them to perform their job of carrying blood gases.

---

### TEST YOURSELF 4-4

1. Of the thousands of different proteins that a cell could make, how many does it actually produce? Why?
2. Where does protein synthesis begin?
3. What is a nucleotide and how is it structured?
4. Compare and contrast the structures of DNA and RNA.
5. What are the nucleotides found in DNA? In RNA?
6. What is the term for mRNA formation?
7. What are codons and what role do they play in transcription?
8. Can you describe the events that occur in translation?
9. When in the cell cycle does DNA replication occur?

---

## CLINICAL APPLICATION

### Cancer

The word *cancer* is frightening to many of us. It is mysterious in its ability to affect some animals and people and not others. Sharks, for example, rarely develop cancer, whereas certain breeds of dogs, such as Boxers, are considered "tumor factories" by many veterinarians. Why is it that some of us have had or will have cancer, but others of us will not?

The causes of cancer are complex. Many factors influence the development of a normal cell and transform it into a killer. Environmental pollutants, certain food additives, radiation, some kinds of viruses, and certain chemicals have all been known to be carcinogenic (cancer causing). Also, certain genes have been linked to cancer in humans, and we see indications of this in animals as well. Rats, for example, carry a high risk of developing mammary carcinoma, and large dogs are far more likely to develop osteosarcoma, a tumor of bone, than small dogs.

Cancer develops when cells lose their normal control over cell division. Any cell can become cancerous and can divide unchecked in any tissue anywhere in the body. When cells proliferate excessively, they form abnormal masses called *neoplasms*, which are classified as either benign *(kind)* or malignant *(mal* meaning *bad)*. Benign neoplasms are well circumscribed and may be encapsulated. Because they do not spread to other parts of the body and tend to grow slowly, they are rarely of danger to the patient as long as they are not affecting vital organs. Some benign neoplasms, such as lipomas, are common in older animals and are often found in the subcutaneous fat layer.

Malignant neoplasms, on the other hand, are invasive, aggressive, and can spread to other parts of the body and form secondary tumors. Malignant cells are less sticky than normal cells and therefore tend to break away from the primary tumor. These cells are carried through blood and lymph to other parts of the body, where they may establish secondary tumors. This process is called *metastasis,* and the secondary tumors are called *metastatic masses.* In animals, primary lung cancer is extremely rare because animals do not smoke, which is the leading cause of lung cancer in humans. Thus, when an animal is found to have lung cancer, every effort is made to find another tumor—the primary tumor—somewhere else in the body. Malignant cells form disorganized clumps, rather than the neatly arranged rows of cells seen in normal tissue. Because they have lost their sense of contact inhibition, malignant cells invade the surrounding normal tissue by "walking over" the normal cells. In contrast, benign cancer cells tend to push the normal cells away. The invasive nature and ability to metastasize make complete surgical removal of malignant cancer difficult. Cancer cells also tend to be immature in nature and tend to be larger and less differentiated than their normal adult counterparts.

So how do the carcinogenic chemicals, viruses, and genes actually cause cancer? The answer is deceptively simple: they cause mutations in the DNA which alter the expression of certain genes. Genes that were permanently turned off may be

*Continued*

turned on, and genes that should be turned on may be turned off. The cell is unable to perform normally because the programming has been altered. A *proto-oncogene* is a gene with fragile parts that are easily broken off or damaged by carcinogens. When the gene is damaged, it becomes known as an

*oncogene* and provides incorrect instructions to the cell. Not all cancers are attributed to the formation of oncogenes, but their discovery has offered greater insight into the important relationship between carcinogens and genetics in the development of cancer.

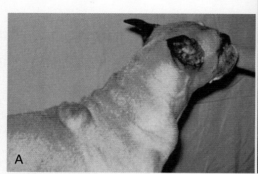
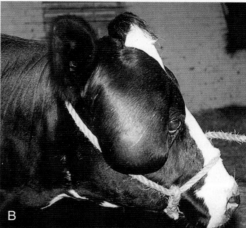

**A,** This dog has a mast cell tumor and multiple subcutaneous nodules on the withers. **B,** Holstein cow with large fibrosarcoma mass on the face. (**A,** from Scott DW, Miller WT Jr, Griffin CE: Muller and Kirk's small animal dermatology, ed 6, St Louis, 2001, Saunders; **B,** from Melling M, Alder M: Bovine practice, ed 2, St Louis, 1998, Saunders.)

## Chemotherapeutic Drugs

Many drugs are currently used to fight cancer in animals. These drugs are called *chemotherapeutic* drugs, and they work by blocking cell division and protein synthesis. With such treatments the cancerous cell cannot repair itself or divide, and it subsequently dies without leaving behind daughter cells. Chemotherapeutic drugs may be either specific for a certain phase of cell division or nonspecific, affecting all phases of cell division. These drugs are particularly effective against rapidly dividing cells, such as tumor cells, but may affect rapidly dividing normal cells as well. For example, cells that line the intestinal tract, young blood cells that form in bone marrow, and the active cells in hair follicles are all normal cells that are often affected by chemotherapeutic drugs. Therefore it is not surprising that some of the side effects of chemotherapy include nausea, diarrhea, hair loss, and decreased production of blood cells. Unfortunately, some tumors that do not grow quickly are not as affected by chemotherapeutic agents. In these cases, chemotherapy may need to be extended for long periods, or the veterinarian may consider using other forms of cancer treatment, such as surgery and radiation therapy.

Some chemotherapeutic drugs are extremely toxic to the tissues that lie outside of blood vessels, so technicians must be very careful when administering the drugs intravenously. Placing a catheter in the vein is a good way to ensure that the chemotherapeutic agent is administered properly. Extravascular administration of vincristine, for example, will cause

necrosis (tissue death) and sloughing of the perivascular tissue. Any attempt to irrigate the tissue or dilute the drug by injecting saline only spreads the drug, increasing the amount of tissue that will subsequently die.

There are six major classes of chemotherapeutic drug: alkylating agents, antimetabolites, plant alkaloids, antibiotics, hormonal agents, and miscellaneous agents.

### How Do They Work?

Alkylating agents such as cyclophosphamide (Cytoxan), cisplatin (Platinol), carboplatin (Paraplatin), chlorambucil (Leukeran), and melphalan (Alkeran) stop cell division by causing strands of DNA to cross-link and, in doing so, they inhibit DNA replication because a cell cannot divide or make proteins if the DNA is abnormally linked together. Without the necessary proteins and enzymes required for metabolic function, the cell quickly dies. The antibiotic doxorubicin (Adriamycin) works in a similar manner, as it binds DNA and inhibits mitotic activity.

Antimetabolites such as cytosine arabinoside, 5-fluorouracil, and methotrexate are analogs of the DNA bases purine and pyrimidine. Antimetabolites are incorporated into the DNA molecule during DNA replication and subsequently inhibit protein and enzyme synthesis.

Plant alkaloids, such as vincristine, are phase specific and affect only the M phase of the cell cycle by inhibiting mitosis. Plant alkaloids bind to the proteins in microtubules and interrupt the formation of the mitotic spindle. Without a spindle, the chromosomes cannot be separated properly, cell division is halted, and the cell subsequently dies.

In high doses, corticosteroids, such as prednisone and prednisolone, interfere with the cell division of lymphocytes. This lympholytic activity makes them particularly useful in treating lymphoid cancers such as lymphoma. They have an added benefit of increasing appetite and therefore are often used in conjunction with other chemotherapeutic agents.

The best known miscellaneous agent in veterinary use is asparaginase, which, as its name implies, is an enzyme that breaks down asparagine, an amino acid used by cancer cells. It has no effect on normal cells and usually is used in combination with other chemotherapeutic drugs.

### Example

A chemotherapeutic treatment protocol for a cat with lymphosarcoma might include vincristine, prednisone, and Cytoxan. Can you explain why each of these drugs is used?

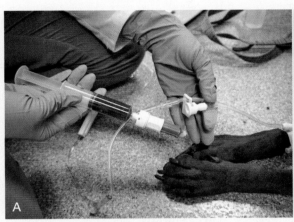
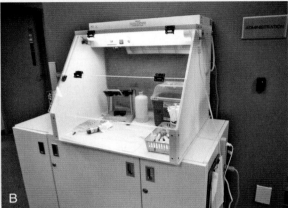

**A,** Be careful when administering chemotherapy. Use universal precautions such as wearing a cap, mask, gloves, and protective clothing when working with chemotherapeutic agents. A needle-less system is also helpful to ensure that chemotherapeutic agents are not inadvertently injected into a veterinary technician. **B,** An oncology hood is used by veterinary technicians to draw up chemotherapeutic products safely. (From Bassert JM, Thomas JA: McCurnin's clinical textbook for veterinary technicians, ed 8, St Louis, 2014, Elsevier.)

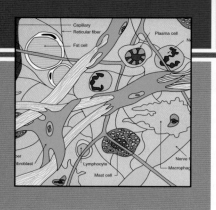

# Tissues: Living Communities $\boxed{5}$

*Joanna M. Bassert*

## OUTLINE

## LEARNING OBJECTIVES

*When you have completed this chapter you will be able to:*
1. List the four major tissue types.
2. Describe the functions of epithelial tissues.
3. Differentiate among the three major types of cellular junction found between epithelial cells.
4. Describe the structure of the basement membrane.
5. List and describe the characteristics used to classify different epithelial tissues.
6. List and describe the characteristics used to classify different glands.
7. List and describe the components of connective tissues.
8. Differentiate between areolar, adipose, and reticular connective tissues.
9. Differentiate between dense regular, dense irregular, and elastic connective tissues.
10. Differentiate between hyaline cartilage, elastic cartilage, and fibrocartilage.
11. List and describe the components of bone.
12. Describe each of the three types of muscle.
13. List the components of the neuron.
14. List and describe each of the phases of healing.

## VOCABULARY FUNDAMENTALS

*Absorptive cell*  ahb-**sohrp**-tihv sehl
*Acinar gland*  **ah**-sihn-ahr glahnd
*Adipose*  **ahd**-ih-pōs
*Adipose cell*  **ahd**-ih-pōs sehl
*Alveolar gland*  ahl-**vē**-ō-lahr glahnd
*Amorphous*  ah-**mohr**-fuhs
*Apical surface*  ā-pihck-ahl **suhr**-fihs
*Apocrine gland*  **ahp**-ō-krihn glahnd

*Areolar connective tissue*  ah-**rē**-ō-lahr kuh-**nehck**-tihv
   **tihsh**-yoo
*Articular cartilage*  ahr-**tihck**-yuh-lər **kahr**-tih-lihj
*Ascites*  ah-**sī**-tēz
*Avascular*  ā-**vahsk**-yoo-lahr
*Axon*  **ahck**-sohn
*Basal surface*  bās-sahl **suhr**-fihs
*Basement membrane*  bās-mehnt **mehm**-brān

*Blast* blahst

*Blood* bluhd

*Bone* bōn

*Broad ligament* brawd **lihg**-ah-mehnt

*Brown adipose tissue* broun **ahd**-ih-pōs **tihsh**-yoo

*Brush border* bruhsh **bohr**-dər

*Calcified* **kahl**-sih-fīd

*Canaliculi* kahn-ahl-**ihck**-ū-lī

*Cardiac muscle* **kahr**-dē-ahck **muhs**-uhl

*Cartilage* **kahr**-tih-lihj

*Chondroblast* **kohn**-drō-blahst

*Chondrocyte* **kohn**-drō-sīt

*Chondroitin sulfate* kohn-**droy**-tihn **suhl**-fāt

*Chondronectin* kohn-drō-**nehck**-tihn

*Cilia* **sihl**-ē-ah

*Collagenous fiber* kohl-**lahj**-ehn-uhs **fī**-bər

*Compound gland* **kohm**-pohwnd glahnd

*Connective tissue* kuh-**nehck**-tihv **tihsh**-yoo

*Connective tissue proper* kuh-**nehck**-tihv **tihsh**-yoo **praw**-pər

*Connexon* keh-**nehck**-sohn

*Cuboidal cell* **kyoo**-boy-dahl sehl

*Cuboidal epithelium* **kyoo**-boy-dahl ehp-ih-**thē**-lē-uhm

*Cutaneous membrane* kyoo-**tā**-nē-uhs **mehm**-brān

*Cyte* sīt

*Dendrite* **dehn**-drīt

*Dense fibrous connective tissue* dehnz **fī**-bruhs kuh-**nehck**-tihv **tihsh**-yoo

*Dense irregular connective tissue* dehnz ihr-**rehg**-ū-lər kuh-**nehck**-tihv **tihsh**-yoo

*Dense regular connective tissue* dehnz **rehg**-ū-lər kuh-**nehck**-tihv **tihsh**-yoo

*Dermis* **dər**-mihs

*Desmosome* **dehz**-mō-sōm

*Diapedesis* dī-ah-peh-**dē**-sihs

*Duct* duhckt

*Edema* eh-**dē**-mah

*Effusion* ē-**fū**-shuhn

*Elastic cartilage* eh-**lahs**-tihck **kahr**-tih-lihj

*Elastic connective tissue* eh-**lahs**-tihck kuh-**nehck**-tihv **tihsh**-yoo

*Elastic fiber* eh-**lahs**-tihck **fī**-bər

*Endocrine gland* **ehn**-dō-krihn glahnd

*Endocrine system* **ehn**-dō-krihn **sihs**-tehm

*Endothelium* ehn-dō-**thē**-lē-uhm

*Epidermis* ehp-ih-**dər**-mihs

*Epithelial tissue* ehp-ih-**thē**-lē-ahl **tihsh**-yoo

*Epithelialization* ehp-ih-**thē**-lē-ahl-ih-zā-shuhn

*Erythrocyte* ē-**rihth**-rō-sīt

*Excretion* ehck-**skrē**-shuhn

*Excretory duct* ehck-skreh-tohr-ē duhckt

*Exocrine gland* **ehcks**-ō-krihn glahnd

*Extracellular fiber* ehcks-trah-**sehl**-ū-lahr **fī**-bər

*Extracellular matrix* ehcks-trah-**sehl**-ū-lahr **mā**-trihks

*Exudate* **ehcks**-ū-dāt

*Fascia* **fahsh**-ē-ah

*Fibrin* **fī**-brihn

*Fibrinogen* fī-**brihn**-ō-jehn

*Fibroblast* fī-brō-blahst

*Fibrocartilage* fī-brō-**kahr**-tih-lihj

*Fibrous adhesion* fī-bruhs ahd-**hē**-shuhn

*First-intention healing* fihrst ihn-**tehn**-shuhn **hē**-lihng

*Fixed cell* fihkst sehl

*Gap junction* gahp **juhngk**-shuhn

*Glandular epithelium* **glahnd**-ū-lahr ehp-ih-**thē**-lē-uhm

*Glycosaminoglycan* glī-kōs-ah-mē-nō-**glī**-kahn

*Goblet cell* **gohb**-leht sehl

*Granulation tissue* grahn-ū-lā-shuhn **tihsh**-yoo

*Gristle* **grihs**-ehl

*Ground substance* ground **suhb**-stuhnz

*Haversian canal* hah-**vər**-zhehn kuh-**nahl**

*Hemidesmosome* hehm-ē-**dehs**-mō-sōm

*Hemorrhaging* **hehm**-ohr-rihdj-ihng

*Hemothorax* hēm-ō-**thorh**-ahx

*Heparin* **hehp**-ahr-ihn

*Hibernate* **hī**-bər-nāt

*Hibernating gland* hī-bər-**nāt**-ihng glahnd

*Histamine* **hihs**-tah-mēn

*Histiocyte* **hihs**-tē-ō-sīt

*Histology* hihs-**tohl**-ō-jē

*Holocrine gland* **hō**-leh-krihn glahnd

*Homogeneous* hō-mō-**jē**-nē-uhs

*Hormone* **hohr**-mōn

*Hyaline cartilage* **hī**-ahl-ihn **kahr**-tih-lihj

*Hyaluronic acid* hī-ah-lū-**rohn**-ihck **ah**-sihd

*Hyaluronidase* hī-ah-lū-**rohn**-ih-dāz

*Immunoglobulin* ihm-ū-nō-**gloh**-bū-lihn

*Infection* ihn-**fehck**-shuhn

*Inflammatory process* ihn-**flahm**-ah-tohr-ē **proh**-sehs

*Innervated* ihn-**nər**-vāt-ehd

*Integument* ihn-**tehg**-gū-mehnt

*Intermediate filament* ihn-tər-mē-dē-eht **fihl**-ah-mehnt

*Junctional complex* **juhnck**-shuhn-ahl **kohm**-plehkx

*Keratin* **keər**-ah-tehn

*Keratinized stratified squamous epithelium* **keər**-ah-teh-nīzd **straht**-eh-fīd **skwey**-muhs ehp-ih-**thē**-lē-uhm

*Kupffer cell* **koopf**-fər sehl

*Lacunae* lah-**kyoo**-nē

*Lamina propria* **lahm**-ihn-ah **prō**-prē-ah

*Leukocyte* **loo**-kō-sīt

*Loose connective tissue* loos kuh-**nehck**-tihv **tihsh**-yoo

*Lumen* **loo**-mehn

*Macrophage* **mah**-krō-fāj

*Mast cell* mahst sehl

*Merocrine gland* **mər**-ō-krihn glahnd

*Mesoderm* **mē**-sō-dərm

*Mesothelium* mē-sō-**thē**-lē-uhm

*Microanatomy* **mī**-krō-ah-**naht**-ah-mē

*Microbe* **mī**-krōb
*Microglial cell* mī-krō-**glē**-ahl sehl
*Microvilli* mī-krō-**vihl**-lī
*Mixed exocrine gland* mihckst **ehcks**-ō-krihn glahnd
*Mucin* **myoo**-sihn
*Mucosae* myoo-**kō**-sē
*Mucous membrane* **myoo**-kuhs **mehm**-brān
*Mucous secretion* **myoo**-kuhs seh-**krē**-shuhn
*Muscle tissue* **muhs**-uhl **tihsh**-yoo
*Myoepithelial cell* **mī**-ō-ehp-ih-**thē**-lē-ahl sehl
*Nephrosis* nehf-**rō**-sihs
*Nervous tissue* **nər**-vuhs **tihsh**-yoo
*Neuroglial cell* nər-**ohg**-lē-ahl sehl
*Neuron* **nər**-ohn
*Nonstriated involuntary muscle* nohn-**strī**-ā-tehd
    ihn-**vohl**-uhn-teər-ē **muhs**-uhl
*Omentum* ō-**mehn**-tuhm
*Osteoblast* **ohs**-tē-ō-**blahst**
*Osteoclast* **ohs**-tē-ō-**klahst**
*Oviduct* **ō**-vih-duhckt
*Paralyzed* **peər**-ahl-īzd
*Paramecium* peər-ah-**mē**-cē-uhm
*Paretic* pah-**reht**-ihck
*Parietal layer* pah-**rī**-eh-tahl **lā**-ər
*Pathogen* **pahth**-ō-jehn
*Pericardial fluid* peər-ih-**kahr**-dē-ahl **floo**-ihd
*Perichondrium* peər-ih-**kohn**-drē-uhm
*Perikaryon* peər-ih-**keər**-ē-ohn
*Peristalsis* peər-eh-**stahl**-sihs
*Peritoneal fluid* peər-ih-tō-**nē**-ahl **floo**-ihd
*Peritonitis* peər-ih-tehn-**ī**-tihs
*Phagocytize* **fāhg**-ō-sih-**tīz**
*Pitting edema* **piht**-tihng eh-**dē**-mah
*Plaque* plahck
*Plasma* **plahz**-mah
*Platelet* **plāt**-leht
*Pleural fluid* **ploor**-ahl **floo**-ihd
*Polar* **pō**-lahr
*Proteoglycan* **prō**-tē-ō-**glī**-kahn
*Proud flesh* proud flehsh
*Pseudostratified columnar epithelium* **soo**-dō-**straht**-eh-fīd
    koh-**luhm**-nahr ehp-ih-**thē**-lē-uhm
*Reproductive system* rē-prō-**duhck**-tihv
    **sihs**-tehm
*Reticular cell* reh-**tihck**-ū-lahr sehl
*Reticular connective tissue* reh-**tihck**-ū-lahr kuh-**nehck**-tihv
    **tihsh**-yoo
*Reticular fiber* reh-**tihck**-ū-lahr **fī**-bər
*Sebaceous gland* seh-**bā**-shuhs glahnd

*Second-intention healing* **sehk**-uhnd ihn-**tehn**-shuhn
    **hē**-lihng
*Secretion* seh-**krē**-shuhn
*Secretory unit* **sē**-kreh-tohr-ē **ū**-niht
*Serosae* seh-**rō**-sē
*Serous membrane* **seer**-uhs **mehm**-brān
*Serous secretion* **seer**-uhs seh-**krē**-shuhn
*Simple ciliated columnar epithelium* **sihmp**-ehl
    **sihl**-ē-ā-tehd koh-**luhm**-nahr ehp-ih-**thē**-lē-
    uhm
*Simple columnar epithelium* **sihmp**-ehl koh-**luhm**-nahr
    ehp-ih-**thē**-lē-uhm
*Simple cuboidal epithelium* **sihmp**-ehl **kyoo**-boyd-ahl
    ehp-ih-**thē**-lē-uhm
*Simple epithelium* **sihmp**-ehl ehp-ih-**thē**-lē-uhm
*Simple gland* **sihmp**-ehl glahnd
*Simple squamous epithelia* **sihmp**-ehl **skwey**-muhs
    ehp-ih-**thē**-lē-ah
*Skeletal muscle* **skehl**-ih-tahl **muhs**-uhl
*Smooth muscle* smooth **muhs**-uhl
*Specialized connective tissue* **spehsh**-uh-līzd kuh-**nehck**-tihv
    **tihsh**-yoo
*Squamous cell* **skwey**-muhs sehl
*Stratified cuboidal epithelium* **straht**-eh-fīd **kyoo**-boyd-ahl
    ehp-ih-**thē**-lē-uhm
*Stratified epithelium* **straht**-eh-fīd ehp-ih-**thē**-lē-uhm
*Stratified squamous epithelium* **straht**-eh-fīd **skwey**-muhs
    ehp-ih-**thē**-lē-uhm
*Striated muscle* **strī**-āt-ehd **muhs**-uhl
*Stroma* **strō**-mah
*Submucosa* suhb-myoo-**kō**-sah
*Synovial membrane* sih-**nō**-vē-ahl **mehm**-brān
*Thrombocyte* **throhm**-bō-sīt
*Thyroxine* thī-**rohck**-zihn
*Tight junction* tīt **juhngk**-shuhn
*Tissue* **tihsh**-yoo
*Tonofilament* toh-nō-**fihl**-ah-mehnt
*Transitional epithelium* trahn-**sihsh**-ihn-ahl
    ehp-ih-**thē**-lē-uhm
*Transudate* trahn-soo-**dāt**
*Tubular gland* **too**-būl-ahr glahnd
*Tubuloacinar* **too**-būl-ō-**ah**-sihn-ahr
*Tubuloalveolar* **too**-būl-ō-ahl-**vē**-ō-lahr
*Unicellular exocrine gland* ū-nih-**sehl**-ū-lər **ehcks**-ō-krihn
    glahnd
*Vascularized* **vahs**-kyoo-lahr-īzd
*Visceral layer* **vih**-sər-ahl **lā**-ər
*Voluntary muscle* **vohl**-uhn-teər-ē **muhs**-uhl
*White adipose tissue* whīt **ahd**-ih-pōs **tihsh**-yoo

A unicellular organism, such as a **paramecium**, can live as an individual. It can feed itself, respire, grow, and produce or find all of the biochemical substances that it needs without the assistance of other cells. The cells that compose multicellular organisms, however, cannot survive independently. These cells have *differentiated* to form a wide range of cell types, each with its own characteristic structural features and distinct function. In the course of their differentiation, they have lost the ability to perform all of the metabolic functions required to sustain life as an isolated entity. Consequently, the cells that compose animals and all multicellular organisms exist within cooperative living communities.

Many different types of community are found in any individual animal. These communities differ from one another based on the types of cells that compose them and on the role that they play in the organism as a whole. In this way, cells of similar type and function are clustered into layers, sheets, or groups called **tissues**. Tissues are classified into the following four primary types:

- Epithelial tissue
- Connective tissue
- Muscle tissue
- Nervous tissue

Although each classification is divided further into subgroups, each with its own special purpose, we can summarize the main functions of each tissue classification. In general, **epithelial tissue** *covers* and *lines*, **connective tissue** *provides support*, **muscle tissue** *enables movement*, and **nervous tissue** *controls work*. Because each type completes a specific purpose, the tissues must work collaboratively to meet the vital needs of the animal as a whole. Thus tissues are clustered to form organs, such as the liver, spleen, or kidney. All four tissue types can be found in most organs. The heart, for example, is a powerful *muscle* that moves blood throughout the body. Blood vessels, such as the coronary arteries, provide pathways for blood to reach the heart muscle. The vessels are composed of *connective* and *epithelial tissues*. Nerves and *nervous tissue* are threaded throughout the muscle of the heart to govern coordinated contractions of the ventricular and atrial chambers. These chambers are covered and lined with layers of *epithelia*. In this chapter, epithelial and connective tissues are the primary focus. Muscle and nervous tissues are discussed in greater detail in subsequent chapters.

## GROSS AND MICROSCOPIC ANATOMY

**Gross anatomy** is the study of anatomic structures that can be seen with the naked eye, and includes learning the names and locations of bones, muscles, arteries, veins, and nerves. Therefore anatomists must have excellent memories, because hundreds if not thousands of isolated structures can be examined. The study of the microscopic structures of tissues and organs is called **histology** or **microanatomy**. This chapter represents an introduction to the study of microanatomy, a discipline that beautifully complements the study of gross anatomy and gives a structural basis for understanding the physiology of each anatomic system.

## EPITHELIAL TISSUE

Epithelial tissue is composed of sheets of cells that cover and line other tissues. For example, it lines the bladder, mouth, blood vessels, thorax, and all of the body cavities and ducts in the body. Although well grounded to underlying structures, epithelia have an exposed surface that affords access to the surrounding environment or to the inner openings of chambers and ducts. Epithelial tissue acts as an interface layer that separates and defines the beginning and ending of different types of tissues. It is protective of underlying tissues and frequently acts as a filter of biochemical substances. In addition, epithelia may be absorptive; for example, the epithelia that line the gastrointestinal tract absorb nutrient molecules from the gut, which are then placed into circulation. Epithelia can detect changes in the environment and play an important role in the reception of sensory input. Epithelial cells on the tongue, for example, are sensitive to touch, temperature, and taste. The eyes, ears, and nasal passages also are assisted by the presence of specialized epithelia that provide the sensations of sight, sound, and smell. The sensory information collected by these cells is conveyed to the nervous system.

Another common function of epithelial tissue is the secretion or excretion of biochemical substances. Epithelia that engage in the manufacture and release of substances are called **glandular epithelia**. Glandular epithelial cells may occur as individuals, such as the **goblet cells** found in the intestine, or they may occur as organized glands, such as those found in the pancreas. Some of the substances produced by glandular epithelia lubricate parts of the body, such as the mucus secreted in the colon, whereas others play a vital role in producing biochemical substances that influence physiologic events. Hormones, enzymes, milk, sweat, and musk are all examples of substances produced by glandular epithelia. Substances that ultimately leave the body, such as sweat, urine, and feces, are called **excretions**, and substances that remain within the body, such as regulatory molecules and mucus, are termed **secretions**.

Epithelia perform vital functions in the bodies of animals. The functions of epithelial tissue are summarized as follows:

- Protects, covers, and lines
- Filters biochemical substances
- Absorbs nutrients
- Provides sensory input
- Manufactures secretions
- Manufactures excretions

## GENERAL CHARACTERISTICS OF EPITHELIA

Epithelial cells are organized into tightly packed groups that form sheets of tissue. These sheets may be composed of either a single layer or multiple layers of cells, depending on where they are located in the body. Although the size and shape of the cells vary, epithelia share certain common characteristics.

1. Epithelial cells are **polar**, that is, they have a sense of direction relative to surrounding structures. Each epithelial cell has an **apical surface** and a **basal surface**, which are quite different from one another. The apical surface is the side of the cell that faces the **lumen** or body cavity, and the basal surface is the side of the cell that faces the underlying connective tissue.
2. Epithelial cells have lateral surfaces that are connected to neighboring cells by **junctional complexes**. These junctions bring the cells into close apposition to one another, leaving little room for extracellular matrix. The matrix that surrounds epithelia therefore exists in very small quantities, if at all.
3. All epithelial cells lack blood vessels or capillaries. They are **avascular** and rely on underlying connective tissue to provide oxygen and nutrients.
4. Although some epithelia lack nerves, such as those in the stomach, intestines, and cervix, most epithelial cells are **innervated** and provide valuable sensory input.

## CELLULAR ATTACHMENTS

Epithelial cells are held together in many ways. Their lateral surfaces, for example, are wavy and fit together like pieces of a jigsaw puzzle. Between the plasma membranes of adjacent cells are matrix-filled channels, which transport nutrients from underlying connective tissue. These passages act as distribution routes for biologic supplies and as elimination routes for waste. The plasma membranes of epithelial cells are joined to form specialized attachments, called **junctional complexes**, that give epithelial tissue surprising strength, even though the attachments only involve a small portion of the cell membrane. Three major types of cellular junction found between epithelial cells are *tight junctions, desmosomes,* and *gap junctions* (Figure 5-1).

A **tight junction** is formed by the fusion of the outermost layers of the plasma membranes of adjoining cells. The matrix-filled space between cells is lost at the site of a tight junction. For centrally placed cells, the fusion occurs as a strip that wraps around the entire circumference of the cell, like a belt. In this way, an impenetrable barrier is formed that prevents the passage of substances from the luminal end to the basal end

of the cell and vice versa. Only by passing through the body of the cell can substances pass through the epithelial layer. Tight junctions are found in tissues in which there can be no leaks, such as in the urinary bladder, where urine is held, or in the digestive tract, where they play a critical role in preventing the leakage of digestive enzymes into the bloodstream.

A **desmosome** is a strong, welded **plaque** or *thickening*, which connects the plasma membranes of adjacent cells. The bond is a mechanical coupling formed by filaments that interlock with one another, just as plastic fibers do in Velcro. In addition to these linkages **intermediate filaments** called **tonofilaments** extend from the plaque into the cytoplasm of each cell like anchors, forming stabilizing bases for the membrane junction. Since desmosomes form tough bonds between cells they are found most commonly in tissues that undergo repeated episodes of tension and stretching, such as the skin, heart, and uterus. Junctions that look like half of a desmosome are called **hemidesmosomes**, and these link epithelial cells to the basement membrane.

Cells that are connected by **gap junctions** are linked by tubular channel proteins called **connexons** (ko-NEK-sonz), which extend from the cytoplasm of one cell to the cytoplasm of the other. These *transmembrane* proteins allow the exchange and passage of ions and nutrients, such as nucleotides, sugars, and amino acids, from one cell to the other. Gap junctions are most commonly found in intestinal epithelial cells, the heart, and smooth muscle tissue. Although the exact function of gap junctions in epithelial cells is not yet fully understood, their role in cardiac and smooth muscle cells centers around their ability to transport electrical signals quickly from one cell to another. In this way, they coordinate the contraction of cardiac and smooth muscle.

## BASEMENT MEMBRANE

The **basement membrane** is the foundation of the epithelial cell. It is a nonliving meshwork of fibers that cements the epithelial cell to the underlying connective tissue. Its strength and elasticity help prevent the cell from being torn off by intraluminal pressures, such as stretching or erosion caused by the rubbing of luminal material. The basement membrane (also called *basal lamina*) is manufactured and laid down by epithelial cells in varying degrees of thickness. The basement membrane in skin, for example, is thin, but in the trachea it is much thicker. Oxygen and nutrient molecules are supplied to the epithelial cells by diffusing through the basement membrane from capillaries in the underlying connective tissue. Similarly, nutrient substances that are absorbed and waste that is excreted by the epithelium diffuse across the basement membrane into the blood supply of the connective tissue. In this way, the basement membrane acts as a partial barrier between the epithelial cell and the underlying connective tissue. Cancerous epithelia do not respect this boundary and aggressively invade the connective tissue layer underneath.

## SURFACE SPECIALIZATION

The surfaces of epithelial cells vary depending on where the epithelium is located in the body and, more importantly,

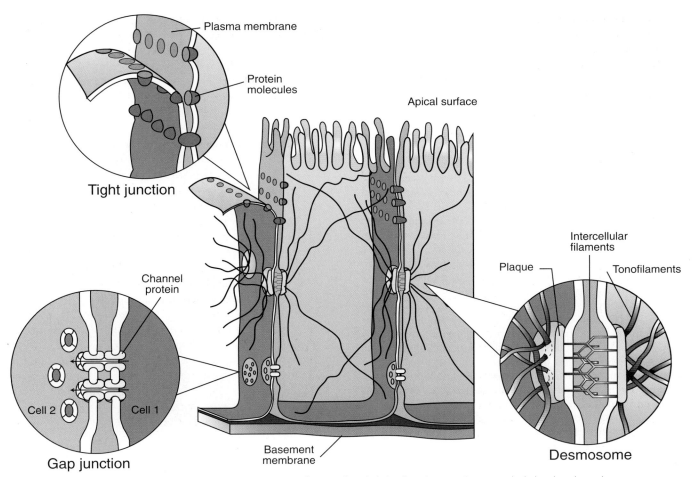

**FIGURE 5-1** Intercellular junctions. An interesting feature of epithelial cells is the varied way in which they bond together. These intercellular junctions are both functionally and structurally different from one another. Three main types of intercellular connection are *tight junctions, gap junctions,* and *spot desmosomes.* A simplified form of these junctions is depicted here.

what role it plays in the function of the tissue. The epithelia that line blood vessels, for example, have smooth surfaces to allow the easy passage of blood cells. However other epithelia have irregular surfaces and may be covered with many fingerlike projections, called **microvilli**, or thousands of tiny hairs, called **cilia** (Figure 5-2).

The surface of a cell covered with microvilli is called the **brush border**. The brush border greatly increases the surface area of the cell, thereby increasing the absorptive ability of the cell. For this reason, microvilli usually occur on cells that are involved in absorption or secretion, such as the epithelia in the intestinal and urinary tracts. Remarkably, a cell with microvilli has about *20 times* the surface area of a cell without them.

Cilia are also found on the free surface of cells, usually in the respiratory and urogenital tracts. In the trachea, for example, the cilia help to propel mucus and debris up and away from the lungs toward the mouth. In the opening of the **oviduct**, called the *infundibulum,* cilia encourage newly expelled ova into the oviduct. Ciliary movement occurs in coordinated "beats," which enable the efficient transport of material. This coordinated action is brought about by an electrical potential that moves through junctional complexes connecting adjacent cells. The movement crosses the entire epithelial surface as a perfectly synchronized wave.

Epithelial cells of the skin become filled with a protective, waterproof substance called **keratin**. The accumulation of keratin occurs as the cell matures and moves from the basal layer to the superficial layer of the integument. These cells are called *keratinized epithelium* and are discussed in greater detail in Chapter 6.

> ✓ **TEST YOURSELF 5-1**
> 1. What are the four primary types of tissue?
> 2. What is histology?
> 3. List seven functions performed by epithelial cells.
> 4. What four attributes characterize epithelial tissue in general?
> 5. List four types of cellular junction. Can you describe them?
> 6. How does the basement membrane act as a partial barrier between the epithelial cell and the underlying connective tissue?
> 7. Why do some epithelial cells have cilia and microvilli? What role do they play? Where are the cells with these specialized surfaces found in the body?

## CLINICAL APPLICATION

Parvovirus: Killer of Intestinal Epithelia

**Feline panleukopenia** and **canine parvoviral enteritis** are life-threatening diseases that affect cats and dogs respectively. **Parvoviruses**, which cause both diseases, are highly contagious and are carried on clothing, shoes, and toys. They are shed in the feces and other excretions of affected animals and can be easily tracked into your house or veterinary office on the soles of your shoes. Fortunately, most cats and dogs are immunized against parvovirus and therefore never contract the disease. However, because of the highly contagious nature of these viruses, veterinary practices should isolate suspected carriers.

For animals that do contract parvovirus, mortality is high if untreated, particularly in young animals. The virus attacks and kills cells that are actively engaged in mitosis. Thus tissues that are continually renewing themselves, such as epithelial tissue, may be devastated by parvovirus. The small intestine, for example, is lined with epithelial tissue that helps to absorb nutrient molecules from the lumen of the gut. During parvovirus infections, the epithelial cells die and slough in sheets and animals develop diarrhea, vomit, and can become severely dehydrated in a short time. The sudden loss of epithelial tissue causes bleeding into the intestine, which creates a distinctively noxious, foul-smelling, hemorrhagic diarrhea. A simple laboratory test on the stool may indicate the presence of the virus and offer a definitive diagnosis.

Treatment centers on combating dehydration and includes intravenous fluid therapy with electrolyte supplements, antibiotics, and anti-vomiting medications. Animals that remain alive after 3 to 4 days of illness generally survive but continue to shed the virus for several months. Because of the highly contagious nature of parvoviral diseases, some veterinary personnel who own young animals change their clothes and shoes before entering their homes.

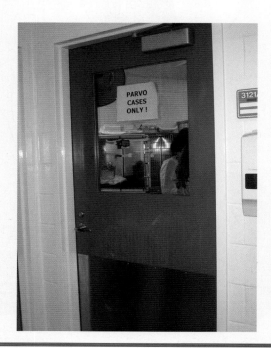

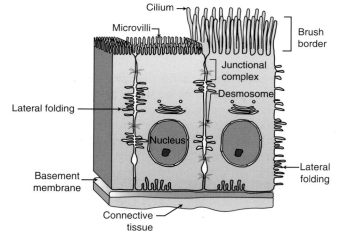

**FIGURE 5-2** Epithelial cell specializations. In addition to forming unique intercellular connections, epithelial cells vary in their cell surfaces. Some cells are smooth and flat, whereas others have elaborate brush borders of microvilli designed to expand surface area to maximize the absorption or secretion of substances. In addition, epithelial cells may be covered with long, hairlike structures called *cilia* that beat in a rhythmic fashion to propel mucus and other materials across the cell's apical border. Elaborate folds of plasma membrane are also evident along the lateral sides of the cell, as well as on the surface. These are important in providing space for those materials that pass within cells from the apical to basal ends and vice versa.

## CLASSIFICATIONS OF EPITHELIA

Epithelial tissue is classified according to the following three characteristics (Figure 5-3):

1. *Number of layers of cells.* If there is only a single layer of epithelial cells, the tissue is classified as *simple.* If there is more than one layer of cells, the tissue is called *stratified.* **Simple epithelia** provide little protection to the underlying connective tissue and therefore are found in protected areas of the body, such as internal compartments, ducts, vessels, and passageways. **Stratified epithelia**, on the other hand, are thicker and stronger and are found in areas of the body that are subjected to mechanical and chemical stress.

2. *Shape of the cells.* In cross section, epithelial cells may take on many shapes, such as squamous, cuboidal, and columnar. In stratified epithelium, many different cell shapes are visible within the same tissue, but the classification is based on the shape of the cell that resides on the exposed or *luminal* surface of the tissue. In **stratified squamous epithelium**, for example, **cuboidal cells** are visible near the basement membrane, but **squamous cells** are found at the luminal surface; therefore, the tissue is called *stratified squamous,* not stratified cuboidal.

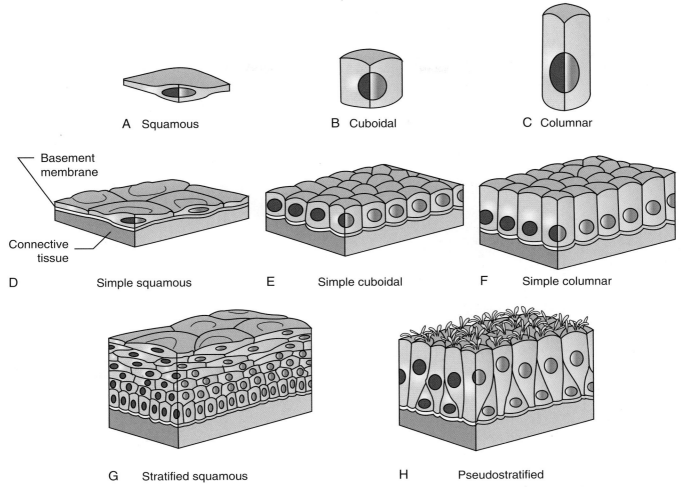

A   Squamous

B   Cuboidal

C   Columnar

Basement membrane

Connective tissue

D     Simple squamous

E     Simple cuboidal

F     Simple columnar

G     Stratified squamous

H     Pseudostratified

**FIGURE 5-3** Classification of epithelia. Epithelial tissues are classified according to the shape of the cell and the way in which the cells are arranged. *Stratified* epithelial tissues are composed of many layers of cells, and each layer of cells may have a different shape. In these cases, tissue is classified according to the shape of the cells on the surface, in the outermost layer. (From Patton KT, Thibodeau GA: Anatomy & physiology, ed 8, St Louis, 2013, Mosby.)

3. *Presence of surface specializations.* Terms for surface specializations, such as "cilia" and "keratinized," may be added to the classifications of epithelia to indicate an increased level of specialization. Stratified squamous epithelium, for example, may be classified as **keratinized stratified squamous epithelium** (found in the skin) or nonkeratinized stratified squamous epithelium (found in the lining of the mouth).

## TYPES OF EPITHELIA
### SIMPLE SQUAMOUS EPITHELIUM

**Simple squamous epithelia** are delicate and thin. They are often found lining surfaces involved in the passage of either gas or liquid, for example in the inner lining of the lung, where oxygen is absorbed and carbon dioxide released, and in the filtration membranes of kidneys, where water and other small molecules are excreted as urine (Figure 5-4). The fragile nature of simple squamous epithelium requires that it occur only in protected regions of the body, such as in the lining of

the chest and abdominal cavities. Because simple squamous epithelia are flat and smooth, they are important in reducing friction and are found in the lining of blood and lymphatic vessels. Simple squamous epithelia have been given special names depending on where they are located in the body. For example, the epithelium that lines the pleural (chest), pericardial (around the heart), and peritoneal (abdominal) cavities is called **mesothelium.** The epithelium that lines blood and lymphatic vessels is called **endothelium**.

### SIMPLE CUBOIDAL EPITHELIUM

**Simple cuboidal epithelium** is composed of a single layer of cubic cells (Figure 5-5). On microscopic examination, their round, dark-staining nuclei are seen to be aligned in a single row that resembles a string of pearls. Like simple squamous epithelium, simple **cuboidal epithelium** provides little protection from abrasion. Therefore it occurs in sheltered regions of the body, where secretion and absorption take place. It is found on the surface of ovaries, in the secretory portions of glands, such as the thyroid, and in the lining of

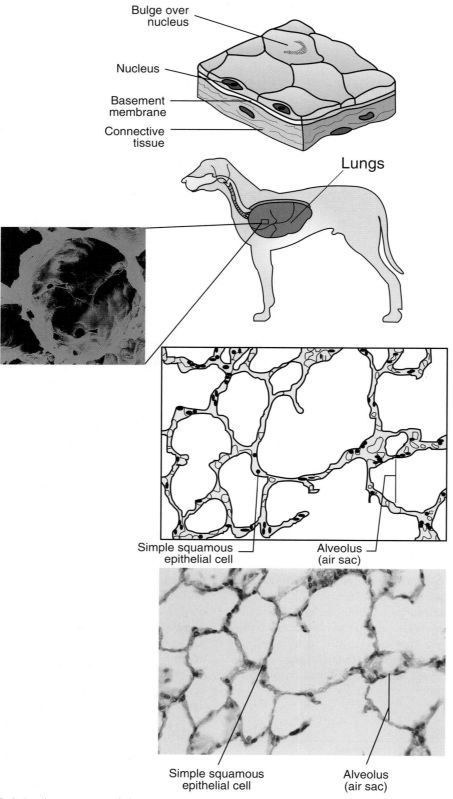

**FIGURE 5-4** Simple squamous epithelium. *Description:* A single layer of flattened, hexagon-shaped cells. The nuclei are disc shaped and centrally located. They often appear as raised bumps in the center of the flattened cell, giving cells a "fried-egg" appearance. *Location:* Alveoli of lungs, lining in blood and lymphatic vessels, lining in heart and major body cavities, filtration units *(glomeruli)* in kidney. *Function:* In regions of the body where protection is not important, simple squamous epithelium allows diffusion, filtration, secretion, and absorption. *Microanatomy:* Photomicrograph and sketch of simple squamous cells that compose the walls of air sacs in the lung. The scanning electron micrograph depicts the three-dimensional nature of living lung tissue. (Courtesy Barbara Cousins and Ed Reschke.)

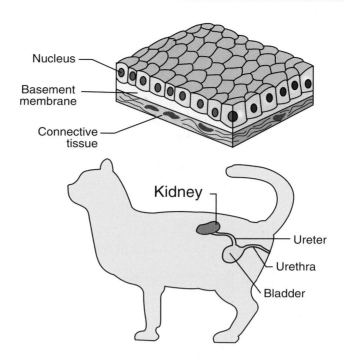

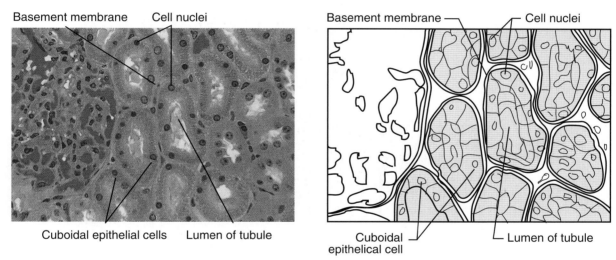

**FIGURE 5-5** Simple cuboidal epithelium. *Description:* A single row of tightly packed, cubelike cells, each of which contains a round, centrally located nucleus. *Location:* Tubules of kidney; terminal bronchioles in lungs; choroid plexus of brain, glands, and their ducts; surface of ovaries. *Function:* Cells in kidney are engaged in absorption and secretion; cells in bronchioles are ciliated and assist with movement of particles away from lungs. Cells in choroid plexus and in glands secrete substances. *Microanatomy:* Photomicrograph and sketch of micrograph show a layer of simple cuboidal epithelium lining the lumen of tubules in the kidneys. (Courtesy Robert Calentine.)

the ducts of the liver, pancreas, kidney, and salivary glands. Some simple cuboidal epithelia in kidney tubules are covered with microvilli, attesting to their absorptive function. Others are smooth surfaced and associated with secretory glands.

Simple cuboidal epithelium plays an important role in both endocrine and exocrine tissues. Exocrine ducts lined with simple cuboidal epithelium, for example, carry saliva from the salivary gland to the oral cavity, and enzymes secreted by the pancreas are transported to the duodenum. In addition the thyroid gland, an endocrine structure, contains chambers lined by a single row of cuboidal cells and

secretes the hormone **thyroxine**, which is carried throughout the body via the bloodstream.

## SIMPLE COLUMNAR EPITHELIUM

**Simple columnar epithelia** are elongated and closely packed together, making the epithelia relatively thick and more protective than the simple squamous and cuboidal epithelia (Figure 5-6). The nuclei are not centrally located, as they are in cuboidal cells, but rather are aligned in a row at the base of the cell near the basement membrane. Simple columnar epithelia line the length of the gastrointestinal tract from the

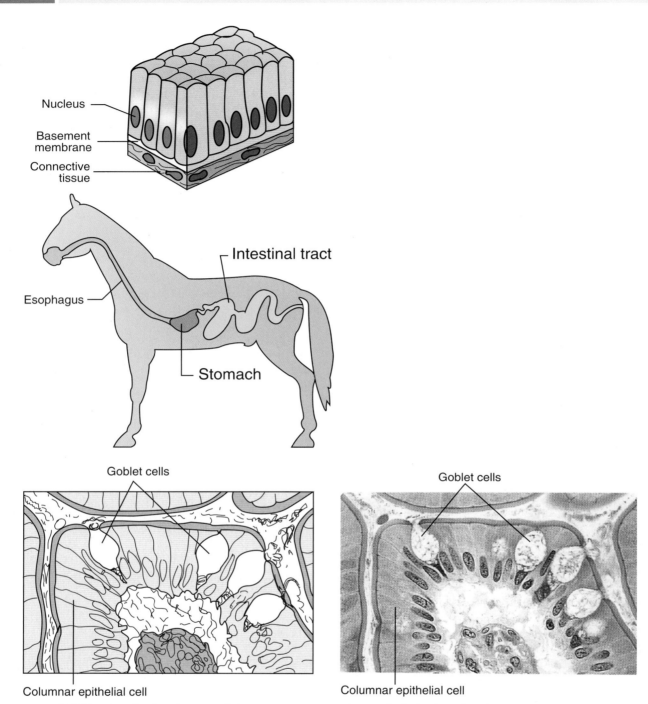

**FIGURE 5-6** Simple columnar epithelium. *Description:* A single row of tall, slender cells with oval nuclei. The surface may or may not be ciliated. Goblet cells can be seen interspersed among the cells. *Location:* The nonciliated variety lines the digestive tract from stomach to rectum, including the gallbladder and the excretory ducts of some glands; ciliated cells are found in uterine tubes, uterus, and small bronchi of the lungs. *Function:* Absorption in intestine and secretion in stomach, glands, and intestines. Ciliated cells assist with movement of particles out of the lungs and with movement of the oocyte through uterine tubes. *Microanatomy:* Photomicrograph and sketch of micrograph show simple columnar epithelium lining the stomach. Notice the goblet cells, which produce mucus. (Courtesy Ed Reschke.)

stomach to the rectum. Like simple cuboidal, they are associated with absorption and secretion and are found in many **excretory ducts,** as well as in the digestive tract.

Two types of cell make up the gut lining. The most numerous is the **absorptive cell,** whose apical surface is blanketed by dense microvilli that maximize absorption by increasing surface contact with the nutrient-filled lumen. The other cell is called a **goblet cell** because of its wineglass shape. Goblet cells manufacture and store lubricating mucus that is secreted onto the luminal surfaces of the epithelia.

Some less common epithelia are covered with cilia on their apical surfaces. These cells are called **simple ciliated columnar epithelia**, and they line the uterine tubes and respiratory tracts.

## STRATIFIED SQUAMOUS EPITHELIUM

**Stratified squamous epithelium** consists of various cell layers (Figure 5-7). It occurs in regions of the body that are subject to mechanical and chemical stresses, such as the linings of the mouth, esophagus, vagina, and rectum. The epithelial cells that make up the outer surface are continually being worn away or sheared off, but they are replaced at an equal rate by cells from deeper layers. Cuboidal cells form the base of stratified squamous epithelium. They are attached to the basement membrane and are continually dividing to keep up with the cell losses from the luminal surface. As the young cuboidal cells mature, they are progressively pushed to the surface, away from the nutrient sources provided by the underlying connective tissue. During this movement, the cells lose their cytoplasm and nuclei, take on a squamous shape, and eventually become paperlike sheets that slough.

## STRATIFIED CUBOIDAL EPITHELIUM

**Stratified cuboidal epithelium** generally occurs as two layers of cuboidal cells and is found primarily along large excretory ducts, such as those of sweat glands, mammary glands, and salivary glands (Figure 5-8). This type of epithelium is important in protecting the delicate tissues in deeper layers.

## STRATIFIED COLUMNAR EPITHELIUM

Stratified columnar epithelium is rare and is found only in select parts of the respiratory, digestive, and **reproductive systems** and along some excretory ducts (Figure 5-9).

## PSEUDOSTRATIFIED COLUMNAR EPITHELIUM

*Pseudo-* means "false," therefore **pseudostratified columnar epithelium** is an epithelial layer that is *not* truly stratified. The epithelial cells appear to be stratified because the nuclei are found at different levels across the length of the tissue layer. However, not all of the cells reach the luminal surface, so cells *appear* to be at different levels as though stratified. In reality, each cell forms a distinct attachment, however subtle, with the basement membrane. In this way, pseudostratified columnar epithelium forms a single layer and therefore is considered a *simple* epithelium (Figure 5-10).

Most pseudostratified columnar epithelium is ciliated and is found in the respiratory tract and in portions of the male reproductive tract. In the trachea, for example, the epithelium is coated with a layer of mucus that is propelled by cilia across the luminal surface toward the mouth. This assists in preventing debris from entering the lungs. The mucus is also fortified with protective **immunoglobulins**, which are disease-fighting molecules that help to protect animals from **pathogens** (bacteria and viruses) that have been inhaled.

## TRANSITIONAL EPITHELIUM

**Transitional epithelium** has the remarkable ability to stretch. It is found in regions of the body that are required to expand and contract as part of their normal function. Thus transitional epithelium is found in portions of the urinary tract where great changes in volume occur, such as the urinary bladder, ureters, urethra, and calyxes of the kidney. The histologic appearance of transitional epithelia varies, depending on how much it is stretched. For example, in an empty bladder the epithelium is thick, multilayered, and has rounded, domelike cells on the luminal surface. When the bladder is filled, greater pressure is applied to the epithelial layer, making it stretch and thin out. The extent to which the membrane stretches depends on how full the bladder is and how much force is applied to the epithelium. As epithelia stretch, they may thin out from six to three cell layers, and the apical cells become flattened and squamous. The ability of transitional cells to change shape in the urine-holding tissues allows greater volumes of urine to be transported, stored, and excreted (Figure 5-11).

In addition to its ability to stretch, transitional epithelium forms a leak-proof membrane that prevents the diffusion of potentially scalding urine into the delicate environment of the abdominal cavity.

---

### ✔ TEST YOURSELF 5-2

1. Epithelial tissue is characterized as simple, stratified, or pseudostratified. What does this mean?
2. What are the three basic shapes of epithelial cell?
3. Draw a picture of each of the following types of epithelia and give an example of where each of them can be found in the body.
   - Simple squamous
   - Simple cuboidal
   - Simple columnar
   - Stratified squamous
   - Pseudostratified columnar
   - Transitional

---

## GLANDS

A *gland* is a cell or group of cells that have the ability to manufacture and discharge a secretion. **Secretions** are specialized protein molecules that are produced in the rough endoplasmic reticulum, packaged into granules by the Golgi apparatus, and discharged from the cell. Thus typical glandular epithelial cells are recognized by their prominent endoplasmic reticulum, Golgi apparatus, and secretory granules. Some of the secretions produced by glandular epithelia are used locally, whereas others are needed in distant regions of the body.

During embryonic development, multicellular glands form from an infolding layer of epithelial cells. Initially, these invaginations form ducts and tubules that maintain contact with the surface epithelium. In the course of development, some of the glands lose the ducts and become separated from

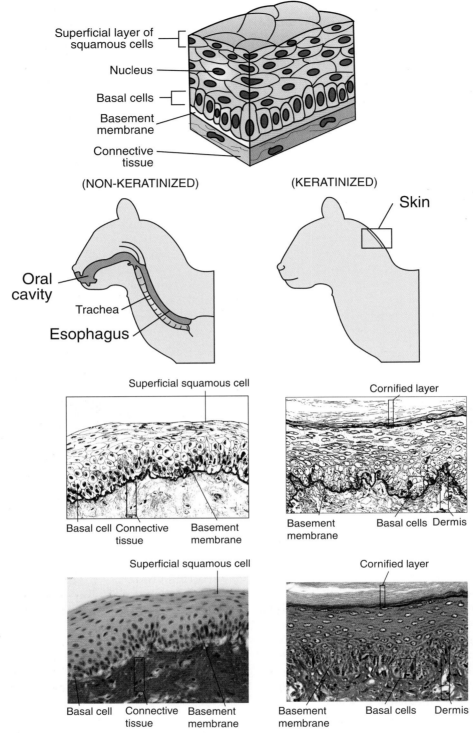

**FIGURE 5-7** Stratified squamous (keratinized and nonkeratinized) epithelium. *Description:* A multilayered tissue in which cells along the basement membrane are metabolically active and dividing. These basal cells are cuboidal or columnar, and as they mature they are pushed to the surface, lose their organelles, and flatten into thin flakes. In skin, maturing cells fill with keratin. *Location:* Nonkeratinized epithelium is found lining the mouth, esophagus, and vagina. Keratinized cells are found in epidermis, the superficial layer of the skin. *Function:* In areas that are prone to abrasion, stratified squamous epithelium protects underlying tissues. *Microanatomy:* Photomicrograph and sketch of micrograph show nonkeratinized squamous epithelium lining the mouth and esophagus in a cat. Photomicrograph and sketch of micrograph show keratinized stratified squamous epithelium in the epidermis of skin. (Courtesy Ed Reschke.)

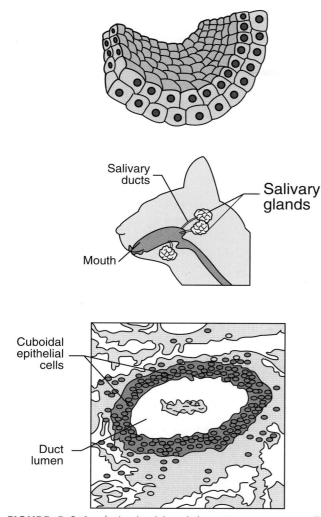

**FIGURE 5-8** Stratified cuboidal epithelium. *Description:* Generally, two layers of cuboidal cells. *Location:* Ducts of mammary glands, sweat glands, and salivary glands. *Function:* Secretion, absorption, and protection. *Microanatomy:* The sketch shows stratified cuboidal epithelia in a salivary gland.

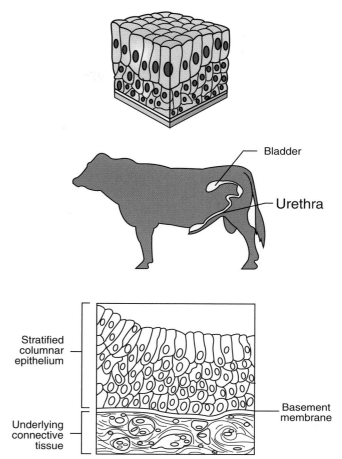

**FIGURE 5-9** Stratified columnar epithelium. *Description:* Several layers of cells in which basal cells are cuboidal and superficial cells are columnar. *Location:* Large ducts of mammary glands and small portion of the urethra of some male animals. This type of epithelium is rare. *Function:* Secretion and protection. *Microanatomy:* Stratified columnar epithelium in the urethra.

the parent epithelial sheet (Figure 5-12). In this way, glands are derived from epithelium.

Glands can be classified in many ways. For example, we can organize them based on the following factors:

1. Presence or absence of ducts (endocrine or exocrine).
2. Number of cells that compose them (unicellular or multicellular).
3. Shape of the secreting ducts (simple or compound).
4. Complexity of the glandular structure (tubular, acinar, or tubuloacinar).
5. Type of secretion they produce (mucoid or serous).
6. Manner in which the secretion is stored and discharged (merocrine, apocrine, or holocrine).

Each of these classifications is discussed.

## ENDOCRINE GLANDS

Glands that do not have ducts or tubules and whose secretions are distributed throughout the body are called **endocrine glands**. They produce and secrete regulatory chemicals, known as **hormones**, into the bloodstream or the lymphatic system, where they are carried to many regions of the body. Endocrine glands are part of a complex, biochemical network known as the **endocrine system**. The pituitary gland in the brain and the adrenal gland near the kidney are examples of endocrine glands. The endocrine system and the glands it includes are discussed in detail in Chapter 11.

## EXOCRINE GLANDS

With the exception of the goblet cell, **exocrine glands** possess ducts. They are more common than endocrine glands and act by discharging secretions via their ducts directly into nearby areas where they may, for example, cover cell surfaces or empty into body cavities. Unlike those of endocrine glands, the secretions of exocrine glands act locally and do not normally enter the circulation. A wide variety of exocrine glands are found in animals, including hepatoid, musk, sweat, and salivary glands. Other examples can be found in the liver and pancreas, where exocrine glands secrete bile

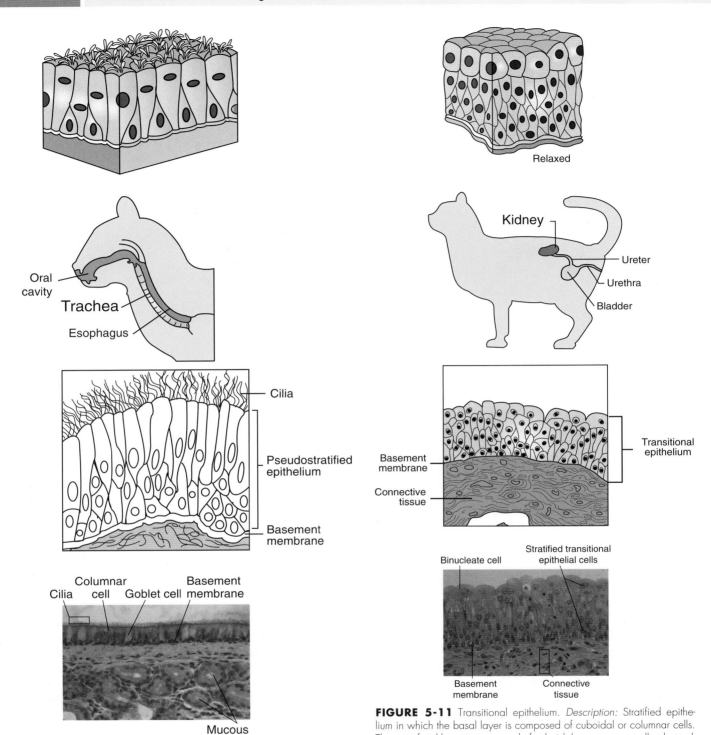

**FIGURE 5-10** Pseudostratified epithelium. *Description:* Pseudostratified epithelia appear stratified but are not. Each cell is attached to basement membrane, but not all of them reach the luminal surface. Cells vary in shape and height. Their nuclei occur at different distances from the basement membrane. Cells are generally ciliated and are often associated with goblet cells. *Location:* Respiratory tract, including nasal cavity, larynx, pharynx, trachea, and bronchi. *Function:* Surface layer of mucus traps particles, which are moved away from the lungs by beating cilia. *Microanatomy:* Photomicrograph and sketch of micrograph show ciliated pseudostratified epithelium lining the trachea. Note the goblet cells that secret protective mucus. (Courtesy Robert Calentine.)

**FIGURE 5-11** Transitional epithelium. *Description:* Stratified epithelium in which the basal layer is composed of cuboidal or columnar cells. The superficial layer is composed of cuboidal or squamous cells, depending on level of distension of the tissue. *Location:* Urinary bladder, ureters, and urethra. *Function:* Transitional epithelium is flexible to accommodate fluctuations in amount of urine in bladder, ureters, and urethra. It forms a permeable barrier that holds liquid and protects underlying tissues from caustic effects of urine. *Microanatomy:* Photomicrograph and sketch of micrograph show transitional epithelium in the bladder of a cat. Notice that the shape of the cells is highly variable and that the superficial layers do not touch the basement membrane, making this a type of stratified epithelium. The epithelium changes (transitions) and is compressed as the bladder fills. (Courtesy Ed Reschke; from Thibodeau GA, Patton KT: Anatomy & physiology, ed 6, St Louis, 2007, Mosby.)

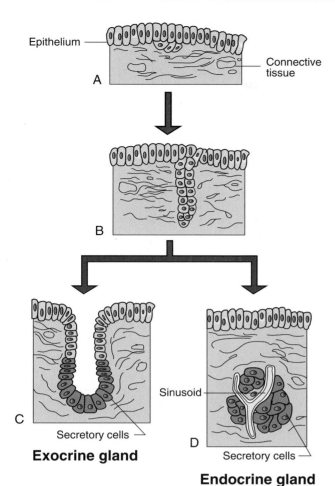

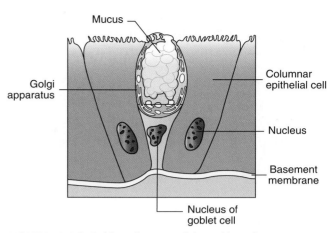

**FIGURE 5-13** Goblet cell. A unicellular goblet cell occurs among simple and pseudostratified epithelia that line the respiratory and digestive tracts. Mucus is contained within the cytoplasm at the luminal end of the cell, and the nucleus is located in the basal end of the cell, near the basement membrane. A goblet cell releases its stored mucus onto the tissue surface.

**FIGURE 5-12** Development of glands. **A** and **B**, Exocrine and endocrine glands develop from epithelium during the maturation of a fetus. Surface epithelial cells grow down into the underlying connective tissue. Exocrine glands develop when the connections between deep and superficial layers of cells form a duct. **C**, The deepest cells become secretory. Endocrine glands form when connecting cells die. **D**, Secretions of the gland are transferred to sinusoids and then into the circulatory system, rather than through a duct.

and digestive enzymes, respectively. The pancreas possesses endocrine and exocrine properties because it is responsible for producing many hormones and for secreting digestive enzymes.

**UNICELLULAR EXOCRINE GLANDS.** The only example of a **unicellular exocrine gland** is the ductless goblet cell, so named because of its resemblance to a drinking goblet (Figure 5-13). The goblet cell is a modified columnar epithelial cell and is found interspersed among the *columnar cells* of the respiratory and digestive tracts and in the conjunctiva of the eye. Goblet cells secrete **mucin**: a thick, sticky mixture of glycoproteins and **proteoglycans** that when mixed with water becomes mucus. The mucus functions in two ways: it helps protect the apical surface of the epithelial layer, and it assists with the entrapment of microorganisms and foreign particles.

**MULTICELLULAR EXOCRINE GLANDS.** *Multicellular exocrine glands* are made up of two distinct components: a **secretory unit** in which secretions are produced by secretory cells and a **duct** that carries the secretion to the deposition site. In most glands the secretory unit is surrounded by connective tissue that is rich in blood vessels and nerve fibers. It not only nourishes the secretory unit but also provides structural support and may extend into the gland to form distinct lobes. In some exocrine glands the secretory unit is surrounded by contractile cells called **myoepithelial cells** that assist with the discharge of secretions into the glandular duct. The rate of secretion production and discharge is controlled by hormonal and nervous influences.

We begin the classification of exocrine glands with examination of the glandular ducts (Table 5-1). If the main duct is *unbranched*, the gland is considered a **simple gland.** If the main duct is *branched*, the gland is called a **compound gland**. Next, we examine the secretory portions of glands. If the secretory cells form a long channel of even width, the gland is called a **tubular gland** (Figure 5-14). If the secretory unit forms a rounded sac, the gland is called an **alveolar gland** or an **acinar gland**. Glands with secretory units that possess both tubular and alveolar qualities are called **tubuloalveolar** or **tubuloacinar** (Figure 5-14).

Glands are classified further according to the way in which they secrete their products. How much of the cell is sacrificed in the act of secretion determines whether the gland is *merocrine, apocrine,* or *holocrine* (Figure 5-15). The majority of glands package their secretions into granular units and release them via exocytosis as they are manufactured. These glands are called **merocrine glands** because the secretory cells remain intact during the secretory process. The pancreas, sweat glands, and salivary glands are examples of merocrine glands. Secretion in **apocrine glands** involves the loss of the top part of the cell, called the *apex* of the secretory cell. The secretory cells in apocrine glands do not

| TABLE 5-1 | Structural Classification of Exocrine Glands | | | |
|---|---|---|---|---|
| **SHAPE** | **COMPLEXITY+** | **TYPE** | **EXAMPLE** | |
| Tubular (single, straight) | Simple | Simple tubular | Intestinal glands | |
| Tubular (coiled) | Simple | Simple | Sweat glands | |
| Tubular (multiple) | Simple | Simple branched tubular | Gastric (stomach) glands | |
| Alveolar (single) | Simple | Simple alveolar | Sebaceous (skin oil) glands | |
| Alveolar (multiple) | Simple | Simple branched alveolar | Sebaceous glands | |
| Tubular (multiple) | Compound | Compound tubular | Mammary glands | |
| Alveolar (multiple) | Compound | Compound alveolar | Mammary glands | |
| Some tubular; some alveolar | Compound | Compound tubuloalveolar | Salivary glands | |

(From Patton KT, Thibodeau GA: Anatomy & physiology, ed 8, St Louis, 2013, Mosby.)

release their granules as they are manufactured. Instead, they store the granules until the apex of the cell is full. Then the cell pinches in two and releases the apex into the duct system. Later, the cell repairs the damage and repeats the process. Apocrine glands can be found in mammary tissue and are represented by some sweat glands.

Like apocrine glands, **holocrine glands** also store granules in the secretory cells until they are needed. However, in holocrine glands, the entire secretory cell is destroyed in the act of releasing its secretory product. The subsequent degeneration of the cell allows the release of the granules. Holocrine secretion occurs principally in **sebaceous glands**.

We can also categorize glands according to the type of secretion they produce. **Serous secretions** are watery and contain a high concentration of enzymes, whereas **mucous**

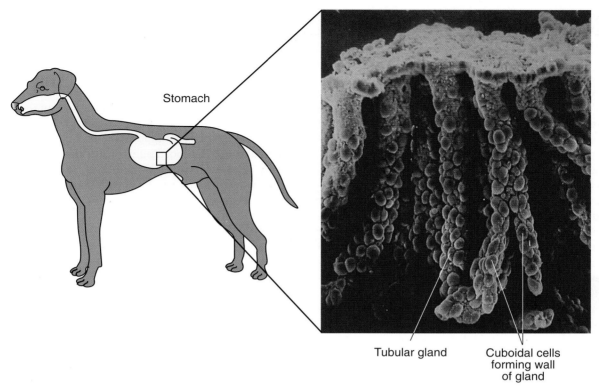

Tubular gland    Cuboidal cells forming wall of gland

**FIGURE 5-14** Tubular exocrine glands in the canine stomach. Exocrine glands are structured in many different ways and occur in diverse regions of the body. In the lining of the stomach exocrine glands occur as simple straight, simple coiled, and compound (or *branched*) tubular glands. These gastric glands produce a mixture of water, enzymes, acid, and mucus, which together form an important digestive "juice."

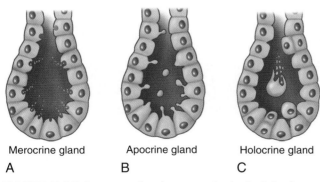

Merocrine gland    Apocrine gland    Holocrine gland
A                  B                 C

**FIGURE 5-15** Secretion styles of exocrine glands. **A,** Cells of **merocrine** glands store substances intended for excretion in vesicles in their cytoplasm. The vesicles are transported to the surface of the cell, where they release their contents. A cell can continue to produce and excrete substances throughout its life and is not in any way harmed by the secretory process. **B,** Cells of **apocrine** glands also store secretory substances within vesicles. However, secretion occurs as the luminal end of the cell is detached from the basal portion. Cytosol, inclusions, and other cytoplasmic components are discharged along with the secretory vesicles. The cell must take time to regrow lost portions of itself before it can secrete again. **C,** Holocrine secretion involves release of the entire contents of the cell. In this process, the cell is killed and is replaced by new cells that have moved up from deeper layers. (From Patton KT, Thibodeau GA: Anatomy & physiology, ed 8, St Louis, 2013, Mosby.)

**secretions** are thick, viscous, and composed of glycoproteins. Secretory cells that manufacture both types of secretion are common in the digestive and respiratory tracts. **Mixed exocrine glands** contain both mucous and serous components.

✓ **TEST YOURSELF 5-3**
1. What is a gland?
2. How do glands develop embryologically?
3. What is the difference between endocrine and exocrine glands? Can you give examples of each?
4. Where are goblet cells found? What type of secretion do they produce?
5. In general, how are multicellular exocrine glands constructed?
6. Can you describe merocrine, apocrine, and holocrine glands? How do they differ from one another?
7. How are serous and mucous secretions different?

## CONNECTIVE TISSUE
### GENERAL CHARACTERISTICS

Connective tissue is found everywhere in the body and represents the most abundant tissue type by weight. Some organ systems, such as the skeletal and integumentary systems, are composed almost exclusively of connective tissue, whereas others, such as the neurologic system, contain very little. Connective tissue is derived from **mesoderm** and, unlike epithelial tissue, is composed primarily of nonliving extracellular matrix. The matrix surrounds and separates the cells, and it provides important structural and nutritional support that enables connective tissue cells to exist farther apart than epithelial cells. In addition, unlike epithelial tissue, which has no direct blood supply, connective tissue is **vascularized** although the level of vascularity varies among different connective tissue types. Loose connective tissue and **adipose connective tissue**, for example, possess good blood supplies, whereas dense connective tissue is poorly vascularized.

All connective tissue is composed of three distinct components: **extracellular fibers**, **ground substance**, and cells. The mixture of fiber and ground substance is called the **extracellular matrix**. Variations in the ground substance, fibers, and cellular components have given rise to a wide range of connective tissue types (Figure 5-16). Blood, tendon, fat, cartilage, and even bone are all examples of connective tissue, though their textures and appearances are different. Variations in the type of ground substance and in the type of fiber enable the tissue to take on many different qualities. It can be elastic and flexible, rigid, semisolid, or liquid. Blood, for example, is a highly cellular connective tissue with a liquid matrix containing relatively little fiber. In contrast, bone is composed of a solid **calcified** matrix. Tendon contains a matrix that is primarily fibrous with little ground substance. These variations give connective tissue the ability to withstand a wide range of forces, such as direct pressure, abrasion, and shearing forces that would destroy other tissue types.

As with all living structures, form and function are intertwined. Thus the plethora of forms that characterize connective tissue give rise to a wide range of functions. In general, as its name implies, connective tissue forms metabolic and structural connections between other tissues; however it serves many other important roles as well. For example, connective tissue forms a protective sheath around organs and helps insulate the body. It acts as a reserve for energy, provides the frame that supports the body, and composes the medium that transports substances from one region of the body to another. In addition, connective tissue plays a vital role in the healing process and in the control of invading microorganisms.

## COMPONENTS OF CONNECTIVE TISSUE

The major components of connective tissue are summarized in Box 5-1.

### GROUND SUBSTANCE

The **ground substance** in connective tissue is an **amorphous**, **homogeneous** material that ranges in texture from a liquid or gel to a calcified solid. In soft connective tissues, it

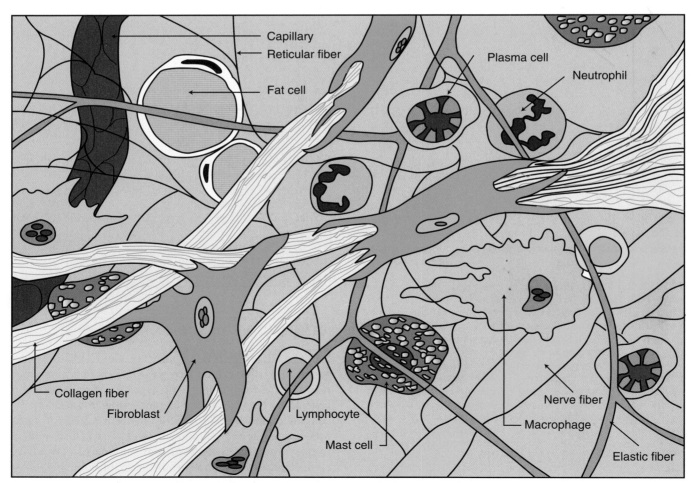

**FIGURE 5-16** Loose or areolar connective tissue. Loose or *areolar* tissue is a model-type of connective tissue because it contains all three types of fiber (elastic, collagen, and reticular) and a wide variety of cells (lymphocytes, mast cells, neutrophils, fibroblasts, adipocytes, and plasma cells) suspended in ground substance. These three components—fibers, cells, and ground substance—are found in varying amounts in all connective tissue.

**Ground Substance**
Ranges from liquid to gel to solid

**Fibers**
Collagenous
Reticular
Elastic

**Cells**
Fixed cells
    Fibroblasts
    Adipocytes (fat cells)
    Reticular cells
Wandering cells
    Mast cells
    Leukocytes (white blood cells)
    Macrophages (fixed and wandering)

is composed of unbranched chains of glycoproteins called **glycosaminoglycans (GAGs)**. The most commonly found GAG in connective tissue is hyaluronic acid combined with 2% protein. These large molecules help to orient the formation of fibers within the tissue.

Ground substance is the medium through which cells exchange nutrients and waste with the bloodstream. It acts as a shock-absorbing cushion and helps to protect the more delicate cells that it envelops. In addition, its thick texture serves as an effective obstacle for invading microorganisms, although some microbes have developed the ability to produce the enzyme hyaluronidase, which degrades hyaluronic acid and enables the **microbe** to move with greater ease through the tissue.

## FIBERS OF CONNECTIVE TISSUE

Connective tissue contains three types of fiber: *collagenous*, *reticular*, and *elastic*. Although these fibers exist in all connective tissue, their proportions vary from one type of connective tissue to another. Collagenous fibers are by far the most commonly found in the body.

**Collagenous fibers** are strong, thick strands composed of the structural protein collagen. Collagen fibers are organized into discrete bundles of long, parallel fibrils, which in turn are composed of bundled microfibrils. Because they possess tremendous tensile strength, enabling them to resist pulling forces, collagenous fibers are found in tendons and ligaments that are continually being pulled and stretched. When not under tension, collagenous fibers look wavy. The fiber itself is white, and the tissue it forms when the fibers are packed closely together is also white. Therefore it is not surprising that collagenous fibers are sometimes known as the *white fibers*.

The density and arrangement of collagen fibers can vary depending on the function of the tissue as a whole. Collagenous connective tissue can range from loose, as in the loose connective tissue that surrounds and protects organs, to

dense arrangements seen in tendons. The tissue forms when collagen proteins are secreted into the extracellular environment, where they are arranged into formation. If subjected to heat, collagen denatures and turns into a soft gel. This is why meat, which is rich with collagenous fibers, softens when cooked for long periods in soups and stews. At the same time, collagen can be fortified with tannic acid, as is evident in leather that has been strengthened by tanning.

**Reticular fibers**, like collagenous fibers, are composed of collagen, but they are not thick. Instead, they are thin, delicate, and branched into complicated networks. Reticular fibers form a kind of "mist net" (*rete* is Latin for *net*) that provides support for highly cellular organs, such as endocrine glands, lymph nodes, spleen, bone marrow, and liver. Reticular fibers are also found around blood vessels, nerves, muscle fibers, and capillaries.

**Elastic fibers** are composed primarily of the protein elastin. Like reticular fibers, elastic fibers are branched and form complex networks, but they lack the tensile strength of collagenous fibers. Elastic fibers are composed of bundles of microfibrils, and because they are coiled, they can stretch and contract like a rubber band. Therefore elastic fibers tend to occur in tissues that are commonly subjected to stretching, such as the vocal cords, lungs, skin, and walls of blood vessels. Because of their color, elastic fibers are sometimes referred to as the *yellow fibers*.

## MAJOR CELL TYPES

Although connective tissue contains a wide variety of cell types, they can be organized into two major categories: those that remain in the connective tissue, called *fixed cells*, and those that pass in and out of the connective tissue, called *transient cells*. Fixed cells remain in the connective tissue and are usually involved in the production and maintenance of the matrix. Transient cells, however, do not have a permanent residence in the tissue but move in and out of it as needed. Transient cells generally are involved in the repair and protection of the tissue.

*FIXED CELLS.* The most noteworthy **fixed cell** is the **fibroblast**. These are large, irregularly shaped cells that manufacture and secrete both the fibers and the ground substance characteristic of their particular matrix. Fibroblasts can reproduce and are metabolically very active. Each type of connective tissue is characterized by a predominant fibroblast. For example, cartilage contains **chondroblasts**, bone contains **osteoblasts**, and connective tissue contains fibroblasts. As the cells mature and the matrix is formed, the cells adopt a less active role. When this occurs, the name of the cell adopts the suffix -**cyte**, for example **chondrocyte**, **osteocyte**, or **fibrocyte**, depending on the tissue in which they are found. If additional matrix is required later, the cells can convert back to the -**blast** form.

Fat cells are found throughout connective tissue and are known as **adipose cells** or **adipocytes**. As young cells, adipocytes resemble fibroblasts, but as they mature, they fill with lipid and become swollen, with their nuclei pushed to one side. When adipocytes cluster into groups, they become a tissue in their own right, known as *adipose tissue*. Adipose tissue is found throughout the body but is particularly evident under the skin (particularly on the ventrum between the hind legs in cats), behind the eyes, around the kidneys, and in the omentum of the abdominal cavity.

**Reticular cells** are flat, star-shaped cells with long, outreaching arms that touch other cells, forming netlike connections throughout the tissue they compose. The function of reticular cells is debated, but most agree that they are involved in the immune response and in the manufacture of reticular fibers. It is not surprising therefore that reticular cells are found primarily in tissues that are part of the immune system, such as lymph nodes, spleen, and bone marrow.

**WANDERING CELLS.** There are many types of wandering cell that move in and out of connective tissue as needed. In this section, three common types of wandering cells are discussed: leukocytes, mast cells, and macrophages.

Commonly known as *white blood cells,* **leukocytes** are found in blood and move into connective tissue in large numbers during times of infection. Although they are relatively large and round compared to red blood cells, they can squeeze through the walls of tiny blood vessels to enter the surrounding tissue. This process is called **diapedesis**. Leukocytes are important members of the defensive immune system. There are five different types of leukocyte, but most protect the body by engulfing and digesting invading microbes. Other kinds, however, defend against infection by manufacturing antibodies that attach to microbes and destroy them.

**Mast cells** are oval cells that are easily identified by the large number of dark-staining granules stored in the cytoplasm. These granules contain **histamine** and **heparin**, potent biochemicals that initiate an inflammatory response when released into the tissue. Histamine increases blood flow to the area by making the capillaries leaky, and heparin prevents blood from clotting and ensures that the pathways for increased blood flow remain open. Mast cells tend to be found near blood vessels, where they can release their contents directly into the bloodstream and where they can most effectively guard against foreign proteins or microbes. When stimulated by the presence of these invaders, mast cells burst open, releasing hundreds of stored granules. This begins the complex events of allergic and inflammatory reactions, a process discussed in greater detail later in this chapter.

**Macrophages** are massive, irregularly shaped phagocytizing scavengers that may be either fixed or transient in connective tissue. They engulf microbes, dead cells, and debris that are subsequently digested in the macrophage's lysosomes. Mobile macrophages are drawn to sites of infection or inflammation, where they move aggressively through the affected area to engulf microinvaders. In this way, they are an important part of the immune system and help tissues fight infection. Macrophages are given different names

depending on the tissue. For example, they are called **Kupffer cells** in the liver, **microglial cells** in the brain, and **histiocytes** in loose connective tissue.

---

✓ *TEST YOURSELF 5-4*

1. How are connective tissue and epithelial tissue similar? How are they different?
2. What are the three basic constituents of connective tissue?
3. List seven functions of connective tissue.
4. What are GAGs and what role do they play in connective tissue? Why do you suppose animals with joint injuries are sometimes given dietary supplements of GAGs?
5. Compare and contrast collagenous, reticular, and elastic fibers.
6. What are fibroblasts and what role do they play in connective tissue?
7. Can you give three examples of cells that are transient in connective tissue? Can you describe their form and function?

---

## TYPES OF CONNECTIVE TISSUE

As already mentioned, all connective tissue is made up of three major components:

- Ground substance
- Cells
- Fibers

Many different types of connective tissue are formed by the variety of textures of ground substance, the number and type of cells, and the number and type of fibers present in the tissue. By varying the three major constituents, a wide range of connective tissue types is generated.

In general, connective tissue is divided into two broad categories: **connective tissue proper** and **specialized connective tissue**.

### CONNECTIVE TISSUE PROPER

*Connective tissue proper* is the largest classification and contains every subtype of connective tissue except bone, cartilage, and blood. The two subclasses of connective tissue proper are *loose connective tissue* and *dense connective tissue*. **Loose connective tissue** includes *areolar, adipose,* and *reticular* tissue; **dense connective tissue** includes *dense regular, dense irregular,* and *elastic* tissue.

### LOOSE CONNECTIVE TISSUE

*AREOLAR TISSUE.* **Areolar connective tissue** is a beautiful tangle of randomly placed fibers and cells suspended in a thick, translucent ground substance (Figure 5-17). The tissue appears relaxed with a myriad of round and star-shaped cells placed among crisscrossing fibers. The predominant cell is the fibroblast, a large spindle-shaped cell that manufactures the elastic, reticular, and collagenous fibers found throughout the tissue. Areolar tissue acquires its name from the Latin *areola,* which means *small, open space.*

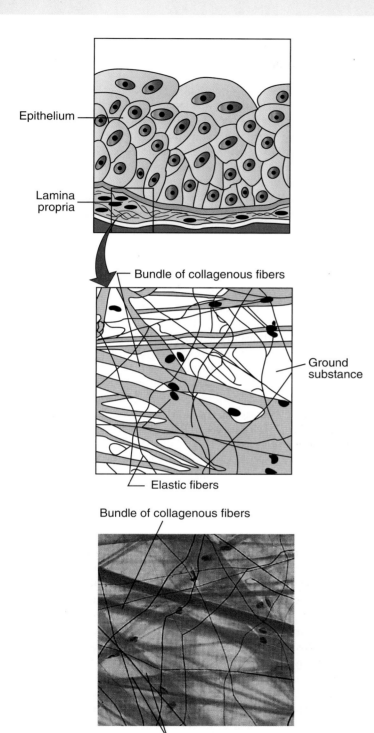

Epithelium

Lamina propria

Bundle of collagenous fibers

Ground substance

Elastic fibers

Bundle of collagenous fibers

Elastic fibers

**FIGURE 5-17** Loose or areolar connective tissue. *Description:* Loose array of fibers suspended in gel-like ground substance. Includes all three types of fiber and many cells, such as macrophages, fibroblasts, mast cells, and some white blood cells. *Location:* Throughout the body, under epithelial basement membranes; between glands, muscles, and nerves; surrounding capillaries and many organs. It is also found under skin and helps to attach it to underlying tissues. *Function:* Provides nutrients to tissues that it surrounds and supports. Important as a loose packing material. *Microanatomy:* Photomicrograph and sketch of loose areolar tissue, which serves as soft padding for many organs. The staining turns the collagen fibers pink and the elastin fibers purple. (Courtesy Ed Reschke.)

Areolar tissue is the most common type of connective tissue and is found everywhere in the body. It acts generally as packing material to support and cushion organs and other delicate structures of the body. It surrounds every organ; forms the subcutaneous layer that connects skin to muscle; envelops blood vessels, nerves, and lymph nodes; and is present in all mucous membranes as the **lamina propria** and submucosa. It is supportive to body structures but is flexible and soft to enable organs the freedom to move within their position. Thus areolar tissue is moderately elastic but tears easily compared with the other types of connective tissue.

The small, open spaces in areolar tissue are filled with a mixture of body fluids and ground substance. The ground substance is thick and is composed primarily of **hyaluronic acid**, which serves as a medium through which nutrients, gases, and waste can be easily transported to and from the bloodstream. In addition, the viscous texture of the ground substance is an effective barrier against most invading microorganisms, because it inhibits their movement through the tissue. Some white blood cells have developed the ability to produce **hyaluronidase**, an enzyme that liquefies the matrix and allows white blood cells to pass through with greater ease. This adaptation has improved the ability of white blood cells to perform their duties in loose connective tissue. Unfortunately, some microbes have also developed the ability to produce hyaluronidase, which facilitates the spread of infection throughout the tissue.

During trauma or other pathologic states, the spaces in loose connective tissue can fill with an excessive amount of body fluid. This condition is called **edema**, and the connective tissue is said to be *edematous*. You can see this condition in cats that have a swollen paw caused by an insect bite or in dogs that have fractured a bone in their leg. Sometimes, the edema will remain compressed in an area after pressing on it with your thumb. This is called **pitting edema** because the tissue, rather than springing back after being compressed, leaves impressions or pits in the tissue.

*ADIPOSE TISSUE.* **Adipose** tissue is commonly known as *fat*. It is areolar tissue in which adipocytes or fat cells predominate (Figure 5-18). Adipose tissue is found beneath the skin, in spaces between muscles, behind the eyeballs, on the surface of the heart, surrounding the joints, in bone marrow, and in the omentum of the abdomen. Its cells expand and wither depending on the amount of lipid that is being stored within them. Not surprisingly, the rate of lipid storage and use is based on the amount of calories being consumed by the animal relative to the amount of energy exerted. In addition the sympathetic nervous system, certain hormones, and genetic influences may also profoundly affect fat metabolism. Adipose tissue is highly vascularized so that the lipid droplets contained within adipocytes are accessible to the enzymes responsible for triglyceride breakdown and to a bloodstream that readily transports the glycerol and free fatty acid products to other parts of the body. Thus adipose tissue represents an important energy store for animals. It also acts as a thermal insulator under the skin, prevents heat

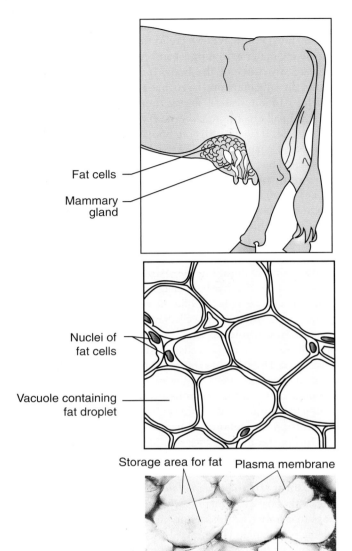

Fat cells

Mammary gland

Nuclei of fat cells

Vacuole containing fat droplet

Storage area for fat    Plasma membrane

Nucleus of adipose cell

**FIGURE 5-18** Adipose tissue. *Description:* Adipose tissue is fat. The tissue has little extracellular material and is composed primarily of closely packed adipocytes filled with lipid. The nucleus is pushed to the periphery of each cell to accommodate sizable lipid stores. *Location:* Throughout the body, under skin, around heart and kidneys, within mesenteries and omentum, and around the colon. *Function:* Thermoinsulator; protects organs and other tissues it surrounds. *Microanatomy:* Photomicrograph and sketch of adipose tissue, which is composed of fat cells. Notice that the nuclei of the cells are pushed to the perimeter as the cytoplasm fills with triglyceride (fat). (Photomicrograph from Dennis Strete.)

eccentrically placed nuclei. As the cells swell, the cytosol is compressed into a thin, barely visible rim that surrounds the lipid droplet. Despite the compact condition of the cytoplasm, it continues to house all of the organelles normally found in cells. During tissue preparation for microscopic examination, the lipid content of the adipocyte is extracted, leaving a large unstained space in the center of the cell. This, combined with the densely cellular nature of adipose tissue, lends itself to the chicken-wire appearance that is evident microscopically.

**Brown adipose tissue** is found in newborn animals and in animals that **hibernate** during the winter. It is a highly specialized form of adipose tissue and plays an important part in temperature regulation, because it is a site of heat production. In brown fat, as in white adipose tissue, the nucleus is eccentrically placed; however the cytoplasm in brown fat is clearly visible, and lipid is stored in multiple small vesicles rather than in a single large droplet. The energy derived from the oxidation of lipids and released from electron transport is dissipated as *heat* in brown fat, rather than adenosine triphosphate (ATP). For this reason, brown fat contains an exceptionally high number of mitochondria (the site of electron transport), which become darkly stained in the cytoplasm. This dark coloration gives brown fat its name. Brown fat is also more vascular than white fat and this rich vascular network helps to dissipate the heat to many areas of the body. In this way, neonatal animals and hibernating animals can generate enough body heat during the vulnerable periods after birth and during the winter to survive. Histologically, brown fat looks glandular and therefore is sometimes called the **hibernating gland**.

*RETICULAR CONNECTIVE TISSUE.* **Reticular connective tissue** is composed of a complex, three-dimensional network of thin reticular fibers (Figure 5-19). It resembles areolar connective tissue in that it contains loosely arranged fibers and many fibroblasts suspended in a supportive ground substance. Unlike areolar connective tissue, however, reticular connective tissue contains only one type of fiber: *reticular fibers.* Together, the cellular and matrix components form a network called **stroma**, which constitutes the framework of several organs, such as the liver, spleen, lymph nodes, and bone marrow. Although reticular fibers are found throughout the body, reticular connective tissue is found in a limited number of sites.

## DENSE FIBROUS CONNECTIVE TISSUE

**Dense fibrous connective tissue** is characterized by its densely packed arrangement of collagen fibers. Because little room is available for ground substance and cells, these are found in smaller quantities than in loose connective tissue. Nevertheless, as in loose connective tissue, fibroblasts can be found intermingled with fibers, where they play out their important role of manufacturing fibers and ground substance. The three major types of *dense fibrous connective tissue* are *dense regular, dense irregular,* and *elastic.*

loss from the body, and acts as a mechanical shock absorber around organs, such as the kidneys.

The two main types of adipose tissue are *white adipose tissue* and *brown adipose tissue.* **White adipose tissue** is found throughout the body, particularly in the deep layers of the skin. Initially, white adipocytes resemble fibroblasts, but as they fill with lipid, the organelles and nuclei are pushed to one side and the cells become large spheres with

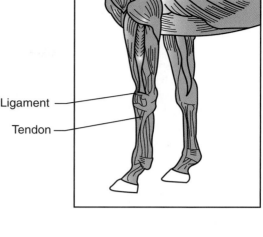

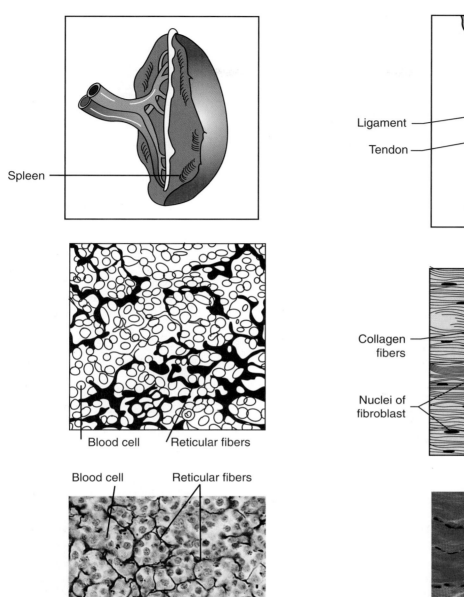

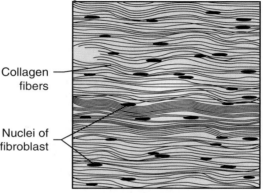

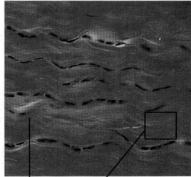

**FIGURE 5-19** Reticular connective tissue. *Description:* Reticular cells supported by a fine network of irregularly arranged reticular fibers. *Location:* Spleen, lymph nodes, and bone marrow. *Function:* Provides internal skeleton for hematopoietic and lymphatic tissue. *Microanatomy:* Photomicrograph and sketch of reticular fibers, which stain darkly. They surround and support cells in the spleen. (Courtesy Ed Reschke.)

**FIGURE 5-20** Dense regular connective tissue. *Description:* Primarily parallel collagen fibers. Occasional fibroblast interspersed among the fibers. *Location:* Tendons and ligaments. Tendons attach muscle to bone, and ligaments attach bones to one another. *Function:* Resists strong pulling forces. Has great capacity for stretch resistance in the direction of the fibers. *Microanatomy:* Photomicrograph and sketch of dense regular connective tissue in the tendon of a horse. Notice that the collagen fibers are arranged in parallel, tight bundles. (Courtesy Phototake.)

**DENSE REGULAR CONNECTIVE TISSUE. Dense regular connective tissue** is composed of tightly packed, parallel collagen fibers (Figure 5-20). The fibers lie in the direction of the force that is exerted on them, thereby giving the overall tissue tremendous tensile strength, but only in one direction. Dense regular connective tissue is silvery or white. It is relatively avascular and therefore is very slow to heal, because restorative nutrients and building molecules have difficulty reaching the damaged tissue. Fibroblasts form rows along the crowded fibers and devote most of their energy to the manufacture of fibers. Little ground substance is produced.

Dense connective tissue makes up the tendons that attach muscles to bone and the ligaments that hold bones together at joints. It also composes the broad, fibrous ribbons that sometimes cover muscles or connect them to other structures. In addition, dense connective tissue can be found in fascial sheets that cover muscles. These sheets are stacked into layers, one on top of another, but the direction of the fibers in one fascial layer may be different from the direction of the fibers in another layer. This helps to create an overall structure or **fascia** that can withstand forces from more than one direction.

### DENSE IRREGULAR CONNECTIVE TISSUE.

**Dense irregular connective tissue** is composed primarily of collagen fibers that are arranged in thicker bundles than those found in dense regular connective tissue (Figure 5-21). The fibers are interwoven randomly to form a single sheet that can withstand forces from many different directions. It is found in the **dermis** of the skin and in the fibrous coverings of organs such as the kidney, testes, liver, and spleen. It also forms the tough capsule of joints.

### ELASTIC CONNECTIVE TISSUE.

Ligaments can stretch more than tendons because of the larger number of elastic fibers contained within them. The massive nuchal ligament in the neck of horses, for example, has a particularly high concentration of elastic fibers and is therefore extremely flexible, enabling horses to lower their heads for long periods while grazing. Dense connective tissue that is primarily composed of elastic fibers, rather than collagen fibers, is called **elastic connective tissue**.

Elastic connective tissue is found in relatively few regions of the body, such as in the spaces between vertebrae in the backbone. It also occurs in regions of the body that require stretching, such as in the walls of arteries, stomach, large airways (bronchi), bladder, and regions of the heart. It lies beneath the transitional epithelium in the urinary tract and in the ligament suspending the penis. As its name implies, elastic connective tissue consists primarily of yellow elastic fibers. These fibers may be arranged in parallel or in an interwoven pattern with fibroblasts and collagenous fibers interspersed.

### SPECIALIZED CONNECTIVE TISSUE

**CARTILAGE.** **Cartilage** is a tough, specialized connective tissue that is commonly called **gristle**. It is more rigid than dense connective tissue but is more flexible than bone (Figure 5-22). Cartilage is found in joints and helps to prevent the sensitive outer layers of bone from rubbing against one another. Because cartilage does not contain nerves, it can tolerate a great deal of compression without causing pain to the animal. (Imagine the compressive forces in the legs of an elephant!) In addition to joints, cartilage is found in the ear, nose, and vocal cords and forms a vital framework on which bone is formed in growing animals.

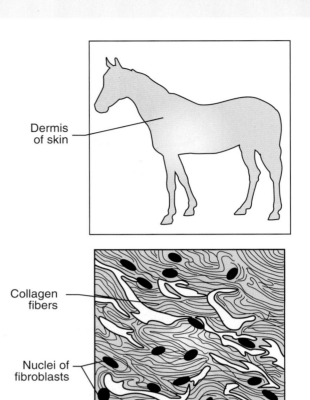

Dermis of skin

Collagen fibers

Nuclei of fibroblasts

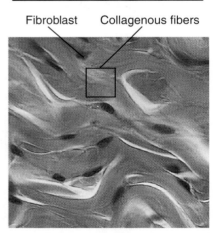

Fibroblast    Collagenous fibers

**FIGURE 5-21** Dense irregular connective tissue. *Description:* Sheets of collagen that run in different directions or sheets of parallel fibers stacked in alternating directions. *Location:* Dermis of skin, organ capsules, submucosa of digestive tract. *Function:* Designed to withstand pulling forces in all directions. *Microanatomy:* Photomicrograph and sketch of dense irregular connective tissue found in the dermis of a cat. Notice that the pink collagen fibers and dark purple staining fibroblast cell nuclei are arranged in a swirling pattern. (Courtesy Ed Reschke.)

Like other forms of connective tissue, cartilage is composed of cells and matrix. The cells, called **chondrocytes**, live in hollowed-out pockets in the matrix, called **lacunae**. The ground substance of the matrix is a firm gel containing two different types of glycosaminoglycans (**chondroitin sulfate** and hyaluronic acid) and an adhesion protein called **chondronectin**. It also contains an unexpectedly large amount of tissue fluid. The fluid is held within the matrix and is

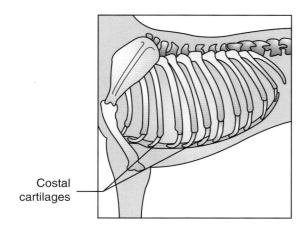

Costal
cartilages

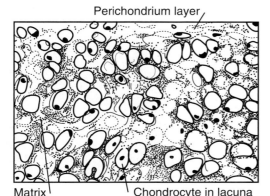

Perichondrium layer

Matrix    Chondrocyte in lacuna

Perichondrium layer

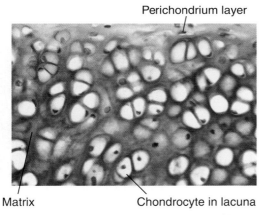

Matrix    Chondrocyte in lacuna

**FIGURE 5-22** Hyaline cartilage. *Description:* Collagen fibers are evenly distributed throughout a rigid matrix. Cartilage cells or chondrocytes sit in spaces within the matrix called *lacunae*. *Location:* Articulating surfaces of bones; costal cartilages of ribs; cartilages in nose, trachea, and larynx; most of embryonic skeleton. *Function:* Provides both structural rigidity and flexibility simultaneously. Cushions joints against compressive forces. *Microanatomy:* Photomicrograph and sketch of hyaline cartilage from the chondral region of the sternum in a horse. (Courtesy Robert Calentine.)

important in transporting nutrients to the chondrocytes. It also gives cartilage its flexible resiliency and its ability to withstand compression. Collagen fibers are most commonly found in the matrix, but elastic fibers are also present in varying amounts.

Cartilage is avascular and therefore is very slow to heal. It receives its nutrition from a surrounding membrane, called the **perichondrium**, which is rich in tiny blood vessels. Nutrients diffuse from the perichondrium through the matrix to the chondrocytes. Therefore the chondrocytes that are farthest away from the perichondrium are potentially less well nourished than cells closer to it. For this reason, the thickness of cartilage is limited.

Three types of cartilage that vary from one another on the basis of the type of fiber found in the matrix are *hyaline cartilage, elastic cartilage,* and *fibrocartilage.*

*HYALINE CARTILAGE.* **Hyaline cartilage** is the most common type of cartilage found in the body. It is composed of closely packed collagen fibers that make it tough but more flexible than bone. Grossly, hyaline cartilage resembles blue–white, frosted, ground glass. It is found as **articular cartilage** at the ends of long bones in joints and connects the ribs to the sternum. In addition, it forms supportive rings in the trachea and composes most of the embryonic skeleton. In growing animals, it is found in the growth plates of long bones, where it supports continued bone development and the extension of the length of the bone. Hyaline cartilage is the most rigid type of cartilage and is enclosed within a perichondrium.

*ELASTIC CARTILAGE.* Histologically, **elastic cartilage** is similar to hyaline cartilage but contains a plethora of elastic fibers, which form dense, branching bundles that appear black microscopically (Figure 5-23). These fibers give elastic cartilage tremendous flexibility so that it can withstand repeated bending. Elastic cartilage is found in the epiglottis of the larynx and in the pinnae (external ears) of animals.

*FIBROCARTILAGE.* **Fibrocartilage** usually is found merged with hyaline cartilage and dense connective tissue (Figure 5-24). It contains thick bundles of collagen fibers, like hyaline cartilage, but it has fewer chondrocytes and lacks a perichondrium. Fibrocartilage is particularly well designed to take compression and therefore is found in the spaces between vertebrae of the spine, between bones in the pelvic girdle, and in the knee joint.

*BONE.* Bone or *osseous connective tissue* is the hardest and most rigid type of connective tissue (Figure 5-25). Its specialized matrix is a combination of organic collagen fibers and inorganic calcium salts, such as calcium phosphate and calcium carbonate. The calcium salts alone would render bone brittle, but when combined with collagen fibers, bone becomes more flexible and has greater strength.

Despite the rigidity of its matrix, bone, unlike cartilage, is well vascularized. A central **Haversian canal** contains both a vascular and a nerve supply. In addition, tiny channels exist within the matrix that support the passage of blood vessels into deeper portions of the tissue. Bone cells, such as **osteoblasts** and **osteoclasts**, collaborate to remodel bone in response to the stresses placed on them. This involves a

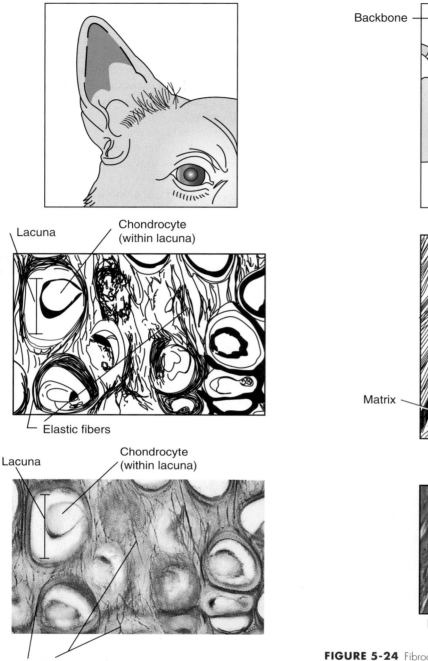

**FIGURE 5-23** *Elastic cartilage. Description:* Elastic fibers suspended in firm matrix. Chondrocytes arranged in lacunae. *Location:* External ear (pinna), auditory tubes, and epiglottis. *Function:* Provides support and even more flexibility than hyaline cartilage. *Microanatomy:* Photomicrograph and sketch of elastic cartilage of the canine ear. Notice the chondrocytes situated within the lacunae and surrounded by a matrix filled with elastic fibers. (Courtesy Ed Reschke.)

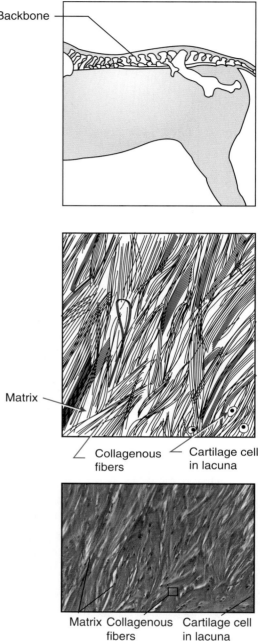

**FIGURE 5-24** Fibrocartilage. *Description:* Similar to hyaline cartilage, but collagen fibers are more numerous and are arranged in thicker bundles. The matrix is less firm. *Location:* Pubic symphysis, intervertebral discs, discs in stifle and knee joints. Also found in temporomandibular joint of jaw. *Function:* Withstands compressive forces. *Microanatomy:* Photomicrograph and sketch of fibrocartilage from the spine of a horse. Notice that the strong, dense fibers are good at absorbing shock, particularly in the direction of the fibers. (Courtesy Robert Calentine.)

well-orchestrated combination of laying down new bone and taking away bone that is not needed. Osteoblasts, like other fibroblasts, manufacture the fibers that are part of the matrix. Although mature osteocytes reside individually in chambers called *lacunae*, they possess long, cellular

extensions that pass through tiny threadlike channels called **canaliculi**, which radiate away from the lacunae. These chambers and canals are created as the osteoblasts surround themselves with the bony matrix they manufacture. Later they mature to become osteocytes. In this way, the cells not

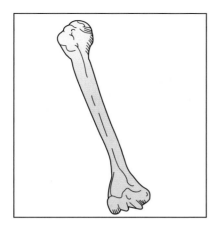

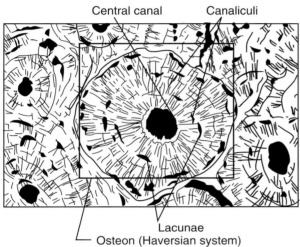

Central canal   Canaliculi

Lacunae
Osteon (Haversian system)

Canaliculi   Osteon (Haversian system)   Central canal

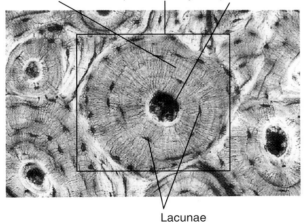

Lacunae

**FIGURE 5-25** Compact bone. *Description:* Hard matrix dominates this tissue and is organized into concentric rings that surround a central canal. Chambers called *lacunae* and tunnels called *canaliculi* form spaces in hard matrix to accommodate bone cells (osteocytes) and their long cytoplasmic projections. *Location:* Bones of skeleton. *Function:* Provides support and protection; blood is produced in bone marrow; provides storage depot for calcium and other types of minerals. *Microanatomy:* Photomicrograph and sketch of compact bone. Notice the osteocytes located in lacunae within the Haversian canal system. (Courtesy Phototake.)

only create their own living spaces but also maintain connections with other cells.

Bone forms the skeletal frame of animals. It protects vital organs, such as the brain and heart, and acts as a calcium reserve for the body. In addition, bone marrow is the site of blood cell production and fat storage. A discussion of the development, structure, and function of bone is found in Chapter 7.

**BLOOD.** The red fluid that passes through vessels and that carries nutrient molecules and gases throughout the body is the most atypical connective tissue (Figure 5-26). The liquid component of blood is called **plasma** and constitutes the matrix. The fibrous component of the matrix is an array of protein molecules suspended in solution and visible only when blood clots. Blood is rich with a variety of cell types, such as **erythrocytes** (red blood cells), **leukocytes** (white blood cells), and **thrombocytes**, also known as **platelets**. Blood is discussed in greater detail in Chapter 12.

Table 5-2 summarizes the organization of connective tissue.

> ✓ *TEST YOURSELF 5-5*
> 1. Connective tissue is divided into two broad categories. What are they?
> 2. What are the components of areolar tissue?
> 3. What is the common term for adipose tissue?
> 4. In terms of its form and function, how is brown fat different from white fat?
> 5. What are three subtypes of dense connective tissue?
> 6. Give three examples of specialized connective tissue. How are they similar to connective tissue proper? How are they different?
> 7. Why is cartilage limited in thickness and slow to heal?
> 8. Describe three types of cartilage. What are their differences and similarities?
> 9. Even though blood and bone appear to be grossly different, they both represent types of connective tissue. Why?

## MEMBRANES

Epithelial and connective tissue may be collaboratively linked to form membranes in the body. Membranes are thin, protective layers that line body cavities, separate organs, and cover surfaces. They are composed of a multicellular epithelial sheet that is bound to an underlying layer of connective tissue proper. Commonly, the epithelium is bathed in a wet solution of liquid mucus or in the case of the bladder, in urine. Four common types of epithelial membranes are *mucous, serous, cutaneous,* and *synovial* (Figures 5-27 and 5-28, Table 5-3).

### MUCOUS MEMBRANES

**Mucous membranes,** or **mucosae,** are characterized by their position in the body, because they are always found

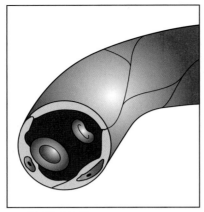

Erythrocyte

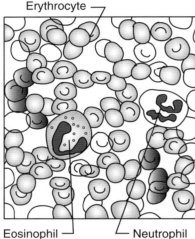

Eosinophil —        ⌐ Neutrophil

Erythrocyte

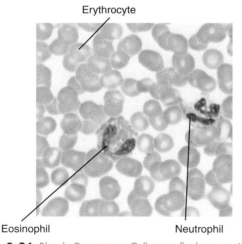

Eosinophil                    Neutrophil

**FIGURE 5-26** Blood. *Description:* Cells in a fluid matrix. *Location:* Found in blood vessels and heart. *Function:* Carries oxygen and nutrients to tissues; transports waste products and gases for disposal. *Microanatomy:* Photomicrograph and sketch of a blood smear. Notice that mature red blood cells (erythrocytes) have no nuclei and are biconcave. They appear lighter in their center where they are thinner. White blood cells (leukocytes) are larger than erythrocytes and have dark-staining nuclei. The leukocyte with the large pink granules in the cytoplasm is called an *eosinophil* and the other one is called a *neutrophil.* (From Thibodeau GA, Patton KT: Anatomy & physiology, ed 6, St Louis, 2007, Mosby.)

lining the organs that have connections to the outside environment. These organs are part of the digestive, respiratory, urinary, and reproductive tracts and include the mouth, esophagus, stomach, intestines, colon, nasal passages, trachea, bladder, and uterus, to name a few. The epithelial layer in mucous membranes is usually composed of either stratified squamous or simple columnar epithelium, and it covers a layer of loose connective tissue called the **lamina propria**. Another connective tissue layer, called the **submucosa**, usually connects the mucosa to underlying structures.

With the exception of the mucosae of the urinary tract, mucosae in general can produce large quantities of protective and lubricating mucus. Goblet cells or multicellular glands may be found throughout the tissue. These structures are responsible for the production and secretion of mucus, which consists primarily of water, electrolytes, and a protein called **mucin**. The mucus is slippery and therefore can decrease friction and assist with the passage of food or waste. Because of its rich supply of antibodies and viscous consistency, the mucus produced by the mucosae is also helpful in the entrapment and disposal of invading pathogens and foreign particles. This is particularly apparent in the nasal passages, where microorganisms and debris are inhaled and trapped by mucus. We may find, for example, accumulations of black debris in our noses after we have been near a sooty campfire. When we have a cold, we find that the amount of mucus produced and secreted by the mucosae increases and a runny nose develops.

Some mucosae can absorb as well as secrete. For example, the epithelial layer in the intestine is specially designed for rapid and efficient transfer of nutrient molecules from the intestinal lumen to the underlying connective tissue and its blood supply. The mucous membranes therefore play an important role in monitoring and controlling what enters the body and form an important barrier between the outside environment and the delicate inner workings of underlying tissues. Their secretory and absorptive qualities make them particularly well suited for this role.

### SEROUS MEMBRANES

**Serous membranes** are also called **serosae**. They line the walls and cover the organs that fill closed body cavities, such as the chest cavity or thorax and the abdominal and pelvic cavities (see Figures 5-27 and 5-28). Serosa is characterized as a continuous sheet that is doubled over to form two layers with a narrow space in between. The portion of the membrane that lines the cavity wall is called the **parietal layer**, and the portion that covers the outer surfaces of the organs is called the **visceral layer**.

The serosa is composed of a sheet of simple squamous epithelium bound to an underlying layer of loose connective tissue. This histologic organization allows a great deal of permeability and enables interstitial fluid to pass through the membrane into the narrow spaces between the serosal layers. In this way, serosal fluid is a **transudate** and, unlike the mucoid thick secretion of mucous membranes,

| TABLE 5-2 | Types of Connective Tissue | | |
|---|---|---|---|
| **TYPE** | **TISSUE** | **LOCATION** | **FUNCTION** |
| **Connective Tissue Proper** | | | |
| Loose connective tissue | Areolar<br> | Between other tissues and organs<br>Superficial fascia | Connection |
| | Adipose (fat)<br> | Under skin. Padding at various points | Protection, insulation, support, food reserve, regulation of other tissues |
| | Reticular<br> | Inner framework of spleen, lymph nodes, bone marrow | Support, filtration, blood production, immunity |
| Dense connective tissue | Dense regular<br> | Tendons, ligaments, aponeuroses | Flexible but strong connection |
| | Dense irregular<br> | Deep fascia, dermis, scars, capsule of kidney, spleen lymph nodes, and so on | Connection, support |
| | Elastic<br> | Walls of some arteries | Flexible, elastic support |

*Continued*

| TABLE 5-2 | Types of Connective Tissue—cont'd | | |
|---|---|---|---|
| **TYPE** | **TISSUE** | **LOCATION** | **FUNCTION** |
| **Specialized Connective Tissue** | | | |
| Cartilage | Hyaline cartilage | Part of nasal septum, covering articular surfaces of bones larynx, rings in trachea and bronchi | Firm but flexible support; connection between structures; resistant to compression, but flexible; protects the ends of long bones in synovial joints; found in the stifle, hip, elbow, and shoulder |
| | Elastic cartilage | External ear, Eustachian or auditory tube | Highly flexible cartilage found in tissues the require regular bending such as the nose and pinna |
| | Fibrocartilage | Discs between vertebrae, pubic symphysis | Tough inflexible cartilage that resists compressive forces and protects underlying bone |
| Bone | Compact Skeleton (outer shell of bone) | | Support, protection, calcium reservoir |
| **Tissue** | | | |
| Bone | Cancellous Skeleton (inside bones) | Found inside various bones and particularly abundant inside the ends of long bones | Provides framework for blood production |
| Blood | In blood vessels | In blood vessels and capillaries | Transportation, hydration, immunity and defense |

(Images from Patton KT, Thibodeau GA: Anatomy & physiology, ed 8, St Louis, 2013, Mosby.)

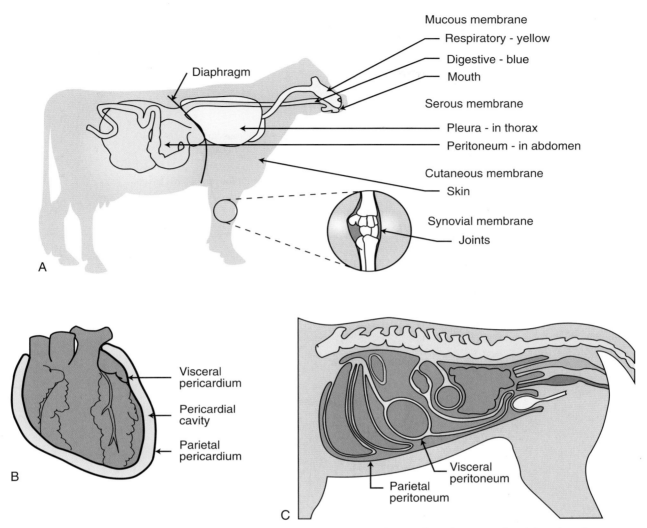

**FIGURE 5-27** Types of membrane. **A,** Mucous, serous, cutaneous, and synovial membranes are found throughout the body. *Mucous* membranes line body cavities that are exposed to the outside, such as the anus, mouth, and nares. Membranes often contain glands, which secrete mucus. *Serous* membranes line body cavities that have no connection with the outside. Although they do not contain glands, they secrete serous fluid, which helps lubricate and prevent adhesions within body cavities. The *cutaneous* membrane is the dermis, or skin, which covers the outer region of the body. *Synovial* membranes line cavities that surround joints. **B,** The heart is covered by a serous membrane called the *pericardium*. The pericardium folds back on itself, forming two layers with a space or cavity in between. The layer closest to the heart is called *visceral pericardium,* whereas the outer layer is called the *parietal pericardium.* **C,** The serous membrane in the abdominal cavity is called the **peritoneum**. Visceral peritoneum covers organs, and parietal peritoneum lines the peritoneal, or abdominal, cavity.

is thin and watery. It contains electrolytes but no mucin. By coating the parietal and visceral layers, serosal fluid creates a moist and slippery surface, which reduces friction between adjacent organs and between the organs and the cavity wall. Transudates take on different names depending on where they are located in the body. A transudate in the thorax, for example, is called **pleural fluid**; in the abdomen, **peritoneal fluid**; and in the region around the heart, **pericardial fluid**.

The consistency of serous fluid may vary and change in pathologic conditions. For example, if an animal fractures a rib, blood cells and fluid may leak from ruptured capillaries into the pleural space, creating a **hemothorax.** When cells, protein, and other solid material mix with serous fluid, it becomes denser than a transudate and is called an **exudate**.

Normally, the amount of serous fluid found in body cavities is small, but during trauma or some pathologic conditions, such as in hemothorax, the amount of fluid may become excessive. When an abnormally large amount of fluid enters a body cavity, the fluid is known as an **effusion**. **Ascites**, for example, is the presence of an effusion in the peritoneal space of the abdominopelvic cavity and can be caused by a wide range of pathologic conditions, such as congestive heart failure, **nephrosis**, malignant neoplastic disease, and **peritonitis**.

When the serous membranes are damaged, production of serous fluid may be impeded and abnormal connections called *adhesions* may form between the parietal and visceral layers. These connections may alter the normal function of the organs involved and can cause excruciating discomfort

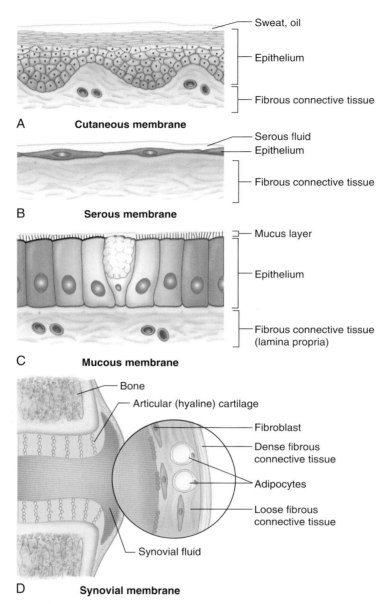

A    **Cutaneous membrane**

— Sweat, oil

— Epithelium

— Fibrous connective tissue

B    **Serous membrane**

— Serous fluid
— Epithelium

— Fibrous connective tissue

C    **Mucous membrane**

— Mucus layer

— Epithelium

— Fibrous connective tissue (lamina propria)

D    **Synovial membrane**

— Bone
— Articular (hyaline) cartilage
— Fibroblast
— Dense fibrous connective tissue
— Adipocytes
— Loose fibrous connective tissue
— Synovial fluid

**FIGURE 5-28** Structure of membranes. Epithelial membranes (contain epithelium): **A,** Cutaneous membrane (skin); **B,** serous membrane (serosa: "pleura" in the thoracic cavity, "peritoneum" in the abdominal cavity); and **C,** mucous membrane (mucosa: epithelium that lines body orifices). Connective tissue membranes (do not contain epithelium): **D,** synovial membrane (line mobile joints and bursae, produce synovial fluid). (From Patton KT, Thibodeau GA: Anatomy & physiology, ed 8, St Louis, 2013, Mosby.)

to the patient, particularly if the adhesions occur in the pleural space of the thoracic cavity.

In the abdominopelvic cavity, the visceral layers of serosa merge to form supportive ligaments called *mesenteries*. These ligaments secure organs to the body wall and form a framework for the passage of blood vessels and nerves. The stomach, for example, is connected to the abdominal wall by mesentery called the **omentum**, and the uterus is similarly attached via the **broad ligament**.

## CUTANEOUS MEMBRANES

The **cutaneous membrane** is also called the **integument**, or, more simply, *skin*. It is an organ that is perpetually exposed to the outside environment and therefore possesses unique features that distinguish it from the other membrane types. It is composed of an outer **keratinized stratified squamous epithelium**, or **epidermis**. **Keratin** is a waxy substance that fills the cells of the **epidermal** layer as they make their developmental migration from the basement membrane to the outermost layer. It is responsible for the waterproof quality of skin and aids in the prevention of desiccation. Keratinized squamous epithelium is also durable and is partly responsible for the skin's ability to withstand abrasive forces.

The epidermis is attached to an underlying layer of dense irregular connective tissue called the **dermis**. The

| TABLE 5-3 | Membranes in Animals | | | | | |
|---|---|---|---|---|---|
| **TYPE** | **SUPERFICIAL LAYER** | **DEEP LAYER** | **LOCATION** | **FLUID SECRETION** | **FUNCTION** |
| **Epithelial** | | | | | |
| **Cutaneous**<br>Example:<br>Integument | Keratinized stratified squamous epithelium (epidermis) | Dense irregular fibrous connective tissue (dermis) | Directly exposed to external environment | Sweat; sebum (skin oil) | Protection, sensation, thermoregulation |
| **Serous**<br>Examples:<br>Lining of thorax (plura) and abdomen (peritoneum) | Simple squamous epithelium | Fibrous connective tissue | Lines body cavities that are not open to the external environment | Serous fluid | Lubrication |
| **Mucous**<br>Examples:<br>Gums, vulva, and anus | Various types of epithelium | Fibrous connective tissue (lamina propria) | Lines tracts that open to the external environment | Mucus | Protection, Lubrication |
| **Connective** | | | | | |
| **Synovial**<br>Examples:<br>Lining of knee, elbow, and shoulder joints | Dense fibrous connective tissue | Loose fibrous connective tissue (in movable joints) | Lines joint cavities lubricates, cushions | Synovial fluid | Helps hold joint together |

From Patton KT, Thibodeau GA: Anatomy & physiology, ed 8, St Louis, 2013, Mosby.

dermis is rich in collagenous, reticular, and elastic fibers, which enable skin to be both strong and elastic. The structural and functional properties of skin are discussed further in Chapter 6.

## SYNOVIAL MEMBRANES

**Synovial membranes** line the cavities of joints. Unlike the other membrane types, synovial membranes have no epithelium. They are composed exclusively of connective tissue. Grossly, the synovial membrane is smooth, shiny, and white. Histologically, the membrane is composed of loose connective tissue and adipose tissue covered by a layer of collagen fibers and fibroblasts. Synovial membranes manufacture the synovial fluid that fills the joint spaces and, together with hyaline cartilage, reduces friction and abrasion at the ends of the bones.

## CLINICAL APPLICATION

Mucous Membranes: Keys to a Diagnosis

When animals are sick, they show signs of illness in many ways. We know that they may become depressed and lethargic. They may stop eating and drinking, may vomit, have diarrhea or bloody urine, or stop urinating entirely. Animals may show signs of illness through changes in the appearance of their mucous membranes. The easiest mucous membranes to examine are those located on the inside of the mouth and on the gums. Here, a veterinarian or veterinary technician can gain clues about the general state of the animal. For example, dehydrated animals have dry, tacky mucous membranes. Animals with wet mouths are less likely to be dehydrated.

The *color* of mucous membranes is also very important. A yellow tinge, for example, may indicate elevation of bilirubin in the blood. This condition is known as **icterus**, and the yellow appearance of an animal is called **jaundice**. There are many causes of increased levels of bilirubin, such as liver failure and **hemolytic anemia**. For this reason, additional tests are needed to determine the cause of the jaundice. Blue mucous membranes occur in animals that cannot provide their tissues with adequate amounts of oxygen. These animals develop a condition called **hypoxia** (*hypo* meaning *below* [normal] and *oxia* meaning *oxygen*). Animals with tracheal obstruction, severe pneumonia, or circulatory collapse may all show signs of hypoxia. Bright red mucous membranes may be evident in animals that are *hyperperfused*, a condition in which blood flow to peripheral tissues is increased. Febrile and hypertensive animals and animals undergoing an allergic reaction may have **hyperemia** or bright red mucous membranes. In contrast, pale or white mucous membranes may indicate anemia, shock, or hypothermia.

Finally, the clinician may gain additional clues about the state of the circulatory system by examining the gums. If pressed firmly, the pink region of a animal's gum blanches white. When released, the gum changes from white back to pink relatively quickly. The time that it takes for blood to return to the capillaries and turn the gum pink again is called the **capillary refill time** (**CRT**). Normal CRT is 1 to 2 seconds. In animals that have compromised cardiac output, low blood pressure, or severe peripheral vasoconstriction, the CRT will be prolonged. Animals with high blood pressure and those in hypercompensatory states may have shortened CRTs, lasting less than 1 second.

Thus examination of the mucous membranes in an animal is very important and may lead to a greater understanding of the animal's condition.

*Continued*

**CLINICAL APPLICATION—cont'd**

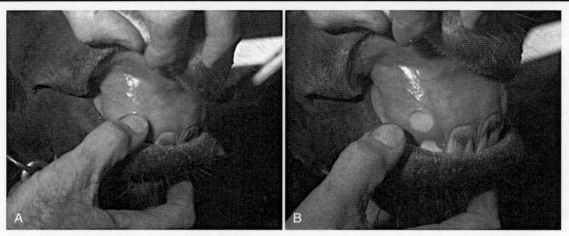

Capillary refill time (CRT). **A,** If you press firmly on the pink region of a horse's gum, the gum blanches white. **B,** When you remove your finger, you will notice that the gum changes from white back to pink relatively quickly. The time that it takes for blood to return to the capillaries, and turn the gum pink again, is called the CRT. (From Speirs VC: Clinical examination of horses, St Louis, 1997, Saunders.)

---

 **CLINICAL APPLICATION**

Histopathology: An Introduction

Histopathology is the microscopic study of disease in tissues (*histo-* means *tissue* and *pathology* is the study of disease). The normal microanatomy of tissues is altered by pathologic disorders in many ways. For example, in mammary tissue that contains a malignant tumor, abnormally large, immature mammary cells may be evident microscopically. The nuclei of these cells are abnormally large, and many of the cells may be actively dividing. Other diseases, such as viral and bacterial infections, may cause cell death and create regions within the tissue that are dead or **necrotic**. Still other diseases may cause the abnormal accumulation of fluid, leading to a condition called **edema**, or may involve the accumulation of a waxlike glycoprotein called **amyloid**. Thus pathologic conditions may be evident microscopically as an increase or decrease in cell numbers, cell size, and changes in the cell's shape and in the architecture of the tissue's support structures.

Although the pathologic nature of diseased tissue is often evident under microscopic examination, grossly the tissue may appear normal. For this reason, a definitive diagnosis often can be made only through the microscopic examination of tissue by taking a biopsy. Occasionally, aspirating cells from the tissue can lead to a diagnosis also.

A **biopsy** is the removal of a small piece of tissue from an organ or mass. This may involve the insertion of a special kind of biopsy needle into the tissue, or it may involve cutting out, or **excising**, a piece of tissue with a scalpel. Some biopsy samples are obtained using special grasping attachments on the exploratory end of endoscopes; others may be acquired using a cookie-cutter type of instrument called a *biopsy punch*. Biopsy samples are harvested from the normal–abnormal tissue borders if possible. In addition, because the tissues are delicate, they should be cut with sharp instruments, such as scalpels, and maneuvered with **tissue forceps**, not **dressing forceps**, so that the microanatomy is not crushed.

No matter how the sample is obtained, it must be handled with care and specially prepared before it can be examined. Samples should be sliced so that each piece is no thicker than 1 cm, and these should be placed in a fixative solution of 10% buffered formalin. **The ratio of the volume of formalin solution to the volume of tissue should be approximately 10:1**, so the specimen can absorb enough fixative to preserve it in its thickest regions. For example, if a large section of heart from a Doberman Pinscher is stuffed into a small container of formalin, the fixative may not be able to penetrate the tissue adequately and the heart will degenerate. Thus the architecture of the muscle will be lost, and a potential diagnosis of dilated cardiomyopathy, for example, will be impossible to confirm. Encapsulated or very fibrous tissues are also difficult to fix. A good rule of thumb is to make sure that the tissue is freely mobile in the container of formalin. Conversely, samples that are extremely small are sometimes invisible within a sea of formalin and are seemingly lost. In these cases, reports stating "no sample found" are returned to the clinician. Therefore, minute specimens should be placed in small, labeled cassettes.

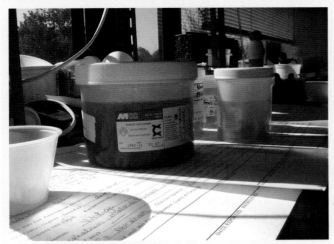

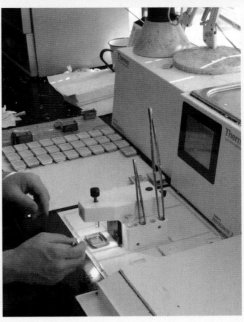

Preparation of tissues for histopathologic evaluation. Tissue is placed in formalin-filled, leak-proof containers. The ratio of the volume of formalin to tissue is about 10:1. Once received by the laboratory, the tissue is examined and sectioned. Sections are placed into tissue cassettes, which are numbered with the patient's surgical *accession number*. Sections are then placed in an automatic tissue processor to be treated overnight. Under a vacuum system, the tissues are dehydrated with progressively higher concentrations of alcohol. Tissues are then cleared with xylene, which is a solvent capable of dissolving **paraffin**. Cassettes are put through a series of xylene–paraffin solutions in which the concentration of paraffin increases until the tissue becomes infiltrated, which facilitates thin slicing.

Tissues are individually transferred to rectangular metal molds, which are filled with liquid paraffin.

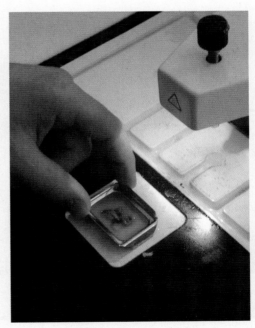

The paraffin hardens into a soft white wax.

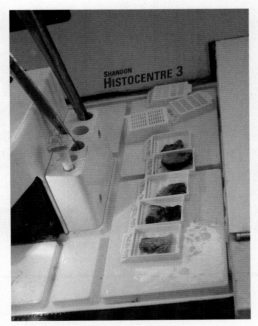

Tissue cassettes are removed from the processor.

*Continued*

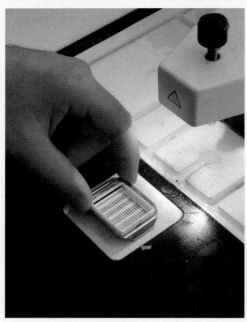

Before the paraffin hardens completely, the cassette cover with the correct identification is placed over the mold.

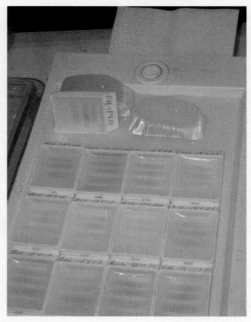

Paraffin provides support to the tissue and enables it to be sliced into very thin sections. Just before being sliced, the paraffin is chilled further with ice to make it easier to slice.

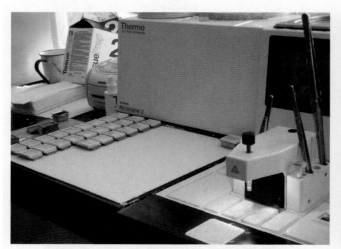

The molds are then arranged and ordered for slicing.

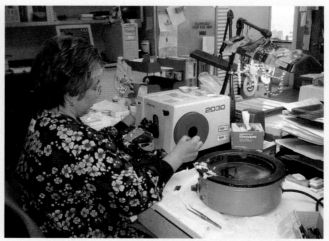

Extraordinarily thin slices (4 to 8 μm) are cut from the chilled paraffin blocks using a special cutting device called a **microtome**.

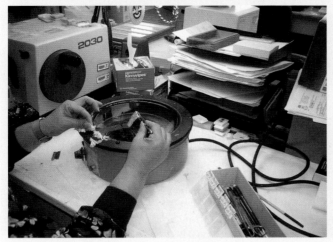

Several serial slices form a paper-thin strip, which is floated on the surface of a water bath.

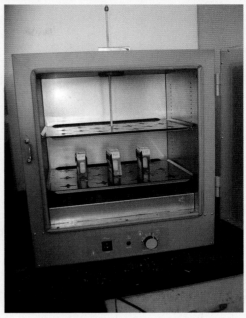

Slides are stood vertically to drip dry and are then transferred to a warm incubator, such as the one pictured, to speed drying and help tissue adhere to the slide.

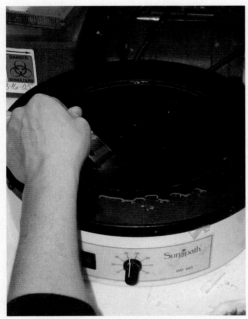

Carefully, these thin sections are collected onto labeled glass microscope slides.

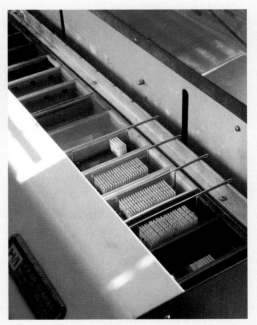

In preparation for staining, tissue sections are de-paraffinized and rehydrated so that aqueous stains can react with them. Laboratories that process large numbers of slides daily use automated staining machines such as the one pictured. After being stained, tissues are again dehydrated with progressively higher concentrations of alcohol and then cleared with xylene.

*Continued*

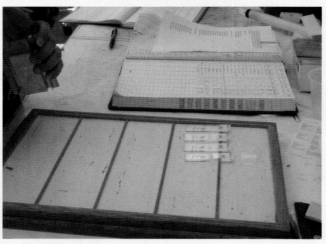

Finally, a protective glass cover slip is applied to each slide with Permount (a type of glue) sandwiched in between the two glass layers. Finished slides are logged in a journal before being examined microscopically by a veterinary pathologist.

---

✓ **TEST YOURSELF 5-6**

1. Membranes are composed of what two tissue types?
2. Where are mucous membranes found? What functions do they perform?
3. What portion of a serous membrane covers the outer surface of organs?
4. What is an effusion? What is ascites?
5. What is another name for *cutaneous membrane*?
6. Where are synovial membranes found? How are they different from other membrane types?

## MUSCLE TISSUE

Muscle cells, or muscle *fibers*, are uniquely designed for contraction. The fibers are composed of specialized proteins called *actin* and *myosin,* which are arranged into microfilaments. Contraction, or shortening, of the muscle cell occurs when the microfilaments slide over one another, like the bars in an old-fashioned slide ruler. In this way, the cells change shape and can be made shorter or longer. As the muscles contract, they move the bones, blood, and soft tissue structures that are associated with them. Thus blood is circulated, legs are made to run, and food is moved slowly through the intestine. There are three types of muscle tissue: *skeletal, smooth,* and *cardiac* (Figure 5-29).

### SKELETAL MUSCLE

**Skeletal muscle** contains numerous large cells that may be a foot or more in length. Because of their large size and heavy metabolic requirements, the cells contain hundreds of nuclei and mitochondria needed to maintain cellular

homeostasis. Skeletal muscle is responsible for an animal's ability to walk, run, kick, bite, and show facial expression. Unlike cardiac and smooth muscle, skeletal muscle is usually controlled through conscious effort and therefore is called **voluntary muscle**. In other words, the animal can control its movement through conscious thought. In addition, skeletal muscle cells are *striated*, or striped, because histologically they have alternating bands of light and dark across them. Thus skeletal muscle is referred to as *voluntary, striated muscle*.

The cells of skeletal muscle are essentially fibers that are clustered into bundles and held together by loose connective tissue. The collagen fibers that surround the cells merge with the collagen fibers in tendons to attach muscle firmly to bone. Muscle cells are stimulated to contract by the action of nerve fibers attached to them, located throughout the entire muscle belly. If the nerves are damaged, the ability of the muscle to contract is impaired, and the muscle is said to be **paretic**, or **paralyzed**. In this way, all of the actions that an animal can normally control, such as walking, running, eating, and moving the head and arms, depend on a healthy nervous system as well as a healthy muscular system.

### SMOOTH MUSCLE

**Smooth muscle** is composed of small, spindle-shaped cells that lack striations or bands and therefore appear smooth. Like skeletal muscle, smooth muscle may be stimulated to contract by the action of nerves but, unlike skeletal muscles, the contractions cannot be consciously controlled. Smooth muscle is therefore called **nonstriated, involuntary muscle**. It is found in the walls of hollow organs, such as blood vessels, urinary bladder, uterus, intestines, and stomach and is also found in exocrine glands and along the respiratory

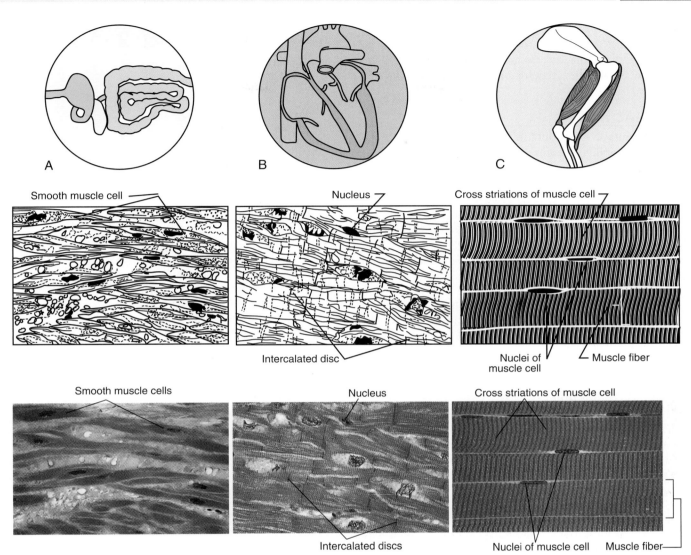

**FIGURE 5-29** Types of muscle tissue. **A**, Smooth muscle. *Description:* Nonstriated, involuntary; composed of small, spindle-shaped cells that lack striations or bands and therefore appear "smooth." Each cell has a centrally located nucleus. *Location:* In the walls of hollow organs such as the esophagus, stomach, intestine, colon, blood vessels, and bladder; also in skin attached to hair and in the iris of the eye. *Function:* Moves food through the digestive tract, regulates the size of an organ, controls light entering the eye, moves fluid through vessels, and causes hair to stand erect. *Microanatomy:* Photomicrograph and sketch of smooth muscle cells. **B**, Cardiac muscle. *Description:* Striated, involuntary; cells are cylindrical and branched with a single, centrally located nucleus. Cells form an intricate network and are connected by intercalated discs in a specialized type of gap junction. *Location:* Found only in the heart. *Function:* Pumps blood through the vascular system. *Microanatomy:* Photomicrograph and sketch of cardiac muscle cells. Notice the intercalated discs unique to the cardiac cell. Each cell contains only one, centrally located, nucleus. **C**, Skeletal muscle. *Description:* Striated, voluntary; cells are striped, long, and cylindrical, each one with multiple, eccentrically placed nuclei. *Location:* Attached to bone and occasionally to skin, eyeballs, and upper part of the esophagus. *Function:* Voluntary movement of body, including movement of the eyes and the initial part of swallowing. *Microanatomy:* Photomicrograph and sketch of skeletal muscle cells. Notice that each cell contains multiple nuclei, which are found along the cell membrane. (**A**, Courtesy Carolina Biological Supply Company/Phototake. **B** and **C**, Courtesy Ed Reschke.)

tract. It is responsible for **peristalsis** in the gastrointestinal tract, for the constriction of blood vessels, and for the emptying of the bladder. Because smooth muscle cells are relatively small, they require only one centrally located nucleus.

## CARDIAC MUSCLE

**Cardiac muscle** exists only in the heart and possesses the remarkable ability to contract even when neural input has been altered. Specialized pacemaker cells within the heart muscle supply the signal for the heart to contract at regular intervals. This input is entirely involuntary and is responsible for initiating the pumping force, which propels blood through blood vessels. Thank goodness we do not need to *concentrate* on keeping our hearts beating!

As in smooth muscle, the cells of cardiac muscle are relatively small and contain only one nucleus. However, unlike smooth or skeletal muscle, cardiac muscle branches to form a complex network. The cardiac muscle cells are striated and are connected to one another at each end via a specialized intercellular junction called an **intercalated disc**. These discs occur only in cardiac muscle. Thus cardiac muscle is classified as an *involuntary, striated* tissue.

## NERVOUS TISSUE

Nervous or *neural* tissue is uniquely designed to receive and transmit electrical and chemical signals throughout the body (Figure 5-30). It is found in the brain, spinal cord, and peripheral nerves and is composed primarily of two general cell types: *neurons* and supporting *neuroglial* cells.

**Neurons** are the longest cells in the body and may reach up to a meter in length. They are composed of three primary parts: a cell body called a **perikaryon**, short cytoplasmic extensions called **dendrites**, and a long, single extension called an **axon**. The cell body contains the nucleus, which controls the metabolism of the cell. The dendrites *receive* impulses from other cells, whereas the axon conducts impulses *away* from the cell body. The neuron forms connections with many other tissues, such as muscle, viscera, glands, and other neurons. In this way, a complex network is formed that controls and regulates many body functions. The neuron is exquisitely sensitive to electrical and chemical changes in its environment and may respond by transmitting nerve impulses along its axon to other tissues. These electrical impulses, which carry information and instructions, are transmitted through conductive membranes on the neurons.

**Neuroglial cells** are found in greater numbers in neural tissue than are neurons. They do not transmit impulses but rather serve to support the neurons. Some specialized types of neuroglial cells function to isolate the conductive membranes, others provide a supportive framework that helps bind the components of neural tissue together, and still others **phagocytize** or *digest* debris, or they help supply nutrients to neurons by connecting them to blood vessels.

| BOX 5-2 | Summary of Tissues |
| --- | --- |

I. Epithelial tissue
  A. Simple squamous
  B. Simple cuboidal
  C. Simple columnar
  D. Stratified squamous
  E. Stratified cuboidal
  F. Stratified columnar
  G. Transitional
  H. Pseudostratified
II. Connective tissue
  A. Connective tissue proper
    1. Loose connective tissue
      a. Areolar tissue
      b. Adipose tissue
      c. Reticular tissue
    2. Dense connective tissue
      a. Dense regular
      b. Dense irregular
      c. Elastic tissue
  B. Specialized connective tissue
    1. Cartilage
      a. Hyaline cartilage
      b. Elastic cartilage
      c. Fibrocartilage
    2. Bone
      a. Compact
      b. Cancellous
    3. Blood
III. Muscle tissue
  A. Skeletal (striated, voluntary)
  B. Cardiac (striated, involuntary)
  C. Smooth (nonstriated, involuntary)
IV. Nervous tissue

The gross anatomy and physiology of nervous tissue are discussed in Chapter 9.

Box 5-2 summarizes tissues.

## TISSUE HEALING AND REPAIR

Injuries occur in many ways. Animals may experience trauma from being hit by a car or from falling out a window. They may be bitten, scratched, or kicked by other animals and may experience broken bones and wounds that later become infected by pathogens. The body's initial response to these injuries is *inflammation,* a series of events that develop quickly to limit further damage and eliminate any harmful agents. Repair occurs more slowly and involves the *organization* of granulation tissue and the *regeneration* of lost tissue or the formation of scar tissue. Many of these processes occur simultaneously, making the injured area a busy workplace for cells. We will take a closer look at what is happening during the healing process. A summary of tissue repair is illustrated in Figure 5-31.

Neuron

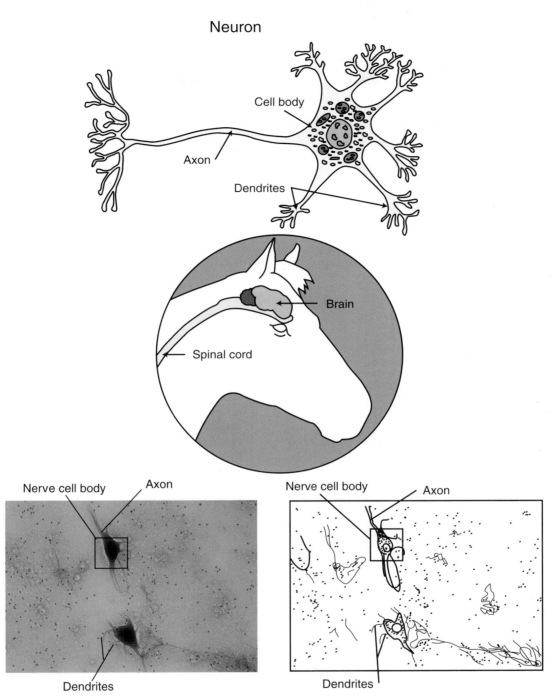

**FIGURE 5-30** Nervous tissue. *Description:* Composed of neurons and supportive neuroglial cells. A neuron may be multipolar (as shown) or unipolar. Each multipolar neuron is composed of a cell body, which contains a nucleus; multiple short, branched dendrites; and a single long axon. A unipolar neuron is composed of a cell body and one branched axon. *Location:* Brain, spinal cord, and nerves. *Function:* To conduct electrical signals, store information, and evaluate data; to transmit sensory information to spinal cord and brain. *Microanatomy:* Photomicrograph and sketch of tissue from a spinal cord. Notice the cell body (soma) from which multiple dendrites and a single axon emerge. (Photomicrograph from Thibodeau GA, Patton KT: Anatomy & physiology, ed 6, St Louis, 2007, Mosby.)

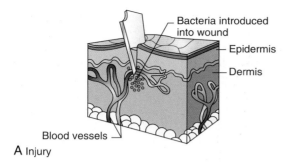

A Injury

Bacteria introduced into wound
— Epidermis
— Dermis
Blood vessels

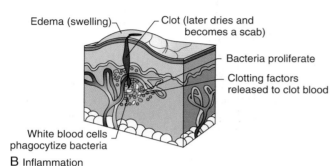

B Inflammation

Edema (swelling)
Clot (later dries and becomes a scab)
Bacteria proliferate
Clotting factors released to clot blood
White blood cells phagocytize bacteria

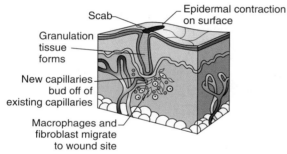

C Organization

Scab
Epidermal contraction on surface
Granulation tissue forms
New capillaries bud off of existing capillaries
Macrophages and fibroblast migrate to wound site

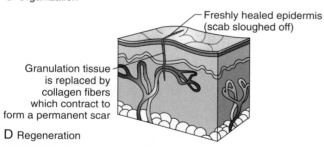

D Regeneration

Freshly healed epidermis (scab sloughed off)
Granulation tissue is replaced by collagen fibers which contract to form a permanent scar

**FIGURE 5-31** Tissue repair of minor skin wound. **A,** Injury. A piece of glass causes a cut in the skin. **B,** Inflammation. Blood vessels dilate and become more permeable, causing redness in the tissue around the wound. Fluid leaks into the tissue from dilated capillaries and causes swelling. A blood clot, which later becomes a scab, forms at the wound opening. Pressure of fluid on nerve endings causes pain. **C,** Organization. Granulation tissue forms below the scab. Fibroblasts lay down collagen fibers while macrophages engulf foreign debris and invading microorganisms. **D,** Regeneration or fibrosis. Epithelial cells around the wound edges proliferate and cover the granulation tissue. The scab is pushed off. Granulation tissue becomes fibrous scar tissue, which contracts and pulls the wound edges together.

## INFLAMMATION: THE FIRST STAGE

Whenever a tissue is injured, it causes an immediate inflammatory response. The affected area becomes red, swollen, hot, and tender. Sometimes there is decreased function of the injured body part. Inflammation is the body's attempt to isolate the area, limit the damage caused by the injury, and prevent further damage. *Note that inflammation does not imply infection.* **Infection** is inflammation caused by viruses, bacteria, and fungi. Injuries such as chemical burns, broken bones, and pulled muscles do not necessarily involve the invasion of these microorganisms. Inflammation therefore is a nonspecific reaction to injury or disease. The **inflammatory process** is the same regardless of the type of disease or injury. The extent of inflammation, however, depends on the type of tissue involved and on the severity of the injury or illness.

## STEPS IN THE PROCESS OF INFLAMMATION

1. Inflammation begins with a 5- to 10-minute period of *vasoconstriction*, followed by a sustained period of *vasodilation*. The initial constriction occurs in the small vessels of the injured tissue and aids in the control of **hemorrhage**. Histamine and heparin molecules subsequently are released from mast cells, which stimulate vasodilation and increase permeability of the capillaries. Blood flow to the area is increased, which in turn causes the clinical signs of heat and redness. It also increases the supplies of oxygen and nutrients to the active cells of the damaged tissue.

2. Fluid from plasma, composed of enzymes, antibodies, and proteins, pours into the affected area, causing swelling of the soft tissue structures. This swelling irritates delicate nerve endings and causes pain and tenderness in the affected area.

3. Clot formation begins to take place, which slows bleeding. The clot also helps to isolate the wound from the invasion of pathogens and helps to prevent bacteria and toxins from spreading to surrounding soft tissue structures. A clot first forms when platelets become sticky and clump together. **Fibrinogen**, which is found in large quantities in the swollen tissue, is converted to an insoluble protein called **fibrin**. The fibrin is woven into a netlike structure that surrounds the platelets and provides support and stability to the newly formed clot. It also forms a framework to support the movement of cells throughout the site. Clots that form on external surfaces, such as skin, eventually dry to become scabs.

4. Large cells such as macrophages and **neutrophils**, a type of white blood cell, move through blood vessels and squeeze through dilated capillaries to assist in the removal of debris and microinvaders. These *phagocytic* cells are short lived, however, and can function for only a few hours before dying. Pus, which is an accumulation of dead and degenerated neutrophils and macrophages, may therefore collect in the injured area.

5. With increased blood flow, histamine and heparin are dispersed, and their levels drop in the affected area. The decrease in these molecules causes the return of normal capillary size and permeability. When capillaries return to normal size, blood flow and fluid leakage into the affected area abate. Swelling, heat, and redness begin to subside.

## ORGANIZATION: THE FORMATION OF GRANULATION TISSUE

Wound repair begins soon after the injury occurs and continues while dead cells and debris are removed from the area. In wounds that are infected, neutrophils and macrophages play a particularly critical role in the healing process, because they are responsible for phagocytizing and disposing of invasive microorganisms. The presence of pathogens inhibits healing.

As macrophages work to clear debris, a new, bright pink tissue, called **granulation tissue**, forms beneath the overlying blood clot or scab. Granulation tissue is composed of a layer of collagen fibers that have been manufactured by fibroblasts. It is richly infiltrated with small permeable capillaries that have branched off from existing capillaries in the deeper layers of the damaged tissue. These tiny new vessels push up into the bed of collagen fibers and provide rich supplies of nutrients and oxygen to the hard-working fibroblasts, macrophages, and neutrophils. Grossly, the capillaries appear to be minute *granules* and therefore account for the name. Granulation tissue produces bacterium-inhibiting substances, which make it highly resistant to infection.

In some cases, granulation tissue becomes *too* thick and stands out above the epithelial layer. This is known as **proud flesh** and may be surgically cut down to facilitate closure of the epithelial layer. Proud flesh is commonly seen in horses that have sustained skin wounds.

## REGENERATION OR FIBROSIS
### EPITHELIALIZATION AND SCAR TISSUE

While organization is occurring, epithelial cells around the wound edges actively divide to lay down a new layer of epithelial tissue over the granulation tissue. This process is called **epithelialization**. Connections between the scab and the thickening epithelial layer are weakened, and the scab subsequently falls off. Fibroblasts in the granulation tissue continue to manufacture collagen fibers and ground substance, which are used to replace lost tissue and bridge the wound. Slowly, the granulation tissue is completely replaced by fibrous scar tissue, which contracts and assists in pulling the wound closed. When epithelialization is complete, the underlying scar may or may not be visible, depending on the severity of the injury and on the extent of scar formation.

Although scar tissue is strong, it is less flexible than normal tissue and cannot perform the function of the damaged tissue. With time, scar tissue shrinks, but its presence can still have detrimental effects on the organ as a whole. For example, if scar tissue forms in the wall of the heart, it can interrupt electrical pathways, weaken contractile

capability, and result in decreased cardiac function. Similarly, if it occurs in the wall of the intestine or esophagus, it can decrease the diameter of the lumen and lead to obstruction or occlusion. For this reason, dogs that have undergone esophageal surgery to remove a foreign body are likely to have a repeated episode. The site of the first incision in the esophagus often heals with a thick, fibrous scar, which narrows the esophageal lumen and increases the possibility that another foreign body, such as a piece of bone or chew toy, will once again become lodged.

In the abdominal and thoracic cavities, healing is often associated with the formation of **fibrous adhesions** and tags, which cover organs and form connections between multiple structures. Reentry into the abdomen to repeat a surgical procedure or to correct a complication therefore can be more difficult because of the formation of adhesions. Adhesions can reduce the visibility of important structures. They can restrict normal shifting of bowel loops and can bind organs to the body wall or to the omentum. In addition, adhesions can be painful to the animal if they cause tension between well-innervated structures.

## CLASSIFICATIONS

Wound repair may be classified as first or second intention, depending on the mechanism of healing and the proximity of the wound edges. Wounds that heal via first intention are those in which the edges of the wound are held in close apposition. These wounds may be superficial scratches or wounds that have been sutured or held closed with special

 **CLINICAL APPLICATION**

The Clinical Patient and Healing

Some tissue types heal more readily than others. Epithelial tissues such as skin and mucous membranes heal rapidly but smooth muscle and dense regular connective tissue have limited regenerative ability. Cardiac muscle and nervous tissue in the brain and spinal cord regenerate extremely slowly if at all and are often replaced by scar tissue. In addition, some patients heal more easily than other patients. Old, **immunosuppressed**, debilitated, or sick animals heal more slowly than young, healthy, well-nourished animals. In this way, the age, overall health, and nutrition of patients are important factors in the rate and extent of healing. This is why elective surgery is avoided in unhealthy animals and why intravenous nutrition may be used in critically ill patients. Some diseased or otherwise stressed animals, for example, may produce too much cortisol, which can inhibit the animal's ability to heal; incision sites may take weeks rather than days to close, and wounds from even superficial injuries may become chronic nightmares. In addition, some drugs, such as prednisone, can also delay healing if blood levels are high. Thus the clinician must consider the overall health and medical history of an animal before carrying out any procedure that subsequently requires the healing of tissue.

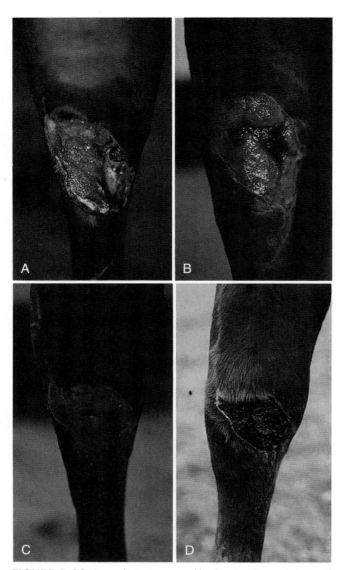

bandages. During **first-intention healing**, the skin forms a primary union without the formation of granulation tissue or significant scarring. **Second-intention healing** occurs in wounds in which the edges are separated from one another, in which granulation tissue forms to close the gap, and in which scarring results (Figure 5-32).

**FIGURE 5-32** Second-intention wound healing in a horse. **A,** Wound on the anterior aspect of the hock in a gelding. Note the granulation tissue evident in **B** and **C** and the epithelial contraction that followed (**D**). Scarring remained after the wound healed, but this is well concealed in animals because of coverage by the hair coat. (From Melling M, Alder M: Equine practice, ed 3, Philadelphia, 1998, Saunders.)

---

✓ **TEST YOURSELF 5-7**

1. In what ways are muscle fibers uniquely adapted for contraction?
2. List three types of muscle. How do they differ from one another?
3. What are the two basic cell types that make up neural tissue?
4. What is the most important function of neural tissue?
5. Describe the process of inflammation. What causes the clinical signs of heat, swelling, redness, and tenderness?
6. When does the healing process begin?
7. What is granulation tissue? Why is it important in the healing process?
8. Describe first- and second-intention wound repair.

# 6 The Integument and Related Structures

*Joanna M. Bassert*

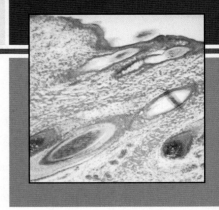

## OUTLINE

## LEARNING OBJECTIVES

*When you have completed this chapter you will be able to:*

1. List the cell types that comprise the epidermis and describe the function of each cell type.
2. List the five layers of the epidermis.
3. Describe the process of keratinization.
4. List the structures that comprise the dermis and describe the function of each.
5. List the structures that comprise the hypodermis.
6. Describe the unique features of the paw pads and *planum nasale.*
7. Describe the parts of the hair follicle and explain how hair grows.
8. List and describe the three types of hair.
9. Describe the structure and location of sebaceous glands.
10. Differentiate between eccrine and apocrine sweat glands.

## VOCABULARY FUNDAMENTALS

*Anagen phase* **ahn**-eh-jehn fāz
*Anal sac* **ān**-ehl sahck
*Angle* **ahng**-uhl
*Apocrine sweat gland* **ahp**-ō-krihn sweht glahnd
*Arrector pili muscle* ahr-**rehck**-tər **pī**-lē **muhs**-uhl
*Catagen phase* **kaht**-ah-jehn fāz
*Central sulcus* **sehn**-trahl **suhlck**-uhs
*Chestnut* **chehs**-nuht
*Coffin bone* **kaw**-fihn bōn
*Collateral sulcus* kō-**laht**-ər-ahl **suhlck**-uhs
*Compound follicle* **kohm**-pohwnd **fohl**-ih-kuhl
*Corium* **kohr**-ē-uhm
*Coronary band* **kohr**-ah-nər-ē bahnd
*Coronary corium* **kohr**-ah-nər-ē **kohr**-ē-uhm
*Cortex* **kohr**-tehx
*Cuticle* **kyoo**-tih-kuhl

*Defecation* dehf-eh-**kā**-shuhn
*Dermal papillae* **dər**-mahl pah-**pihl**-lī
*Dermis* **dər**-mihs
*Dewclaw* **dyoo**-klahw
*Digital cushion* **dihj**-ih-tahl **kuhsh**-uhn
*Distal phalanx bone* **dihs**-tahl **fah**-lahngks bōn
*Eccrine gland* **ehk**-rihn glahnd
*Epidermal orifice* ehp-ih-**dər**-mahl **ohr**-uh-fihs
*Epidermis* ehp-ih-**dər**-mihs
*Ergot* **ər**-goht
*Frog* frawg
*Frog corium* frawg **kohr**-ē-uhm
*Hair bulb* hᵊr buhlb
*Hair follicle* hᵊr **fohl**-ih-kuhl
*Heel* hēl
*Hoof* hoof

*Hoof wall*  hoof wahl

*Horn tube*  hohrn toob

*Horn*  hohrn

*Hypodermis (subcutaneous layer)*  hī-pō-**dǝr**-mihs (suhb-kyoo-**tā**-nē-uhs **lā**-ǝr)

*Hypophysis*  hī-**pohf**-uh-sihs

*Implantation angle*  ihm-plahn-**tā**-shuhn **ahng**-uhl

*Infraoribital pouch*  ihn-frah-**ohr**-bih-tahl pouch

*Inguinal pouch*  **ihn**-gwih-nahl pouch

*Integument*  ihn-**tehg**-ū-mehnt

*Integumentary system*  ihn-tehg-ū-**mehn**-tahr-ē **sihs**-tehm

*Interdigital pouch*  ihn-tǝr-**dij**-eh-tahl pouch

*Keratin*  **keǝr**-ah-tehn

*Keratinization*  **keǝr**-ah-tehn-eh-zā-shuhn

*Keratinocyte*  **keǝr**-ah-tehn-ō-sīt

*Laminae*  **lahm**-eh-nē

*Laminar corium*  **lahm**-eh-nahr **kohr**-ē-uhm

*Laminitis*  **lahm**-eh-nī-tihs

*Langerhans cell*  **lahng**-ǝr-hahnz sehl

*Lanolin*  **lahn**-ō-lihn

*Lateral cartilage*  **laht**-ǝr-ahl **kahr**-tih-lihj

*Matrix*  **mā**-trihks

*Medulla*  meh-**duhl**-ah

*Meissner's corpuscle*  **mīz**-nǝrz **kohr**-puhs-ehl

*Melanin*  **mehl**-ah-nihn

*Melanocyte*  mehl-**ahn**-ō-sīt

*Melanocyte stimulating hormone (MSH)*  mehl-**ahn**-ō-sīt **stihm**-ū-lā-tihng **hohr**-mōn

*Melanosome*  mehl-**ahn**-ō-sōm

*Merkel cell*  **mǝr**-kehl sehl

*Merkel disc*  **mǝr**-kehl dihsk

*Metacarpal bone*  meht-ah-**kahr**-pahl bōn

*Navicular bone*  neh-**vihck**-ū-lahr bōn

*Notoedres*  nōt-ō-**ehd**-rēz

*Pacinian corpuscle*  peh-**sihn**-ē-ahn **kohr**-puhs-ehl

*Papilla*  pah-**pihl**-lah

*Papillary layer*  pah-pihl-**leǝr**-ē **lā**-ǝr

*Perioplic corium*  peǝr-ē-**ōp**-lihck **kohr**-ē-uhm

*Phalangeal bone*  fah-**lahn**-jē-ahl bōn

*Pheomelanin*  fē-ō-**mehl**-ah-nihn

*Pigmentation*  pihg-muhn-**tā**-shuhn

*Planum nasale*  **plā**-nehm **nāz**-ahl-ē

*Planum nasolabiale*  **plā**-nehm **nāz**-ō-**lā**-bē-ah-lē

*Point*  poynt

*Polled breed*  pōld brēd

*Primary hair*  **prī**-meǝr-ē heǝr

*Pruritus*  proo-**rīt**-uhs

*Quarter*  **kwahr**-tǝr

*Reticular layer*  reh-**tihck**-ū-lahr **lā**-ǝr

*Root*  root

*Root hair plexus*  root heǝr **plehck**-suhs

*Sebum*  **sē**-buhm

*Secondary hair*  **sehk**-uhn-dahr-ē heǝr

*Shaft*  shahft

*Sinus hair*  **sī**-nuhs heǝr

*Sole*  sōl

*Sole corium*  sōl **kohr**-ē-uhm

*Squamous cell carcinoma*  **skwey**-muhs sehl **kahr**-sih-nō-mah

*Stratum basale*  **strā**-tuhm bā-**sā**-lē

*Stratum corneum*  **strā**-tuhm **kohr**-nē-uhm

*Stratum germinativum*  **strā**-tuhm **jǝr**-mihn-ah-tī-vehm

*Stratum granulosum*  **strā**-tuhm **grahn**-ū-lō-suhm

*Stratum lucidum*  **strā**-tuhm **loo**-sihd-uhm

*Stratum spinosum*  **strā**-tuhm spī-**nō**-suhm

*Sweat gland*  sweht glahnd

*Tactile hair*  **tahck**-tihl heǝr

*Tail gland*  **tā**-uhl glahnd

*Tactile elevation*  **tahck**-tihl ehl-eh-**vā**-shuhn

*Telogen effluvium*  **tē**-lō-jehn ih-**floo**-vē-uhm

*Telogen phase*  **tē**-lō-jehn fāz

*Toe*  tō

*Tylotrich hair*  **tī**-lō-trihck heǝr

*Tyrosine melanin*  **tī**-rō-sēn **mehl**-ah-nihn

*Ungula*  **uhng**-yuh-lah

*Ungulate*  **uhng**-yoo-lāt

*Velvet skin*  **vehl**-veht skihn

*Vitamin D*  **vī**-ta-mihn D

*White line*  whīt līn

*Wool-type hair*  wool tīp heǝr

The **integument** is one of the largest and most extensive organs in the body. Composed of all four tissue types, it covers and protects underlying structures and forms a critical barrier between the delicate inner workings of the body and the harsh elements of the external world. Its surface is constantly being rubbed, scratched, attacked by microbes, irritated by external parasites, and subjected to environmental chemicals and ultraviolet radiation. The skin, together with related structures such as horns, hooves, claws, glands and hair, form the **integumentary system** or *common integument*. This system involves every inch of the external animal and is contiguous with the mucous membranes that line the mouth, anus, and nostrils. It is frequently injured, but possesses a remarkable ability to regenerate and heal.

Although derived from living germinal layers, the outer shell of an animal or person is entirely dead. Remarkably, everything you see, from the hair to the skin, is composed of the remains of dead cells. Once alive, in histologically deeper layers and in earlier stages of development, these cells gave up vital organelles and nuclei to make room for the tough, protective substance called **keratin**. It is during this process, called **keratinization**, that the cells expire and in doing so form the vital protective barrier that helps enable an animal's survival.

## INTEGUMENT

The integument carries out a plethora of protective and regulatory duties. One of its most important functions is to prevent desiccation and rampant infection. In addition, it assists in the maintenance of normal body temperature and excretes water, salt, and organic wastes. It is an important sensory organ that takes in information from the environment via touch and pressure and conveys this input to regions of the central nervous system. It is also engaged in the synthesis of **vitamin D** and in the storage of nutrients.

The thickness of skin varies among species and according to its location in the body. The thinnest skin, for example, tends to occur around the eyes and the scrotum, whereas some of the thickest layers can be found in the center of the back, between the shoulder blades, and on the paw pads.

Histologically, skin forms two distinct layers: the **epidermis** and the underlying **dermis**, which is also known as the *corium*. These layers are separated by an epithelial basement membrane. In some species, this membrane is wavy and undulating, creating infoldings and outpouchings. The downward folds of the epidermis interdigitate with the upward projections of the dermis, which are called **dermal papillae**. These interdigitations help cement the epidermis and the dermis together and are therefore most pronounced in areas where there is a great deal of friction.

The epidermis is composed of keratinized stratified squamous epithelium and forms an outer waterproof shield. The majority of skin, however, is composed of the underlying dermis, which is a tough, leathery layer made of dense fibroelastic connective tissue. Only the dermis contains blood vessels. The epidermis is avascular but is provided with nutrient molecules by interstitial fluid that diffuses up from the underlying dermis.

A third layer, the **hypodermis** or **subcutaneous layer**, is found below the dermis and is composed primarily of adipose tissue, which acts as a thermoinsulator and a mechanical shock absorber.

Figure 6-1 offers an overview of the structure of skin, which includes the dermis and epidermis, and of the hypodermis with its accessory structures. Let us examine these layers in greater detail.

### EPIDERMIS
#### CELLS OF THE EPIDERMIS

Several different kinds of cell are found in the epidermis. The principal ones are *keratinocytes, melanocytes, Merkel cells*, and *Langerhans cells*. The majority of cells found in the epidermis are **keratinocytes**, which produce a tough, fibrous, waterproof protein called **keratin** that gives skin its resiliency and strength. Keratinocytes located along the basement membrane are well nourished by the blood supply of the underlying dermis, therefore these cells can grow and divide. As daughter cells are produced, they push older cells away from the life-sustaining nutrients of the dermis and toward the outer layers of the epidermis. As the older cells travel from the basal to the superficial layers, they undergo profound changes: They fill with keratohyaline granules, lose their nuclei, cytosol, and organelles, and ultimately become lifeless sheets of keratin. This process is called **keratinization**, and it enables millions of dead cells to rub off or exfoliate daily at no expense to the health of the animal. Remarkably, an entirely new epidermis forms in humans every 7 to 8 weeks.

The pigment found in skin is produced by another type of cell, the **melanocyte**, which is found in the deepest epidermal layers. The melanocyte is octopus-like and possesses long projections that extend outward to all of the keratinocytes in the basal layer. As its name implies, the melanocyte produces **melanin**, a dark pigment stored in membrane-bound granules called **melanosomes**. The melanosomes are transported to the tips of the cellular projections, where they are released into the intracellular space and ultimately absorbed by keratinocytes. The keratinocytes use the melanin to protect themselves from exposure to damaging ultraviolet rays.

The **Langerhans cell** is a macrophage specific to the epidermis. Like other macrophages, it originates in bone marrow and subsequently migrates to the skin, where it

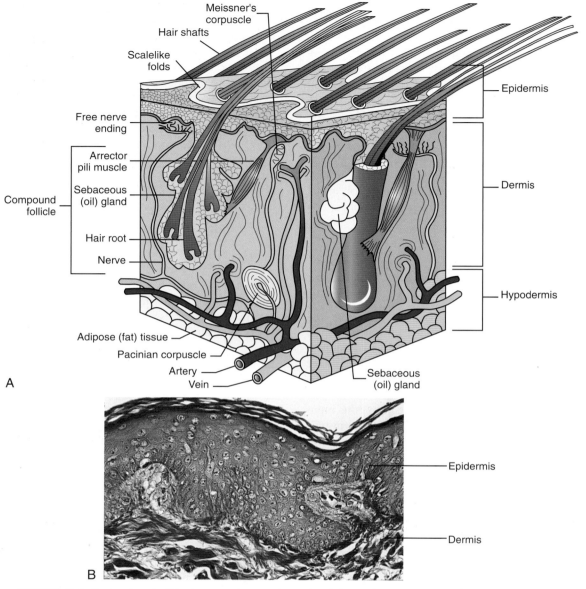

**FIGURE 6-1** Canine skin. **A,** Cubed section of canine skin and underlying subcutaneous tissue, showing many structural details discussed in this chapter. Notice that the epidermis of canine skin includes folds from which compound hairs arise. **B,** Photomicrograph of skin showing the many cellular layers of the epidermis, the basement membrane, and the underlying dermis. (**B,** Courtesy Ed Reschke.)

phagocytizes microinvaders and plays an important role in helping to stimulate other aspects of the immune system.

At the epidermal–dermal junction, **Merkel cells** can be found in small numbers. These are always associated with a sensory nerve ending and are thought to aid in the sensation of touch, taking on a half-dome shape, which perfectly complements the half-dome shape of the sensory nerve ending. Together, these components form what is called a **Merkel disc**.

## LAYERS OF THE EPIDERMIS

Early histologists examined sections of human skin and found five distinct layers in the epidermis (Figure 6-2). These

layers were given Latin names and are used today to describe the epidermis in other mammalian species. The deepest layer is the **stratum germinativum**, but it is also known as the **stratum basale** or *basal layer*. For the most part, this layer consists of a single row of keratinocytes, which are firmly attached to the epithelial basement membrane and are actively engaged in cell division. The daughter cells move from the stratum basale to more superficial layers as they mature, to replace epithelial cells that have exfoliated at the skin's surface. Merkel cells, melanocytes, and keratinocytes are found in the basal layer.

The next layer is the **stratum spinosum** or *spiny layer*, so named because when the cells of this epidermal layer are

## Skin Cancer

With the increasing deterioration of the protective ozone layer that surrounds the earth, people are becoming more aware of the growing risk of skin cancer and the importance of protecting the skin from excessive exposure to the sun. However, we are less likely to consider skin cancer in animals, though cancer of the skin, particularly in certain species and breeds, is very common.

Because cancer is the *aberrant growth of cells*, skin cancer can stem from any of the cell types found in the epidermis or dermis. As you have learned, many different cell types make up these layers; however, three types of particular importance in cancer are the *squamous cells, melanocytes*, and *basal cells.*

Abnormal changes in the genetic programming of melanocytes, for example, can induce a deadly form of skin cancer called *malignant melanoma.* Malignant melanoma commonly occurs in aged gray horses and initially appears as nodules under the tail base, in the perianal area, and in the scrotum. Later, these nodules will grow, ulcerate, and spread to multiple internal locations in the horse. Although melanomas may appear on any area of the body in dogs and cats, they are most malignant in the oral cavity. Among pigs in general the disease is rare, but malignant melanoma commonly occurs in the Duroc-Jersey breed.

**Squamous cell carcinoma** is another deadly form of skin cancer, because it spreads rapidly to local lymph nodes and is aggressively invasive locally. It tends to form circular, ulcerated lesions that seem to eat away the surrounding tissue. Squamous cell carcinoma commonly appears on the eyeball, nictitating membrane, and surrounding the eyelids of cattle and horses. It is also seen on the planum nasale, earflaps, and nose of white cats and in the vulvar regions of Merino ewes. It is one of the most common skin tumors in dogs over the age of 5. Areas of skin that receive prolonged sun exposure are most vulnerable to squamous cell carcinoma.

The *basal cell tumor* stems from the cells found in the basal layer of the epidermis, in hair follicles, and in sebaceous glands. They do not spread to other areas of the body and therefore are considered benign; however, they do recur after removal. Basal cell tumors grow slowly and are found on the head and neck in dogs. They are thought to be one of the most common tumors found in cats but account for only 6% of the neoplasms in dogs.

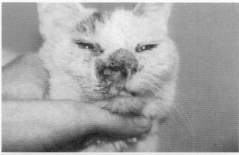
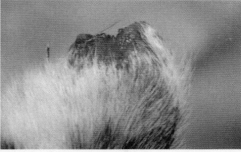

White cats are more vulnerable to developing squamous cell carcinoma. A common location for the tumor to appear is on the nose *(top)* and on the tips of the ears *(bottom)*. (From Scott DW, Miller WT Jr, Griffin CE: *Muller and Kirk's small animal dermatology,* ed 6, Philadelphia, 2001, Saunders.)

---

fixed for histologic examination, they contract into spiculated masses that resemble sea urchins. These cells are sometimes called *prickle cells*; however, their cellular projections do not occur naturally, and the cells are normally smooth in situ. Unlike the stratum basale, the stratum spinosum contains several layers of cells that are held together by desmosomes. Although cell division is dramatic in the stratum basale, infrequent divisions are seen in the stratum spinosum. Langerhans cells are found in greater abundance in the spinosum layer, where their slender projections form a weblike frame around the keratinocytes.

The **stratum granulosum** or *granular layer* is the middle layer of skin. It is composed of two to four layers of flattened, diamond-shaped keratinocytes. The cytoplasm of these cells begins to fill with keratohyaline and lamellated granules, which in turn leads to the dramatic degeneration of the nucleus and other organelles. Without these vital parts, the cell quickly dies. The lamellated granules contain waterproofing glycolipids and are transported to the periphery of the cell, where their contents are discharged into the extracellular space. These glycolipids play an important role in waterproofing the skin and in slowing water loss across the epidermis.

The **stratum lucidum** or *clear layer* is only found in very thick skin, so most skin lacks this layer. Microscopically, the stratum lucidum appears as a translucent layer composed of a few rows of flattened, dead cells. In this clear layer and in the outermost epidermal layer, the sticky contents of the keratogranules combine with intracellular tonofilaments to form keratin fibrils.

The **stratum corneum** or *horny layer* is the outermost layer and dominates the epidermis. It constitutes up to three quarters of the total epidermal thickness and is composed of 20 to 30 rows of keratinocytes. Viewed in a sagittal section, the keratinocytes have a paper-thin, almost two-dimensional appearance, yet when viewed from above, they appear hexagonal. Keep in mind that these are really only the remnants of keratinocytes, because the actual cell died in the stratum

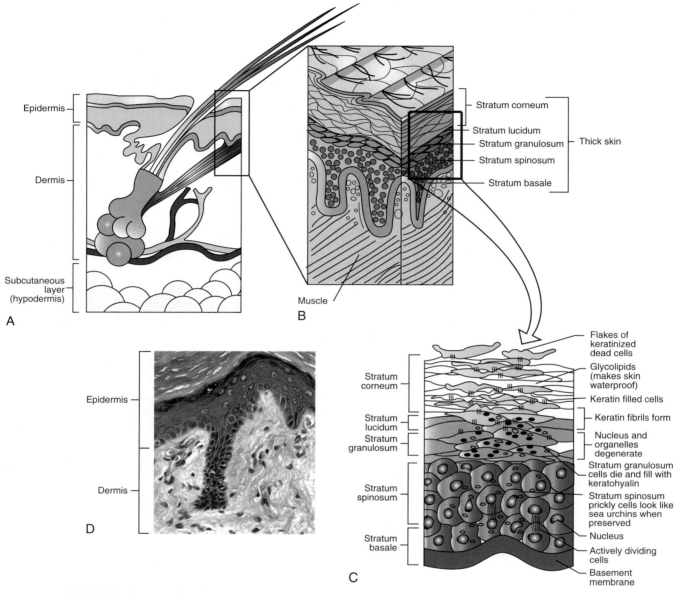

**FIGURE 6-2** Layers of epidermis. **A,** Epidermis is the outermost layer of skin. **B,** Thick regions of skin are composed of five layers, whereas thinner regions may contain only three. **C,** Layers of the epidermis. Skin cells actively divide in the stratum basale, where they are supplied with nutrients from blood vessels in the dermis immediately below. As new cells are produced, older ones are pushed into more superficial layers. During this migration, cells lose their organelles, fill with keratin, and die. By the time they arrive at the skin's surface, they have become little more than thin flakes of keratin. **D,** Light photomicrograph of integument. (**D,** Courtesy Joanna Bassert.)

granulosum. These remnants are sometimes called *horny* or *cornified cells*, but are better known as *dandruff*.

## EPIDERMIS OF HAIRY SKIN

Humans are unusual in their degree of hairlessness, because most mammals are covered with fur. Unlike the epidermis of people and other relatively hairless animals, skin covered with fur usually consists of three epidermal layers, rather than five. These layers are the *stratum basale, stratum spinosum*, and *stratum corneum*. The stratum granulosum and stratum lucidum in general are missing. However, a few regions of five-layered epidermis are found in furry

mammals, but these are usually seen in regions where the keratinization process has slowed and the skin is very thick.

The surface of hairy skin is covered in scalelike folds. Hair emerges from beneath the scales and is directed away from the opening. In dogs the hair is organized in clusters of three follicles per scale.

Interspersed throughout the surface of the epidermis are knoblike elevations called **tactile elevations**, or *epidermal papillae*. Each tactile elevation is usually associated with a **tactile hair**. These special hairs are called **tylotrich hairs**, and they are important in the perception of touch (Figure 6-3).

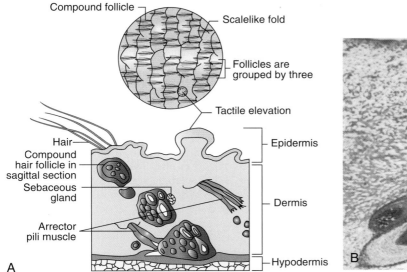

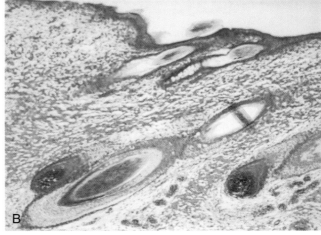

**FIGURE 6-3** Tactile elevation and tylotrich hair. **A,** Compound hairs in dogs are organized into groups of three. Interspersed among these groups are tactile elevations, which are prominent, knoblike extensions of epidermis. They are found in most mammalian species and often are associated with specialized sensory hairs called *tylotrich hairs.* Hair may be found medial, lateral, cranial, or caudal to a tactile elevation. It is thought that this arrangement enables animals to detect subtle pressure, such as the light touch and movement of insects on their skin. **B,** Photomicrograph of skin showing hair follicles on the dermis. (Courtesy Joanna Bassert.)

## DERMIS

The **dermis** makes up the greatest portion of the integument and is responsible for most of the structural strength of the skin. Unlike the epidermis, which is primarily cellular, the dermis is highly fibrous. It is composed of dense irregular connective tissue that contains collagen, elastic, and reticular fibers. Hair follicles, nerve endings, glands, smooth muscle, blood vessels, and lymphatic channels are all found in the dermis as well, creating a rich and interesting tissue community. Fibroblasts, adipocytes, and macrophages also are present and represent the most commonly found cellular elements in the dermis.

The dermis is a tough layer that binds the superficial epidermis to the underlying tissues. It represents the "hide" of the animal and is the layer often used to make leather. The dermis is composed of two layers: the thin, superficial

---

 **CLINICAL APPLICATION**

### What is Mange Anyway?

Mange is an inflammation of the dermis and epidermis *(dermatitis)* caused by tiny mites that live on or in the skin. The mites cause irritation, itchiness **(pruritus)**, and hair loss *(alopecia).* Animals often rub and scratch themselves to the point of causing deep scratches in their skin *(excoriations),* which ooze serum and blood. The skin thickens *(hyperkeratosis)* and becomes flaky. Bloody exudates from vigorous scratching harden and form crusts, making the swollen red integument vulnerable to secondary bacterial infection *(pyoderma).*

The distribution of the red, hairless patches and the way in which the mange spreads depend on the species of the host and the type of mite involved. The type of mange can be identified by scraping the skin with a dull scalpel blade, transferring the scrapings to a microscope slide, and examining the slide under a microscope. Mites that live in the hair follicles and sebaceous glands are called *Demodex.* These are long, thin mites with short stubby legs. *Demodex* are normally found in small numbers on many mammals, but in young or immunosuppressed animals the population of mites can go unchecked and increase to abnormal levels, causing visible patches of hair loss. Infestations of *Sarcoptes* mites are particularly itchy, because they like to burrow into the oozing excoriations of the skin. In contrast to *Demodex, Sarcoptes* mites have round bodies. They are drawn initially to areas that are relatively hairless such as the edges of the ears and elbow caps. From these locations, the mange spreads in dogs onto the face, neck, and up and down the legs. Sarcoptic mange is agonizingly itchy, and affected dogs are often miserable and unable to sleep. *Sarcoptes scabiei* is the species of mite that causes *scabies* or mange in people, dogs, foxes, horses, and cattle.

*Notoedres* is the mite most commonly linked to mange in cats, rats, and rabbits. It looks and behaves like *Sarcoptes* but is smaller. It often begins on the ears in cats, then spreads over the face, to the paws during grooming, and then to the hind legs because of the position the animal assumes when sleeping.

*Continued*

Because mites can spread from humans to other animals and from animals to humans, it is important to identify the mite involved in the infestation correctly. Performing a skin scraping is essential in any suspected mange case. For example, Mimi was a 3-year-old, female spayed domestic shorthair cat. Her owner brought her to the clinic because of hair loss on Mimi's face. The hair loss had occurred progressively during the previous 3 weeks and was getting worse. Given the species of the host (felid) and the location of the alopecia, *Notoedres cati* was high on the list of probable causes for the hair loss; however, when a skin scraping was performed, Mimi had scabies, not *Notoedres*. When the owner was asked if she had any red, itchy rashes, she pulled up her shirt to show a rash under the waistband of her pants. It was later shown that the woman had infected the cat, not the other way around.

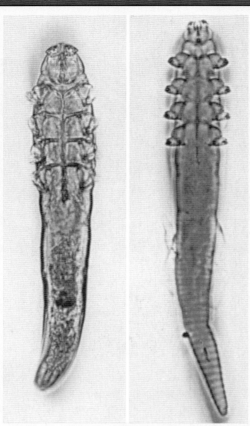

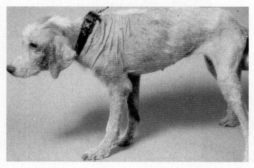

Dog with extensive scabies. (From Scott DW, Miller WT Jr, Griffin CE: Muller and Kirk's small animal dermatology, ed 6, Philadelphia, 2001, Saunders.)

*Demodex canis (left)* and *D. cati (right)* (×390). (From Bowman DD: Georgis' parasitology for veterinarians, ed 8, Philadelphia, 2003, Saunders.)

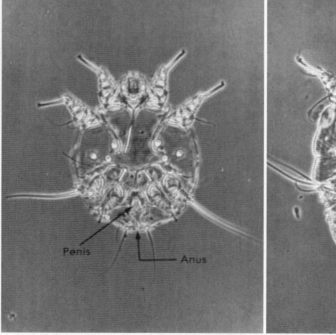

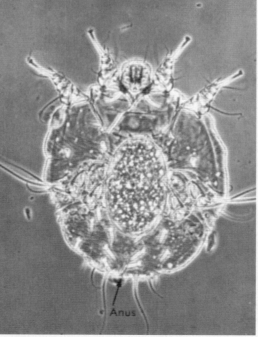

*Sarcoptes* male (*left*, ×140) and female (*right*, ×140). (From Bowman DD: Georgis' parasitology for veterinarians, ed 8, Philadelphia, 2003, Saunders.)

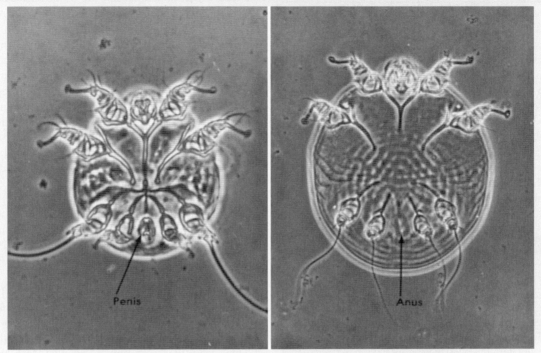

*Notoedres* male (*left*, ×250) and female (*right*, ×290). (From Bowman DD: Georgis' parasitology for veterinarians, ed 8, Philadelphia, 2003, Saunders.)

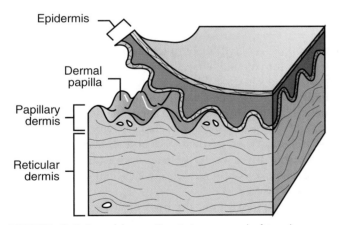

**FIGURE 6-4** Dermal layers. Dermis is composed of two layers: a papillary layer and a deeper, reticular layer. Projections called *dermal papillae* help cement the epidermis and dermis together. In addition, dermal papillae provide extra surface area for exchange of nutrients and waste, and for temperature regulation.

*papillary layer* and the thick, deeper *reticular layer* (Figure 6-4). The **papillary layer** lies just beneath the epithelial layer of the epidermis and is composed of loose connective tissue with loosely woven fibers and ground substance. In most regions of the skin, the papillary layer of the dermis forms nipplelike projections called **dermal papillae**, which rise up into the epidermis. These help to cement the

epidermis and the dermis together. In addition, looping blood vessels are found in the papillary layer, which provide nourishment to the active cells of the stratum basale in the epidermis. The vessels also help to remove waste products and assist with temperature control of the body. Nerve endings or pain receptors and touch receptors called **Meissner's corpuscles** can also be found within the papillary layer. Receptors sensitive to temperature changes are present also.

The deeper **reticular layer**, which consists of dense irregular connective tissue, accounts for 80% of the dermis. The boundary between these two layers is indistinct, because bundles of collagen fibers from the papillary layer blend into those of the reticular layer. The majority of fibrous bundles tend to run parallel to one another, and their orientation depends on the direction of the stress placed on them. Separations between the bundles represent tension lines in the skin. Tension lines are important to surgeons because the healing of an incision occurs best if the incision is made parallel to the direction of the collagen bundles, so fewer collagen fibers are disrupted, and less scar tissue is needed for healing. Wounds or incisions made perpendicular to the tension lines tend to gape open, particularly if that portion of the body bends or flexes. In regions where a great deal of bending occurs, such as around joints, dermal folds or flexure lines can be found. Here the dermis is tightly secured to underlying tissue.

## HYPODERMIS OR SUBCUTANEOUS LAYER

The hypodermis is a thick layer that resides below the dermis. It is a loose layer of areolar tissue that is rich with adipose cells, blood and lymphatic vessels, and nerves. In addition, it contains a type of touch receptor called the **Pacinian corpuscle**. Meissner's corpuscle in the dermis is sensitive to light touch, whereas the Pacinian corpuscle in the hypodermis is sensitive to heavier pressure. The fibers of the hypodermis and those of the dermis are continuous with one another, blurring the distinction between these two layers. The hypodermis is important because it permits the skin to move freely over underlying bone and muscle without putting tension on the skin that would result in tearing.

---

✓ **TEST YOURSELF 6-1**

1. Why is skin important? Can you think of six important functions of skin?
2. What is keratinization and why is it an important process?
3. Can you list all five layers of the epidermis? What is happening in each layer?
4. How is the skin of hairy animals different from that of humans?
5. How is the dermis different from the epidermis?

---

## SPECIAL FEATURES OF THE INTEGUMENT

### PIGMENTATION

Some regions of skin, mucous membranes, hooves, and claws are darkly pigmented, whereas other areas are not. **Pigmentation** is caused by the presence or absence of melanin granules in the armlike extensions of the melanocytes. Grossly, no pigmentation is apparent if the granules are concentrated around the nucleus in the cell body of the melanocyte. As the granules move into the cellular "arms" and into the surrounding tissue, pigmentation becomes grossly apparent. The more granules in the arms of the melanocyte and surrounding tissue, the darker the pigmentation. The dispersion of the granules is controlled by the release of **melanocyte-stimulating hormone** (MSH), which in turn is controlled by the intermediate lobe of the **hypophysis**. The melanosomes are transported to the tips of the cellular projections, where they are released into the intracellular space and ultimately absorbed by keratinocytes. The keratinocytes arrange the melanin on the side of the cell that has the greatest amount of sun exposure. In this way, the pigment acts to protect the keratinocytes from exposure to damaging ultraviolet rays.

### PAW PADS

The feet of many animals are padded and quiet. Thick layers of fat and connective tissue form the foundation of the digital pads that bear the weight of the animal. The pad's outer surface is the toughest and thickest skin on the body.

It is often pigmented and is composed of all five epidermal layers. Of these five layers, the outermost epidermal layer, the stratum corneum, is thicker than all of the others combined. The insulating fat and tough outer skin form a protective barrier against abrasion and thermal variation, enabling the animal to walk on rough surfaces, hot roads, and cold snow. The surface of the pad feels rough, and an uneven surface is visible with the naked eye. On close inspection, minute conical papillae can be seen covering the entire pad (Figure 6-5). Sometimes the central surface of the pad is worn smooth from walking on rough surfaces such as concrete. In this case, the central papillae are rounded or flattened rather than conical, and the papillae on the periphery of the pad maintain their conical shape and are more grossly evident.

Many species have multiple footpads. These include (1) the *carpal pads*, which reside on the caudal surfaces of the "wrist," (2) the *metacarpal* and *metatarsal pads*, which are the central weight-bearing pads of the foot, and (3) the *digital pads*, which protect each of the digits.

In addition to thick adipose layers, the pad is composed of *exocrine sweat glands* and *lamellar corpuscles*. Histologically, the ducts from these sweat glands can be seen passing through the dermis to the stratum basale of the epidermis. Their glandular excretion is expelled onto the surface of the pad.

### PLANUM NASALE

It is not uncommon for people to judge their pet's health by the animal's nose. An alarmed client, for example, may telephone her veterinarian because her dog's nose is too warm, too wet, too dry, or "just not right." The top of the nose in cats, pigs, sheep, and dogs is called the **planum nasale** (Figure 6-6). In the cow and horse, the nose is commonly called the *muzzle* and is technically referred to as the **planum nasolabiale**. Like paw pads, the planum nasale represents an unusual form of skin. Although abnormalities in the appearance of the planum nasale can indicate certain illnesses, its wetness or dryness is usually not an indicator of the health of the animal as a whole. Normal animals can have wet, dry, moist, hot, or cold noses. Let's take a look at the planum nasale in greater detail.

On close inspection, the nose of a dog appears to be composed of polygonal plates packed together. Although usually pigmented and appearing as a tough, thick region of integument, the planum nasale in dogs is composed of only three epidermal layers; the stratum lucidum and stratum granulosum are not present. The outermost layer, the stratum corneum, is composed of only four to eight cell layers, which is surprisingly thin considering the exposed location of the nose and its heavy use, particularly in dogs. The epidermal surface is divided by deep surface grooves, which give it the appearance of being composed of multiple plaques. As with other regions of the skin, the dermis and epidermis interdigitate to form an irregular line of attachment that includes dermal papillae. Although often moist from nasal secretions and licking, the planum nasale in dogs contains no glands in

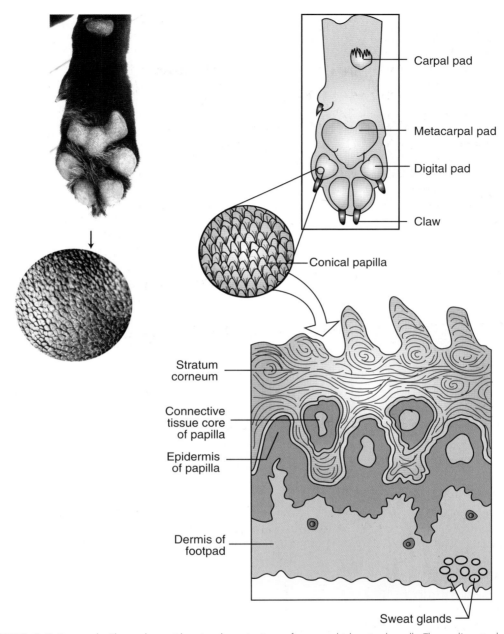

**FIGURE 6-5** Paw pads. The pads provide a tough, protective surface on which animals walk. The pad's outer layer is the thickest skin in the body and is composed of thousands of conical papillae. Papillae arise from stratum corneum, the outermost layer of epidermis.

the epidermis or dermis; however, in sheep, pigs, and cattle tubular glands are found.

## ERGOTS AND CHESTNUTS

*Ergots* and *chestnuts* are dark, horny structures found on the legs of horses, ponies, and other members of the equine family. **Chestnuts** are usually dark brown and are found on the inside of each leg at the carpus (knee) of the forearm and at the tarsus or hock of the hind leg (Figure 6-7). **Ergots** are similar but much smaller and are often overlooked, because they are usually buried in the long, caudal hairs of the fetlock. The horse walks only on the third digit, though its ancestors walked on multiple toes much like dogs today. In the course of its evolutionary path, the horse progressively lost digits to become a faster runner. Chestnuts are thought to be vestiges of carpal and tarsal pads of the first digit, and ergots are thought to be vestiges of the second and fourth digits. Visible remnants of a fifth digit do not exist.

✓ **TEST YOURSELF 6-2**
1. What causes pigmentation of skin?
2. How are paw pads and the planum nasale different from other regions of skin?

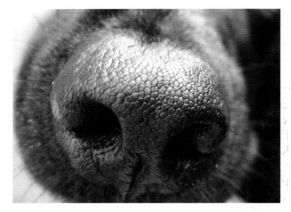

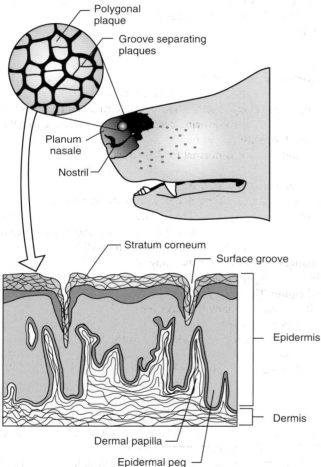

**FIGURE 6-6** Planum nasale. The planum nasale is composed of polygonal plaques separated by epidermal grooves. Unlike footpads, the epidermis in the planum nasale is surprisingly thin and contains three layers rather than five.

## CUTANEOUS POUCHES IN SHEEP

Cutaneous pouches are infoldings of the skin found in sheep. Their three primary locations are in front of the eyes, between the digits above the hooves, and in the groin (Figure 6-8). Respectively, these pouches are technically called the **infraorbital**, **interdigital**, and **inguinal pouches**. Each of these pouches contains fine hairs and numerous sebaceous and oil glands. The glands secrete a fatty yellow substance that dries and sticks to the skin, covering it.

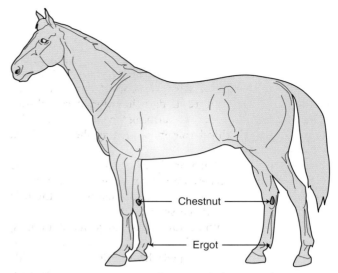

**FIGURE 6-7** Location of ergots and chestnuts in horses.

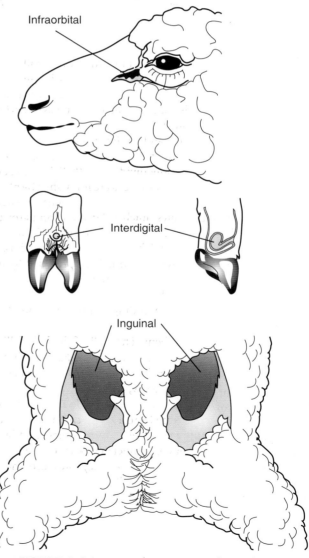

**FIGURE 6-8** Locations of cutaneous pouches in sheep.

## RELATED STRUCTURES OF THE INTEGUMENT

### HAIR

For most animals, hair is essential for survival. By trapping insulating layers of air, hair plays an important role in maintaining body temperature. If dark in color, it can absorb light, which further assists in warming the animal. Coat color may also play a critical role in protecting the animal via camouflage.

In most species of mammal, hair occurs as fur. Marine mammals such as whales, domestic pigs, human beings, and relatively few other species are exceptional in that the hair covering their bodies is sparse and thin. Such species have evolved to survive without fur. For the majority of animals, however, thick fur covers the greater surface of their bodies. Only the hooves, lips, paw pads, horns, nipples, inner folds of genitalia, and nasal regions may be devoid of hair. Animals' coats tend to be thickest on the most exposed regions of the body, such as on the back and sides, whereas the abdomen and inner sides of the proximal limbs are less densely covered.

### HAIR STRANDS AND THEIR FOLLICLES

The part of hair that is visible above the skin is called the **shaft**, and the portion buried within the skin is called the **root**. Hair is anchored by the **hair follicle**, which is an invagination of the epidermis that extends from the skin surface to the dermis or, occasionally, to the hypodermis. The deepest part of the hair follicle expands to form a **hair bulb**. At the base of the bulb is a mound of dermal cells called the **papilla**, which is covered with rapidly dividing epithelial cells called the **matrix** (Figure 6-9, A). These cells are nourished by blood flow from vessels in the underlying papilla. Nourishment of the epithelial cells stimulates much cell division and growth. As the cells divide, older cells are pushed upward into the tunnel away from the papilla. These cells become keratinized, and as they lose contact with the nutrition provided by the papilla, they die and become part of the developing hair. In this way hair is constructed from dead epithelial cells.

A web of sensory nerve endings called the **root hair plexus** envelops the root, making it an important touch receptor when the hair is bent. The wall of the hair follicle is composed of three layers: an *internal epithelial* root sheath, an *outer epithelial* root sheath, and a *dermal* or *connective tissue* root sheath (see Figure 6-9, B and C).

Animals with fur often have **compound follicles** in which multiple hair strands emerge from a single **epidermal orifice** or *pore*, although each strand has its own follicle and bulb. As many as 15 hairs may be associated with one pore. In compound follicles a single, long **primary hair**, also known as a *guard hair* or *cover hair*, is usually surrounded by shorter **secondary hairs**, also called *satellite hairs*. In dogs, three compound follicles are usually grouped together to emerge from the same epidermal fold.

Hair is formed in three concentric layers (see Figure 6-9, D). The innermost layer and central core is called the **medulla**. It is composed of two to three layers of loosely arranged cells that are separated by spaces filled with liquid or air. The cells themselves contain flexible *soft keratin* similar to that found in the stratum corneum of the epidermis. Surrounding the medulla is the **cortex**. Unlike the flexible medulla, the cortex is stiff and rigid because it is composed of *hard keratin* and is the thickest of the three layers. A single layer of cells arising from the edge of the papilla forms the hair surface, which is called the **cuticle**. It is also composed of hard keratin. The cells of the cuticle are layered like shingles on a roof, which prevents the hairs from sticking together and forming mats. However in some animals, such as sheep, the edges of the cells in the cuticle are raised, enabling them to "grab onto" the cuticle cells from other hair strands. Because of this, wool threads can be created by twisting and pulling clumps of hair.

### GROWTH CYCLES OF HAIR

However unconsciously, we are all aware that hair undergoes a cycle of growing and falling out. When we remove a wad of hair from a clogged sink, when we vacuum up hair left behind by the dog on his favorite chair, and when we can cover the barn floor with a layer of hair from our horse after brushing, we know that it is normal for hair to fall out. Hair is shed to make room for the production of new strands. The volume of shedding is influenced by genetics and by the environment. For example, shedding is heaviest in the spring and fall for animals that live outside. Longhaired animals may shed more than shorthaired animals, and animals kept indoors may shed less than animals kept outdoors. In addition, hormonal changes may influence shedding. For example, many bitches lose a large percentage of their total hair volume at once after whelping. The technical term for this phenomenon is **telogen effluvium**, but many breeders refer to it as *blowing the coat*. Whether an animal is undergoing routine shedding or blowing its coat, hair is lost to make room in the follicles for the production of new hair strands. How does this happen?

When a hair is produced, dead keratinized epithelial cells push up and away from the dermal papilla and are organized into the layers that make up the hair shaft and root (Figure 6-10). As more cells are added at the base of the root, the hair lengthens. During this time of growth, the hair is said to be in the **anagen phase**. As one would expect, the maximum length achieved by the anagen hair is genetically predetermined. In this way, some species and breeds of animals have long coats, whereas others have short coats. When the maximum length of hair is achieved, the hair stops growing, the hair follicle shortens, and the hair is held in a resting phase. This quiescent period is called the **telogen phase**, which can last from weeks to years depending on the location, type of hair, and species involved. The period of transition between the anagen and telogen phases is called the **catagen phase**.

### HAIR COLOR

Pigment in the cortex and medulla gives hair its color. Genetically programmed melanocytes located at the base of the

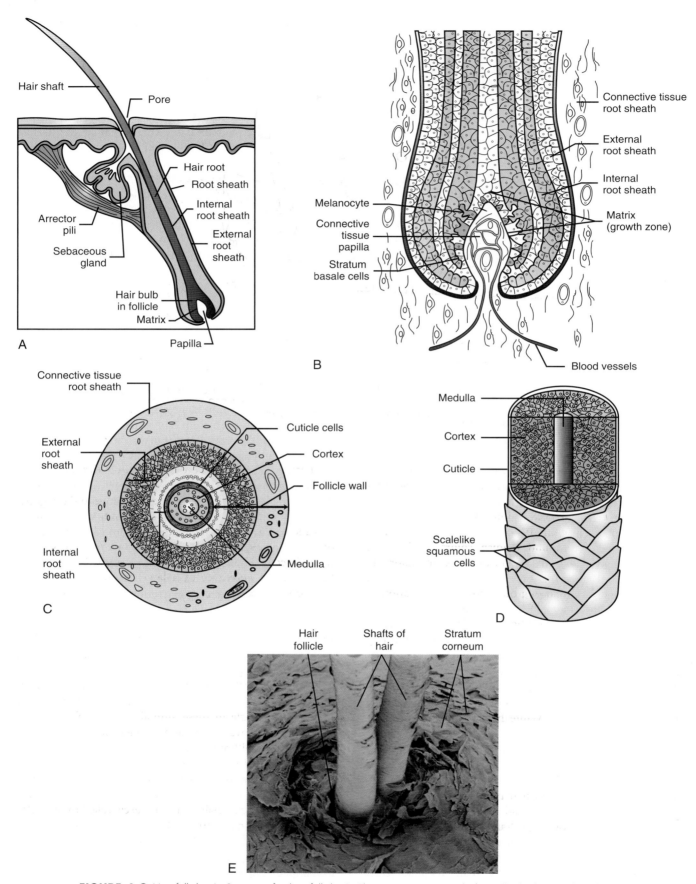

**FIGURE 6-9** Hair follicle. **A,** Structure of a hair follicle. **B,** The matrix is composed of rapidly dividing epidermal cells that are supplied with important nutrients from the blood vessels in the **connective tissue papilla**. A strand of hair is formed as daughter epithelial cells mature, fill with keratin, and move away from the papilla and its blood supply. Cells subsequently die and become part of the hair. **C,** The root sheath is composed of three layers: *connective tissue* root sheath, *external* root sheath, and *internal* root sheath. **D,** Dead epithelial cells make up the hair. Each strand is organized into three layers: *cuticle, cortex,* and *medulla.* **E,** Scanning electron micrograph of two hair shafts. (Copyright © by David Scharf, 1986, 1993.)

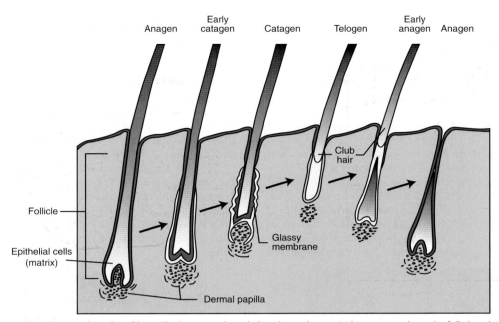

**FIGURE 6-10** Growth cycles of hair. The hair growth cycle has three phases. In the *anagen* phase the follicle is longest. The *catagen* phase occurs with the appearance of a thick, glassy membrane and a shortening of the hair follicle. Thickening of the basement membrane in the matrix separates epidermal cells from the dermal papilla. In the *telogen* phase the hair follicle is very short, and the dermal papilla is separated from the bulb. The hair strand is rounded and resembles a club and is therefore called a *club* hair.

hair follicle produce melanin, which is transferred to the cortical and medullary cells that form the hair strand. Different colors are achieved depending on the quantity and type of melanin incorporated into the hair. Horses, for example, produce only one type of melanin, whereas dogs produce two. Yellowish and reddish colors in dogs are achieved with **pheomelanin**, and the brown–black colors are formed by the presence of **tyrosine melanin**. In horses, all colors are achieved by varying the amount and location of the melanin, not the type. Darker colors are generally achieved with greater quantities of melanin than lighter shades. In addition, pigmentation may occur uniformly throughout the hair to form a solid color, or it may be concentrated at just the base or just the tip of the strand to form agouti-type coloration.

As animals age, melanin production decreases, and the hair begins to turn gray. White hair is formed when the cortex loses its pigment entirely and the medulla becomes completely filled with air.

## TYPES OF HAIR

Animals possess a variety of hair types. In general, hair has been categorized into three broad groups: *primary* or *guard hairs*, *secondary* or **wool-type hairs**, and *tactile* or **sinus hairs**. **Primary hairs** are generally straight or arched and are thicker and longer than secondary hairs. They are the dominant hairs in a complex hair follicle. As already mentioned, the complex hair follicle in dogs consists of one primary hair surrounded by numerous secondary hairs. **Secondary hairs** are softer and shorter than primary hairs. They are generally wavy or bristled in dogs and are the predominant hair type

in species with wool-type coats. **Tactile hairs** are used as probes and feelers. They are well supplied with sensory endings that make them particularly sensitive to the slightest bending or touch. These hairs are commonly known as *whiskers* and can be found around the mouth and on the muzzle of many species, as well as mixed intermittently throughout the hair coat. The tactile hair is also called the **sinus hair** because of the presence of a large blood sinus, which is located in the connective tissue portion of the follicle.

## ARRECTOR PILI MUSCLES

In most animals, hair slopes from the nose to the tail. In some species or breeds of animal, the hair is more erect than in others. The degree of erection is called the **implantation angle**. The summer coats of horses, for example, are short and lie flat against the surface of the skin, therefore the implantation angle in these animals is relatively low. Dog breeds tend to have implantation angles that range from 30 to 40 degrees, although the Chow, Airedale, and Scottish Terrier have angles as high as 45 degrees.

When frightened or cold, animals can make their hair stand up beyond the normal implantation angle. This is due to the presence of a small, smooth muscle called the **arrector pili muscle**, which is attached to each hair follicle and is innervated by the sympathetic nervous system. When the muscle contracts, it pulls the hair to an erect position. Perhaps you have seen a frightened cat "puff up." This reaction is a defense mechanism designed to make the animal appear bigger and therefore less vulnerable to potential predators. In addition, hair that stands erect can better trap insulating layers of air than nonerect hair. So animals with erect

### Allergies: Itchy Business

When cats and dogs develop allergies, they do not usually develop congested sinuses and runny eyes and noses the way people do. Instead, dogs and cats develop itchy skin and ears. Like people, animals can develop an allergy to just about anything, including human dander. Imagine finding out your pet is allergic to *you*!

Allergies to inhalant particles such as pollen, dust, and mold spores are common. This type of allergy is called *atopy* and can cause seasonal itchiness, as in the case of ragweed pollen, or year-round itchiness like that caused by house dust. Atopic dogs tend to rub their faces on the carpet, scratch in the axillae (armpits) with their hind feet, and lick the tops of their paws. Food allergies and allergies to ectoparasites, such as fleas, are also very common. Dogs with flea allergies tend

to "corncob chew" the base of their tail and the medial sides of their hind legs. Cats rarely chew but exhibit itchiness by excessive licking, grooming, and scratching their face with a hind leg. Facial excoriations are evident in the photo on the left, and excessive grooming causes hair loss and redness on the abdomen of a cat in the photo on the right. Notice the lines of normal skin, which fall into folds when the cat is curled to lick its abdomen.

To some extent the veterinarian can distinguish between the various types of allergies by the pattern of *pruritus* or itchiness on the body. Areas that have been scratched or licked excessively will be excoriated, raw, and hairless. In chronic cases the skin may become *hyperpigmented* and turn black, or areas of white fur may exhibit *salivary staining* by turning the hairs yellow.

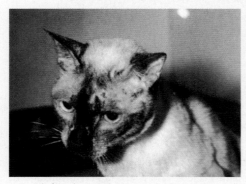

Feline atopy with facial excoriations. (From Scott DW, Miller WT Jr, Griffin CE: Muller and Kirk's small animal dermatology, ed 6, Philadelphia, 2001, Saunders.)

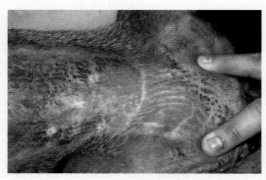

Feline atopy with plaques and alopecia. (From Scott DW, Miller WT Jr, Griffin CE: Muller and Kirk's small animal dermatology, ed 6, Philadelphia, 2001, Saunders.)

---

### ✓ TEST YOURSELF 6-3

1. Draw and label the parts of a hair follicle.
2. How does hair form and grow?
3. What are the three cycles of hair growth?
4. Why does hair turn gray and then white as animals age?
5. What factors stimulate contraction of the arrector pili muscle? Why is this muscle important?

hair coats stay warmer than animals with flat coats. In humans, contraction of the arrector pili muscles causes goose bumps. The arrector pili muscle also is responsible for forcing sebum from the sebaceous gland, which helps keep the integument moist and supple.

## GLANDS OF THE SKIN
### SEBACEOUS GLANDS

Sebaceous glands are generally found all over the body except in certain specialized regions, such as paw pads and the planum nasale. The glands are located in the dermis and may be simple or complex alveolar structures. Although most sebaceous glands have a single duct that empties into a hair

follicle, others have ducts that empty directly onto the surface of the skin. This latter group of sebaceous glands is found at the mucocutaneous junctions of the lips, labia vulvae, penis, prepuce, anus, eyelid, and in the ear canal. In sheep, sebaceous glands empty directly onto the surface of the skin in the infraorbital pouches, interdigital pouches, and inguinal pouches. The sebaceous glands associated with hair follicles are found in the triangle formed by the surface of the skin, the hair follicle, and the arrector pili muscle.

Sebaceous gland alveoli are lined with epithelial cells that manufacture and store an oily, lipid substance composed primarily of glycerides and free fatty acids. Eventually, the cells become so full that they rupture and release their contents, together with cellular debris, into the center of the alveolus. This white, semiliquid mixture is called **sebum**. In sheep, sebaceous glands produce a substance that ultimately becomes **lanolin**. Because the epithelial cell is lost in the process of secretion, the sebaceous gland is classified as a holocrine structure.

When the arrector pili muscle contracts, it compresses the sebaceous gland, and the sebum is forced from the alveolus through the duct into the hair follicle. Here sebum coats the base of the hair and the surrounding skin and plays an important role in trapping moisture to prevent excessive drying. In this way, the skin and hair are kept soft, pliant, and somewhat waterproof. Sebum also possesses some antibacterial and antifungal properties, which reduce the skin's risk of infection. The sebaceous gland is sensitive to changes in levels of sex hormones and therefore is most productive during puberty in humans. Excessive amounts of sebum can clog the openings of hair follicles, forming whiteheads. With time, the sebum turns black and forms blackheads, which are also called *comedones*. If untreated, comedones may develop into pimples or pustules. This process occurs in animals as well as in humans.

## SWEAT GLANDS

**Sweat glands** are also called *sudoriferous glands* and are found over the entire body of most domestic species, including pigs, horses, cattle, dogs, and sheep. As we all know, sweat is a watery, transparent liquid that helps cool the body through evaporation. Although sweat glands are numerous in most domestic species, only the horse produces a profuse sweat, which sometimes works itself into a white froth. The two types of sweat glands are *eccrine* and *apocrine* (Figure 6-11).

### ECCRINE SWEAT GLANDS. The excretory portion of
the **eccrine gland** consists of a simple coiled tube located in the dermis or hypodermis. It is connected to the surface of the skin by a long duct. In dogs, eccrine sweat glands are found only in the deep layers of fat and in the connective tissue of footpads.

### APOCRINE SWEAT GLANDS. Like eccrine sweat
glands, **apocrine sweat glands** have a coiled, excretory portion buried in the dermis or hypodermis with a single excretory duct. However, unlike eccrine sweat glands, apocrine glands empty into hair follicles, rather than onto the surface of the skin. In dogs, apocrine glands are located in the external ear canal. Interestingly, dogs with long hair have more sebaceous and apocrine glands in their external ear canals than do dogs with short hair. Dogs with more hair in their ear canals have an increased incidence of *otitis externa*, which is an infection of the ear canal.

## TAIL GLANDS

Most felids (cats) and canids (dogs) possess an oval region at the dorsal base of their tails called the **tail gland** (Figure 6-12). The tail gland is thought to assist with the recognition and identification of individual animals, and may be grossly recognizable by the presence of coarse, oily hairs. Apocrine and sebaceous glands are especially large in this region. Like sebaceous glands, apocrine glands are sensitive to changes in sex hormone levels, and therefore they become particularly active during puberty and estrus. The tail gland is thought to assist animals in identifying one another.

## ANAL SACS

**Anal sacs** and other related musk glands are famous for their powerful, foul-smelling secretions. Although skunks

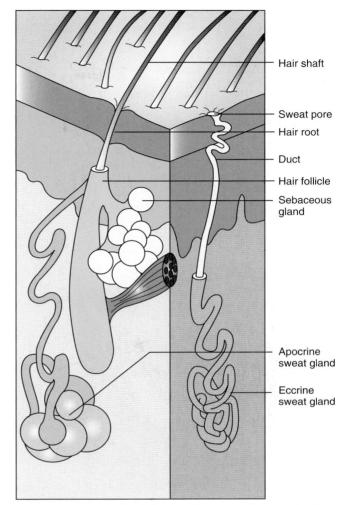

**FIGURE 6-11** Glands of the skin. Two types of sweat gland are *apocrine glands*, with ducts that connect to hair follicles, and *eccrine glands*, which empty directly onto the skin surface. Sebaceous glands are also depicted.

are shy and not often seen in the wild, it is not uncommon to catch the noxious odor of a skunk's spray from our car as we drive down a suburban or rural road. The odor can linger in the region for days. Cats and dogs have anal sacs similar to musk glands that are located at the 5 and 7 o'clock positions relative to the anus. They are connected to the lateral margin of the anus by a small, single duct. The anal sac is lined with sebaceous and apocrine glands and acts as a reservoir for the secretions that are produced from these glands. When the animal defecates or becomes frightened, some or all of the anal sac contents are expressed, feces become coated with the secretions stored in the anal sac, and the unique smell of the animal is transferred to the environment. Thus **defecation** serves the purposes of elimination, marking territory, and attracting a mate. Sometimes the small duct of the anal sac clogs and can become infected if left untreated. Animals with irritated or impacted anal sacs often drag their rumps along the ground to help alleviate the discomfort.

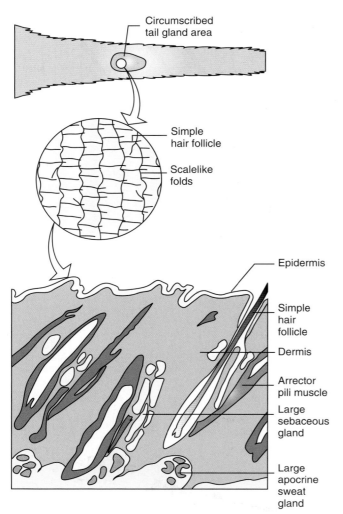

**FIGURE 6-12** Tail gland area. The tail gland region in dogs and cats is rich with apocrine and sebaceous glands, which become particularly productive when sex hormone levels are high. Simple, coarse hairs predominate, making the region look grossly different from surrounding areas.

---

✓ TEST YOURSELF 6-4

1. Name two types of sweat gland. How are they different from one another?
2. Where are anal sacs found and what is their importance to animals?

---

## CLAWS AND DEWCLAWS

Many animals have **claws**, which are the hard, often pigmented outer coverings of the distal digits. Claws are important for maintaining good traction while running, walking, and climbing and serve as lifesaving tools for defense and for catching prey. In most animals claws are nonretractable, although, with the exception of the cheetah, cats can retract their claws (Figure 6-13). Interestingly, the claws of cats cannot be separated from the **distal phalanx bones**. A declaw

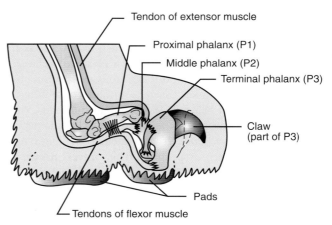

**FIGURE 6-13** Cat claw. The claw on a cat is an extension of the third phalanx. Declaw procedures involve complete amputation of this bone.

procedure therefore necessitates amputation of the entire third phalanx. Fortunately, this procedure is usually limited to the front feet.

**Dewclaws** are the remains of digits that have regressed in the course of evolution. In dogs, the dewclaw is the first digit, but actual bones are only found in the dewclaws of the forelimbs. In cattle, pigs, and sheep, the medial and lateral dewclaws are the second and fifth digits, respectively. Of these three species only pigs have dewclaws that contain bones. Both the **metacarpal bones** and **phalangeal bones** are present in the dewclaws of pigs, just as they are in the weight-bearing digits.

## THE HOOF

We all know what hooves are, but we might not know that the technical name for the **hoof** is **ungula** and that hoofed animals are called **ungulates**. Ruminants have four hooves per foot, and each one covers a digit; however, weight is carried only on two of the four hooves in many ungulates such as sheep, cattle, and goats. The weight-bearing hooves represent the third and fourth digits. Imagine walking only on your middle and ring fingers. In essence, that is what these farm animals are doing. Although their evolutionary ancestors had five toes, the "thumb" or first digit has disappeared, and the "index finger" and "pinky"—the second and fifth digits—have regressed into what we call the *dewclaws*. These digits are found on the caudal aspect of the foot behind the weight-bearing hooves. As mentioned, a horse, remarkably, walks on only one digit of each foot, that being the third digit, which is equivalent to our middle finger or toe. (See Figure 6-14 for an illustration of the equine foot.)

Both claws and hooves rest on underlying sensitive tissue called the **corium**. The corium is firmly attached to the periosteum of the third phalanx and is rich with blood vessels that provide nutrient molecules to the developing cells in the inner layers of the hoof. Thus the outer hoof is a modified

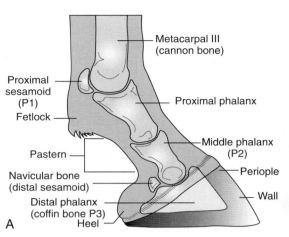

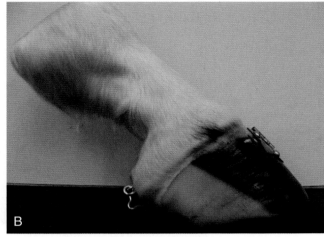

**FIGURE 6-14** Bones of the equine foot. **A,** The skeletal foot of the horse includes the distal part of the second phalanx; the distal sesamoid bone, or *navicular bone;* and the entire third phalanx, commonly known as the *coffin bone.* **B,** Photograph of equine foot.

epithelial layer, and the corium is modified dermis. The corium is well innervated and sensitive to pain, whereas the outer layers of the wall, sole, and frog have no sensation. In addition, the corium is divided into regions based on the portion of the hoof that it produces and/or maintains. There are five types of corium in the equine foot: laminar, perioplic, coronary, sole, and frog.

1. **Laminar corium** consists of primary and secondary lamina and is located between the hoof wall and the third phalanx. It provides nutrients to the stratum internum. **Laminitis** is a serious condition in horses in which the laminar corium becomes inflamed (Figure 6-15).
2. **Perioplic corium** is located in the perioplic sulcus and supplies nutrients to the overlaying periople.
3. **Coronary corium** is found in the coronary sulcus and provides nutrients to the stratum externum and stratum medium.
4. **Sole corium** is located superior to the sole and provides nutrients to the sole.
5. **Frog corium** is located superior to the frog and provides nutrients to the frog.

The hoof grows from the **coronary band** downward. Growth of the hoof is continuous, and hooves that are not trimmed can become so long that they curl up like the shoes worn by elves. In wild horses the abrasion caused by running on rough surfaces is an important part of maintaining normal hoof length. Domestic horses, however, rely on a farrier to trim their hooves. Horses are used for work: to carry heavy riders; pull loads; and carry packs, often on hard roads and surfaces. This puts the equine hoof at greater risk for cracking or chipping, which in turn causes lameness and renders the horse unable to work. Long ago, it was discovered that nailing a rigid metal shoe to the plantar and palmar surface of the hoof increased the integrity of the wall and strengthened the foot. A horseshoe prevents excessive expansion of

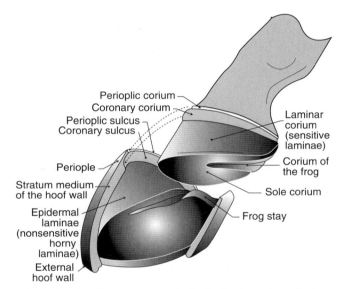

**FIGURE 6-15** Equine laminae. The hoof is held onto the coffin bone by delicate, interdigitating laminae. When these laminae become inflamed during a painful condition called *laminitis,* the connection between the hoof and the coffin bone is weakened. Consequently, the coffin bone may slip and rotate downward.

the hoof when the animal carries weight. It also improves traction, creates an additional barrier between the hoof and the ground, and allows horses to be kept in working condition with greater regularity.

The skeletal foot of the horse includes the distal part of the second phalanx; the distal sesamoid bone, which is called the **navicular bone;** and the entire third phalanx, which is commonly known as the **coffin bone.** The coffin bone is cloaked in a layer of corium, which in turn is covered by the cornified hoof. The hoof and the corium form an

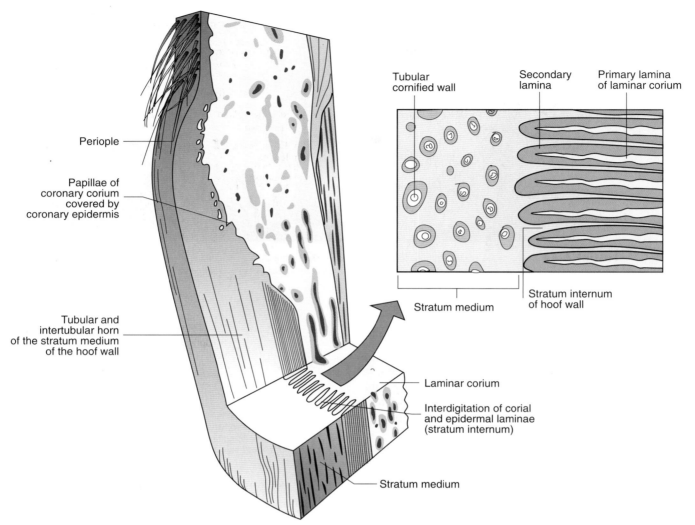

**FIGURE 6-16** Longitudinal cross section of the hoof wall.

elaborate array of interdigitations called **laminae**. The laminae consist of primary and secondary extensions, which increase the contact area between the corium and the **hoof wall**. These important interdigitations form the attachment between the hoof and the coffin bone (Figure 6-16).

The equine hoof is generally divided into three parts: the *wall*, the *sole*, and the *frog*. Let's examine each of these parts.

### THE WALL

The wall is the convex, external portion of the hoof that is visible from the anterior, lateral, and medial views. It is divided into three regions: the *toe*, the *quarters*, and the *heels* (Figure 6-17). The **toe** is the front of the foot, and the **quarters** make up the lateral aspects. The **heel** is the portion of the wall that tapers downward and wraps around the back of the foot. The hooves of the front feet are angled at about 50 degrees, and those in the back are angled at about 55 degrees. Minute, vertical lines representing **horn tubes** may be evident running from the coronary band to the ground,

and rings or ridges can be seen wrapping around the hoof. Like the rings in tree trunks, these lines or ridges represent periods of growth in the hoof.

### THE SOLE

The **sole** is the plantar or palmar surface of the hoof. It is concave and fills the space bordered by the wall and the bars. The part of the sole that immediately surrounds the bars is called the **angle**. Like other external portions of the hoof, the outer layers of the sole are avascular and lack innervation. Deeper layers of the corium provide nutrient molecules and contain nervous input. The corium connects the sole to the underside of the coffin bone. A thin strip called the **white line** is formed at the junction of the sole and the hoof wall.

### THE FROG

The insensitive **frog** is a triangular, horny structure located between the heels on the underside of the hoof. The **point** or apex of the frog faces the toe, and the base runs across the

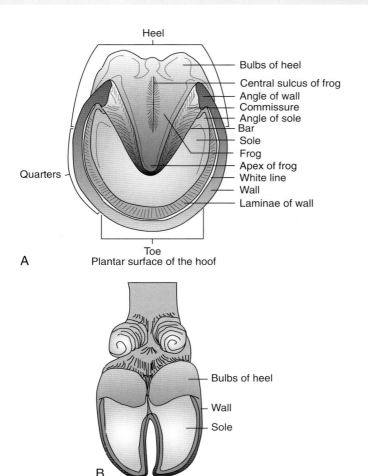

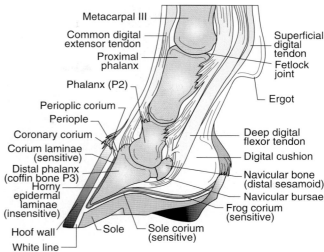

**FIGURE 6-18** Longitudinal section of equine foot showing internal anatomic structures.

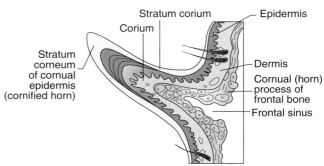

**FIGURE 6-19** Cross section through a horn.

**FIGURE 6-17** Anatomy of volar region of equine and bovine hooves. A, Equine hoof. B, Bovine hoof.

caudal aspect of the foot between the heels. The frog is divided by a central depression known as the **central sulcus** or *cleft* of the frog. The frog is separated from the bars on the lateral and medial sides by a deep, concave region called the **collateral sulcus**. A thick pad of fat and fibrous tissue, called the **digital cushion**, lies beneath the sensitive frog.

Two large bands of cartilage called the **lateral cartilages** extend proximally from the distal phalanx and form an important structural support for the equine foot. These bands, together with the frog and digital cushion, work as a kind of circulatory pump to assist blood flow through the foot. As the horse bears weight, the frog is compressed against the bars, and the heel of the foot expands (Figure 6-18). In addition, the digital cushion is compressed against the lateral cartilages and the frog, which forces blood out of the corium, away from the foot, and into the digital veins. Shifting weight off of the foot releases the compressive force and enables blood to flow back into the corium via the digital arteries.

## HORNS

Like hooves, **horns** are epidermal in origin and are structurally similar to hair. They emerge from the horn processes of

the frontal bones and take on diverse shapes and sizes in ruminating ungulate species such as sheep, goats, cattle, buffalo, and antelope. In adults the horn is generally hollow and communicates directly with the frontal sinus (Figure 6-19). Like the hoof, the horn is a mass of horny keratin. The corium lies at the root of the horn and is bound to the horn process by periosteum. In addition, long, slender papillae of corium interdigitate with one another to form critical attachments that bind the outer horn to the underlying periosteum. The body of the horn is composed of tubules, which are packed close together to form a single mass. Although externally the diameter of the horn is larger at the base and forms a point at the apex, the wall of the horn is actually thinner at the base than at the apex. In fact, the apex of the horn is considerably stronger and denser than the horn base (Figure 6-20).

With the exception of the American Pronghorn, which sheds its horns annually, horns grow continuously throughout the life of the animal and can reach great lengths. Many domestic species of sheep, goats, and cattle are dehorned when young to facilitate their management by the farmer (Figure 6-21). Several different instruments and methods can be used to dehorn an animal, depending on the age and

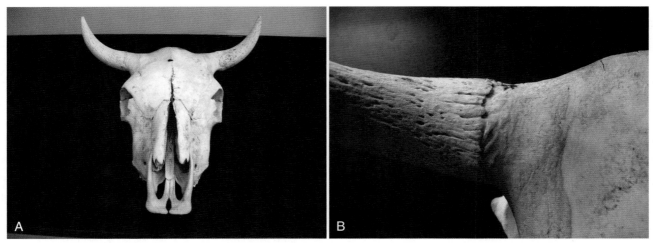

**FIGURE 6-20** **A,** Horns are found on male and female cattle, sheep, and goats and are made of highly keratinized stratum corneum of the epidermis. The medullary cavity of the horn is continuous with the frontal sinus in the skull. Variations in nutrition affect the rate at which horns grow. **B,** Horns form from the *os cornua* or *horny process,* which is an outgrowth of the frontal bone. The horny process is covered with a thick layer of modified dermis called *corium,* which gives rise to the epidermal cells that make up the horn.

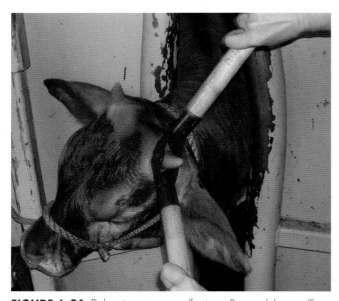

**FIGURE 6-21** Dehorning a young calf using a Barnes dehorner. (From McCurnin DM, Bassert JM: Clinical textbook for veterinary technicians, ed 6, St Louis, 2006, Saunders.)

species involved. The standard procedure is to remove the horn or horn bud and to destroy the corium, usually via cauterization, to prevent further growth. Some species of domestic animals have been bred to be horn free. These breeds are called **polled breeds**. In nonpolled breeds, horns are found on both males and females. Unlike antlers, they are not sex specific.

In contrast to horns, antlers are found primarily on males, are dermal in origin, and arise as bony protuberances from the skull. They grow and are shed annually. Antlers lack a central core and internal blood supply but are nourished externally by a soft, velvetlike tissue. When the antler has completed its growth, a dense ring of connective tissue forms at the base of the antler, which restricts blood supply to the outer **velvet skin**, causing it to die and subsequently be scraped off by the animal. Loss of the velvet allows the antler to harden and become a formidable weapon, a status symbol, and an attractive male secondary sex characteristic. With time, the bony connection between the antler and the skull breaks down, the antlers fall off, and new growth begins.

 **CLINICAL APPLICATION**

## Laminitis: A Painful Health Risk to Horses

*Laminitis,* or *founder* as it is commonly called, is an excruciatingly painful disorder that affects the feet—primarily the front feet—of horses and ponies. As its name implies, laminitis is inflammation of the delicate laminae that attach the hoof wall to the underlying coffin bone. As with all inflammation, laminitis involves swelling; however, the outer wall of the hoof is rigid and cannot expand to accommodate the swelling of the inner foot, so the laminae become compressed. Blood flow and circulation within the foot are inhibited, and the laminae degenerate. Because the laminae attach the coffin bone to the outer hoof, their degeneration may cause the distal phalanx or coffin bone to pull away from the hoof wall. Under the weight of the animal, the bone may rotate downward and push against the sole of the hoof. With very severe rotation, the distal phalanx can actually perforate the sole, and this will lead to the death of the animal. Chronic laminitis causes abnormal hoof growth.

## CLINICAL APPLICATION—cont'd

Because laminitis is acutely painful, affected animals are often recumbent for extended periods, standing only to urinate, defecate, and access water and food. When standing, horses with laminitis tend to shift their weight away from the front feet to their hind legs to alleviate pressure in the toe. Their gait is slow and hesitant, and their heart rate and respiratory rate may be elevated because of the pain. A mild tap on the toe with hoof testers can elicit a strong pain response from the horse.

In cases of chronic laminitis, external changes to the hoof become evident. Circumferential rings in the outer hoof wall become pronounced, marking previous aberrations in hoof growth. The angle of the hoof is reduced, and the hoof consequently appears flattened. If rotation has occurred, the sole may appear "dropped." With corrective trimming of the hoof, change in diet, and good management techniques, some of these aberrant changes can be corrected.

Predisposing factors for laminitis include the following:
- Engorgement of foods high in carbohydrates
- Any systemic illness or condition that might lead to endotoxemia
- The postoperative period
- Retained placentas in mares
- Adverse reaction to drugs

Ponies, in particular, are prone to developing laminitis, particularly if they are permitted to graze on lush pasture or are fed diets rich in carbohydrates such as corn, molasses, and grains. Treatment is designed to decrease swelling, relieve pain, and increase circulation in the feet. Prevention by adherence to a strict, low-carbohydrate diet is essential in ponies and horses that are sensitive to carbohydrate levels.

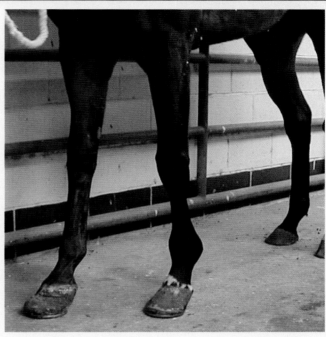

Gross pathologic photograph of sagittal section of both front feet of a horse with bilateral laminitis that has undergone coffin bone rotation. (From McCurnin DM, Bassert JM: Clinical textbook for veterinary technicians, ed 6, St Louis, 2006, Saunders.)

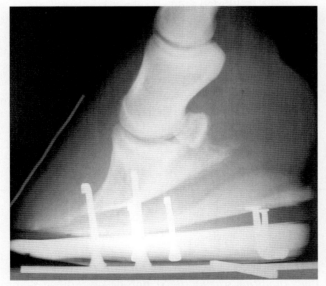

Lateral radiograph of the front foot of a horse with laminitis that shows evidence of coffin bone rotation. (From McCurnin DM, Bassert JM: Clinical textbook for veterinary technicians, ed 6, St Louis, 2006, Saunders.)

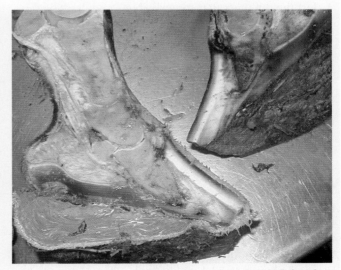

Abnormal hoof growth in a horse with chronic laminitis in both front feet. (From McCurnin DM, Bassert JM: Clinical textbook for veterinary technicians, ed 6, St Louis, 2006, Saunders.)

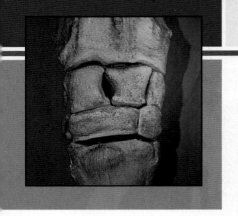

# The Skeletal System

*Thomas Colville*

## LEARNING OBJECTIVES

*When you have completed this chapter you will be able to:*

1. List the cell types that comprise bone and describe the function of each cell type.
2. List the functions of bone.
3. Differentiate between cancellous and compact bone.
4. Describe the process of endochondral bone formation and growth.
5. Describe the process of intramembranous bone formation.
6. List and describe the four bone shapes.
7. Differentiate between yellow and red bone marrow.
8. List and define the terms used to describe shape and surface features of bone.
9. List the components of the axial and appendicular skeletons.
10. Name the internal and external bones of the face and cranium.
11. List the divisions of the spinal column.
12. Describe the structure of the ribs and sternum.
13. Name the bones of the thoracic and pelvic limbs.
14. List and describe the three classifications of joints.

## VOCABULARY FUNDAMENTALS

*Abduction* ahb-**duhck**-shuhn
*Acetabulum* ahs-eh-**tahb**-yuh-luhm
*Adduction* ahd-**duhck**-shun
*Amphiarthrosis* **ahm**-fih-ahrth-rō-sihs
*Anconeal process* ahn-**kō**-nē-ahl **proh**-sehs
*Antebrachium* ahn-tē-**brā**-kē-uhm
*Appendicular skeleton* ahp-ehn-**dihck**-ū-lər **skehl**-ih-tuhn
*Arthrodial joint* **ahrth**-rō-dē-ahl joynt
*Articular cartilage* ahr-**tihck**-yuh-lər **kahr**-tih-lihj
*Articular process* ahr-**tihck**-yuh-lər **proh**-sehs
*Articular surface* ahr-**tihck**-yuh-lər **suhr**-fihs

*Asternal rib* ā-**stuhrn**-ahl rihb
*Atlas* **aht**-lehs
*Axial skeleton* **ahck**-sē-ahl **skehl**-ih-tuhn
*Axis* **ahck**-sihs
*Ball-and-socket joint* bahl *and* **sohck**-eht joynt
*Body condition scoring (BCS)* **boh**-dē kohn-**dihsh**-shuhn **skohr**-ihng
*Bone cortex* bōn **kohr**-tehx
*Bone marrow* bōn **meər**-ō
*Bone of the cranium* bōn *of the* **krā**-nē-uhm
*Bone of the ear* bōn *of the* ēr
*Bone of the face* bōn *of the* fās

*Brachium* **brā**-kē-uhm
*Brachycephalic* brahck-ē-seh-**fahl**-ihck
*Calcaneal tuberosity* kahl-**kān**-ē-ahl too-buh-**rohs**-ih-tē
*Calciotropic* kahl-sē-ah-**trōp**-ihck
*Calcitonin* kahl-sih-**tō**-nihn
*Canaliculi* kahn-ahl-**ihck**-yoo-lī
*Cancellous bone* kahn-**sehl**-uhs bōn
*Cannon bone* **kahn**-nuhn bōn
*Carpal bone* **kahr**-puhl bōn
*Carpus* **kahr**-puhs
*Cartilaginous* kahr-tih-**lahj**-ehn-uhs
*Cervical vertebrae* **sihr**-vihck-ahl **vərt**-eh-brā
*Circumduction* sihr-kuhm-**duhck**-shuhn
*Coccygeal vertebrae* kohck-**sihj**-ē-ahl **vərt**-eh-brā
*Coccyx* **kohck**-sihcks
*Collateral* kō-**laht**-ər-ahl
*Compact bone* **kohm**-pahckt bōn
*Condyle* **kohn**-dīl
*Costal cartilage* **kohst**-ahl **kahr**-tih-lihj
*Costochondral junction* kohst-ō-**kohn**-drahl **juhngk**-shuhn
*Cranium* **krā**-nē-uhm
*Cribriform plate* **krihb**-reh-fohrm plāt
*Dens* dehnz
*Dewclaw* **doo**-klaw
*Diaphysis* dī-**ah**-fih-sihs
*Diarthrosis* dī-ahrth-**rō**-sihs
*Digit* **dihj**-iht
*Distal sesamoid bone* **dihs**-tahl **sehs**-ah-moyd bōn
*Dolichocephalic* dō-lih-kō-seh-**fahl**-ihck
*Endochondral bone formation* ehn-dō-**kohn**-drahl bōn fohr-**mā**-shuhn
*Endosteum* ehnd-**ohs**-tē-uhm
*Epiphyseal fracture* ehp-ih-fihz-**ē**-ahl **frahck**-chər
*Epiphyseal plate* ehp-ih-fihz-**ē**-ahl plat
*Epiphysis* ē-**pihf**-eh-sihs
*Ethmoid bone* **ehth**-moyd bōn
*Ethmoidal sinus* **ehth**-moyd-ahl **sī**-nuhs
*Extension* ehck-**stehn**-shuhn
*External acoustic meatus* ehcks-**tər**-nahl ah-**koo**-stihck mē-**ā**-tuhs
*Fabella* fah-**behl**-lah
*Facet* **fah**-seht
*Femur* **fē**-mər
*Fetlock joint* **feht**-lohck joynt
*Fibrous joint* **fī**-bruhs joynt
*Fibula* **fihb**-ū-lah
*Flat bone* **flaht** bōn
*Flexion* **flehck**-shuhn
*Floating rib* **flō**-tihng rihb
*Foramen* fohr-**ā**-mehn
*Foramen magnum* fohr-**ā**-mehn **mahg**-nuhm
*Fossa* **fohs**-ah
*Frontal bone* **fruhn**-tahl bōn
*Frontal sinus* **fruhn**-tahl **sī**-nuhs
*Ginglymus joint* **gihng**-gluh-muhs joint
*Glenoid cavity* **glē**-noyd **kahv**-ih-tē

*Gliding joint* **glī**-dihng joynt
*Growth plate* **grōth** plāt
*Hard palate* hahrd **pahl**-iht
*Haversian canal* hah-**vər**-zhehn kuh-**nahl**
*Haversian system* hah-**vər**-zhehn **sihs**-tehm
*Head* hehd
*Hematopoiesis* hē-**mah**-tō-poy-**ē**-sihs
*Hematopoietic tissue* hē-**mah**-tō-poy-**eh**-tihck **tihsh**-yoo
*Hinge joint* **hihnj** joynt
*Hip dysplasia* hihp dihs-**plā**-zhuh
*Hock* hohck
*Humerus* **hū**-mər-uhs
*Hyoid apparatus* **hī**-oyd ahp-uh-**raht**-uhs
*Hyoid bone* **hī**-oyd bōn
*Ilium* **ihl**-ē-uhm
*Incisive bone* ihn-**sī**-sihv bōn
*Incus* **ihng**-kuhs
*Interparietal bone* ihn-tər-pah-**rī**-eh-tahl bōn
*Intervertebral disc* ihn-tər-**vər**-teh-brahl dihsk
*Intramembranous bone formation* ihn-trah-**mehm**-bruh-nuhs bōn fohr-**mā**-shuhn
*Irregular bone* ihr-**rehg**-ū-lər bōn
*Ischium* **ihs**-kē-uhm
*Joint* joynt
*Joint capsule* joynt **kahp**-sehl
*Joint cavity* joynt **kahv**-ih-tē
*Joint space* joynt spās
*Lacrimal bone* **lah**-kreh-mahl bōn
*Ligament* **lihg**-ah-mehnt
*Long bone* **lohng** bōn
*Lumbar vertebrae* **luhm**-bahr **vərt**-eh-brā
*Malleus* **mahl**-ē-uhs
*Mandible* **mahn**-dih-buhl
*Mandibular symphysis* mahn-**dihb**-ū-lahr **sihm**-fih-sihs
*Manubrium* mah-**noo**-brē-uhm
*Maxillary bone* **mahck**-seh-leər-ē bōn
*Maxillary sinus* **mahck**-seh-leər-ē **sī**-nehs
*Meniscus* meh-**nihs**-kuhs
*Metacarpal bone* meht-ah **kahr**-pahl bōn
*Metatarsal bone* meht-ah **tahr**-sahl bōn
*Nasal bone* **nāz**-ahl bōn
*Nasal conchae* **nāz**-ahl **kohng**-kē
*Nasal septum* **nāz**-ahl **sehp**-tuhm
*Navicular bone* nuh-**vihck**-ū-lər bōn
*Neck* nehck
*Nutrient foramen* **noo**-trē-ehnt fohr-**ā**-mehn
*Obturator formen* **ohb**-tər-ā-tər fohr-**ā**-mehn
*Occipital bone* ohck-**sihp**-eh-tahl bōn
*Occipital condyle* ohck-**sihp**-eh-tahl **kohn**-dīl
*Olecranon process* ō-**lehck**-reh-nohn **proh**-sehs
*Os cordis* ohz **kohr**-dihs
*Os penis* ohz **pe**-nihs
*Os rostri* ohz **rohs**-trī
*Ossicle* **ohs**-eh-kuhl
*Ossification* **ohs**-eh-fih-**kā**-shuhn
*Osteoblast* **ohs**-tē-ō-blahst

*Osteoclast* **ohs**-tē-ō-klahst
*Osteocyte* **ohs**-tē-ō-sīt
*Palatine bone* **pahl**-ah-tīn bōn
*Palpation* pahl-**pā**-shuhn
*Paranasal sinus* pahr-ah-**nā**-sahl **sī**-nehs
*Parathyroid hormone* pahr-ah-**thī**-royd **hohr**-mōn
*Parietal bone* pah-**rī**-eh-tahl bōn
*Patella* pah-**tehl**-ah
*Patellar ligament* pah-**tehl**-ahr **lihg**-ah-mehnt
*Pelvic limb* **pehl**-vihck lihm
*Pelvic symphysis* **pehl**-vihck **sihm**-fih-sihs
*Pelvis* **pehl**-vihs
*Periosteum* peər-ē-**ohst**-ē-uhm
*Phalanges* fah-**lahn**-jēz
*Phalanx* **fah**-lahngks
*Pituitary fossa* pih-**too**-ih-teər-ē **fohs**-ah
*Pivot joint* **pihv**-eht joynt
*Primary growth center* **prī**-mahr-ē grōth **sehn**-tər
*Process* **proh**-sehs
*Proximal sesamoid bone* **prohck**-sih-mahl **sehs**-ah-moyd bōn
*Pterygoid bone* **teər**-ih-goyd bōn
*Pubis* **pyoo**-bihs
*Radius* **rād**-ē-uhs
*Ramus of the mandible* **rā**-muhs *of the* **mahn**-dih-buhl
*Red bone marrow* rehd bōn **meər**-ō
*Rib* rihb
*Rotation* rō-**tā**-shuhn
*Sacral vertebrae* **sā**-krahl **vərt**-eh-brā
*Sacroiliac joint* **sā**-krō-**ihl**-ē-ahck joynt
*Sacrum* **sā**-kruhm
*Scapula* **skahp**-ū-luh
*Secondary growth center* **sehk**-uhn-dahr-ē grōth **sehn**-tər
*Sesamoid bone* **sehs**-ah-moyd bōn
*Shaft of the mandible* shahft *of the* **mahn**-dih-buhl
*Short bone* shohrt bōn
*Skull* skuhl
*Sphenoid bone* **sfē**-noyd bōn
*Sphenoidal sinus* **sfē**-noyd-ahl **sī**-nuhs
*Spheroidal joint* sfeer-**oyd**-ahl joynt

*Spinal canal* **spī**-nahl kuh-**nahl**
*Spinal column* **spī**-nahl **kohl**-uhm
*Spinous process* **spī**-nuhs **proh**-sehs
*Splint bone* **splihnt** bōn
*Stapes* **stā**-pēs
*Sternal rib* **stər**-nahl rihb
*Sternebrae* **stər**-neh-brā
*Sternum* **stər**-nuhm
*Stifle joint* **stī**-fuhl joynt
*Suture* **soo**-chər
*Synarthrosis* sihn-ahrth-**rō**-sihs
*Synovial fluid* sihn-ō-vē-ahl **floo**-ihd
*Synovial joint* sihn-ō-vē-ahl joint
*Synovial membrane* sihn-ō-vē-ahl **mehm**-brān
*Tarsal bone* **tahr**-sahl bōn
*Tarsus* **tahr**-suhs
*Temporal bone* **tehm**-pohr-ahl bōn
*Temporomandibular joint* **tehm**-pohr-ō-mahn-**dihb**-ū-lahr joynt
*Thoracic limb* thohr-**ah**-sihck lihm
*Thoracic vertebrae* thohr-**ah**-sihck **vərt**-eh-brā
*Tibia* **tih**-bē-ah
*Tibial crest* **tih**-bē-ahl krehst
*Transverse process* trahnz-**vərs proh**-sehs
*Trochoid joint* **trō**-koyd joynt
*Turbinate* **tuhr**-buh-nāt
*Tympanic membrane* tihm-**pahn**-ihck **mehm**-brān
*Ulna* **uhl**-nah
*Ungual process* **uhng**-gwuhl **proh**-sehs
*Vertebra* **vərt**-eh-brah
*Vertebral column* vər-**tēh**-brahl **kohl**-uhm
*Visceral skeleton* **vih**-sər-ahl **skehl**-ih-tuhn
*Volkmann's canal* **vawhlk**-mahnz kuh-**nahl**
*Vomer bone* **vō**-mər bōn
*Xiphoid* **zī**-foyd
*Yellow bone marrow* **yehl**-lō bōn **meər**-ō
*Zygomatic arch* zī-gō-**maht**-ihck ahrch
*Zygomatic bone* zī-gō-**maht**-ihck bōn

## INTRODUCTION

Try to imagine what an animal's body would be like without a skeleton. Picture a furry sac of semisoft, gelatin-like material lying on the ground twitching. That is about what it would look like. The other connective tissues would hold the cells together, and the muscles would still contract and attempt to move the body; however, without bones to support it and give the muscles leverage, the body would lie on the ground, unable to accomplish anything useful.

The skeleton is the framework of bones that supports and protects the soft tissues of the body. Besides making up the skeleton, the bones also serve a variety of other important functions. Before discussing the parts of the skeleton, let us take a look at bone—what it is, what it does, and some of its common characteristics.

# BONE

## BONE TERMINOLOGY

The terms *os* and *osteo-* generally refer to bone. For example, the *os penis* is a bone in the penis of dogs and *osteo*cytes are bone cells.

## BONE CHARACTERISTICS

Bone is one of the most fascinating body tissues. It is the second hardest natural substance in the body—only the enamel of the teeth is harder. Despite its dead, rocklike appearance, bone is a vital, living tissue with an excellent capacity to repair itself after injury. All that is usually necessary for broken bones to heal is for the broken ends to be brought together in some reasonable sort of alignment and then kept from moving for a few weeks or months. (See the Clinical Application on fracture repair for more information.)

Bone is composed of a sparse population of cells embedded in a hard intercellular substance called the *matrix*. The cells that produce bone are called *osteoblasts*: the suffix *blast* indicates a cell that produces something. Osteoblasts secrete the matrix, which is initially soft and composed of collagen fibers embedded in a gelatin-like ground substance made of protein and complex carbohydrates called *polysaccharides*.

The osteoblasts then harden the matrix through a process called **ossification**. When ossification takes place, the matrix is infiltrated with calcium and phosphate in the form of hydroxyapatite crystals. These hydroxyapatite crystals give bone its characteristic hardness. As they create areas of bone, the osteoblasts become trapped in spaces in the ossified matrix called *lacunae*. Once they are surrounded by bone, the former osteoblasts get a new identity (kind of like people in the Witness Protection Program). They are now called *osteocytes* or *bone cells*.

Osteocytes live out their days in their little cell-like lacunae. Their only contact with each other or with their blood supply is through threadlike, cellular processes in tiny channels through the bone called **canaliculi**. The canaliculi are like slots in the jail cell doors through which the osteocytes get food and communicate with each other.

## FUNCTIONS OF BONES

### SUPPORT

The most basic function of bone is to support the animal body. The cells and tissues that make up the rest of the body are fairly soft and do not have much inherent strength, so the bones serve as a sort of scaffolding to support them. The rest of the body either hangs from the bones or is attached directly to them.

### PROTECTION

Bones also have an important protective function. Their firm strength protects many delicate, vital organs and tissues by surrounding them partially or completely. For example, the bones of the skull protect the brain and the delicate structures of the eyes and ears.

### LEVERAGE

Bones act as levers for the skeletal muscles to move the body. Attachment of skeletal muscles to bones via the tendons allows the muscles to move the joints. This lets the animal move around in its environment.

### STORAGE

Bones act as storage sites for minerals, particularly calcium. They act as reservoirs or "banks" for this important mineral. They enable the body to deposit and withdraw calcium as needed to control its level in the bloodstream precisely.

Calcium is involved in many important body functions, including muscle contraction, blood clotting, milk secretion, and skeleton formation and maintenance. Its level in the blood must be kept within a narrow range for these functions to proceed without difficulty. Two hormones, **calcitonin** from the thyroid gland and **parathyroid hormone** from the parathyroid glands, act as "cashiers" at the calcium bank. Calcitonin helps prevent *hypercalcemia*, which is too high a level of calcium in the blood. Parathyroid hormone does the opposite: it helps prevent *hypocalcemia*.

 **CLINICAL APPLICATION**

### The Role of Bones in Calcium Homeostasis

Calcium homeostasis is regulated by two calciotropic hormones, each of which has effects on bones. (**Calcitropic** means they are involved in the regulation of calcium levels in the body.)

When the level of calcium in the blood begins to rise too high, the hormone calcitonin is secreted by the thyroid glands. This encourages calcium to be deposited in the bones by **osteoblasts**, inhibits bone reabsorption by **osteoclasts**, and increases the amount of calcium excreted by the kidneys into the urine. All of these actions help decrease the amount of calcium in the blood.

When the level of calcium in the blood drops too low, parathyroid hormone is released from the parathyroid glands. This hormone inhibits calcium deposition in bones by osteoblasts, encourages osteoclasts to withdraw calcium from bones, and causes calcium to be retained by the kidneys by decreasing the amount excreted in the urine. These actions all serve to increase the amount of calcium in the blood.

This depositing and withdrawal of calcium from the bones goes on constantly as the body's needs and the contents of its food supply change. (Chapter 11 explains this process more fully.)

### BLOOD CELL FORMATION

Some of the bones serve as sites for blood cell formation—which is called **hematopoiesis**—in the bone marrow that fills their interiors. This will be covered in more depth later.

## BONE STRUCTURE

The two main types of bone are light, spongy, **cancellous bone** and heavy, dense, **compact bone**.

## CANCELLOUS BONE

*Cancellous bone* is sometimes called *spongy bone* because it looks like a sponge (Figures 7-1 and 7-2). It consists of tiny spicules of bone that appear randomly arranged with lots of spaces between them, like a bunch of pick-up-sticks that have been tossed into a pile. The spaces between the spicules are occupied by bone marrow. To the naked eye, the many spicules and spaces give cancellous bone its spongy appearance. It is light but amazingly strong and helps reduce the weight of the bones of the skeleton without significantly reducing their strength. The organization of the spicules of cancellous bone appears random, but they are actually arranged to stand up to the forces the bone is subjected to. Muscles, gravity, and other bones all push and pull on bones constantly. The makeup of cancellous bone helps keep the bones light while also preventing them from being damaged by all the forces acting on them.

## COMPACT BONE

*Compact bone* is very heavy, dense, and strong. It makes up the shafts of long bones and the outside layer of all bones. It is composed of tiny, tightly compacted cylinders of bone called **Haversian systems** (see Figure 7-2). Each Haversian system runs lengthwise to the bone and consists of a

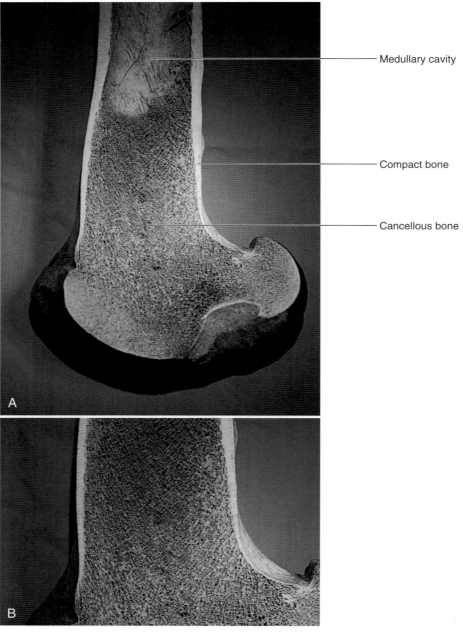

Medullary cavity

Compact bone

Cancellous bone

**FIGURE 7-1** Bone structure. **A,** Cut surface of distal end of horse femur. **B,** Close-up view showing detail of cancellous bone structure.

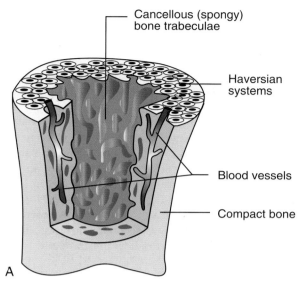

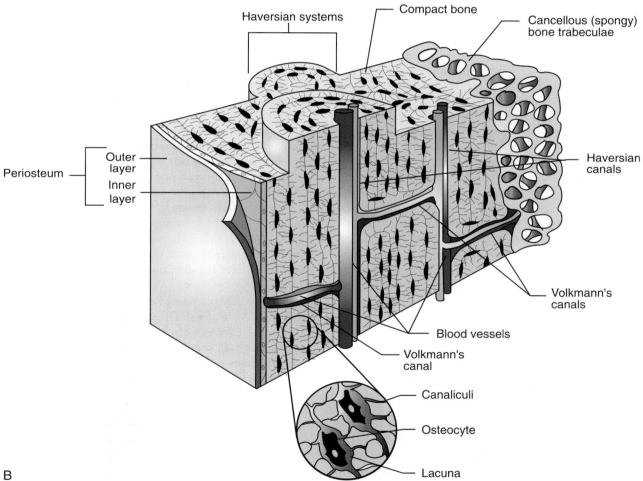

**FIGURE 7-2** Structure of compact and cancellous bone. **A,** Section through the long bone showing outer compact and inner cancellous bone. **B,** Enlarged view showing components of each type of bone.

multilayered or *laminated* cylinder composed of concentric layers of ossified bone matrix arranged around a central **Haversian canal**. The Haversian canal contains blood vessels, lymph vessels, and nerves that supply the osteocytes. The osteocytes are located at the junctions between the layers of bone that make up each Haversian system. In cross section, these layers of bone look like the growth rings of a tree. Tiny channels through the bone, called *canaliculi*, allow osteocytes to contact each other and exchange nutrients and wastes.

Except for their *articular* or *joint* surfaces, the outer surfaces of bones are covered by a membrane called the **periosteum**. The outer layer of the periosteum is composed of fibrous tissue, and its inner layer contains bone-forming cells (osteoblasts). This inner, bone-forming layer enables bones to increase in diameter. It is also involved in the healing of bone fractures. Another membrane, the **endosteum**, lines the hollow interior surfaces of bones. The endosteum also contains osteoblasts.

## BONE CELLS

Three types of cell that make up bone are *osteoblasts, osteocytes*, and *osteoclasts*. **Osteoblasts** are the cells that form bone. They secrete the matrix of bone and then supply the minerals necessary to harden it. Once the osteoblasts become trapped in the ossified matrix they have created, they are called **osteocytes**. Talk about painting yourself into a corner! Osteocytes are always ready to revert to their former lives as osteoblasts and form new bone if an injury makes that necessary.

**Osteoclasts** are like the "evil twins" of osteoblasts; instead of forming bone, they eat it away. Actually, they are not evil at all. Bones are dynamic structures that must be remodeled constantly. Osteoclasts are necessary for remodeling to take place by removing bone from where it is *not* needed, and osteoblasts form new bone in areas where it *is* needed. Osteoclasts also allow the body to withdraw calcium from the bones when it is needed to raise the calcium level in the blood.

> ✔ **TEST YOURSELF 7-1**
>
> 1. Besides supporting the other tissues of the body, what else do bones do?
> 2. What happens to bones when the level of calcium in the blood falls too low? What happens when it rises too high?
> 3. What are the three kinds of bone cell? What role does each play in the life of a bone?
> 4. What is the matrix of bone made of? What makes it so hard?
> 5. What are the main differences between the structures of cancellous bone and compact bone? Why does the body need these two different types of bone?

## BLOOD SUPPLY TO BONE

Most of the blood supply to bones comes from countless tiny blood vessels that penetrate in from the periosteum. The vessels pass through tiny channels in the bone matrix called **Volkmann's canals**. Volkmann's canals come in at right angles to the long axis of the bone and at right angles to the Haversian canals. The blood vessels in Volkmann's canals join with the blood vessels in the Haversian canals to bring nutrition to the osteocytes in the Haversian systems.

Large blood vessels, along with lymph vessels and nerves, also enter many large bones—especially long bones— through large channels called **nutrient foramina**. These large vessels primarily carry blood into and out of the bone marrow. The locations of the larger nutrient foramina on long bones are fairly predictable. Seen from the side on a radiograph (x-ray picture), a nutrient foramen can resemble a crack-type fracture of the **bone cortex**. This is a good example of why a thorough knowledge of anatomy is necessary to interpret radiographs properly.

## BONE FORMATION

Bone is formed in the body by one of two mechanisms: it either grows into and replaces a cartilage model, called *endochondral* or *cartilage bone formation*; or it develops from fibrous tissue membranes, called *intramembranous* or *membrane bone formation*.

Most bones in the body develop by **endochondral bone formation**. When bones form by this method, the body first creates a cartilage "template" that is subsequently replaced by bone. Most bones start out as rods of cartilage in the developing fetus. These cartilage rods are prototypes of the bones that will eventually replace them. In long bones, such as the **femur** or thigh bone, bone begins developing in the shaft or **diaphysis** of the cartilage rod in what is called the **primary growth center**. Cartilage is removed gradually as bone is created and the growth center expands. Additional growth centers called **secondary growth centers** develop in the ends or **epiphyses** of the bone. By the time an animal is born, most of the cartilage prototypes have been replaced by bone.

Just two areas of a long bone remain as cartilage when an animal is born: these are two *plates* of cartilage, located between the shaft, or diaphysis, of the bone and the ends, or epiphyses, of the bone. They are called **epiphyseal plates** or **growth plates** (Figures 7-3 and 7-4). They are the sites where the creation of new bone allows the long bones to lengthen as the animal grows. In each growth plate, cartilage cells create new cartilage on the outside or *epiphyseal* surface of the plate, and osteoblasts replace the cartilage on the inside or *diaphyseal* surface of the plate with bone. By this mechanism, the bone gradually gets longer as the animal grows. When the bone has reached its full size, the epiphyseal plates completely *ossify*; that is, all of the cartilage is replaced by bone. This stops the growth of the bone. Remodeling continues to take place, but the bone is as long as it is going to get.

**Intramembranous bone formation** occurs only in certain skull bones. Bone forms in the fibrous tissue membranes that cover the brain in the developing fetus. This process creates the flat bones of the **cranium**, which surround the brain.

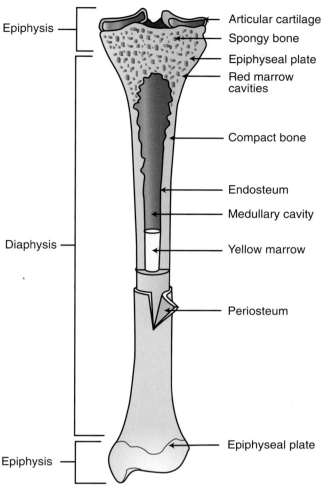

Epiphysis

Diaphysis

Epiphysis

Articular cartilage
Spongy bone
Epiphyseal plate
Red marrow cavities

Compact bone

Endosteum
Medullary cavity

Yellow marrow

Periosteum

Epiphyseal plate

**FIGURE 7-3** Long bone. Structure of long bone (tibia).

## BONE SHAPES

Bones come in four basic shapes: *long, short, flat,* and *irregular.*

## LONG BONES

As their name implies, **long bones** (Figure 7-5, *A*) are longer than they are wide. Most bones of the limbs are long bones. The basic parts of a long bone are illustrated in Figure 7-3. Each long bone has a proximal epiphysis and a distal epiphysis, which consist primarily of light, cancellous bone covered by a thin layer of compact bone. The main part of a long bone is the diaphysis, which is composed of strong, compact bone. In a young animal, the epiphyseal plates of cartilage found between the epiphyses and the diaphysis are commonly called the *growth plates* because they are the sites of bone growth that allow long bones to get longer as the animal grows. They are also weak areas of the bone. Fractures through epiphyseal plates, called **epiphyseal fractures,** are common in young animals. When an animal reaches its full adult size, the epiphyseal plates ossify to become solid bone.

## SHORT BONES

**Short bones** are shaped like small cubes or marshmallows. They consist of a core of spongy bone covered by a thin

layer of compact bone. Examples include the carpal (Figure 7-5, *B*) and tarsal bones.

 **CLINICAL APPLICATION**

### Fracture Repair

Bones are among the best healing tissues in the body. When bones are broken, three things are necessary for optimal healing to occur: *alignment, immobilization,* and *time.* The fractured ends must be brought close together in reasonable alignment and must be kept from moving apart until healing processes have had adequate time to effect new bone growth. Alignment of the fractured fragments is called *setting* or *reducing* the fracture; immobilization is called *fixation* of the fracture.

External fixation devices such as splints and casts may be used, as can internal devices such as pins, wires, screws, or plates, which must be surgically implanted. The length of time that the fixation device must be kept in place varies with the type and location of the fracture and must take into consideration the physical characteristics of the animal. Factors such as species, age, physical condition, and size of the animal affect the speed of healing. In a small, young animal, the whole process might only take a couple of weeks; in an older or larger animal, it might take several months or more.

Regardless of the type and location of the fracture, the basic healing processes are the same. The large blood supply of bones results in considerable bleeding (hemorrhage) at the fracture site. After the blood begins to clot, forming what is called the *fracture hematoma,* the bone is gradually infiltrated by healing cells and tissues over the next few weeks and months. Osteoblasts from the area form the healing tissue, called the **callus,** that gradually bridges the fracture gap. The callus can be felt as a lump at the fracture site, and the size of the callus is an indicator of how much movement has been occurring between the fracture fragments. The less movement, the smaller the callus. Fractures with small calluses generally heal faster, which is usually our treatment goal. Once the callus is fully formed and mineralized, the basic healing of the fracture is complete; however, what occurs after that is very important. Over the next few months, the body slowly remodels the bone at the fracture site according to the mechanical stresses that are placed on it. Ideally, this gradual remodeling will return the bone to its original size, shape, and strength.

## FLAT BONES

**Flat bones,** as their name implies, are relatively thin and flat. Their structure is like a cancellous bone sandwich that consists of two thin plates of compact bone separated by a layer of cancellous bone. Many of the skull bones are flat bones, as are the **scapulae,** or shoulder blades (Figure 7-5, *C*), and the pelvic bones.

## IRREGULAR BONES

The term **irregular bone** is the anatomist's version of a miscellaneous category. Irregular bones do not fit into the long, short, or flat categories. They either have characteristics of more than one of the other categories, or they have a truly

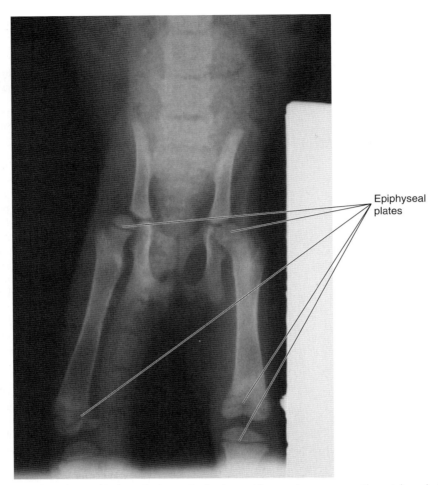

Epiphyseal plates

**FIGURE 7-4** Epiphyseal (growth) plates. Radiograph of pelvis and femurs of a young cat. The epiphyseal plates appear dark because they are made up largely of cartilage, which is relatively transparent to x-rays. Note that the bones appear paler, because they absorb most of the x-rays.

irregular shape. The **vertebrae**, which are the bones of the spine (Figure 7-5, *D*), are irregular bones; so are some of the strangely shaped skull bones. **Sesamoid bones** are also included in this category. Sesamoid bones got their name because early anatomists thought their shapes resembled sesame seeds. (You have to give the early anatomists credit for their creative imaginations.) Sesamoid bones are present in some tendons where they change direction markedly over the surfaces of joints. The kneecap or **patella** is the largest sesamoid bone in the animal body, but several others are also found. We will discuss some of the clinically important sesamoid bones in the section on the appendicular skeleton.

## BONE MARROW

**Bone marrow** fills the spaces within bones. This includes the spaces between the spicules of cancellous bone and the large spaces within the diaphyses of long bones. Bone marrow comes in two basic types: *red bone marrow* and *yellow bone marrow.*

### RED BONE MARROW

**Red bone marrow** is **hematopoietic tissue.** *Hemato* refers to blood, and *poiesis* means to form something. Red bone

marrow forms blood cells. It makes up the majority of the bone marrow of young animals but represents only a small portion of the marrow of older animals. In older animals it is confined to a few specific locations, such as the ends of some long bones and the interiors of the pelvic bones and sternum. (See Chapter 12 for more information on blood cell formation.)

### YELLOW BONE MARROW

**Yellow bone marrow** consists primarily of adipose connective tissue, which is better known as *fat*. It is the most common type of marrow in adult animals. Yellow bone marrow does not produce blood cells, but it can revert to red bone marrow if the body needs to produce larger than normal numbers of blood cells. This might be necessary if, for example, an animal were suffering from chronic, low-level blood loss due to numerous blood-sucking parasites.

## COMMON BONE FEATURES

The roles that particular bones play often become clear when their lumps, bumps, grooves, and holes are examined. These

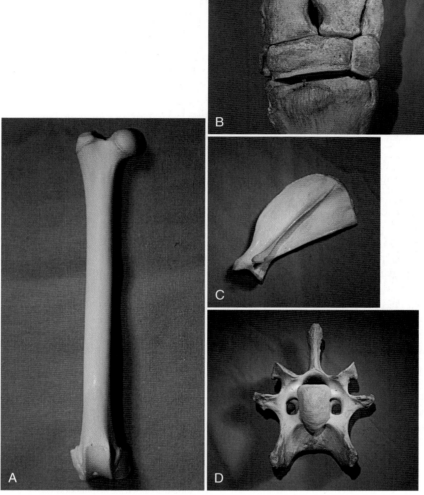

**FIGURE 7-5** Bone shapes. **A,** Long bone. Feline femur. **B,** Short bones. Equine carpus. **C,** Flat bone. Canine scapula. **D,** Irregular bone. Bovine cervical vertebra.

✓ *TEST YOURSELF 7-2*

1. What is the difference between a *Haversian canal* and a *Volkmann's canal*?
2. By which mechanism of bone formation do most bones in the animal body develop before birth, and how does the process take place?
3. What is the difference between the primary growth center of a bone and a secondary growth center?
4. Where would you find an epiphyseal plate, and what would you find it doing?
5. What is bone marrow, and what is the difference between the red kind and the yellow kind?

features show us where bones form joints with each other, where muscles attach to move them, where tendons press on their surfaces, and where they are pierced by blood vessels and nerves. We can learn a lot about a bone just by looking at its shape and surface features.

## ARTICULAR SURFACES

**Articular surfaces** are joint surfaces: smooth areas of compact bone where bones come in contact with each other to form **joints**. Each articular surface is covered by a smooth, thin layer of hyaline cartilage called **articular cartilage.** The smooth articular surface and its smooth, slightly softer articular cartilage covering help reduce friction and wear in joints.

***CONDYLE.*** A **condyle** is usually a large, round articular surface. Condyles have, in the creative imagery of anatomists, a somewhat cylindrical shape. The major condyles of the body are located on the distal end of the humerus (see Figure 7-25) and femur (see Figure 7-34, *A* and *B*) and on the occipital bone of the skull (see Figure 7-12, *C*), where the skull joins the spinal column to attach the head to the neck.

**HEAD.** A **head** is a somewhat spherical articular surface on the proximal end of a long bone. Heads are found on the proximal end of the humerus, femur, and ribs. The heads of the humerus (see Figure 7-25) and femur (see Figure 7-34, *A* and *B*) form the ball portion of the ball-and-socket shoulder and hip joints. The head of a bone is united with the main shaft portion of the bone by an often narrowed region called the **neck**.

**FACET.** A **facet** is a flat articular surface. The joint movement between two facets is a kind of rocking motion. Facets are found on many bones, such as carpal and tarsal bones, vertebrae, and long bones such as the radius and ulna.

### PROCESSES

The term **process** includes all the lumps, bumps, and other projections on a bone. Some processes, such as heads and *condyles*, have joint-forming functions; they have very smooth surfaces. Other processes are not parts of joints; they have rough, irregular surfaces. These are usually sites where muscles—or more accurately, tendons—attach. In general, the larger the process, the more powerful the muscular pull on that area of the bone. This can help us figure out how and in what directions the bone usually moves and how powerful the movement usually is. This principle is often used by paleontologists to explain the functions that fossilized dinosaur bones probably had when the animals were alive.

Unfortunately, processes are given a variety of names depending on their location. Sometimes they are simply called *processes*, such as the spinous process of a vertebra (see Figure 7-16). On other bones they have a variety of names, such as trochanter on the femur (see Figure 7-34, *A* and *B*), tubercle on the humerus (see Figure 7-25), tuberosity on the ischium (see Figure 7-33, *A*), spine on the scapula (see Figure 7-24), crest on the tibia (see Figure 7-35), and wing on the atlas (see Figure 7-17). Such is the complex language of anatomy.

### HOLES AND DEPRESSED AREAS

**FORAMEN.** A hole in a bone is called a **foramen** (plural, *foramina*). Usually something important, such as a nerve or blood vessel, passes through a foramen in a bone, but there are exceptions. For example, no major structures pass through the two large obturator foramina of the pelvis (see Figure 7-33); they merely exist to lighten the pelvis.

**FOSSA.** A **fossa** is a depressed or sunken area on the surface of a bone (see Figure 7-24). Fossae are usually occupied by muscles or tendons. Paleontologists use the fossae of dinosaur bones to infer the sizes and actions of some of the animals' tendons and muscles.

### AXIAL SKELETON

The bones of the skeleton can be conveniently divided into two main groups: the *bones of the head and trunk* and the *bones of the limbs*. Because the bones of the head and trunk

are located along the central axis of the body, they are referred to as the **axial skeleton**. The limbs are appendages of the trunk and their bones are collectively called the **appendicular skeleton**. Some animals may have a third category of bones called the **visceral skeleton**. These are bones formed in the *viscera* or soft organs, which are discussed in more detail later. Figure 7-6 is a generic, "word" skeleton that shows the locations of the main bones of the axial and appendicular portions of the skeleton. Figures 7-7 and 7-8 show the bones that make up the skeletons of the horse and dog.

The components of the axial skeleton are the skull, the hyoid bone, the spinal column, the ribs, and the sternum. All the bones of the axial skeleton lie on or near the median plane of the body.

### SKULL

The **skull** is the most complex part of the skeleton. At first glance it looks like one big bone—two if you count the mandible—but in most domestic animals it consists of 37 or 38 separate bones. Most of the skull bones are united by jagged, immovable, fibrous joints called **sutures**. Only the **mandible** or lower jaw is connected to the rest of the skull by a freely movable **synovial joint**. Figures 7-9 through 7-12 show the externally visible skull bones of horses, cattle, cats, and dogs.

*Author's suggestion:* If you have access to a skull and a live animal of the same species, locate each of the external skull bones on the skull and find the comparable regions on the head of the live animal. Anatomy is a lot more fun and useful if we find the structures we are discussing on live animals.

Because of the skull's complexity, we group the skull bones into regions: the *bones of the cranium*, the *bones of the ear*, and the *bones of the face*. Table 7-1 lists the skull bones in each region.

| **TABLE 7-1** | Skull Bones* | |
|---|---|
| **EXTERNAL BONES (LANDMARKS)** | **INTERNAL BONES (HIDDEN)** |
| **Bones of the Cranium** | |
| Frontal bones (2) | Ethmoid bone (1) |
| Interparietal bones (2) | Sphenoid bone (1) |
| Occipital bone (1) | |
| Parietal bones (2) | |
| Temporal bones (2) | |
| **Bones of the Ear** | |
| None | Incus (2) |
| | Malleus (2) |
| | Stapes (2) |
| **Bones of the Face** | |
| Incisive bones (2) | Palatine bones (2) |
| Lacrimal bones (2) | Pterygoid bones (2) |
| Mandible (1 or 2) | Turbinates (4) |
| Maxillary bones (2) | Vomer bone (1) |
| Nasal bones (2) | |
| Zygomatic bones (2) | |

*Bones are listed in alphabetical order.

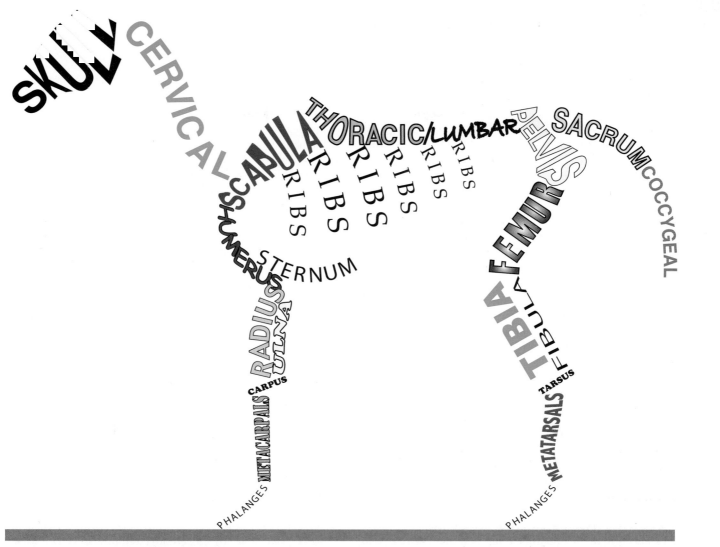

**FIGURE 7-6** Word skeleton. The main bones of axial and appendicular portions of the skeleton.

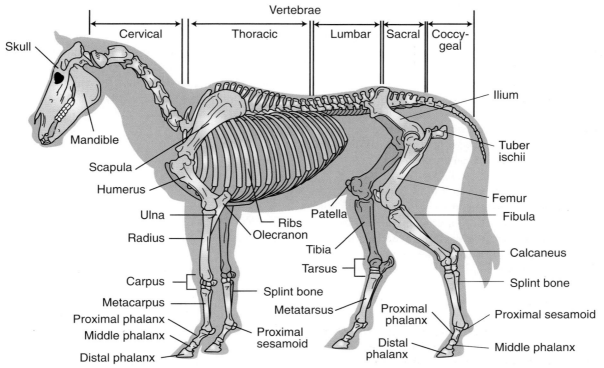

**FIGURE 7-7** Equine skeleton. (Modified From McBride DF: Learning veterinary terminology, ed 2, St Louis, 2002, Mosby.)

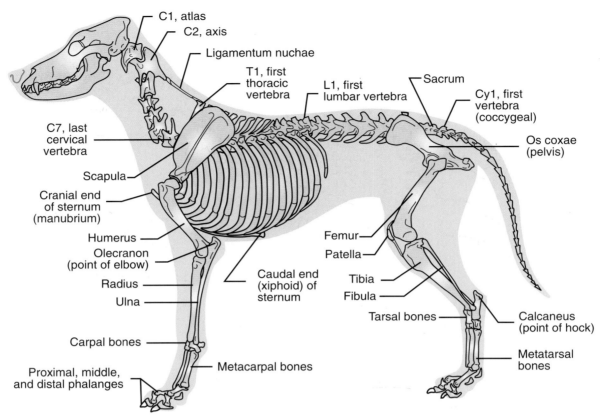

C1, atlas
C2, axis
Ligamentum nuchae
T1, first thoracic vertebra
L1, first lumbar vertebra
Sacrum
Cy1, first vertebra (coccygeal)
Os coxae (pelvis)
C7, last cervical vertebra
Scapula
Cranial end of sternum (manubrium)
Humerus
Olecranon (point of elbow)
Radius
Ulna
Caudal end (xiphoid) of sternum
Femur
Patella
Tibia
Fibula
Tarsal bones
Calcaneus (point of hock)
Carpal bones
Metacarpal bones
Metatarsal bones
Proximal, middle, and distal phalanges

**FIGURE 7-8** Canine skeleton.

## EXTERNAL BONES OF THE CRANIUM

The **cranium** is the portion of the skull that surrounds the brain. In most domestic animal species, 11 bones form the cranium. To make things a little easier, we can divide the bones of the cranium into external and internal bones. External bones are at least partially visible on the surface of an intact skull. We can use them as landmarks to describe the locations of features on the heads of living animals. Internal bones are hidden and cannot be seen without disassembling the skull.

Starting at the rear or *caudal* end of the skull and working our way forward or *rostral*, the external bones of the cranium are the *occipital bone*, the *interparietal bones*, the *parietal bones*, the *temporal bones*, and the *frontal bones*.

### OCCIPITAL BONE.
The **occipital bone** is a single bone that forms the *caudoventral* portion or base of the skull. It is the most caudal skull bone and is very important because (1) it is where the spinal cord exits the skull and (2) it is the skull bone that articulates (forms a joint) with the first cervical (neck) vertebra. A large hole, the **foramen magnum**, is in the center of the occipital bone: this is where the spinal cord exits the skull. On either side of the foramen magnum are the **occipital condyles**: articular surfaces that join with the first cervical vertebra, called the **atlas**, to form the atlantooccipital joint, which is the joint that connects the head with the neck. As you might imagine, injuries to the occipital

bone are serious because of its location and the vital structures it encloses. Fortunately, it is well protected by muscles, tendons, and ligaments, so injuries to the occipital bone are rare.

### INTERPARIETAL BONES.
The **interparietal bones** are two small bones located on the dorsal midline between the occipital bone and the parietal bones. They are usually clearly visible in young animals. In older animals, they may fuse together into one bone, or they may fuse to the parietal bones and become indistinguishable.

### PARIETAL BONES.
The two **parietal bones** form the dorsolateral walls of the cranium. They are large and well developed in dogs, cats, and humans but are relatively small in horses and cattle.

### TEMPORAL BONES.
The two **temporal bones** are located below or *ventral to* the parietal bones. The temporal bones are important for several reasons: they form the lateral walls of the cranium, they contain the middle and inner ear structures, and they are the skull bones that form the **temporomandibular joints (TMJs)** with the **mandible** (lower jaw). The ear structures are contained within the temporal bone, and most are not visible from the outside. The only ear structure that is visible from the outside is the **external acoustic meatus**—the bony canal that leads into the middle

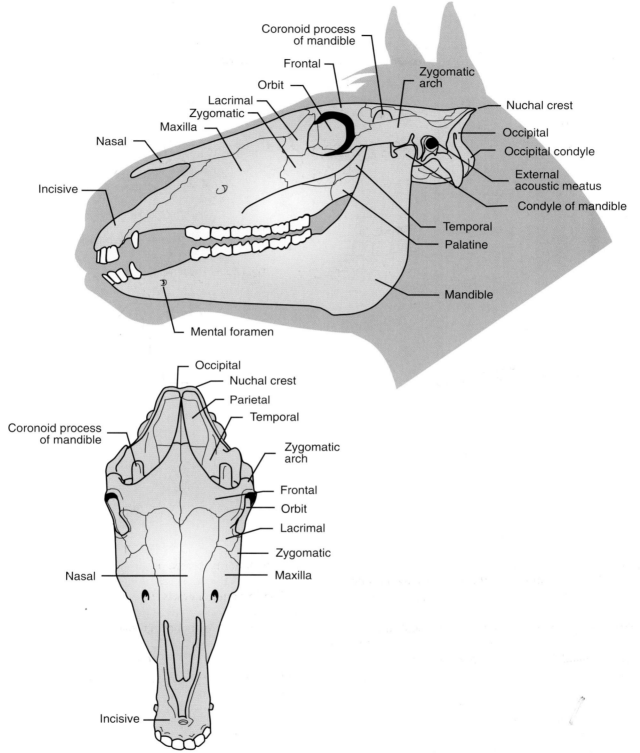

**FIGURE 7-9** Skull of the horse.

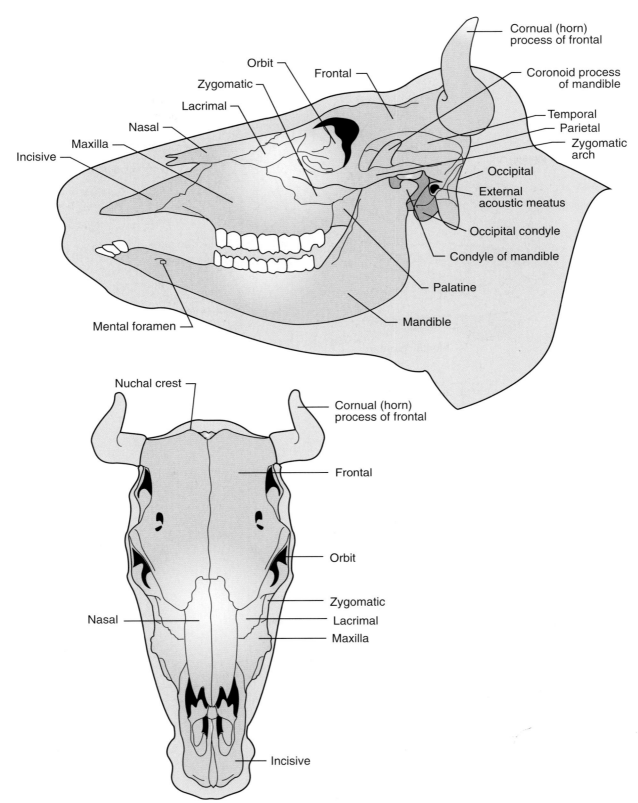

**FIGURE 7-10** Skull of the cow.

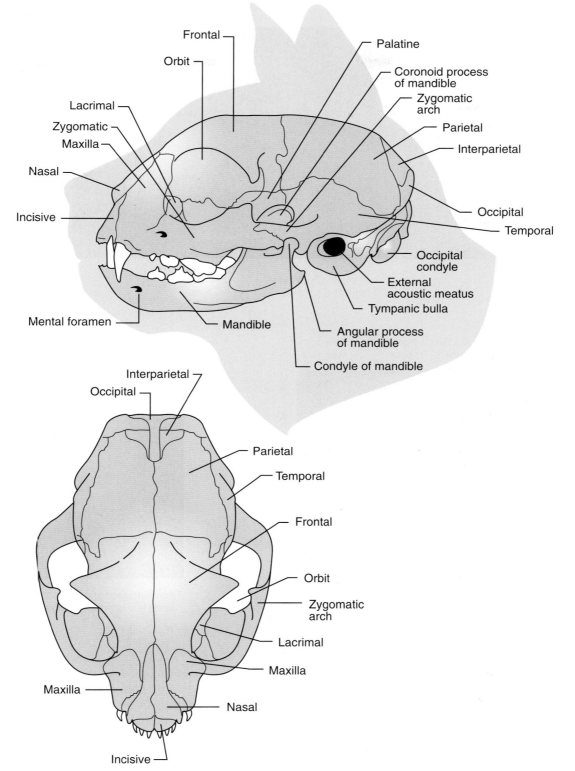

**FIGURE 7-11** Skull of the cat.

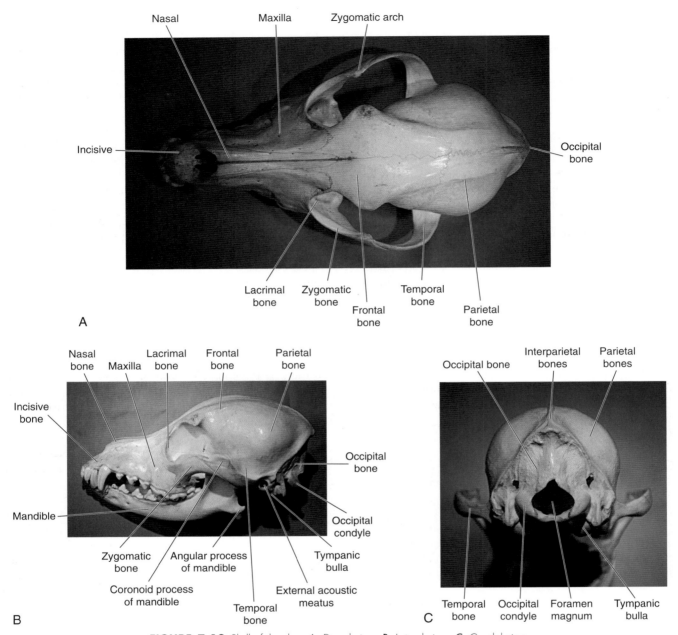

**FIGURE 7-12** Skull of the dog. **A,** Dorsal view. **B,** Lateral view. **C,** Caudal view.

and inner ear cavities. In the living animal it contains the external ear canal. By looking into the external acoustic meatus, we can see the middle ear cavity. Ventral to (below) the external acoustic meatus on each side is the concave articular (joint) surface that receives the condyle of the mandible to form the TMJ. These articular surfaces are located on the ventral (bottom) surface of each of the temporal bones.

**FRONTAL BONES.**  The **frontal bones** form the forehead region of the skull. They are located just *rostral to* (in front of) the parietal bones, and they form the rostrolateral portion of the cranium and a portion of the orbit, which is the concave socket that holds the eye. A large **paranasal sinus,** the **frontal sinus,** is contained within the frontal bone. In horned breeds

of cattle, the cornual process of the frontal bone is the horn core around which the horn develops. This process is hollow and communicates with the frontal sinus. When adult cattle are dehorned, the cornual processes are sawed off and we can look right down into the frontal sinus. This is a really good reason to dehorn cattle when they are young, before the horn buds have united with the frontal bones.

### INTERNAL BONES OF THE CRANIUM
The two hidden bones of the cranium are the *sphenoid bone* and the more rostral *ethmoid bone.*

**SPHENOID BONE.**  A single **sphenoid bone** forms the ventral part (bottom) of the cranium and contains a depression—the **pituitary fossa**—that houses the pituitary gland, which is an important *endocrine* (hormone-producing) gland. The sphenoid bone is located just rostral to (in front of) the occipital bone. If removed from the skull and examined, the sphenoid bone looks like a bat with its wings and legs extended. The sphenoid bone of most animals contains a paranasal sinus called the **sphenoidal sinus**.

**ETHMOID BONE.** The **ethmoid bone** is a single bone located just rostral to (in front of) the sphenoid bone. It contains the sievelike **cribriform plate**, through which the many branches of the olfactory (sense of smell) nerve pass from the upper portion of the nasal cavity to the olfactory bulbs of the brain. Horses and humans have a small paranasal sinus, the **ethmoidal sinus**, in the ethmoid bone.

## BONES OF THE EAR

The three tiny but very important pairs of ear bones are hidden away in the middle ear. Known as the **ossicles**, these bones are—starting from the outside—the **malleus** or hammer, the **incus** or anvil, and the **stapes** or stirrup. Their function is to transmit vibrations from the **tympanic membrane** (eardrum) across the middle ear cavity to an inner ear structure called the *cochlea*. In the cochlea, receptor cells for hearing convert the vibrations to nerve impulses that are interpreted by the brain as sound. The characteristics and functions of the ossicles are covered more completely in Chapter 10.

## EXTERNAL BONES OF THE FACE

The **bones of the face** make up the rest of the skull. We can also divide them into external, *landmark bones* and internal, *hidden bones*.

Starting at the rostral (front) end of the skull and working caudally (toward the rear), the external bones of the face are the *incisive bones*, the *nasal bones*, the *maxillary bones*, the *lacrimal bones*, the *zygomatic bones*, and the *mandible*.

**INCISIVE BONES.** The two **incisive bones**, sometimes called the *premaxillary bones*, are the most rostral (forward) skull bones. In all common domestic animals except ruminants such as cattle, sheep, and goats, the incisive bones house the upper incisor teeth. Our ruminant friends do not have upper incisor teeth; they have a hard dental pad instead.

**NASAL BONES.** The two **nasal bones** form the bridge of the nose, which is the dorsal or upper part of the nasal cavity. Considerable variety is seen in the relative size and shape of the nasal bones, depending on the species and breed of animal. The length of the animal's face is the main influence on the nasal bones. In animals with long faces, such as horses, and **dolichocephalic** or long-faced dog breeds, such as collies, the nasal bones are long and thin. In animals with short faces, such as cats and **brachycephalic** or short-faced breeds of dogs, such as Pekingese, the nasal bones are short and more triangular.

**MAXILLARY BONES.** The two **maxillary bones** make up most of the upper jaw. (The incisive bones make up the rest.) The maxillary bones house the upper canine teeth, all of the upper cheek teeth (premolars and molars), and the **maxillary sinuses**. Along with the palatine bones, the maxillary bones form the **hard palate**, which is the bony separation between the mouth and the nasal cavity that we call the *roof* of the mouth. The maxillary bones form the rostral (forward) portion of the hard palate, and the palatine bones form the caudal (rear) part.

**LACRIMAL BONES.** The **lacrimal bones** are two small bones that form part of the medial portion of the orbit of the eye. A space within each lacrimal bone houses the lacrimal sac, which is part of the tear drainage system of the eye.

**ZYGOMATIC BONES.** The two **zygomatic bones** are also known as the *malar bones*. They form a portion of the orbit of the eye and join with a process from the temporal bones to form the **zygomatic arches** on either side of the skull. The caudal-facing (rear-facing) temporal process of the zygomatic bone joins with the rostral-facing (forward-facing) zygomatic process of the temporal bone (do you sense a pattern here?) to form the zygomatic arch on each side. The zygomatic arches are easily palpable, bony landmarks below and behind the eyes that form the widest part of the skull in dogs and cats.

**MANDIBLE.** The **mandible** is the lower jaw (Figure 7-13). It houses all the lower teeth and is the only movable skull bone. It forms the TMJ with the temporal bone on each side. In some species, such as dogs, cats, and cattle, the two sides of the mandible are separate bones united by a cartilaginous joint, the **mandibular symphysis**, at their rostral (front) ends. Because the symphysis is the weakest part of the mandible, separation of the bones can occur at that site from blunt-force trauma to the face. This is called a *mandibular symphyseal fracture*. It is the most common type of

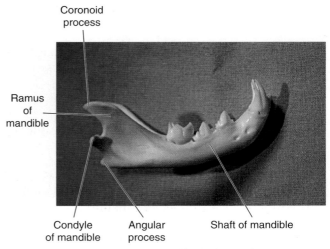

**FIGURE 7-13** Cat mandible. Right lateral view.

Coronoid process

Ramus of mandible

Condyle of mandible

Angular process

Shaft of mandible

mandibular fracture in dogs and cats. Fortunately, it usually is easy to repair. In adult horses and swine, the two halves of the mandible fuse together into one solid bone.

The two main regions of the mandible are the *shaft* and the *ramus*. The **shaft of the mandible** is the horizontal portion that houses all the teeth. At its caudal end is the vertical portion of the mandible, called the **ramus of the mandible**. This is where the powerful jaw muscles attach and where the articular condyles that form the TMJs with the temporal bones are located.

## INTERNAL BONES OF THE FACE

The internal bones of the face are the *palatine bones*, the *pterygoid bones*, the *vomer bone*, and the *turbinates*.

**PALATINE BONES.** The two **palatine bones** make up the caudal portion of the hard palate (the bony part of the roof of the mouth), which separates the mouth from the nasal cavity. The rest of the hard palate (the rostral portion) is made up of part of the maxillary bones.

**PTERYGOID BONES.** The two small **pterygoid bones** support part of the lateral walls of the *pharynx* (throat).

**VOMER BONE.** The single **vomer bone** is located on the midline of the skull and forms part of the **nasal septum**, which is the central "wall" between the left and right nasal passages.

**TURBINATES.** The **turbinates** are also called the **nasal conchae** (Figure 7-14). They are four thin, scroll-like bones that fill most of the space in the nasal cavity. Each side has a dorsal and a ventral turbinate. The turbinates are covered by the moist, very vascular soft tissue lining of the nasal passages. The scroll-like shape of the turbinates forces air inhaled through the nose around many twists and turns as it passes through the nasal cavity. This helps warm and humidify the air and also helps trap any tiny particles of

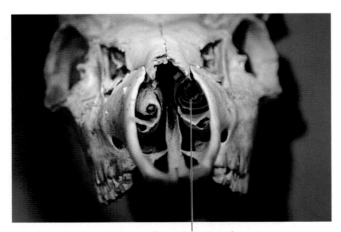

Rostral portion of
turbinate removed to
show interior detail

**FIGURE 7-14** Turbinates. Rostral view of deer skull.

inhaled foreign material in the moist surface of the nasal epithelium. This process helps condition the inhaled air before it reaches the delicate lungs. (I'll bet you didn't know you had air conditioners in your nose.)

> ✓ **TEST YOURSELF 7-3**
>
> 1. Name the skull bones that make up each of these groups:
>    External bones of the cranium
>    Internal bones of the cranium
>    Bones of the ear
>    External bones of the face
>    Internal bones of the face
> 2. In which skull bones are each of the following structures found?
>    Cribriform plate
>    External acoustic meatus
>    Foramen magnum
>    Frontal sinus
>    Lacrimal sac
>    Lower teeth
>    Pituitary fossa
>    Upper incisor teeth
>    Upper cheek teeth
> 3. Which would likely be a greater threat to an animal's well-being: a fracture of the mandible or a fracture of the occipital bone? Why?

## HYOID BONE

The **hyoid bone,** also called the **hyoid apparatus** (Figure 7-15), looks somewhat like the letter H with its two legs bent back to form a U-shaped structure. It is located high in the neck, just above the larynx, between the caudal ends of the mandible. It supports the base of the tongue, the pharynx, and the larynx and helps the animal swallow. It is usually referred to as a *single bone*, but it is composed of several individual portions united by cartilage. It is attached to the temporal bone by two small rods of cartilage. Some authors include the hyoid bone as a skull bone for convenience, but its location and attachments seem to indicate that it is a separate bone of the axial skeleton.

## SPINAL COLUMN

The **spinal column,** also called the **vertebral column,** is made up of a series of individual irregular bones called **vertebrae** (*singular,* **vertebra**) that extend from the skull to the tip of the tail. The spinal column is divided into five regions: *cervical* (neck), *thoracic* (chest), *lumbar* (abdomen), *sacral* (pelvis), and *coccygeal* (tail). Most vertebrae do not have individual names. Instead, they are numbered within each region from cranial to caudal. A shorthand way of referring to particular vertebrae uses the abbreviation for the region— *C* for cervical, *T* for thoracic, *L* for lumbar, *S* for sacral, and *Cy* for coccygeal—followed by the number of the vertebra within that region, starting at the cranial end. For example, *C5* is the fifth cervical vertebra, and *L2* is the second lumbar vertebra. The usual numbers of vertebrae within each region,

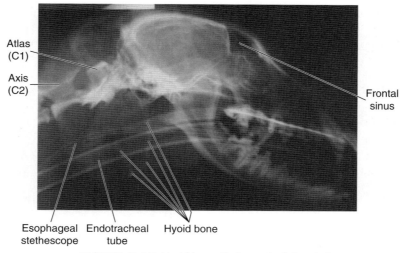

**FIGURE 7-15** Hyoid bone. Radiograph of dog skull.

| TABLE 7-2 | Vertebral Formulas for Some Common Species | | | | |
|---|---|---|---|---|---|
| | **CERVICAL** | **THORACIC** | **LUMBAR** | **SACRAL** | **COCCYGEAL** |
| Cat | 7 | 13 | 7 | 3 | 5-23 |
| Cattle | 7 | 13 | 6 | 5 | 18-20 |
| Dog | 7 | 13 | 7 | 3 | 20-23 |
| Goat | 7 | 13 | 7 | 5 | 16-18 |
| Horse | 7 | 18 | 6 | 5 | 15-21 |
| Human | 7 | 12 | 5 | 5 | 4-5 |
| Pig | 7 | 14-15 | 6-7 | 4 | 20-23 |
| Sheep | 7 | 13 | 6-7 | 4 | 16-18 |

called *vertebral formulas*, are listed in Table 7-2 for some common species.

## VERTEBRAL CHARACTERISTICS

A typical vertebra consists of a *body*, an *arch*—sometimes called the *neural arch*—and a group of *processes* (Figure 7-16). The body of a vertebra is the main, ventral portion of the bone. It is the strongest, most massive portion. The bodies of adjacent vertebrae are separated by the **intervertebral discs**, made of fibrocartilage, which act as little shock-absorbers.

Dorsal to the body of a vertebra is the hollow arch. When the arches of all the vertebrae are lined up, they form a long, flexible tunnel called the **spinal canal**, which houses and protects the spinal cord.

Vertebrae usually have some combination of three kinds of processes. The single, dorsally projecting **spinous process** and the two laterally projecting **transverse processes** vary in size among vertebrae. These act as sites for muscle attachment and provide leverage to move the spine and trunk. The **articular processes** are located on the cranial and caudal ends of the vertebral arches and help form the joints between adjacent vertebrae. Each intervertebral joint allows only very limited movement but, taken as a whole, the entire spinal column has considerable flexibility. Cats demonstrate this flexibility by the strange positions they can get their bodies

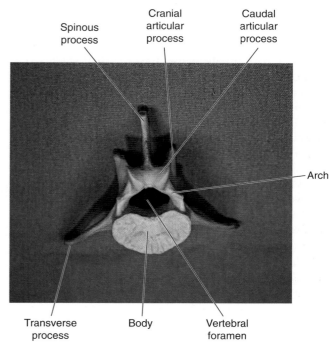

**FIGURE 7-16** Basic anatomy of a vertebra. Caudal view of dog L4 vertebra.

into, especially while lying in a sunbeam. *Author's note:* As I was writing this section, one of our cats, Bogie, was doing a spinal flexibility demonstration beside my computer by lying on his back with his front end facing one direction and his back end facing the other.

## CERVICAL VERTEBRAE

The **cervical vertebrae** are in the neck region. A quick look at Table 7-2 will show that seven cervical vertebrae are found in all common domestic animals and in humans. Actually, nearly all mammals have seven cervical vertebrae. Even the long-necked giraffe has only seven v-e-r-y l-o-n-g cervical vertebrae. This is the only group of vertebrae that has a constant number across most species.

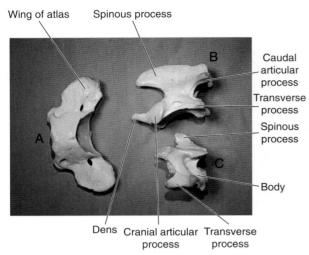

**FIGURE 7-17** Cervical vertebrae of the dog. **A**, Atlas (C1), dorsal view. **B**, Axis (C2), lateral view. **C**, Fourth cervical vertebra (C4), lateral view.

The first two cervical vertebrae are somewhat unusual in shape and have specific names (Figure 7-17). The first, C1, is called the **atlas** because, like the mythical figure Atlas who holds up the world, this vertebra "holds up" the head. The atlas has two large, winglike transverse processes called the *wings of the atlas* that can be **palpated** (felt) just behind the skulls of most animals. The next time you are around a dog or cat, feel the wings of the atlas right behind the skull. The atlas is unique in that it has no vertebral body: it consists only of a bony ring that the spinal cord passes through with the two wings sticking out laterally. Just caudal to the atlas is the second cervical vertebra, C2, which is called the **axis**. Its most prominent features are its large, bladelike spinous process that projects up dorsally and the pegike **dens** that fits into the caudal end of the atlas to help form the atlantoaxial joint. The rest of the cervical vertebrae are fairly normal looking and are numbered like the rest of the vertebrae.

 **CLINICAL APPLICATION**

### Fun Facts About Human Intervertebral Discs

Because we walk upright, gravity compresses our intervertebral discs slightly when we are up and moving around during the day. At night when we lie down and sleep, the compression stops and the discs expand back to their original size. The compression and expansion of each individual disc are very slight but, when combined, the variation in the total length of the spine is measurable. As a result, we are tallest in the morning—by as much as an inch! We proceed to get shorter throughout the day. For astronauts living in the microgravity environment of space, the result is even more impressive: after just a few days in space, their spines can expand up to 2 inches or more. Some astronauts report back pain during the first few days in space because this spinal expansion stretches the muscles around the spinal column. This dramatic increase in height is temporary, and astronauts quickly return to their normal, terrestrial height when they return to earth.

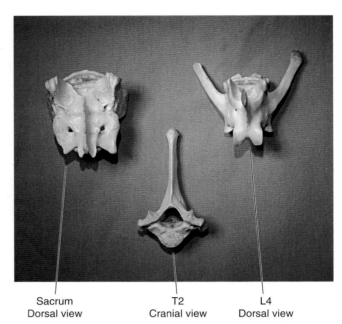

Sacrum Dorsal view     T2 Cranial view     L4 Dorsal view

**FIGURE 7-18** Thoracic, lumbar, and sacral vertebrae of the dog.

## THORACIC VERTEBRAE

The **thoracic vertebrae** are located dorsal to the thorax. Their number varies among species and can even vary within a species. Usually, however, the number of thoracic vertebrae is the same as the number of pairs of ribs the animal has. The most characteristic features of thoracic vertebrae are their tall, spinous processes and their lateral articular facets, which form joints with the heads of the ribs (Figure 7-18).

 **CLINICAL APPLICATION**

### Intervertebral Disc Disease

Normal intervertebral discs have a soft, cushioning center of gelatinous material called the *nucleus pulposus*, which is surrounded by tough fibrocartilage. On their sides and bottoms, intervertebral discs are surrounded by tough ligaments and dense muscles that support the spinal column and join the vertebrae together. The only thing dorsal to these discs is the spinal cord, which is tightly encased in the bony spinal canal.

Intervertebral disc disease results when one or more discs degenerate. When a disc becomes diseased, normal mechanical forces on the spine often result in degenerated disc material being squeezed out. The ligaments and muscles on the sides and bottom of the disc prevent the material from moving in any of those directions, so the only direction it can protrude is dorsally, up into the spinal canal, where it presses on the spinal cord. Because the spinal cord is surrounded by bone, it has no way to escape the pressure when the protruded disc material compresses it, which causes the common clinical signs of intervertebral disc disease: pain, numbness, weakness, and paralysis.

Intervertebral disc disease can occur in any species of animal but is seen most often in dogs, particularly long-backed breeds such as Dachshunds. It usually occurs in one

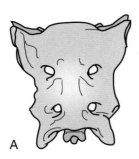
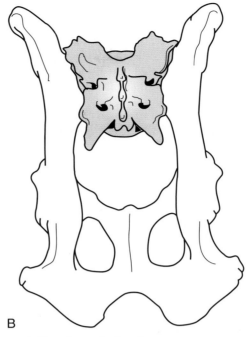

**FIGURE 7-19** Canine sacrum. **A,** Ventral view. **B,** Dorsal view.

 **CLINICAL APPLICATION—cont'd**

of two sites: the cervical region or the thoracolumbar region. Cervical disc disease usually causes severe pain. The neck muscles go into spasm, and the animal holds its head and body very rigidly and does not like being touched. Disc disease in the mid back usually causes weakness, sometimes called *paresis*, and numbness of the hind legs that can progress to complete paralysis. Treatment options include exercise restriction or cage rest, medical treatment with drug therapy to reduce pressure on the spinal cord, and surgery to decompress the spinal cord directly. The prognosis depends on the location, extent, and duration of the damage to the spinal cord.

*Author's note:* I once had a Dachshund patient with thoracolumbar disc disease whose rear legs remained paralyzed despite weeks of intensive treatment. The dog's owners reluctantly decided to **euthanize** him and have him buried in a nearby pet cemetery. The afternoon before the scheduled euthanasia, a representative from the pet cemetery came to our hospital to measure the dog for a coffin. This apparently got his attention, because the next morning, when the time came to do the regrettable deed, we noticed some slight rear-leg movement. We canceled the euthanasia and the dog went on to make a full recovery. Apparently, he had only needed the proper motivation.

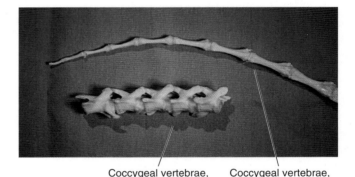

Coccygeal vertebrae, cranial end of tail    Coccygeal vertebrae, caudal end of tail

**FIGURE 7-20** Coccygeal vertebrae of the dog.

## LUMBAR VERTEBRAE

The **lumbar vertebrae** are dorsal to the abdominal region. Like the thoracic vertebrae, their number varies among species and even within a species. The lumbar vertebrae are the most massive-looking bones of the spinal column. Their bodies are large and bulky, because they have to support all the weight of the abdominal organs and structures without the aid of the ribs, which help support the thoracic contents (see Figure 7-18).

## SACRAL VERTEBRAE

The **sacral vertebrae** are unique in that they fuse to form a single, solid structure called the **sacrum** (Figures 7-18 and 7-19). The number of vertebrae fused in the sacrum varies among species (see Table 7-2). The sacrum is located dorsal to the pelvic region and forms a joint with the pelvis on each side in what is called the **sacroiliac joint.**

## COCCYGEAL VERTEBRAE

The **coccygeal vertebrae** are the bones of the tail (Figure 7-20). Their number varies greatly not just between species but even within a species. Their appearance also varies quite a bit, even within an individual animal. The first few coccygeal vertebrae have the usual characteristics of vertebrae, such as bodies, arches, and processes, but nearer the tip of the tail they are reduced to simple little rods of bone. In humans the coccygeal vertebrae are fused into a single bone called the **coccyx** or, more commonly, the *tailbone*.

## CLINICAL APPLICATION

### Wobbler Syndrome

Wobbler syndrome occurs most commonly in certain breeds of dog—Basset Hounds, Borzois, Doberman Pinschers, and Great Danes—and horses, particularly Thoroughbreds. It results from a narrowing of the spinal canal in the cervical region that compresses the spinal cord. This narrowing can result from physical abnormalities (malformations) of cervical vertebrae or improper joints (malarticulations) between them. The precise cause is not known, but inherited factors and nutritional factors seem to be involved. Clinical signs typically develop slowly and gradually, starting with weakness and incoordination, called *ataxia*. The name *wobbler syndrome* comes from the wobbly, uncoordinated gait seen in affected animals, and the disease can progress to complete paralysis. Medical treatments may be attempted to decrease the compression of the spinal cord, but surgery is often necessary. The prognosis for recovery is usually guarded at best.

## CLINICAL APPLICATION

### The Anticlinal Vertebra

In most veterinary practices, dogs are the animal species in which intervertebral disc disease is most commonly seen. As a result, veterinary personnel take a lot of spinal radiographs of dogs. The bones of the spine can be confusing to look at. When trying to identify the precise location of a lesion, the *anticlinal vertebra* is a convenient landmark. The eleventh thoracic vertebra, T11, is called *anticlinal* because its spinous process, unlike those of the surrounding vertebrae, projects straight up. The spinous processes of the first 10 thoracic vertebrae all recline caudally, and the last two, T12 and T13, incline cranially, so T11 looks out of place and is easily identified. The anticlinal vertebra in cats is also T11, but in horses it is T16; in cattle and sheep it is T13, and it is T10 in swine.

## RIBS

The **ribs** are flat bones that form the lateral walls of the thorax (Figures 7-21 to 7-23). The number of pairs of ribs usually equals the number of thoracic vertebrae the animal has. At their dorsal ends, the heads of the ribs form joints with the thoracic vertebrae. These freely movable joints help the process of ventilation, which is the movement of air in and out of the lungs. By swivelling the ribs at their dorsal ends, the ventilatory muscles can enlarge or diminish the size of the thorax, depending on the direction of the muscle contraction.

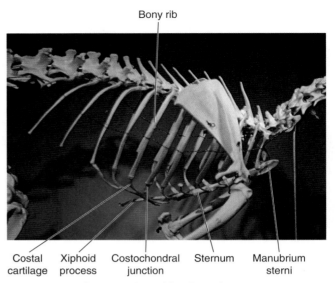

**FIGURE 7-21** Rabbit ribs and sternum.

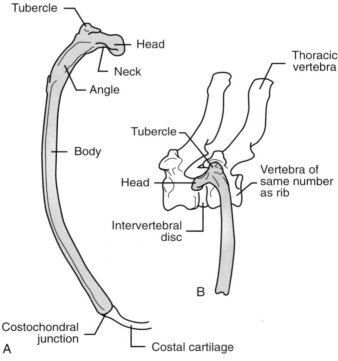

**FIGURE 7-22** Canine rib. **A,** Caudal view of rib. **B,** Lateral view of rib articulating with vertebrae.

The ventral ends of the ribs are a lot more variable. Each rib actually has two parts: a *dorsal* part, made of bone, and a *ventral* part, made of cartilage. The term for *rib* is *costal*, so the cartilaginous part is called the **costal cartilage**, and its junction with the bony part is called the **costochondral junction**. The costal cartilages either join the sternum directly or join the costal cartilage ahead of them (see Figure 7-23). The ribs whose cartilages join the sternum are called **sternal ribs** and make up the cranial part of the thorax. The

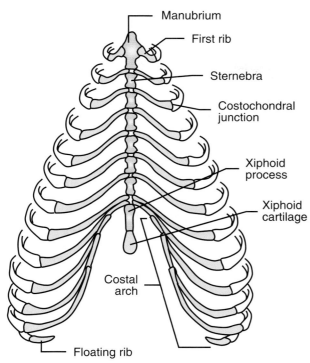

Manubrium

First rib

Sternebra

Costochondral junction

Xiphoid process

Xiphoid cartilage

Costal arch

Floating rib

**FIGURE 7-23** Canine costal cartilages and sternum. Ventral view.

| TABLE 7-3 | Bones of the Limbs (Proximal to Distal) |
| THORACIC LIMB | PELVIC LIMB |
| --- | --- |
| Scapula | Pelvis |
| | Ilium |
| | Ischium |
| | Pubis |
| Humerus | Femur |
| Radius | Tibia |
| Ulna | Fibula |
| Carpal bones (carpus) | Tarsal bones (tarsus) |
| Metacarpal bones | Metatarsal bones |
| Phalanges | Phalanges |

ones that join the adjacent costal cartilage are called **asternal ribs** and make up the caudal part of the thorax. The cartilages of the last ribs, the two on each side, may not join anything at all; they may just end in the muscles of the thoracic wall. These unattached ribs are called **floating ribs**.

## STERNUM

The **sternum**, also called the *breastbone*, forms the floor of the thorax. It is made up of a series of rodlike bones called **sternebrae** (see Figures 7-21 and 7-23). Only the first and last sternebrae are named and used as landmarks. The others are numbered from cranial to caudal. The first, most cranial

sternebra is called the **manubrium** or *manubrium sterni*. The last, most caudal sternebra is called the **xiphoid** or *xiphoid process*. A piece of cartilage, known as the *xiphoid cartilage*, extends caudally from the xiphoid process and is easily felt in most animals at the caudal end of the sternum.

## APPENDICULAR SKELETON

The appendicular skeleton is made up of the bones of the main appendages of the animal body, that is, the limbs. In anatomical terms, the front leg is the **thoracic limb**, and the hind leg is the **pelvic limb** (Table 7-3).

*Author's suggestion:* Find the bones discussed in the following section on skeletons, and identify the bones in living animals. Sometimes they are not where we think they are.

## THORACIC LIMB

In common domestic animals, the thoracic limb has no direct, bony connection with the axial skeleton. This is in contrast with primates, such as humans, that have a collarbone or *clavicle* that joins the scapula with the sternum. Instead, the forelegs support the weight of the body by a slinglike arrangement of muscles and tendons. Some animals, such as dogs and cats, may have a small remnant of the clavicle embedded in a tendon in the shoulder region, but it does not articulate with the axial skeleton and is of little or no clinical significance.

### SCAPULA

The **scapula** (Figure 7-24) is the most proximal bone of the thoracic limb. It is a flat, somewhat triangular bone with a prominent, longitudinal ridge on its lateral surface, which is referred to as the *spine* of the scapula. At its distal end, it forms the socket portion of the ball-and-socket shoulder joint. This fairly shallow, concave articular surface is called the **glenoid cavity**. It is connected with the main body of the scapula by a narrowed area known as the *neck*.

### HUMERUS

The **humerus** (Figure 7-25) is the long bone of the upper arm or **brachium**. On its proximal end is the ball portion of

TEST YOURSELF 7-4

1. Which groups of vertebrae make up the spinal column dorsal to the following regions?
   Abdomen
   Neck
   Pelvis
   Tail
   Thorax
2. What are the three kinds of processes found on vertebrae and what are their characteristics?
3. Where in a vertebra is the spinal cord located?
4. What are the names of the first two cervical vertebrae and what are their distinguishing characteristics?
5. What is the difference between a *sternal rib*, an *asternal rib*, and a *floating rib*?
6. What is the manubrium?
7. What is the xiphoid?

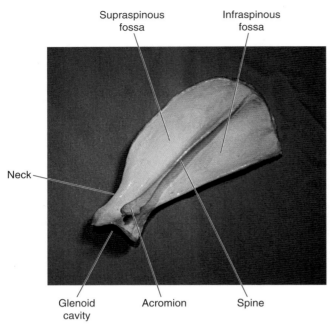

Supraspinous fossa

Infraspinous fossa

Neck

Glenoid cavity

Acromion

Spine

**FIGURE 7-24** Canine left scapula. Lateral view.

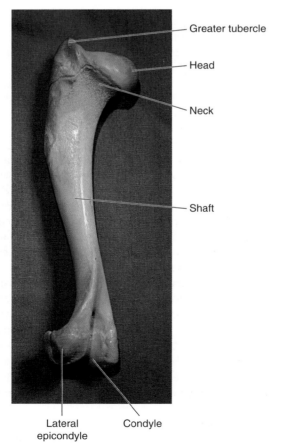

Greater tubercle

Head

Neck

Shaft

Lateral epicondyle

Condyle

**FIGURE 7-25** Canine left humerus. Lateral view.

the ball-and-socket shoulder joint: the head of the humerus, which is joined to the shaft by a neck. Opposite the head on the proximal end are some large processes called *tubercles*, where the powerful shoulder muscles attach. The largest one is called the *greater tubercle*. The shaft of the humerus extends down to the distal end that forms the elbow joint with the radius and ulna. The distal articular surfaces of the humerus are referred to collectively as the *condyle*. To be more precise, the medial articular surface is the *trochlea*, which articulates with the ulna, and the lateral one is the *capitulum*, which articulates with the radius. Just above the condyle on the back surface of the humerus is a deep indentation called the *olecranon fossa*, which will be discussed later with the ulna. The nonarticular "knobs" on the medial and lateral surfaces of the condyle are called the *medial* and *lateral epicondyles*. These are easily palpated and can be used as landmarks on living animals.

*Author's note:* Note the spelling of *humerus*. It looks a lot like the word *humorous*, which might lead you to believe that it is the "funny bone." It is not. Actually, the "funny bone" is not a bone at all, but the ulnar nerve, which is located fairly superficially as it passes through the elbow joint region. When we bump it, we experience that distinctive, funny-bone tingle.

## ULNA

Two bones form the forearm or **antebrachium**: the *ulna* and the *radius*. The **ulna** (Figure 7-26) forms a major portion of the elbow joint with the distal end of the humerus. Several interesting structures can be found on its proximal end. The large **olecranon process** forms the point of the elbow, where the tendon of the powerful *triceps brachii* muscle attaches. The *trochlear notch* is a half-moon shaped, concave articular surface that wraps around part of the humeral condyle to help make the elbow joint a tight, secure joint. At the proximal end of the trochlear notch is a beak-shaped process known as the **anconeal process**. When the elbow is extended into a straightened position, the anconeal process tucks into the *olecranon fossa* on the distal end of the humerus. At the distal end of the trochlear notch are the medial and lateral *coronoid processes*. They are located on the medial and lateral ends of the horizontal, concave facet on the proximal end of the ulna that articulates with the radius. The shaft of the ulna extends down to the carpus in all common species except for the horse. Its shape parallels the straight or curved shape of the radius. In the horse the ulna consists only of the proximal portion, which joins with the radius about midshaft. In other species, the distal end of the ulna consists of a pointed process, called the *styloid process*, that articulates with the carpus.

## RADIUS

The **radius** (Figure 7-27) is the main weight-bearing bone of the antebrachium. On its proximal end, the radius has facets that articulate with the proximal end of the ulna and a large, concave articular surface, where it joins with the distal end of the humerus. The shaft of the radius varies from fairly straight in cats and cattle to somewhat bowed in dogs, horses, and swine. At its distal end, the radius has several

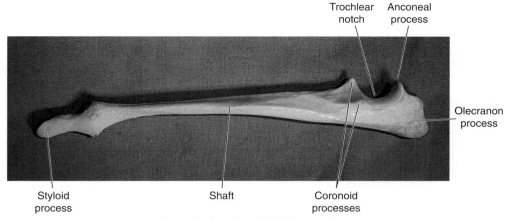

FIGURE 7-26 Canine left ulna. Lateral view.

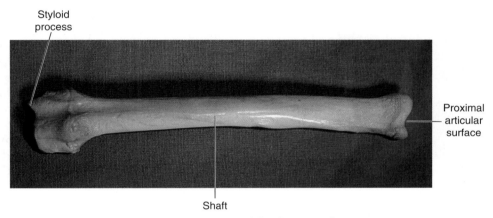

FIGURE 7-27 Canine left radius. Cranial view.

 **CLINICAL APPLICATION**

## Ununited Anconeal Process in the Dog

The anconeal process of the ulna develops from a secondary growth center that is separate from the primary growth center in the ulnar shaft. In dogs it normally fuses to the rest of the ulna by about 6 months of age. Sometimes, particularly in large and giant dog breeds, mechanical forces in the elbow break down the fusing tissues and prevent the anconeal process from uniting with the rest of the bone. This results in elbow joint instability that damages the joint surfaces and leads to secondary **osteoarthritis**, and the affected animal gradually becomes lame. The diagnosis can be confirmed by taking a lateral radiograph of the elbow in the flexed position, which will show the unattached process. Treatment usually involves surgical removal of the ununited anconeal process.

facets and a pointed process called the *styloid process* that articulate with the carpus.

## CARPAL BONES

The **carpus** (Figure 7-28) consists of two rows of **carpal bones**. The two rows of bones are arranged parallel to each other in a proximal row and a distal row. In humans the carpus is our *wrist*, but in horses it is referred to as the *knee*. Considerable variety is seen among the species in the precise makeup of the carpus, but a basic naming convention holds true across species lines. The bones of the proximal row are given individual names. All common species have a *radial carpal bone*, an *ulnar carpal bone*, and, protruding backward on the lateral side of the carpus, an *accessory carpal bone*. Some species also have an *intermediate carpal bone*. The bones of the distal row of the carpus are given numbers instead of names, starting at the medial side and working laterally. Figure 7-29 shows the distal bones of the horse leg from the carpus down, and Figure 7-30 shows comparable bones of the dog.

## METACARPAL BONES

The **metacarpal bones** extend distally from the distal row of carpal bones to the proximal phalanges of the digits. In humans, metacarpal bones are the bones of our hands. They extend from our wrists down to our first knuckles and are numbered from medial to lateral. The metacarpal of our thumb is *metacarpal I*, and that of our little finger is *metacarpal V*. The flexibility of the joint between the metacarpal bone of our thumb and our wrist makes our thumb apposable with the rest of our hand, which gives us a great grasping advantage over many other animal species. In other animals the appearance of the metacarpal bones is determined largely by what kind of foot the animal has.

Horses have a simple foot consisting of only one digit or toe. Therefore they have only one large metacarpal bone

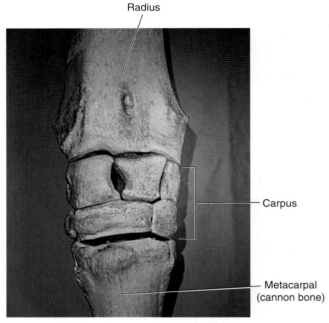

Radius

Carpus

Metacarpal
(cannon bone)

**FIGURE 7-28** Equine left carpus. Cranial view.

supporting their weight in each leg (see Figure 7-29). This large metacarpal bone is commonly referred to as the cannon bone. Actually, a horse has three metacarpal bones in each leg: one *large metacarpal* and two smaller *vestigial metacarpal* bones known as the **splint bones**. According to fossil evidence, ancestors of the modern horse had multiple toes. Over many millennia, those animals became increasingly specialized for speed and eventually developed into the modern horse that walks on only one toe. Figure 7-31 shows a modern horse digit alongside the fossilized distal leg bones of *Parahippus leonensis*, a small, three-toed horse considered to be an ancestor of the modern horse. The large metacarpal bone of the horse is assumed to be what is left of *metacarpal III*, and the smaller splint bones on either side of it are designated as *metacarpals II and IV*. There is no remnant of the first or fifth digits.

The splint bones do not support any weight and only extend one-half to two-thirds of the way down the shaft of the large metacarpal. They do, however, sometimes cause problems for horses, because they can suffer various kinds of injury including fractures. Most commonly, though, the ligaments joining them to the large metacarpal bone become inflamed. This condition is referred to as *splints*, and it can be quite painful for the horse. Treatment ranges from rest to surgery.

The feet of cattle are like horse feet split in two (Figure 7-32). Cattle walk on two toes. Accordingly, they have two metacarpal bones, *bones III and IV*, but these are

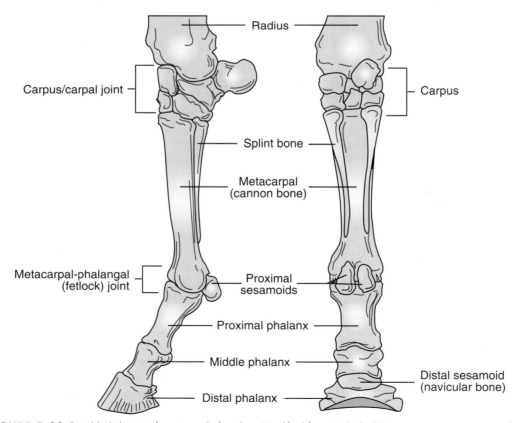

Radius

Carpus/carpal joint

Carpus

Splint bone

Metacarpal
(cannon bone)

Metacarpal-phalangal
(fetlock) joint

Proximal
sesamoids

Proximal phalanx

Middle phalanx

Distal sesamoid
(navicular bone)

Distal phalanx

**FIGURE 7-29** Distal limb bones of equine right front leg. (Modified from McBride DF: *Learning veterinary terminology,* ed 2, St Louis, 2002, Mosby.)

Medial

Lateral

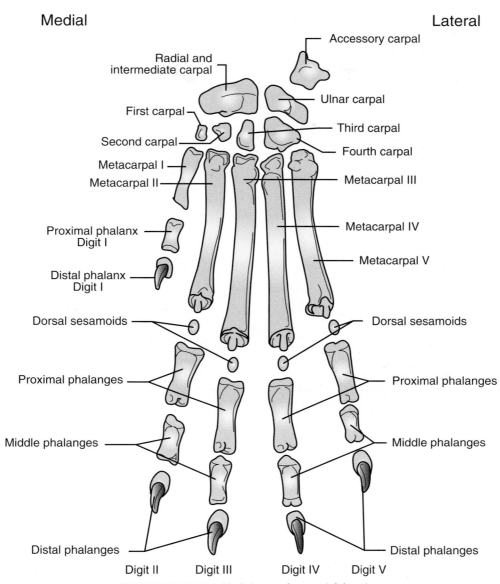

Accessory carpal

Radial and
intermediate carpal

Ulnar carpal

First carpal

Third carpal

Second carpal

Fourth carpal

Metacarpal I

Metacarpal II

Metacarpal III

Proximal phalanx
Digit I

Metacarpal IV

Metacarpal V

Distal phalanx
Digit I

Dorsal sesamoids

Dorsal sesamoids

Proximal phalanges

Proximal phalanges

Middle phalanges

Middle phalanges

Distal phalanges

Distal phalanges

Digit II    Digit III        Digit IV    Digit V

**FIGURE 7-30** Distal limb bones of canine left front leg.

fused into a single bone. A longitudinal groove running down the metacarpal bone clearly shows its two-bone origin, however.

Dogs and cats have paws that are structurally similar to our hands. They typically have five digits or toes making up their front paws. Figure 7-30 shows the bones of the canine forepaw. The bones of the cat are quite similar. Note that, like us, dogs have five metacarpal bones that are numbered from medial to lateral. *Metacarpal I* is part of what is usually termed the **dewclaw**, and the others are numbered *II, III, IV,* and *V. Metacarpal V* is the lateral-most metacarpal.

## PHALANGES

We need to clarify and differentiate a couple of terms used to describe animal feet. The anatomical term **digit** means the same as the common term *toe* (and, in our case, *finger*). Each

digit is made up of two or three bones called **phalanges** (singular, **phalanx**). So the phalanges are the individual bones that make up the digits.

Horses have one digit on each limb. It is composed of three phalanges and three sesamoid bones. The phalanges are named according to their position: they are the *proximal phalanx*, commonly called the *long pastern bone*; the *middle phalanx*, commonly called the *short pastern bone*; and the *distal phalanx*, commonly known as the *coffin bone*. In some older anatomy texts, the phalanges are numbered from proximal to distal instead of being named. This method works okay for horses, since they have only one digit, but it becomes confusing in animals with multiple digits that are already numbered. For clarity, we ignore that particular identification scheme.

The digit of the horse also contains two *proximal sesamoid bones* and one *distal sesamoid bone*. You will recall

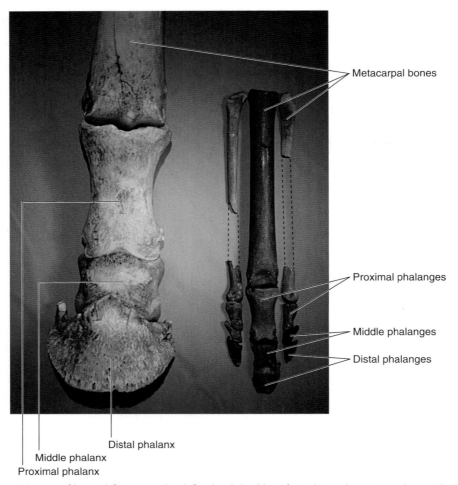

Metacarpal bones

Proximal phalanges

Middle phalanges

Distal phalanges

Distal phalanx

Middle phalanx

Proximal phalanx

**FIGURE 7-31** Digit of horse *(left)* compared with fossilized distal leg of *Parahippus leonensis (right)*. *Parahippus* was a primitive, three-toed horse that lived over 13 million years ago. Considered to be an ancestor of the modern horse, it was about the size of a large dog. It had a large, central hoof that bore most of its weight and two "side hooves." All that is left of those extra toes in the modern horse are the splint bones. (*Parahippus* fossils from the author's collection.)

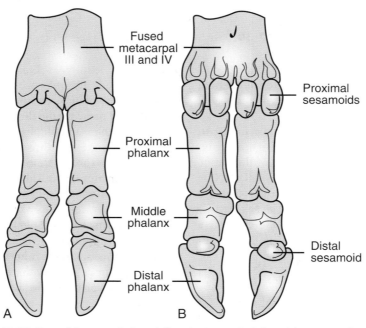

Fused metacarpal III and IV

Proximal sesamoids

Proximal phalanx

Middle phalanx

Distal phalanx

Distal sesamoid

A          B

**FIGURE 7-32** Digit of the cow. **A,** Dorsal *(front/top)* view. **B,** Palmar/plantar *(rear/bottom)* view.

that sesamoid bones are irregular bones found in some tendons where they change direction suddenly over the surfaces of joints. They act as bearings over the joint surfaces to allow muscles to exert powerful forces on the bones without the tendons wearing out from the constant, back-and-forth movement over the joint. The sesamoid bones of the horse digit are important in allowing the spindly little horse foot to support and propel the large horse body around. The two **proximal sesamoid bones** are located behind the joint between the large metacarpal bone and the proximal phalanx in the large digital flexor tendons. This joint is commonly referred to as the **fetlock joint**. The **distal sesamoid bone** is located deep in the hoof behind the joint between the middle and distal phalanges, where the digital flexor tendon attaches to the distal phalanx. Some imaginative early anatomist thought this distal sesamoid bone resembled a tiny boat, which led to its common name: the **navicular bone**. Proximal and distal sesamoid bones are found in both the front and hind digits of the horse.

Cattle have four digits on each limb: the third and fourth support the body weight, and the second and fifth are vestiges. The two vestigial digits are called the **dewclaws**, and each contains one or two small bones that do not articulate with the rest of the bones of the foot. Figure 7-32 shows the structure of the weight-bearing bones of the bovine foot. As you can see, each digit has a proximal, middle, and distal phalanx, as well as two proximal sesamoid bones and one distal sesamoid bone.

Dog and cat forepaws contain bones that are very similar to our fingers. Figure 7-30 clearly shows that digit I—the dewclaw—contains only two bones: a *proximal phalanx* and a *distal phalanx*. This is similar to our thumb, which contains only two phalanges. Digits II to V each contain three bones: a *proximal phalanx*, a *middle phalanx*, and a *distal phalanx*. Each distal phalanx contains a pointed **ungual process** that is surrounded by the claw. The digits of dogs and cats also contain tiny sesamoid bones, but they are rarely of clinical significance except in performance dogs, such as racing Greyhounds, and heavy large-breed dogs, such as St. Bernards. These heavy breeds can fracture sesamoid bones by jumping.

---

**TEST YOURSELF 7-5**

1. Name the bones of the thoracic limb from proximal to distal.
2. What is the anatomical name for the shoulder blade?
3. What are the brachium and the antebrachium, and which bones form them?
4. On which bone is the olecranon process found? What is its purpose?
5. What are the anatomical names for the cannon bone and the splint bones in a horse?
6. Which digit is the dewclaw on the front leg of a dog?
7. What is the common name for the distal sesamoid bone in the horse?

---

 **CLINICAL APPLICATION**

## Navicular Disease in the Horse

Because of its location deep in the hoof, where powerful forces are placed on it with each step, the navicular or *distal sesamoid* bone is subject to chronic wear and injury. This is particularly true in the front feet because of their more upright position. When the bone starts to undergo chronic, painful degeneration, the condition is called *navicular disease.*

Navicular disease is not one specific disease with one specific cause; it is a complex syndrome that involves many factors, including damage to the bone itself, damage to the bone's blood supply, and damage to surrounding structures, such as bursas, tendons, and ligaments. The net result is a lameness that begins intermittently and progressively gets worse. The animal tries to shift weight off the heel area of the affected foot where the damaged navicular bone is located. This changes the animal's gait and can lead to secondary problems.

The signs of navicular disease can sometimes be managed, but the condition is usually not curable. Some pain relief sometimes can be provided with corrective hoof trimming and shoeing and with drug therapy.

---

## PELVIC LIMB

Unlike the thoracic limb, the **pelvic limb** is directly connected to the axial skeleton through the sacroiliac joint that unites the ilium of the pelvis with the sacrum of the spinal column. This eliminates the need for large, slinglike muscles in the rear quarters to support the weight of the caudal part of the body and allows room for all the reproductive, urinary, and digestive system structures that lie between and behind the rear legs.

### PELVIS

The **pelvis** is sometimes referred to anatomically as the *os coxae*. It starts developing as three separate bones on each side that eventually fuse into a solid structure. The two halves of the pelvis are joined ventrally by a cartilaginous joint called the **pelvic symphysis**. The pelvis joins the axial skeleton dorsally at the left and right sacroiliac joints.

Even though the bones that make up the pelvis fuse together, the names of the individual bones are still used to designate the main regions of the pelvis: the *ilium*, the *ischium*, and the *pubis* (Figure 7-33).

***ILIUM.*** The **ilium** is the cranial-most bone of the pelvis. When we put our hands on our hips, the ilium on each side is the bone each hand rests on. It projects up in a dorsocranial direction and is the bone that forms the sacroiliac joints with the sacrum. In dogs and cats, the smooth "wing" of the ilium projects forward and is easily felt as a landmark in living animals. In cattle and horses, the cranial end of the ilium on each side has large medial and lateral processes. The *tuber sacrale* projects medially and joins with the *sacrum* to

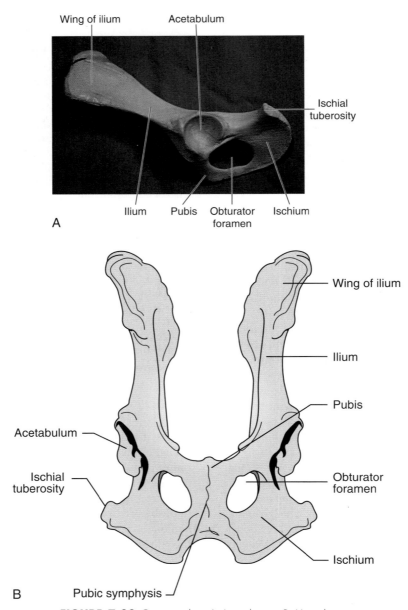

**FIGURE 7-33** Canine pelvis. **A**, Lateral view. **B**, Ventral view.

form the *sacroiliac joint*. The *tuber coxae* projects laterally and is called the *point* of the hip.

**ISCHIUM.** The **ischium** is the caudal-most pelvic bone. If you are sitting down as you are reading this, you are sitting on your ischia. The main, rear-projecting process of the ischium is the *ischial tuberosity*.

**PUBIS.** The **pubis** is the smallest of the three pelvic bones. It is located medially and forms the cranial portion of the pelvic floor, while the ischium forms the caudal part.

The three bones that make up each side of the pelvis come together at the socket portion of the ball-and-socket hip joint in a concave area called the **acetabulum**. The acetabulum is a deep socket that tightly encloses the head of the femur to form the relatively stable hip joint.

Located on either side of the pelvic symphysis are two large holes known as the **obturator foramina**. Usually a big hole in a bone would allow something large and important to pass through it; however, that is not the case here. Nothing but a few small blood vessels and nerves pass through the obturator foramina. Their primary function is to lighten the pelvis. Drag racers use this same principle when they drill numerous holes in many of the chassis components of their race cars to lighten them.

**FEMUR**

The **femur** (Figure 7-34) is the long bone of the thigh. On its proximal end is the ball portion of the ball-and-socket hip joint, called the *head of the femur*, which is attached to the shaft by a neck. In contrast to the large, round head of the humerus, the head of the femur is smaller and more

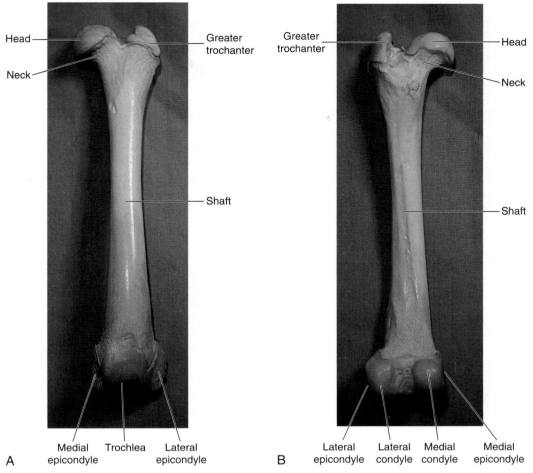

Head — Greater trochanter

Neck

Shaft

Medial epicondyle  Trochlea  Lateral epicondyle

**A**

Greater trochanter — Head

Neck

Shaft

Lateral epicondyle  Lateral condyle  Medial condyle  Medial epicondyle

**B**

**FIGURE 7-34** Canine left femur. **A,** Cranial view. **B,** Caudal view.

spherical. It normally fits very deeply and securely into the acetabulum of the pelvis.

Opposite the head on the proximal end are some large processes, the trochanters, where strong hip and thigh muscles attach. The largest one is called the *greater trochanter.* The shaft of the femur is fairly straight and extends down to the distal end to form the **stifle joint,** which is equivalent to our knee, with the patella and tibia. The three articular surfaces on the distal end of the femur are the two condyles caudally and the trochlea cranially. The medial and lateral condyles articulate with the condyles on the proximal end of the tibia. The trochlea is a smooth articular groove in which the patella rides. Like the humerus, the femur has nonarticular "knobs" medial and lateral to the condyles; these are called the *medial* and *lateral epicondyles,* and they are easily palpated and can be used as landmarks on living animals.

## PATELLA

The **patella** or *kneecap* is the largest sesamoid bone in the body. It is formed in the distal tendon of the large quadriceps femoris muscle on the cranial aspect of the stifle joint. It helps protect the tendon as it passes down over the trochlea of the femur to insert on the tibial crest.

## FABELLAE

The medial and lateral **fabellae** are two small sesamoid bones located in the proximal *gastrocnemius* or *calf muscle* tendons just above and behind the femoral condyles of dogs and cats. They are not present in cattle or horses.

## TIBIA

The **tibia** (Figure 7-35) is the main weight-bearing bone of the lower leg. It forms the **stifle joint** with the femur above it and the **hock** with the tarsus below it. When viewed from above, the proximal end of the tibia appears triangular with the apex of the triangle facing forward. The tibial condyles on top of the proximal end articulate with the condyles of the femur. The forward-facing point of the triangle is the *tibial tuberosity,* which continues distally as a ridge called the **tibial crest.** The patellar ligament attaches to the tibial tuberosity. The shaft of the tibia is triangular at the proximal end and fairly round further distally. At its distal end, the articular surface of the tibia consists of grooves that articulate with the tibial tarsal bone. Medial to the distal articular surface of the tibia is a palpable process called the *medial malleolus,* which is the "knob" on the medial side of our ankle at the distal end of our tibia. If you start at the tibial crest just below

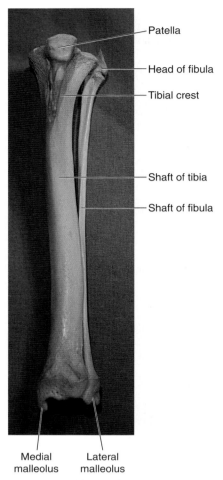

- Patella
- Head of fibula
- Tibial crest
- Shaft of tibia
- Shaft of fibula

Medial malleolus    Lateral malleolus

**FIGURE 7-35** Canine left tibia, fibula, and patella. Cranial view.

the front of your knee, you can trace down the tibia or *shinbone* to your medial malleolus.

## FIBULA

The **fibula** (see Figure 7-35) is a thin but complete bone in dogs and cats that parallels the tibia and consists of a *proximal extremity*, a *shaft*, and a *distal extremity*. It does not support any significant weight but mainly serves as a muscle attachment site. In horses and cattle, only the proximal and distal ends of the fibula are present—the shaft is not. At its distal end, the fibula forms a palpable process called the *lateral malleolus*. The lateral knob of our ankle is our lateral malleolus.

## TARSAL BONES

The **tarsus** (Figure 7-36) is what we call our ankle. In a four-legged animal, it is commonly called the **hock**. It consists of two rows of short bones known as the **tarsal bones**. Like the carpus, the proximal row of bones is named, and the distal row is numbered. The two largest proximal tarsal bones are the *tibial tarsal bone* and the *fibular tarsal bone*. A smaller, *central tarsal bone* is tucked behind the two larger bones. The tibial tarsal bone has a large trochlea that articulates with the distal end of the tibia to form the most movable part of the hock joint. The **calcaneal tuberosity** of the fibular tarsal bone projects upward and backward to form the point of the hock. It acts as the point of attachment for the tendon of the large gastrocnemius muscle and corresponds to our heel. The distal row of tarsal bones is numbered from medial to lateral, much like the distal row of carpal bones.

## CLINICAL APPLICATION

### Canine Hip Dysplasia

Canine **hip dysplasia** is an abnormal looseness or laxity of the hip joints of some dogs that leads to joint instability and degenerative bony changes. Many factors contribute to its development, including overnutrition that leads to too rapid growth, exercise, and genetic factors. Puppies of dysplastic parents are more likely to develop hip dysplasia than are puppies of normal parents, and larger breeds are affected more often than smaller breeds.

In a dysplastic animal, the normally tight-fitting hip joint is much looser, allowing the femoral head to "rattle around" in the acetabulum. This damages the joint surfaces and leads to degenerative changes and osteoarthritis. Movement of the diseased hips is painful, especially after exercise. Definitive diagnosis of canine hip dysplasia usually requires pelvic radiographs, and treatment can range from weight reduction and exercise restriction, to medical treatments with anti-inflammatory drugs, to a variety of surgical procedures. The best treatment for canine hip dysplasia is to attempt to prevent its development by only breeding hip dysplasia-free parents.

## CLINICAL APPLICATION

### Patellar Luxation in Dogs

Normally the patella rides securely in the deep groove of the trochlea on the distal end of the femur. The pull of the quadriceps tendon is normally directly in line with the trochlea. Sometimes physical abnormalities cause the pull of the tendon to be off-line, or one rim of the trochlear groove may not be high enough to hold the patella securely in place. When that occurs, the patella can *luxate* or pop out of the trochlea, usually toward the medial side. The most common type of patellar luxation occurs in small and miniature dog breeds and results in the patella popping out of the medial side of the trochlear groove when the foot is planted. This causes pain when the animal tries to flex the stifle joint to take its next step, and so it will often carry or hold up the affected leg for a step or two until the patella pops back into place. This causes a periodic, skipping-type gait that is characteristic of this disorder. The condition is easily diagnosed by extending the stifle joint and palpating the easily displaced patella. Treatment usually consists of any of several types of surgical correction.

## METATARSAL BONES

The **metatarsal bones** (see Figure 7-36) are almost exactly the same as the metacarpal bones. The only major differences

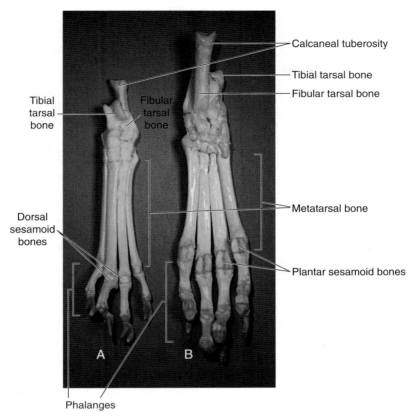

Calcaneal tuberosity

Tibial tarsal bone

Fibular tarsal bone

Tibial tarsal bone

Fibular tarsal bone

Metatarsal bone

Dorsal sesamoid bones

Plantar sesamoid bones

A    B

Phalanges

**FIGURE 7-36** Left feline and canine tarsus, metatarsals, and phalanges **A,** Feline, dorsal view. **B,** Canine, plantar view.

are in the dog and cat. Usually only four digits make up the paw on each hind leg, so there are usually only four metatarsal bones: metatarsals II through V. Like the front leg, horses have a large metatarsal bone—the cannon bone—and two small metatarsal bones—the splint bones—on each hind leg. Our metatarsal bones are the bones of our feet.

## PHALANGES

The phalanges of the pelvic limb (see Figure 7-36) are almost exactly like the phalanges of the thoracic limb. The only major difference is, again, in dogs and cats. Usually only four digits make up the paw on each hind leg: digits II through V.

## CLINICAL APPLICATION

### Using External Skeletal Landmarks in Body Condition Scoring

**Body condition scoring (BCS)** uses a numerical scale to indicate the amount of fat in an animal's body. The details of different BCS systems vary, but most use either a 9-point or 5-point scoring system. In each case the middle of the range, 5 out of 9 (BCS = 5/9) or 3 out of 5 (BCS = 3/5), is the desired body condition status. An animal with a low BCS is too thin: a BCS of 1/5 or 1/9 means the animal is emaciated. An animal with a high BCS is overweight: one with a BCS of 5/5 or 9/9 is obese.

Regardless of the BCS system being used, the basic technique involves visually assessing the animal's body shape, and palpating (feeling) external skeletal landmarks to determine how much fat is around them. Common skeletal landmarks used in body condition scoring include ribs, vertebrae (wings of atlas, spinous processes, transverse processes), shoulder (greater tubercle of humerus, spine of scapula),

elbow (olecranon process of ulna, epicondyles of humerus), pelvis and hip (ilium, ischium, greater trochanter of femur), and stifle (patella, epicondyles of femur).

The more prominent these skeletal landmarks are, the lower the amount of fat in the animal's body, and the lower the BCS. Conversely, the more difficult these landmarks are to feel, the greater the amount of fat in the body, and the higher the BCS.

*Author's note*: Precise BCS criteria vary from species to species. (Enter "Body Condition Scoring" into your favorite internet search engine to see some examples.) But the basic concepts can be applied to virtually any animal species. At the zoo I am often asked by zookeepers to assess their animals' body conditions. They use those values along with body weights to judge whether the animals' diets are appropriate. On a given day I may evaluate the BCS of a chinchilla weighing less than a pound, and that of a camel weighing a ton. The same basic principles apply to each.

✓ *TEST YOURSELF 7-6*

1. Name the bones of the pelvic limb from distal to proximal.
2. What three pairs of bones make up the pelvis? What region of the pelvis does each form?
3. What is the largest sesamoid bone in the animal body?
4. Which bone is larger and supports more of an animal's weight, the tibia or the fibula?
5. On which bone of the pelvic limb is the calcaneal tuberosity found? What is its purpose?
6. Is an animal with a body condition score (BCS) of 3/9 too fat or too skinny?

## VISCERAL SKELETON

The **visceral skeleton** consists of bones that form in soft organs or *viscera*. It is the strangest division of the skeleton and the most variable. Not all animals have visceral bones. As a matter of fact, they are pretty unusual. Three examples include the *os cordis*, *os penis*, and *os rostri*. The **os cordis** is a bone in the heart of cattle and sheep that helps support the valves of the heart. The **os penis** (Figure 7-37) is a bone in the penis of dogs, beavers, raccoons, and walruses that partially surrounds the penile portion of the urethra. The urethral groove on the ventral surface of the bone encloses the dorsal portion of the urethra. The **os rostri** is a bone in the nose of swine that strengthens the snout for the rooting behavior of pigs, whereby they dig into the ground with their snouts. In Europe, pigs are used to find and root out rare and expensive truffles, a type of underground fungus used in gourmet cooking.

## JOINTS

**Joints** are the junctions between bones. Some of them are completely immovable, some are slightly movable, and some are freely movable. When we think of joints, we usually think of freely movable joints, such as the elbow or the hip; however, the immovable sutures that hold most of the skull bones together are joints also.

### JOINT TERMINOLOGY

The terms *arthro-* and *articular* refer to joints. For example, the study of joints is *arthrology*, and the smooth bony

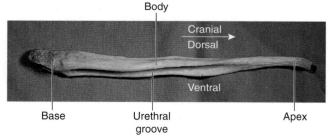

Body

Cranial →

Dorsal

Ventral

Base     Urethral        Apex
         groove

**FIGURE 7-37** Canine os penis. Lateral view.

 **CLINICAL APPLICATION**

### Canine Os Penis Problems

The most common clinical problem associated with the os penis in dogs occurs when urinary calculi, called *stones*, lodge in the urethra where it enters the narrow urethral groove at the base of the bone. The lodged calculi can obstruct the flow of urine, and surgery may be required to remove them.

*Author's note:* I once saw a fractured os penis in a Labrador-type dog. The dog was very weak and nearly comatose when it was presented by the owners. They reported lethargy, vomiting, and progressive weakness over the previous several days. Abdominal radiographs showed fluid in the dog's abdomen and a complete fracture through the body of the os penis. When I explored the abdomen surgically, I found a sizeable tear in the wall of the urinary bladder and a large quantity of urine free in the abdominal cavity. The fractured os penis had apparently obstructed the flow of urine through the urethra, which resulted in the urinary bladder filling to the point that it burst. The dog became very ill after waste products from the urine in its abdomen were absorbed back into the bloodstream. I removed the urine, repaired the urinary bladder, and sutured a urethral catheter into place until the fracture healed. Happily, the dog went on to make a complete recovery.

surfaces that come together to form freely movable joints are called *articular* surfaces.

The terminology of arthrology can be confusing because the meanings of many anatomical terms used to describe types of joint are obscure and cryptic to many of us. In our discussions of joints, we use the clearer terms commonly used in clinical veterinary medicine. The more complex anatomical terms are mentioned in case you wish to consult other, more in-depth anatomical references.

### TYPES OF JOINT

The three general classifications of joint in the animal body are the immovable *fibrous joints*, the slightly movable *cartilaginous joints*, and the freely movable *synovial* joints.

#### FIBROUS JOINTS

The anatomical term for **fibrous joints** is **synarthroses**. (See what I mean about that obscure terminology?) Fibrous joints are immovable in that the bones are firmly united by fibrous tissue. Some examples include the sutures that unite most of the skull bones (Figure 7-38) and the fibrous union of the splint bones of horses with the large metacarpal and metatarsal bones.

#### CARTILAGINOUS JOINTS

Slightly movable, **cartilaginous joints** are termed **amphiarthroses**. They are capable of only a slight rocking movement. Examples include the intervertebral joints (containing the discs) between the bodies of adjacent vertebrae in the spine and the symphyses between the two halves of the pelvis and

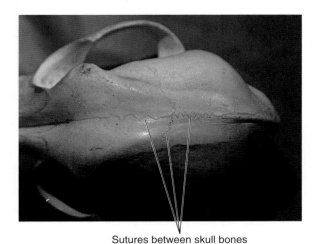

Sutures between skull bones

**FIGURE 7-38** Fibrous joints. Dorsal view of sutures between canine skull bones.

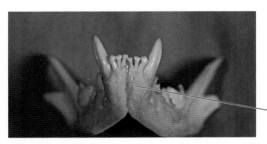

Mandibular symphysis

**FIGURE 7-39** Cartilaginous joint. Rostral view of feline mandibular symphysis.

between the two sides of the mandible (Figure 7-39) in some animals.

## SYNOVIAL JOINTS

**Synovial joints** are what we usually think of when we hear the word *joint*. They are freely movable joints, such as the shoulder joint and the stifle joint. The anatomical term for synovial joints is **diarthroses**.

The rest of our discussion of joints centers on synovial joints.

**SYNOVIAL JOINT CHARACTERISTICS.** Synovial joints all share some common characteristics. These include articular surfaces on the bones, articular cartilage covering the articular surfaces, and a fluid-filled **joint cavity** enclosed by a **joint capsule**. Firm connective tissue bands called *ligaments* may help stabilize the bones and hold the joint together.

Articular surfaces are the very smooth joint surfaces of bones, where they rub together in a joint. They consist of a smooth, thin layer of compact bone over the top of cancellous bone.

Articular cartilage is a thin, smooth layer of hyaline cartilage that lies on top of the articular surface of a bone. The articular cartilage functions like a Teflon coating on the joint surfaces to aid the smooth movement between them to reduce friction.

The joint cavity, also called the **joint space** clinically, is a fluid-filled potential space between the joint surfaces. A multilayered joint capsule surrounds it. The outer layer of the joint capsule is fibrous tissue, and the lining layer is called the **synovial membrane**. The synovial membrane produces the **synovial fluid** that lubricates the joint surfaces. Synovial fluid is normally transparent and has the viscosity of medium-weight motor oil. When joint disease is suspected, a joint "tap" is often done. This involves doing a presurgical skin prep, inserting a sterile needle into the joint cavity, and withdrawing synovial fluid for examination, analysis, and possible bacterial culture.

**Ligaments** are bands of fibrous connective tissue that are present in and around many synovial joints. They are similar to tendons but differ in that they join bones to other bones. Tendons join muscles to bones. Ligaments are not present in all synovial joints, but when they are present, they are often vital to the joint's effective operation.

The stifle joint, which is equivalent to our knee, offers an excellent model of how important ligaments can be to normal joint function. Consult Figure 7-40 as we look at the components of the stifle joint. The arrangement of the joint surfaces of the stifle joint, between the distal end of the femur and the proximal end of the tibia, makes it an inherently unstable joint. No deep sockets or closely fitting heads are present to hold it together or to allow only the desired hingelike movements between the bones. The round condyles of the femur sit on top of the flattish condyles of the tibia, supported only by two shallow, concave, half-moon–shaped fibrocartilage structures, which are the medial **meniscus** and the lateral meniscus.

The stifle joint normally only bends and straightens like a hinge. Bend and straighten your knee and you will see the normal movement of the joint. A large tendon and a group of four ligaments provide the stability that allows the stifle joint to function properly. The large tendon is the distal tendon of the large quadriceps femoris (cranial thigh) muscle that passes over the cranial surface of the stifle joint and attaches to the proximal end of the tibia at the tibial tuberosity. The patella, or kneecap, is embedded in this tendon. The tendon is called the quadriceps femoris tendon until it reaches the patella. Distal to the patella its name changes to the **patellar ligament**. Same structure, different name. The patellar ligament provides support on the front of the stifle joint. On the medial and lateral sides of the joint, two straplike **collateral**—which means *on both sides*—ligaments connect the femur and the tibia, and prevent sideways movement of the bones. Inside the joint are two ligaments that cross each other like the letter X. They are called the *cranial* and *caudal cruciate* (X-shaped) *ligaments*. They help prevent the bones of the stifle from sliding forward and backward as the joint bends and straightens.

**SYNOVIAL JOINT MOVEMENTS.** The movements possible in synovial joints are illustrated in Figures 7-41 and 7-42. They are **flexion**, **extension**, **adduction**, **abduction**, **rotation**, and **circumduction**.

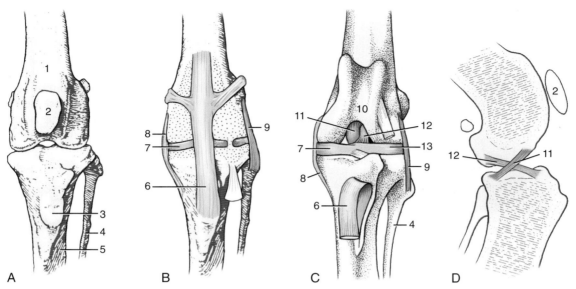

**FIGURE 7-40** Left stifle joint of the dog. **A-C,** Cranial views. **A** shows just the bones. The extent of the joint capsule is shown in **B**. The patella has been removed in **C**. **D** shows the crossing of the cruciate ligaments in a medial view. *1,* Femur; *2,* patella; *3,* tibial tuberosity; *4,* fibula; *5,* tibia; *6,* patellar ligament; *7,* medial meniscus; *8,* medial collateral ligament; *9,* lateral collateral ligament; *10,* trochlea; *11,* caudal cruciate ligament; *12,* cranial cruciate ligament; *13,* lateral meniscus. (Adapted from Dyce KM, Sack WO, Wensing CJG: Textbook of veterinary anatomy, ed 4, St Louis, 2010, WB Saunders Company.)

 **CLINICAL APPLICATION**

### Cranial Cruciate Ligament Rupture

Sometimes, particularly in dogs, a wrong step can result in a *rupture* or tearing of the cranial cruciate ligament (CCL), which is damaged more often than other ligaments. This injury can occur in athletic dogs if they plant a foot wrong while running and turning, or it can occur in overweight, sedentary dogs if they land wrong as they jump off the couch. The result is instability of the stifle joint. Instead of hinging on each other like they are supposed to, the femur and tibia also slide forward and backward relative to each other. This can damage other joint structures, such as the menisci, and can lead to osteoarthritis in the joint.

Rupture of the CCL is diagnosed by palpating the stifle joint and producing what is called *anterior drawer movement*, which is an abnormal forward and backward movement of the femur and tibia relative to each other. Therapy for CCL rupture can range from exercise restriction, weight reduction, and physical therapy to any of several surgical repair techniques.

Flexion and extension are opposite movements. **Flexion** decreases the angle between two bones. Picking a horse's front foot up for examination flexes the carpus joint. **Extension** is the opposite movement, and it increases the angle between two bones. Straightening a bent (or flexed) elbow joint extends the joint.

Adduction and abduction are also opposite movements. They involve movement of extremities relative to the median plane of the body. **Adduction** is the movement of an extremity toward the median plane, and **abduction** is a movement away from the median plane. One way to avoid confusion is to remember that to *abduct* something is to take it *away*.

**Rotation** is a twisting movement of a part on its own axis. If you hold your arm out with your palm down and move it so your palm is up, that movement is rotation.

**Circumduction** is the movement of an extremity so that the distal end moves in a circle. You can produce this movement by extending your arm and moving your hand in a circle.

**TYPES OF SYNOVIAL JOINT.** Synovial joints can be categorized according to the type of joint surfaces and the movements that are possible. Most of the joints of the body can be classified into one of four basic joint types: *hinge joints, gliding joints, pivot joints,* and *ball-and-socket* joints.

**HINGE JOINTS.** **Hinge joints** are also called **ginglymus joints**. One joint surface swivels around another. The only movements possible are flexion and extension. The elbow joint (Figure 7-43) is a good example of a hinge joint, as is the atlantooccipital joint (Figure 7-44) between the occipital bone in the skull and the first cervical vertebra. Flexion and extension of the atlantooccipital joint moves the skull up and down in a nodding, "yes" motion.

**GLIDING JOINTS.** The complicated name for **gliding joints** is **arthrodial joints**, but *rocking joints* would be more

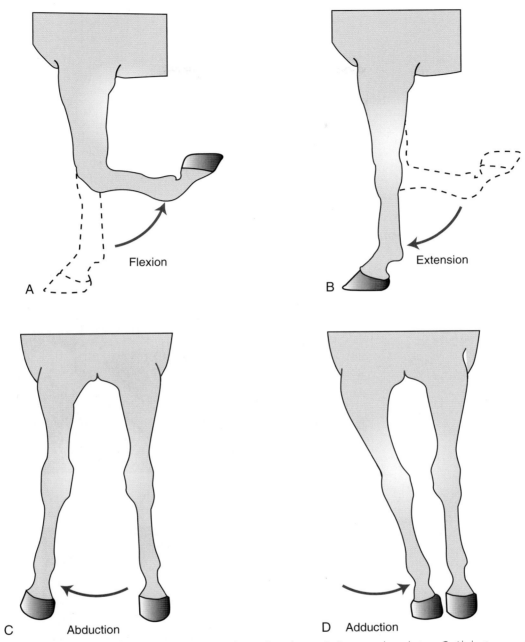

**FIGURE 7-41** Movements of equine front leg. **A,** Flexion, lateral view. **B,** Extension, lateral view. **C,** Abduction, cranial view. **D,** Adduction, cranial view.

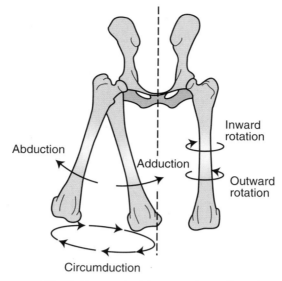

**FIGURE 7-42** Movements of the canine femur. Cranial view.

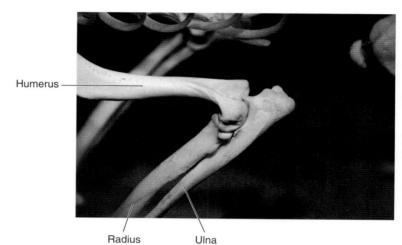

**FIGURE 7-43** Hinge-type synovial joint. Canine left elbow, lateral view.

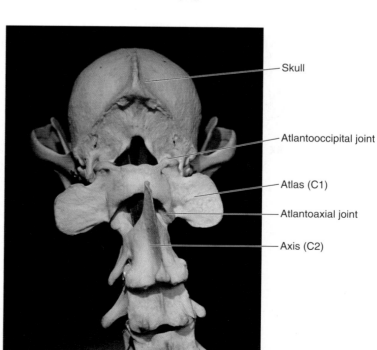

**FIGURE 7-44** Hinge-type and pivot-type synovial joints. Canine atlantooccipital (hinge) joint and atlantoaxial (pivot) joint. Canine skull and cervical vertebrae, caudal view.

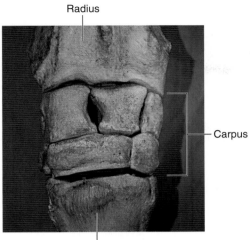

FIGURE **7-45** Gliding-type synovial joint. Equine carpus, cranial view.

Radius

Carpus

Large metacarpal bone (cannon bone)

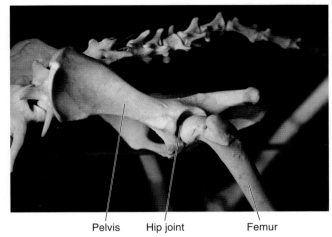

Pelvis    Hip joint    Femur

FIGURE **7-46** Ball-and-socket synovial joint. Canine left hip joint, craniolateral view.

descriptive. The joint surfaces of a gliding joint are relatively flat. The movement between them is a rocking motion of one bone on the other. The main movements possible are flexion and extension, but some abduction and adduction may also be possible. The *carpus* or *wrist* (Figure 7-45) is a good example of a gliding joint. Note that you can flex and extend your wrist, but you can also move your hand side to side (abduction and adduction). Most four-legged animals can do only the flexion and extension part.

*PIVOT JOINTS.* **Pivot joints** are also known as **trochoid joints.** One bone *pivots* or *rotates* on another. The only movement possible is rotation. Only one true pivot joint is found in the bodies of most animals, that being the joint between the first and second cervical vertebrae— the atlantoaxial joint (see Figure 7-44). Some anatomists with a sense of humor refer to this as the *no* joint, because the only movement it allows is a rotation of the head back and forth in a "no" movement. The movement is actually occurring between the vertebrae, but the head goes along with the first cervical vertebra as it pivots on the second cervical vertebra.

## BALL-AND-SOCKET JOINTS

**Ball-and-socket joints** are also called **spheroidal joints.** They allow the most extensive movements of all the joint types and allow all the synovial joint movements. Ball-and-socket joints permit flexion, extension, abduction, adduction, rotation, and circumduction. The shoulder and hip joints (Figure 7-46) are ball-and-socket joints.

### ✓ TEST YOURSELF 7-7

1. What are the main characteristics of fibrous joints, cartilaginous joints, and synovial joints?
2. What is synovial fluid and why is it important to the functioning of a synovial joint?
3. What is the difference between a *tendon* and a *ligament*?
4. Make the following joint movements with your own body: abduction, adduction, circumduction, extension, flexion, and rotation.
5. Name some examples of each of these kinds of synovial joint:
   Ball-and-socket joint
   Gliding joint
   Hinge joint
   Pivot joint

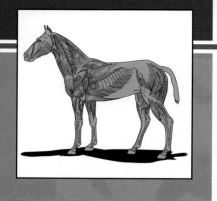

*Joann Colville*

## OUTLINE

## LEARNING OBJECTIVES

*When you have completed this chapter you will be able to:*

1. List the three types of muscle and describe the general characteristics of each type.
2. Describe the structure and function of tendons, aponeuroses, and ligaments.
3. Differentiate between prime mover, antagonist, synergist, and fixator muscles.
4. List the locations and actions of muscles of the head and neck.
5. List the locations and actions of muscles of the abdomen, thoracic limb, and pelvic limb.
6. List the locations and actions of muscles of respiration.
7. Describe the microscopic anatomy of skeletal muscle, smooth muscle, and cardiac muscle cells.
8. List the components of a neuromuscular junction and describe the function of each component.
9. List and describe the roles of the connective tissues in skeletal muscles.
10. Describe the events that occur in skeletal muscle cells during muscle contraction and relaxation.
11. Differentiate between visceral smooth muscle and multi-unit smooth muscle.

## VOCABULARY FUNDAMENTALS

*A band* A bahnd
*Abductor muscle* ahb-**duhck**-tohr **muhs**-uhl
*Actin filament* **ahck**-tihn **fihl**-ah-mehnt
*Adductor muscle* ahd-**duhck**-tohr **muhs**-uhl
*Adenosine diphosphate (ADP)* ah-**dehn**-ō-sēn dī-**fohs**-fāt
*Adenosine triphosphate (ATP)* ah-**dehn**-ō-sēn trī-**fohs**-fāt
*Aerobic metabolism* ər-**rō**-bihck meh-**tahb**-uh-lihz-ehm
*Agonist* **ahg**-uh-nihst
*Anaerobic metabolism* ahn-ər-**rō**-bihck meh-**tahb**-uh-lihz-ehm
*Antagonist* ahn-**tahg**-uh-nihst
*Aponeuroses* ahp-uh-noo-**rō**-sēz
*Brachium* **brā**-kē-uhm
*Cardiac muscle* **kahr**-dē-ahck **muhs**-uhl
*Creatine phosphate (CP)* **kree**-ah-tēn **fohs**-fāt
*Cross-bridge* krohs brihj
*Cutaneous muscle* kyoo-**tā**-nē-uhs **muhs**-uhl

*Dense body* dehnz **boh**-dē
*Diaphragm* **dī**-ah-frahm
*Endomysium* ehn-dō-**mī**-sē-uhm
*Epimysium* ehp-ih-**mī**-sē-uhm
*Expiratory muscle* ehcks-**spīr**-uh-tohr-ē **muhs**-uhl
*Fascicle* **fahs**-ih-kuhl
*Fixator* **fihck**-sā-tər
*H band* H bahnd
*I band* I bahnd
*Inspiratory muscle* ihn-**spīr**-uh-tohr-ē **muhs**-uhl
*Intercalated disc* ihn-**tər**-kuhl-lā-tehd dihsk
*Intramuscular* ihn-trah-**muhs**-kyoo-lər
*Involuntary muscle* ihn-**vohl**-uhn-teər-ē **muhs**-uhl
*Involuntary striated muscle* ihn-**vohl**-uhn-teər-ē **strī**-ā-tehd **muhs**-uhl

*Lactic acid* lahck-tihck **ah**-sihd
*Linea alba* lihn-ē-ah **ahl**-bah
*Motor unit* mō-tər ū-niht
*Multi-unit smooth muscle* **muhl**-tī-ū-niht smooth
   **muhs**-uhl
*Muscle* **muhs**-uhl
*Myofibril* mī-ō-**fī**-brihl
*Myoglobin* mī-ō-glō-bihn
*Myosin filament* mī-ō-sihn **fihl**-ah-mehnt
*Neuromuscular junction* nər-ō-**muhsk**-ū-**lahr**
   juhngk-shuhn
*Nonstriated involuntary muscle* nohn-**strī**-ā-tehd
   ihn-**vohl**-uhn-teər-ē **muhs**-uhl
*Perimysium* peər-ih-**mihz**-ē-uhm
*Sarcolemma* **sahr**-kō-lehm-ah
*Sarcomere* **sahr**-kō-mēr
*Sarcoplasm* **sahr**-kō-plahz-ehm

*Sarcoplasmic reticulum* **sahr**-kō-plahz-mihck
   reh-**tihck**-ū-luhm
*Sinoatrial node* sī-nō-ā-trē-ahl nōd
*Skeletal muscle* **skehl**-ih-tahl **muhs**-uhl
*Skeletal muscle fiber* **skehl**-ih-tahl **muhs**-uhl
   **fī**-bər
*Smooth muscle* smooth **muhs**-uhl
*Synergist* **sihn**-ər-jihst
*Tendon* **tehn**-dohn
*Transverse tubule (T tubule)* trahnz-vərs **too**-byool
*Twitch contraction* twihtch kohn-**trahck**-shuhn
*Viscera* **vih**-sər-ah
*Visceral smooth muscle* **vih**-sər-ahl smooth
   **muhs**-uhl
*Voluntary striated muscle* **vohl**-uhn-teər-ē **strī**-ā-tehd
   **muhs**-uhl
*Z line* Z līn

## INTRODUCTION

When we think about an animal's body moving, it all seems so simple and automatic. The animal wants to move forward, so it moves its legs appropriately to walk, trot, or run in that direction. At the same time, things are moving inside its body, too. Blood is being pumped through the blood vessels, food is being moved along the digestive tract, and little adjustments are being made all over to help keep the body operating smoothly. All this just seems to happen, but all these activities and many more are produced by the work of the muscular system.

**Muscle** is one of the four basic tissues of the body (epithelial tissue, connective tissue, and nervous tissue are the other three). It is made up of muscle cells with four common characteristics (1) excitability: they can respond to a stimulus such as a nerve impulse, (2) contractibility: they shorten in length when stimulated, (3) extensibility: they will stretch when pulled, and (4) elasticity: they will return to their original shape and length after contraction or extension. In the body, muscles have three primary functions: to provide motion, maintain posture, and generate heat.

When we hear the word *muscle* we usually think of large muscles, like the biceps or gluteal muscles. Actually, three different types of muscle make up the muscular system: *skeletal muscle* (the most familiar kind), *cardiac muscle,* and *smooth muscle* (Table 8-1). **Skeletal muscle** is controlled by the conscious mind and moves the bones of the skeleton so that the animal can move around. This type is what we usually think of as muscle. The other two types are a little less obvious.

**Cardiac muscle** is found only one place in the body—the heart. It makes up most of the structure of the heart. It starts the entire heart beating long before an animal is born and keeps it going until the animal dies. It has some interesting features, which we will discuss later in this chapter.

| TABLE 8-1 | Comparison of Muscle Features | | |
|---|---|---|---|
| **FEATURE** | **SKELETAL MUSCLE** | **CARDIAC MUSCLE** | **SMOOTH MUSCLE** |
| Location | Skeletal muscles | Heart | Internal organs, blood vessels, eye |
| Action | Move the bones, generate heat | Pump blood | Produce movements in internal organs and structures |
| Nuclei | Multiple | Single | Single |
| Striations | Present | Present | Absent |
| Cell shape | Long, thin fiber | Branched | Spindle |
| Nerve supply | Necessary for function | Modifies activity, not necessary for function | Visceral—modifies activity, not necessary for function |
| | | | Multi-unit—necessary for function |
| Control | Voluntary | Involuntary | Involuntary |

**Smooth muscle** is found all over the body in places such as the eyes, the air passageways in the lungs, the stomach and intestines, the urinary bladder, the blood vessels, and the reproductive tract. It carries out most of the unconscious, internal movements that the body needs to maintain itself in good working order.

In general the nervous system gives the orders, and the muscular system carries them out. This is certainly true of the skeletal muscles, although things are different for cardiac muscle and smooth muscle. They do not require stimulation from nerves to carry out their basic functions; instead, this kind of activity is "built in" to the cardiac and visceral smooth muscle cells. The nervous system can influence cardiac and visceral smooth muscle cells, but only to adjust and modify their basic activities, not to start them.

Like most parts of the body, the muscular system is associated with some strange and unique terminology. The prefix *myo-* refers to muscle generally, and *sarco-* more specifically refers to muscle cells. For example, *myo* logy is the study of muscles, and *myo* sitis is inflammation of muscle tissue. Down at the cellular level, the cytoplasm of a muscle cell is called the *sarco* plasm. We will use these terms fairly often in this chapter.

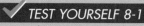

**TEST YOURSELF 8-1**
1. What is muscle?
2. What are the three types of muscle and what are some of the general characteristics of each type?

## SKELETAL MUSCLE

**Skeletal muscle** is the type that usually comes to mind when we hear the word *muscle.* It is called *skeletal muscle* because it moves the bones of the skeleton, which in turn move the animal around. You might also hear it referred to by an old name—**voluntary striated muscle** (called *voluntary* because it is under the control of the conscious mind). However, not every movement an animal makes is a conscious one. That would be very cumbersome because so many movements are going on all the time. Actually, many skeletal muscle movements, such as maintaining balance and an upright posture, are governed by built-in "cruise control" settings that involve sensory structures, the central nervous system, nerve fibers, and muscle fibers. This kind of system allows animals to breathe, swallow, and stand upright without having to think consciously about each part of the process. And yet animals can voluntarily change their breathing, swallowing, or standing position. To illustrate this yourself, try consciously to control your breathing—how often you breathe, how much air you take in with each breath, how long you hold it in, and how much air you exhale. Pretty soon the process of breathing becomes a chore. The antidote is to think about other things and let the cruise control kick back in. By the time you read the next few paragraphs, your breathing cruise control will probably have taken over again.

The **striated** part of skeletal muscle's alias (voluntary striated muscle) comes from its microscopic appearance. Even under low-power magnification, skeletal muscle cells are obviously striped (striated) (see Figure 5-29, *A*). Alternating, crosswise, dark and light bands run the length of each cell. Under higher magnification, the pattern of bands appears more complex than just dark and light bands. We will look into what gives skeletal muscle that appearance when we discuss its microscopic anatomy.

### GROSS ANATOMY OF SKELETAL MUSCLE

By *gross anatomy* we mean those features that can be seen with the unaided eye; that is, without microscopes or magnifying glasses. (Some people think all anatomy is gross, but that's another story.)

A skeletal *muscle* is a well-defined group of muscle *cells* surrounded by a fibrous connective sheath called the **epimysium.** Skeletal muscles come in a variety of shapes and sizes, but they usually have a thick central portion called the *belly* and two or more attachment sites that join them to whatever structures they move when they contract.

### SKELETAL MUSCLE ATTACHMENTS

Most skeletal muscles are attached to bones at both ends by tough, fibrous connective tissue bands called **tendons** that are a continuation of the epimysium. However, as usual, a few oddballs exist. Instead of connecting to bandlike tendons, some muscles are attached to bones or to other muscles by broad sheets of fibrous connective tissue called **aponeuroses.** The most prominent aponeurosis is the **linea alba** *(white line)* (Figure 8-1) that runs lengthwise between the muscles on an animal's ventral midline. It connects the abdominal muscles from each side together and is a common site for surgical entry into the abdomen (see the Clinical Application on abdominal incisions).

One of a skeletal muscle's attachment sites is generally more stable (moves less) than the other. This more stable site is called the **origin of the muscle.** It does not move much when the muscle contracts. The **insertion of the muscle** is the site that undergoes most of the movement when a muscle contracts. For example, the origin of the *gastrocnemius* muscle (the muscle on the back of your calf) is on the femur; its insertion is on the calcaneal tuberosity of the fibular tarsal bone (the point of the hock). When the gastrocnemius muscle contracts, it pulls on the calcaneal tuberosity. In a standing animal contraction of the gastrocnemius muscle flexes the knee and extends the tarsus, which helps propel the animal forward (Figure 8-2).

**TEST YOURSELF 8-2**
1. What is the difference between a *tendon* and an *aponeurosis?*
2. What is the origin of a muscle? The insertion?
3. Why might it be of clinical importance to know the origin and insertion of a muscle?

### SKELETAL MUSCLE ACTIONS

A skeletal muscle does only one thing, but it does it really well. When stimulated by a nerve impulse, a muscle contracts (shortens). By pulling on its attachment sites (its origin and insertion), the contraction of the muscle produces movement of bones and other structures. Skeletal muscles rarely act alone. They usually work in groups, with certain muscles producing most of the desired movement

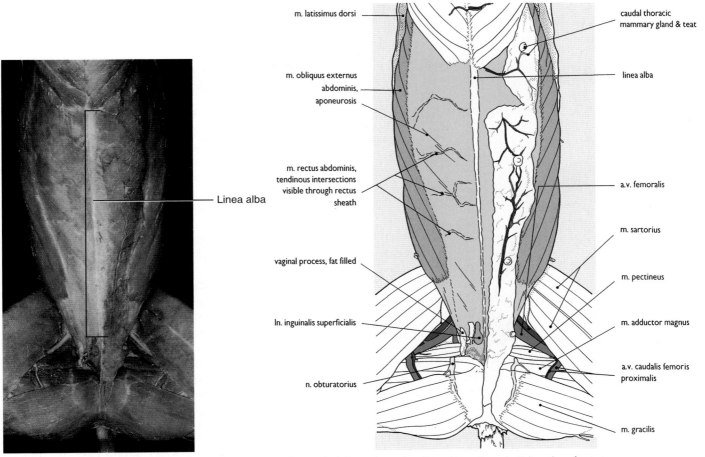

m. latissimus dorsi

caudal thoracic
mammary gland & teat

m. obliquus externus
abdominis,
aponeurosis

linea alba

m. rectus abdominis,
tendinous intersections
visible through rectus
sheath

a.v. femoralis

m. sartorius

vaginal process, fat filled

m. pectineus

ln. inguinalis superficialis

m. adductor magnus

a.v. caudalis femoris
proximalis

n. obturatorius

m. gracilis

Linea alba

**FIGURE 8-1** Linea alba. The aponeurosis of several abdominal muscles. (From Done S et al: Color atlas of veterinary anatomy, vol 3, St Louis, 2009, Elsevier Ltd.)

and others stabilizing nearby joints and providing smooth control over body movements. The term **agonist** (or **prime mover**) is used to describe a muscle or muscle group that directly produces a desired movement.

An **antagonist** is a muscle or muscle group that directly opposes the action of an agonist. Through partial contractions, antagonists can help smooth out the movements of agonists, or they can contract forcefully at the same time as the agonist, resulting in rigidity and lack of motion. For example, the *biceps brachii* muscle that flexes (bends) the elbow and the *triceps brachii* muscle that extends (straightens) the elbow can each act as an agonist or antagonist, depending on the movement desired.

A **synergist** is a skeletal muscle that contracts at the same time as an agonist and assists it in carrying out its action. For example, the *deep digital flexor* muscle flexes the digits of the front limb and at the same time the *superficial digital flexor* muscle acts as a synergist to aid the motion. **Fixator** muscles stabilize joints to allow other movements to take place. For example, some of the muscles that flex the digits also can flex the carpus, or wrist. If a muscle that extends the carpus contracts at the same time as a digital flexor muscle, it fixes the carpus in place (prevents it from moving) while the digits are pulled into a flexed position. You can demonstrate this by

starting with the fingers of one of your hands extended and then tightly squeezing them into a fist while feeling your forearm muscles with your other hand. You will be able to feel the muscles on the underside of your forearm contracting to flex your fingers, but you will also feel muscles on the top of your forearm contracting to stabilize your wrist (carpus).

Movements of the body are complex, so each skeletal muscle may fulfill all four of these roles at one time or another. For one type of movement a muscle may act as the agonist, but for others it may act as an antagonist, a synergist, or a fixator.

## MUSCLE-NAMING CONVENTIONS

Among the biggest causes of misery for students of anatomy are the odd and seemingly random names given to muscles. Surely anatomists must be sadistic ogres who delight in thinking up the most obscure and complicated names possible for body structures, especially muscles? Actually, there is logic behind the names given to most muscles. They are often named for physical characteristics, such as the following:

- Action: A portion of a muscle's name is often related to its function. Muscles that flex a joint are often called *flexor muscles*. For example, the action of the *superficial digital*

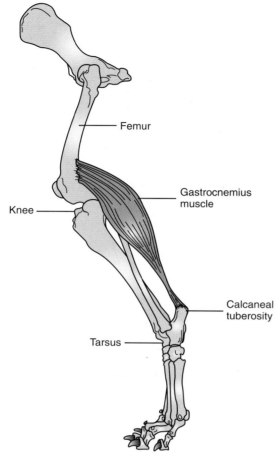

**FIGURE 8-2** The gastrocnemius muscle. When the muscle contracts it pulls on the calcaneal tuberosity, causing the knee joint to flex and the tarsal joint to extend. (From Cunningham JG: Texbook of veterinary physiology, ed 4, St Louis, 2007, Elsevier.)

*flexor* muscle is fairly apparent from its name. It flexes the digits when it contracts. Extensor muscles do the opposite in that they extend joints.

- Shape: A muscle's name can reflect its distinctive shape, such as with the *deltoid* muscle. "Deltoid" means triangular. The *deltoid* muscle is a triangular muscle that is located in the shoulder region.
- Location: A muscle's name can indicate its physical location in the body. For example, the *biceps brachii* muscle is located in the brachial (upper "arm") region.
- Direction of fibers: The term "rectus" means straight. The *rectus abdominis* muscles are two straplike muscles on either side of the linea alba on the ventral abdomen. (When someone who lifts weights is referred to as having "six-pack abs," the *rectus abdominis* muscles are being noticed.) The fibers of the rectus muscles run straight lengthwise with the long axis of the body and parallel to each other.
- Number of heads or divisions: The number of heads refers to the number of attachment sites that a muscle has to its origin. From the term "cephal," meaning head, comes the combining form -cep. We can then deduce that the *biceps brachii* muscle has two heads, the *triceps brachii*

muscle has three heads, and the *quadriceps femoris* muscle has four heads.
- Attachment sites: Origin and insertion sites are used to name some muscles. For example, the origin of the *sternocephalicus* muscle is the sternum, and its insertion is (the back of) the head.

## SELECTED SKELETAL MUSCLES

Animals have several hundred muscles in their bodies. Complete descriptions of each of them can be found in larger anatomy textbooks. Rather than attempting to catalog all the muscles in the common domestic animal species, we will discuss only muscles that are of clinical importance or those that can be used as reference points or landmarks on an animal's body. Figure 8-3 shows the locations of many of the superficial muscles in the horse. The general arrangement of muscles in other species is similar.

**CUTANEOUS MUSCLES.** Have you ever watched an animal twitch its skin to get rid of an annoying insect? If so, you have seen that animal contracting one of its **cutaneous (skin) muscles**. Actually, the muscles are not in the skin itself but are in the connective tissue *(fascia)* just beneath it. Unlike most skeletal muscles, the cutaneous muscles have little or no attachment to bones. They are thin, broad, and superficial and serve only to twitch the skin. (It's a pity we humans lack cutaneous muscles. They could save us a lot of swatting during mosquito season.)

**HEAD AND NECK SKELETAL MUSCLES.** The muscles of the head have many roles. They control facial expression, enable chewing *(mastication)*, and move sensory structures such as the eyes and ears. The muscles of the neck help support the head and allow the neck to flex, extend, and move the head laterally. The large *masseter* muscle in the cheek area of the skull is the most powerful of the chewing muscles. Its main action is to close the jaw. Two of the main muscles that extend (raise) the head and neck are the *splenius* and *trapezius* muscles, which are located on the dorsal (upper) part of the neck. Another muscle that extends the head and neck and also pulls the front leg forward is the *brachiocephalicus* muscle. It is a fairly large, straplike muscle that runs from the proximal area of the humerus (brachio-) up to the base of the skull (cephalicus). Neck flexor muscles are located on the ventral (lower) portion of the neck. The *sternocephalicus* muscle is a smaller, straplike muscle that extends from the sternum to the base of the skull and acts to flex (lower) the head and neck. Flexors of the head and neck do not have to be particularly large or strong because gravity helps them lower the head and neck.

**ABDOMINAL SKELETAL MUSCLES.** The most obvious function of the abdominal muscles is to support the abdominal organs. However, that's not all they do. They also help flex (arch) the back and participate in various functions that involve straining, such as expulsion of feces from the

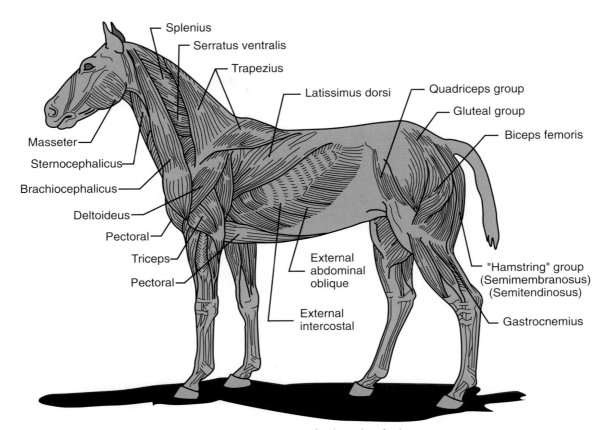

**FIGURE 8-3** Major superficial muscles of a horse.

rectum *(defecation),* urine from the bladder *(urination),* a fetus from the uterus *(parturition),* and the processes of vomiting and regurgitation. Abdominal muscles also play a role in respiration. We discuss their respiratory role more in the section on respiratory muscles.

The abdominal muscles are arranged in layers. From outside in, they are the *external abdominal oblique* muscle, the *internal abdominal oblique* muscle, the *rectus abdominis* muscle, and the *transversus abdominis* muscle. The left and right parts of each muscle come together on the ventral midline at the linea alba (the aponeurosis that extends from the xiphoid process [caudal end] of the sternum to the cranial brim of the pubis).

The oblique muscles are given that name because their fibers run in an oblique (slanting) direction to the long axis of the body and opposite to each other. The fibers of the *external abdominal oblique* muscle run in a caudoventral (backward and downward) direction. The *internal abdominal oblique* muscle fibers run in the opposite direction, which is cranioventral, or forward and downward. The *rectus abdominis* muscle forms the floor (ventral portion) of the muscular abdominal wall. It consists of two straplike muscles on either side of the linea alba that run from the ribs and sternum back to the brim of the pubis. The *transversus abdominis* muscle is the deepest of the abdominal muscles. Its fibers run directly downward in a ventral direction to insert on the linea alba.

**THORACIC LIMB SKELETAL MUSCLES.** The muscles of the thoracic (front) limb function mainly in locomotion, thereby allowing the animal to walk and run and generally move around its environment. The primary muscles we will discuss are the large muscles of the shoulder and brachial (upper "arm") regions, although we do touch on the smaller, but very important, muscles of the lower leg.

The superficial muscles of the shoulder region are the *latissimus dorsi* muscle, the *pectoral* muscles, and the *deltoid* muscle. The *latissimus dorsi* muscle is a broad, triangular muscle that extends from the spinal column down to its insertion on the humerus. It flexes the shoulder, which helps propel the body forward. Usually two *pectoral* muscles, one superficial and one deep, are located on each side of the sternum. They both extend from the sternum to the humerus and act as ***adductor muscles*** *(inward movers)* of the front leg. Adductor muscles help keep the front legs under the animal and prevent them from splaying out to the sides. The *deltoid* muscle is also triangular and extends from the lateral portion of the scapula down to the humerus. It is an ***abductor muscle*** *(outward mover)* and flexes the shoulder joint.

As mentioned earlier, the names of the *biceps brachii* muscle and *triceps brachii* muscles reveal their general location and basic physical appearance. Both are muscles of the **brachium**, or upper "arm" region, and they have opposite actions on the elbow joint. The *biceps brachii* muscle has two proximal head attachments and extends from the distal end of the scapula to the proximal end of the radius. When it contracts, it flexes the elbow joint. The *triceps brachii* muscle has three proximal head attachments and extends from the distal scapula and proximal humerus down to the olecranon process of the ulna (the point of the elbow). When it contracts, it extends the elbow joint.

The muscles distal to the elbow joint are an important collection of carpal and digital flexors and extensors that play important roles in locomotion. Their names often reveal their actions and something about their location. They have names like *extensor carpi radialis* (extends the carpus and is located over the radius), and *deep digital flexor* (flexes the digit and is located beneath some of the other digital flexor muscles). Despite the general similarities in these muscles among species, their precise locations, names, and actions vary greatly. Consult more in-depth anatomic references if you need more information about these muscles.

**PELVIC LIMB SKELETAL MUSCLES.** Like the thoracic limb muscles, the pelvic limb muscles are involved mainly in locomotion. The large *gluteal* muscles and the *hamstring* muscle group are extensor muscles of the hip joint. These powerful muscles help propel the body forward by extending the hip joint (pulling the leg backward). The gluteal muscles extend from the bones of the pelvis down to the trochanters of the femur. The hamstring muscle group is three muscles

located on the caudal part of the thigh region: the *biceps femoris* muscle, the *semimembranosus* muscle, and the *semitendinosus* muscle. They not only help extend the hip joint but also are the main flexors of the stifle joint.

The *quadriceps femoris* muscle is the main extensor muscle of the stifle joint. It is located in the cranial part of the thigh region. When an animal has taken a stride with its hind leg, the quadriceps femoris muscle helps bring the leg forward to prepare for the next stride. As its name implies, it is composed of four heads.

The flexors and extensors of the tarsus and digits are similar to the flexors and extensors of the carpus and digits of the front legs. One important landmark muscle in some species is the *gastrocnemius* muscle, which is the equivalent of our main calf muscle. It extends from the caudal portion of the distal end of the femur and inserts on the calcaneal tuberosity of the fibular tarsal bone (the point of the hock). The distal gastrocnemius tendon in humans attaches to our heel and is called the *Achilles tendon*. The *gastrocnemius* muscle is a powerful extensor muscle of the hock. It also helps propel the body forward as an animal takes a stride.

**SKELETAL MUSCLES OF RESPIRATION.** The muscles of respiration increase and decrease the size of the thoracic cavity to draw air into, and push air out of, the lungs. Because drawing air into the lungs is called *inspiration*, the

 **CLINICAL APPLICATION**

### Abdominal Incisions

Abdominal surgery is commonly performed on veterinary patients. From rumenotomies in cattle to ovariohysterectomies (*spays*) in dogs, abdominal surgical procedures have one thing in common—the surgeon must make an incision somewhere in the abdominal muscles to expose the contents of the abdomen. The location of the incision is usually carefully selected to offer maximum exposure of the required organ or structure. It will also allow a secure closure when the surgical procedure is over and the incision is sutured shut.

The positions and arrangements of the abdominal muscles and the direction in which their fibers run are important considerations when choosing the site for an abdominal incision. The most common abdominal incision site is the *ventral midline,* where the linea alba is located. It offers several advantages over other sites, such as excellent exposure of abdominal organs, easy closure, and few sensory nerves. Nearly all abdominal organs and tissues can be reached through a ventral midline incision. Also, because all of the abdominal muscles come together at the linea alba, an incision through it opens the abdomen in one cut. When it is time to close the abdomen, one layer of sutures (stitches) in the linea alba can effectively and securely close the abdominal cavity. The linea alba contains fewer sensory nerves than the adjacent muscles, therefore less postoperative pain is involved with a ventral midline incision than with other abdominal incision sites. The only real disadvantage of a ventral midline incision is that the weight of all the abdominal contents presses on it during the healing process, so it must be closed with very secure sutures.

At times, however, a ventral midline incision is not practical, such as when a cesarean section must be performed on a cow. The complicated digestive system of a ruminant animal like a cow can make it dangerous to position the animal on its back for a surgical procedure. Therefore abdominal surgery in cattle is often done with the animal standing and wide awake. Local anesthetic blocks are used to numb the flank (side) area. The incision is usually made in an up-and-down (dorsal–ventral) direction in the flank area. This means that three layers of muscle—the *external abdominal oblique, internal abdominal oblique,* and *transversus abdominis muscles*—must be cut to gain access to the abdominal cavity. To minimize trauma and allow normal function after surgery, many surgeons suture each muscle layer individually according to the direction that its fibers run. Optimal closure of this type of incision requires a separate layer of sutures for each muscle layer that was incised, which entails a lot more work than suturing closed a ventral midline incision.

Several other common abdominal incisions can be used, such as the paramedian incision (parallel to, but beside, the ventral midline), the paracostal incision (parallel to, and just behind, the last rib), and the transverse incision (crosswise, perpendicular to the linea alba). The abdominal muscles present at each incision site determine how the abdominal cavity should be entered and how it can be sutured most securely. (See, this anatomy stuff is important even after you're done with your anatomy class!)

muscles that increase the size of the thoracic cavity when they contract are called **inspiratory muscles**. Pushing air out of the lungs is called *expiration,* so the muscles that decrease the thoracic cavity size are called **expiratory muscles**.

The main inspiratory muscles are the **diaphragm** and the *external intercostal* muscles. The diaphragm is a thin, dome-shaped sheet of skeletal muscle that separates the thoracic cavity from the abdominal cavity. The convex surface of its dome shape protrudes into the thoracic cavity. The caudal-most lobes of the lungs are in contact with the diaphragm, and the liver is just behind (caudal to) it. When the diaphragm contracts, it flattens out somewhat. This pushes the abdominal organs caudally. It also increases the size of the thoracic cavity, causing air to be drawn into the lungs.

The *external intercostal* muscles have the same general inspiratory effect, but they accomplish it by a different mechanism. The word *intercostal* means *between ribs.* Animals have two sets of intercostal muscles, located between each pair of adjacent ribs. The *external intercostal* muscles are inspiratory muscles, and the deeper, *internal intercostal* muscles are expiratory muscles. The difference is the orientation of their fibers. The fibers of the external intercostal muscles are directed in an oblique direction so that when they contract they rotate the ribs upward and forward. This increases the size of the thoracic cavity and causes air to be drawn into the lungs.

Expiration (pushing air out of the lungs) does not require as much effort as inspiration, because mechanical forces, such as gravity, and the elastic nature of the lungs help collapse the rib cage and push air out. Nonetheless, two sets of expiratory muscles that aid the process are the *internal intercostal* muscles and the *abdominal* muscles. The fibers of the internal intercostal muscles run at right angles to those of the external intercostal muscles. When the internal intercostal muscles contract, they rotate the ribs backward, which decreases the size of the thorax and pushes air out of the lungs. When abdominal muscles contract, they push the abdominal organs against the caudal side of the diaphragm. This pushes the diaphragm back into its full dome shape and decreases the size of the thorax. The contributions of the abdominal muscles to breathing become important mainly when animals are breathing hard and fast, such as when they are exerting themselves physically.

## MICROSCOPIC ANATOMY OF SKELETAL MUSCLE

### SKELETAL MUSCLE CELLS

Skeletal muscle cells are large cells. They are not very wide, but they are quite long. Most body cells are a few micrometers ($\mu$m) in length or diameter (1 $\mu$m = 0.001 millimeter [mm]). Skeletal muscle cells can be several *inches* long. An inch is equal to about 25 mm, or 25,000 $\mu$m, which is

---

 **CLINICAL APPLICATION**

### Intramuscular Injection Sites

Because skeletal muscles have large blood supplies, drugs injected into them are absorbed into the bloodstream and quickly carried off to the rest of the body. This method of drug administration is called an **intramuscular injection (IM injection)**, and it is commonly used, particularly when a rapid drug effect is desired. An intravenous injection (IV injection), into a vein, provides the fastest method of drug distribution. An IM injection is the next fastest.

In theory we should be able to use any skeletal muscle for an intramuscular injection. In practice, however, only a few muscles are suitable in each species. Many muscles are either too small or too thin to allow such an injection; others have prominent structures nearby, such as nerves that could be damaged by the injection. To be useful for an intramuscular injection, a muscle must be fairly large, must be easily accessible, and must have a sufficiently thick "belly" into which we can deposit the drug.

The following are some common intramuscular injection sites used in domestic animals.

**Cats and Dogs**
**Pelvic Limb**
Gluteal muscles
Quadriceps femoris muscle
Gastrocnemius muscle
Hamstring group (biceps femoris, semimembranosus, and semitendinosus muscles)

**Thoracic Limb**
Triceps brachii muscle

**Cattle and Goats**
**Pelvic Limb**
Gluteal muscles
Hamstring group

**Thoracic Limb**
Triceps brachii muscle

**Neck**
Trapezius muscle

**Horses**
**Pelvic Limb**
Gluteal muscles
Hamstring group

**Thoracic Limb**
Triceps brachii muscle

**Neck**
Trapezius muscle

**Chest**
Pectoral muscles

**Swine**
**Pelvic Limb**
Semitendinosus muscle

**Neck**
Brachiocephalicus muscle
Trapezius muscle

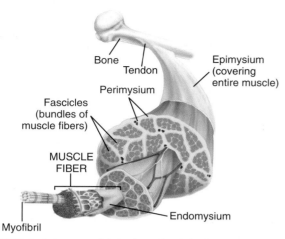

**FIGURE 8-4** Structure of skeletal muscle. Skeletal muscle is composed of bundles of muscle fibers called fascicles. Each bundle is surrounded by the connective tissue perimysium. A single muscle fiber is surrounded by the connective tissue endomysium and is made up of smaller myofibrils. (From Thibodeau G, Patton K: Structure and function of the body, ed 14, St Louis, 2012, Elsevier.)

really large on a cellular scale. Despite being so long, skeletal muscle cells are very thin (up to 80 μm in diameter). This gives them an overall threadlike or fiberlike shape. In fact, skeletal muscle cells are usually called *fibers* rather than *cells* (Figure 8-4).

Aside from their large size, skeletal muscle fibers have some other unique characteristics. Instead of having just one nucleus, like most cells, skeletal muscle fibers have many. Large fibers can have 100 or more nuclei per cell, all located out at the edge of the cell just beneath the **sarcolemma** (muscle cell membrane). This reflects the fiber's development from numerous primitive muscle cells that fused. The interior of a muscle fiber is even more interesting. Most of the volume of one skeletal muscle fiber is made up of hundreds or thousands of smaller **myofibrils** packed together lengthwise, which are themselves composed of thousands of even tinier protein filaments. Prominent organelles between the myofibrils in a muscle fiber include many energy-producing mitochondria, an extensive network of **sarcoplasmic reticulum** (a storage organelle for calcium ions), and a system of tubules called **transverse tubules**, or **T-tubules**, that extend in from the sarcolemma (cell membrane) (Figure 8-5). We will look at the important roles that these organelles play in muscle cells when we discuss how they contract.

As mentioned above, one myofibril is made up of a series of protein filaments. These filaments form the contractile units of a myofibril. Each one of these contractile units is called a **sarcomere** and is the basic contracting unit of skeletal muscle. There are many sarcomeres laid end to end in one myofibril. Each sarcomere has a disc on each end called the **Z line** or **Z disc.** Sarcomeres share discs, so there is one common disc between adjacent sarcomeres. Within a sarcomere there are two primary protein filaments that are responsible for contraction. There are thin protein filaments called **actin** that attach to the Z lines and extend toward the

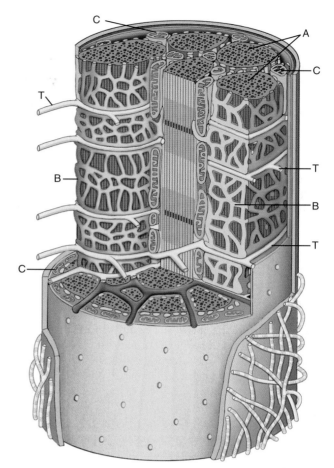

**FIGURE 8-5** A three-dimensional view of the internal structure of a muscle fiber. **A,** Myofibril. **B,** Sarcoplasmic reticulum. **C,** Mitochondria. **T,** Transverse tubules (T-tubules).

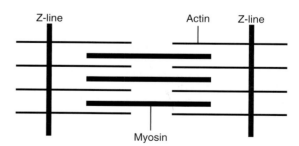

**FIGURE 8-6** A sarcomere. (From Cunningham JG: Textbook of veterinary physiology, ed 4, St Louis, 2007, Elsevier.)

center of the sarcomere, but don't meet. There are also thick protein filaments called **myosin** that appear to float in the middle of the sarcomere between parallel actin fibers. They don't connect to the Z lines (Figure 8-6).

Looking at a myofibril at a higher magnification we can see large light-colored bands (Figure 8-7). These are called **I bands** and are made up of the thin actin filaments. Each I band extends from one end of the thick myosin filaments in one sarcomere across the Z line to the beginning of the myosin fibers in the next sarcomere. In the center of the I band is the dark Z disc or line that is the attachment site for the actin filaments. From one Z line to the next Z line is one sarcomere. Between the light I bands are darker bands called **A bands**. They are areas where the thick myosin filaments and thin actin filaments overlap. The **H band** is the light-colored area located in the middle of the A band. It is made up of myosin filaments only, with no overlapping actin filaments, so the H band doesn't cover the entire width of the myosin filament.

Looking at one sarcomere you can see that the myosin filaments don't extend all the way from one Z line to the next. There is part of an I band between the end of the A band and the Z line. The I band crosses the Z line and continues until it comes to the beginning of the next myosin filament, where the A band begins again.

The actin fibers are actually two strands of protein twisted together to form a helical structure similar in appearance to a DNA molecule. The myosin molecule has a twisted tail attached to two globular heads that form **cross-bridges** to actin and interact with the actin to shorten the sarcomere during muscle contraction (Figure 8-8).

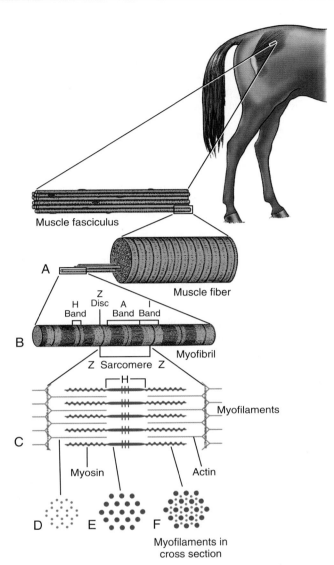

**FIGURE 8-7** Ultrastructure of a sarcomere. **A,** One muscle fiber with an extended myofibril. **B,** One myofibril composed of four sarcomeres (each one runs from Z line to Z line). **C,** One sarcomere composed of actin (thin) filaments and myosin (thick) filaments. **D,** A cross section of the I band (actin filaments only). **E,** A cross section of the H band (myosin filaments only). **F,** A cross section of the A band (actin and myosin filaments). (From Hodgson D, McGowan C, McKeever K: The athletic horse: principles and practice of equine sports medicine, ed 2, St Louis, 2014, Saunders. Adapted with permission from Gloom W, Fawcett DW: A textbook of histology, Philadelphia, 1986, Saunders.)

---

✓ **TEST YOURSELF 8-3**

1. Describe a skeletal muscle cell in terms of cell size, shape, number of nuclei, and appearance under the microscope.
2. What are the differences among a skeletal muscle fiber, a skeletal muscle myofibril, and a skeletal muscle protein filament?
3. Which contractile protein filaments make up the dark bands of skeletal muscle cells? Which make up the light bands?
4. What is a sarcomere and what are its components?

## NEUROMUSCULAR JUNCTION

Skeletal muscle is under conscious, voluntary control. Unless it receives nerve impulses, it does not do anything. If a skeletal muscle's nerve supply is interrupted for a lengthy period as a result of injury, the muscle will not only lack the ability to function, it will shrink down through a process called *atrophy.*

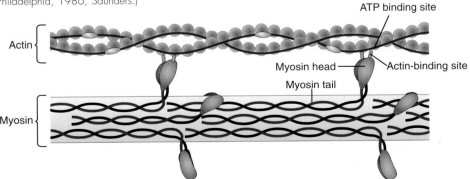

**FIGURE 8-8** Actin and myosin. Note the cross-bridges formed between the heads on the myosin tails and the actin filament.

Sites where the ends of motor nerve fibers connect to muscle fibers are called **neuromuscular junctions**. However, the word *connect* is not accurate, because a very small space—called the *synaptic space*—exists between the end of the nerve fiber and the sarcolemma (cell membrane) of the muscle fiber (Figure 8-9 *A*). Within the end of a nerve fiber in a neuromuscular junction are tiny sacs called *synaptic vesicles* that contain the chemical neurotransmitter *acetylcholine*. When a nerve impulse comes down the motor nerve fiber, it causes the release of acetylcholine, which quickly diffuses across the synaptic space and binds (attaches) to receptors on the sarcolemma. This starts the process that leads to the contraction of the muscle fiber. (We explore this process more fully in the section on skeletal muscle physiology.) The effect of acetylcholine on its receptor is very short. The enzyme acetylcholinesterase found in the synaptic space quickly removes the acetylcholine molecule from its sarcolemma receptor and splits it apart. This ends the effect of that nerve impulse. If the body needs to contract the muscle fiber again, it must send down another nerve impulse.

Each nerve fiber *innervates* (sends impulses to) more than one muscle fiber. The number of muscle fibers per nerve fiber determines how small a movement will result from a nerve stimulus. The term **motor unit** is used to describe one nerve fiber and all the muscle fibers it innervates (Figure 8-9 *B*). Muscles that must make very small, delicate movements, such as the muscles that position the eyes, have only a few muscle fibers per nerve fiber in each motor unit. On the other hand, large, powerful muscles, such as leg muscles, may have a hundred or more muscle fibers per motor unit. This allows the nervous system to control the activities of the skeletal muscles in an economical manner. If each nerve fiber attached to only one skeletal muscle fiber, immense numbers of nerve impulses would be constantly necessary to control the muscles' activities. That would require so much work that the nervous system would not be able to do anything else.

### CONNECTIVE TISSUE LAYERS

Because they exert a lot of force when they contract, skeletal muscle fibers must be securely fastened together and securely fastened to the structures (usually bones) they move. A delicate connective tissue layer called the **endomysium** surrounds each individual skeletal muscle *fiber*. It is composed of fine, reticular fibers. Groups of skeletal muscle fibers, called **fascicles**, are bound together by a tougher connective tissue layer, called the **perimysium**, which is composed of reticular fibers and thick collagen fibers. Groups of muscle fascicles are surrounded by **epimysium**, a fibrous connective tissue layer composed largely of tough collagen fibers. The epimysium is the outer covering of the entire muscle (see Figure 8-4). These three connective tissue layers are continuous with the tendons or aponeuroses that connect the muscle to bones or other muscles. So they not only hold the components of the muscle together but also help fasten the muscle firmly to its attachment mechanisms.

Aside from holding the muscle firmly together and attaching it to the appropriate structures, the connective tissue layers of a muscle also contain the blood vessels and nerve fibers that supply the muscle fibers. They commonly contain varying amounts of adipose tissue, or fat. The fat deposits are often grossly visible in meat and are called ***marbling***.

## PHYSIOLOGY OF SKELETAL MUSCLE
### INITIATION OF MUSCLE CONTRACTION AND RELAXATION

When a nerve impulse travels down a motor nerve fiber and reaches the end bulb at the neuromuscular junction, acetylcholine is released into the synaptic space. The acetylcholine molecules bind to receptors on the surface of the sarcolemma (cell membrane) of the muscle fiber, which starts an impulse that travels along the sarcolemma and through the T-tubules to the interior of the cell. When the impulse reaches the sarcoplasmic reticulum, it causes the release of stored calcium ions ($Ca^{2+}$) into the **sarcoplasm** *(cytoplasm)*. As the $Ca^{2+}$ diffuses into the myofibrils, it turns on the contraction process, which is powered by high-energy molecules of **adenosine triphosphate (ATP)**. ATP's function of providing cells with energy was discussed with cell metabolism in Chapter 2. We will discuss its role in muscle contraction later, in the section on the chemistry of muscle contraction.

Almost as soon as the sarcoplasmic reticulum releases its $Ca^{2+}$ into the sarcoplasm, it begins pumping it back in again. This pulls the $Ca^{2+}$ out of the myofibrils, and the contraction process shuts down. The elasticity of the muscle fiber then restores it to its original length, relaxing the fiber. Pumping the $Ca^{2+}$ back into the sarcoplasmic reticulum requires energy, which is also supplied by ATP molecules. So not only does muscle *contraction* require energy, but muscle *relaxation* does too.

The amount of calcium in the muscle fiber is determined largely by the level of calcium in the bloodstream. If the blood calcium level is too high or too low, abnormalities in skeletal muscle function can result. (See Chapter 11 for a discussion of the hormones calcitonin and parathyroid hormone, which control the blood calcium level, as well as the Clinical Application on hypocalcemia.)

### MECHANICS OF MUSCLE CONTRACTION

When a muscle fiber is in a relaxed state, the actin and myosin filaments overlap only a little. When the fiber is stimulated to contract, the globular heads attached to the tails of the myosin filaments, called cross-bridges, which are in contact with the actin filaments, ratchet back and forth and pull the actin filaments on both sides toward the center of the myosin filaments. This sliding of the filaments over each other shortens the sarcomere. The combined shortening of all the end-to-end sarcomeres in a muscle fiber results in what we call a *muscle contraction*. Microscopically the H band becomes narrower as the actin filaments are pulled toward the center of the sarcomere and the band of overlapping of actin and myosin filaments (the A band) becomes wider.

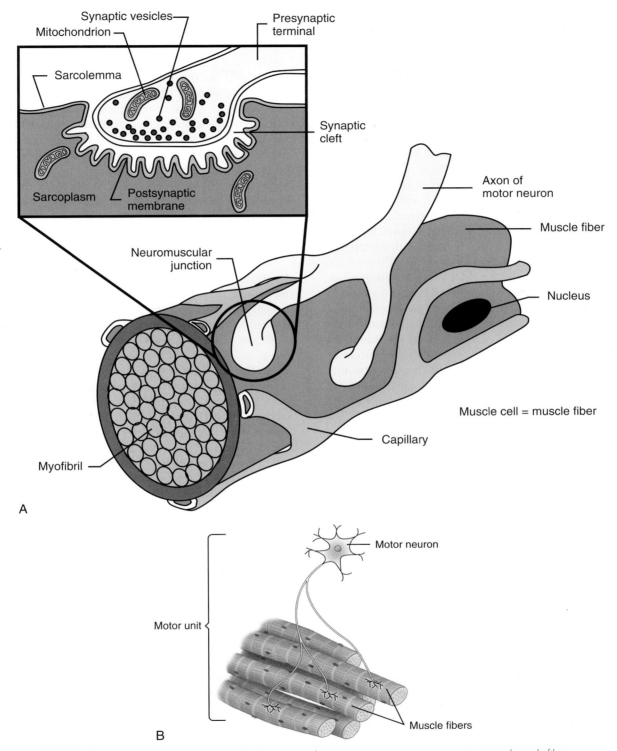

**FIGURE 8-9** A, A neuromuscular junction. B, A motor unit showing one motor neuron innervating several muscle fibers.

## CHARACTERISTICS OF MUSCLE CONTRACTION

An individual muscle fiber either contracts completely when it receives a nerve impulse, or it does not contract at all. This is known as the **all-or-nothing principle**. We know this is not true of whole muscles, so how does the body produce movements that vary in range and strength when individual muscle fibers are doing all or nothing? It does so by carefully controlling the *number* of muscle fibers it stimulates for a particular movement. Small, fine movements require only a few muscle fibers to contract. Larger, more powerful movements require the contraction of many muscle fibers. The nervous system is calling the shots; therefore, it must predict how large and powerful a movement needs to be, and then it must send the appropriate nerve impulses down to the appropriate muscle fibers in the appropriate muscle(s). This results in what we refer to as the "muscle memory" necessary to perform learned repetitive activities skillfully, such as knitting, shooting a basketball, or walking.

Getting down to the basics of muscle contraction, a single muscle fiber contraction (called a **twitch contraction**) can be divided into three phases: (1) the *latent phase,* (2) the *contracting phase,* and (3) the *relaxation phase.* The latent phase is the brief hesitation between the nerve stimulus and the beginning of the actual contraction. It lasts about 0.01 second (10 milliseconds [ms]). The contracting phase lasts about 0.04 second (40 ms), and the relaxation phase lasts about 0.05 second (50 ms). The entire contraction cycle takes about 0.1 second (100 ms). So maximum contraction efficiency occurs if nerve impulses arrive about 0.1 second apart. This results in a series of complete muscle fiber twitches.

Whole muscles rarely contract by twitching, so how do they contract smoothly? They do so mainly by careful timing of the nerve impulses to the various motor units of the muscle. Twitches of individual muscle fibers are stimulated out of phase with each other; that is, they each occur at slightly different times. Some muscle fibers are contracting while others are relaxing. When all the muscle fiber activity is averaged out, smooth, sustained muscle contractions result. Pretty tricky, eh?

## CHEMISTRY OF MUSCLE CONTRACTION

The considerable mechanical work of muscle contraction must be powered by a plentiful supply of energy. The immediate energy source that powers the sliding of the actin and myosin filaments is adenosine triphosphate (ATP), which is produced by the many mitochondria in muscle fibers. ATP molecules are like tiny batteries that can release energy and then be recharged so that they can do it again. As their name implies, ATP molecules have three phosphate groups attached to a central adenosine core. When one of the phosphate groups is split off (forming **adenosine diphosphate [ADP]**), a considerable amount of energy is released, which powers the sliding of the actin and myosin filaments. This also "discharges" the ATP molecule. Another energy source has to reattach the phosphate group to "recharge" the ATP to get it ready to supply energy again.

The "battery charger" that converts ADP back to ATP is another compound in the muscle fiber called **creatine phosphate (CP)**. When the CP molecule splits, the energy that is released adds a phosphate group to the ADP, converting it back to ATP. The newly recharged ATP molecule is ready to provide energy for further muscle contraction or relaxation (by helping to pump $Ca^{2+}$ back into the sarcoplasmic reticulum).

The ultimate source of energy used to produce ATP and CP and keep the whole system operating comes from the *catabolism* (breakdown) of nutrient molecules. The two main compounds involved are *glucose* and *oxygen.* Glucose is a sugar molecule that is the primary energy source for most body cells, including the muscle cells. The muscles have a very large blood supply that constantly brings new supplies of glucose and oxygen to the muscle fibers.

When the supplies are plentiful and the cells are fairly inactive, muscle fibers can also store glucose and oxygen for future needs. Glucose is stored in the fibers in the form of glycogen, and oxygen is stored attached to large protein molecules called **myoglobin**. Like hemoglobin, myoglobin is red and can store and release large quantities of oxygen. When strenuous muscle contractions begin to deplete the oxygen supply to a muscle fiber, myoglobin can release its stash of oxygen molecules to resupply the fiber. As long as the oxygen supply is adequate to keep up with the energy needs of the fiber, the process is known as **aerobic** *(oxygen-consuming)* **metabolism**, and the maximum amount of energy is extracted from each glucose molecule.

Sometimes, particularly during periods of strenuous activity, the need for oxygen exceeds the available supply, and muscle fibers must shift to what is called **anaerobic** *(non–oxygen-dependent)* **metabolism** to produce the energy required for continued activity. Anaerobic metabolism is not as efficient as aerobic metabolism and results in **lactic acid** formation as a by-product of incomplete glucose breakdown. The lactic acid can accumulate in the muscle tissue and cause discomfort. (Have your muscles have ever felt sore after physical activities that were more strenuous than you were used to? That was lactic acid making its presence known.) After the burst of activity is over, some of the lactic acid diffuses into the bloodstream and goes to the liver, where it is converted back to glucose by a process that requires oxygen. So, after a strenuous burst of exercise, an animal may continue to breathe heavily for a while as its body repays its so-called "oxygen debt."

---

### ✓ TEST YOURSELF 8-4

1. What ion, released from the sarcoplasmic reticulum by a nerve impulse, starts the contraction process in a muscle fiber?
2. What molecules in muscle act as the "batteries" to power the sliding of the actin and myosin filaments? What molecules function as the "battery chargers"?
3. If individual muscle fiber contractions obey the all-or-nothing principle, how does an animal control the size and strength of its muscular movements?
4. What is myoglobin and why is it important?
5. Why does an animal breathe heavily for a while after heavy exercise?

---

## HEAT PRODUCTION

Like all machines, muscles are less than 100% efficient at converting energy to useful work (or in this case, motion). A considerable amount of the energy produced in muscles is in the form of heat. In fact, muscular activity is one of the major heat-generating mechanisms that the body uses to maintain a constant internal temperature. If heat production exceeds body needs, the excess must be eliminated by

## CLINICAL APPLICATION

### Rigor Mortis

The term used to describe the stiffness of skeletal muscles that occurs shortly after an animal dies is *rigor mortis*, which is Latin for "stiffness of death." It would seem more sensible for the muscles to go limp after death, because all nerve stimulation ceases, but chemical reactions at the cellular level send things in another direction.

When the animal dies, lack of oxygen to the cells causes normal activities and barriers within the cells to break down. One of the things that happens in skeletal muscle cells is that most of the $Ca^{2+}$ spills out of the sarcoplasmic reticulum. This causes contraction of many of the muscle fibers, fueled by the last of the ATP molecules in the sarcoplasm. However, all the ATP is used up in the contraction, and no more is being made; therefore no energy source is available to relax the muscles. The result is that the muscles get stuck in the contracted position. Rigor mortis is not a permanent condition. As soon as the muscle fibers begin to decompose, the cross-bridges between the myosin and actin filaments break down and the muscles go into a relaxed state. When this happens rigor mortis has passed and the body becomes limp.

Forensic experts can use the onset of rigor mortis and the subsequent muscle relaxation to help establish the time of death.

---

mechanisms such as panting or sweating. Under cold conditions, the body may need to increase the production of heat to avoid *hypothermia* (too low a body temperature). It often does this by producing the small, spasmodic muscle contractions we know as *shivering*.

## CARDIAC MUSCLE

Cardiac muscle is also known as **involuntary striated muscle**. It is called *involuntary* because its contractions are not under conscious control. The *striated* part of the name is given because under the microscope its cells have the same kind of striped appearance as skeletal muscle cells.

## GROSS ANATOMY OF CARDIAC MUSCLE

Cardiac muscle is found in only one place in the body—the heart. It forms most of the volume of the heart and makes up the majority of the walls of the cardiac chambers (the atria and the ventricles). Instead of being organized into distinct muscular structures, like skeletal muscle, cardiac muscle cells form elaborate networks around the cardiac chambers. The arrangement and physical characteristics of cardiac muscle allow it to start contracting early in the embryonic period before birth and to continue contracting without a rest until the animal dies. To get a feel for how amazing that is, make a fist and, for the next minute or two, clench it tightly and then relax it about once per second. Before too long, the forearm muscles that tighten your fist will become fatigued. The heart does this same kind of work, but it gets no rest periods.

## MICROSCOPIC ANATOMY OF CARDIAC MUSCLE

Cardiac muscle cells are striated (striped) like skeletal muscle cells, and they contain many of the same organelles and intracellular structures, such as myofibrils. However, cardiac muscle cells and skeletal muscle cells are otherwise very different. Cardiac muscle cells are *much* smaller than skeletal muscle cells and have only one nucleus per cell. They are not shaped like the long, thin fibers of skeletal muscle. They are longer than they are wide and often have multiple branches. They are securely attached to each other end to end to form intricate, branching networks of cells. The firm, end-to-end attachments between cardiac muscle cells are visible under the microscope as dark, transverse lines between the cells (see Figure 5-29, *B*). These attachment sites are called **intercalated discs**. The intercalated discs securely fasten the cells together and also transmit impulses from cell to cell to allow large groups of cardiac muscle cells to contract in a coordinated manner. In fact, the networks of cardiac muscle cells around the cardiac chambers function as if they were each a large, single unit instead of a whole bunch of individual cells.

## PHYSIOLOGY OF CARDIAC MUSCLE

### MUSCLE CONTRACTIONS

If we looked through a microscope at individual cardiac muscle cells growing in a tissue culture flask, we would see something amazing. Each cell would be contracting rhythmically with no external stimulation at all. Furthermore, each cell would be contracting at a constant rate set by its own internal metronome—some rapidly and others more slowly. However, if two cells touch, the slower contracting cell adopts the faster cell's contraction rate. This demonstrates two unique and important things about cardiac muscle: (1) it contracts without any external stimulation, and (2) groups of cardiac muscle cells adopt the contraction rate of the most rapid cell in the group.

These self-starting and self-controlling aspects of cardiac muscle enable the heart to function as a very efficient pump. Rather than large numbers of muscle cells contracting at the same time, as in skeletal muscle, cardiac muscle cells contract in a rapid, wavelike fashion. The impulse that coordinates the contractions spreads from cell to cell across the intercalated discs like a wave. These rapid, wavelike contractions effectively squeeze blood out of the cardiac chambers, much like milk being squeezed out of a dairy cow's teat at milking time.

For these wavelike contractions of cardiac muscle to move blood effectively through the chambers and valves of the heart and out into the rest of the body, they must be carefully initiated and controlled. This is the role of the heart's internal impulse conduction system, which functions like a "mini nervous system." This impulse conduction system consists entirely of cardiac muscle cells. The impulse that starts each heartbeat begins in the heart's "pacemaker," the **sinoatrial (SA) node**, located in the wall of the right atrium (see Figure 14-17).

Why does the SA node have so much control over things? The reason goes back to that business about cardiac muscle cells adopting the contraction rate of the most rapidly contracting cells in the group. The contraction rate of the cardiac muscle cells in the SA node is faster than those in the walls of the atria or ventricles, therefore its rate takes precedence. The impulse that starts in the SA node follows a carefully controlled path through the conduction system of the heart. Structures in the system transmit, delay, and redirect each impulse so that the cardiac muscle cells in the walls of the heart chambers contract in the coordinated, effective manner necessary to pump blood around the body. Details of the cardiac impulse conduction system can be found in Chapter 14.

### NERVE SUPPLY

Although it is not needed to *initiate* the contractions of cardiac muscle, the heart does have a nerve supply that can *modify* its activity. We know from successful heart transplants that the heart's nerve supply is not essential to its function. (The nerves to the heart are severed when it is removed from the donor.) So what role does the heart's nerve supply play in controlling the heartbeat?

The nerves to the heart are from both divisions of the autonomic portion of the nervous system; that is, the *sympathetic* and *parasympathetic* systems. Sympathetic fibers stimulate the heart to beat harder and faster as part of the fight-or-flight response that kicks in when an animal feels threatened. Parasympathetic fibers do the opposite in that they inhibit cardiac function, thereby causing the heart to beat more slowly and with less force when the body is relaxed and resting. The two opposing systems strike a balance that keeps the heart's activity appropriate for what is going on inside and outside the animal at any particular time. More information about the autonomic portion of the nervous system and its effect on cardiac function can be found in Chapters 9 and 14.

---

✓ **TEST YOURSELF 8-5**

1. Describe a cardiac muscle cell in terms of size, shape, number of nuclei, and appearance under the microscope.
2. What are intercalated discs and why are they important to the functioning of cardiac muscle?
3. Describe the effect of a cardiac muscle's nerve supply on its functioning.
4. What is the general effect of sympathetic nervous system stimulation on cardiac muscle? What is the effect of parasympathetic nervous system stimulation?

---

## SMOOTH MUSCLE

Smooth muscle is also called **nonstriated involuntary muscle**, or sometimes just **involuntary muscle**. Like cardiac muscle, it is called *involuntary* because its contractions are not under conscious control. The *smooth* part of the name is because its cells do not have the striped appearance under

the microscope that skeletal muscle and cardiac muscle cells have (see see Figure 5-29 *C*). Nonstriated involuntary muscle is really very different from the other two types of muscle.

### GROSS ANATOMY OF SMOOTH MUSCLE

Smooth muscle is found all over the body but not in distinct structures like skeletal muscles and the heart. Rather, it is found in two main forms: (1) as large sheets of cells in the walls of some hollow organs (**visceral smooth muscle**) and (2) as small, discrete groups of cells (**multi-unit smooth muscle**) (Figure 8-10).

### MICROSCOPIC ANATOMY OF SMOOTH MUSCLE

Smooth muscle cells are small and spindle shaped (tapered at the ends) with a single nucleus in the center. They have a smooth, homogeneous appearance under the microscope because their filaments of actin and myosin are not arranged in parallel myofibrils as in skeletal and cardiac muscle. Rather, small, contractile units of actin and myosin filaments crisscross the cell at various angles and are attached at both ends to **dense bodies** that correspond to the Z lines of skeletal muscle (Figure 8-11). When these contractile units shorten, they cause the cell to ball up as it contracts. Because their contractile units are not organized into regular, parallel sarcomeres, individual smooth muscle cells can shorten to a greater extent than skeletal or cardiac muscle cells.

### PHYSIOLOGY OF SMOOTH MUSCLE
### VISCERAL SMOOTH MUSCLE

Visceral smooth muscle is found in the walls of many internal soft organs, which are also known by the general name **viscera**. The muscle cells are linked to form large sheets in the walls of organs such as the stomach, intestine, uterus, and urinary bladder. Fine movements are not possible with visceral smooth muscle; rather, it experiences large, rhythmic waves of contraction. These contractions can be quite strong, as in the peristaltic contractions that move food along the

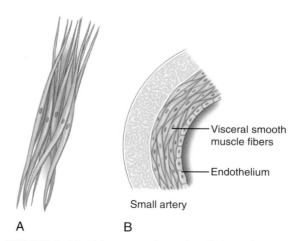

Visceral smooth muscle fibers

Endothelium

Small artery

A          B

**FIGURE 8-10** Multi-unit smooth muscle cells **(A)** and visceral smooth muscle cells **(B)**.

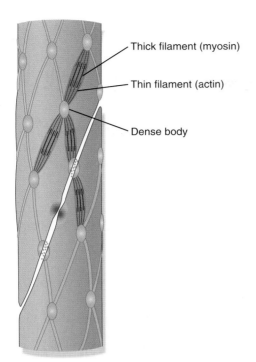

- Thick filament (myosin)
- Thin filament (actin)
- Dense body

**FIGURE 8-11** Smooth muscle cells. (From Koeppen B, Stanton B: Berne & Levy physiology [updated], ed 6, St Louis, 2010, Mosby.)

gastrointestinal tract and the uterine contractions that push the newborn animal out into the world at parturition (birth).

Like cardiac muscle, visceral smooth muscle contracts without the need for external stimulation. It does react to stretching, however, by contracting more strongly. This is useful in the gastrointestinal tract, where the presence of food in the lumen stretches the organ and the smooth muscle in its wall responds with increased contractions that help move the food along. Something similar happens in the urinary bladder; however, the slow, gradual stretching of the bladder wall caused by urine accumulation does not trigger contraction of the smooth muscle in its wall until the bladder is nearly full.

In the pregnant uterus it is very important that the smooth muscle in its wall *does not* contract as the fetus grows and stretches the uterine wall. The would result in a premature loss of the fetus and termination of the pregnancy. The uterus must be kept quiet as the fetus enlarges and develops. This is accomplished through the activity of hormones, such as progesterone, that inhibit the smooth muscle in the uterine wall from contracting during pregnancy. When the time comes to give birth, the level of progesterone in the bloodstream drops dramatically. This removes the inhibition of the uterine smooth muscle, and a combination of factors, including rising levels of other hormones (such as estrogens and oxytocin), stimulates the smooth muscle to contract. This starts the process of labor.

Like cardiac muscle, visceral smooth muscle has a nerve supply that is not necessary to initiate contractions but serves to modify them. Also like cardiac muscle, the nerve supply to smooth muscle consists of the sympathetic and parasympathetic divisions of the autonomic nervous system. However, the effects of the two are the reverse of what is seen in cardiac muscle. Sympathetic stimulation *decreases* visceral smooth muscle activity, and parasympathetic stimulation *increases* it. This makes sense if we think about sympathetic and parasympathetic functions. Sympathetic stimulation prepares an animal for intense physical activity. Blood is diverted away from the viscera and redirected to the heart, skeletal muscles, and brain to help deal with whatever threat initiated the fight-or-flight response. Decreasing gastrointestinal motility as a part of this response makes sense. Digestion is not a priority at this point. On the other hand, when the animal is relaxed and resting, the parasympathetic system predominates and enhances functions such as gastrointestinal activity to help supply nutrients to the body cells during this "down time." As with the heart, the two opposing autonomic divisions strike a balance to keep smooth muscle activity at an appropriate level for the body's ever-changing needs.

## MULTI-UNIT SMOOTH MUSCLE

Whereas visceral smooth muscle is large and relatively powerful, multi-unit smooth muscle is small and delicate. Instead of being formed into large sheets that function as a single, large unit, multi-unit smooth muscle is made up of individual smooth muscle cells or small groups of cells. It is found where small, delicate contractions are needed, such as the iris and ciliary body of the eye, the walls of small blood vessels, and around small air passageways in the lungs. Also unlike visceral smooth muscle, contractions of multi-unit smooth muscle are not automatic. They require specific impulses from autonomic nerves to contract.

The actions of multi-unit smooth muscle are specific and carefully controlled. This allows fine control of actions, such as adjusting the size of the pupil of the eye or the accommodation (focusing) of the lens. It also allows delicate control of blood flow throughout the body and airflow through the lungs by adjusting the size of blood vessels and air passageways according to the body's needs.

---

✓ **TEST YOURSELF 8-6**

1. Describe a smooth muscle cell in terms of its size, shape, number of nuclei, and appearance under the microscope.
2. What are the main differences between *visceral* smooth muscle and *multi-unit* smooth muscle?
3. Describe the effect of nerve stimulation on the functioning of visceral smooth muscle vs. multi-unit smooth muscle.
4. What is the general effect of sympathetic nervous system stimulation on visceral smooth muscle? What is the effect of parasympathetic nervous system stimulation?
5. What are the main differences in the structures and functions of skeletal muscle, cardiac muscle, and smooth muscle?

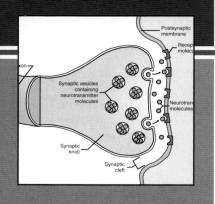

# Nervous System

9

*Thomas Colville*

## OUTLINE

## LEARNING OBJECTIVES

*When you have completed this chapter you will be able to:*

1. Describe the structures and functions of neurons and neuroglia.
2. Differentiate between white matter and gray matter.
3. Describe the functions of afferent and efferent nerves.
4. List the components of the central nervous system and the peripheral nervous system.
5. Differentiate between the autonomic and somatic nervous systems.
6. Describe the process of depolarization and repolarization of neurons.
7. List excitatory and inhibitory neurotransmitters and describe their role in the conduction of nerve impulses.
8. Describe the structures and functions of the cerebrum, cerebellum, diencephalon, and brainstem.
9. Describe the connective tissue layers that surround the brain and spinal cord.
10. Explain the functions of the cerebrospinal fluid.
11. List the cranial nerves and describe their functions.
12. Differentiate between the sympathetic and parasympathetic divisions of the autonomic nervous system.
13. Differentiate between autonomic and somatic reflexes.
14. Describe the components of a reflex arc.
15. Describe the stretch reflex, withdrawal reflex, crossed extensor reflex, palpebral reflex, and pupillary light reflex.

*Acetylcholine* ah-sēt-ehl-**kō**-lēn

*Acetylcholinesterase* ah-sēt-ehl-kō-luh-**nehs**-tuh-rās

*Adrenergic neuron* ahd-reh-**nər**-jihk **nər**-ohn

*Afferent* ā-fər-ehnt

*Afferent nerve* ā-fər-ehnt nərv

*All-or-nothing principle* awl or **nuhth**-ihng **prihn**-suh-puhl

*Alpha₁-adrenergic receptor* **ahl**-fuh wuhn ahd-reh-**nər**-jihk reh-**sehpt**-ər

*Anesthesia* ahn-uhs-**thē**-zhuh

*Antiparasitic drug* ahn-tē-peər-uh-**siht**-ihck druhg

*Arachnoid* ah-**rahck**-noyd

*Autonomic nervous system* aw-tō-**noh**-mihck nərv-uhs **sihs**-tehm

*Autonomic reflex* aw-tō-**noh**-mihck **rē**-flehcks

*Axon* **ahck**-sohn

*Beta₁-adrenergic receptor* **bāt**-ah wuhn ahd-reh-**nər**-jihk reh-**sehpt**-ər

*Beta₂-adrenergic receptor* **bāt**-ah too ahd-reh-**nər**-jihk reh-**sehpt**-ər

*Blood–brain barrier* bluhd brān **beər**-ē-ər

*Brainstem* brān stehm

*Catecholamine* kaht-ih-**kōl**-ih-mēn

*Central canal* **sehn**-trahl kuh-**nahl**

*Central nervous system* **sehn**-trahl nər-vuhs **sihs**-tehm

*Cerebellum* sehr-eh-**behl**-luhm

*Cerebral cortex* seh-**rē**-brahl **kohr**-tehx

*Cerebral hemisphere* seh-**rē**-brahl **hehm**-ih-sfeer

*Cerebrospinal fluid* seh-rē-brō-**spī**-nahl **floo**-ihd

*Cerebrum* seh-**rē**-bruhm

*Cholinergic neuron* kō-luh-**nər**-jihk **nər**-ohn

*Cholinergic receptor* kō-luh-**nər**-jihk reh-**sehpt**-ər

*Conduction of the action potential* kuhn-**duhck**-shuhn *of the* **ahk**-shuhn puh-**tehn**-shuhl

*Contralateral reflex* kohn-trah-**laht**-ər-ahl **rē**-flehcks

*Contrast radiography* **kohn**-trahst rā-dē-**ohg**-rah-fē

*Corpus callosum* **kohr**-pahs kal-**lō**-suhm

*Cranial nerve* **krā**-nē-ahl nərv

*Cranial–sacral system* **krā**-nē-ahl **sā**-krahl **sihs**-tehm

*Crossed extensor reflex* krohst ehck-**stehn**-sohr **rē**-flehcks

*Dendrite* **dehn**-drīt

*Depolarization* dē-pō-lər-uh-**zā**-shuhn

*Diencephalon* dī-ehn-**sehf**-uh-lohn

*Dopamine* **dō**-puh-mēn

*Dorsal horn* **dohr**-sahl hohrn

*Dorsal nerve root* **dohr**-sahl nərv root

*Dura mater* **duhr**-ah **mah**-tər

*Effector cell* ē-**fehck**-tər sehl

*Efferent* ē-**fər**-ehnt

*Efferent nerve* ē-**fər**-ehnt nərv

*Endocrine system* **ehn**-dō-krihn **sihs**-tehm

*Enzyme* **ehn**-zīm

*Epidural anesthesia* ehp-ih-**duhr**-ahl ahn-uhs-**thē**-zhuh

*Epinephrine* ehp-ih-**nehf**-rihn

*Excitatory neurotransmitter* ehcks-sī-tuh-**tōr**-ē nər-ō-**trahnz**-miht-ər

*Fenestration* fehn-ih-**strā**-shuhn

*Fight-or-flight response* fīt *or* flīt reh-**spohns**

*Fissure* **fihsh**-ər

*GABA* **gah**-buh

*Gamma-aminobutyric acid* **gahm**-uh ah-mē-nō-byoo-**tihr**-ihck **ah**-sihd

*Ganglion* **gahng**-glē-uhn

*General anesthesia* **jehn**-ər-ahl ahn-uhs-**thē**-zhuh

*Glial cell* **glē**-ahl sehl

*Glycine* **glī**-sēn

*Gray matter* grā **maht**-ər

*Gyrus (plural gyri)* **jī**-ruhs (*plural* **jī**-rī)

*Hormone* **hohr**-mōn

*Hypermetria* hī-pər-**mē**-trē-uh

*Hyperreflexive* hī-pər-rē-**flehcks**-ihv

*Hyporeflexive* hī-pō-rē-**flehcks**-ihv

*Hypothalamus* hī-pō-**thahl**-uh-muhs

*Inhibitory neurotransmitter* ihn-**hihb**-ih-tohr-ē nər-ō-**trahnz**-miht-ər

*Interneuron* ihn-tər-**nər**-ohn

*Ipsilateral reflex* ihp-sih-**lah**-tər-ahl rē-**flehcks**

*Ivermectin* ī-vər-**mehck**-tihn

*Lobe* lōb

*Local anesthesia* lō-kuhl ahn-uhs-**thē**-zhuh

*Longitudinal fissure* lohn-jih-**tūd**-ihn-ahl **fihsh**-ər

*Medulla oblongata* meh-**duhl**-uh ohb-lohng-**gah**-tah

*Meninges* meh-**nihn**-jēz

*Midbrain* **mihd**-brān

*Mixed nerve* mihckst nərv

*Motor nerve* **mō**-tər nərv

*Motor neuron* **mō**-tər **nər**-ohn

*Muscarinic receptor* muhs-kuh-**rihn**-ihck reh-**sehpt**-ər

*Muscle spindle* **muhs**-uhl **spihn**-duhl

*Myelin* **mī**-eh-lihn

*Myelin sheath* **mī**-eh-lihn shēth

*Myelography* mī-ehl-**ohg**-rahf-ē

*Nerve impulse* nərv **ihm**-puhls

*Nerve* nərv

*Nerve fiber* nərv **fī**-bər

*Neuroglia* nər-**ōg**-lē-ah

*Neuron* **nər**-ohn

*Neurotransmitter* nər-ō-**trahnz**-miht-ər

*Nicotinic receptor* nihck-uh-**tihn**-ihck reh-**sehpt**-ər

*Node of Ranvier* nōd *of* rohn-**vē**-ā

*Norepinephrine* nohr-ehp-ih-**nehf**-rihn

*Nuclei* noo-**klē**-ī

*Oligodendrocyte* ohl-ih-gō-**dehn**-drō-sīt

*Palpebral reflex* pahl-**pē**-brahl **rē**-flehcks

*Parasympathetic nervous system* peər-uh-sihm-puh-**theht**-ihck nər-vuhs **sihs**-tehm

*Perikaryon* peər-ih-**keər**-ē-ohn

*Peripheral nervous system* puh-**rihf**-ər-uhl nər-vuhs **sihs**-tehm

*Pia mater* **pē**-ah **mah**-tər

*Pituitary gland* pih-**too**-ih-teər-ē glahnd

*Pons* pohnz

*Postganglionic neuron* pōst-gahng-glē-**ohn**-ihck **nər**-ohn
*Postsynaptic neuron* pōst-sih-**nahp**-tihck **nər**-ohn
*Preganglionic neuron* prē-gahng-glē-**ohn**-ihck **nər**-ohn
*Presynaptic neuron* prē-sih-**nahp**-tihck **nər**-ohn
*Pupillary light reflex (PLR)* **pyoo**-peh-leər-ē līt rē-flehcks
*Receptor* reh-**sehpt**-ər
*Reflex* rē-flehcks
*Reflex arc* rē-flehcks ahrk
*Refractory period* rē-**frahck**-tər-ē **peer**-ē-uhd
*Repolarization* rē-pō-lər-uh-**zā**-shuhn
*Resting membrane potential* rehs-tihng **mehm**-brān puh-**tehn**-shuhl
*Resting state* rehs-tihng stāt
*Saltatory conduction* **sahl**-tuh-tohr-ē kuhn-**duhck**-shuhn
*Schwann cell* shwahn sehl
*Sensory nerve* **sehn**-sər-ē nərv
*Sensory neuron* **sehn**-sər-ē **nər**-ohn
*Sensory receptor* **sehn**-sər-ē reh-**sehpt**-ər
*Sodium–potassium pump* sō-dē-uhm puh-**tahs**-ē-uhm puhmp
*Soma* **sōm**-uh
*Somatic nervous system* sō-**maht**-ihck **nər**-vuhs **sihs**-tehm
*Somatic reflex* sō-**maht**-ihck rē-flehcks
*Spinal nerve* **spī**-nahl nərv

*Stretch reflex* strehch rē-flehcks
*Sulcus (plural sulci)* **suhlck**-uhs (*plural* **suhlck**-ī)
*Sympathetic ganglion chain* sihm-pah-**theht**-ihck **gahng**-glē-uhn chān
*Sympathetic nervous system* sihm-pah-**theht**-ihck **nər**-vuhs **sihs**-tehm
*Synapse* **sih**-nahps
*Synaptic cleft* sih-**nahp**-tihck klehft
*Synaptic end bulb* sih-**nahp**-tihck ehnd buhlb
*Synaptic knob* sih-**nahp**-tihck nohb
*Synaptic transmission* sih-**nahp**-tihck trahnz-mihsh-uhn
*Target* **tahr**-giht
*Telodendron* tēl-uh-**dehn**-drohn
*Terminal bouton* tər-muh-nuhl boo-**tawn**
*Thalamus* **thahl**-uh-muhs
*Thoracolumbar system* **thohr**-ah-kō-**luhm**-bahr **sihs**-tehm
*Threshold* **threhsh**-ōld
*Threshold stimulus* **threhsh**-ōld **stihm**-ū-luhs
*Ventral horn* **vehn**-trahl hohrn
*Ventral nerve root* **vehn**-trahl nərv root
*Wave of depolarization* wāv *of* dē-pō-lər-uh-**zā**-shuhn
*White matter* whīt **maht**-ər
*Withdrawal reflex* wihth-**draw**-uhl rē-flehcks

# INTRODUCTION

An animal's body is enormously complex, whether we are talking about something small, like a 1-pound chinchilla, or something large, like a 2000-pound camel. In order to maintain homeostasis, and therefore health, all those cells, tissues, organs, and systems have to be able to communicate with each other, and their functions have to be coordinated and controlled. Fortunately the body has two communication and control systems that help keep things working properly: the nervous system and the **endocrine system**. Both use chemicals to carry their messages, but they do it by different means, and on different timescales. The nervous system's chemical messengers are called **neurotransmitters**, and they are produced only by **neurons** (nerve cells). The neurotransmitters travel only very short distances, across spaces between nerve cells called **synapses**. This allows the system to react quickly, but the limited supplies of neurotransmitters in the cells do not allow it to sustain individual activities for long periods of time. The chemical messengers of the endocrine system, on the other hand, called **hormones**, are secreted directly into the bloodstream, where they travel comparatively long distances to reach their **targets**. The hormone targets, therefore, react more slowly to changes, but hormones can be secreted for long periods of time, so they can sustain individual activities for long periods of time. We discuss the endocrine system in Chapter 11. This chapter is about the nervous system.

The nervous system is the rapid response, boss of bosses, communication and control system in the animal body. It monitors what's going on inside and outside the animal, and directs activities to maintain well-being. Understanding how the nervous system is organized and how it functions can help us appreciate what is going on in an animal that is anesthetized, intoxicated with a neurotoxin (poison affecting the nervous system), or unable to move properly because of trauma (hit by a car, intervertebral disc rupture, and so on).

Structurally the nervous system has two main divisions: the *central nervous system (CNS)* and the *peripheral nervous system (PNS)*. The **central nervous system** is composed of the brain and spinal cord, and the **peripheral nervous system** consists of cordlike **nerves** that link the central nervous system with the rest of the body.

Functionally, the nervous system's activities fall into three main categories: (1) *sensory functions*, (2) *integrating functions*, and (3) *motor functions*. The nervous system senses changes from within the body or from outside the body and conveys this information to the spinal cord and brain. In the brain and spinal cord, the sensory information is received, analyzed, stored, and integrated to produce a response. A motor response instructs the body to do something, such as contract a muscle or cause a gland to secrete its product(s).

The branch of science that studies the nervous system is called *neurology; neuro-* refers to the nervous system, and *logos* means *study of.*

## NEURONS AND SUPPORTING CELLS

**Neurons** (nerve cells) are the stars of the nervous system show. They are the basic, functional units of the system. That means they are the smallest pieces of the nervous system that show basic nervous system functions, such as responding to stimuli and conducting impulses from one part of the cell to another.

Like many Hollywood stars, neurons are high maintenance. They have a very high requirement for oxygen; they can't live without it for more than a few minutes. That is why cardiopulmonary resuscitation must be started within a few minutes of cardiac arrest. The heart may start beating again after that, but there could be brain damage if the neurons have been without oxygen for too long.

Shortly after an animal is born, its neurons lose their ability to reproduce, but they can regenerate cell processes if the cell body remains intact. The lack of reproductive ability is why serious nervous system injuries, such as strokes and spinal cord damage, are often so debilitating and have such long-lasting effects. Emerging research suggests that it may be possible to turn neurons' reproductive ability back on. This holds great promise for the future of patients with neurologic deficits.

Also, like Hollywood stars, neurons need a great supporting cast and crew to be successful. The **neuroglia**, or **glial cells** (from the Greek *glia,* meaning *glue*), structurally and functionally support and protect the neurons. They outnumber neurons about 10 to 1, but they are not directly involved in the transmission of information or impulses through the nervous system. Rather they are important parts of the infrastructure necessary for the neurons to do their jobs. The neurons are the stars of the nervous system show, and the glial cells are the supporting actors, tech crew, and minions that surround and support them.

Although neurons in different parts of the nervous system vary somewhat in appearance, their basic structure is the same (Figure 9-1). Structurally a neuron can be divided roughly into the central cell body, also called the **soma** or **perikaryon**, and the two different types of processes (extensions) from the cell body, called *dendrites* and *axons.*

**Dendrites** receive stimuli, or impulses, from other neurons and conduct this stimulation to the cell body. They can be referred to as **afferent** processes, because they conduct impulses toward the cell body (*ad* means "toward," and *ferre* means "to carry"). Dendrites also may be modified into **sensory receptors** that receive, or sense, stimuli such as heat, cold, touch, pressure, stretch, or other physical changes from inside or outside the body. Dendrites tend to be short, numerous, and have many branches. (The word *dendro* is derived from the Greek word for branch because, when examined under a microscope, dendrites resemble the branches of a tree.)

The axon is the other type of process from the neuron cell body. **Axons** conduct nerve impulses away from the cell body

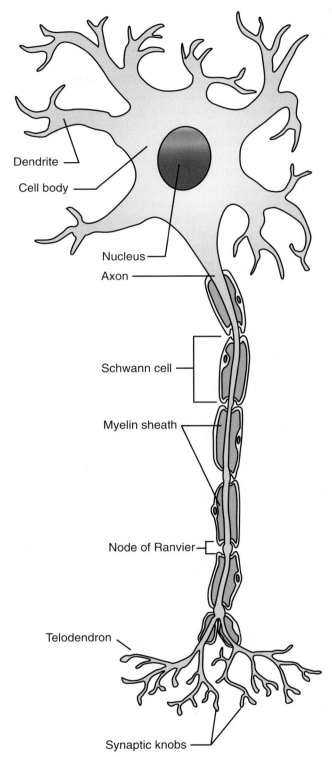

**FIGURE 9-1** Structure of neuron.

toward another neuron or an **effector cell** (a cell that does something when stimulated, such as a muscle or gland cell). They can be called **efferent** processes, because they conduct impulses away from the cell body (*ex,* "away"; *ferre,* "to carry"). In contrast to the short, numerous, branched dendrites, the axon is a single process that can be very long. For example, a single axon in the horse may extend for several feet—from the spinal cord all the way to the lower leg. *Note:* axons are sometimes referred to by another name, **nerve fibers**. When we're talking about the components of nerve cells, the term *axon* is usually used. When we're talking about the bundles of axons that make up cordlike nerves in the body, they are usually called *nerve fibers.* "Axons" and "nerve fibers" are two different names for the same thing. Think of them as aliases for each other.

Axons are often covered by a sheath of a fatty substance called **myelin**. Myelin grossly (without magnification) appears white. For that reason, nervous tissue containing many myelinated axons is often referred to as **white matter**. (Conversely, nervous tissue that is made up largely of neuron cell bodies appears darker and is called **gray matter**.) The **myelin sheath** is actually made of the cell membranes of specialized glial cells called **oligodendrocytes** in the brain and spinal cord, and **Schwann cells** in the nerves outside of the brain and spinal cord. These special glial cells wrap themselves around the axon like a thin pancake tightly wrapped around a hot dog. Because the axon of most neurons is fairly long, it takes multiple Schwann cells or oligodendrocytes lined up end to end to cover the entire length of the axon. Between adjacent glial cells are small gaps in the myelin sheath called **nodes of Ranvier**. The myelin sheath and nodes of Ranvier work together to enhance the speed of conduction of nerve impulses along the axon. Myelinated axons conduct nerve impulses faster than unmyelinated axons (Figures 9-2 and 9-3).

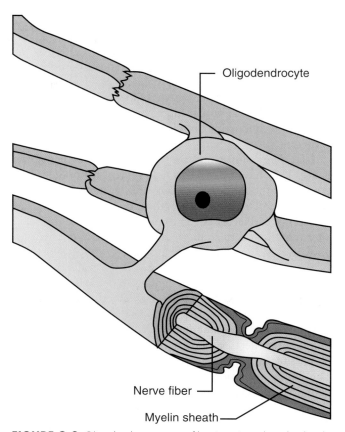

**FIGURE 9-2** Oligodendrocyte, nerve fiber (axon), and myelin sheath. Oligodendrocytes wrap around nerve fibers in the central nervous system to form myelin sheaths.

---

### ✔ TEST YOURSELF 9-1

1. How do basic communication and control functions differ between the nervous system and the endocrine system?
2. How are the functions of neurons and neuroglia different from each other?
3. Name the parts of a typical neuron.
4. How are the dendrites and axons different in structure and function?
5. What is the difference between gray matter and white matter?
6. What is the relationship between the myelin sheath and the nodes of Ranvier?

---

## ORGANIZATION OF THE NERVOUS SYSTEM

Many schemes are used to describe the anatomic or functional organization of the nervous system. Because the organizational terminology sets the foundation for our discussion about the nervous system, let's first look at how this terminology is used.

### ANATOMIC LOCATION: CNS VERSUS PNS

A simple way to organize the nervous system anatomically is to think of it as being divided into two components: the

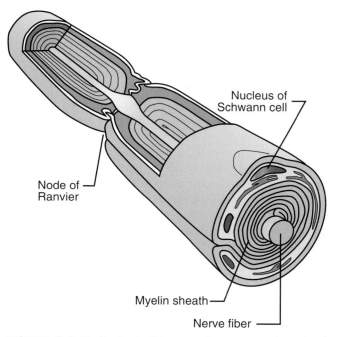

**FIGURE 9-3** Myelin sheath. Schwann cells wrap around peripheral nerve fibers (axons) to form thick myelin sheaths.

*central nervous system (CNS)* and the *peripheral nervous system (PNS)*. As the name implies, the CNS is anatomically composed of the brain and the spinal cord, which are found along the central axis of the body. *Peripheral* means "to the side" or "*away* from the center." Therefore the peripheral nervous system (PNS) is made up of those components of the nervous system that extend away from the central axis outward, toward the periphery of the body. **Cranial nerves** are those few nerves of the PNS that originate directly from the brain. Most PNS nerves are **spinal nerves** that emerge from the spinal cord.

## DIRECTION OF IMPULSES: AFFERENT VERSUS EFFERENT

Some nerve fibers conduct electrical impulses from the periphery toward the CNS, and other nerve fibers conduct impulses in the opposite direction, from the CNS toward the periphery. These two functional types of nerve fiber are called *afferent nerve fibers* and *efferent nerve fibers*. **Afferent nerve fibers** conduct nerve impulses *toward* the CNS, whereas **efferent nerve fibers** conduct nerve impulses *away* from the CNS.

Because afferent nerve fibers conduct sensations from the sensory receptors in the skin and other locations in the body to the CNS, afferent nerve fibers are usually called **sensory nerve fibers**. In contrast, efferent nerve fibers conduct impulses from the CNS out toward muscles and other organs. Because the efferent impulses are the ones that, among other things, cause skeletal muscle contraction and movement, efferent nerve fibers are usually called **motor nerve fibers**. The cranial and spinal nerves in the PNS and *nerve tracts* (bundles of axons) in the CNS may be made up of nerve fibers that are sensory or motor, or a combination of both. A nerve that contains only sensory nerve fibers is called a sensory nerve. A nerve that contains only motor nerve fibers is called a motor nerve. Nerves that contain both kinds of nerve fibers are called mixed nerves. Most nerves in the PNS are mixed nerves.

## FUNCTION: AUTONOMIC VERSUS SOMATIC

When an animal turns its head in response to its name being called by its owner, efferent (outgoing) motor impulses from the brain are consciously sent to the muscles in the neck to turn the head toward the sound. This conscious, or voluntary, control of skeletal muscles is referred to as a **somatic nervous system** function. Because the action of the animal turning its head was caused by voluntary initiation of efferent impulses, this function would be classified as a *somatic motor function*. Impulses being sent to the CNS from receptors in the muscles, skin, eyes, or ears would be classified as *somatic sensory functions*, because they are consciously perceived by the brain.

In contrast to the voluntary movement of the somatic nervous system function, animals do not consciously have to think to contract their intestines, increase their heart rate in response to a threat, or stimulate release of digestive juices in response to ingestion of a meal. The animal also does not

have to be consciously aware of blood pressure receptors informing the body that the blood pressure is too low or of stretch receptors indicating that the lungs have inflated. The part of the nervous system that controls and coordinates these automatic functions is called the **autonomic nervous system** (*auto* means "self," and *nomos* means "law," so the autonomic nervous system is the *self-regulating* system).

Like the somatic (voluntary) system, the autonomic system also has motor nerves and sensory nerves. However, instead of these motor nerves going to skeletal muscle to cause voluntary limb or body movement, the autonomic motor nerves send impulses to smooth muscle, cardiac muscle, and glands to regulate a wide variety of automatic body functions. Autonomic sensory nerves receive the afferent sensory impulses from sensory receptors that are used automatically to regulate these body functions.

---

✓ *TEST YOURSELF 9-2*

1. What are the anatomic differences between the CNS and the PNS?
2. Which are afferent nerve fibers: motor nerve fibers or sensory nerve fibers? Which are efferent?
3. Identify each of the following as being controlled by the autonomic or the somatic nervous system and as being either sensory or motor:
   Conscious movement of the forelimb
   Slowing of the heart rate in response to an increased blood pressure
   Constriction of blood vessels in the skin in response to cold temperatures
   Perception of pain from an injection of antibiotics
   Perception of the amount of acidity present in the duodenum.

---

## NEURON FUNCTION: DEPOLARIZATION AND REPOLARIZATION

It is often said that a nerve "fires," or that an impulse is conducted from one end of a neuron to the other. What actually is occurring in the neuron when this happens? If we understand the concepts of *depolarization* and *repolarization* it is easier to understand how drugs such as local anesthetics can prevent nerves from firing or how imbalances of sodium or potassium in the body can adversely affect nerve function.

### RESTING STATE, POLARIZATION, AND RESTING MEMBRANE POTENTIAL

When a neuron is not being stimulated, it is said to be in a **resting state**. However, even when the neuron is resting, it is still working to maintain its resting state. The cell membranes of neurons are electrically polarized at rest, like tiny charged batteries. Specialized molecules located in the neuron's cell membrane pump sodium ions ($Na^+$) from the inside of the neuron to the outside and pump potassium ions ($K^+$) from the outside to the inside. This specialized molecule is called the **sodium–potassium pump** (Figure 9-4).

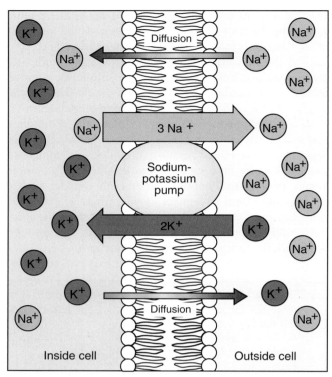

**FIGURE 9-4** Sodium–potassium pump. This cellular mechanism is located in the cell membrane and actively pumps sodium ions (Na+) out of the neuron and potassium ions (K+) into the neuron.

Sodium (Na⁺) cannot readily diffuse or leak through the cell membrane on its own. Because sodium cannot diffuse across the membrane, the action of the sodium–potassium pump causes a higher concentration of sodium to accumulate *outside* the cell. The action of the sodium–potassium pump and the negative charges inside the cell cause a higher concentration of potassium to accumulate *inside* the cell. By keeping the sodium on one side of the membrane (outside) and the potassium on the other (inside), the cellular membrane separating the two is said to be *polarized* (because it has two distinct poles of ions on either side of the membrane).

The distribution of positive and negative charges from sodium, potassium, proteins, and other charged ions on either side of the neuronal membrane creates a difference in electrical charge across the membrane, with the inside of the neuron being more negatively charged than the outside. This electrical difference in charges across the membrane is called the **resting membrane potential**. The net negative resting membrane potential usually is stated as a certain negative number of millivolts (for example, −70 mV), indicating the net negative charge within the cell. By selectively pumping sodium out and potassium in, the sodium–potassium pump maintains this negatively charged, resting membrane potential—the cell membrane "battery" is charged (Figure 9-5, *A*).

## DEPOLARIZATION

When an impulse from an adjoining neuron or from a specific type of external stimulus (such as heat, touch, or taste)

stimulates a neuron, a set of specific steps occurs, resulting in the nerve "firing" or depolarizing. At the point where the stimulus occurs on the neuron, a specialized molecular structure on the neuron cell membrane called a *sodium channel* opens (Figure 9-5, *B*). This sodium channel allows *only* sodium ions (Na⁺) to pass through it. Because a higher concentration of sodium ions exists outside the cell than inside the cell, the sodium ions readily flow through the open sodium channels from the outside to the inside by passive diffusion. Not only is the sodium driven into the cell by the concentration gradient (the differences in concentration between the outside and inside), but the positive sodium (Na⁺) ions are attracted into the cell by the net negative charge inside the cell. Remember, opposite charges attract each other, and therefore the positive Na⁺ ions are attracted to the relative negative charge within the cell.

**Depolarization** refers to this opening of the sodium channels and the sudden influx of many sodium ions into the cell. It is called *de*polarization, because the sodium influx results in the loss of the two distinct poles of sodium and potassium on either side of the membrane. If we hooked an electric meter to the neuron, we would see the inside of the neuron go from a negatively charged resting membrane potential to a net positive charge during depolarization. This shift inside the cell from negative to positive makes sense when we consider the positive sodium ions flooding into the neuron. This significant change in electric charge from negative to positive is also referred to as an **action potential**.

## REPOLARIZATION

Within a fraction of a second after sodium begins to flood into the cell during depolarization, the sodium channels snap shut, halting the influx. Almost simultaneously, specialized potassium channels open up in the cellular membrane (Figure 9-5, *C*). Analogous to the sodium channels, the potassium channels only allow potassium ions to pass through them.

With the potassium channels open, the potassium ions (K⁺) passively diffuse out of the cell, propelled by both the potassium concentration gradient (a high concentration inside and a lower concentration outside) and the strong positive charge brought into the cell by the influx of sodium ions. Remember that *like* charges repel, therefore the positive potassium ions are repelled by the relatively positive charge inside the neuron caused by the sodium influx. This outflow of potassium ions continues until these specialized potassium channels snap shut a split second after they have opened (Figure 9-5, *D*). Because the potassium ions (K⁺) are positive, the exodus of potassium ions from the neuron causes the charge inside the cell to swing back in the negative direction.

This change of the cell's charge back toward the net negative resting membrane potential is called **repolarization**. The cell is said to be *re*polarized, because the sodium and potassium ions are once again on opposite sides (opposite poles) of the cell membrane. The only difference between the end of the repolarization phase and the resting state is that

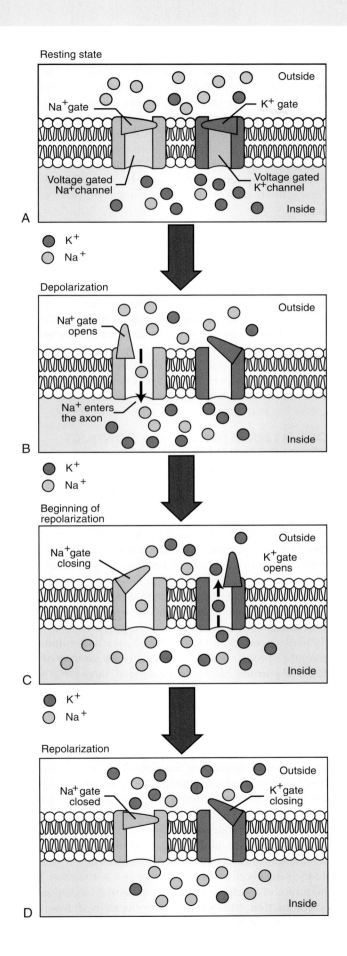

A, Resting state
B, Depolarization
C, Beginning of repolarization
D, Repolarization

K+
Na+

**FIGURE 9-5** Depolarization and repolarization. **A,** Resting state. Sodium has been pumped out of the cell and potassium has been pumped in, producing a net negative electrical charge inside the cell membrane compared to the outside. **B,** Depolarization. A stimulus has caused the gate on the sodium channel to open, allowing sodium ions to flow into the cell. This produces a net negative charge on the *outside* of the cell membrane—the opposite of the resting state. **C,** Beginning of repolarization. The gate on the sodium channel is closing and the gate on the potassium channel is opening to allow potassium ions to flow out of the cell. **D,** Repolarization. A sufficient outflow of potassium ions has restored the net negative charge to the inside of the cell, but the sodium and potassium ions are on opposite sides of the cell membrane from where they started. Therefore, sodium ions are pumped out of the cell and potassium ions are pumped into the cell. The regain of the resting state is shown in Figure 9-4.

the sodium and potassium ions are on the opposite sides from where they began. To restore the sodium and potassium to their original locations on either side of the membrane, the sodium–potassium pump quickly moves the misplaced sodium and potassium ions back to their original sides (see Figure 9-4).

*Note:* It may seem as though the acts of depolarization and repolarization must involve a molecular tidal wave of ions moving back and forth. The truth is that relatively few sodium and potassium ions move at each point of the depolarization–repolarization cycle, which explains why the cycle is completed rapidly and why even minor imbalances in sodium or potassium in the body can greatly affect normal neuron function.

## DEPOLARIZATION THRESHOLD, NERVE IMPULSE CONDUCTION, AND ALL-OR-NOTHING PRINCIPLE

Not every depolarization stimulus results in the complete depolarization–repolarization cycle. The initial stimulus must be sufficient to make the neuron respond. When the stimulus is strong enough to cause complete depolarization, it is said to have reached the **threshold**, and this causes the cell to depolarize or "fire." A stimulus of sufficient intensity to generate a nerve impulse is called a **threshold stimulus**.

To understand how this works, let's use an example in which a neuron with sensory receptors on its dendrites receives a very weak stimulus. The weak stimulus results in only a few sodium channels opening and therefore only a small influx of sodium ions into the neuronal cell. Because of this, we would only see a slight positive change in neuron charge from the resting membrane potential. Because the charge was not very significant, the cell did not reach the threshold, and the few sodium channels that opened would close without causing further effect on other sodium channels. The sodium–potassium pump would quickly move the few displaced sodium ions from inside back to the outside, and the neuron would go back to its resting state. In this case, the stimulus failed to depolarize the neuron, and the information from the sensory receptors in the dendrites was not transmitted to the brain.

If, however, the stimulus on these sensory receptors had been larger, more sodium channels would have opened, and a larger number of sodium ions would have entered the neuronal cell. This would have produced a significant positive change in the membrane potential in the immediate area of the cellular membrane. If the change had been sufficient to reach the threshold, sodium channels adjacent to this area would also open. This would allow sufficient sodium influx into these adjacent areas to reach the threshold, causing further adjacent sodium channels to open. In other words, the initial stimulus would cause a spreading wave of opening sodium channels to travel along the cell membrane of the entire neuron. This wave of sodium channels opening to allow sodium influx is called the **wave of depolarization**. As you recall, the strong influx of sodium ions during depolarization was called the *action potential;* therefore this wave of depolarization can also be called **conduction of the action potential**. In clinical terms, however, this wave of depolarization or conduction of the action potential along the cell membrane is most commonly called a **nerve impulse**.

In the simplest terms, a nerve impulse is conducted along a nerve fiber by the "flipping" of the electric charges across the cell membrane (depolarization), followed quickly by the "unflipping" of the electric charges (repolarization). That process stimulates the adjacent area of the cell membrane in the direction of impulse conduction (remember that dendrites conduct impulses toward the cell body, and axons conduct impulses away from the cell body) to flip and unflip, which stimulates the adjacent area, and so on. If we were very tiny and could watch the cell membrane in one area of the neuron while a nerve impulse was being conducted, we could watch the flipping and unflipping of charges happen as the impulse passed by us.

Regardless of how strong the initial stimulus was, if it were sufficient to achieve the threshold for a neuron to fire (depolarize), the nerve impulse (action potential) would be generated and conducted along the entire neuron with uniform strength. This phenomenon is called the **all-or-nothing principle**, because either the complete neuron depolarizes to its maximum strength, or it does not depolarize at all. This is an important concept! A nerve impulse is a nerve impulse is a nerve impulse. They are all basically the same. What makes one nerve impulse signify the color red, another represent a particular odor, and a third cause a muscle fiber to contract? It depends on where the impulse is going. Sensory (afferent) nerve impulses go to particular areas of the brain, where they are interpreted as the appropriate sensation. Motor (efferent) nerve impulses go to *effector organs,* which are stimulated to perform particular actions.

## REFRACTORY PERIOD

For a very brief period during and after a neuron has generated a nerve impulse, it cannot generate another impulse. This is called the neuron's **refractory period**. If a second threshold stimulus arrives at the dendrites or on the neuron cell body while the sodium channels are open or while the

potassium molecules are moving rapidly through their open channels, the stimulus will not cause a second depolarization. Because cells in the depolarization and early repolarization phases are already in the process of executing the depolarization–repolarization cycle (firing), they can't depolarize (fire) again until the cycle is completed. Thus, any stimulus arriving at that point in the depolarization–repolarization cycle would die out. The neuron is said to be in a **refractory period** because it is refractory or "insensitive" to new stimuli until it recovers from the previous nerve impulse.

The period of sodium influx and early potassium outflow is a part of the refractory period during which no stimulus, no matter how strong, can cause the cell to depolarize again. This period is called the *absolute refractory period* because the cell absolutely cannot respond. However, if a very strong stimulus comes during the tail end of the time the membrane is repolarizing and restoring the resting membrane potential, it may be possible to stimulate another depolarization. Therefore, during this part of the refractory period, the cell may depolarize again if the stimulus is much stronger than normal. This period is called the *relative refractory period,* because the cell is still refractory to stimuli of normal intensity but may respond to very strong stimuli.

## HOW MYELINATED AXONS CONDUCT ACTION POTENTIALS QUICKER: SALTATORY CONDUCTION

If all neurons sent their wave of depolarization or their conduction of action potentials from one sodium channel to the next in a series of tiny steps, the transmission of the nerve impulse from one end of a neuron to the other would be relatively slow. Think of the sodium channels as a set of tiny dominos set up in a line several feet long. When we tip over the first domino, we know that it is going to take some time for the last domino to fall. The same thing happens if each sodium channel opening stimulates the opening of the adjacent channel.

If, however, our domino line tipped over 10 dominoes at a time, the speed at which we would reach the end of the domino line would be greatly accelerated. In neurons with axons wrapped in a myelin sheath, a similar effect happens with the depolarization wave. Like a rubber coating on an electrical wire that prevents electrical shorts, the myelin sheath prevents sodium ions from flowing across the neuronal cell membrane. Therefore depolarization in myelinated axons can only take place at the gaps in the myelin sheath that occur at the nodes of Ranvier. Thus, when the sodium influx at one node is sufficient to open adjacent sodium channels, the next available sodium channel is at the next node of Ranvier. The depolarization wave in the myelinated axon skips from one node of Ranvier to the next, greatly accelerating the rate at which the depolarization wave moves from the neuron cell body to the other end of the axon. This rapid means of conducting an action potential is called **saltatory conduction** (the word *saltatory* is derived from the Latin *saltare,* which means "to leap") (Figure 9-6).

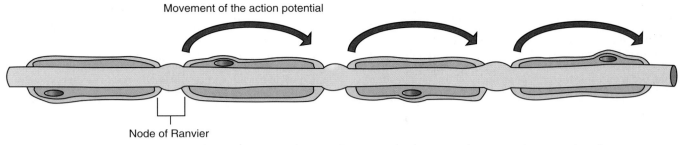

Movement of the action potential

Node of Ranvier

**FIGURE 9-6** Saltatory conduction. A nerve impulse jumps from one node of Ranvier to the next, producing rapid conduction of the nerve impulse.

 **CLINICAL APPLICATION**

### Local Anesthetics

Local anesthetics are drugs that are injected into superficial areas of the body to block the conduction of sensations from that area. You may have experienced this form of anesthesia if your dentist administered a local anesthetic to numb an area of your mouth. Local anesthetic drugs such as *lidocaine* prevent sensory nerves from depolarizing despite stimulation from the dental or surgical procedure. If these sensory nerves do not depolarize, the brain is unaware of any sensation from that area of the body, therefore you do not feel pain. Lidocaine prevents the sensory neuron from depolarizing by blocking the sodium channels through which sodium ions usually flood into the neuronal cell. If the sodium channels are plugged by the local anesthetic molecule, no sodium can flood into the cell despite the channels being stimulated to open. No sodium influx means that no positive charge occurs in the neuron, threshold is not attained, and the stimulus is not turned into

a depolarization wave. Any nerve impulse that has been generated stops at that point.

*Anesthesia* means *without sensitivity*. If a sensory nerve does not depolarize, the animal's brain does not perceive sensations from that area of the body. Local anesthetics are used not only to anesthetize areas of the body for minor surgical procedures, but also to aid in identifying sources of pain that cause lameness in horses. In a lame horse, a local anesthetic may be injected around selected sensory nerves to prevent them from transmitting impulses. If injection around a particular nerve improves the horse's movement or reduces the lameness, the veterinarian knows that the source of the problem is in the area of the leg or hoof whose sensations are supplied by the "blocked" nerve. If the "nerve block" does not improve the lameness, the veterinarian injects another specific sensory nerve and repeats the process until the horse appears to have less pain.

The rapid conduction of impulses along myelinated neurons by saltatory conduction makes processes such as vision and fine motor control possible in larger animals such as humans and many domestic animal species. The importance of the myelin sheath and saltatory conduction to normal functioning can be illustrated by the symptoms of demyelinating diseases (diseases that damage or destroy myelin) such as multiple sclerosis

### HOW NEURONS COMMUNICATE: THE SYNAPSE

Once the nerve impulse, or action potential, has been successfully conducted to the end of the axon, it must be transmitted to the next neuron or to the cells of the target organ or tissue. Because two adjacent neurons do not physically touch each other, this process cannot be accomplished by directly continuing the depolarization wave. Instead, the neuron must release a chemical that stimulates the next neuron or cell. This perpetuation of the nerve impulse from one neuron to the next cell is called **synaptic transmission**.

The *synapse* is the junction between two neurons or a neuron and a target cell. The synapse consists of a physical

gap between the two cells called the **synaptic cleft**. The neuron bringing the nerve impulse to the synapse and releasing the chemical to stimulate the next cell is called the **presynaptic neuron**. The chemical released by the presynaptic neuron is called the **neurotransmitter**, and the neuron that contains the receptors that receive the neurotransmitter is the **postsynaptic neuron** (Figure 9-7).

If we look closely at the end of the axon on the presynaptic neuron, we see a branched structure called the **telodendron**. Each branch of the telodendron ends in a slightly enlarged bulb called the **terminal bouton** (*bouton* meaning "button"), **synaptic end bulb**, or **synaptic knob**. The synaptic knobs contain many mitochondria that provide energy for the processes that occur there, and also many vesicles (small sacs) that contain the neurotransmitter. When the axon's wave of depolarization reaches the synaptic knob, calcium channels open in the knob's cellular membrane, resulting in an influx of calcium into the synaptic knob. This influx of calcium causes the vesicles containing neurotransmitters to fuse with the knob's cellular membrane and dump their contents into the synaptic cleft. These neurotransmitters diffuse rapidly across the tiny synaptic cleft toward the postsynaptic membrane.

## Multiple Sclerosis

Multiple sclerosis, also known as MS, is a disease of humans that results in damage to the myelin sheaths of nerve fibers in the brain and spinal cord. Nerve fibers whose myelin sheaths have been damaged conduct impulses abnormally, or not at all. Because both sensory and motor nerve fibers can be affected, the clinical signs of MS can be sensory and/or motor.

Sensory effects include tingling, numbness, visual problems, and difficulties with coordination and balance. Motor effects include muscle weakness, muscle spasms, difficulty moving, and problems with speech and swallowing. The exact cause of MS is not known, but it is believed to be caused, at least in part, by the person's own immune system attacking the nervous system.

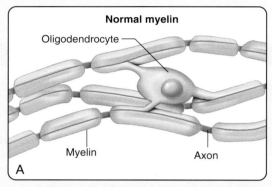

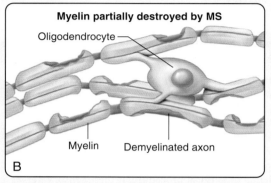

Effects of multiple sclerosis (MS). **A,** A normal myelin sheath allows rapid conduction. **B,** In MS, the myelin sheath is damaged, disrupting nerve conduction. (From Thibodeau G, Patton K: Structure and function of the body, ed 14, St Louis, 2012, Mosby.)

---

### ✓ TEST YOURSELF 9-3

1. During depolarization, what ion channels open and what ion moves? Where does it move?
2. During repolarization, what ion channels open and what ion moves? Where does it move?
3. What normally maintains the resting membrane potential of a neuron during the resting state?
4. What is threshold? What role does threshold play in the all-or-none principle?
5. What is the difference between the *absolute* and the *relative* refractory periods?
6. Explain why waves of depolarization are conducted faster in myelinated axons than in unmyelinated ones.

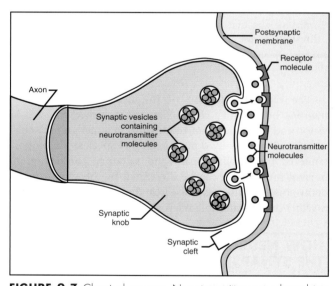

**FIGURE 9-7** Chemical synapse. Neurotransmitters are released into the synaptic space, where they combine with receptors on the postsynaptic membrane (another neuron or an effector cell).

On the postsynaptic membrane are specialized proteins called **receptors**. The neurotransmitter molecules released by the synaptic knob bind to these receptors and trigger a change in the postsynaptic cell. However, the postsynaptic membrane receptors are very specific about which neurotransmitters they will bind. If the neurotransmitter and receptor are not matched, they will not bind to each other, and no change will be triggered in the postsynaptic cell. An analogy that illustrates this concept is that of a lock and key. Only certain keys (types of neurotransmitter) will fit in a lock (the receptor) and cause the lock to open (the receptor to trigger cellular changes). Thus, synaptic transmission is only effective if receptors to the neurotransmitter exist on the postsynaptic cell's membrane.

## TYPES OF NEUROTRANSMITTER AND THEIR EFFECT ON POSTSYNAPTIC MEMBRANES

Many different types of neurotransmitter are associated with synapses in both the CNS and PNS. Generally, we can classify these neurotransmitters into two categories: *excitatory neurotransmitters* and *inhibitory neurotransmitters*. As their name implies, **excitatory neurotransmitters** have an excitatory effect on the postsynaptic membrane when they combine with their specific receptors. Specifically, excitatory neurotransmitters usually cause an influx of sodium so that the postsynaptic membrane moves toward threshold. If the postsynaptic membrane is stimulated sufficiently by enough excitatory neurotransmitter, then threshold will be reached and depolarization of the postsynaptic membrane will occur, beginning a new nerve impulse.

In contrast to excitatory neurotransmitters, **inhibitory neurotransmitters** tend to hyperpolarize the postsynaptic membrane, making the inside of the cell more negative instead of positive and moving the charge within the postsynaptic cell farther away from threshold. When inhibitory neurotransmitters combine with their specific receptors on the postsynaptic side, they may cause chloride channels or potassium channels to open up on the postsynaptic membrane. This allows the negatively charged chloride ions ($Cl^-$) to enter the postsynaptic cell and allows potassium ($K^+$) ions to leave the cell, making the inside of the cell more negatively charged (a change in charge that is *opposite* from that needed to reach threshold).

Neurotransmitters usually can be classified as excitatory or inhibitory based on the effect they have on the postsynaptic cell. Some neurotransmitters, however, can have an excitatory effect on some cells and an inhibitory effect on others, so it is difficult in most cases to make sweeping statements about whether a given neurotransmitter is one or the other.

**Acetylcholine** is one of the most commonly studied neurotransmitters in the body. It can be either an excitatory or inhibitory neurotransmitter depending on its location in the body. At the junction between somatic motor neurons and the muscles they supply, acetylcholine is an excitatory neurotransmitter that stimulates muscle fibers to contract. However, at the site where **parasympathetic** nerves synapse with the heart, acetylcholine has an inhibitory effect that slows the heart rate.

*Norepinephrine, dopamine,* and *epinephrine* are all neurotransmitters that belong to a group called **catecholamines**. **Norepinephrine** is associated with arousal and fight-or-flight reactions of the sympathetic nervous system. **Epinephrine** is released primarily from the adrenal medulla (center of the adrenal gland) and therefore plays more of a role as a hormone in the fight-or-flight reactions of the sympathetic nervous system. **Dopamine** is found in the brain, where it is involved with autonomic functions and muscle control. Humans with a decreased number of functioning dopamine neurons show the muscle tremors and shaky gait associated with Parkinson's disease.

**Gamma-aminobutyric acid (GABA)** and **glycine** are two neurotransmitters that are inhibitory. GABA is found in the brain, and glycine is found in the spinal cord. Some groups of tranquilizers, such as diazepam (Valium), work by increasing the GABA effect on the brain, thus inhibiting activity in the brain and producing tranquilization (reduced anxiety) with sedation (drowsiness).

One postsynaptic membrane may have multiple types of presynaptic neurons across the synaptic cleft. For example, a postsynaptic motor neuron in the brain may have some presynaptic neurons that release the excitatory neurotransmitter acetylcholine into the synaptic cleft and other presynaptic neurons that release the inhibitory neurotransmitter GABA into that same synaptic cleft. Depending on which set of neurons is more active—the excitatory, acetylcholine-releasing neurons or the neurons releasing the GABA inhibitory neurotransmitter—the postsynaptic motor neuron may either be stimulated or inhibited.

By having both inhibitory and excitatory neurotransmitters, the nervous system can selectively increase or decrease

 **CLINICAL APPLICATION**

### Poisons That Affect the Nervous System

Every year, animals are injured or killed by nervous system poisons in the form of insecticides (flea products, bug sprays, agricultural chemicals), rodenticides (mice and rat killers), poisonous plants, or other chemical poisons that disrupt the function of the nerve synapse. Many of these poisons act by combining with or blocking the neurotransmitter receptors on the postsynaptic membranes. To combine with the receptors, these poisons must have a similar molecular structure to the natural neurotransmitters in the body.

Many of these poisons bind to the receptors just like the natural neurotransmitters do, thereby stimulating the postsynaptic cell or neuron. In these cases of poisoning, we see an overstimulation of some aspect of the nervous system or the tissues innervated by that part of the nervous system. Animals may show signs of seizures or muscle tremors, indicating stimulation of the somatic motor system or overstimulation of the autonomic nervous system, resulting in vomiting or changes in respiration, heart rate, or other autonomic functions.

In some cases, the poison can combine with the receptor, but it does *not* produce an effect. In this case, the poison would *prevent* the natural neurotransmitter from combining with the receptor to produce its normal effect. Because the poison acts as a blocker of that receptor, we would see a suppression of that part of the nervous system. A classic example of this effect is curare, the nerve poison found on the skin of the brightly colored poison dart frogs in South America. Curare combines with the receptors on skeletal muscles and prevents the presynaptic neuron's neurotransmitter from stimulating the muscle to contract; thus, curare paralyzes the animal's muscles. South American natives use this toxin to coat the tips of their hunting darts, arrows or spears to paralyze their quarry. In this way, the animals are easily captured, even if the wound itself is not fatal.

We use a similar effect medically to paralyze the normal respiratory movements of animals during open chest surgery. By paralyzing the respiratory muscles, we can more easily mechanically ventilate, or breathe for, an animal without fighting its body's own contraction of the diaphragm and rib cage muscles.

the activity of specific parts of the brain or spinal cord. Drugs or poisons that imitate inhibitory or excitatory neurotransmitters will cause CNS depression or increased CNS activity, respectively. For example, ivermectin, a commonly used antiparasitic drug (it kills parasites), causes an increased inhibitory neurotransmitter effect. In animals receiving an overdose of ivermectin, the main clinical signs are severe depression, loss of normal control of voluntary movements, and coma, all of which reflect inhibition of the neuronal activity in the brain.

## STOPPING AND RECYCLING THE NEUROTRANSMITTER

If the neurotransmitter were released, combined with its corresponding receptor, and allowed to remain in the synapse or on the postsynaptic receptor, the postsynaptic cell would either continue to be excited or continue to be inhibited depending on the type of receptor being stimulated. Therefore the body must have a way of stopping the effect of the neurotransmitter quickly so that this does not occur.

In the case of acetylcholine, the neurotransmitter is broken down quickly by an enzyme found on the postsynaptic membrane called **acetylcholinesterase**. The *-ase* suffix tells us that this compound is an enzyme that acts on acetylcholine. The broken-down components of acetylcholine are reabsorbed by the synaptic knob, reassembled into new acetylcholine molecules, and repackaged into vesicles for release with the next wave of depolarization. If acetylcholinesterase is prevented from working, acetylcholine will not be broken down and acetylcholine receptors will continue to be stimulated. This is what happens when animals are exposed to poisonous levels of flea products containing organophosphate insecticides. In organophosphate poisoning, the insecticide combines with the acetylcholinesterase and inactivates it. The small amount of acetylcholine normally released by presynaptic neurons causes overstimulation of acetylcholine receptors, resulting in diarrhea, vomiting, difficulty in breathing, and constricted pupils.

After the release of norepinephrine from the presynaptic neuron, the norepinephrine is rapidly taken back into the synaptic knob, where it is broken down into its components by the enzyme monoamine oxidase (MAO). Any norepinephrine not reabsorbed by the synaptic knob is degraded by another enzyme called *catechol-O-methyl transferase* (COMT). Compared with acetylcholinesterase, the activity of MAO and COMT is relatively slow, which helps to explain why effects of these excitatory neurotransmitters can linger for a while after their release. One of the mechanisms by which some human antidepression medications work is by blocking MAO or COMT, which allows norepinephrine to prolong its excitatory effect on the brain.

Because drugs and poisons encountered in veterinary medicine often produce their effects by increasing or decreasing excitatory or inhibitory neurotransmitter effects or by affecting the enzymes that terminate these effects, it's important to understand the concepts of synaptic function and neurotransmitter release and termination.

---

> ✓ **TEST YOURSELF 9-4**
>
> 1. What role do the synaptic cleft, presynaptic neuron, neurotransmitter, and postsynaptic neuron play in the continuation of a depolarization wave from one nerve to another?
> 2. What is the functional relationship between a neurotransmitter and a receptor? Will any neurotransmitter stimulate any receptor?
> 3. What is the difference between an *excitatory* and an *inhibitory* neurotransmitter?
> 4. How is acetylcholine different from acetylcholinesterase?
> 5. What are catecholamines?
> 6. What are GABA and glycine?

---

## THE CENTRAL NERVOUS SYSTEM—BRAIN AND SPINAL CORD

To the unaided eye, the central nervous system (CNS) consists of the brain and the spinal cord. At the microscopic level, however, the main components of the CNS are neuron cell bodies, myelinated and uynmyelinated nerve fibers, and glial cells. The **gray matter** of the CNS contains most of the neuron cell bodies, and appears a dark brownish-gray color grossly. It is usually thought of as the "thinking" part of the CNS. The **white matter** contains most of the myelinated nerve fibers and appears white because of all the myelin. It is the "wiring" that connects the various components of the brain. It has been estimated that the white matter of the human brain makes up a network of some 100,000 miles of nerve fibers. (See "Secrets of the Brain" in the February 2014 issue of National Geographic.)

Neurologic disease or disorders affecting the brain produce clinical signs that sometimes can be identified as belonging to specific areas of the brain. Although knowing all the centers or nuclei (clusters of neurons within the CNS) of the brain is not essential, the veterinary technician should be familiar with what the main parts of the brain do, to better understand the effect of neurologic disease and medications that affect the CNS (Figure 9-8).

In general, we can think of the brain as being divided into four different sections: the *cerebrum, cerebellum, diencephalon,* and *brainstem.* Each section of the brain has its own particular functions. The brainstem and diencephalon are the more primitive parts of the brain; the cerebellum coordinates motor control; and the centers of higher learning and intelligence are found in the cerebrum. Therefore disease in each part of the brain produces different clinical signs.

### CEREBRUM

The **cerebrum** is made up of gray matter in the **cerebral cortex** (the outer-most superficial layer of the brain) and white matter beneath the cortex, including the **corpus**

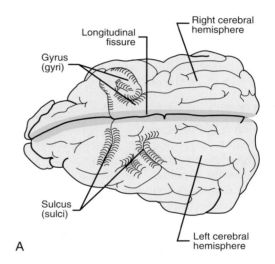

**FIGURE 9-8** Anatomy of the central nervous system.

**callosum** (a set of fibers that connects the two halves of the cerebral cortex). The cerebrum is the largest part of the brain in domestic animals and constitutes the area of the brain responsible for those functions most commonly associated with higher-order behaviors, such as learning, reasoning, and intelligence. The cerebrum receives and interprets sensory information, initiates conscious (voluntary) nerve impulses to skeletal muscles, and integrates neuron activity that is normally associated with communication, expression of emotional responses, learning, memory and recall, and other behaviors associated with conscious activity.

The surface of the cerebrum is covered by "wrinkles" which serve to increase the area of the cerebral cortex, therefore making more room for gray matter. The wrinkled appearance is made up of folds called **gyri** (plural of **gyrus**) separated by deep grooves called **fissures** and more shallow grooves called **sulci** (plural of **sulcus**). The most prominent groove is the **longitudinal fissure**, which divides the cerebrum into right and left **cerebral hemispheres** (Figure 9-9). Each hemisphere is divided by sulci into **lobes**. Different lobes of the cerebral hemispheres specialize in certain functions. For example, a section of lobes in the front half of the brain contains the organized areas that initiate voluntary motor functions, whereas the lobe immediately posterior to this section contains the area that identifies the locations of sensations in or on the body.

If neurons of certain lobes of the cerebrum begin to fire spontaneously as a result of drugs, cellular damage, or neurotransmitter imbalance, the animal can exhibit spontaneous movements, seizure activity, abnormal behaviors, or hallucinations, depending on which lobes are affected. If parts of the cerebrum become damaged and nonfunctional from lack of oxygen, poisonous substances, or blood clots (strokes), the animal may lose the perception of specific sensations, may experience loss of voluntary movement, or may be unable to retain or recall information (unable to learn).

## CEREBELLUM

The **cerebellum**, located just caudal to the cerebrum, is the second largest component of the brain. It also has a

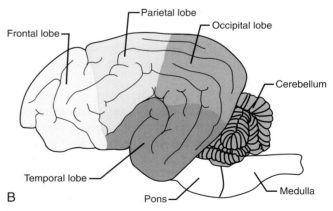

**FIGURE 9-9** Sulci and gyri of the cerebrum. **A,** Top view. **B,** Side view.

wrinkled-appearing surface, and a gray matter cortex with white matter beneath it. The cerebellum allows the body to have coordinated movement, balance, posture, and complex reflexes. Essentially, the cerebellum compares the movement the body intends to make with the actual position of muscles and joints to determine whether the intentions of the cerebral cortex are actually being carried out. If the movements are not being carried out accurately, the cerebellum will stimulate or inhibit muscles to fine-tune the movements.

For example, if you flex your arm, you can feel your biceps muscle contract while the opposing triceps muscle relaxes. When your arm begins to flex, stretch receptors associated with the muscles send feedback to the cerebellum to keep it informed of the position of the arm. The cerebellum then sends impulses to both the cerebral cortex and the muscles involved in the arm movement so that adjustments in the contraction can be made. In addition to making the voluntary body movements smooth and accurate, the cerebellum also uses this same sensory feedback from the muscles to maintain posture and balance.

Damage or disease involving the cerebellum results in **hypermetria**, a condition in which voluntary movements become jerky and exaggerated. A condition like this occurs in pigs with cerebellar disease and causes the affected animals to exhibit a goose-step gait in which the lifting and placing of the foot become exaggerated. Similar abnormal gaits can be seen in the young of other species born with an incompletely developed cerebellum or in animals with viral or bacterial disease that affects the cerebellum.

## DIENCEPHALON

The **diencephalon** is not as physically defined as the cerebrum and cerebellum. It does not have clearly visible layers of gray matter and white matter. It serves as a nervous system passageway *between* the primitive brainstem and the cerebrum. That gives rise to its common name: the *between brain*. Although many structures are associated with the diencephalon, veterinary technicians need to be familiar with three major ones:
1. The **thalamus** acts as a relay station for regulating sensory inputs to the cerebrum.
2. The **hypothalamus** is an interface between the nervous system and the endocrine system.
3. The **pituitary** is the endocrine "master gland" that regulates production and release of hormones throughout the body.

The hypothalamus also plays major roles in temperature regulation, hunger, thirst, and components of rage and anger responses. Disease or drugs that result in fever *(hyperthermia)* or compulsive eating or drinking often involve centers within the hypothalamus.

## BRAINSTEM

The **brainstem** is the connection between the rest of the brain and the spinal cord. Its name comes from its appearance as a stem on which the other parts of the brain (the cerebrum, cerebellum, and diencephalon) sit. It is the most primitive part of the brain and is composed of the **medulla oblongata**, the **pons**, and the **midbrain**. Like the diencephalon, the brainstem does not have clearly visible layers of gray matter and white matter.

The brainstem's role is to maintain basic support functions of the body, so it operates at the subconscious level. It is heavily involved in autonomic control functions related to

the heart, respiration (including coughing, sneezing, and hiccupping), blood vessel diameter *(vasomotor control)*, swallowing, and vomiting. Many of the cranial nerves (see later text) originate from this area of the brain. Because functions related to the heart, blood vessel diameter, and respiration are critical to life, damage to the brainstem can result in the animal dying rapidly from respiratory failure or cardiovascular collapse. Fortunately, the brainstem is well protected by the skull, so brainstem injury rarely occurs unless there is major damage to the skull.

> ### ✓ TEST YOURSELF 9-5
> 1. What part of the brain is responsible for conscious thought and perception of sensations?
> 2. What are the correct names for the bumps and fissures that make the cerebral cortex appear wrinkled?
> 3. What part of the brain is critical for coordination, posture, and fine motor control? How does this part of the brain accomplish these responsibilities?
> 4. What part of the brain serves as a relay station for impulses going to and from the cerebrum?
> 5. Which part of the brain controls many autonomic functions related to cardiovascular, respiratory, and gastrointestinal functions?

## OTHER CLINICALLY IMPORTANT STRUCTURES OF THE BRAIN

Other structures in the brain are important for the veterinary technician to be aware of because of their role in how drugs or disease affect the brain or their role in diagnostic procedures used in veterinary medicine.

### MENINGES

The **meninges** are a set of connective tissue layers that surround the brain and spinal cord (Figure 9-10). The three

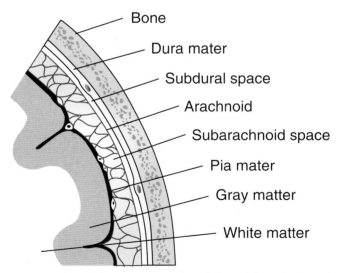

Bone
Dura mater
Subdural space
Arachnoid
Subarachnoid space
Pia mater
Gray matter
White matter

**FIGURE 9-10** The meninges. (Adpated from Gilbert S: Pictorial anatomy of the cat, Seattle, 1975, University of Washington Press.)

layers of the meninges—from outside to the innermost layer—are the tough, fibrous **dura mater**, the delicate, spiderweb-like **arachnoid**, and the very thin **pia mater**, which lies directly on the surface of the brain and spinal cord. These connective tissue layers contain a rich network of blood vessels that supply nutrients and oxygen to the superficial tissues of the brain and spinal cord. The fluid, fat, and connective tissue found between the layers of the meninges also provide some cushioning and distribution of nutrients for the CNS. Inflammation of these meningeal membranes resulting from viral or bacterial infections is called *meningitis.*

## CEREBROSPINAL FLUID

The brain and spinal cord are bathed and protected from the hard inner surfaces of the skull and spinal column by a fluid called the **cerebrospinal fluid (CSF)**. The clear, slippery CSF circulates between layers of the meninges and through cavities (canals and ventricles) inside the brain (ventricles) and the spinal cord (central canal). In addition to its cushioning function, the CSF's chemical composition may be involved in the regulation of certain autonomic functions, such as respiration and vomiting. For example, if the pH of the CSF becomes more acidic, the respiratory center in the brainstem will increase the respiratory rate.

Because the CSF circulates throughout the CNS, infection, inflammation, or cancer in the brain or spinal cord can cause changes in the amount of protein contained in the CSF; they can also cause changes in the composition of the CSF cells, including white blood cells or cancer cells. Veterinarians can diagnose certain nervous system diseases or cancers by taking a sample of the CSF, called a *CSF tap,* and examining it for particular types of cells or for specific changes in composition.

## BLOOD–BRAIN BARRIER

The **blood–brain barrier** is a functional barrier separating the capillaries in the brain from the nervous tissue itself. Unlike other capillaries in the body that have small openings between the cells of the capillary walls, the cells that make up the capillary walls in the brain are aligned tightly together without these openings, or **fenestrations**. In addition, the capillaries in the brain are covered by the cell membranes of glial cells. Thus, the tightly constructed capillary wall and the additional glial cell membranes result in a cellular barrier that prevents many drugs, proteins, ions, and other molecules from readily passing from the blood into the brain. In this way, the blood–brain barrier protects the brain from many poisons circulating in the bloodstream. For example, the heartworm preventive drug ivermectin is poisonous to

---

 **CLINICAL APPLICATION**

### Epidural Anesthesia

We sometimes inject anesthetic agents into the space outside the spinal cord dura mater—the outermost layer of the meninges—to produce large areas of local anesthesia. Anesthetic drugs introduced in this way block depolarization waves through spinal nerves as they emerge from the dura mater and thus remove the perception of pain from the part of the body

they supply. This is called **epidural anesthesia**, because the anesthetic is injected into the space between the dura mater and the surrounding bone. *Epidurals* have the advantage of decreasing the perception of pain without having to anesthetize the brain. By not anesthetizing the brainstem and diencephalon, the body can more readily maintain its normal autonomic function during this type of anesthesia.

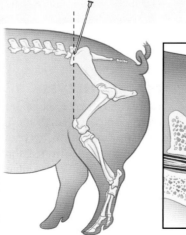
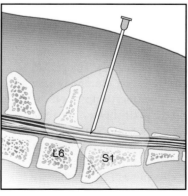

Needle placement for epidural anesthesia in the pig. L6 is the sixth lumbar vertebra, and S1 is the first sacral vertebra. (Redrawn from William WM, III, Hubbell J: Handbook of veterinary anesthesia, ed 5, St Louis, 2013, Mosby.)

## CLINICAL APPLICATION

### Myelogram

We can use the spaces between the meninges in veterinary medicine when an animal is suspected of having spinal trauma due to intervertebral disc disease. For example, Dachshunds often suffer from rupture of intervertebral discs, so-called *slipped discs,* between the cranial lumbar vertebrae and/or caudal thoracic vertebrae. The rupture of an intervertebral disc forces the gelatinous material inside the disc through the fibrous ring of the disc dorsally, where it presses on the spinal cord. The pressure exerted by the gelatinous material compresses, or closes off, the space between the meninges on the ventral side (the underside) of the spinal cord at the point of disc rupture. To identify the existence of this material pushing up against the spinal cord, we can inject a radiopaque dye—a dye that shows up white on x-rays—into the subarachnoid space in the spinal cord, which is the space just beneath the arachnoid membrane. The subsequent radiograph will show places along the spinal cord where the dye did not flow. These areas are where the gelatinous disc material is pressing against the spinal cord and causing damage. This procedure is a form of **contrast radiography** called **myelography.**

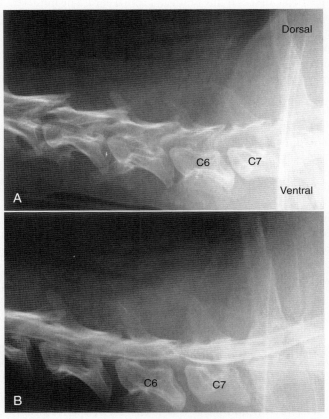

**A,** Plain radiograph. Cervical region of a 6-year-old Doberman Pinscher with a sudden onset of stumbling and weakness in the rear limbs, and mild cervical pain. **B,** Myelogram. The addition of the white-appearing myelography contrast media shows the normal smooth line of the spinal cord being compressed from the ventral side at the junction of vertebrae C6 and C7. Surgery revealed a large amount of ruptured disc material ventral to the spinal cord at this site. (From Nelson R, Couto C: Small animal internal medicine, ed 4, St Louis, 2009, Mosby.)

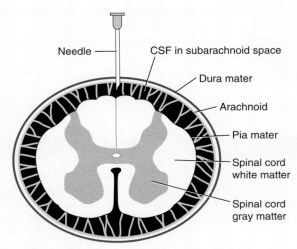

Transverse section showing the relationship among the meninges, the cerebrospinal fluid (CSF), and the spinal cord. The tip of the needle is in the subarachnoid space, as it would be for myelography. (Redrawn from Nelson R, Couto C: Small animal internal medicine, ed 4, St Louis, 2009, Mosby.)

insects and parasites but, at the proper dose, does not adversely affect the dogs and cats that receive it. The reason for this *selective toxicity* of ivermectin is that mammals have a blood–brain barrier that prevents ivermectin from reaching target receptors on cells within the brain; however, insects and parasites do not have such a barrier, so the ivermectin can readily reach target receptors throughout the nervous system.

The blood–brain barrier can also prevent drugs that we administer from penetrating into the brain. If we want to treat an infection in the brain, for example, we must choose an antibiotic that is capable of crossing the blood–brain barrier and reaching the site of the infection.

### CRANIAL NERVES

Cranial nerves are a special set of 12 nerve pairs in the peripheral nervous system that originate directly from the brain. Each pair of cranial nerves is conventionally numbered in Roman numerals from I through XII (1 through 12). The cranial nerve itself may contain axons of motor neurons, axons of sensory neurons, or combinations of both. Cranial nerve I (CN I, olfactory nerve) and cranial nerve II (CN II, optic nerve) are both examples of pure *sensory* cranial nerves. The olfactory nerve is responsible for conveying sensory impulses from receptors in the nose to the brain for the sense of smell, and the optic nerve is responsible for perception of light and vision. Unlike CN I and CN II, CN III is the oculomotor nerve and, as the name implies, it is a *motor* cranial nerve that controls eye movement. Other cranial nerves include CN V (trigeminal nerve), which controls muscles of the jaw for chewing and also conveys sensations from the nose, mouth, and part of the throat. Thus, CN V is an example of a cranial nerve that serves both sensory and motor functions. See Table 9-1 for a list of the different functions of the 12 cranial nerves.

Table 9-2 shows two mnemonic devices (memory aids) that can be used for remembering the names of the cranial

nerves and their functions (sensory, motor, or both). In the first mnemonic, each word of the saying begins with the same letter as the corresponding cranial nerve. Of course, you have to remember which O represents which cranial nerve in the first three cranial nerves, but the saying still helps students remember the names of the cranial nerves more readily.

The second mnemonic tells whether the cranial nerve in question is a sensory nerve, a motor nerve, or both sensory and motor. In the saying, the words beginning with *S* indicate that the corresponding nerve is primarily sensory. If the word begins with *M*, the corresponding nerve is primarily a motor nerve; and if the word begins with *B*, the nerve is both sensory and motor.

## SPINAL CORD

The spinal cord is the caudal continuation of the brainstem outside the skull that continues down the bony spinal canal formed by the vertebrae. It conducts sensory information and motor instructions between the brain and the periphery of the body, but it is not simply a "cable" of nerve fibers. It

---

✔ **TEST YOURSELF 9-6**

1. What are the protective membranes that surround, support, and protect the CNS?
2. What is the fluid called that bathes, cushions, and aids in transport of materials to and from the CNS?
3. What helps keep dangerous poisons and certain drugs from leaving the blood and entering the brain? Describe this structure.
4. What are the 12 cranial nerves? Which nerves are motor, which are sensory, and which are both?

---

| TABLE 9-1 | Functions of the 12 Cranial Nerves | | | |
|---|---|---|---|---|
| **NUMBER** | **NAME** | **TYPE** | **KEY FUNCTIONS** | |
| I | Olfactory | Sensory | Smell | |
| II | Optic | Sensory | Vision | |
| III | Oculomotor | Motor | Eye movement, pupil size, focusing lens | |
| IV | Trochlear | Motor | Eye movement | |
| V | Trigeminal | Both sensory and motor | Sensations from the head and teeth, chewing | |
| VI | Abducent | Motor | Eye movement | |
| VII | Facial | Both sensory and motor | Face and scalp movement, salivation, tears, taste | |
| VIII | Vestibulocochlear | Sensory | Balance, hearing | |
| IX | Glossopharyngeal | Both sensory and motor | Tongue movement, swallowing, salivation, taste | |
| X | Vagus (*wanderer*) | Both sensory and motor | Sensory from gastrointestinal tract and respiratory tree; motor to the larynx, pharynx, parasympathetic; motor to the abdominal and thoracic organs | |
| XI | Accessory | Motor | Head movement, accessory motor with vagus | |
| XII | Hypoglossal | Motor | Tongue movement | |

---

| TABLE 9-2 | Mnemonic Devices for Cranial Nerve Names and Functions | | | |
|---|---|---|---|---|
| **CRANIAL NERVE** | **NERVE NAME** | **WORD OF THE SAYING** | **TYPE OF NERVE** | **WORD OF THE SAYING** |
| I | Olfactory | On | Sensory | Six |
| II | Optic | old | Sensory | sailors |
| III | Oculomotor | Olympus' | Motor | made |
| IV | Trochlear | towering | Motor | merry, |
| V | Trigeminal | top, | Both sensory and motor | but |
| VI | Abducent | a | Motor | my |
| VII | Facial | fine, | Both sensory and motor | brother |
| VIII | Vestibulocochlear | vocal | Sensory | said, |
| IX | Glossopharyngeal | German | Both sensory and motor | "Bad |
| X | Vagus | viewed | Both sensory and motor | business, |
| XI | Spinal accessory | some | Motor | my |
| XII | Hypoglossal | hops | Motor | man" |

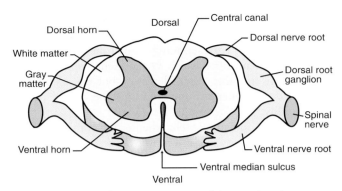

**FIGURE 9-11** Cross section of the spinal cord.

contains many neuron cell bodies (in the gray matter) and extensive synapses (connections) between ascending nerve fibers conducting sensory information toward the brain and descending nerve fibers conducting motor information to muscles and other organs. A considerable amount of processing and modification of nerve impulses between the brain and the peripheral nerves takes place in the spinal cord. This is important to remember when we are trying to prevent or treat severe pain in our patients. (See the Clinical Application on Preventing Windup in Chapter 10.)

The positions of the gray matter and white matter of the spinal cord are reversed from the arrangement in the cerebrum and cerebellum of the brain. In cross section (Figure 9-11), the gray matter of the spinal cord is located in the medulla (inner part) and takes the shape of a butterfly with the CSF-containing **central canal running its length** in the center. The white matter of the spinal cord forms the cortex (outer part) that surrounds the gray matter. As in the brain, the gray matter contains many neuron cell bodies, and the white matter consists mainly of myelinated nerve fibers.

Between each pair of adjacent vertebrae, the spinal cord sends off dorsal and ventral nerve roots from each side that combine to form left and right spinal nerves; these link the spinal cord with peripheral nerves. The **dorsal nerve roots** contain sensory (afferent) fibers, and the **ventral nerve roots** contain motor (efferent) fibers. So, sensory information comes into the spinal cord via the dorsal nerve roots, and motor instructions go out to the body via the ventral nerve roots. The neurons that process and carry sensory (afferent) nerve impulses to the brain or other parts of the spinal cord are located in what are called the **dorsal horns** of the spinal cord's gray matter "butterfly" (see Figure 9-11). The neurons that process and carry motor (efferent) nerve impulses to the spinal nerves are located in the **ventral horns** of the gray matter.

## THE AUTONOMIC NERVOUS SYSTEM

As mentioned previously, the autonomic nervous system controls many functions of the body at a subconscious level. These automatic functions are performed by two divisions of the autonomic nervous system: the **sympathetic nervous system** and the **parasympathetic nervous system**. These two systems generally have opposite effects on organs or tissues, and whichever system dominates at any given moment determines how excited or relaxed things are in the body.

## STRUCTURE

The first anatomic difference between these two systems is where the peripheral nerves of each system emerge from the CNS. The nerves for the sympathetic nervous system emerge from the thoracic and lumbar vertebral regions in the back. Thus, the sympathetic system is often referred to as the **thoracolumbar system**. In contrast, the parasympathetic system emerges from the brain and the sacral vertebral regions and therefore is called the **cranial–sacral system**.

The efferent motor nerves of both the sympathetic and parasympathetic nervous systems are composed of a sequence of two neurons. The first neuron has its cell body in the brain or spinal cord and extends its axon out from the CNS to a cluster of neuronal cell bodies outside of the CNS called an autonomic **ganglion**. Here the first neuron synapses with one or more second neurons, which then connect to the target organ (e.g., endocrine gland, smooth muscle). The first neuron is called the **preganglionic neuron**, because it is before the ganglion. The second neuron is the **postganglionic neuron**, because it carries the impulse from the ganglia to the target organ.

The sympathetic and parasympathetic systems also differ anatomically in the length of the preganglionic and postganglionic neurons (Figure 9-12). The sympathetic preganglionic neuron originates in the thoracic and lumbar segments of the spinal column. Outside the thoracolumbar area of the spinal column are a series of autonomic ganglia (many ganglions) that form a chain called the **sympathetic ganglion chain**. The sympathetic preganglionic neuron extends out from the spinal cord and either synapses with a neuron within the ganglion chain or passes through the ganglionic chain and synapses with a neuron located beyond the sympathetic chain. Each sympathetic preganglionic neuron usually synapses with many postganglionic neurons in a wide variety of locations in the sympathetic chain or in ganglia outside the sympathetic chain. This helps explain why sympathetic nervous system responses are usually spread throughout the body and involve several organs simultaneously.

The sympathetic postganglionic neuron extends the remaining distance to the target organ. Therefore, the sympathetic postganglionic neuron is much longer than its corresponding preganglionic neuron.

Unlike the short sympathetic preganglionic neuron, the parasympathetic preganglionic neuron is quite long and originates from the **nuclei** (clusters of neurons in the brain) of several cranial nerves and from the sacral region of the spinal cord. Thus the parasympathetic system is called the *cranial–sacral division* of the autonomic nervous system.

In contrast to the sympathetic preganglionic neuron, which terminates close to the spinal cord, the parasympathetic preganglionic neuron travels directly from the

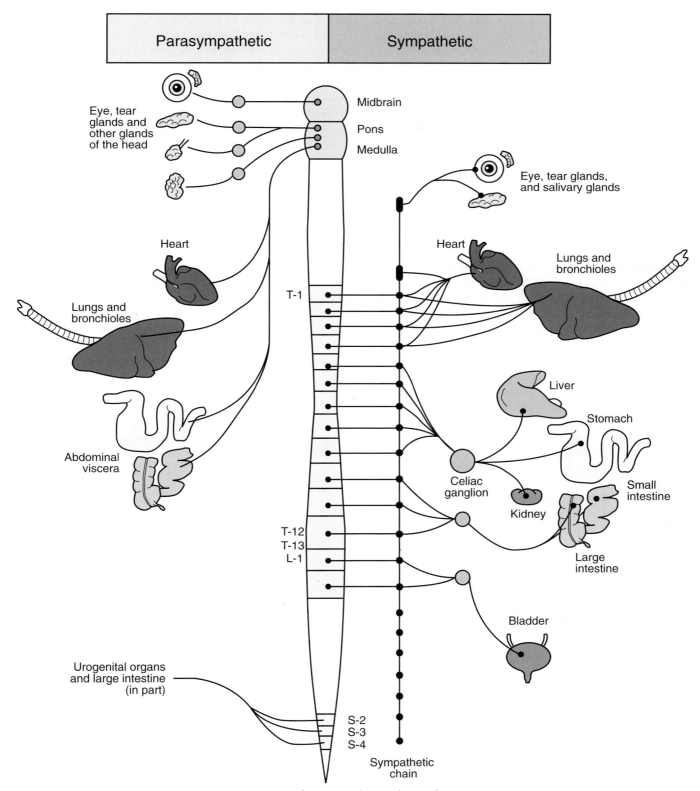

**FIGURE 9-12** Structure of parasympathetic and sympathetic nervous systems.

CNS to its target organ, where it synapses with a short post-ganglionic neuron in the target organ. Thus the parasympathetic preganglionic neuron is relatively long compared with the short postganglionic neuron.

## GENERAL FUNCTIONS

The sympathetic nervous system is often called the *fight-or-flight system,* meaning that this is the system that helps the body cope with emergency situations in which an animal might have to defend itself (fight) or escape (flight). In contrast, the parasympathetic nervous system could be called the *rest-and-restore system* because of its ability to decrease the strong excitatory effects of the fight-or-flight system (bring the body back to resting state) and its ability to facilitate all the processes that will replace those body resources used up during the emergency (restore).

Using this simple model of fight or flight or rest and restore, we can make sense of the clinical signs observed with stimulation of either part of the autonomic nervous system. Table 9-3 summarizes these effects. In a fight-or-flight situation, the animal needs to move rapidly, therefore the muscles are going to be working vigorously. To meet the needs of the muscles, the bronchioles (airway passages) increase in diameter *(bronchodilation)* to allow a greater exchange of oxygen and carbon dioxide. Once the oxygen leaves the lungs and enters the blood, it must be delivered rapidly. Therefore heart rate and the force of cardiac contractions increase, which increases the rate at which blood is moved around the body. Finally, to deliver more blood into the working muscles, the small blood vessels (arterioles) supplying the muscles dilate *(vasodilation).*

In contrast to the dilation of skeletal muscle blood vessels under sympathetic stimulation, the small blood vessels supplying the skin, gastrointestinal tract (GI tract), and the kidney constrict, thereby reducing blood flow to these areas so that blood can be redirected to the muscles. During this time, when blood is redirected away from these organs, the digestive and absorptive functions of the GI tract and the filtering function of the kidney are temporarily suspended or decreased until the crisis passes. The decreased blood supply to the skin also means that superficial wounds will bleed less.

Why would eye pupil dilation be of benefit to an animal in a fight-or-flight situation? Opening up the pupil admits more light, but an additional benefit may be an increase in peripheral vision (you can see more "out of the corner of the eye"). Thus the sympathetic nervous system may allow the animal to take in a wider field of vision and see better under low-light conditions.

It's pretty easy to see how the parasympathetic nervous system antagonizes (works against) many but not all of the sympathetic nervous system effects. The parasympathetic system causes the GI tract to increase its activity, thus digesting and absorbing nutrients that are needed to replenish the energy resources used during the fight-or-flight situation. The parasympathetic system also reduces the heart rate and reduces the sympathetic system's dilation of the bronchioles. Except for the GI tract, the parasympathetic system has little effect on the blood vessels in most parts of the body, so the return to normal vessel diameter is handled by other regulatory mechanism.

## TABLE 9-3    Effects of Sympathetic and Parasympathetic Nervous Systems

|  | SYMPATHETIC SYSTEM EFFECT | PARASYMPATHETIC SYSTEM EFFECT |
|---|---|---|
| Heart rate | Increases | Decreases |
| Force of heart contraction | Increases | No significant effect |
| Diameter of bronchioles | Increases (dilates) | Decreases (constricts) |
| Diameter of pupil | Increases (dilates) | Decreases (constricts) |
| Gastrointestinal motility, secretions, and blood flow | Decreases | Increases |
| Diameter of skin blood vessels | Decreases | No significant effect |
| Diameter of muscle blood vessels | Increases | No significant effect |
| Diameter of blood vessels to kidney | Decreases | No significant effect |

### 🔍 CLINICAL APPLICATION

#### The Sympathetic Nervous System Response to Shock or Blood Loss

One of the key roles of the sympathetic nervous system is to maintain arterial blood pressure. The arterial blood pressure can drop to a point where the brain may not be receiving adequate blood flow in situations involving a loss of blood volume; a loss of fluid in the blood, as with dehydration; or a large-scale dilation of blood vessels throughout the body, as in the case of shock. The body responds to this loss of arterial blood pressure by causing massive stimulation of the sympathetic nervous system. The heart pounds rapidly and fiercely in the chest to increase the output of blood into the arteries; simultaneously, the small blood vessels, or arterioles, in the skin, GI tract, kidney, and other areas constrict. The increased cardiac output and arteriole vasoconstriction result in an increased arterial blood pressure and more blood directed to the brain.

The increase in blood arterial pressure from the increased cardiac output and vasoconstriction would be like the increase in air pressure within a rubber tube if you blew forcefully into the tube while simultaneously pinching the far end. The narrowing of the small blood vessels supplying the skin also explains why the skin and mucous membranes of people or animals with a sudden decrease in blood pressure appear so pale.

Drugs or diseases that imitate, stimulate, or inhibit either the parasympathetic or sympathetic nervous system produce physiologic changes that mimic one of these branches of the autonomic system. Therefore the veterinary professional should know how and why the sympathetic and parasympathetic nervous systems affect the body.

## NEUROTRANSMITTERS AND RECEPTORS

The sympathetic nervous system primarily uses norepinephrine as its neurotransmitter. As stated previously, norepinephrine, epinephrine, and dopamine are all part of a group of neurotransmitters and hormones called *catecholamines.* Because epinephrine and norepinephrine used to be called *adrenaline* and *noradrenaline,* respectively, the neurons that release norepinephrine are said to be **adrenergic** neurons. *Note:* The terms adrenaline and noradrenaline are still used in some countries. In addition to the release of norepinephrine from postganglionic adrenergic neurons, the body's sympathetic response also comes from the release of epinephrine and norepinephrine from the medulla (inner part) of the adrenal gland. The adrenal medulla acts like a cluster of adrenergic neurons releasing the epinephrine and norepinephrine directly into the bloodstream, where they are quickly distributed to receptors throughout the body.

Neurotransmitters can only work on cells that contain specific receptors capable of binding to the particular neurotransmitter molecules. So, blood vessels in the skin, the GI tract, and the skeletal muscle must have adrenergic receptors for epinephrine or norepinephrine. What we find is that there are actually different types of adrenergic receptors in the tissues or organs affected by the sympathetic nervous system. **Alpha$_1$-adrenergic receptors** typically are found on blood vessels and cause the vasoconstriction of the skin, GI tract, and kidney associated with sympathetic stimulation. The increases in heart rate and force of contraction are the result of stimulation of **beta$_1$-adrenergic receptors**, and the bronchodilation associated with sympathetic stimulation results from **beta$_2$-adrenergic receptor** stimulation.

The effects and side effects of drugs that mimic the sympathetic nervous system can be explained by the specificity (selectiveness) of the drug molecule for alpha$_1$, beta$_1$, or beta$_2$ receptors. Therefore it is important for the veterinary professional to remember the different adrenergic receptors and the organs or tissues with which they are associated.

The neurons associated with the parasympathetic nervous system secrete acetylcholine as their neurotransmitter. Therefore these neurons often are referred to as **cholinergic neurons.** Even though norepinephrine is the neurotransmitter associated with sympathetic nervous system effects, the preganglionic neuron (the neuron that emerges from the CNS and synapses with the postganglionic neuron) in both the sympathetic and parasympathetic nervous system is a cholinergic neuron that releases acetylcholine. That may seem a little strange, but remember the ultimate effect of the sympathetic and parasympathetic systems is determined by their postganglionic neurons.

Like the adrenergic receptors of the sympathetic nervous system, the **cholinergic receptors** for acetylcholine also come in different types. The two types of acetylcholine receptor are called *nicotinic* and *muscarinic.* The **nicotinic**

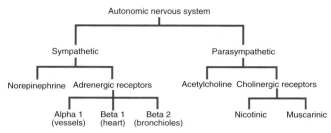

**FIGURE 9-13** Simplified concept map for the autonomic nervous system.

**receptors** are found primarily on the postganglionic neurons of both the sympathetic and parasympathetic nervous system, as well as between motor neurons and muscle in the somatic (voluntary) motor system (Figure 9-13). The **muscarinic receptors** are found on the target organs and tissues supplied by the postganglionic neurons of the parasympathetic nervous system. Certain toxins (e.g., nicotine or plants containing nicotine-like compounds) may selectively stimulate the nicotinic receptors more than the muscarinic receptors, whereas others may selectively affect the muscarinic receptors. The clinical signs of the toxicities reflect which receptors have been stimulated.

---

> ✓ *TEST YOURSELF 9-7*
>
> 1. Which part of the autonomic nervous system is responsible for the fight-or-flight response and which is responsible for the rest-and-restore system?
> 2. Compare and contrast the sympathetic and parasympathetic nervous systems. Include in your comparison the preganglionic and postganglionic neurons; the origin of preganglionic neurons; the neurotransmitters; and each system's impact on the heart, GI tract, blood vessels, bronchiole diameters, and the size of the pupil of the eye.
> 3. With which branch of the autonomic nervous system are the alpha$_1$, beta$_1$, and beta$_2$ receptors associated? What happens to the body when these particular receptors are stimulated?
> 4. With which branch of the autonomic nervous system are muscarinic and nicotinic receptors associated?

---

## REFLEXES AND THE REFLEX ARC

Reflexes are rapid, automatic responses to stimuli designed to protect the body and maintain homeostasis. Reflexes can be **somatic reflexes**, which involve contraction of skeletal muscles, or **autonomic reflexes**, which regulate smooth muscle, cardiac muscle, and endocrine glands.

Regardless of whether the reflex is somatic or autonomic, all reflexes have the same basic structure, called the **reflex arc**. The reflex arc originates from a sensory receptor, which detects a change either in the external environment or within the body itself. Once stimulated to threshold, the sensory receptor sends an action potential (nerve impulse) along the **sensory neuron** to the gray matter of the spinal cord or brainstem. In the CNS gray matter, the sensory neuron synapses with other **interneurons**, which serve to integrate the incoming sensory impulse with other impulses from other sensory neurons. Finally, the integrated response of the reflex is sent out from the spinal cord or brainstem by the **motor neuron**, which ends at the target organ (muscle or endocrine gland). If the motor neuron is a somatic neuron, the reflex arc ends in contraction or inhibition of skeletal muscle. If it is an autonomic neuron, the reflex arc ends in smooth muscle within an organ or blood vessel, cardiac muscle, or endocrine gland.

Stimulation of skeletal muscle (somatic) reflex arcs is commonly used in veterinary medicine to aid in the diagnosis of spinal cord trauma, peripheral nerve damage, or muscle disease. Various types of somatic reflex are evaluated by the veterinarian, including the *stretch reflex,* the *withdrawal reflex,* and the *extensor reflex.* Understanding how these somatic reflex arcs function and are regulated is important for comprehending how normal and abnormal reflexes can indicate disease or damage in the nervous system or musculoskeletal system.

## STRETCH REFLEX

The **stretch reflex** is considered a simple, *monosynaptic* or two-neuron reflex arc, because it involves only a sensory neuron and a motor neuron (with only one synapse between them) without any interneurons (Figure 9-14). The sensory receptor in the stretch reflex arc is a specialized structure within the muscle called the **muscle spindle**. If a muscle is stretched, the muscle spindle also stretches and sends impulses via the somatic sensory neuron to the spinal cord. At the spinal cord, the sensory neuron synapses with the motor neuron that innervates the *same* muscle. Stimulation of the motor neuron causes that muscle to contract in response to the stretching of the muscle. In this way, the body can maintain the tension or tone of a muscle to meet an increased force applied to stretch the muscle, or it can prevent an overstretching of a muscle caused by contraction of opposing muscles.

You may have had this reflex tested in your own doctor's office, when your patellar ligament (located just below your kneecap) was tapped. In this situation, the force against the ligament slightly stretched the large quadriceps femoris muscle on your thigh, stimulating a reflex arc that resulted in contraction of the quadriceps and the subsequent extension—a slight kick—of the lower leg.

When stimulated by the stretch receptor, the afferent somatic sensory neuron from the muscle spindle does more than just cause the stretched muscle to contract. Branches off the sensory neuron will synapse with another reflex arc to cause the opposing muscles to relax. Therefore, when the stretch receptor in your quadriceps femoris muscle initiated the stretch reflex arc, a branch of the sensory neuron also synapsed with an *inhibitory* interneuron in the spinal cord. This inhibitory interneuron released inhibitory neurotransmitters at a synapse with the motor neuron to the semimembranosus and semitendinosus (hamstring) muscles, the muscles that normally oppose the quadriceps femoris muscle. By inhibiting stimulation of these opposing muscles, the quadriceps femoris muscle could contract without *antagonism,* or without being worked against by the opposing muscle.

Finally, another branch off the stretch receptor's sensory neuron enters the spinal cord and goes up to the brain so that the cerebellum can coordinate the movement and the conscious sensory centers in the cerebral cortex can be informed of the stimulation and subsequent limb movement. *Note:* The patellar tap reflex is a pure reflex that cannot be overridden by conscious effort. Even if you tighten up your leg muscles and do your best not to kick when the patellar ligament is tapped, you cannot completely prevent that kick from occurring.

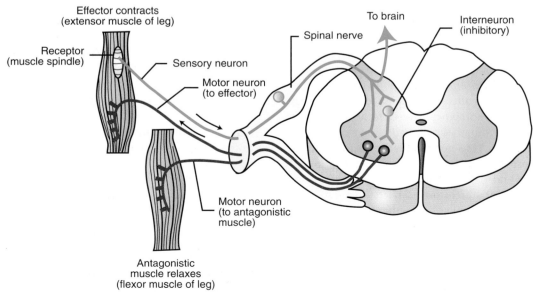

**FIGURE 9-14** Basic reflex arc as illustrated by simple stretch reflex.

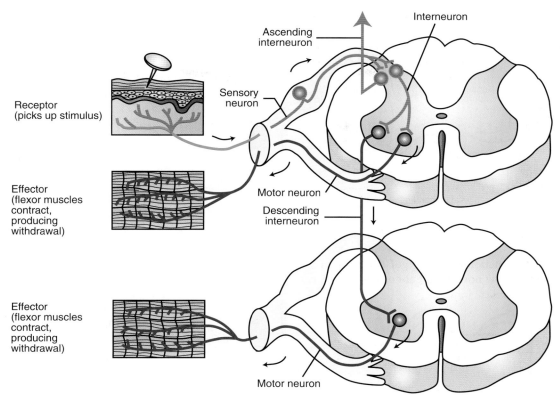

**FIGURE 9-15** Flexor (withdrawal) reflex. The reflex arc involves several spinal segments. Some branches of the spinal reflex arc extend to motor nerves in other spinal segments, resulting in relatively complex reflex movement.

## WITHDRAWAL REFLEX

The **withdrawal reflex**, also called the *flexor reflex,* happens when you rapidly withdraw a limb or flex the joints after accidentally touching a hot stove or stepping on a sharp object with your bare foot (Figure 9-15). In both of these situations, a strong stimulus to a receptor causes the sensory somatic neuron to send impulses to the spinal cord. Unlike the simpler stretch reflex, the withdrawal reflex involves synapses with several interneurons. Some of these interneurons will synapse with motor neurons that will cause contraction of a specific set of muscles responsible for pulling the limb away from the painful stimulus. Other interneurons will inhibit those opposing muscle groups so that the withdrawal of the limb is rapid and complete. This reflex can be complicated, because many different muscles may be involved in the withdrawal from the painful stimulus.

Even though the reflex arc may involve several interneurons, several motor neurons, and several different segments of the spinal cord, the reflex occurs without the brain being aware of the incident. In other words, the limb has been withdrawn from the painful stimulus before the brain becomes consciously aware of the painful stimulus.

## CROSSED EXTENSOR REFLEX

If you step on a sharp tack, which results in the leg being withdrawn rapidly before the brain is aware of what is going on, you should fall over. The reason you don't is that when the withdrawal reflex arc is stimulated, the afferent somatic sensory neuron also synapses with another set of interneurons that cause extensor muscles in the opposite leg to contract and support the full weight of your body when the other leg flexes. This reflex is called the **crossed extensor reflex**, because the afferent sensory impulse crosses to the other side of the spinal cord and stimulates the muscles that extend the opposite limb (Figure 9-16).

Reflexes that start on one side and travel to the opposite side of the body are said to be **contralateral reflexes**; the crossed extensor reflex is one example. Reflexes like the stretch reflex are called **ipsilateral reflexes**, because the stimulus and response are on the same side of the body. The veterinary technician needs to be familiar with the terms *contralateral* and *ipsilateral* because they are used for a variety of applications in veterinary medicine and do not pertain only to reflexes.

## THE ROLE OF THE UPPER CNS IN MODERATING REFLEXES

An animal with severe spinal cord damage in the area of the first or second lumbar vertebrae (L1 or L2) can still have reflexes in the hind limbs. Even though sensory impulses from the hind limbs are blocked from reaching the brain, and conscious motor impulses from the brain to the hind limbs are blocked by the damaged section of the spinal cord, the reflex arcs in the lumbar spinal cord segments caudal to

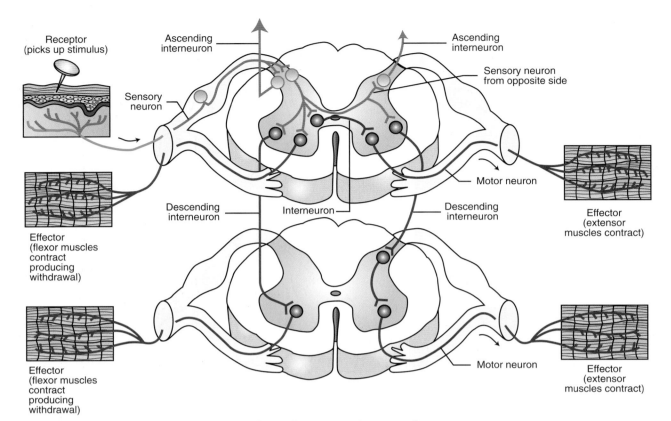

**FIGURE 9-16** Crossed extensor reflex.

the trauma are still intact and can still function. The animal, however, is unaware that the hind limbs are moving, because it cannot receive any sensory information as a result of the spinal cord damage at L1 to L2.

Not only are the reflex arcs functioning in the hind limbs despite the damage to the spinal cord at L1 to L2, but the reflex responses are **hyperreflexive**. This means when the veterinarian taps on the patellar ligament, the quadriceps muscles contract with more force and produce more limb movement than normal. This illustrates an important concept used by veterinarians to diagnose location of spinal cord injuries. The upper CNS normally produces a dampening or inhibitory effect on the reflex arcs. Thus, under normal conditions, the patellar ligament stretching usually only produces a relatively small kick because of the dampening effect of the upper CNS. With spinal cord trauma, this dampening effect from the upper CNS is blocked, and any intact reflex arcs caudal to the spinal cord trauma are now exaggerated, or *hyperreflexive.*

If spinal cord trauma occurs where the reflex arc enters or leaves the spinal cord, or if the sensory nerve or motor nerve of the reflex arc is damaged, the reflex will be less than normal (**hyporeflexive**) or absent altogether. In other words, if the arc is damaged or broken anywhere, the reflex will either not function, or it will function weakly.

By stimulating different somatic reflex arcs, knowing through which spinal cord segments the reflex arc travels, and observing whether the response is normal,

hyperreflexive, or hyporeflexive, the veterinarian can localize the area of the spinal cord in which trauma or disease has occurred.

## OTHER CLINICALLY SIGNIFICANT REFLEXES

Many reflexes are used to assess the clinical condition of patients in veterinary medicine. Most are complex reflexes relating to posture, gait, the animal's ability to right itself, and the placement of limbs. Two other reflexes that the veterinary technician should understand are the **palpebral reflex** and the **pupillary light reflex (PLR)**. These two reflexes are routinely used when assessing an animal for depth of anesthesia and when performing a physical examination.

The palpebral reflex arc originates from receptors on the eyelid margins, travels via sensory neurons in CN V to the pons (brainstem), synapses with neurons in the pons, then travels via CN VII to the muscles that blink the eyelids. If the reflex is active, a light tap on the medial canthus of the eye (the medial corner of the eye, where the top and bottom eyelids meet) produces a blink of the eyelids. When an animal is anesthetized, the neurons in the pons become less responsive. Therefore, as anesthesia deepens, the palpebral reflex (also called the *palpebral blink reflex*) becomes less responsive and provides an indication of the animal's depth of anesthesia.

The PLR is a test for a reflex arc that includes the retina (light-sensing layer of the eye), the optic nerve (CN II), neuron clusters in the diencephalon of the brain, and motor neurons of CN III (which supply the muscle of the iris that constricts the size of the pupil). A normal response to shining light in the eye of an animal is for the iris in *both* eyes to constrict, thus making the pupil smaller. Normally, this pupillary constriction would reduce the amount of light entering the eye and protect the retina against bright light. Because shining the light in one eye causes a constriction in both eyes, the reflex arc must cross over to the other side of the body. By examining the PLRs in both eyes, a veterinarian can evaluate each reflex arc and identify whether an animal has a visual problem in the retina, the optic nerve, or the motor nerve. Note that the PLR does *not* assess vision. An animal with damage to the visual centers in the cerebral cortex can be blind and still have normal PLRs in both eyes.

## CLINICAL APPLICATION

### Dachshund With Intervertebral Disc Disease

Gretchen was an 8-year-old, spayed, female Miniature Dachshund brought in when it became apparent that she was suddenly unable to move her hind legs. On examination, the veterinarian observed that Gretchen could not stand on her rear legs and did not yelp when the skin on her rear toes was pinched. She did, however, react to firm squeezing of the toes themselves. The veterinarian concluded that spinal cord trauma was interfering with the sensory impulses reaching the brain and with conscious motor impulses from the brain reaching the muscles of the hind limb.

Given the history and Gretchen's breed, spinal trauma from the rupture of an intervertebral disc seemed the most likely cause. In these situations, the material from the disc between vertebrae can rupture forcibly against the adjacent spinal cord, producing severe trauma and swelling that renders the spinal cord at that segment nonfunctional.

Before ordering radiographs, the veterinarian must localize the area of the spinal cord where the trauma is most likely to have occurred. In this way, the radiograph can be focused directly over the suspected site with the vertebrae lined up to allow a better view of disc material in the spinal canal and any narrowing of the affected disc space.

Gretchen's veterinarian tested some somatic reflexes—withdrawal and crossed extensor among them—in the hind limb and determined that the reflexes that travel through segments of spinal cord caudal to L3 were all hyperreflexive. This indicated that the reflex arcs were functional but were not being dampened by the upper CNS. Therefore the veterinarian could conclude that these spinal cord segments were caudal to the spinal cord trauma. The reflex arcs that traveled through L1, L2, and L3 were all hyporeflexive or nonexistent. The reflex arcs at these spinal cord segments were broken because of the trauma to the spinal cord segments. The reflexes that involved spinal cord segments cranial to T13 were normal, so these spinal cord segments were unaffected and still had communication with the upper CNS.

The veterinarian ordered the radiographs centered over L2 on Gretchen. The radiographs indicated narrowed disc space between vertebrae L1 and L2. Because Gretchen's owner rushed her in quickly, the veterinarian could arrange emergency surgery to relieve the pressure on the spinal cord by removing part of the vertebral bone over the affected areas. Gretchen slowly recovered over several days, until she could walk with 90% of her normal strength and control.

## TEST YOURSELF 9-8

1. What are the differences between an autonomic reflex and a somatic reflex?
2. What roles do the sensory receptor, sensory neuron, interneuron, and motor neuron play in the reflex arc?
3. What is the sensory receptor in the stretch reflex? What results from the stretch reflex arc stimulation? Is this an ipsilateral or contralateral reflex?
4. What happens in a withdrawal reflex? Is this reflex more or less complex than the stretch reflex?
5. How is the crossed extensor reflex tied in with the withdrawal reflex? Is the crossed extensor reflex an ipsilateral or contralateral reflex?
6. What is the role of the upper CNS in the reflex arc? If the CNS influence is removed or blocked, do reflexes become hyporeflexive or hyperreflexive?
7. If trauma occurs in the segment of the spinal cord through which a particular reflex arc passes, will the reflex arc be hyperreflexive or hyporeflexive?
8. What is the palpebral reflex? How is it used in veterinary medicine?
9. What is the result of a normal PLR?

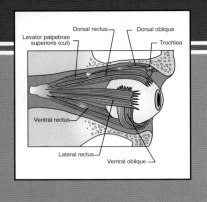

Levator palpebrae superioris (cut), Dorsal rectus, Dorsal oblique, Trochlea, Ventral rectus, Lateral rectus, Ventral oblique

# Sense Organs  10

*Thomas Colville*

## OUTLINE

## LEARNING OBJECTIVES

*When you have completed this chapter you will be able to:*

1. List the four general types of stimulus that can trigger a response from sensory receptors.
2. List and describe the visceral senses.
3. Differentiate between superficial and central temperature sensors.
4. List and describe the processes that contribute to nociception.
5. Describe the structure of the taste buds.
6. List and describe the special senses.
7. Describe the structure and function of the components of the ear.
8. Describe the processes that contribute to the sense of equilibrium.
9. Describe the structure and function of the components of the eyeball.
10. Describe the structure of the conjunctiva and eyelids.
11. Describe the origin of tears and explain how tears flow onto and drain from the eye.

## VOCABULARY FUNDAMENTALS

*Accommodation* uh-kohm-uh-**dā**-shuhn
*Ampulla* ahm-**pyoo**-luh
*Analgesia* ahn-ahl-**jē**-zhuh
*Anesthesia* ahn-uhs-**thē**-zhuh
*Anterior chamber* ahn-**teer**-ē-ər **chām**-bər
*Aqueous compartment* ā-kwē-uhs kuhm-**pahrt**-mehnt
*Aqueous humor* ā-kwē-uhs **hyoo**-mər
*Bulbar conjunctiva* **buhl**-bər kohn-**juhnck**-tih-vah
*Canal of Schlemm* kuh-**nahl** *of* shlehm
*Canthus* **kahn**-thuhs
*Choroid* **kohr**-oyd
*Ciliary body* sihl-ē-ahr-ē **boh**-dē
*Ciliary muscle* sihl-ē-ahr-ē **muhs**-uhl
*Cochlea* **kōk**-lē-ah
*Cochlear duct* **kōk**-lē-ahr duhckt
*Cone* kōn
*Conjunctiva* kohn-**juhnck**-tih-vah
*Conjunctival sac* kohn-**juhnck**-tih-vahl sahck
*Cornea* **kohr**-nē-uh
*Crista* **krihs**-tuh

*Cupula* **kuh**-pū-luh
*Eardrum* **ēr**-druhm
*Endolymph* **ehn**-dō-lihmf
*Equilibrium* ē-kwuh-**lihb**-rē-uhm
*Eustachian tube* yoo-**stā**-shehn toob
*External auditory canal* ehcks-**tər**-nahl **ahw**-dih-tohr-ē kuh-**nahl**
*External ear* ehcks-**tər**-nahl ēr
*Extraocular eye muscle* ehcks-trah-**ah**-kyoo-lahr ī **muhs**-uhl
*Eyelid* **ī**-lihd
*Fundus* **fuhn**-duhs
*General anesthesia* jehn-ər-ahl ahn-uhs-**thē**-zhuh
*General sense* jehn-ər-ahl sehns
*Gustatory sense* **guhs**-tuh-tohr-ē sehns
*Hearing* **hihr**-ihng
*Heatstroke* **hēt**-strōk
*Hyperthermia* hī-pər-**thuhr**-mē-uh
*Hypothermia* hī-pō-**thuhr**-mē-uh
*Incus* **ihn**-kuhs

*Inner ear* **ihn**-ər ēr
*Lacrimal apparatus* **lah**-kreh-mahl ahp-uh-**raht**-uhs
*Lacrimal gland* **lah**-kreh-mahl glahnd
*Lacrimal puncta* **lah**-kreh-mahl **puhngk**-tuh
*Limbus* **lihm**-buhs
*Local anesthesia* **lō**-kuhl ahn-uhs-**thē**-zhuh
*Macula* **mahck**-ū-lah
*Malleus* **mahl**-ē-uhs
*Meibomian gland* mih-**bō**-mē-ahn glahnd
*Middle ear* **mihd**-uhl ēr
*Modulation* **mohd**-ū-lā-shuhn
*Nasolacrimal duct* **nā**-zō-**lahck**-rihm-ahl duhckt
*Nictitating membrane* **nihck**-tih-**tā**-tihng **mehm**-brān
*Nociception* nō-sih-**sehp**-shuhn
*Nociceptor* nō-sih-**sehp**-tuhr
*Olfactory sense* ohl-**fahck**-tuh-rē sehns
*Optic disc* **ohp**-tihck dihsk
*Organ of Corti* **ohr**-gahn *of* **kōr**-tē
*Ossicle* **ohs**-eh-kuhl
*Otolith* **ō**-tō-lihth
*Oval window* **ō**-vahl **wihn**-dō
*Pain* pān
*Palpebral conjunctiva* pahl-**pē**-brahl kohn-**juhnck**-tih-vah
*Perception* puhr-**sehp**-shuhn
*Perilymph* **peər**-ih-lihmf
*Photoreceptor* fō-tō-reh-**sehpt**-ər
*Pinna* **pihn**-nuh
*Posterior chamber* pō-**steer**-ē-ər **chām**-bər
*Pressure* **prehsh**-ər
*Proprioception* **prō**-prē-ō-**sehp**-shuhn
*Pupil* **pū**-puhl

*Retina* **reh**-tih-nuh
*Rod* rohd
*Round window* round **wihn**-dō
*Saccule* **sahck**-ūl
*Sclera* **skleər**-uh
*Semicircular canal* seh-mē-**suhr**-kyoo-lər kuh-**nahl**
*Sensory receptor* **sehn**-sər-ē reh-**sehpt**-ər
*Smell* smehl
*Special sense* **spehsh**-uhl sehnz
*Stapes* **stā**-pēs
*Suspensory ligament* suh-**spehn**-suh-rē **lihg**-ah-mehnt
*Tactile sense* **tahck**-tihl sehns
*Tapetum* tah-**pē**-duhm
*Tapetum lucidum* tah-**pē**-duhm **loo**-sihd-uhm
*Tarsal gland* **tahr**-sahl glahnd
*Taste* tāst
*Tectorial membrane* tehck-**tohr**-ē-uhl **mehm**-brān
*Temperature sense* **tehm**-pər-uh-chər sehns
*Third eyelid* thihrd **ī**-lihd
*Touch* tuhch
*Transduction* trahnz-**duhck**-shuhn
*Transmission* trahnz-**mihsh**-uhn
*Tympanic membrane* tihm-**pahn**-ihck
   **mehm**-brān
*Utricle* **ū**-trih-kuhl
*Uvea* **ū**-vē-uh
*Vestibule* **vehs**-tuh-byool
*Visceral sensation* **vih**-sər-ahl sehn-**sā**-shuhn
*Vitreous compartment* **vih**-trē-uhs kuhm-**pahrt**-mehnt
*Vitreous humor* **vih**-trē-uhs **hyoo**-mər
*Wind-up* **wīnd**-uhp

## INTRODUCTION

The old expression "perception is reality" is nowhere as true as it is for the sensory system. The world that animals, including us humans, live in exists only as it is perceived in their (our) brains. Colors are merely different wavelengths of electromagnetic radiation that stimulate photoreceptors in the eye to send nerve impulses to the brain that are perceived as what we call "colors." If there is no brain to interpret nerve impulses from the appropriate photoreceptors, colors do not independently exist. So the correct answer to the old question, "If a tree falls in a forest and there is no one (or nothing) present with a sense of hearing, does it make a sound?" would be "No." What the brain perceives as sound is vibrations of air molecules. If there are no receptors present to detect those vibrations and send impulses to a brain that can perceive them as sounds, sound does not independently exist. This may seem like a strange concept, but it is an important one. The world that the animals we work with live in is determined by the sensory receptors they are equipped with, and how their brains interpret the nerve impulses created by those receptors. The world they perceive is different from the world

we perceive—sometimes slightly and sometimes greatly. Awareness of those differences makes it much easier for us to work with them in a useful manner.

Okay, let's get down to basics. How many senses do animals have? Tradition says five: *hearing, seeing, feeling, smelling,* and *tasting.* Anatomy and physiology concepts, however, say they have more than that. Coming up with a precise number is difficult, because so many different kinds of sensations can be identified, and the total number depends on how we separate or group them. However, the total is definitely more than five.

Before we sort through the sensory numbers game, let's look at what sense organs are. In simplest terms, they are extensions of the central nervous system (CNS) that allow it to monitor what is going on inside and outside the animal. At the heart of all sense organs are various kinds of specially modified nerve endings (dendrites), called **sensory receptors**. When triggered by an appropriate stimulus, a sensory receptor generates nerve impulses that travel to the CNS and are interpreted (perceived) as a particular sensation.

The sensory receptors of common domestic animals are sensitive to only four general types of stimulus:

1. Mechanical stimuli (e.g., touch, hearing, balance).
2. Thermal stimuli (e.g., hot and cold).
3. Electromagnetic stimuli (e.g., vision).
4. Chemical stimuli (e.g., taste and smell).

All of the sensations that an animal can perceive start with one or more of these four types of stimuli. Therefore the CNS has to do a lot of work to interpret the resulting sensory nerve impulses correctly. For instance, one type of mechanical stimulus is a pesky cat rubbing against a dog's leg. Another type of mechanical stimulus is the sound of a can opener being used to open a can of dog food. The distinction is important to a hungry dog. Fortunately, its CNS is preprogrammed to perceive the many sensory nerve impulses it receives correctly.

So how many senses are there? Would you believe 10? That's right; we are going to discuss 10 senses, or categories of sensation, in this chapter—five *general senses* and five *special senses*. These are listed in Table 10-1.

| TABLE 10-1 | General and Special Senses | |
|---|---|---|
| **SENSE** | **WHAT IS SENSED** | **TYPE OF STIMULUS** |
| **General Senses** | | |
| Visceral sensations | Hunger, thirst, hollow-organ fullness | Chemical, mechanical |
| Touch | Touch and pressure | Mechanical |
| Temperature | Heat and cold | Thermal |
| Pain | Intense stimuli of any type | Mechanical, chemical, or thermal |
| Proprioception | Body position and movement | Mechanical |
| **Special Senses** | | |
| Taste | Tastes | Chemical |
| Smell | Odors | Chemical |
| Hearing | Sounds | Mechanical |
| Equilibrium | Balance and head position | Mechanical |
| Vision | Light | Electromagnetic |

## GENERAL SENSES

The **general senses** are *visceral sensations, touch, temperature, pain,* and *proprioception.* Some of them are not exactly household terms, but as their category name implies, general senses are distributed generally throughout the body. Their receptors tend to be fairly simple structures, and they transmit sensory information to the CNS through peripheral and autonomic nerve fibers. Because their receptors tend to be widespread on the inside and outside of the body, the general senses keep the CNS informed about the overall prevailing conditions both inside and outside the body.

Although they are important to the well-being of an animal, with the exception of pain the general senses are rarely involved in clinical disease or treatment. So we will give them a quick once-over, but we will not discuss them in detail. Additional information about the general senses can be found in more in-depth anatomy and physiology references.

## VISCERAL SENSATIONS

**Visceral sensations** make up a somewhat miscellaneous category of interior body sensations. Most are vague and poorly localized. They include the sensations of hunger and thirst, which indicate deficiencies of nutrients and water. The result of such sensations is the initiation of actions designed to secure the needed substances and restore nutrient and fluid balance (homeostasis) in the body.

Other visceral sensations originate in internal organs, particularly hollow organs such as the gastrointestinal tract and portions of the urinary system. Interestingly, these organs have only certain, specific kinds of receptors, particularly stretch receptors. Anything that stretches the wall of the organ, such as a bubble of gas in the intestine or a stone (calculus) in the ureter, can be intensely painful. On the other hand, these same organs can be handled, cut, or crushed without any apparent pain. This can be a problem on those rare occasions when an abdominal surgical incision breaks down (called *surgical wound dehiscence*) and internal organs come out through the defect. The animal actually can traumatize its own organs without feeling any apparent discomfort.

The urinary bladder is an exception to the rule that stretching causes severe pain, which holds true for most other hollow internal organs. The job of the urinary bladder is to store urine as it is produced by the kidneys and release it periodically to the outside. The sensation of a filling bladder reaches the conscious mind, but it is not an acutely painful event. Rather, it triggers reflex centers in the spinal cord that cause the smooth muscle in the wall of the bladder to contract. Urination may then take place, or it can be delayed if the animal contracts the voluntary sphincter muscle that surrounds the neck of the bladder.

The pleura and peritoneum (membranes that line and cover the contents of the thorax and abdomen, respectively) are well supplied with sensory receptors. As long as conditions are normal and the pleural and peritoneal surfaces slide over each other smoothly, no sensation is felt. However, if the surfaces become roughened by inflammation and/or infection, the resulting pleuritis or peritonitis is very painful. Pleuritis and peritonitis most often result from penetrating wounds from the outside or from ruptures or perforations of internal organs. When opening thoracic or abdominal organs surgically, we must be very careful to suture them closed securely to prevent leakage, which could lead to pleuritis or peritonitis.

## TOUCH

We include **touch** and **pressure** together, even though they are sometimes classified as separate senses. Touch, also known as the **tactile sense**, is the sensation of something being in contact with the surface of the body. It can be difficult to differentiate touch from pressure, which is the sense of something pressing on the body surface. Different kinds of specific touch and pressure receptor produce sensations of light contact, deep pressure, vibration, or hair movement. The overall effect is to give the CNS a picture of what, where, and to what extent objects from the outside environment are physically in contact with the surface of the body. The touch and pressure sensations operate almost at an unconscious level, unless the contact is abrupt or the pressure severe. Once physical contact or pressure is initially sensed, it quickly fades into the sensory background unless it changes or is extreme.

If you are sitting down while reading this, take a moment to think about where the chair is contacting your body—probably in the areas of your lower back, your buttocks, and the backs of your thighs. Until you thought about those areas, you probably were not consciously aware of the pressure on them, unless you are sitting in a very uncomfortable chair. The CNS has too much information to process to keep track of everything that is, or is not, in contact with every square millimeter of the skin's surface. Usually, only when things change, or are extreme, do the sensations of touch and pressure rise to the level of the conscious mind.

## TEMPERATURE

The **temperature sense** is the monitoring half of the body's temperature control (temperature homeostasis) system. Temperature receptors detect increases or decreases in body temperature and transmit the information to the CNS. The CNS can activate mechanisms to correct conditions of **hypothermia** (too low a body temperature) or **hyperthermia** (too high a body temperature).

Temperature receptors fall into two categories: *superficial* and *central*. Superficial temperature receptors are located in the skin and detect upward or downward changes in skin temperature. Heat receptors increase their generation of nerve impulses when the temperature increases, and cold receptors increase theirs when the temperature falls. These increased impulses get the attention of the conscious mind and let it know that things are out of balance. At constant temperatures, the receptors generate steady, low-level streams of nerve impulses that are sensed at the subconscious level and do not intrude on the conscious mind.

Central temperature receptors keep track of the core (interior) temperature of the body by monitoring the temperature of the blood. Central temperature receptors are located in the hypothalamus, a small but very important area of the brain. (See Chapters 9 and 11 on the nervous and endocrine systems for information on other important functions of the hypothalamus.) An animal's rectal temperature indicates its core temperature.

By monitoring the temperature of the body both superficially and centrally, the nervous system can initiate corrective actions if things become too hot or cold. By controlling functions such as blood flow in and beneath the skin, sweating, piloerection (hairs standing on end to increase insulation by trapping air), shivering, and even thyroid hormone production, the nervous system can set in motion mechanisms that can help bring body temperature back into balance. It can also initiate actions to help heat or cool the animal as needed. If the animal is too hot, it may seek out shade or cool water. If it is too cold, it might seek out warmth or increase its muscular activity to generate more heat.

### CLINICAL APPLICATION

#### Heatstroke and Hypothermia

Normal cellular functions in warm-blooded animals depend on the core body temperature remaining fairly constant. This is because chemical reactions, including all the metabolic reactions that occur in the body, are temperature dependent. Higher temperatures speed up chemical reactions, and lower temperatures slow them down. Significant variations in the core temperature of the body, such as might occur in **heatstroke** (significantly elevated body temperature) or hypothermia (significantly decreased body temperature), can have serious consequences and endanger the life of the animal.

Heatstroke can result from prolonged exposure to high environmental temperatures. The core temperature of the affected animal climbs to dangerously high levels. Early on, the animal typically appears weak and confused; as things progress, it may lapse into unconsciousness that can lead to convulsions and even death. The very rapid heart and respiratory rates that occur in affected animals are signs of the abnormally accelerated metabolic reactions in the body. If the animal is not cooled in time, the distorted metabolic reactions, particularly in the brain, can reach a point at which brain damage and possibly death can result. The maximum body temperature compatible with life is about 10° F (5° C) above the animal's normal body temperature level.

Hypothermia results from an abnormally low body temperature that slows all the metabolic processes. The heart and respiratory rates of affected animals slow as their core temperatures drop. If not warmed, affected animals can lose consciousness and die. Hypothermia can result from prolonged exposure to cold environmental temperatures, but it can also occur in the veterinary hospital in animals under general anesthesia. Most general anesthetic drugs anesthetize the temperature control centers in the brain along with the conscious mind. This often results in a slow fall in body temperature during anesthetic procedures that can be accelerated by contact with cold environmental surfaces, such as metal surgery tables. The falling core temperature slows metabolic reactions in the animal's body, including those that metabolize or eliminate the anesthetic agent at the end of the procedure and allow the animal to wake up. This can prolong the time it takes for the animal to recover from the anesthetic. For this reason, we generally try to keep anesthetized and recovering animals warm through means such as table and cage warmers, towels, blankets, and hot water bottles.

## PAIN

**Pain** receptors, also called **nociceptors**, are the most common and widely distributed sensory receptors inside and on the surface of the body. They are found almost everywhere. They range from simple, free nerve endings that respond to intense stimuli of all types, to more specialized structures that detect mechanical forces, temperature, and so on. Their purpose is to protect the body from damage by alerting the CNS to potentially harmful stimuli. Interestingly, the only place in the body where pain receptors are *not* found is the brain. It is not uncommon for certain types of human brain surgery to be performed on wide-awake patients who have had local anesthesia to allow the brain to be exposed.

The process of experiencing pain is called **nociception**. It seems like it should be a straightforward, simple process. A painful stimulus should generate a sensory nerve impulse that goes to the brain and is perceived as pain, right? Actually the process is more complicated than that, and our growing understanding of the processes involved is enabling us to provide more effective pain management to veterinary patients.

Four processes contribute to nociception (Figure 10-1). Some fit our logical preconceptions, and at least one adds some new wrinkles to our thinking. The first step in nociception has the strange name of **transduction**. This is the conversion of the painful stimulus to a nerve impulse, which occurs at the sensory nerve ending. **Transmission** of the nerve impulse up the sensory nerve fibers to the spinal cord is the next step. So far, everything is as we expected. The next step in the process, however, has only recently been fully appreciated. The spinal cord does not simply relay the sensory nerve impulses up to the brain. **Modulation** (changing) of the sensory nerve impulses can occur in the spinal cord, and this can significantly influence the information the brain receives, particularly in cases of chronic or severe pain. This modulation process can amplify (make more severe)

or suppress (make less severe) sensory impulses through synapses between neurons in the dorsal horns of the spinal cord. We can influence this modulation process through therapy with several different classes of drugs. This can enhance our ability to prevent and treat chronic and severe pain in our patients.

The last step in the nociception process is **perception** of the painful impulses by several areas of the brain. Conscious perception occurs in the cerebral cortex, but other areas of the brain are involved also. These include areas involved with the autonomic nervous system (fight or flight), fear and anxiety, memory, arousal, and behavior and emotion. Severe or chronic pain can have far-reaching negative effects on an animal's well-being that can extend beyond just the unpleasant conscious discomfort of pain.

Pain can be classified in a number of ways. One useful system classifies pain as *superficial* (affecting the skin and subcutaneous areas), *deep* (involving muscles and joints), and *visceral* (relating to the internal organs). Another system classifies pain as *acute* (sharp and intense) or *chronic* (dull and aching).

We cannot get inside the head of a dog or a horse to find out precisely how they perceive pain, but behavioral and physiologic responses suggest that they experience pain much the same way we do. The difference is often in how they *react* to the pain. We humans often tend to dwell on pain we are experiencing, which can make the overall experience even more stressful, whereas nonhuman animals seem to accept the current situation as how things are supposed to be. This is not to say that they do not suffer pain; rather, they just do not seem to have the same kind of emotional reaction to it that we humans do. They often seem to hide it well, which can be a problem for us clinically when we are trying to assess the degree of pain a patient is experiencing. Actually, hiding signs of pain is a survival instinct for most animals. An animal that shows signs of pain is showing signs of weakness that might encourage other animals, including predators, to attack it.

Visible reactions to pain vary greatly among species, breeds, and individual animals. Some animals are very sensitive to pain and become stressed by even mildly painful stimuli. Others hardly seem to react at all until pain becomes severe. Prevention and relief of pain are becoming increasingly important in veterinary medicine, as we learn more about its harmful effects and how to prevent them. Research studies are providing the knowledge necessary to detect the subtle signs of pain that many animals show. This information is allowing us to become more proactive in our efforts to prevent and treat pain in ill and injured patients.

## PROPRIOCEPTION

Without looking at them, can you tell what positions your arms and legs are in? Of course you can, although precisely how you do it may not be clear. You just seem to know where all your body parts are. Actually, you are making use of your sense of **proprioception**, which is the sense of body position and movement. This sense operates largely at the subconscious level and is very important in allowing an

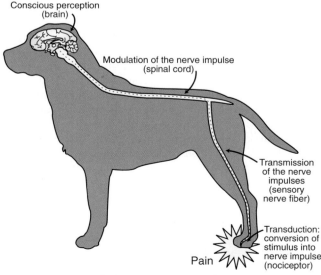

Conscious perception
(brain)

Modulation of the nerve impulse
(spinal cord)

Transmission
of the nerve
impulses
(sensory
nerve fiber)

Transduction:
conversion of
stimulus into
nerve impulse
(nociceptor)

Pain

**FIGURE 10-1** Pain pathways.

animal to stand upright and make accurate, purposeful movements as it interacts with its environment. During the examination of an animal with suspected nervous system damage, a veterinarian may evaluate proprioception by curling the animal's foot under so that it is upside down, and seeing how long it takes the animal to right it. Animals with normal proprioception almost immediately bring the foot up into a normal standing position.

The heart of the proprioception sense is the variety of stretch receptors located in skeletal muscles, tendons, ligaments, and joint capsules. These receptors keep the CNS informed about the movements of limbs, the positions of joints, the state of contraction of muscles, and the amount of tension being exerted on tendons and ligaments. This information is important to the CNS so that it can send out the right combination of motor nerve impulses, which are appropriate in range and strength, to produce smooth body movements.

## SPECIAL SENSES

The **special senses** include four of the traditional senses—taste, smell, hearing, and vision—plus the important sense of equilibrium. In contrast with the general senses, the special senses are organized into specific, often complex sensory organs and structures that are all located in the head. Because of their locations, structures, and functions, the special sense organs often are involved in clinical illnesses and injuries.

## TASTE

The sense of **taste**, also called the **gustatory sense**, is a chemical sense. Its receptors are located in the mouth in structures called *taste buds*. When they detect chemical substances dissolved in the saliva, the taste receptors generate nerve impulses that travel to the brain and are interpreted as tastes.

---

 **CLINICAL APPLICATION**

### Anesthesia and Analgesia

The ability to perceive sensations, or to feel things, is known as *esthesia*. (The study of the sensory system is called *esthesiology*.) **Anesthesia** is the loss of esthesia, or the complete loss of sensation. In clinical veterinary medicine, we use two basic types of anesthesia to carry out procedures that would be painful for patients: *general anesthesia* and *local anesthesia*.

**General anesthesia** involves a complete loss of sensory perception accompanied by loss of consciousness. The animal is placed into a controlled sleep that prevents it from feeling painful procedures. We produce this sleep by administering general anesthetic drugs either by injecting them or by having animals breathe them from an inhalant anesthesia machine. Animals under general anesthesia must be monitored closely, because the drugs depress cardiovascular and respiratory functions along with the CNS.

**Local anesthesia** produces loss of sensation from a specific, localized area of the body without affecting consciousness. It is produced by injecting a local anesthetic drug into an area through which sensory nerve fibers pass. The drug blocks the transmission of nerve impulses through the site, which prevents sensory information from reaching the central nervous system. This can allow potentially painful procedures to be performed without having to render the animal unconscious.

**Analgesia** is a related state in which the perception of pain is decreased but not completely absent. The pain is dulled but not completely gone. A drug that produces analgesia is called an *analgesic* drug. Aspirin, carprofen (Rimadyl[R]), and morphine are all examples. Analgesic drugs are often used to make animals with severe pain (postsurgical patients for example) more comfortable.

---

 **CLINICAL APPLICATION**

### Preventing Wind-Up

We used to believe that potentially painful procedures we carried out on an animal under general anesthesia, such as surgery, had no long-lasting effects. After all, properly administered general anesthetics effectively block the perception of painful impulses by the conscious part of the brain. We now know that the other three nociceptive processes—transduction, transmission and modulation—are still operating full-bore in an anesthetized animal during surgery, and they can significantly affect the animal's level of pain once they wake up from the anesthetic.

Most important, we now understand that the neurons of the spinal cord are bombarded with painful stimuli during surgical procedures despite the fact that the conscious mind is temporarily disconnected from the process by the general anesthetic. Because the spinal cord is capable of changing (modulating) the information it forwards on to the brain, this sensory assault during surgery can cause the pain signals going to the brain to be amplified once the animal wakes up from

the general anesthesia. This can make the animal's postoperative pain level even more severe than the tissue damage caused by the surgery would seem to warrant. This exaggerated pain response is referred to as **wind-up**, and it can cause significant stress on a postsurgical patient.

Wind-up is much easier to prevent than it is to treat. It is difficult to bring the exaggerated pain response produced by wind-up under control with drugs. On the other hand, if we can decrease the painful stimuli received by the spinal cord during surgery, we can often prevent wind-up from developing in the first place. This can be done by administering analgesic and possibly local anesthetic drugs before, and even during, surgery. Using small amounts of several drugs with different analgesic/anesthetic mechanisms is often more effective than using a large dose of a single drug. This strategy of heading off the effects of severe surgical pain before it occurs can make pain control during the postoperative period much more effective, and it can actually speed a patient's recovery from surgery.

The majority of the taste buds are located on the sides of certain small, elevated structures on the tongue called *papillae,* although a few can be found in the lining of the mouth and throat (pharynx). As seen in Figure 10-2, taste buds are tiny, rounded structures made up of gustatory (sensory) cells and supporting cells. Tiny openings on the surface of each taste bud, the *taste pores,* allow dissolved substances to enter the taste buds and contact the sensory receptors. The sensory receptors are tiny, hairlike processes (modified dendrites) from the gustatory cells that project up into the taste pores. When appropriate chemical substances dissolved in the saliva come in contact with the sensory processes, nerve impulses are generated that travel to the brain and are interpreted as particular tastes.

In humans the four primary taste sensations are sweet, sour, salty, and bitter. Each has a particular area of the tongue that responds most strongly to that taste. The ability to detect many different kinds of taste is due to combinations of the four basic taste sensations and interactions with the sense of smell. We cannot know if nonhuman animals experience tastes in the same way, but taste sensations most likely vary among animal species.

## SMELL

The sense of **smell** is also called the **olfactory sense**. It is a chemical sense very similar to taste. The sense of smell is more important in most nonhuman animals than it is in humans. We live in a sight-oriented world. Although we have a decent sense of smell, our keen vision is more important to us as we interact with our environment. In contrast, many nonhuman animals have less sensitive eyesight but a highly sensitive sense of smell. They live in more of a smell-oriented world. This can be difficult for us to relate to, but dogs obtain a huge amount of information from sniffing the air or an object such as a fire hydrant (this can be thought of as reading their "pee-mail"). For reasons we will discuss shortly, dogs probably do not see colors like we do, but they can smell "colors" that we cannot even imagine. So the next time you are walking a dog and it decides to stop and do a thorough sniff-examination of something, do not immediately yank on its leash to get it moving. It is busy reading messages left for it by every other dog that has visited there and left a pee-mail message. Take a moment to appreciate the amazing communication process you are witnessing. The dog will appreciate it, and may add a "reply to all" message of its own by leaving a small amount of urine!

The sense of smell is organized in two patches of olfactory epithelium located up high in both nasal passages. Figure 10-3 shows the location and some of the structure of the olfactory epithelium. Sensory (olfactory) cells are mixed with supporting cells in these epithelial patches. Hairlike processes (modified dendrites) from the surfaces of the olfactory cells project up into the mucous layer that covers the nasal epithelium. When odor molecules dissolve in the mucus and contact the sensory processes, nerve impulses are generated that travel to the brain and are interpreted as particular smells.

## HEARING

**Hearing**, also called the *auditory sense,* is a mechanical sense that converts vibrations of air molecules into nerve impulses that are interpreted by the brain as sound. The ear, the organ of hearing, can be divided into three physical and functional areas: the *external ear,* the *middle ear,* and the *inner ear.* The **external ear** acts as a funnel to collect sound wave vibrations and direct them to the eardrum. The **middle ear** amplifies and transmits the vibrations from the eardrum to the inner ear. The **inner ear** contains the actual sensory receptors that convert the mechanical vibrations to nerve impulses, along with receptors for the equilibrium sense.

Most of the ear structures are housed within the temporal bones of the skull. The external ear canal, the middle ear cavity, and the inner ear structures all occupy hollowed-out areas in the temporal bones that are lined with soft tissue membranes. The processes of collecting, transmitting, and converting sound wave vibrations all take place within these membrane-lined bony cavities. Figure 10-4 shows the main structures of the external, middle, and inner portions of the ear.

### EXTERNAL EAR

The external ear consists of structures that collect sound waves and transmit them to the middle ear. Its main parts

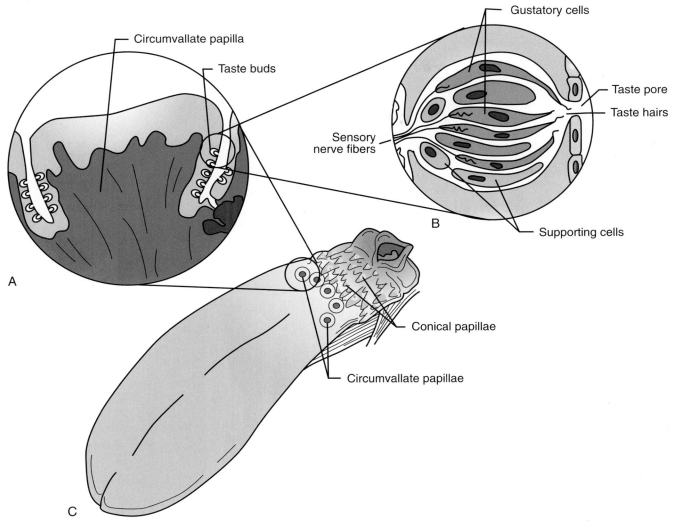

**FIGURE 10-2** Taste buds on the tongue. **A,** One magnified papilla showing locations of taste buds. **B,** Taste bud structure. **C,** Tongue showing a few of the many papillae containing taste buds.

---

### CLINICAL APPLICATION

#### Upper Respiratory Tract Infections

Upper respiratory tract infections are caused by disease-causing organisms, such as viruses and bacteria. They affect primarily the nasal passages and pharynx (throat) and result in coughing, sneezing, sore throat, and discharges from the eyes and nose. The common cold is a human upper respiratory tract infection. What sometimes makes upper respiratory tract infections dangerous for domestic animals is their effect on the animals' sense of smell—these infections effectively eliminate it. Think back to your last cold. You probably did not have much of a sense of smell, which rendered most foods bland and tasteless.

The effect on animals that live in a smell-oriented world is even more drastic. They often stop eating and drinking completely, because they cannot smell anything. If this continues for very long, they can be in real danger from dehydration. Therefore we often have to administer fluids, either orally or by injection, to animals with upper respiratory tract infections. By keeping them properly hydrated while we provide other necessary medical and nursing care, we often can help them fight off the infection.

---

are the *pinna,* the *external auditory canal,* and the *tympanic membrane (eardrum).*

The **pinna** is the part of the ear that we can see from the outside. It is a funnel-like structure composed mainly of elastic cartilage and skin that collects sound wave vibrations and directs them into the external auditory canal. In many animals, the pinna is very mobile and can be aimed in the direction of a sound. For instance, watch the ears of a horse in a strange environment. Its ears will probably be scanning the area like a couple of little radar

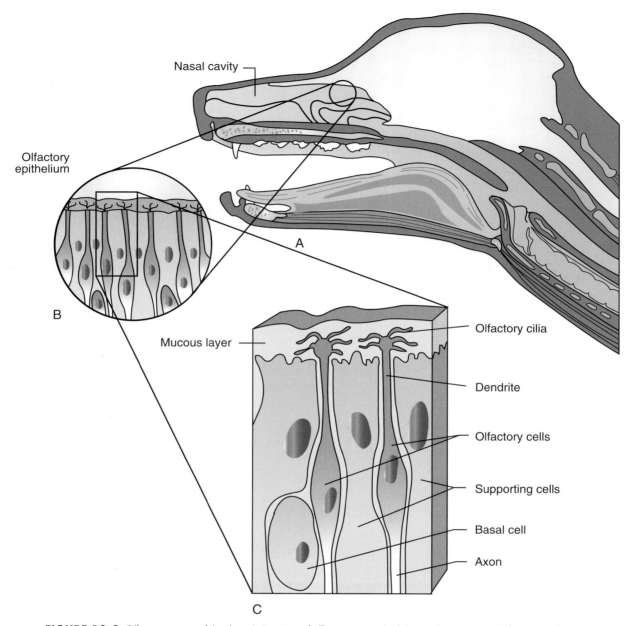

Nasal cavity

Olfactory
epithelium

A

B

Mucous layer

Olfactory cilia

Dendrite

Olfactory cells

Supporting cells

Basal cell

Axon

C

**FIGURE 10-3** Olfactory region of the dog. **A,** Location of olfactory region high in nasal passage. **B,** Olfactory epithelium. **C,** Detail of olfactory epithelium showing olfactory cilia projecting up into overlying mucous layer.

dishes. This ability is particularly useful in animals with erect ears.

The **external auditory canal** is a soft, membrane-lined tube that begins at the base of the pinna and carries sound waves to the tympanic membrane (eardrum). In most domestic animal species, it is somewhat L-shaped with an outer, vertical portion and an inner, horizontal portion. It ends blindly at the tympanic membrane.

The **tympanic membrane** is commonly called the **eardrum**. It is a paper-thin connective tissue membrane that is tightly stretched across the opening between the external auditory canal and the middle ear cavity. When sound wave vibrations strike it, the tympanic membrane vibrates at the same frequency through a process called *sympathetic*

*vibration.* (*Author's note:* Another example of sympathetic vibration is the annoying audible vibration of a snare drum that occurs when certain notes are played by a band or orchestra. If you have ever been in a band or orchestra you are probably familiar with that sound.)

## MIDDLE EAR

The middle ear cavity is a hollowed-out area of the temporal bone that is lined by soft tissue membranes. It is filled with air and contains three small bones called **ossicles** and the opening of the **Eustachian tube**, which connects it with the pharynx (throat). Laterally it is separated from the external ear by the tympanic membrane, and medially it is separated

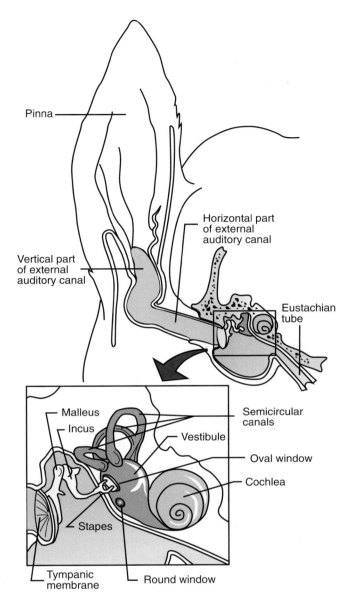

Pinna

Horizontal part
of external
auditory canal

Vertical part
of external
auditory canal

Eustachian
tube

Malleus

Incus

Vestibule

Semicircular
canals

Oval window

Cochlea

Stapes

Tympanic
membrane

Round window

**FIGURE 10-4** Cross section of dog's ear structures with middle and inner ear regions enlarged.

from the inner ear by the membranes that cover the oval and round windows of the cochlea.

Three small bones called ossicles link the tympanic membrane with the **cochlea** of the inner ear, where the receptors for hearing are located. The individual ossicles are named for some past anatomist's fanciful impression of their shapes. The outermost bone, the **malleus** (hammer), is attached to the tympanic membrane. The malleus forms a complete synovial joint with the middle bone, the **incus** (anvil), which in turn forms a joint with the medial-most bone, the **stapes** (stirrup). The other end of the stapes is attached to the membrane that covers the oval window of the cochlea. How this attachment to the cochlea contributes to hearing is described further in the section on the inner ear.

The ossicles act as a system of levers that transmit the sound wave vibrations from the tympanic membrane to the

cochlea. In doing so, they decrease the amplitude (size) of the vibrations but amplify their force. This helps transmit the vibrations accurately to the supersensitive receptor structures in the cochlea, ideally without causing any damage. Another mechanism that helps prevent damage to the hearing receptors is a tiny muscle, the *tensor tympani,* that attaches to the malleus. It adjusts the tension of the tympanic membrane and helps deaden the transmission of extremely loud sound vibrations to the cochlea. Another tiny muscle, the *stapedius,* assists the damage-control process by restricting the movement of the stapes in response to loud sounds.

The Eustachian tube, also called the *auditory tube,* connects the middle ear cavity with the pharynx. Its purpose is to equalize the air pressure on the two sides of the tympanic membrane. Without this structure, every time the atmospheric (barometric) pressure changed (as it often does; watch the next weather forecast), the tympanic membrane would bulge in or out, depending on whether the pressure increased or decreased. This would be painful, because the tympanic membrane is liberally supplied with pain receptors, and it would decrease sound wave transmission. Fortunately, the Eustachian tube comes to the rescue. The slitlike opening of the tube in the pharynx is stretched open whenever the animal swallows or yawns. This allows air to enter or leave as necessary to equalize the pressure in the middle ear cavity with that of the outside air. (Note how this system is put to the test when we engage in activities that rapidly change the pressure on the outside of the tympanic membrane, such as flying or scuba diving. Consciously swallowing or yawning often helps correct the resulting pressure imbalance.)

### CLINICAL APPLICATION

#### Ear Hematomas

The pinna of the ear consists of elastic cartilage and small blood vessels covered by skin. Sometimes irritation in the ear canal (such as with *otitis externa*) will cause an animal to shake its head vigorously (see the Clinical Application on otitis externa). In some animals, particularly floppy-eared dogs, this movement can rupture small blood vessels under the skin of the pinna, usually on the inside surface. The resulting bleeding between the cartilage and skin can cause an accumulation of blood, called an *ear hematoma,* which is an abnormal accumulation of free blood between the cartilage and skin of the pinna.

An ear hematoma usually is not dangerous or even painful, but it is heavy and swollen and often seems to bother the animal. If left untreated, the blood will be reabsorbed slowly, but the ear probably will be permanently deformed by scar tissue, resulting in what is called a *cauliflower ear.* Treatment of ear hematomas usually involves surgically draining the material from the hematoma and placing sutures through the pinna to hold the skin tight against the cartilage and prevent fluid from reaccumulating. The underlying cause of the head shaking needs to be determined and treated also to prevent recurrence.

### Otitis Externa

Otitis externa is an inflammation of the skin of the external ear canal that occurs most commonly in dogs, cats, and rabbits. It is often caused by parasites such as ear mites, foreign bodies, or microorganisms such as bacteria and yeasts. The irritation in the ear canal causes redness, pain, itching, and fluid accumulation. The owner usually notices that the animal shakes its head a lot and spends time scratching at its ears. When the affected ear is examined, the ear canal is usually red, moist, swollen, and painful, and often has a characteristic pungent odor.

The basic anatomy of the external ear canal adds a challenge to the treatment of otitis externa. Gravity makes inflammatory fluids drain downward and accumulate in the horizontal portion of the canal next to the tympanic membrane. Because topical medications are usually part of the treatment of otitis externa, the ear canals must be cleaned thoroughly and carefully to remove discharges before the medications are instilled. Because the ear canals are often swollen and painful, this process can be difficult for at least the first few days. Therapy for otitis externa often must be continued for many weeks to bring the condition under control.

### INNER EAR

The inner ear is made up of structures that contribute to both hearing and equilibrium. The hearing portion of the inner ear is contained in a snail shell-shaped spiral cavity in the temporal bone called the *cochlea* (Figures 10-4 and 10-5). Within the hollowed-out bony cavity of the cochlea is a soft, multilayered, fluid-filled portion that contains the receptor organ of hearing—the **organ of Corti**. The organ of Corti runs the length of the cochlea in a long tube called the **cochlear duct**, which is filled with a fluid called **endolymph**. A U-shaped tube containing another fluid, **perilymph**, lies on either side of the cochlear duct. Membrane-covered openings at the ends of the "U," called the **oval window** and the **round window**, are located at the base of the cochlea. The bottom of the U is located at the tip of the cochlea. Nothing lies against the round window, but the stapes (one of the ossicles) is attached to the oval window.

The organ of Corti runs along the cochlear duct, on a shelf called the *basilar membrane,* like a long ribbon. Its main parts are *hair cells, supporting cells,* and the **tectorial membrane**. The hair cells are the receptor cells of hearing. They have tiny, hairlike projections (modified dendrites) on their surfaces. The gelatin-like tectorial membrane lies gently on top of the hairs like a long, soft strip lying on top of a broad series of brush bristles. As their name implies, the supporting cells provide physical support to the hair cells.

Sound wave vibrations cause the tympanic membrane and the ossicles in the middle ear to vibrate. As the stapes vibrates back and forth, it alternately pushes and pulls on the membrane covering the oval window of the cochlea. This causes the perilymph around the cochlear duct to vibrate

back and forth (the membrane covering the round window acts as a pressure relief mechanism by alternately bulging in and out as the fluid moves back and forth). This process is summarized in Figure 10-6. The movement of the perilymph causes the cochlear duct to move, which causes the tectorial membrane and the hair cells of the organ of Corti to rub against each other. This bends the sensory hairs, which generate nerve impulses that travel to the brain and are interpreted as sound.

Different frequencies of sound wave vibration stimulate different areas along the length of the organ of Corti. Areas near the oval window respond best to high-frequency (high-pitched) sounds, and areas at the tip of the cochlea respond best to low-frequency (low-pitched sounds). This physical process generates nerve impulses in different parts of the organ and helps the brain differentiate high- and low-pitched sounds.

---

✔ *TEST YOURSELF 10-3*

1. Which skull bone houses the middle and inner ear structures?
2. Why would keen hearing be important to the survival of a potential prey animal? Why would it be important to a predator?
3. How would the rupture or perforation of an eardrum affect hearing?
4. How would arthritis in the tiny joints of the ossicles affect hearing? Could this possibly affect the hearing of older animals?
5. How would an animal probably feel if they had a middle ear infection that caused the opening of the Eustachian tube to swell closed?
6. How might repeated exposure to loud sounds lead to progressive hearing loss?

---

### Recovery from General Anesthesia

The importance of head position to overall body posture and balance can be seen in an animal that is recovering from general anesthesia. One of the first things that a recovering animal tries to do as it regains consciousness is to raise its head into an upright position and steady it there. It has to get its head into that position before it can start trying to raise its body. Primitive instincts for survival prompt many animals to try and stand before they are steady and coordinated enough to support themselves. This can lead to stumbling and falling, which can cause injury.

By taking advantage of our knowledge of the sense of equilibrium, we can prevent an animal from trying to get up prematurely by gently holding its head down in a horizontal position until it has enough strength and coordination to rise. This can be particularly important for larger animals, such as horses. By holding a recovering horse's head down with a gentle hand or knee on the dorsal part of its neck just behind the skull, we can keep the animal from trying to get up too soon. Once we feel it has regained enough strength, we can allow it to raise its head and prepare to help steady it as it rises to its feet.

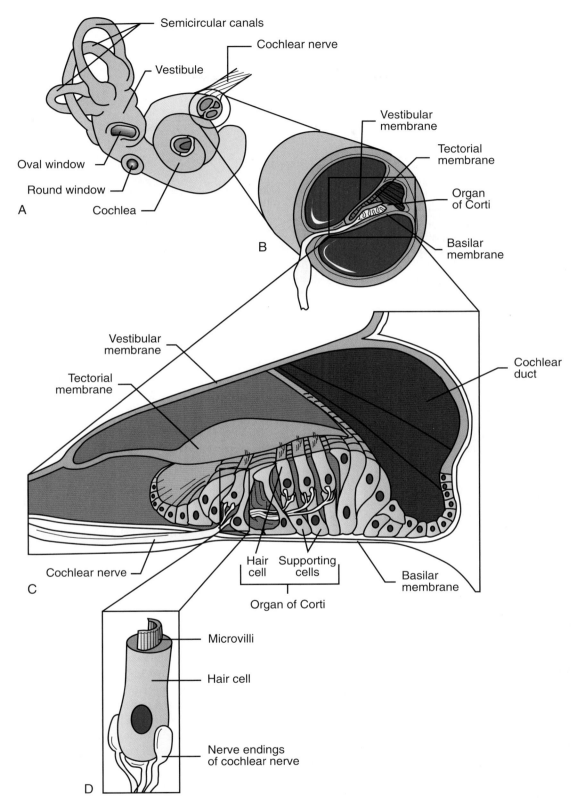

**FIGURE 10-5** Inner ear structures, with detail of cochlear anatomy. **A,** Inner ear structures. **B,** Enlarged cross section of cochlea. **C,** Detail of organ of Corti. **D,** Greatly enlarged, single sensory hair cell.

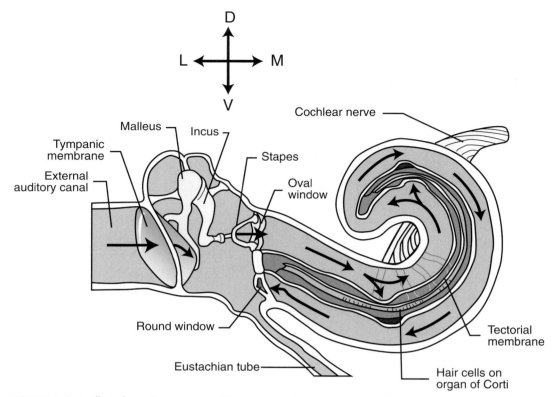

**FIGURE 10-6** Effect of sound waves on cochlear structures. Sound waves cause the tympanic membrane and ossicles to vibrate. As the stapes vibrates back and forth, it pushes and pulls on the membrane covering the oval window of the cochlea. This sets the fluid in the cochlea in motion, which causes the hair cells and tectorial membrane to rub against each other. This bends sensory hairs, generating nerve impulses that are transmitted to the brain and interpreted as sound.

## EQUILIBRIUM

As the head goes, so goes the rest of the body. At least that is the principle behind the sense of **equilibrium**. This mechanical sense helps the animal maintain its balance by keeping track of the position and movements of the head. The receptors are located in portions of the inner ear called the *vestibule* and the *semicircular canals*.

Actually, maintaining balance is a complicated process that involves information from the equilibrium receptors, as well as from the eyes and the proprioceptors around the body. (See the Clinical Application on motion sickness for an explanation of what happens when the information from these various sources does not agree.)

## VESTIBULE

The **vestibule** is the portion of the inner ear that is located between the cochlea and the semicircular canals. It is made up of two saclike spaces, called the **utricle** and the **saccule**, that are continuous with the cochlear duct of the cochlea and are filled with the same endolymph fluid. Like the cochlear duct, the utricle and saccule are surrounded by perilymph.

In each utricle and saccule is a patch of sensory epithelium called the **macula** (Figure 10-7). It consists of hair cells and supporting cells covered by a gelatinous matrix that contains tiny crystals of calcium carbonate called **otoliths**. (The word *otolith* literally means "ear stone.") The hair cells

here are similar to the hair cells of the organ of Corti in the cochlea. They have hairlike processes (modified dendrites) on their surfaces that the gelatinous matrix sits on. Gravity causes the otoliths and the gelatinous matrix to put constant pressure on the hairs as long as the head stays still. Movement of the head bends the sensory hairs, which generates nerve impulses that give the brain information about the position of the head.

## SEMICIRCULAR CANALS

The **semicircular canals** are located on the other side of the vestibule from the cochlea. Each canal is semicircular and oriented in a different plane at right angles to the other two. If you are indoors in a room with square walls, look up in a corner where two walls and the ceiling come together. Each of the walls and the ceiling is in a different plane, at right angles to the other two. This is the basic arrangement of the semicircular canals.

Within each bony semicircular canal is an endolymph-filled membranous tube that is surrounded by perilymph. (Each of the endolymph-filled structures in the inner ear is continuous with the others, as are the perilymph-filled structures.) Near the utricle end of each semicircular canal is an enlargement, called the **ampulla**, that contains the receptor structure, called the *crista ampullaris*, or simply the **crista**.

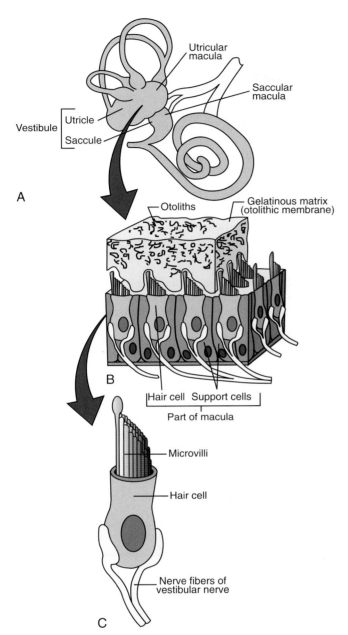

**FIGURE 10-7** Inner ear structures, with detail of vestibular anatomy. **A,** Inner ear structures. Note the utricle and saccule, which make up the vestibule, and locations of the macula (sensory epithelium) in each. **B,** Enlarged view of macula showing sensory hair cells, gelatinous matrix, and otoliths. **C,** Greatly enlarged sensory hair cell.

The crista is similar to the macula of the vestibule. It consists of a cone-shaped area of supporting cells and hair cells with their processes (modified dendrites) sticking up into a gelatinous structure called the **cupula** (Figure 10-8). However, there are no otoliths to weigh down the cupula. It functions as a float that moves with the endolymph in the membranous canal.

When the head moves in the plane of one of the semicircular canals, inertia causes the endolymph to lag behind the movement of the canal itself. The same principle is at work if you quickly rotate a glass containing liquid and ice cubes.

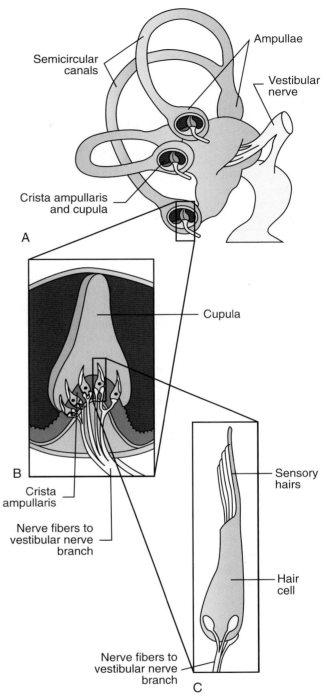

**FIGURE 10-8** Semicircular canals, with detail of ampulla and crista ampullaris. **A,** Semicircular canals, showing locations of ampullae. **B,** Enlarged view of crista ampullaris in an ampulla, showing sensory hair cells and cupula. **C,** Greatly enlarged sensory hair cell.

The glass turns, but the liquid and ice cubes lag behind. The relative movement of the endolymph pulls on the cupula, which bends the hairs. This generates nerve impulses that give the brain information about motion of the head, particularly rotary motion.

So the vestibular system senses rotary motion of the head with the semicircular canals, and linear motion and the position of the head with the vestibule. By integrating this information, the brain forms a picture of what is happening to the animal's head and, by extension, to its body as a whole.

---

**TEST YOURSELF 10-4**

1. How is the functioning of the vestibule and the semicircular canals similar? How is it different?
2. What are otoliths and why are they important to the equilibrium sense?
3. What is the difference between *ossicles* and *otoliths?*
4. How is the physical concept of inertia important to the functioning of the semicircular canals?
5. What is the basic cause of motion sickness?

---

## VISION

The eyes have a lot in common with digital cameras. They have lens covers (the eyelids), a "window" on the front to let light in (the cornea), an adjustable diaphragm to control the amount of light that enters (the iris), a lens that can be focused, an image sensor on which the image is formed (the retina), and connections (the optic nerves) to carry the images to a memory device (the brain) for storage.

As complicated as the eye seems, most of its components exist to help *form* an accurate visual image, not to *detect* one. The actual **photoreceptors** that detect the image and generate visual nerve impulses are in a single layer of cells in the **retina** (the structure that lines the back of the eyeball). In our discussion of vision, we'll deal mostly with the image-formation structures of the eye.

### TERMINOLOGY

Two general terms are used to refer to the eye: the word *ocular* and the combining form *ophthalm/o.* For example, *ocular anatomy* refers to the anatomy of the eye, *ophthalmic medications* are used to treat the eye, and *ophthalmology* is the study of the eye.

### MAJOR LAYERS OF THE EYEBALL

The eyeball consists of three major layers: the outer *fibrous layer,* the middle *vascular layer,* and the inner *nervous layer.* Figure 10-9 illustrates the main structures of each layer.

**FIBROUS LAYER.** The outer, fibrous layer of the eye admits light to its interior and gives strength and shape to the eyeball. Its two components are the *cornea* and the *sclera.* The **cornea** is the transparent "window" that admits light to the interior of the eye. It consists of an orderly arrangement of collagen fibers and contains no blood vessels. Its transparency is maintained by careful control of the amount of water it contains. Too much water (corneal edema) or too little water (corneal dehydration) causes the cornea to become cloudy and opaque. The cornea is richly supplied with pain receptors, making it one of the most sensitive tissues of the body.

**CLINICAL APPLICATION**

### Motion Sickness

The brain relies on the vestibular system, the eyes, and the proprioceptors around the body for information about how and where the body is moving so that it can keep the animal upright and maintain balance. Usually the information the brain receives from these sources agrees—the animal is either moving, or it is not. This is fine as long as it is standing or moving around on the ground (assuming the ground is not moving). But when we put an animal into a moving car, boat, airplane, or space vehicle, things become more complicated. The eyes look around the interior of the vehicle and see that nothing is apparently moving, but the equilibrium receptors and proprioceptors detect motion (or, in the case of space travel, the absence of gravity).

This disagreement between the sensory receptors can result in the unpleasant sensations of motion sickness, such as headache, nausea, and vomiting. This often occurs in animals that travel by car, truck, boat, or plane. Medications often can be used to prevent motion sickness, but they usually must be administered before traveling. Motion sickness is easier to prevent than it is to treat in mid journey. Veterinary clinics may dispense anti–motion-sickness medications to clients who must travel with animals that are prone to motion sickness.

A form of motion sickness is common in astronauts as well. *Space adaptation syndrome* occurs in a high percentage of astronauts, particularly during the first few days of a space flight. It causes symptoms similar to normal motion sickness, such as headache, nausea, and cold sweats. The symptoms often disappear after a day or two, indicating that the brain has adjusted to the conflicting signals. Ongoing research is focused on finding ways to prevent this annoying and sometimes debilitating disorder. It seems more complicated to deal with than traditional earth-bound motion sickness.

---

The **sclera** is the "white" of the eye. Like the cornea, it consists mainly of collagen fibers and makes up the majority of the outer fibrous layer of the eye. The junction of the cornea and the sclera is called the **limbus.** It can be used as a landmark to describe the position of lesions (abnormalities) on the cornea or sclera.

**VASCULAR LAYER.** The middle, vascular layer is also called the **uvea.** It has several parts, including the *choroid,* the *iris,* and the *ciliary* body.

The **choroid** is sandwiched between the sclera and the retina. It consists mainly of pigment and blood vessels that supply blood to the retina. Most of the pigment is dark melanin, but in most domestic animals, except swine, the choroid forms a highly reflective area in the rear of the eye called the **tapetum lucidum** or, more commonly, the **tapetum.** (See Figure 10-12.) The tapetum is like a brightly colored mirror, and it is responsible for the bright light that seems to shine from an animal's eyes in the dark, when a light is directed into them. Its purpose seems to be to act as

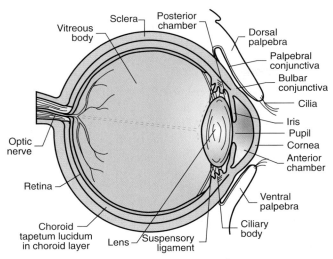

**FIGURE 10-9** Sagittal section of an eye.

for vision, the rods and cones. (We discuss the retina in more detail shortly.) The term **fundus** is sometimes used to describe the caudal interior surface of the eye. The retina is the main component of the fundus, along with the optic disc, which we discuss below.

a light amplifier to aid low-light vision. After light has passed through the photoreceptors (the rods and cones in the retina), it reflects off the tapetum and passes back through the photoreceptors again, stimulating them a second time. Therefore most animals can see better in dim light than we can. Humans and pigs do not have a tapetum.

At the front of the eye, the middle vascular layer is modified into the iris and the ciliary body. The **iris** is the colored part of the eye. If we speak of an animal as having blue eyes, it is the iris color we are talking about. The iris is a pigmented muscular diaphragm that controls the amount of light that enters the posterior part of the eyeball. The opening at its center is called the **pupil**. The pupil enlarges in low-light conditions and gets smaller in bright light. Two types of multiunit smooth muscle fiber make up the iris: *radially arranged fibers* (oriented like the spokes of a wheel) that enlarge the pupil when they contract, and *circularly arranged fibers* that constrict the pupil when they contract. The nerve supply for the smooth muscle cells of the iris comes from the autonomic nervous system.

The **ciliary body** is a ring-shaped structure located immediately behind the iris. It contains the tiny muscles that adjust the shape of the lens to allow near and far vision. The muscles of the ciliary body (the **ciliary muscles**) are also multiunit smooth muscles. They are contained within small processes (called the *ciliary processes*) that are attached to the periphery of the lens by tiny **suspensory ligaments**. The ciliary muscle fibers are oriented so that when they are relaxed the suspensory ligaments pull on the periphery of the lens, stretching it into a flattened shape. When they contract, they move the ciliary body forward and inward. This action takes tension off the suspensory ligaments, allowing the lens to assume its natural, more rounded shape. (We discuss this focusing process more in the section on the lens.)

**NERVOUS LAYER.** The inner, nervous layer is the retina, which lines the back of the eye. It is like the image sensor in the camera of the eye. It contains the actual sensory receptors

## MAJOR COMPARTMENTS OF THE EYEBALL

The interior of the eyeball is made up of two fluid-filled compartments: one in front of the lens and ciliary body and the other behind it. The **aqueous compartment** is in front of the lens and ciliary body and contains a clear, watery fluid called **aqueous humor**. The **vitreous compartment** is behind the lens and ciliary body and contains a clear fluid with the consistency of soft gelatin, called **vitreous humor**. The term *humor* is an old anatomical term meaning *fluid*. The eye is the only part of the body for which this archaic term is still commonly used.

When we look into an animal's eye, we are looking into its aqueous compartment. Actually, to be more precise, we are looking into the anterior chamber of its aqueous compartment. The aqueous compartment is subdivided into two parts by the iris. The space in front of the iris is the **anterior chamber**, and the space behind the iris and in front of the lens is the **posterior chamber**. The anterior chamber is the only portion of the eye's interior that we can see clearly without special instruments.

Within the aqueous compartment, aqueous humor is constantly being produced and drained. It is produced in the posterior chamber by cells of the ciliary body. It then passes very slowly through the pupil into the anterior chamber, where it is drained by the **canal of Schlemm** and the fluid is returned to the bloodstream. The canal of Schlemm is a ringlike structure located way out at the periphery of the anterior chamber at the angle where the iris and the cornea meet (Figure 10-10).

The vitreous compartment of the eye is considerably larger than the aqueous compartment. It fills the whole back of the eyeball behind the lens and ciliary body. It contains vitreous humor (sometimes called the *vitreous body*), which is a clear fluid that has a soft, gelatinous consistency.

## LENS

The lens of the eye is a soft, transparent structure made up of layers of microscopic fibers that are arranged like the

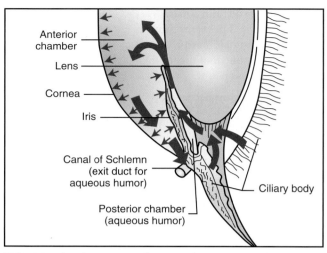

**FIGURE 10-10** Formation of aqueous humor. Aqueous humor *(large arrows)* is formed in the posterior chamber by cells of the ciliary body. It slowly circulates through the pupil into the anterior chamber and is drained by the canal of Schlemm, located at the junction between the cornea and the iris. The pressure of the aqueous humor is indicated by small arrows.

 **CLINICAL APPLICATION**

### Glaucoma

Glaucoma is not one simple disease. Rather, it is a group of diseases characterized by increased intraocular pressure (pressure within the eye) that causes pain and can lead to blindness. In domestic animals, glaucoma is most often diagnosed in dogs, partly because it is seen fairly often in that species but partly because other species are not commonly tested for it. An instrument called a *tonometer* is used to test for glaucoma by measuring the intraocular pressure.

Glaucoma can have many origins, but the basic mechanism is that aqueous humor is being produced at a faster rate than it is being drained from the eye. This causes the intraocular pressure to rise. Most often the problem is due to insufficient drainage of aqueous humor, rather than overproduction. Therapy for glaucoma usually involves medical or surgical treatments designed to increase the rate at which aqueous humor drains from the anterior chamber.

The treatment of glaucoma usually is not as successful in domestic animals as it is in humans, because glaucoma is often in a very advanced stage when veterinary patients are presented for treatment. Unfortunately, glaucoma comes on very slowly and gradually with few, if any, clinical signs noticed early in the process, when treatment would be most beneficial. By the late stages, when the eyeball becomes noticeably enlarged and painful, it is often too late to save the animal's vision. In many cases, the affected eye must be surgically removed.

layers of an onion. It is elastic and biconvex (meaning it bulges out on both sides). Its normal shape is fairly rounded, but it can be pulled into a flatter shape if tension is applied equally around its equator. The front (rostral) surface of the lens is in contact with aqueous humor, and its back (caudal) surface is in contact with vitreous humor.

The main role of the lens is to help focus a clear image on the retina regardless of whether the object being viewed is close up or far away. It does this with the help of the muscles of the ciliary body through a process called **accommodation**.

Accommodation is the process whereby the shape of the lens is changed to allow close-up and distant vision. When the muscle fibers of the ciliary body are relaxed, the suspensory ligaments that attach it to the periphery of the lens exert tension on the lens, pulling it into a flattened shape that allows clear distant vision (greater than about 20 feet). For close-up vision, the ciliary muscles must contract to take tension off the suspensory ligaments. This allows the lens to assume its natural, more rounded shape. So close-up vision requires muscle contractions in the ciliary body, but distant vision does not. This explains why we often suffer eyestrain when we do close-up work for long periods (like reading this book, for example). Fortunately, we can take advantage of our knowledge of how accommodation works to relieve the eyestrain; that is, we just need to look off into the distance periodically to give our ciliary muscles a break.

 **CLINICAL APPLICATION**

### Cataracts

A cataract is an abnormal condition of the eye whereby the lens becomes opaque. Instead of having a normal transparent appearance, a cataract lens appears milky. This impairs vision, particularly in dim light. Cataracts can be a normal part of the aging process. As a result, they are often seen in older animals, in which they can lead to total or near-total blindness. In younger animals, they can be genetically inherited or develop secondary to conditions such as infection, trauma, diabetes mellitus, or excessive exposure of the eyes to ionizing radiation (such as x-rays). Usually the only effective treatment for a cataract is surgical removal of the affected lens.

### RETINA

The **retina** is the business end of the eye—the image sensor in the camera, so to speak. It is where the visual image is formed, sensed, and converted to nerve impulses that are decoded in the brain to re-form the image in the conscious mind. The whole reason the rest of the eye structures exist is to produce as accurate and clear an image as possible on the retina.

The retina is a complex, multilayered structure that lines most of the vitreous compartment of the eye. Its main components are three layers of neurons, the outermost (closest to the outside of the eyeball) of which is the actual layer of sensory cells. Figure 10-11 is a diagram of the major layers of the retina. From outside in, the layers of the retina are a thin *pigment layer,* the *photoreceptor layer,* the *bipolar cell layer,* the *ganglion cell layer,* and a *nerve fiber layer* that proceeds to the optic nerve. The bipolar cells and ganglion cells are neurons that integrate and relay nerve impulses from the photoreceptor

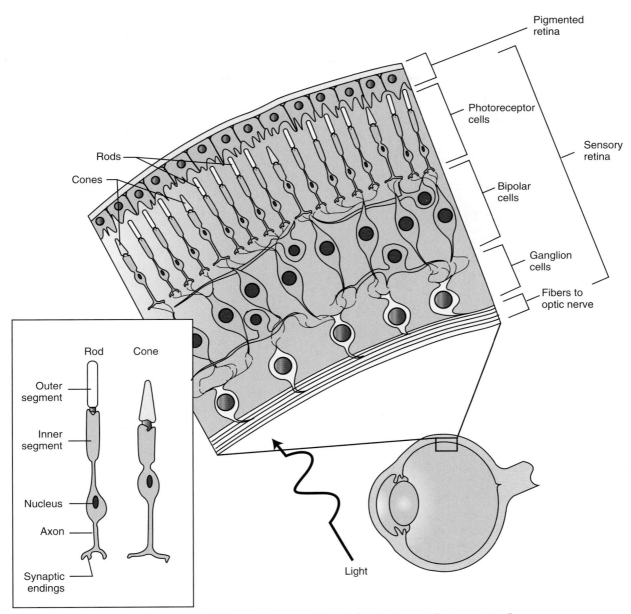

**FIGURE 10-11** Cell layers of retina, with detail of rod and cone (photoreceptor) cells.

cells to the optic nerve. Because the photoreceptor cells form the outermost (deepest) layer of neurons, light rays (which approach the retina from the inside of the eye, having entered through the cornea and lens) must pass through the other, more superficial layers before reaching them. Fortunately, these layers are basically transparent to light.

The nerve fibers on the inside surface of the retina all converge at the **optic disc**. This is where they leave the eye to form the optic nerve that carries visual information to the brain. The optic disc contains only nerve fibers and a few blood vessels but no photoreceptor cells (so no visual images are formed there). It is the blind spot of the eye. See Figure 10-12.

The resolution of a digital photograph is determined by how many tiny dots (aka *pic*tur*e* *el*ements or *pixels*) make it

up. In the digital camera of the eye, the photoreceptors form the pixels that make up the image that is perceived by the brain. Photoreceptor cells are neurons, but their dendrites have been modified into the actual sensory receptors for light. Two receptors, with different shapes and characteristics, are found among the photoreceptor cells: thin, rod-shaped receptors and thicker, cone-shaped receptors. They are usually referred to as **rods** and **cones** and actually have different sensory roles (Table 10-2).

Rods are more sensitive to light than are the cones, but the rods produce a somewhat coarse image in shades of gray. The cones are more sensitive to color and detail than are the rods, but they do not function well in dim light. So rods are the main receptors for low-light vision, and cones perceive color and detail. (The next time you are in dimly lit

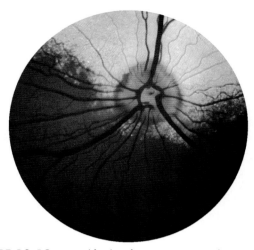

**FIGURE 10-12** Normal fundus of canine eye. Note the ivory-colored optic disc, the blue tapetum, and the dark red retinal blood vessels. (From Dziezyc J: Color atlas of canine and feline ophthalmology, Philadelphia, 2005, WB Saunders Company.)

| TABLE 10-2 | Photoreceptor Characteristics | | |
|---|---|---|---|
| **RECEPTOR** | **SENSITIVITY TO LIGHT** | **SENSITIVITY TO DETAIL** | **SENSITIVITY TO COLOR** |
| Rods | High | Low | Absent |
| Cones | Low | High | High |

conditions, notice that you see little or no color and that things do not appear very sharp. Your rods are doing most of the work.)

Domestic animals are often said to be color blind. This is not really an accurate way to describe their vision, because color blindness implies a defect in color reception that sometimes occurs in humans. Most domestic animals *can* see colors to some extent, but because most have a lot of rods and not as many cones, colors probably appear washed out to them. Their color vision probably looks like an old color photograph that has been exposed to too much direct sunlight; the colors are there, but are they are pale and faded. Recent research has shown that different animal species may perceive certain colors more intensely than others.

Domestic animals also do not perceive detail as sharply as we do for another physical reason. Humans and other primates have a dense accumulation of cones in a small depression called the *fovea centralis* in the center of the retina. This is the area of clearest vision and the one you are using to read these words. Domestic animals do not have a fovea, so their vision is apparently less sharp. Focus your eyes on the center of this page. The way the top, bottom, and sides of the page appear to you is probably as sharp as the world appears to many animals. That might seem like a severe handicap to us sight-oriented humans, but that's not a good way to think of it. Remember that animals are equipped with sense organs that are appropriate for them. To other animals, our limited sense of smell would seem as much of a handicap as their visual limitations seem to us.

## CLINICAL APPLICATION

### The Blind Spot of the Eye

To detect the blind spot of your eye, mark an *X* on a piece of paper, and about 2 inches to the right of that mark an *O*. Now close or cover your left eye, focus your right eye on the *X*, and hold the paper about 12 inches from your face. Slowly move the page toward your eye. At some point, the *O* will disappear. When that happens, it has fallen on your optic disc, where there are no photoreceptors. So its image disappears! Interestingly, the brain normally fills in the blind spot area, so the conscious mind is not usually aware of that "hole" in the visual field.

## FORMATION OF A VISUAL IMAGE

For the eye to transmit a clear visual image to the brain, a clear image must be formed on the retina. This is done by structures in the eye that refract (bend) light rays so they come into focus on the retina. *Refraction* is the bending of light rays that occurs as the rays pass into a medium of a different optical density, which affects the speed of light transmission. The more oblique the angle, the greater the degree of refraction. Because eye structures are curved, most light rays (except those directly in the center) strike the ocular surfaces at an angle.

Four refractive media in the eye help form a clear image on the retina: the *cornea,* the *aqueous humor,* the *lens,* and the *vitreous humor.* All contribute to the creation of a clear visual image, but the cornea does the majority of the refractive work. Its curved shape and the extreme difference between its optical density and that of the air in front of it result in significant refraction of light rays as they pass through it. The other refractive media, even the adjustable lens, only fine-tune the image that the cornea has formed. Interestingly, the image formed on the retina by these refractive structures is upside down. The brain somehow inverts the image so the conscious mind sees everything right side up.

### ✔ TEST YOURSELF 10-6

1. Where is aqueous humor produced? Where is it drained from the aqueous compartment of the eye?
2. Which type of vision requires more muscular effort: close-up vision or far-away vision? Why?
3. Why is the optic disc the blind spot of the eye?
4. What kind of vision do the rods in the retina perceive? What do cones perceive?
5. What is the main refractive structure of the eye? Why?

## EXTRAOCULAR STRUCTURES

Extraocular structures are not part of the eye itself, but they play important roles in its protection and functioning. They include the conjunctivae, the eyelids, the tear-production and drainage system, and the muscles that delicately move and position the eyeballs. Figure 10-13 shows many of the externally visible extraocular structures.

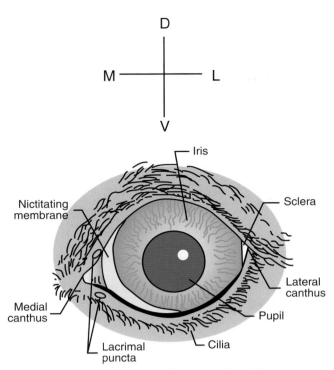

**FIGURE 10-13** External view of a dog's left eye.

### CLINICAL APPLICATION

#### Conjunctivitis

Conjunctivitis is inflammation of the conjunctiva of the eye. It is one of the most common eye diseases and occurs in all common domestic animal species. Signs include redness (hyperemia) and swelling (chemosis) of the conjunctiva, accompanied by ocular discharge and discomfort. The ocular discharge seen with conjunctivitis can range from watery (serous) to bloody (sanguineous) or pus-like (purulent). Causes include bacterial and viral infections, as well as physical and chemical irritants. Conjunctivitis is often seen in dogs that have been swimming in pools containing chlorinated water or hanging their heads out of car windows. Often the precise cause (etiologic factor) is not known. In mild cases of conjunctivitis, medical treatment may not be necessary. In more severe cases, antibiotic ointments or drops, which often contain corticosteroids to lessen the inflammation, are administered topically. Most cases of conjunctivitis respond well to treatment.

**CONJUNCTIVA.** The **conjunctiva** is a thin, transparent membrane that covers the front portion of the eyeball and lines the interior surfaces of the eyelids. The portion covering the front of the eyeball is called the **bulbar conjunctiva** (*bulbar* refers to the eyeball), and the portion lining the eyelids is called the **palpebral conjunctiva** (*palpebral* refers to the eyelids). The transparency of the conjunctiva allows the underlying tissues to show through, so it can be used as a window to see the blood vessels that are hidden elsewhere in the body by opaque structures, such as the skin. By looking through the conjunctiva at the lining of the eyelid, for example, we can often detect abnormalities such as anemia (paleness caused by decreased blood flow), jaundice (yellowish color), and cyanosis (dark purplish color).

The space between the bulbar and palpebral portions of the conjunctiva (between the eyelid and the eyeball) is called the **conjunctival sac**. It is normally only a potential space moistened by tears, but the ventral (bottom) conjunctival sac can be a useful place to deposit ophthalmic medications if the bottom lid is gently pulled out away from the eye before the medication is administered.

**EYELIDS.** The **eyelids** consist of upper and lower folds of skin that are lined by the thin, moist conjunctiva. The lateral and medial corners, where the eyelids come together, are called the lateral and medial *canthi* (**singular, canthus**). Along the margin of each eyelid are the tiny openings of the **tarsal glands**, also known as **meibomian glands**. These can be seen as a line of little dots along the eyelid margin. They produce a waxy substance that helps prevent tears

from overflowing onto the face. Eyelashes *(cilia)* are most prominent on the upper lid of most animals. Lower eyelashes are usually more sparse and thin, if they are present at all.

Domestic animals also have a **third eyelid** (also called the **nictitating membrane**) located medially between the eyelids and the eyeball. It consists mainly of a T-shaped plate of cartilage covered by conjunctiva. On its ocular surface (the surface in contact with the eyeball) are lymph nodules and an accessory lacrimal (tear-producing) gland. No muscles attach to the third eyelid. Its movements are entirely passive.

**LACRIMAL APPARATUS.** The **lacrimal apparatus** includes the structures that produce and secrete tears and the structures that drain them away from the surface of the eye. Tears are an important part of the overall liquid film that moistens and protects the surface of the eye. They are produced by the **lacrimal glands** and the accessory lacrimal glands of the third eyelids. The lacrimal glands are the primary source of tears. They are located dorsal and lateral to each eye inside the bony orbits that protect the eyeballs. Several small ducts from each gland deposit tears in the dorsal conjunctival sacs; from there, tears wash down over the surface of the eyes, aided by blinking movements of the eyelids. Figure 10-14 illustrates the position of the lacrimal glands.

The overall liquid film that moistens and protects the surface of the eye actually is made up of three main layers, only one of which comes from the lacrimal glands. These are an inner *mucous layer,* a middle *tear layer,* and an outer *oily layer.* The inner mucous layer comes from cells in the conjunctiva. It contains antibacterial substances that help protect the eye from infection. The middle tear layer comes from the lacrimal glands and the accessory lacrimal glands of the third eyelids. It serves to keep the cornea moist. The outer oily layer comes from the tarsal (meibomian) glands. It helps

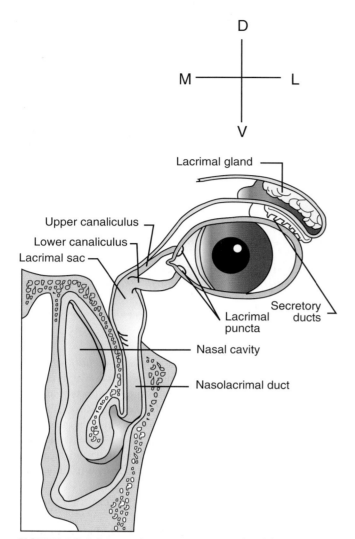

**FIGURE 10-14** Lacrimal apparatus. Tears produced by the lacrimal glands flow down over the surface of eye and drain into the lacrimal puncta. From there, they pass into the lacrimal sac and down the nasolacrimal duct to the nasal passage.

reduce evaporation of the underlying tear layer and prevents tears from flowing over the lid margin.

Tears are constantly being produced, so they must constantly be drained from the surface of the eye to prevent their spilling down the animal's face. The tear-drainage system is illustrated in Figure 10-14. Two small openings, one each in the upper and lower eyelid margins, drain the tears away from the surface of each eye. The openings are called the **lacrimal puncta** (singular, *punctum*), and they are located near the medial canthus of each eye. From the lacrimal puncta on each side, the tears flow down two small ducts to the **lacrimal sacs** and then down single ducts, called the **nasolacrimal ducts**, to the nasal cavity. This is why you get the sniffles when your eyes water: those excess tears have to go somewhere, and they drain down into your nasal cavity.

**EYE MUSCLES.** The **extraocular eye muscles** attach to the sclera of the eye (Figure 10-15). They are the small

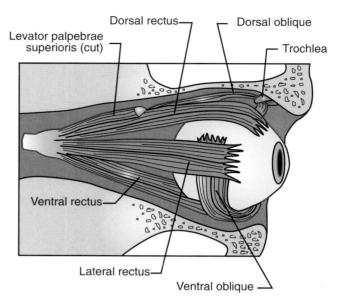

**FIGURE 10-15** Extraocular muscles of the right eye.

skeletal muscles that hold the eyeballs in place and delicately and accurately move them. They are capable of a wide range of movements that allow the eyes to track and examine objects with great precision. As you are reading this, note that your eyes track along the lines of words. If you concentrate, you can cause your eyes to move from letter to letter instead of from word to word. That's pretty delicate muscle control!

Humans share six extraocular muscles with domestic animals: four *straight muscles* and two *oblique muscles*. The four straight muscles are called the *rectus muscles*. (The word *rectus* means "straight.") They include the *dorsal, ventral, medial,* and *lateral* rectus muscles. Their names indicate where they attach to the eyeball. The two oblique muscles are the *dorsal* and *ventral* oblique muscles. Many animals also have a seventh extraocular muscle—the *retractor bulbi muscle*. It retracts the eyeball slightly deeper into the orbit when it contracts. This may assist the activity of the other muscles by enhancing their mechanical advantage. Most movements of the eye involve a combination of several of these muscles contracting together.

---

### ✓ TEST YOURSELF 10-7

1. How might examination of the bulbar and palpebral portions of the conjunctiva be useful as part of the overall physical examination of an animal?
2. An animal can intentionally blink its eyelids. Can it intentionally cover its eye with its third eyelid? Why or why not?
3. How would an animal with a plugged nasolacrimal system appear? Why?
4. If the medial rectus muscle of an animal's eye was damaged and lost its ability to contract, what would the effect be on the positioning of the affected eye? Why?

# 11  Endocrine System

*Thomas Colville*

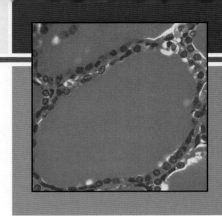

## OUTLINE

## LEARNING OBJECTIVES

*When you have completed this chapter you will be able to:*

- Describe the negative feedback system that controls the production of hormones.
- List the major endocrine glands and the hormones they produce.
- Describe the structure and functions of the pituitary gland.
- Describe the effects of growth hormone, prolactin, thyroid-stimulating hormone, adrenocorticotropic hormone, follicle-stimulating hormone, luteinizing hormone, melanocyte-stimulating hormone, antidiuretic hormone, and oxytocin.

- Describe the structure of the thyroid gland.
- Describe the effects of thyroid hormone, calcitonin, and parathormone.
- Differentiate between $T_3$ (triiodothyronine) and $T_4$ (tetraiodothyronine, or thyroxine).
- List the three categories of hormones produced by the adrenal cortex.
- List the hormones produced by the pancreatic islet cells and describe the effects of each.
- Describe the effects of androgens, estrogens, and progestins.
- List the hormones produced by the kidneys, stomach, small intestine, placenta, thymus, and pineal body.

## VOCABULARY FUNDAMENTALS

*Acromegaly* ahck-rō-**mehg**-ah-lē
*Adrenal cortex* ah-**drē**-nuhl **kohr**-tehx
*Adrenal gland* ah-**drē**-nuhl glahnd
*Adrenal medulla* ah-**drē**-nuhl meh-**duhl**-uh
*Adrenocorticotropic hormone (ACTH)* ah-**drē**-nō-**kohr**-tih-kō-**trō**-pihck **hohr**-mōn
*Aldosterone* ahl-**dohs**-tuhr-ōn
*Alopecia* ahl-ō-pē-shuh
*Anabolism* ah-**nahb**-uh-lihz-ehm
*Androgen* **ahn**-drō-jehn
*Anterior pituitary gland* ahn-**teer**-ē-ər **pih-too**-ih-tə**r**-ē glahnd
*Antidiuretic hormone (ADH)* ahn-tē-dī-ū-**reht**-ihck **hohr**-mōn

*Atrophy* **aht**-ruh-fē
*Calcitonin* kahl-sih-**tō**-nihn
*Calorigenic* kuh-**lohr**-uh-jehn-ihck
*Catabolism* kah-**tahb**-uh-lihz-ihm
*Catecholamine* **kaht**-ih-**kōl**-ih-mēn
*Cell-mediated immunity* sehl **mē**-dē-ā-tehd ihm-**myoo**-nih-tē
*Cholecystokinin* kō-leh-sihs-tō-**kī**-nihn
*Chorionic gonadotropin* kohr-ē-ohn-ihck gō-nahd-uh-**trō**-pihn
*Chyme* kīm
*Corpus luteum* **kohr**-pahs lū-tē-uhm
*Cortex* **kohr**-tehx
*Diabetes insipidus* dī-ah-**bē**-tēs ihn **sihp**-eh-dihs

*Diabetes mellitus*  dī-ah-**bē**-tēs **mehl**-eh-tihs

*Diuresis*  dī-ū-**rē**-sihs

*Duodenum*  doo-ō-**dēn**-uhm

*Dysfunction*  dihs-**fuhngk**-shuhn

*Eclampsia*  ih-**klahmp**-sē-ah

*Endocrine gland*  **ehn**-dō-krihn glahnd

*Endocrinology*  **ehn**-dō-krihn-ohl-uh-jē

*Epinephrine*  ehp-ih-**nehf**-rihn

*Erythropoietin*  ē-rihth-rō-**poy**-eh-tihn

*Estrogen*  **ehs**-trō-jehn

*Exocrine gland*  **ehcks**-ō-krihn glahnd

*Feedback mechanism*  **fēd**-bahck **mehck**-uh-nihz-uhm

*Fight-or-flight response*  fīt *or* flīt reh-**spohns**

*Follicle-stimulating hormone (FSH)*  **fohl**-ih-kuhl
  **stihm**-ū-lā-tihng **hohr**-mōn

*Gastrin*  **gahs**-trihn

*Glucagon*  **gloo**-kah-gohn

*Glucocorticoid hormone*  gloo-kō-**kohr**-tih-koyd
  **hohr**-mōn

*Gluconeogenesis*  gloo-kō-nē-ō-**jehn**-eh-sihs

*Glycosuria*  glī-kōs-**yɘr**-ē-ah

*Gonad*  **gō**-nahd

*Gonadotropin*  **gō**-nahd-uh-**trō**-pihn

*Growth hormone (GH)*  grōth **hohr**-mōn

*Homeostasis*  hō-mē-ō-**stā**-sihs

*Hormone*  **hohr**-mōn

*Hydrophilic*  hī-drō-**fihl**-ihck

*Hydrophobic*  hī-drō-**fō**-bihck

*Hyperadrenocorticism*  hī-pɘr-ah-**drē**-nō-**kohrt**-uh-
  kihz-uhm

*Hypercalcemia*  hī-pɘr-**kahl**-sē-**mē**-ah

*Hyperglycemia*  hī-pɘr-glī-**sē**-mē-ah

*Hyperplasia*  hī-pɘr-**plā**-zhuh

*Hypoadrenocorticism*  hī-pō-ah-**drē**-nō-**kohrt**-uh-
  kihz-uhm

*Hypocalcemia*  hī-pō-**kahl**-sē-mē-uh

*Hypoglycemia*  hī-pō-glī-**sē**-mē-uh

*Hypothalamus*  hī-pō-**thahl-uh-muhs**

*Hypoxia*  hī-**pohx**-ē-ah

*Iatrogenic*  ī-**aht**-rō-**jehn**-ihck

*Insulin*  **ihn**-suh-luhn

*Interstitial cell*  ihn-tɘr-**stihsh**-ahl sehl

*Interstitial cell-stimulating hormone (ICSH)*  ihn-tɘr-
  **stihsh**-ahl sehl **stihm**-ū-lā-tihng **hohr**-mōn

*Lactation*  lahck-**tā**-shuhn

*Luteinizing hormone (LH)*  loo-tē-eh-**nīz**-ihng **hohr**-mōn

*Luteolysis*  loo-tē-ohl-**ī**-sihs

*Medulla*  meh-**duhl**-uh

*Melanocyte-stimulating hormone (MSH)*  mehl-**ahn**-ō-sīt
  **stihm**-ū-lā-tihng **hohr**-mōn

*Melatonin*  mehl-ah-**tō**-nihn

*Metabolism*  meh-**tahb**-uh-lihz-ehm

*Milk fever*  mihlk **fē**-vɘr

*Milk let-down*  mihlk **leht**-doun

*Mineralocorticoid hormone*  **mihn**-ɘr-ahl-ō-**kohr**-tih-koyd
  **hohr**-mōn

*Monoamine hormone*  mohn-ō-ah-**mēn** **hohr**-mōn

*Myoepithelial cell*  mī-ō-ehp-ih-**thē**-lē-ahl sehl

*Myometrium*  mī-ō-**mēt**-rē-uhm

*Neurotransmitter*  nɘr-ō-**trahnz**-miht-ɘr

*Nonsteroidal anti-inflammatory drug (NSAID)*  nohn-
  **steer**-royd-ehl **ahn**-tē-ihn-**flahm**-uh-tohr-ē druhg

*Norepinephrine*  nohr-ehp-ih-**nehf**-rihn

*Oogenesis*  ō-ō-**jehn**-eh-sihs

*Ovary*  **ō**-vɘr-ē

*Oxytocin*  ohck-sē-**tō**-sihn

*Pancreas*  **pahn**-krē-ahs

*Pancreatic islet*  pahn-krē-**aht**-ihck **ī**-leht

*Parathyroid gland*  peɘr-ah-**thī**-royd glahnd

*Parathyroid hormone (PTH)*  peɘr-ah-**thī**-royd
  **hohr**-mōn

*Parturition*  pahr-tuhr-**ih**-shuhn

*Peptide hormone*  **pehp**-tīd **hohr**-mōn

*Pineal body*  **pī**-nē-ahl **boh**-dē

*Pituitary gland*  pih-too-ih-**teɘr**-ē glahnd

*Placenta*  pluh-**sehn**-tah

*Polydipsia*  pahl-ē-**dihp**-sē-ah

*Polyphagia*  pahl-ē-**fā**-jē-ah

*Polyuria*  pahl-ē-**yɘr**-ē-ah

*Portal system*  **pohr**-tehl **sihs**-tehm

*Posterior pituitary gland*  pō-**steer**-ē-ɘr **pih-too-ih-teɘr-ē**
  glahnd

*Precursor*  prē-**kuhr**-sɘr

*Progesterone*  prō-**jehs**-tɘr-ōn

*Progestin*  prō-**jehs**-tihn

*Prohormone*  prō-**hohr**-mōn

*Prolactin*  prō-**lahck**-tuhn

*Prostaglandin*  prohs-tuh-**glahn**-duhn

*Prostate gland*  **prah**-stāt glahnd

*Secretin*  seh-**krēt**-ihn

*Seminal vesicle*  **sehm**-ihn-uhl **vehs**-uh-kuhl

*Sex hormone*  sehx **hohr**-mōn

*Spermatogenesis*  spɘr-mah-tō-**jehn**-eh-sihs

*Steroid hormone*  **steer**-oyd **hohr**-mōn

*Superovulation*  soo-pɘr-**ohv**-ū-lā-shuhn

*Target*  **tahr**-giht

*Testes*  **tehs**-tēs

*Testosterone*  tehs-**toh**-stɘr-ōn

*Tetraiodothyronine (T$_4$)*  teht-ruh-ī-ō-dō-**thī**-rō-nēn
  (tee fohr)

*Thymopoietin*  thī-mō-**poy**-ē-tehn

*Thymosin*  **thī**-mō-suhn

*Thymus*  **thī**-muhs

*Thyroid gland*  **thī**-royd glahnd

*Thyroid hormone*  **thī**-royd **hohr**-mōn

*Thyroid-stimulating hormone (TSH)*  **thī**-royd **stihm**-ū-
  lā-tihng **hohr**-mōn

*Thyroxin*  thī-**rohck**-sihn

*Triiodothyronine (T$_3$)*  trī-ī-ō-dō-**thī**-rō-nēn
  (tee thrē)

*Unsaturated fatty acid*  uhn-**sahch**-ɘr-rā-tihd **faht**-ē
  **ah**-sihd

## INTRODUCTION

The endocrine system and the nervous system share the work of controlling and coordinating all the intricate parts and functions of the animal body. Put most simply, the two systems each help maintain **homeostasis** (balance) in the body. They constantly send instructions to the rest of the body, telling it how to respond to changes in internal and external conditions.

Table 11-1 summarizes the similarities and differences between the endocrine and nervous systems, but let's discuss some of the main ones. Both systems use chemicals to transmit their messages, but they do it by different means. The endocrine system messengers, **hormones**, are produced by **endocrine gland** cells, or modified neurons. They travel through the bloodstream to distant cells and tissues, where they produce their effects. The nervous system messengers, called **neurotransmitters**, are produced only by neurons. They travel very short distances across synaptic spaces to produce their effects. The targets of hormones are all of the cells and tissues in the body. The targets of neurotransmitters are generally only muscle cells, glands, and other neurons. The endocrine system reacts slowly to changes but can sustain its responses for long periods. The nervous system reacts quickly to changes but cannot sustain prolonged responses.

The basic units of the endocrine system are **endocrine glands**. Located throughout the body, endocrine glands secrete tiny amounts of hormones directly into the bloodstream. This method of secretion gives them the nickname *ductless glands*. This feature differentiates them from **exocrine glands (exo means "out" or "external")**,

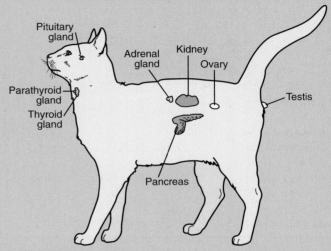

**FIGURE 11-1** Relative locations of major endocrine glands in the cat. (Modified from McBride DF: Learning veterinary terminology, ed 2, St Louis, 2002, Mosby.)

| TABLE 11-1 | Comparison of Endocrine and Nervous System Characteristics | |
| --- | --- | --- |
| **CHARACTERISTIC** | **ENDOCRINE SYSTEM** | **NERVOUS SYSTEM** |
| General function | Regulation of body functions to maintain homeostasis | Regulation of body functions to maintain homeostasis |
| Reaction to stimuli | Slow | Fast |
| Duration of effects | Long | Short |
| Target tissues | Virtually all body cells and tissues | Muscle and glandular tissues |
| Chemical messenger | Hormone | Neurotransmitter |
| Messenger producing cells | Endocrine gland cells or modified neurons | Neurons |
| Distance from chemical message | Long (via bloodstream) production to target | Short (across synaptic space) |

| TABLE 11-2 | Major Endocrine Glands | | |
| --- | --- | --- | --- |
| **GLAND** | **HORMONE** | **TARGET** | **ACTION** |
| Anterior pituitary | Growth hormone | All body cells | Growth, metabolic regulation |
| | Prolactin | Female—mammary gland | Lactation |
| | | Male—no known effect | None |
| | Thyroid-stimulating hormone | Thyroid gland | Thyroid hormone production |
| | Adrenocorticotropic hormone | Adrenal cortex | Adrenocortical hormone production |
| | Follicle-stimulating hormone | Female—ovary (follicles) | Oogenesis |
| | | Male—testis (seminiferous tubules) | Spermatogenesis |
| | Luteinizing hormone | Female—ovary (follicle/corpus luteum) | Ovulation and corpus luteum production |
| | | Male—testis (interstitial cells) | Testosterone production |
| | Melanocyte-stimulating hormone | Unknown | Unknown |
| Posterior pituitary | Antidiuretic hormone | Kidney | Water conservation |
| | Oxytocin | Female—uterus | Contraction at parturition |

*Continued*

| TABLE 11-2 | Major Endocrine Glands—cont'd | | |

| GLAND | HORMONE | TARGET | ACTION |
|---|---|---|---|
| | | Mammary gland | Milk letdown |
| | | Male—no known target | No known effect |
| Thyroid | Thyroid hormone | All body cells | Growth, metabolic regulation |
| | Calcitonin | Bones | Prevents hypercalcemia |
| Parathyroid | Parathyroid hormone | Kidneys, intestines, bones | Prevents hypocalcemia |
| Adrenal cortex | Glucocorticoid hormones | Whole body | Increased blood glucose, blood pressure maintenance |
| | Mineralocorticoid hormones | Kidneys | Sodium and water retention, potassium elimination |
| | Sex hormones | Whole body | Minimal effects |
| Adrenal medulla | Epinephrine and norepinephrine | Whole body | Part of fight-or-flight response |
| Pancreas (islets) | Insulin | All body cells | Movement of glucose into cells and its use for energy |
| | Glucagon | Whole body | Increased blood glucose |
| Testis | Androgens | Whole body | Anabolic effect, development of male secondary sex characteristics |
| Ovary | Estrogens | Whole body | Preparation for breeding and pregnancy |
| | Progestins | Uterus | Preparation for and maintenance of pregnancy |

which secrete their products onto epithelial surfaces through tiny tubes called *ducts*. The hormones produced by the endocrine glands circulate throughout the body in the blood and produce effects whenever they find specific receptors to which they can attach, either in or on cells.

Endocrine glands are found throughout the body, and the list of them grows as we learn more about **endocrinology**. In this chapter we focus mostly on the major endocrine glands. Table 11-2 summarizes the major endocrine glands and their hormones, and Figure 11-1 shows their relative locations in the body. Like many other parts of the body, hormones and endocrine structures are known by more than one name or abbreviation. We use common clinical veterinary usage as our guide, with alternative terms included where appropriate for clarity.

✓ **TEST YOURSELF 11-1**
1. How do endocrine glands differ from exocrine glands?
2. In what ways are the functions and characteristics of the endocrine system similar to those of the nervous system? In what ways are they different?

## HORMONES

### CHARACTERISTICS

Hormones are chemical messengers produced by endocrine glands and secreted directly into blood vessels. They travel in the bloodstream to all parts of the body and produce effects only when they bind to their particular receptors in or on cells. Figure 11-2 shows examples of cell membrane and intracellular receptor binding. Each body cell has specific receptors for a variety of hormones. These receptors are like locks into which only specific keys (hormones) can fit. When a hormone (key) binds to its receptor (lock) in or on a cell, it changes some activity of that cell. If a cell does not have receptors to a particular hormone, that hormone just passes by and has no effect on that cell. A cell that has receptors for a particular hormone is referred to as a **target** of that hormone.

## HORMONE CHEMISTRY

Animal hormones have diverse chemical structures, but they can be categorized into three main groups: peptide hormones, steroid hormones, and monoamine hormones. Box 11-1 shows which major hormones belong to each group.

**Peptide hormones** consist of chains of a few to 200 or more amino acids arranged like pearls in a necklace. They are **hydrophilic** (soluble in water), so they can easily travel in the blood plasma, which is mostly water. Receptors for peptide hormones are located on the cell membranes of their target cells.

**Steroid hormones** are lipids that are synthesized from cholesterol (Figure 11-3). They are **hydrophobic** (insoluble in water), so they must bind to hydrophilic transport proteins in order to travel in the plasma. The portion of hormone molecules that are attached to transport protein molecules is called "bound hormone," and the portion that is not attached is called "unbound, or free, hormone." Only the free form of the hormone can leave the bloodstream and reach a target cell. Receptors for steroid hormones are located within the cell—either in the cytoplasm or the nucleus. The lipid structure of these hormones allows them to pass easily through the cell membrane to reach their receptors.

**Monoamine hormones** are derived from amino acids and retain an amino group, which gives the group its name.

The **catecholamine** hormones (epinephrine and norepinephrine) are hydrophilic, and are transported dissolved in the plasma like the peptide hormones. Thyroid hormones, however, are hydrophobic like the steroid hormones, and require transport proteins. Receptors for catecholamine hormones are located on the cell membranes of their target cells,

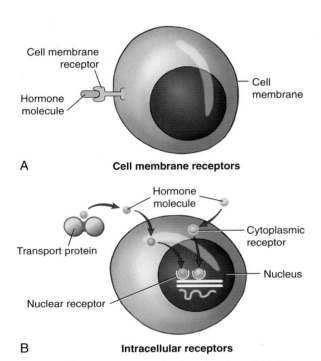

**FIGURE 11-2** Hormone receptor binding. **A,** Water-soluble hormones such as peptides and catecholamines bind to receptors on the cell membrane. **B,** Lipid-soluble hormones such as steroid and thyroid hormones pass through the cell membrane and bind to receptors in the cytoplasm or nucleus.

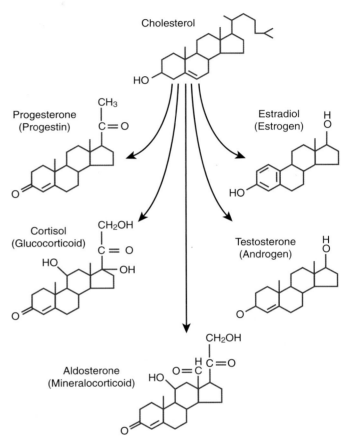

**FIGURE 11-3** Structure of steroid hormones.

---

**BOX 11-1** | Chemical Categories of Hormones

**Monoamine**
- Catecholamines (e.g., epinephrine and norepinephrine)
- Thyroid hormones

**Peptide Hormones**
- Adrenocorticotropic hormone (ACTH)
- Antidiuretic hormone (ADH)
- Calcitonin
- Cholecystokinin
- Chorionic gonadotropin
- Erythropoietin
- Follicle-stimulating hormone (FSH)
- Gastrin
- Glucagon
- Growth hormone (GH)
- Insulin
- Luteinizing hormone (LH)

- Melanocyte-stimulating hormone (MSH)
- Melatonin
- Oxytocin
- Parathyroid hormone (PTH)
- Prolactin
- Relaxin
- Secretin
- Thymic hormones (e.g., thymopoietin)
- Thyroid-stimulating hormone

**Steroid Hormones**
- Androgens (e.g., testosterone)
- Estrogens (e.g., estradiol)
- Glucocorticoid hormones (e.g., cortisol)
- Mineralocorticoid hormones (e.g., aldosterone)
- Progestins (e.g., progesterone)

whereas receptors for thyroid hormones are located in the nucleus, like those for some of the steroid hormones.

## CONTROL OF HORMONE SECRETION

Hormone secretion is commonly controlled by what are called **feedback systems**. This means that the level of hormone in the blood directly or indirectly "feeds back" to the gland that produced it and affects the activity of the gland. If the activity is decreased by rising levels of the hormone, the feedback is said to be *negative feedback*. If the activity is increased by falling levels of the hormone, the feedback is said to be *positive feedback*.

Negative hormonal feedback systems are the most common type in the animal body. They function in a similar fashion to a thermostatically controlled room heater on a cold day. When the heater's thermostat is set to a temperature higher than the current ambient temperature, the heater is turned on to heat the air. When the room's rising temperature reaches the thermostat setting, the heater is turned down or off. Without a source of heat, the air in the room cools. When the temperature falls below the thermostat setting, the heater is turned back on again, and so forth. The rising temperature of the room air *feeds back* to the thermostat and has a *negative* effect on the heater; that is, the heater is turned down or off. This is an example of a negative feedback system.

The secretion of many hormones is controlled in a similar fashion. For example, let's assume the "heater" is the **thyroid gland**, which produces its hormone as a result of stimulation by another hormone, called ***thyroid-stimulating hormone (TSH)***, from the **anterior pituitary gland**. When the level of **thyroid hormone** drops below needed levels—the "thermostat setting"—the anterior pituitary produces more TSH, which stimulates the thyroid gland to produce more of its hormone. This "turns on" the heater (thyroid gland) and tells it to produce more heat (thyroid hormone). The rising level of thyroid hormone in the bloodstream eventually reaches the level required in the body. Once that level is reached, the production of TSH by the anterior pituitary is turned down. This reduces the stimulation of the thyroid gland, causing it to produce less thyroid hormone (the heater has been turned down). When the level of thyroid hormone again drops below what the body needs, the anterior pituitary ramps up its production of TSH, which turns the production of thyroid hormone back up, and the process continues.

Positive feedback systems, in which rising levels of hormone produced by a gland feed back and further increase hormone production, are less common, because of their potential to lead to "vicious cycles" of out-of-control hormone production. Positive feedback systems do play specific, limited roles, for example in the complicated interplay of hormones involved in the female estrous cycle, but the system they are part of prevents vicious cycles of hormone production from developing.

One endocrine gland uses a totally different, non–feedback-related control mechanism for hormone secretion—direct stimulation from the nervous system. The secretion of hormones from the **medulla** of the adrenal gland is directly stimulated by sympathetic nerve impulses when an animal feels threatened. The adrenal medullary hormones that are released into the bloodstream as a result of this stimulation contribute to the whole-body **fight-or-flight response** that prepares the animal's body for intense physical activity. (The adrenal gland is discussed more fully later in this chapter.)

---

### ✓ TEST YOURSELF 11-2

1. What is a hormone?
2. What is a hormone target?
3. What are the three main chemical groups of hormones?
4. Which chemical hormone group(s) bind to receptors on the target cell membrane? In the cytoplasm or nucleus?
5. How does the negative feedback system control the secretion of many hormones?

---

## THE MAJOR ENDOCRINE GLANDS

### THE HYPOTHALAMUS
#### CHARACTERISTICS

The **hypothalamus** is a part of the diencephalon of the brain. It is located in the ventral part of the brain just caudal to the optic chiasma, where the optic nerves partially cross. It has many important nervous system functions, including appetite control, body temperature regulation, and control of wake–sleep cycles. It also links the conscious mind with the rest of the body by connecting higher centers in the cerebral **cortex** with lower brain centers and the endocrine system. This link with the endocrine system is accomplished through the control the hypothalamus has over the activities of the pituitary gland. This makes it a very important bridge between the nervous system and the endocrine system.

#### RELATIONSHIP WITH PITUITARY GLAND

The **pituitary gland** is an endocrine gland that is located ventral to the hypothalamus and is attached to it by a slender stalk. Blood vessels and nerve fibers in the stalk enable the hypothalamus to control the activity of the pituitary gland and therefore most of the rest of the body.

A system of tiny blood vessels called a **portal system** links the hypothalamus with what is called the *anterior portion* of the pituitary gland. Figure 11-4 shows this pituitary portal system. Modified neurons in the hypothalamus secrete hormones into these portal blood vessels. The hormones travel the short distance down to the anterior pituitary and regulate much of its function. These hypothalamic hormones, called *releasing* and *inhibiting factors*, are each specific for a particular anterior pituitary hormone. As their name implies, a releasing factor causes the anterior pituitary to produce and release a particular hormone, and an inhibiting factor has the opposite effect, inhibiting the production and release of a hormone. Because some anterior pituitary hormones influence all of the body's cells, the hypothalamus indirectly affects the whole body by

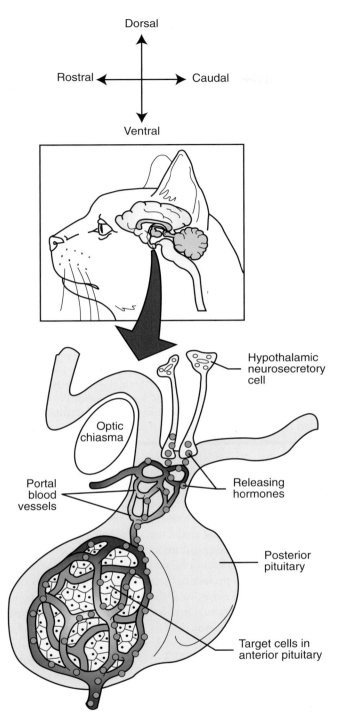

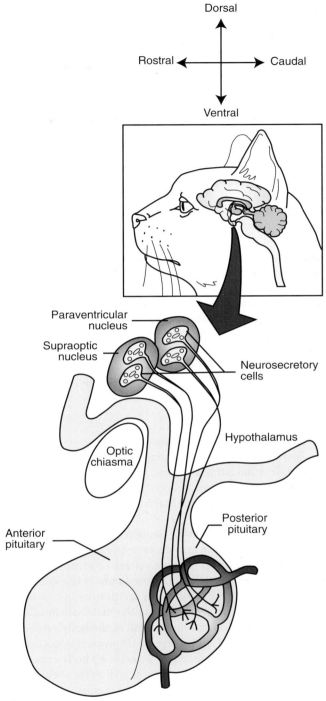

**FIGURE 11-4** Relationship of hypothalamus and anterior pituitary. Releasing and inhibiting hormones from the hypothalamus are secreted into portal blood vessels that carry them to the anterior pituitary. There they stimulate or inhibit release of anterior pituitary hormones.

**FIGURE 11-5** Relationship of hypothalamus and posterior pituitary. Neurosecretory cells (modified neurons) in the hypothalamus produce hormones that are transported down nerve fibers to the posterior pituitary, where they are stored. Their release is controlled by nerve impulses from the hypothalamus.

regulating anterior pituitary gland functions. In part, this is how the state of an animal's mind can influence its susceptibility and reaction to illnesses.

The effect of the hypothalamus on the posterior part of the pituitary gland is more direct. Modified neurons in the hypothalamus produce two hormones, **antidiuretic hormone (ADH)** and **oxytocin**, which are transported down nerve fibers (axons) to the **posterior pituitary gland**, where they are stored.

They are then released into the bloodstream by nerve impulses from the hypothalamus. Figure 11-5 illustrates this process.

## THE PITUITARY GLAND
### CHARACTERISTICS

The pituitary gland (also referred to as the *hypophysis*) is often called the *master endocrine gland* because many of its hormones direct the activity of other endocrine glands around the body. Physically the pituitary gland is tiny, about the size of a small pea or bean. It is connected to the hypothalamus above it by a slender stalk and is securely housed in a small pocket in the sphenoid bone of the skull called the *pituitary fossa.*

Although it looks like one structure, the pituitary gland is actually two separate glands with completely different structures, functions, and embryologic origins. The rostral (front) portion is called the *anterior pituitary,* or the *adeno-hypophysis.* It develops from glandular tissue in an embryo and looks like normal glandular tissue under the microscope. The caudal (rear) portion is called the *posterior pituitary,* or the *neurohypophysis.* It develops from the embryo's nervous system and looks like nervous tissue under the microscope.

The functions of the two parts of the pituitary gland are as different as their appearance. The anterior pituitary produces seven known hormones, when stimulated by the hypothalamus and direct feedback from target organs and tissues. The posterior pituitary does not produce any hormones. Rather, it stores and releases two hormones that are produced in the hypothalamus and transported to the posterior pituitary along nerve fibers.

## THE ANTERIOR PITUITARY

The following are the seven known anterior pituitary hormones:

- Growth hormone
- Prolactin
- Thyroid-stimulating hormone
- Adrenocorticotropic hormone
- Follicle-stimulating hormone
- Luteinizing hormone
- Melanocyte-stimulating hormone

**GROWTH HORMONE.** **Growth hormone (GH)** is also known as *somatotropin* and *somatotropic hormone.* Its name comes from its most obvious effect—the promotion of body growth in young animals, particularly the growth of bone and muscle. It has other important roles in animals of all ages, however. It helps regulate the **metabolism** of proteins, carbohydrates, and lipids in all of the body's cells.

The effect of GH on protein metabolism is to encourage the **anabolism**, or synthesis, of proteins by body cells. This supplies the materials for growth, as well as for the ongoing regeneration and repair of body tissues that have undergone injury or normal wear and tear.

The effects of GH on carbohydrate and lipid metabolism are linked. GH causes the mobilization (release) of lipids from storage in adipose (fat) tissue and their **catabolism** (breakdown) in body cells for energy production. At the same time, it discourages the cells from using carbohydrates, especially glucose, as energy sources. Because less glucose is removed from the blood by the cells, the level of glucose in the blood tends to rise. This is called a *hyperglycemic effect.* This effect is opposite to that of the pancreatic hormone **insulin**, which tends to lower blood glucose levels. Because glucose is such an important energy source

for the body's cells, a balance between GH and insulin is important to maintaining homeostasis of glucose levels in the blood.

### CLINICAL APPLICATION

#### Growth Hormone (GH)

Because of its whole-body effects, deficiencies or excesses of GH can produce some very obvious effects. The most pronounced effect of a GH deficiency is dwarfism, a condition in which a young animal does not grow normally. Other, less dramatic effects of GH deficiency relate to its metabolic effects and interrelationships with other hormones and endocrine glands. These can include **alopecia** (hair loss), thin skin, and development of secondary abnormalities of thyroid, adrenal, and reproductive hormones. Animals with GH deficiencies often respond to the therapeutic administration of GH. An excess of GH can result in a form of gigantism referred to as **acromegaly**. The cause of this condition is often a pituitary gland tumor.

A synthetic GH-like drug is also used to increase milk production in dairy cows. The drug bovine somatotropin (BST) is used for its generalized anabolic effect, which enhances the production of milk by the mammary glands. As is often the case with hormone-related drugs, some potentially serious side effects are associated with the use of BST. The drug is known to elevate animals' body temperatures, reduce conception rates, increase the risk of mammary gland infection (mastitis), and increase the risk of digestive disorders.

**PROLACTIN.** **Prolactin** is named for its effect in the female. It helps trigger and maintain **lactation**, the secretion of milk by the mammary glands. Once lactation has begun, prolactin production and release by the anterior pituitary gland continue as long as the teat or nipple continues to be stimulated by nursing or milking. If nursing or milking ceases, the production of prolactin will cease as well. Without stimulation from prolactin, the mammary gland "dries up," milk production stops, and the mammary gland shrinks back to its nonlactating size. In the male, prolactin has no known specific function.

**THYROID-STIMULATING    HORMONE.** **Thyroid-stimulating hormone (TSH)** is also known as *thyrotropic hormone.* As its name implies, it stimulates the growth and development of the thyroid gland and causes it to produce its hormones. Increased TSH secretion increases thyroid hormone production and vice versa. TSH secretion is regulated by feedback from its target organ—the thyroid gland. This occurs both through direct effects on the anterior pituitary gland and through changes in TSH-releasing factor produced by the hypothalamus. If thyroid hormone levels rise higher than the body needs, TSH production diminishes. With less stimulation, the thyroid gland decreases its hormone production, causing the thyroid hormone level in the bloodstream to drop. If the level drops too low, TSH production increases, stimulating the thyroid gland to increase its hormone production again. Homeostasis of thyroid hormone production is maintained through this interaction among the hypothalamus, anterior pituitary gland, and thyroid gland.

***ADRENOCORTICOTROPIC HORMONE.*** **Adrenocorticotropic hormone (ACTH)** stimulates the growth and development of the cortex (outer portion) of the adrenal gland and the release of some of its hormones. Its production is generally regulated by feedback from the hormones of the **adrenal cortex** in much the same manner as TSH production is regulated by feedback from thyroid hormones. In times of sudden stress to an animal, however, ACTH can be released quickly as a result of stimulation of the hypothalamus by other parts of the brain. When stimulated in this way, the hypothalamus sends a burst of ACTH-releasing factor down to the anterior pituitary through the portal system of blood vessels that links them, which causes ACTH to be released quickly.

***FOLLICLE-STIMULATING HORMONE.*** **Follicle-stimulating hormone (FSH)** is another hormone that is named for its effect in the female. It stimulates the growth and development of follicles in the **ovaries**. Each **follicle** is an "incubator" for a single, large female reproductive cell (the oocyte), which develops and matures as the follicle enlarges. This process is termed **oogenesis**. FSH also stimulates the lining cells of the follicles to produce and secrete **estrogens,** which are the female **sex hormones**. Estrogens are responsible for the physical and behavioral changes that prepare the female for breeding and pregnancy.

In the male, FSH has an effect similar to one of its effects in the female. It stimulates **spermatogenesis**, the development of male reproductive cells, the spermatozoa, in the seminiferous tubules of the **testes**.

### CLINICAL APPLICATION

#### Superovulation

Drugs like FSH are often used to "superovulate" animals in preparation for embryo transfer. They cause the ovaries to produce more follicles and ova than normal. This production of larger than normal numbers of ova is called **superovulation**. Once the animal is bred, the resulting fertilized embryos are retrieved from the uterus (usually by flushing) before they implant in its wall. They can then be transferred to other recipient animals, whose estrous cycles have been synchronized with the donor animal, for the remainder of the gestation (pregnancy) period. This allows females of particularly good genetic stock to produce more offspring in their lifetimes than normal reproductive mechanisms would allow.

***LUTEINIZING HORMONE.*** **Luteinizing hormone (LH)** is yet another hormone whose name is derived from its effect in the female. (Are you seeing a pattern here?) LH completes the process of follicle development in the ovary that was started by FSH. As a follicle grows, it produces increasing amounts of estrogens that feed back to the hypothalamus and anterior pituitary. They cause the production of FSH to decrease and the production of LH to increase. By the time a

follicle is fully mature, LH levels reach a peak. In most animal species, this causes ovulation, or rupture of the mature follicle and subsequent release of the reproductive cell. Once ovulation has occurred, the high LH level stimulates the cells left behind in the empty follicle to multiply and develop into another endocrine structure—the **corpus luteum**. The corpus luteum produces progestin hormones, principally **progesterone**, which will be necessary for the maintenance of pregnancy should it occur. In the male, LH stimulates cells in the testes called **interstitial cells** to develop and produce the male sex hormone **testosterone**. Therefore LH is sometimes called *interstitial cell-stimulating hormone (ICSH)* in the male.

FSH and LH are sometimes grouped together under the term **gonadotropins**, because they stimulate the growth and development of the *gonads*—the ovaries and testes.

***MELANOCYTE-STIMULATING HORMONE.*** Everything in the animal body exists for a reason, although the reason may just be that something is left over from some long-ago time in the species' history. That seems to be the case with our little toe and a horse's splint bones. **Melanocyte-stimulating hormone (MSH)** may be another remnant of an earlier time, but we have no conclusive evidence one way or the other. MSH is associated with control of color changes in the pigment cells (melanocytes) of reptiles, fish, and amphibians—animals that can rapidly change colors and color patterns. Administration of artificially large amounts of MSH to higher mammals can cause darkening of the skin from melanocyte stimulation, but its effect at normal physiologic levels is not known. Does it have some important role that we are not yet aware of? The jury is still out.

### THE POSTERIOR PITUITARY

Unlike the very busy anterior pituitary, the posterior pituitary, also called the *neurohypophysis*, does not produce *any* hormones. Instead, it serves as a place for two hormones produced in the hypothalamus to be stored for periodic release into the bloodstream. Antidiuretic hormone and oxytocin are transported along nerve fibers down to the posterior pituitary and stored there in nerve endings. Nerve impulses from the hypothalamus tell the nerve endings when to release them into the bloodstream.

***ANTIDIURETIC HORMONE.*** The name **antidiuretic hormone (ADH)** tells us what it does. It helps prevent **diuresis**, which is the loss of large quantities of water in the urine. Put more plainly, it helps the body conserve water in times of short supply by acting on the kidneys. ADH causes the kidneys to reabsorb more water from the urine they are producing back into the bloodstream. This makes the resulting urine more concentrated than it would have been otherwise. Concentrated urine has a deeper color and a stronger odor.

ADH is released when the hypothalamus detects a water shortage (dehydration) in the body. When an animal becomes a little dehydrated, the *osmotic pressure* of the blood increases (the blood becomes more concentrated), producing a condition called *hemoconcentration*. Receptors in the hypothalamus detect this change. This triggers nerve impulses that travel down to the posterior pituitary and cause the release of ADH. The ADH travels to its target organ, the kidney, and causes it to conserve water by producing urine that is more concentrated.

An interesting side note is that ADH release is inhibited by alcohol and caffeine. So, if we attempt to relieve thirst by drinking alcoholic beverages or caffeine-containing drinks, such as colas or coffee, we can actually produce the opposite effect. By putting the brakes on ADH release, these substances allow more water to flow out of the body in the urine. This worsens the hemoconcentration, making the thirst worse instead of better in the long run. So your mother's advice is accurate: The best thing to drink when you are thirsty is water! Moms are pretty smart.

A deficiency of ADH in the body causes the disease **diabetes insipidus**. Affected animals produce large quantities of very dilute urine (**polyuria**) and drink large quantities of water (**polydipsia**). Other disease conditions also produce polyuria and polydipsia, therefore a complete diagnostic workup is necessary to confirm the diagnosis of diabetes insipidus. The condition is treated by administering a drug with ADH activity for the rest of the animal's life.

**OXYTOCIN.** The two targets for the hormone oxytocin are the uterus and the mammary glands. In the uterus, oxytocin causes contraction of the **myometrium** (the muscle of the uterus) at the time of breeding and at **parturition**. At the time of breeding, oxytocin induces uterine contractions that aid the transport of spermatozoa up to the oviducts. When parturition (the birth process) begins, oxytocin stimulates strong uterine contractions that aid in the delivery of the fetus and the **placenta**. During a prolonged or difficult labor, oxytocin in the form of an injectable drug is sometimes given to dams to help strengthen weak uterine contractions. However, the myometrium may be "burned out" by overstimulating it with oxytocin, so good clinical judgment must govern its use.

The effect of oxytocin on active (milk-producing) mammary glands is to cause what is called **milk let-down**, or the movement of milk down to the lower parts of the gland. As milk is produced, it accumulates in the *alveoli* (milk-producing structures) and small ducts in the upper part of the mammary gland. Stimulation of the teat or nipple by nursing or milking causes oxytocin to be released into the bloodstream. The oxytocin circulates down to the mammary gland and causes the musclelike **myoepithelial cells** around the alveoli and small ducts to contract. This squeezes milk down into the lower parts of the gland, where it is accessible for nursing or milking. Usually the lag time lasts from a few seconds to a minute or two, from the time teat stimulation starts to when milk flow caused by milk let-down begins. This is how long it takes for the sensory stimulation to reach the brain and signal the hypothalamus to release oxytocin from the posterior pituitary and for the oxytocin to reach the mammary gland via the blood circulation.

Recent studies suggest that oxytocin may play roles in human, and perhaps other animal, behaviors such as social group recognition, pair connection and maternal–neonate bonding. You may hear it referred to as the "cuddle hormone" or the "bonding hormone." This is an emerging area of knowledge that may help us better understand normal and abnormal social and bonding behaviors. Put "oxytocin" into your favorite internet search engine to see what the current state of knowledge is. As always, however, carefully consider the source of internet information before accepting it as factual.

---

✔ **TEST YOURSELF 11-3**

1. Through what mechanisms does the hypothalamus control the production or release of hormones from the pituitary gland? How do its effects on the anterior and posterior portions of the pituitary differ?
2. Why is the pituitary gland referred to as the *master endocrine gland?*
3. Other than promoting growth in young animals, what are some of other effects of GH?
4. What stimulates the continued release of prolactin during lactation?
5. Do FSH and LH play important roles in male animals? If so, what are they?
6. Does ADH help promote or prevent the loss of large amounts of water in the urine? What effect would the inhibition of ADH release have on the body?
7. When milking a cow by hand, why does it take a minute or two of teat stimulation before milk starts to flow freely?

---

## THE THYROID GLAND

### CHARACTERISTICS

The thyroid gland consists of two parts called *lobes* that are located on either side of the larynx. The lobes may be connected by a narrow band called an *isthmus,* depending on the animal species. Figure 11-6 shows how the thyroid glands appear in several species. Microscopically the thyroid gland has an odd appearance (Figure 11-7). It is composed of tens of thousands of tiny *follicles,* where thyroid hormone is produced. Each follicle consists of a little sphere of simple, cuboidal glandular cells surrounding a globule of the thyroid hormone **precursor** (the raw material for thyroid hormone) they have produced. The thyroid hormone precursor in the globule is called *colloid.* The thyroid gland is the only endocrine gland that stores large amounts of hormone precursor for later use.

The thyroid gland produces two hormones: *thyroid hormone,* which mainly helps regulate the body's metabolic rate, and **calcitonin**, which helps regulate blood calcium levels.

### THYROID HORMONE

**Thyroid hormone** is produced when TSH from the anterior pituitary gland stimulates the thyroid gland. It is actually two hormones: $T_4$ (**tetraiodothyronine,** or **thyroxine**), which is considered a **prohormone**, and $T_3$ (**triiodothyronine**), which is the active hormone. Their names are derived from the number

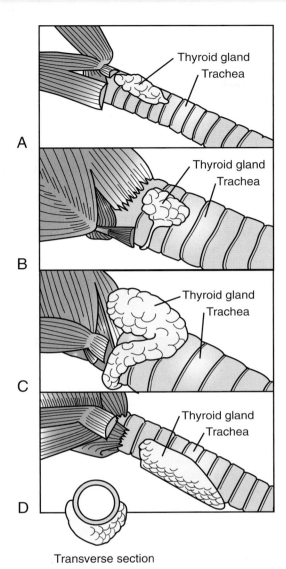

**FIGURE 11-6** The thyroid glands of several species. The inset cross section shows the ventral connection of the thyroid glands in the pig. A, Dog. B, Horse. C, Ox. D, Pig.

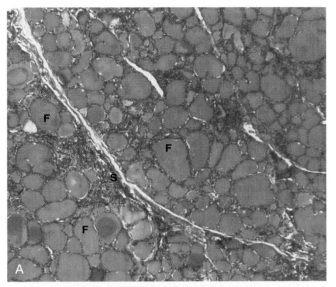

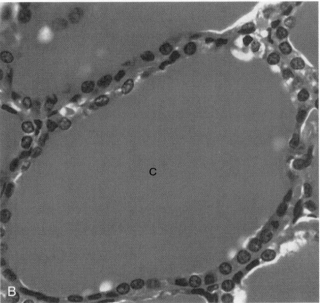

**FIGURE 11-7** Photomicrographs of the thyroid gland at low (**A**) and high (**B**) magnification. C, colloid; F, thyroid follicles; S, connective tissue septa. (From Koeppen B, Stanton B: Berne & Levy physiology [updated], ed 6, St Louis, 2010, Mosby.)

of iodine atoms each molecule of hormone contains. $T_4$ contains four iodine atoms per molecule, and $T_3$ contains three. The thyroid gland produces far more $T_4$ than $T_3$, but $T_3$ is the most biologically active form of thyroid hormone. The $T_4$ functions as a circulating reservoir. It is converted to $T_3$ in peripheral tissues, mainly the liver, kidney and muscle, as needed.

**CALORIGENIC EFFECT.** Thyroid hormone's **calorigenic** effect helps heat the body. It regulates the metabolic rate of all the body's cells, that is, the rate at which they burn nutrients to produce energy. Thyroid hormone's influence over the metabolic rate of the body's cells allows an animal to generate heat and maintain a constant internal body temperature when the temperature of the outside world changes. The production of thyroid hormone increases with exposure to cold temperatures. This response increases the body's metabolic rate, which generates more heat. It also causes

nutrients to be burned at a faster rate; so animals housed outdoors in cold temperatures need to be fed more calories than those kept in warmer temperatures, to prevent significant loss of body weight. The level of thyroid hormone can be thought of as the body's internal "temperature setting."

Thyroid hormone production can be inhibited by emotional or physical stresses on an animal. Under cold conditions, this effect can cause them to have difficulty maintaining their body temperatures. This in turn can compound the stress and open the door to disease. In otherwise healthy animals, cold temperatures alone usually do not cause disease outbreaks. However, if stress is added, animals can become more susceptible and disease outbreaks can occur.

### EFFECT ON PROTEIN, CARBOHYDRATE, AND LIPID METABOLISM.

Thyroid hormone also affects the metabolism of proteins, carbohydrates, and lipids, much like GH does. It encourages the anabolism, or synthesis, of proteins if the animal's diet contains adequate energy sources. If the diet is deficient in energy foods, or if the amount of thyroid hormone is excessive, the opposite can occur— protein catabolism or breakdown. The effect on carbohydrate metabolism is a hyperglycemic effect. Through several mechanisms, thyroid hormone helps maintain homeostasis of the blood glucose level by helping to prevent it from dropping too low. The effect on lipids is to encourage their catabolism, or breakdown.

### EFFECT ON YOUNG, GROWING ANIMALS.

Thyroid hormone is necessary for normal growth and development in young animals. In particular, it influences the development and maturation of the central nervous system and the growth and development of muscles and bones.

## CALCITONIN

**Calcitonin**, the other hormone produced by the thyroid gland, has an entirely different role. It is produced by C cells located between the thyroid follicles. Calcitonin is one of two hormones involved in maintaining homeostasis of blood calcium levels (the other is parathyroid hormone). Calcium is a vital substance in the body. It is involved in many important body functions, such as muscle contraction, blood clotting, milk secretion, and formation and maintenance of the skeleton. The level of calcium in the bloodstream must be kept within a narrow range to allow these functions to take place without any difficulty.

The action of calcitonin is to help prevent **hypercalcemia** (an excessively high blood calcium level) by decreasing the blood calcium level if it gets too high. It does this mainly by encouraging the excess calcium to be deposited in the bones. This is like putting money in the bank, knowing that you can go back and take it out later if you need it. The bones are the body's "calcium bank."

---

 **CLINICAL APPLICATION**

### Thyroid Dysfunction

Because of the thyroid's many important roles, **dysfunction** of this gland can have serious effects on the health and well-being of an animal. Three conditions most commonly seen are *goiter, hypothyroidism,* and *hyperthyroidism.*

Goiter manifests itself as a nonneoplastic (noncancerous), noninflammatory enlargement of the thyroid gland. It usually results from an iodine-deficient diet. Because iodine is an important component of thyroid hormone, a deficiency of iodine results in a deficiency of thyroid hormone. The anterior pituitary attempts to compensate for this by producing more thyroid-stimulating hormone (TSH). The elevated TSH levels overstimulate the thyroid and cause **hyperplasia** (overdevelopment) of the gland. This causes it to enlarge, resulting in what we call *goiter.* Although goiter can be treated with iodine supplementation, it is more easily prevented than treated. In areas known to be iodine deficient, iodized salt should be added to animals' diets.

Hypothyroidism results from a deficiency of thyroid hormone. It is most commonly seen in dogs, although it can be seen in any species. Because thyroid hormone influences the functioning of all cells, organs, and systems, hypothyroidism affects the whole body. This results in clinical signs that are vague and nonspecific. They relate primarily to a slowing of the body's metabolism. Common clinical signs include *alopecia,* or hair loss (usually bilaterally symmetric), dry skin, lethargy, reluctance to exercise, and weight gain without any increase in appetite. Affected animals often seek out sources of heat, because deficient thyroid hormone levels cause the animal to have difficulty maintaining its body temperature. Most cases of hypothyroidism occur in middle-aged animals, but if it occurs in a young animal, dwarfism (impaired growth) and impaired mental development occur along with the other common signs. Hypothyroidism often can be treated effectively by administering thyroid hormone supplements to affected animals. These supplements are usually in the form of the pro-hormone $T_4$, or thyroxine. The body then converts the $T_4$ to the active hormone $T_3$ as needed. Thyroid supplements usually have to be continued for the rest of the animal's life.

Hyperthyroidism is the opposite problem. It results from too much thyroid hormone production. It is most commonly seen in cats, although it is seen occasionally in dogs. Excessive amounts of thyroid hormone speed up cellular metabolism all over the body. This results in signs such as nervousness, excitability, weight loss, increased appetite, tachycardia (abnormally fast heart rate), vomiting, diarrhea, polyuria (excessive urine production), and polydipsia (excessive thirst). Hyperthyroidism is usually treated either by surgical removal of the thyroid gland *(thyroidectomy)* or by long-term administration of a thyroid-inhibiting drug.

---

 **CLINICAL APPLICATION**

### Hypocalcemia

The hypocalcemia-preventing action of parathyroid hormone can sometimes be overwhelmed by the loss of calcium in the milk of lactating animals. The hypocalcemia that results can be a serious, potentially life-threatening condition. The most obvious clinical signs relate to disturbances in skeletal muscle function caused by the lack of calcium. In cattle this condition is called **milk fever**, and it results in generalized muscle weakness. In mild cases, tremors and weakness are seen. As the condition becomes more severe, the animal may lie down and be unable to rise. Such an affected animal is often referred to as a *downer cow.* In dogs and cats, the condition is called **eclampsia**; it can cause muscle tremors and spasms that can progress to full-blown seizures if left untreated. Treatment in both cases is aimed at rapidly increasing the level of calcium in the blood by infusing a calcium solution intravenously.

## THE PARATHYROID GLANDS

### CHARACTERISTICS

The **parathyroid glands** got their name because of their physical relationship with the thyroid gland. They are several small, pale nodules in, on, or near the thyroid glands. Figure 11-8 shows a parathyroid gland on the surface of an animal's thyroid gland. The precise location and appearance of the parathyroid glands vary quite a bit from animal to animal and species to species.

### PARATHYROID HORMONE

**Parathyroid hormone (PTH)** is also conveniently called *parathormone.* It helps maintain blood calcium homeostasis by exerting an effect opposite to calcitonin. PTH helps prevent **hypocalcemia**, a blood calcium level that is too low, by increasing the blood calcium level if it should fall. It does this through its effects on the kidneys, the intestine, and the bones. It causes the kidneys to retain calcium and the intestine to absorb calcium from food, and it withdraws calcium from the calcium bank (the bones).

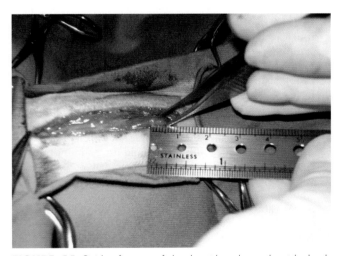

**FIGURE 11-8** Identification of the thyroid and parathyroid glands during surgery. The animal's head is to the right. The forceps are grasping the cranial end of the thyroid gland. The parathyroid gland is the oval structure just adjacent to the end of the ruler and measuring approximately 4 to 5 mm. (From Little S: The cat, Philadelphia, 2012, WB Saunders Company.)

## THE ADRENAL GLANDS

### CHARACTERISTICS

The **adrenal glands** are named for their proximity to the kidneys (*renal* refers to kidneys). The two adrenal glands are located near the cranial ends of the kidneys. (Note their locations in Figure 11-9.) Like the pituitary gland, the adrenals appear to be single structures, but they are actually two glands. In this case, one gland is wrapped around the other like chocolate wrapped around a peanut (Figure 11-10). The two glands, the outer *adrenal cortex* and the inner **adrenal medulla**, come from different embryologic origins and have different structures and functions.

### ADRENAL CORTEX

The **adrenal cortex**, the outer gland, develops from glandular tissue and looks like normal endocrine tissue microscopically. Under the direction of ACTH from the anterior pituitary gland and other mechanisms, the adrenal cortex produces an assortment of hormones that are classified into

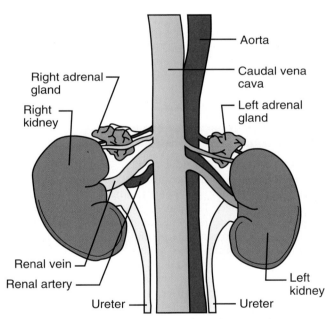

**FIGURE 11-9** Adrenal glands of the dog. Ventral view.

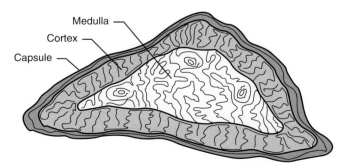

**FIGURE 11-10** Adrenal gland. Cross section showing cortex and medulla.

three main groups: *glucocorticoid hormones, mineralocorticoid hormones,* and *sex hormones.* All are referred to as *steroids* because their chemical structure is based on cholesterol.

### GLUCOCORTICOID HORMONES.

The name for the group of **glucocorticoid hormones** comes from its effect on the blood glucose levels. These hormones—cortisol, cortisone, and corticosterone among them—have a general hyperglycemic effect; that is, they cause the blood glucose level to rise. Several mechanisms are involved, including the breakdown (catabolism) of proteins and lipids. Most of the breakdown products are ultimately converted to glucose in the liver through a process called **gluconeogenesis**. Other effects of glucocorticoids include helping to maintain blood pressure and helping the body resist the effects of stress.

### MINERALOCORTICOID HORMONES.

**Mineralocorticoid hormones** regulate the levels of some important electrolytes (mineral salts) in the body. The principal mineralocorticoid hormone, **aldosterone**, affects the levels of sodium, potassium, and hydrogen ions in the body. Its target is the kidney, where it causes sodium ions to be reabsorbed from the urine back into the bloodstream in exchange for potassium and hydrogen ions, which pass out of the body in the urine. The level of sodium in the body must be maintained at a fairly high level normally, but much less potassium is needed. Potassium actually can be toxic if it accumulates to a level that is too high. Some drug preparations used to euthanize animals contain very high levels of potassium, which stops the beating of the heart. Hydrogen ions affect the body's acid–base balance, which must be

---

 **CLINICAL APPLICATION**

### Glucocorticoid-Related Diseases

A condition that results from too much glucocorticoid hormone being produced by the adrenal cortex is **hyperadrenocorticism**, sometimes called *Cushing's disease.* Initial clinical signs include polyuria (excess urine production), polydipsia (excess water consumption), and **polyphagia** (increased appetite). Long-term signs include hair loss, muscle wasting, and slow wound healing. The signs of naturally occurring hyperadrenocorticism can be mimicked by administration of high doses of corticosteroid drugs.

*Hypoadrenocorticism* (sometimes called *Addison's disease*) is a condition caused by a deficiency of adrenocortical hormones. Clinical signs are somewhat nonspecific, including weakness, lethargy, vomiting, and diarrhea. It is usually a progressive condition that can lead to circulatory problems and kidney failure. The effects of the disease can be mimicked if long-term corticosteroid drug administration is suddenly stopped.

---

 **CLINICAL APPLICATION**

### Glucocorticoid-Related Drugs

Drugs modeled after glucocorticoid hormones are commonly used therapeutically in animals, usually for their anti-inflammatory effect. This general class of drugs is commonly known as *corticosteroids* or *glucocorticosteroids* and includes drugs such as hydrocortisone, prednisone, dexamethasone, and triamcinolone. Because they mimic many of the effects of natural glucocorticoid hormones and are given in amounts much larger than the natural hormones, these powerful drugs have many potential side effects. These include the following:

- *Suppression of the immune response.* This can lower an animal's defenses and make it more susceptible to infection.
- *White blood cell count alteration.* As a result of corticosteroid drug administration, neutrophil numbers go up, and lymphocyte, eosinophil, and monocyte numbers go down. This mimics the body's natural stress response. If we're going to administer corticosteroid drugs to an animal around the time that blood is to be drawn for a complete blood count (CBC), the blood should be drawn *before* the drug is given. This approach avoids confusion in interpreting the results.
- *Slowing of wound healing.* Scar tissue-producing fibroblast cells are inhibited.
- *Catabolic effect.* After long-term corticosteroid drug use, the catabolism (breakdown) of protein can result in thinning of the skin, loss of hair, and a general loss of muscle mass.

- *Premature parturition.* Administration of corticosteroid drugs to pregnant animals can cause abortion of fetuses.
- **Hyperglycemia.** This condition can be significant in an animal with diabetes mellitus, because it can change the animal's insulin requirement.
- *Suppression of adrenal cortex stimulation.* The body's normal feedback mechanisms interpret the high levels of corticosteroid drug in the bloodstream as high levels of glucocorticoid hormones. This causes a cascade effect from the hypothalamus to the anterior pituitary gland to the adrenal cortex. The hypothalamus decreases its production of ACTH-releasing factor, which causes the anterior pituitary gland to decrease its production of ACTH. This results in diminished stimulation of the adrenal cortex. Long-term, high-level corticosteroid drug use actually can cause physical shrinkage (atrophy) of the adrenal cortex. If corticosteroid drug administration were then suddenly withdrawn, the animal would be left with a severe deficiency of glucocorticoid hormones. This would result in signs of **hypoadrenocorticism** (see the Clinical Application on glucocorticoid-related disorders). Therefore long-term use of corticosteroid drugs should not be terminated suddenly but tapered off gradually to give the adrenal cortex a chance to recover.
- **Iatrogenic *hyperadrenocorticism*.** This can result when excessive levels of corticosteroid drugs are administered; *iatrogenic* means *caused by treatment.* Signs mimic naturally occurring hyperadrenocorticism.

controlled carefully. Aldosterone also affects water levels in the body in that water accompanies sodium back into the bloodstream when sodium ions are reabsorbed.

**SEX HORMONES.** The adrenal cortex in both females and males produces small amounts of sex hormones. Both **androgens** (male sex hormones) and **estrogens** (female sex hormones) are produced. The amounts are very small, and their effects are usually minimal.

### ADRENAL MEDULLA

The **adrenal medulla**, the inner gland, develops from nervous tissue and resembles nervous tissue microscopically. Its hormone-secreting cells are modified neurons that secrete directly into the bloodstream. Two very similar hormones are produced: **epinephrine** and **norepinephrine**.

Hormone secretion by the adrenal medulla is under the control of the sympathetic portion of the autonomic nervous system—the threat-control system. When an animal feels threatened, its sympathetic system kicks in, producing what is termed the *fight-or-flight response*. This reaction prepares the body for intense physical activity. Sympathetic nervous system effects include increased heart rate and output, increased blood pressure, dilated air passageways in the lungs, and decreased gastrointestinal function. These effects are produced partly by direct sympathetic nerve stimulation of target tissues and partly by the epinephrine and norepinephrine released into the bloodstream by the adrenal medulla. The adrenal medullary hormones circulate around the body, helping to produce the whole-body fight-or-flight effect. After the threat has passed, it takes the body a while to come down from its excited state. This delay is due to the epinephrine and norepinephrine circulating in the bloodstream. It takes some time for them to be metabolized and removed from circulation. *Author's note:* The next time you suffer a sudden fright that does not actually threaten your well-being, such as riding a roller coaster, notice how long it takes for your accelerated heart and respiratory rates to settle down after the "threat" has passed. That's how long it has taken your body to corral all your fight-or-flight hormones.

---

✔ **TEST YOURSELF 11-5**

1. What three groups of hormones are produced in the adrenal cortex? What are their effects?
2. How are the hormones of the adrenal medulla involved in the fight-or-flight response?

---

### THE PANCREAS

The **pancreas** is a long, flat, abdominal organ located near the **duodenum** (the first portion of the small intestine) that has both exocrine and endocrine functions. Most of its mass is made up of exocrine glandular tissue that produces important digestive enzymes. Its endocrine component makes up only a small percentage of the total volume of the organ, but one of its hormones, insulin, is vital to the life of an animal.

### THE PANCREATIC ISLETS

The endocrine portion of the pancreas is organized into thousands of tiny clumps of cells scattered throughout the organ. These clumps of cells are called **pancreatic islets**, or *islets of Langerhans*. The main endocrine cells of the pancreatic islets are *alpha cells*, which produce the hormone **glucagon**; *beta cells*, which produce insulin; and *delta cells*, which produce somatostatin.

### PANCREATIC HORMONES

Two of the three hormones produced by the pancreatic islets, insulin and glucagon, play important roles in controlling the metabolism and use of glucose, and they have opposite effects. The third hormone, somatostatin, inhibits the secretion of insulin and glucagon, as well as GH, and diminishes the activity of the gastrointestinal tract.

---

 **CLINICAL APPLICATION**

### Diabetes Mellitus

Without sufficient insulin in the body, glucose does not move into body cells. It builds up in the blood, resulting in excessively high blood glucose levels (hyperglycemia), which spill over into the urine, thereby producing **glycosuria**, or glucose in the urine. At the same time, the body's cells are starved of energy, because they cannot absorb and use the glucose that surrounds them.

**Diabetes mellitus** is a disease caused by a deficiency of the hormone insulin. The clinical signs of diabetes mellitus usually develop gradually. They include polyuria, polydipsia, polyphagia, weight loss, and weakness. Laboratory tests reveal hyperglycemia (too *high* a level of glucose in the blood) and glycosuria. The condition can be fatal if left untreated.

Diabetes mellitus is not presently curable, but it often can be controlled effectively through appropriate treatment. This approach usually involves careful management of the animal's diet and amount of exercise, administration of insulin injections once or twice a day, and frequent monitoring of the animal's urine and blood glucose levels. The dose of insulin must be carefully controlled, because an overdose can result in **hypoglycemia** (too *low* a level of glucose in the blood), which can lead to weakness and collapse.

---

**INSULIN.** The hormone insulin is essential for life. It causes glucose, amino acids, and fatty acids in the bloodstream to be absorbed through cell membranes into body cells and used for energy. Because its overall effect on glucose is to move it out of the bloodstream and into cells, insulin acts to lower the level of glucose in the blood.

**GLUCAGON.** Glucagon has an effect opposite to insulin. Insulin lowers the blood glucose level, whereas glucagon raises it. This hyperglycemic effect is accomplished by two main mechanisms: glucagon stimulates liver cells to convert glycogen (a storage form of glucose) to glucose. It also stimulates gluconeogenesis (the conversion of fat and protein breakdown products to glucose). The net effect of both is to raise the level of glucose in the blood. Because other hormones, such as GH (from the anterior pituitary gland) and glucocorticoid hormones (from the adrenal cortex), have similar hyperglycemic effects, a deficiency of glucagon is not as devastating to the body as a deficiency of insulin.

## THE GONADS

The gonads are the reproductive organs—the testes in the male and the ovaries in the female. They produce the male and female reproductive cells and important hormones.

### THE TESTES

The two testes are housed in the scrotum, a sac of skin in the inguinal region. The majority of each testis is made up of coiled seminiferous tubules, where spermatozoa are produced. Scattered between the seminiferous tubules are clumps of endocrine cells, called the *interstitial cells* (Figure 11-11), which produce androgens, the male sex hormones. The production of androgens by the interstitial cells is stimulated by the anterior pituitary hormone luteinizing hormone (LH), also known as **interstitial cell stimulating hormone (ICSH)** in the male. The principal androgen that the interstitial cells produce is testosterone. It is responsible for the development of male secondary sex characteristics, such as the muscular male body shape and the male libido, or sex drive. Testosterone also stimulates the development of

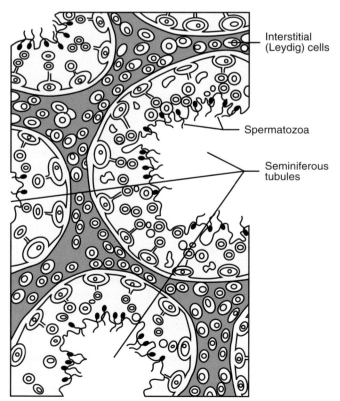

Interstitial
(Leydig) cells

Spermatozoa

Seminiferous
tubules

**FIGURE 11-11** Interstitial cells of testes. Interstitial cells of testes produce androgens, principally testosterone, under stimulation by luteinizing hormone from the anterior pituitary.

the male accessory sex glands, activates spermatogenesis (spermatozoa production), and stimulates the growth of the penis. Testosterone is a steroid hormone with an overall anabolic effect in that it stimulates the buildup of proteins in muscle and bone.

## THE OVARIES

The two **ovaries** are located in the abdomen up near the kidneys. Unlike the testes, which produce spermatozoa and hormones continuously, the ovaries produce the female reproductive cells (ova) and hormones in cycles. The ovarian cycles are controlled by two anterior pituitary hormones: follicle stimulating hormone (FSH) and luteinizing hormone (LH). The main hormone groups produced in the ovaries are *estrogens* and **progestins**. A third hormone, relaxin, may be produced in the ovary late in pregnancy.

**ESTROGENS.** Estrogens, such as estradiol and estrone, are the female sex hormones. They are produced when FSH from the anterior pituitary gland stimulates follicles to develop in the ovaries. Follicles are fluid-filled structures in which the female reproductive cells develop. The cells that make up the follicles produce and release the estrogens into the bloodstream. Estrogens are responsible for the physical and behavioral changes that prepare the female for breeding and pregnancy and signal the male that the time for breeding is approaching.

As an ovarian follicle grows, the amount of estrogens it produces grows as well. The increasing estrogen levels accelerate the physical and behavioral changes that are occurring and feed back to the anterior pituitary gland. The feedback causes the anterior pituitary gland to reduce the production of FSH and increase the production of LH. As the follicle continues to grow, the amount of FSH in the bloodstream gradually decreases and the LH level increases. When the follicle is fully mature, the LH level peaks and, in most animal species, ovulation occurs. Ovulation is the rupture of the blisterlike follicle with release of the ovum into the oviduct. (See Chapter 19 for a more complete description of the whole process of follicle development and rupture.)

**PROGESTINS.** After ovulation has taken place, the high LH level stimulates the cells of the now-empty follicle to multiply and develop into a solid, hormone-producing structure—the *corpus luteum*. The term literally means *yellow body* and derives from its pale yellow color. The corpus luteum produces several hormones that are collectively called **progestins**. The principal progestin is *progesterone*, whose name means *pregnancy-promoting steroid hormone*. Progesterone helps prepare the uterus to receive the fertilized ovum and is necessary for pregnancy to be maintained once the fertilized ovum implants in the uterus.

If the female animal is bred and becomes pregnant, the corpus luteum must continue to be active in the ovary, producing the pregnancy-supporting progestin hormones. Different species have different ways to do this, but the basic mechanism is that a substance produced by the early embryo feeds back to the uterus and ovary, and causes the corpus luteum to be maintained. If pregnancy does not occur, no "we are pregnant" signal is received, and the corpus luteum shrinks up and disappears.

Progestin-related drugs are often used therapeutically, especially in horses. They are most commonly used to delay the onset of estrus (the heat period), to synchronize the estrous periods in a group of mares so that they can be bred at the same time, and to help maintain pregnancy in mares that have deficient natural progesterone levels.

***RELAXIN.*** Late in pregnancy, the hormone **relaxin** causes ligaments between the bones surrounding the birth canal to soften and relax in preparation for parturition (the birth process). It may also play a role in mammary development in some species. Depending on the species, relaxin may be produced by the corpus luteum, the placenta or the uterus.

---

### TEST YOURSELF 11-6

1. Which four hormones have hyperglycemic effects in the body? What is the only hormone that acts to lower the blood glucose level?
2. Which hormone are anabolic steroid drugs related to?
3. How do the basic actions and purposes of estrogens and progestins differ?
4. How does relaxin help prepare a pregnant animal for parturition?

---

## CLINICAL APPLICATION

### Anabolic Steroid Drugs

Anabolic steroid drugs, which are related to testosterone, are used to help debilitated animals regain strength and weight after surgery or long illnesses. Unfortunately, they are sometimes abused by people seeking a shortcut to muscular development and performance enhancement. Because of their similarity to the hormone testosterone, they have many undesirable side effects that alter reproductive functions, behavior, and other body systems.

---

## CLINICAL APPLICATION

### Hormones as Drugs

Because of their powerful and often widespread effects, hormones and hormonelike substances are used as drugs to treat illnesses or to produce particular desired effects in animals. When natural hormone levels are too low, hormones can be given therapeutically to help correct the imbalance. This is often the case with hypothyroidism (deficiency of thyroid hormone), diabetes insipidus (deficiency of antidiuretic hormone), and diabetes mellitus (deficiency of insulin). In other cases, drugs derived from natural hormones are used to produce particular effects, such as an anti-inflammatory effect

## CLINICAL APPLICATION—cont'd

(glucocorticoid-like drugs) or stimulation of uterine contractions (oxytocin), cardiovascular stimulation (epinephrine), or to synchronize estrous cycles (prostaglandin $F_2\alpha$).

Because the production and effects of natural hormones are so interrelated, the therapeutic use of hormones and hormonelike drugs can produce some potent and widespread problems, along with beneficial effects. The amounts of hormones used therapeutically are usually very large compared with the normal physiologic hormone levels in the body, therefore the potential for undesired side effects increases accordingly. For example, use of a hormonelike drug can inhibit production of the natural hormone it mimics. Later, when the drug is to be discontinued, the animal should be gradually weaned off it so that the natural hormone production mechanisms can gradually take over again. Suddenly stopping the drug after long-term administration can produce disastrous results. In general, hormone therapy must be carefully planned and closely monitored so that the benefits outweigh the consequences.

---

## OTHER ENDOCRINE ORGANS

Hormone production is not restricted to the major endocrine glands that we have just discussed. Other organs and tissues produce hormones that also play important roles in maintaining homeostasis in the body. We discuss some of the most important and well-understood ones next.

### THE KIDNEYS

In addition to their blood-filtering duties, the kidneys produce the hormone **erythropoietin**, which stimulates red bone marrow to increase production of oxygen-carrying red blood cells. The production of erythropoietin is stimulated by a decrease in the oxygen content of the blood, a condition called **hypoxia**. As the production of red blood cells increases in response to the erythropoietin, the increased oxygen level in the blood feeds back to the kidneys and slows the production of erythropoietin. This helps maintain the long-term homeostasis of the blood's oxygen-carrying ability.

One of the conditions that often accompanies serious kidney disease or kidney failure is *anemia,* which is a deficiency of red blood cells. It results from the damaged kidneys' inability to produce enough erythropoietin. The deficiency of erythropoietin causes the patient to become increasingly hypoxic, because old, worn-out red blood cells continue to be removed from the bloodstream but not enough new red blood cells are being produced to replace them. Blood transfusions are often necessary to support patients with kidney failure while other forms of therapy are administered. Synthetic forms of erythropoietin are available and are often used therapeutically in human patients with kidney failure. Their high cost limits their use in veterinary medicine.

## THE STOMACH

Cells in the wall of the stomach produce the hormone **gastrin**. It is a somewhat oddball hormone, because it is produced in the stomach wall and acts on the stomach wall, too. Its secretion is stimulated by the presence of food in the stomach. When released, gastrin stimulates gastric (stomach) glands to secrete hydrochloric acid and digestive enzymes, and it encourages muscular contractions of the stomach wall.

## THE SMALL INTESTINE

Cells in the lining of the small intestine produce two hormones when partially digested material from the stomach (**chyme**) enters the first portion of the small intestine (the duodenum). One of the hormones, **secretin**, stimulates the pancreas to secrete fluid rich in sodium bicarbonate into the duodenum to neutralize the acidic chyme from the stomach. The other hormone, **cholecystokinin**, stimulates the release of digestive enzymes from the pancreas into the duodenum. Both secretin and cholecystokinin also act on the stomach to inhibit gastric gland secretions and stomach motility. This slows the movement of chyme into the small intestine. They also stimulate the gallbladder of the liver to contract, sending bile down into the small intestine to aid the digestion and absorption of fats and fat-soluble vitamins.

## THE PLACENTA

The **placenta** is the life support system that surrounds a developing fetus during pregnancy and acts as an interface with the maternal circulation. It is also an important endocrine organ. Its secretions vary among species, but the hormones it produces have the general effect of helping to support and maintain pregnancy. Small amounts of estrogen and progesterone are often produced, as well as significant amounts of **chorionic gonadotropin** in some species, most notably the human and the horse. Detection of chorionic gonadotropin is the basis of over-the-counter pregnancy tests for humans and blood tests for the detection of pregnancy in horses. Other species, such as dogs, cats, and cattle, produce too little chorionic gonadotropin to make it useful as a method of pregnancy diagnosis.

The placenta of some species produces the hormone relaxin late in pregnancy. It helps relax ligaments between the bones around the birth canal in preparation for parturition. Depending on the species it may be produced by the placenta, the uterus, or the corpus luteum of the ovary.

## THE THYMUS

The **thymus** is an organ that helps kick start the immune system early in an animal's life. It shrinks down and nearly disappears when the animal reaches adulthood. In a young animal, the thymus is fairly large. It extends cranially from the level of the heart in the thorax up into the neck region along both sides of the trachea, often to the level of the larynx. After puberty, however, the thymus begins to **atrophy** (shrink). By the time the animal reaches adulthood, it is hard or impossible to find any remnant of the thymus.

The thymus is an important part of the animal's developing immune system—the system that helps fight off foreign invaders, such as disease-causing bacteria and viruses. Part of its functioning seems to involve hormones or hormone-like chemical substances, such as **thymosin** and **thymopoietin**. These substances seem to cause primitive cells in the thymus and other lymphoid organs to be transformed into T (for "thymus-derived") lymphocytes. T lymphocytes are often just called *T cells*. They are an important part of the animal's **cell-mediated immunity**—the portion of the immune system that produces "killer cells" that directly attack foreign invaders (see Chapter 13).

## THE PINEAL BODY

The pineal body is a part of the brain located at the caudal end of the deep cleft that separates the two cerebral hemispheres, and just rostral to the cerebellum. Its functions are not well understood yet, but it is known to influence cyclic activities in the body, or the body's biologic clock. It produces a hormonelike substance called melatonin that seems to affect moods and wake–sleep cycles. It may also play a role in the timing of seasonal estrous cycles in some species. We still have a lot to learn about the roles of the pineal body and its secretions.

# PROSTAGLANDINS

Prostaglandins are hormonelike substances that are derived from unsaturated fatty acids. They are produced and exert their effects within a variety of body tissues. Because they only travel a short distance from where they are produced, prostaglandins are sometimes called *tissue hormones*. Typical hormones regulate the activities of tissues and organs at some distance from where they are produced. Prostaglandins do not go very far from home. They regulate the activities of neighboring cells.

The name *prosta*glandin actually came about by mistake. The first prostaglandin was isolated from semen, and its origin was incorrectly identified as the prostate gland, hence the name *prostaglandin*. We now know that the seminal vesicles, not the prostate, produce that particular compound. (*Vesicular-glandins* apparently isn't as catchy a name as *prostaglandins!*)

Prostaglandins are now known to be produced in a variety of body tissues, including the skin, intestine, brain, kidney, lungs, reproductive organs, and eyes. Based on their molecular structure, they are organized into nine main groups—prostaglandins *A* through *I*. Subscript numbers and Greek letters are added to designate subgroups.

Prostaglandins exert some powerful effects in the body, including influences on blood pressure, gastrointestinal tract function, respiratory function, kidney function, blood clotting, inflammation, and reproductive functions. The E group of prostaglandins (PGEs) is known to play a role in the initiation of inflammation in the body. Nonsteroidal anti-inflammatory drugs, such as meloxicam (Metacam), carprofen (Rimadyl) and ibuprofen, produce some of their effects by inhibiting PGE synthesis.

Another clinically important prostaglandin is prostaglandin $F_2$alpha ($PGF_2$alpha). If administered to a female animal that has a functional corpus luteum in her ovary, $PGF_2$alpha will quickly destroy the corpus luteum. This is called luteolysis, and, depending on the species, it may cause a new estrous cycle to begin. If the animal is in early pregnancy, luteolysis will terminate the pregnancy. Drugs with $PGF_2$alpha activity, such as dinoprost tromethamine (Lutalyse), are commonly used to synchronize estrous cycles in livestock species so that groups of animals can be bred at the same time.

*Note:* Because of their potentially harmful reproductive and other effects in humans, it is recommended that $PGF_2$-alpha drugs be handled with caution; they should not be handled *at all* by pregnant women.

---

### ✓ TEST YOURSELF 11-7

1. Why are patients with kidney failure often anemic?
2. How do the actions of gastrin on the stomach differ from those of secretin and cholecystokinin?
3. Why are prostaglandins referred to as *tissue hormones*?
4. Why do hormonelike drugs generally have a high potential for undesirable side effects?

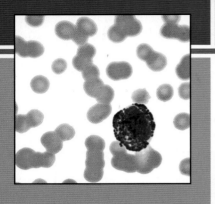

# Blood, Lymph, and Lymph Nodes  12

*Jennifer Maniet, DVM*

## OUTLINE

## LEARNING OBJECTIVES

*When you have completed this chapter you will be able to:*

1. Describe the composition and functions of blood.
2. Explain the difference between plasma and serum.
3. Describe how each type of blood cell is formed.
4. Describe the structure and function of each mature blood cell.
5. Describe the structure of the hemoglobin molecule.
6. Explain the fate of hemoglobin following intravascular and extravascular hemolysis.

7. List and describe the blood cell parameters of the CBC.
8. Describe the indications and goals of transfusion therapy.
9. Describe the two parts of the lymphatic system and the functions of each part.
10. Describe the formation of lymph fluid and its circulation through the lymphatic system.

## VOCABULARY FUNDAMENTALS

*Agranulocyte* ā-**grahn**-ū-lō-sīt
*Anemia* ah-**nē**-mē-ah
*Antibody* **ahn**-tē-boh-dē
*Anticoagulant* ahn-tē-kō-**ahg**-ū-lehnt
*Antigen* **ahn**-teh-jehn
*B cell (B lymphocyte)* bē sehl
  (bē **lihm**-fō-sīt)
*Basopenia* bā-sō-**pē**-nē-ah
*Basophil* **bā**-sō-fihl
*Basophilia* bā-sō-**fihl**-ē-ah
*Chemotaxis* kē-mō-**tahck**-sihs
*Deoxyhemoglobin* dē-**ohck**-sē-**hē**-mō-glō-bihn
*Diapedesis* dī-ah-peh-**dē**-sihs

*Edema* eh-**dē**-mah
*Eosinopenia* ē-ō-**sihn**-ō-**pē**-nē-ah
*Eosinophil* ē-ō-**sihn**-ō-fihl
*Eosinophilia* ē-ō-**sihn**-ō-**fihl**-ē-ah
*Erythrocyte* ē-**rihth**-rō-sīt
*Erythropoiesis* ē-rihth-rō-poy-**ē**-sihs
*Erythropoietin (EPO)* ē-rihth-rō-**poy**-eh-tihn
*Extravascular hemolysis* ehcks-trah-**vahs**-kyoo-lahr
  hēm-**ohl**-eh-sihs
*Fibrin* **fī**-brihn
*Fibrinogen* fī-**brihn**-ō-jehn
*Fibrinolysis* fī-brihn-**ohl**-eh-sihs
*Granulocyte* **grahn**-ū-lō-sīt

*Granulopoiesis* grahn-ū-lō-poy-ē-sihs
*Gut associated lymph tissue (GALT)* guht ah-**sō**-shē-ā-tehd lihmf **tihsh**-yoo
*Haptoglobin* **hahp**-tuh-glō-behn
*Hematocrit* hē-**maht**-ō-kriht
*Hematopoiesis* hē-maht-ō-poy-ē-sihs
*Hemoglobin* **hē**-mō-glō-bihn
*Hemoglobinemia* hē-mō-**glō**-bihn-ē-mē-ah
*Hemoglobinuria* hē-mō-**glō**-bihn-yər-ē-ah
*Hemostasis* **hēm**-ō-**stā**-sihs
*Hypoxia* hī-**pohx**-ē-ah
*Intravascular hemolysis* ihn-trah-**vahs**-kyoo-lahr hēm-**ohl**-eh-sihs
*Leukocyte* **loo**-kō-sīt
*Leukocytosis* loo-kō-sī-**tō**-sihs
*Leukopenia* loo-kō-**pē**-nē-ah
*Leukopoiesis* loo-kō-poy-ē-sihs
*Lymph* lihmf
*Lymphocyte* **lihm**-fō-sīt
*Lymphocytosis* lihm-fō-sī-**tō**-sihs
*Lymphopenia* lihm-fō-**pē**-nē-ah
*Lymphopoiesis* lihm-fō-poy-ē-sihs
*Macrophage* **mah**-krō-fāj
*Mast cell* mahst sehl
*Megakaryocyte* mehg-ah-**keər**-ē-ō-sīt
*Monocyte* **mohn**-ō-sīt
*Monocytopenia* mohn-ō-sī-tō-**pē**-nē-ah
*Monocytosis* mohn-ō-sī-**tō**-sihs
*Monopoiesis* mohn-ō-poy-ē-sihs
*Mononuclear phagocyte system (MPS)* mohn-ō-**noo**-klē-ər **fahg**-ō-sīt **sihs**-tehm
*Natural killer cell (NK cell)* **nahch**-uh-rahl **kihl**-lər sehl
*Neutropenia* noo-trō-**pē**-nē-ah

*Neutrophil* **noo**-trō-fihl
*Neutrophilia* noo-trō-**fihl**-ē-ah
*Opsonin* **ohp**-suh-nuhn
*Opsonization* ohp-suh-nuh-**zā**-shuhn
*Oxyhemoglobin* ohck-sē-**hē**-mō-glō-bihn
*Packed cell volume (PCV)* pahckt sehl **vohl**-ūm
*Peripheral blood* puh-**rihf**-ər-uhl bluhd
*Petechiae* peh-**tē**-kē-ī
*Phagocytosis* fahg-ō-sī-**tō**-sihs
*Phagosome* **fahg**-ō-sōm
*Plasma* **plahz**-mah
*Plasma cell* **plahz**-mah sehl
*Platelet* **plāt**-leht
*Pluripotential stem cell (PPSC)* **ploor**-ē-pō-**tehn**-shuhl stehm sehl
*Polycythemia* pohl-ē-sī-**thē**-mē-ah
*Polymorphonuclear* pohl-ē-**mōhr**-fō-**nū**-klē-ahr
*Postprandial lipemia* pōst-**prahn**-dē-ahl lī-**pē**-mē-ah
*Red bone marrow* rehd bōn **meər**-ō
*Red pulp* rehd puhlp
*Senescence* seh-**nehs**-ehnz
*Serum* **seer**-uhm
*Thrombocyte* **throhm**-bō-sīt
*Thrombocytopenia* throhm-bō-sīt-ō-**pē**-nē-uh
*Thrombocytosis* throhm-bō-sī-**tō**-sihs
*Thrombopoiesis* throhm-bō-poy-ē-sihs
*Thymus* **thī**-muhs
*T cell (T lymphocyte)* tē sehl (tē **lihm**-fō-sīt)
*Vacuole* **vahck**-ū-ōl
*White pulp* whīt puhlp
*Whole blood* hōl bluhd
*Yellow bone marrow* **yehl**-lō bōn **meər**-ō

## INTRODUCTION

In this chapter, we will explore blood—the fluid that flows through arteries and veins, transporting oxygen and nutrients to cells and removing carbon dioxide and other waste products. We will start by examining the components of blood, discuss blood's many functions, and subsequently explore the valuable clinical information about an animal that can be obtained from the analysis of blood. Later in the chapter we will look at the lymphatic system and its role in keeping an animal's immune system healthy.

## BLOOD COMPOSITION

Blood is a fluid connective tissue that flows throughout the entire body. **Whole blood** is the blood contained in the cardiovascular system. **Peripheral blood** is whole blood circulating in blood vessels carrying oxygen, nutrients, and waste materials. When you obtain an animal's blood sample from a vein or artery you are taking peripheral blood.

Grossly, blood is an opaque, deeply red fluid. Microscopically, whole blood is a clear liquid, **plasma**, in which many cellular components are suspended. Plasma is primarily water in which various solutes are dissolved. The cellular components are red blood cells (**erythrocytes**), white blood cells (**leukocytes**), and **platelets** (**thrombocytes**). There are five types of white blood cell: **neutrophils, eosinophils, basophils, lymphocytes,** and

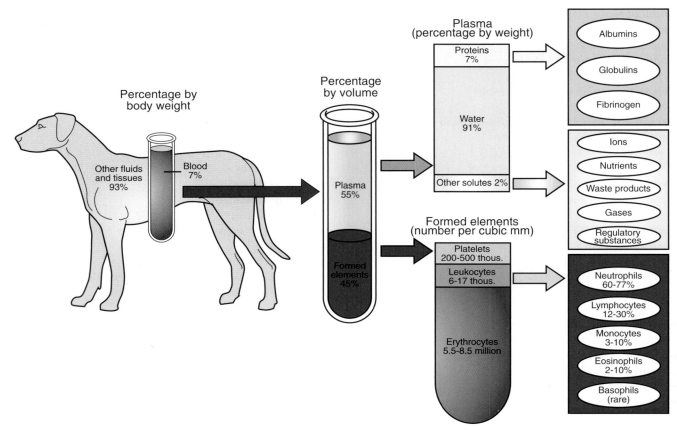

**FIGURE 12-1** Composition of blood. Values are approximate for blood components in normal adult dogs.

**monocytes**. Figure 12-1 illustrates the composition of blood in a healthy adult dog.

In veterinary clinical practice, diagnostic blood tests are routinely performed on sick animals in order to determine the cause of illness. Several different blood samples may be obtained depending on which diagnostic tests are being performed. Whole blood samples are commonly obtained from an animal's vein using a vacuum tube and needle (Figure 12-2), a process called **venipuncture** (for more detail see the Venipuncture section in the Cardiovascular System chapter). The vacuum tubes have differently colored stoppers or tops depending on which **anticoagulant**, if any, they contain. An anticoagulant is a chemical that when added to blood prevents the blood from clotting after it is removed from the body.

 **CLINICAL APPLICATION**

### Anticoagulants, Plasma, and Serum

Blood clotting factors found in plasma need to be present in sufficient quantities for blood to clot. If we want to prevent blood from clotting, we need to add something to it that ties up one of the clotting factors. Substances that tie up clotting factors and prevent blood from clotting are called anticoagulants. (*Coagulation* is another word for clotting.) If an anticoagulant is added to a blood sample in a tube or syringe, the blood will not clot. One of the most common anticoagulants is ethylenediaminetetraacetic acid or EDTA. EDTA prevents clotting by tying up calcium, clotting factor number IV. If even one clotting factor is absent the blood will not clot. No calcium, no clot.

If anticoagulant is added to a blood sample as it is drawn from an animal, the sample will not clot because all the clotting factors are not present. If the blood sample is then centrifuged (spun at a high speed), the fluid that rises to the top of the tube is plasma.

If no anticoagulant is added to a blood sample as it is drawn from an animal, the blood will clot. If the clotted blood is centrifuged, the fluid that rises to the top of the tube is called **serum**. When blood clots, one of the dissolved plasma proteins—fibrinogen—is converted to insoluble fibrin, which precipitates out of solution as a meshwork of tiny fibers (hence its name) and helps make up the framework of the clot. Removing fibrinogen from plasma by allowing it to clot converts plasma to serum.

Many of the diagnostic clinical chemistry tests performed on a patient sample are run on either plasma or serum. After the sample has been centrifuged, the plasma or serum can be drawn off and analyzed or frozen for analysis at a later date. Whole blood cannot be frozen, because blood cells rupture easily during the freezing and thawing processes.

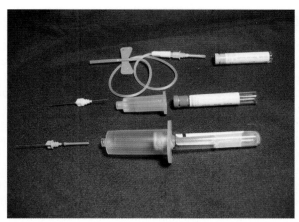

**FIGURE 12-2** Components of a vacutainer, from left to right: a double-pointed needle, a plastic holder or adapter, and a series of vacuum tubes with rubber stoppers of various colors, which indicate the type of additive present. (From Sirois M: Principles and practice of veterinary technology, ed 3, St Louis 2010, Mosby.)

Some blood samples will be collected using a syringe and needle and then transferred from the syringe to a specific tube in order to get a serum, or plasma, sample. If the sample is allowed to clot in a tube that does not contain any anticoagulant, the remaining fluid is **serum**. The clotting factors were removed from the plasma when the blood clotted.

A commonly used diagnostic test in hematology is the complete blood count (CBC) and blood smear. This test uses blood samples that are not allowed to clot so they are collected in a purple-top vacuum tube that contains EDTA (Figure 12-3). The blood sample does not clot because of the presence of (EDTA), which binds calcium ions and prevents the clotting cascade working to clot the blood (more on this later). EDTA is used as the anticoagulant because the blood cells will stay intact. Green-top vacuum tubes contain the anticoagulant heparin. Blood from these tubes is used to analyze blood from very small species such as mice.

If a blood sample in a blood tube with anticoagulant present is centrifuged, it separates into three layers based on the blood components' densities. These layers, from less dense to most dense, are the plasma layer on top containing the clotting proteins, the buffy coat layer in the middle composed of leukocytes (white blood cells) and thrombocytes (platelets), and the erythrocyte (red blood cell) layer on the bottom (Figure 12-4).

The color of plasma varies from colorless to straw to yellow–orange depending on the species, diet and any pathologic condition present. Normal plasma is transparent. The thin middle buffy coat is white or tan in color. The bottom layer is red.

In some cases, a serum sample is needed for analysis so it is collected in a red-top vacuum tube or serum separator tube. These tubes do not contain an anticoagulant; therefore, the blood sample is allowed to clot. If a clotted blood sample is centrifuged, it will separate into two components. The fluid that sits on top is the serum. The clot, composed of all the blood cells entwined in the fibrin clot, is forced to the bottom of the tube (see Figure 12-4).

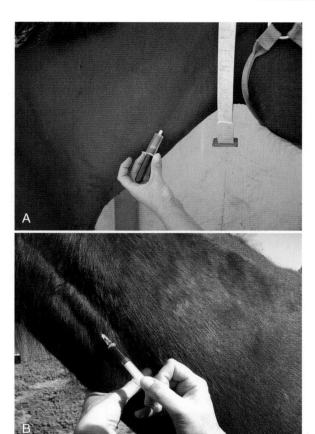

**FIGURE 12-3** Materials needed for blood collection: purple-top tubes with EDTA, needle, and syringe. (From Bassert J, McCurnin D: McCurnin's clinical textbook for veterinary technicians, ed 7, St Louis, 2010, Saunders.)

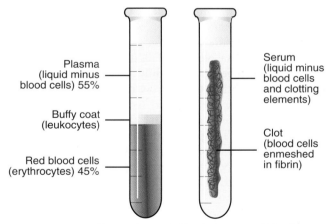

Plasma (liquid minus blood cells) 55%

Buffy coat (leukocytes)

Red blood cells (erythrocytes) 45%

Serum (liquid minus blood cells and clotting elements)

Clot (blood cells enmeshed in fibrin)

**FIGURE 12-4** Difference between blood plasma and blood serum. Plasma is whole blood minus cells; serum is whole blood minus the cells and clotting factors. (From Patton KT, Thibodeau GA: Anatomy & physiology, ed 8, St Louis, 2013, Mosby.)

## FUNCTION

Blood has three main functions: transportation, regulation and defense.

### TRANSPORTATION

- Erythrocytes, or red blood cells, contain **hemoglobin**, which carries oxygen to every cell in the body.

- Nutrients and other essential elements are dissolved in the blood plasma, and are also transported to tissues via arteries and capillaries.
- Blood carries waste products from cellular metabolism via veins to the lungs and kidneys where the waste products are eliminated from the body.
- Blood transports hormones from endocrine glands to target organs; it also transports white blood cells to various sites of activity where they participate in defending the body from infection.
- Blood transports platelets to sites of damage in blood vessel walls to form a plug that will control bleeding; this is a mechanism known as **hemostasis**. Platelets are also involved in activation of the blood-clotting cascade.

## REGULATION

- Blood aids in the regulation of body temperature. Body temperature regulators are located in the brain and are partially influenced by the temperature of the blood that passes through or over them.
- Blood plays a part in tissue fluid content. The composition of body tissue fluid is kept as constant as possible. If an animal is low in tissue fluid or dehydrated because of vomiting, diarrhea, profuse sweating, or some pathologic condition that causes it to lose fluid, some of the plasma will leave the bloodstream and enter the body tissues in an effort to compensate for the fluid loss. This leaves less plasma in the bloodstream, and the cells become more concentrated *(hemoconcentration)*. If an animal has too much body fluid, for example after subcutaneous fluids are administered, the excess fluid will enter the bloodstream. This extra fluid in the plasma dilutes the number of cells *(hemodilution)*.
- Blood aids in the regulation of blood pH (acid–base balance). Normal blood pH falls in a range of 7.35 to 7.45, with the ideal being 7.4 (slightly alkaline). Blood must be maintained within this narrow range for the animal to remain healthy. The pH must remain slightly alkaline to buffer the acidic waste products of cellular metabolism that it carries. The pH of arterial blood is slightly more alkaline than that of venous blood because most of the acidic waste products are carried in venous blood, resulting in lower pH.

## DEFENSE

- Blood carries white blood cells to tissues exposed to foreign invaders. These cells contribute to an animal's immune system to help keep the animal healthy.
- Blood carries platelets to sites of vessel damage to aid in hemostasis so that the animal does not bleed excessively.

### ✓ TEST YOURSELF 12-1

1. What are the main functions of blood?
2. What is the most abundant component of plasma?
3. What is the difference between plasma and serum?
4. What are the three main categories of blood cell?

## HEMATOPOIESIS

Before we take a look at the individual cellular components of blood (erythrocytes, leukocytes, and platelets), let's first look at their origins. **Hematopoiesis** is the production of all blood cells that occurs as a continuous process throughout an animal's life.

In the fetus, hematopoiesis takes place in the liver and spleen. In a newborn animal, this process takes place primarily in the **red bone marrow** located in most of the bones of the body. Many bones are involved because of the high demand for blood cells during growth and development. As the animal matures, the rate of production slows because the animal isn't growing as fast. Some of the red bone marrow becomes less active, is dominated by fat cells, and becomes known as **yellow bone marrow** (Figure 12-5). However, yellow marrow can be reactivated by increased demands from the body. The type of bone marrow is named on the basis of its gross appearance.

In the adult animal, there are various sites of red bone marrow that vary by species. In most species the red marrow sites are the skull, ribs, sternum, vertebral column, pelvis, and the proximal ends of the femurs. On a daily basis, the

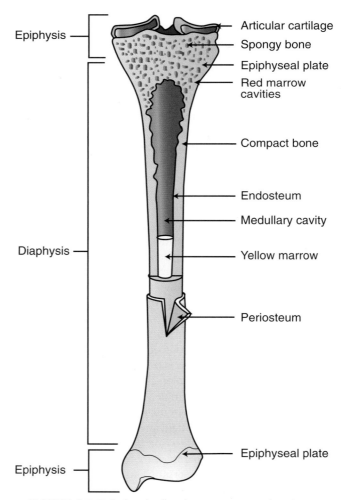

Epiphysis
Articular cartilage
Spongy bone
Epiphyseal plate
Red marrow cavities
Compact bone
Endosteum
Medullary cavity
Diaphysis
Yellow marrow
Periosteum
Epiphyseal plate
Epiphysis

**FIGURE 12-5** Red and yellow bone marrow in a long bone.

red bone marrow produces billions of each cell type. All blood cells grow old and die, or are damaged and can't function properly. These cells must constantly be replaced so an animal can stay alive and remain healthy. The liver and spleen are capable of hematopoiesis in times of great need, but not to the same high capacity as the bone marrow.

In clinical practice, red bone marrow can be obtained via a *needle aspirate* or core biopsy instrument. The bone marrow sample is viewed microscopically to look for abnormalities in the cells or the progression of cell maturation. Cases in which examination of the bone marrow would be helpful include animals with a lower than normal white blood cell count, **anemia**, or when abnormal cells are seen on a blood smear.

All blood cell types are derived from a single primitive stem cell type called a **pluripotential** or **multipotential stem cell** (Figure 12-6). As the name implies, these cells have the potential to replicate and differentiate into many different discrete types of unipotential stem cell. From this stage of development, the unipotential stem cells become committed to developing into specific mature cells through their individual maturation process, that is, **erythropoiesis, leukopoiesis**, or **thrombopoiesis**.

The rate of hematopoiesis is regulated by stimuli called poietins, colony stimulating factors, or interleukins. The fate of the pluripotential stem cells depends upon which chemical or physiologic stimulus acts on the stem cell.

Hematopoiesis is an ongoing process as new cells are made in the bone marrow, become mature, and then travel through the sinuses of the bone marrow and out into the peripheral bloodstream. Here they continue to mature to old age, die, and are eventually removed from the circulation.

## ERYTHROPOIESIS

Erythropoiesis is the process by which red blood cells are created. Unipotential stem cells are stimulated to differentiate into proerythroblasts. The proerythroblasts further divide multiple times through several stages where each stage produces a more mature cell type. At a certain stage the cells will lose their nuclei and stop multiplying. They also start producing hemoglobin. From this stage they have to mature through three more stages to become mature red blood cells

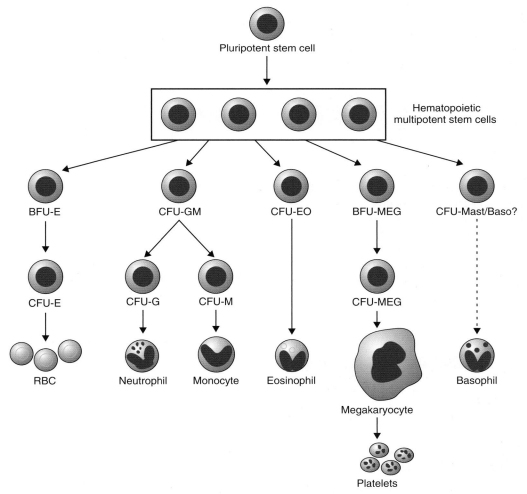

**FIGURE 12-6** Simplified schematic of hematopoiesis. *CFU*, Colony-forming units; *E*, erythroid; *EO*, eosinophils; *GM*, gramulocyte–monocyte; *MEG*, megakaryocyte. (From Withrow SJ, Vail DM, Page RL: Withrow & MacEwen's small animal oncology, ed 5, St Louis, 2013, Saunders.)

(RBCs). The entire process takes about 1 week in the dog, 4 to 5 days in the cow, and 36 hours in birds. The rate of erythropoiesis is controlled by hormones, mainly **erythropoietin (EPO)** and the availability of the materials needed to make red blood cells: iron, folic acid, vitamin B12, and protein.

Erythropoietin is produced primarily by the peritubular interstitial cells of the kidney. The production of erythropoietin is regulated by blood oxygen levels in the kidney. **Hypoxia** is the stimulus for increased erythropoietin production. In many diseases, there may be decreased oxygen available to tissues and, as a result, erythropoietin stimulates erythropoiesis in the red bone marrow.

In cases of severe anemia, nucleated RBCs (NRBCs) may be released. Nucleated RBCs are immature stages of red blood cells that retain their nuclei. They are not fully mature so they aren't as efficient even though they are producing some hemoglobin.

## CLINICAL APPLICATION

### Polychromasia and Nucleated RBCs

Under normal conditions, all but about 1% of the red blood cells in the circulation are mature. If an animal has a sudden loss or destruction of red blood cells, the bone marrow will attempt to compensate by producing more red blood cells in a shorter time. In its hurry to get red blood cells into circulation, the red bone marrow will frequently send out cells that aren't quite mature. These cells still have some metabolic activity going on in their cytoplasm, so when they are stained with a polychomatophilic hematology stain they will pick up some blue stain. There is some hemoglobin present, which will stain red. The result is lavender cytoplasm or *polychromasia.*

Hemoglobin production begins before the cell loses its nucleus. If the bone marrow perceives a great need for oxygen-carrying hemoglobin, it may first send out all its polychromatophilic (lavender), non-nucleated cells and then also start sending nucleated red blood cells. In both cases these are immature cells that don't have their full complement of hemoglobin yet, so they can't carry a full load of oxygen. They can carry some oxygen, though, and that's better than nothing when more RBCs are needed.

The presence of polychromasia and nucleated red blood cells is used as an indication that the bone marrow is responding to a need for more oxygen-carrying capacity of blood. This is a good thing.

## THROMBOPOIESIS

Thrombopoiesis, the production of platelets, begins when a specific stimulant acts on the unipotential stem cell in the red bone marrow, causing it to differentiate into a **megakaryocyte.** The megakaryocyte is a large multinucleated cell that never leaves the bone marrow. Pieces of cytoplasm from the megakaryocyte are released into peripheral blood as platelets. Platelets are also known as thrombocytes. Thrombopoiesis can take up to 7 days to reach completion.

## LEUKOPOIESIS

Leukopoiesis is the general term for the formation of white blood cells. It starts out with the same pluripotential stem cell population that produced proerythroblasts and megakaryocytes. Each specific type of white blood cell has its own stimulus for production.

**Granulopoiesis** is the process by which a pluripotential stem cell differentiates into one of three types of **granulocyte:** neutrophils, eosinophils, or basophils. Early granulocytes are difficult to distinguish from one another because they all appear as large cells with lots of cytoplasm, large round nuclei, and a first set of nonspecific granules. The nonspecific granules are later replaced by specific granules that are unique to each granulocyte type.

Lymphocytes and monocytes each develop from a pluripotential stem cell that has been stimulated by a specific stimulus. They do not contain specific cytoplasmic granules so they are known as **agranulocytes. Lymphopoiesis** is the process that produces lymphocytes, some of which develop outside the bone marrow. **Monopoiesis** is the formation and maturation of monocytes.

### ✓ TEST YOURSELF 12-2

1. What is the difference between red bone marrow and yellow bone marrow?
2. How does one cell population, the pluripotential stem cells, give rise to all the different blood cells?
3. What is the name of the process that produces erythrocytes? Thrombocytes? Leukocytes?
4. What physiologic state of blood acts as the stimulus for erythropoiesis?

## CELLULAR COMPONENTS OF BLOOD: RED BLOOD CELLS

### STRUCTURE

Mature red blood cells (RBCs), also known as erythrocytes, are highly specialized cells that lack a nucleus, mitochondria, and ribosomes, but contain water, hemoglobin, and other structural elements. When viewed microscopically, mature RBCs appear as non-nucleated, biconcave discs with a central zone that is thinner and therefore appears lighter (central pallor) on a stained blood smear (Figure 12-7). Since they have no mitochondria, erythrocytes utilize glucose from plasma for energy. Hemoglobin dissolved in RBC cytoplasm makes them stain red with a polychromatophilic hematology stain.

Different species have differently sized red blood cells. Dogs have the largest red blood cells with a prominent central zone of pallor. Cats, horses, cow, sheep, and goats have smaller red blood cells. The red cells of cats and horses do not have a prominent central zone of pallor. Camelids (llamas, camels, and their relatives) have elliptic or oval red blood cells, and deer have sickle-shaped (like a crescent moon) red blood cells. Birds, fish, amphibians, and reptiles have elliptic red blood cells that are nucleated even when they are mature.

**Red blood cells
(erythrocytes)**

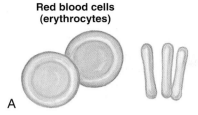

A

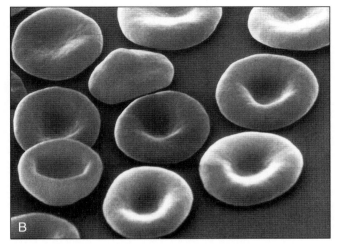

B

**FIGURE 12-7** A, Microscopic view of an erythrocyte. B, Scanning electron photomicrograph of dog erythrocytes. (A, From Thibodeau GA, Patton KT: Anatomy & physiology, ed 5, St Louis, 2003, Mosby. B, From Harvey JW: Veterinary hematology: A diagnostic guide and color atlas, St Louis, 2012, Saunders.)

 **CLINICAL APPLICATION**

### Blood Glucose and RBC Metabolism

Blood is living tissue even after it's been taken from an animal. A fresh blood sample in a tube still contains living red blood cells that utilize plasma glucose for energy. The problem is that there is no way for the glucose to be replenished in a tube after the red blood cells have used it. Clinical laboratory analysis of a blood sample frequently involves measuring blood glucose levels to look for or monitor diseases such as diabetes mellitus. A patient with uncontrolled diabetes will have an elevated blood glucose level. If red blood cells are not removed from the blood sample quickly enough, they could eat up enough glucose to bring an elevated blood glucose level down into the normal range. This could lead to a misdiagnosis and possibly inappropriate treatment. Red blood cells could even utilize enough glucose to take a normal blood glucose level down below normal. Samples that sit around long enough before the red blood cells are removed can have a blood glucose level of zero. Therefore, when the blood glucose level is to be measured, centrifuge the sample and remove the red blood cells soon after the sample is drawn to get an accurate result.

## FUNCTION

The three main functions of red blood cells are:
1. Transporting oxygen to tissues. RBCs are able to perform this function using hemoglobin, a protein that is formed during RBC development. It is made up of four heme

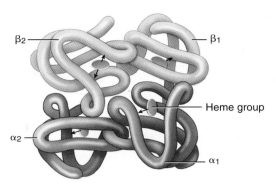

**FIGURE 12-8** Hemoglobin, comprising four globin chains, each with a heme group.

units associated with one globin chain (Figure 12-8). The heme unit is the pigmented portion of hemoglobin. Each heme unit contains an iron atom ($Fe^{2+}$) to which one oxygen molecule can attach. Therefore, one hemoglobin molecule can carry four molecules of oxygen. Hemoglobin that has oxygen bound to it is referred to as **oxyhemoglobin**. When hemoglobin gives up its oxygen to tissues in the body, it is becomes **deoxyhemoglobin**. There are many factors that influence hemoglobin's ability to carry oxygen, including blood pH, body temperature, and blood levels of oxygen and carbon dioxide.
2. Transporting carbon dioxide to the lungs. When the RBCs reach the tissue cells, there is an exchange of oxygen and carbon dioxide. Oxygen is taken from the hemoglobin in the RBCs by the cells in the tissues. At the same time, carbon dioxide, along with other metabolic waste, is released into the blood where it breaks down into ions that are transported to the lungs. Some of the carbon dioxide is taken up by the RBCs but not bound to the iron in the heme molecules.
3. Maintaining cell shape and deformability. It is important for a red blood cell to maintain its biconcave disc shape. This shape provides more membrane surface area for the diffusion of oxygen and carbon dioxide. Also, it allows for a shorter diffusion distance in and out of the cell. Membrane *deformability* refers to the flexibility of the cell membrane, allowing it to change shape to travel through the various blood vessels in the body.

## LIFE SPAN AND DESTRUCTION

The normal life span of a mature red blood cell varies with the species. In dogs, the average life span is 120 days. In cats it is approximately 68 days. Horse and sheep red blood cells live up to 150 days, and those of cows can live as long as 160 days. On the other end of the scale are mice, whose red blood cells live only 20 to 30 days. As red blood cells wear out, age, and die, they are replaced by young red blood cells from the red bone marrow in the never-ending erythropoiesis cycle.

The process of aging is called **senescence**. As a red blood cell becomes senescent, its enzyme activity decreases and the cell membrane loses its deformability by becoming rounder, enclosing a smaller volume. Approximately 1% of aging, dead, or abnormal red blood cells are removed from circulation and destroyed every day. This may occur intravascularly or extravascularly. Oxidative stresses known as free radicals contribute to the rapid aging and destruction of red blood cells. These stresses are exacerbated by certain diseases and toxins present in an animal's body.

## EXTRAVASCULAR HEMOLYSIS

Ninety percent of the destruction of senescent red blood cells occurs by **extravascular hemolysis**, or destruction of red blood cells outside the cardiovascular system. The red blood cells are removed from circulation by macrophages located primarily in the spleen. The membranes of the phagocytized cells are ruptured and hemoglobin is released and degraded into amino acids, iron, and heme. The amino acids are returned to the liver where they are used to build more proteins. The iron is transported to the bone marrow where it will be recycled during erythropoiesis to make new red blood cells. The heme will be further broken down into free or unconjugated *bilirubin*. It will attach to the plasma protein albumin, and be transported to the liver. Here it will be conjugated or bound to a compound called glucuronic acid. Conjugated bilirubin will be excreted into the intestines from the liver as a bile pigment, where it will eventually be converted into *urobilinogen* by intestinal bacteria. Some of this urobilinogen will be reabsorbed and eliminated in the urine as *urobilin*. Some of the urobilinogen will be converted to *stercobilinogen* and excreted in the feces as *stercobilin*. Urobilin and stercobilin are two pigments normally present in urine and feces and are what help give each their normal color.

## INTRAVASCULAR HEMOLYSIS

About 10% of normal red blood cell destruction takes place by **intravascular hemolysis**, or destruction that takes place within blood vessels. While in circulation, a red blood cell is exposed to many oxidative stresses, which can result in red blood cell fragmentation and/or destruction. When the red blood cell membrane ruptures within a vessel, hemoglobin is released directly into the bloodstream. The unconjugated hemoglobin is quickly picked up by **haptoglobin**, a transport protein in plasma, to form a haptoglobin–hemoglobin complex. This complex travels to the macrophages in the liver for further breakdown, similar to what happens with extravascular hemolysis. When haptoglobin is filled with unconjugated hemoglobin, as in cases of severe hemolysis, excess unconjugated hemoglobin appears in the plasma, making it a pink, red, or brown color. This is referred to as **hemoglobinemia**. This excess of unconjugated hemoglobin has no way to get to the liver, so it is carried to the kidney, where it is eliminated in the urine, making it red in color. This is referred to as **hemoglobinuria**.

## COMPLETE BLOOD COUNT

The complete blood count is also known as the hemogram or CBC. It is used to evaluate plasma proteins, red blood cells, white blood cells, and platelets. The CBC is one of the

## CLINICAL APPLICATION

### Jaundice/Icterus

Excess red blood cell breakdown results in an excess amount of unconjugated bilirubin in plasma (hyperbilirubinemia). If the amount of unconjugated bilirubin exceeds the ability of the liver to conjugate it, the excess unconjugated bilirubin will be deposited in tissues. This causes the tissues to turn yellow, a condition called *jaundice* or *icterus*. These two terms are used interchangeably. Clinically, jaundice is most readily seen as a yellowish color of the mucous membranes and the whites *(sclera)* of the eyes.

Jaundice can also be associated with liver diseases that prevent the liver from conjugating even the normal amount of unconjugated bilirubin presented to it. This causes the unconjugated bilirubin from normal red blood cell breakdown to build up in the blood and eventually be deposited in tissues.

In other liver diseases, if the bile ducts are obstructed so the conjugated bilirubin can't be passed with bile into the intestines, conjugated bilirubin will eventually back up into the bloodstream and then into tissues. Jaundice again will result.

## CLINICAL APPLICATION

### Venipuncture and Platelets

Venipuncture is placing a needle into a vein to draw out a blood sample or to administer medication. It makes a hole in the vessel wall. When the needle is removed, the hole will remain and connective tissue will be exposed to the inside of the vessel. This will catch the attention of platelets. The platelets will congregate at the site and form a plug that will prevent loss of blood through the hole. In a healthy animal, this plug will be in place within a couple of minutes. To ensure that the plug is formed as quickly as possible once the needle has been removed from the vein, light pressure should be applied to the venipuncture site. On small animals wrapping a piece of tape around the leg after a cotton ball has been placed on the venipuncture site can help. Don't wipe away the blood that seeps out of the venipuncture site. Every time you rub the area, you disrupt the developing platelet plug and prolong the bleeding time.

most useful clinical evaluations performed on a patient. The health status of an animal and clues as to what may be causing a pathologic condition are commonly reflected in the results of a CBC. The following parameters are normally included in a CBC.

## PACKED CELL VOLUME OR HEMATOCRIT

The **packed cell volume** (PCV), or **hematocrit** (HCT) is the volume of packed erythrocytes measured and expressed as a percentage of a total volume of blood. The two methods for determining the PCV are automated analyzers (blood analyzers) and gross examination of a centrifuged microhematocrit tube. When using microhematocrit tubes, an unclotted blood sample from a lavender-top vacuum tube is used to fill two tubes. The ends of the tubes are plugged with clay (Figure 12-9) and the tubes are spun in a micro-hematocrit centrifuge, causing separation of the blood sample into three components or layers: plasma, buffy coat, and red blood cells (Figure 12-10). To measure the PCV, the microhematocrit tube is placed on a special card (Figure 12-11) so the top of the clay lines up with the 0% line. The tube is rolled along the card until the top of the plasma intersects the 100% line. The line that intersects the top of the red blood cell layer is the PCV value and is reported as a percentage.

Anemia can be the result of an animal's PCV being lower than the normal reference range. This leads to a decreased oxygen-carrying capacity of the blood. There can be several causes of anemia: a low number of circulating mature red blood cells caused by blood loss, increased blood destruction, or decreased red blood cell production.

Some clinical conditions that can result in anemia include hemorrhage, red blood cell parasites, and radiation therapy for cancer. Also, iron deficiency can cause anemia. In this

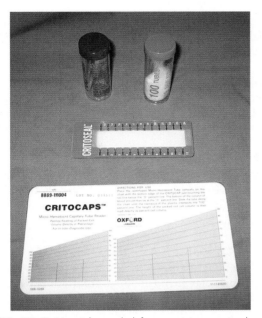

**FIGURE 12-9** Materials needed for examining a microhematocrit tube. (From Busch SJ: Small animal surgical nursing: skills and concepts, St Louis, 2006, Mosby.)

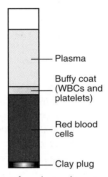

Plasma

Buffy coat (WBCs and platelets)

Red blood cells

Clay plug

**FIGURE 12-10** A centrifuged microhematocrit tube demonstrating the three layers.

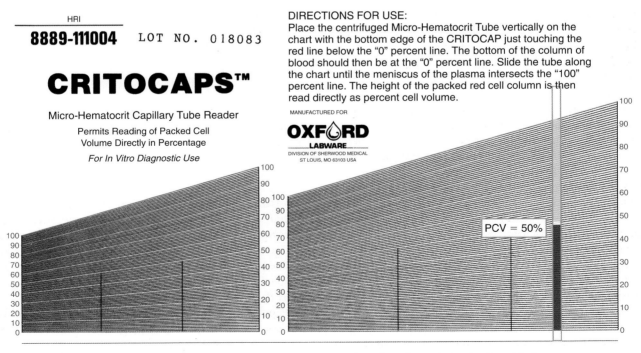

**FIGURE 12-11** Determining the PCV by locating the intersecting line where the packed red cells and buffy coat meet. The PCV is indicated by the black arrow. (From Danaher Corporation, Washington, D.C.)

## Hematocrit and Packed Cell Volume

One of the most important diagnostic screening tests performed on blood is the packed cell volume (PCV), also known as the hematocrit. An anticoagulated blood sample is placed in a small tube and centrifuged at a high speed. This causes cells with a higher specific gravity to settle in the bottom of the tube whereas the plasma, with its lower specific gravity, stays on top. The red blood cells that settle on the bottom will make up 28% to 55% of the sample volume, depending on the species. The height of the column of red blood cells is measured in proportion to the height of the entire sample, which allows the percentage of red blood cells to be determined. This value is called the *packed cell volume* and is expressed as a percentage.

The PCV is a useful test to screen a patient for anemia. The percentage of red blood cells will be smaller if the animal is low on red blood cells or if the red blood cells are smaller than normal, two of the causes of anemia. The PCV can also be used to screen for patient dehydration, which causes relative polycythemia and hemoconcentration because the red blood cells are suspended in less plasma.

Even though most people use the terms *packed cell volume* and *hematocrit* interchangeably, there is a technical difference. The hematocrit is determined by automated hematology analyzers that actually count the number of red blood cells per specific volume of whole blood sample. The hematocrit is also expressed as a percentage of red blood cells in a blood sample, but it is considered more accurate because the red blood cells are counted directly by the analyzer. When a centrifuge is used, we must rely on the efficiency of the centrifuge to pack the cells tightly enough to squeeze all the plasma out from between the cells, but not so tightly that some of the cells rupture. Because of this difference in procedure, sometimes there is a discrepancy between the packed cell volume reported from a centrifuged blood sample and the hematocrit reported from an automated hematology analyzer.

---

case, even though the bone marrow is producing the proper number of red blood cells, there may not be enough hemoglobin produced because of lack of iron to fill each red blood cell. To compensate for the lower hemoglobin production, the red cells produced are smaller than normal.

**Polycythemia** is a condition that results in the animal's PCV being higher than normal, or an increase above normal in the number of red blood cells. There are three types of polycythemia. *Relative polycythemia* is seen when there is a loss of fluid from blood (hemoconcentration), such as when an animal is dehydrated because of vomiting, diarrhea, profuse sweating, or not drinking enough water. *Compensatory polycythemia* is a result of hypoxia. The bone marrow is stimulated to make more red blood cells because the tissues aren't getting enough oxygen. Animals living at high altitudes develop compensatory polycythemia. A patient with congestive heart failure may become polycythemic because the heart isn't pumping enough blood to the tissues. This

causes the kidney to produce more erythropoietin that will stimulate red bone marrow pluripotential stem cells to mature to red blood cells. This is another form of compensatory polycythemia. *Polycythemia rubra vera* is a rare bone marrow disorder characterized by increased production of red blood cells for an unknown reason.

### HEMOGLOBIN

Hemoglobin (Hgb) analysis measures the concentration of hemoglobin contained in the red blood cells in a specific volume of blood.

### RED BLOOD CELL COUNT

The red blood cell count (RBC count) measures the number of red blood cells in a specific volume of blood. It is reported as the RBC count.

### MEAN CORPUSCULAR VOLUME

The mean corpuscular volume (MCV) measures the average volume or size of the individual red blood cells. It is a helpful way to evaluate the erythrocytes in the sample, especially when anemia is present.

### MEAN CORPUSCULAR HEMOGLOBIN CONCENTRATION

Mean corpuscular hemoglobin concentration (MCHC) is another parameter that is clinically helpful to evaluate the erythrocytes in the presence of anemia. It measures the ratio of the weight of hemoglobin to the volume of red blood cells.

### RED CELL DISTRIBUTION WIDTH

Red cell distribution width (RDW) is a numerical expression of variation in red blood cell size. The variation in size from cell to cell in a blood sample is called *anisocytosis*. Marked anisocytosis can be seen in cases of severe anemia where the bone marrow is pumping RBCs out at such a high rate they don't have time to mature fully. These immature RBCs are larger than a fully mature RBC already in circulation.

### RETICULOCYTE COUNT

The reticulocyte count (RETIC) is a count of the number of immature forms of the red blood cells per a specific total number of red blood cells. This count is used to characterize the type of anemia in an animal.

### TOTAL LEUKOCYTE COUNT

The total leukocyte count (WBC count) expresses the total number of white blood cells in a specific volume of blood. The number of each type of white blood cell is also counted either by an automated blood analyzer or by evaluating a stained blood smear.

If there is an increased demand for neutrophils in tissue, red bone marrow will release its reserve stores of mature and, if necessary, immature neutrophils into blood so they can be transported to the site where neutrophils are needed. If a blood sample is drawn while these neutrophils are in transit between the bone marrow and tissue, there will be a higher

## CLINICAL APPLICATION

### Total WBC Count and Differential Count

The total white blood cell count and differential count are used to evaluate a patient for the diagnosis or prognosis of an abnormal condition. For example, if an infection is present in the body, there will be an increased need for neutrophils to kill the invading microorganisms. The bone marrow responds to this need by releasing more neutrophils into the bloodstream that will travel to the infected tissue.

The increased number of neutrophils in the blood will increase the *total white blood cell count*. The total white blood cell count is equal to the sum of each of the individual white blood cell counts. If one cell type increases or decreases, the total white blood cell count will increase or decrease accordingly. Sounds simple, doesn't it? Unfortunately, it's not always that simple. If one cell type increases and another cell type decreases, the net effect could be a normal total white blood cell count. That's the tricky part, so the total white blood cell count is only one of a series of tests performed to evaluate the white blood cells.

To find out which white blood cells are affecting the total white blood cell count, we have to look at a stained smear of the blood. The usual method for evaluating the blood smear is to count the first 100 white blood cells observed microscopically and keep track of the number of each white blood cell type you see. This is called a *differential count,* commonly referred to as "the diff." Because you're counting 100 cells, the number of each cell type you see can be expressed as a percentage. For example, if you count 100 cells and find that 20 of the cells are neutrophils and 80 of the cells are lymphocytes, you would report you saw 20% neutrophils and 80% lymphocytes.

There are automated hematology analyzers that will provide these numbers, but they won't pick up all cellular abnormalities. For this reason, you should always look at a stained blood smear even if you're using an automated analyzer. You don't have to complete a differential count; just look for physical abnormalities.

For every species of common domestic animal, there is a value range that represents a normal white blood cell count. There is also a normal range for individual white blood cell types. For example, a dog will normally have between 6 billion and 17 billion white blood cells per liter of blood, and 60% to 70% of these cells should be neutrophils. Cattle will have between 4 billion and 12 billion white blood cells per liter and only 15% to 45% of the cells should be neutrophils. Taken together, the total white blood cell count and the differential count can provide a lot of information about an animal's state of health.

## CLINICAL APPLICATION

### Leukemia

The word *leukemia* means "white blood." It is caused by an abnormal proliferation of one of the white blood cell types. In response to some unknown stimulus, the stem cells in the bone marrow start producing abnormal cells in one cell line at an increased rate. These abnormal cells show up in peripheral blood in large numbers, many times before they are mature, and cause the total white blood cell numbers to increase dramatically *(leukocytosis)*. Leukemias are considered a form of malignancy or cancer and can be acute or chronic. They are classified by the type of cell involved (e.g., lymphocytic leukemia, monocytic leukemia, eosinophilic leukemia).

of neutrophils, including the immature neutrophils, can be used up faster than the bone marrow can replace them. If this happens, the number of neutrophils in circulation decreases, because the neutrophils are leaving the bloodstream and entering tissue, and there are no cells in the bone marrow to replace them. This condition is called **neutropenia**. The total white blood cell count will also decrease, and this is termed **leukopenia**. The prognosis is poor for an animal that is clinically ill with accompanying neutropenia and leukopenia. Box 12-1 indicates the common abnormalities of each type of leukocyte.

Trauma, fear, and exercise are a few of the stresses that may lead to a temporary transfer of neutrophils from the marginal pool to the circulating pool (discussed later in this chapter). This predictable neutrophil response is part of a larger physiologic reaction called the *stress response.*

### PLATELET COUNT

The platelet count (PLT) measures the total number of platelets (thrombocytes) in a specific volume of blood sample. **Thrombocytosis** and **thrombocytopenia** are used to describe a higher than normal or lower than normal platelet count, respectively. In cats, there may be a false thrombocytopenia due to platelet clumping in the blood sample and/or platelets overlapping with red blood cells, making the two indistinguishable by an automated blood analyzer.

### TOTAL PLASMA PROTEIN

Total plasma protein (TP) measures the amount of protein in the plasma portion of a specific volume of blood. It can be measured by an automated blood analyzer or by using a hand-held refractometer.

### STAINED BLOOD SMEARS

Throughout this chapter you'll read about cells and structures that stain specific colors with specific hematology stains that help identify these cells as they appear when viewed using a microscope. Blood films or smears are made from a patient's blood sample, stained, and evaluated to supplement a CBC. After the smear is stained a veterinary technician can manually count each white blood cell type. This is known as a *differential cell count or diff.*

than normal number of neutrophils in the sample. This is called **neutrophilia**. The increased number of neutrophils will also increase the total number of white blood cells in the sample. This is called **leukocytosis** and usually is detected using an automated blood analyzer or by observing the thickness of the buffy coat in a spun microhematocrit tube.

Leukocytosis with accompanying neutrophilia can indicate an infection somewhere in the animal's body. If the infection is out of control or left untreated, all the reserves

Leukocytosis is an increased number of white blood cells in peripheral blood. It does not indicate which cell or cells are causing the increased number.

Leukopenia is a decreased number of white blood cells in peripheral blood. It does not indicate which cell or cells are causing the decreased number.

Neutrophilia is an increased number of neutrophils in peripheral blood. It can be seen during stressful situations or when there is an increased need for neutrophils in tissue, for example during an inflammatory response.

Neutropenia is a decreased number of neutrophils in peripheral blood. It commonly accompanies a severe pathologic condition where all the mature neutrophils plus the bone marrow reserves have been used before the bone marrow can replace them.

Eosinophilia is an increased number of eosinophils in peripheral blood. It is seen during allergic reactions and with certain parasite infections. The increased numbers are a response to a demand created by a pathologic condition in the animal.

Eosinopenia is a decreased number of eosinophils in peripheral blood. It is difficult to identify because their numbers in peripheral blood are normally low.

Basophilia is an increase in the number of basophils in peripheral blood. It can occur during an allergic response or hypersensitivity reaction in tissue.

Basopenia is a decreased number of basophils in peripheral blood. It is difficult to identify because basophils are so rarely seen in peripheral blood.

Monocytosis is an increased number of monocytes in peripheral blood. It is often associated with a chronic inflammatory condition, such as an infection.

Monocytopenia is a decreased number of monocytes in peripheral blood. It can be difficult to identify because of the low numbers of monocytes normally found in peripheral blood.

Lymphocytosis is an increased number of lymphocytes in peripheral blood. It can be the result of leukemia (a form of cancer of the lymphocytes), chronic infections, or epinephrine release as part of the fight-or-flight response.

Lymphopenia is a decreased number of lymphocytes in peripheral blood. It can be the result of many factors, including decreased production of lymphocytes, the presence of corticosteroids, immune deficiency diseases, or acute viral diseases.

---

Many polychromatophilic hematology stains are a combination of blue and red dyes dissolved in methyl alcohol. One commonly used stain is a Wright's stain, which contains blue and red–orange dyes. The methylene blue dye component will stain acidic structures such as RNA or DNA a blue or purple color. This means nuclei will stain blue or purple. Basic structures such as hemoglobin and some cytoplasmic granules are stained orange or red by the eosin dye component. There are two other commonly used stains. The "Diff-Quik" stain is a modified Wright's stain that is commonly used in clinical practice to stain a blood smear quickly.

New methylene blue stain is a monochromatic stain that will stain only acidic structures. When exposed to new methylene blue stain, ribosomes in the cytoplasm of immature RBCs that are still making hemoglobin are precipitated into the cytoplasm and can be seen as small blue dots or a blue meshlike structure in the cytoplasm. There is no hemoglobin production in mature RBCs so there are no ribosomes present to precipitate (Figure 12-12). There are normally a few reticulocytes in circulating blood, but the number will increase if the bone marrow is releasing the RBCs before they are mature.

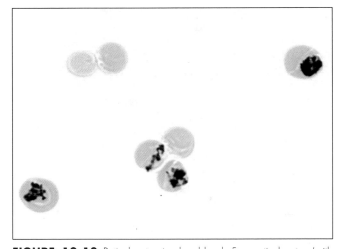

**FIGURE 12-12** Reticulocytes in dog blood. Four reticulocytes (with dark blue-staining material) and three mature erythrocytes in dog blood. New methylene blue reticulocyte stain. (From Harvey JW: Veterinary hematology: A diagnostic guide and color atlas, St Louis, 2012, Saunders.)

## PLATELETS

Platelets are also known as thrombocytes. They are not complete cells, but are pieces of cytoplasm that bud off from giant, multinucleated bone marrow cells called megakaryocytes and are sent into the circulation (Figure 12-13).

### STRUCTURE

On a blood smear, platelets appear non-nucleated, round to oval in shape with clear cytoplasm that contains small blue to purple granules (Figure 12-14). The granules contain clotting factors and calcium, which are necessary for blood to clot. The size of the platelets varies by species. Dog and pig

---

**✓ TEST YOURSELF 12-3**

1. How does a red blood cell carry oxygen to tissues?
2. Where does bilirubin come from? How is it eliminated from the body?
3. What is the difference between anemia and polycythemia?
4. What is a CBC?
5. How can you use the hematocrit to evaluate a patient for anemia?
6. What is the buffy coat?

**Platelets
(thrombocytes)**

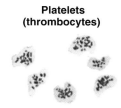

**FIGURE 12-13** Microscopic view of platelets. (From Thibodeau GA, Patton KT: Anatomy & physiology, ed 5, St Louis, 2003, Mosby.)

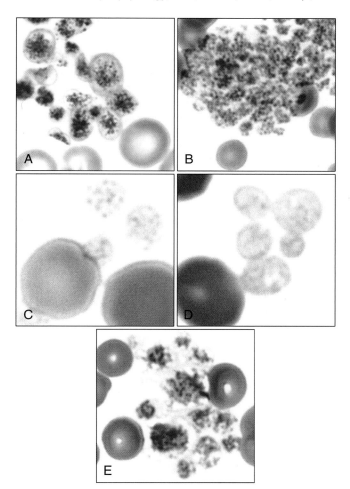

**FIGURE 12-14** Normal platelet morphology in stained blood films from domestic animals. **A,** Dog. **B,** Cow. **C,** Horse. **D,** Horse. **E,** Cat. (From Harvey JW: Veterinary hematology: A diagnostic guide and color atlas, St Louis, 2012, Saunders.)

platelets are similar in size. The cow, horse, sheep, goat, llama, rat, and mouse have small platelets. Of all common species, cats have the largest platelets. Generally, platelets are smaller than RBCs, but giant platelets, called *macroplatelets,* can occasionally be seen. They are more metabolically and functionally active in this larger form. These giant platelets are released into the circulation when there is increased consumption of platelets somewhere in the body.

## FUNCTION

Platelets have many functions in the body, but they are most important for normal hemostasis. Hemostasis is the process

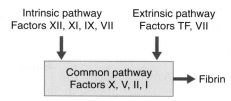

**FIGURE 12-15** The clotting cascade. The intrinsic and extrinsic pathways trigger the common pathway to convert fibrinogen to fibrin.

| TABLE 12-1 | Clotting Factors |
|---|---|
| I | Fibrinogen |
| II | Prothrombin |
| III | Tissue factor |
| IV | Calcium |
| V | Proaccelerin |
| VI | Accelerin |
| VII | Proconvertin |
| VIII | Antihemophilic factor A |
| IX | Christmas factor, antihemophilic factor B |
| X | Stuart–Prower factor |
| XI | Plasma thromboplastin antecedent |
| XII | Hageman factor |
| XIII | Fibrin stabilizing factor |

by which blood is prevented from leaking out of damaged blood vessels. Platelets have specific roles in the clotting process, along with endothelial cells in the blood vessel wall and coagulation factors. The two specific functions of platelets in hemostasis are the formation of a platelet plug and stabilization of the plug, making it irreversible.

When the outer endothelial lining of a blood vessel is damaged, the exposed subendothelium contains proteins, such as collagen, fibronectin, and von Willebrand factor, that attract platelets to adhere to it. This is known as *platelet adhesion.* At the same time, the endothelium produces tissue factors that activate the coagulation cascade to form *thrombin.* In the presence of thrombin, platelets change shape and develop pseudopods that allow them to intertwine with each other. This is known as *platelet aggregation.* The platelets squeeze together to form a primary hemostatic plug. Meanwhile, the formation of thrombin also converts **fibrinogen**, a soluble plasma protein, to insoluble strands of **fibrin**, which will attach to the platelet surface and ultimately help cement the platelets in place.

## COAGULATION CASCADE

The coagulation cascade is a series of reactions that result in inactive enzymes being activated by the preceding enzyme in the cascade. There are 13 different factors that have been identified as necessary for clotting to take place (Table 12-1).

Once a factor is activated, it will cause the activation of the next factor. One reaction leads to another reaction in a cascade effect that will eventually lead to the generation of large quantities of fibrin on the aggregated platelets' surfaces (Figure 12-15). In addition to preventing further escape of blood, the clot also acts as scaffolding for repair of the damaged vessel.

At the same time as the clot is being formed, the endothelium produces substances that will eventually dissolve the clot during **fibrinolysis**, when the endothelium has been repaired.

The absence of platelet adhesion can result in bleeding disorders. If platelets are not present in adequate numbers, large numbers of red blood cells can migrate through the endothelial wall and produce **petechiae**, or small hemorrhages on the skin, around the body.

### LIFE SPAN AND DESTRUCTION

Platelets circulate in the blood for approximately 5 to 7 days. The liver produces thrombopoietin, which regulates the number of platelets circulating in the body. Much like erythrocytes, platelets are removed from the circulation by macrophages because of old age or damage.

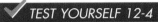

**TEST YOURSELF 12-4**

1. Why are platelets not considered complete cells?
2. What are the main functions of platelets?

## WHITE BLOOD CELLS

White blood cells are also known as WBCs or leukocytes. Mature white blood cells are generally larger than mature red blood cells. There are five types of white blood cell that are normally present in circulating blood (Figure 12-16). They are classified into granulocytes and agranulocytes, based on the presence of cytoplasmic granules when they are stained. Mature granulocytes contain prominent cytoplasmic granules, whereas mature agranulocytes lack obvious granules. The granulocytes are neutrophils, eosinophils, and basophils. The agranulocytes are lymphocytes and monocytes (Table 12-2).

### FUNCTION

The function of all white blood cells is to provide defense for the body against foreign invaders. Each type of white blood cell has its own unique role in this defense. If all the white blood cells are functioning properly, an animal has a good chance of remaining healthy. Individual white blood cell functions will be discussed with each cell type.

The white blood cells use peripheral blood to travel from their site of production in the bone marrow to their site of activity in the tissues. There is a constant flow of white blood cells out of marrow and into tissues in an attempt to control the millions of foreign invaders that attack an animal's body every day. There are two types of defense function: phagocytosis and immunity.

## GRANULOCYTES

The granulocytes are neutrophils, eosinophils, and basophils. They are included in this category because of the prominent appearance of granules in their cytoplasm when viewed on a stained blood smear. Eosinophil granules pick up the acidic stain and appear red, basophil granules pick up the basic stain and appear blue, and neutrophils don't pick up either stain very well, so they appear colorless or faintly violet on a stained blood smear.

**White blood cells (leukocytes)**

**Granular leukocytes**

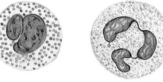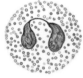

Basophil            Neutrophil            Eosinophil

**Agranular leukocytes**

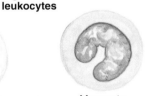

Lymphocyte            Monocyte

**FIGURE 12-16** Microscopic view of each type of leukocyte. (From Thibodeau GA, Patton KT: Anatomy & physiology, ed 5, St Louis, 2003, Mosby.)

| **TABLE 12-2** | White Blood Cells | | | |
|---|---|---|---|---|
| **NAME** | **CYTOPLASMIC GRANULES** | **NUCLEAR SHAPE** | **FUNCTION** | **SITE OF ACTION** |
| Neutrophil | Don't stain well | Polymorphonuclear | Phagocytosis | Body tissues |
| Eosinophil | Stain red | Polymorphonuclear | Allergic reactions, anaphylaxis, phagocytosis | Body tissues |
| Basophil | Stain blue | Polymorphonuclear | Initiation of immune, allergic reactions | Body tissues |
| Monocyte | None | Pleomorphic | Phagocytosis, process antigens (macrophage) | Body tissues or blood |
| B cell (lymphocyte) | None | Mononuclear | Antibody production, humoral immunity | Lymphoid tissue |
| T cell (lymphocyte) | None | Mononuclear | Cytokine production, cell-mediated immunity | Lymphoid tissue and other body tissues |

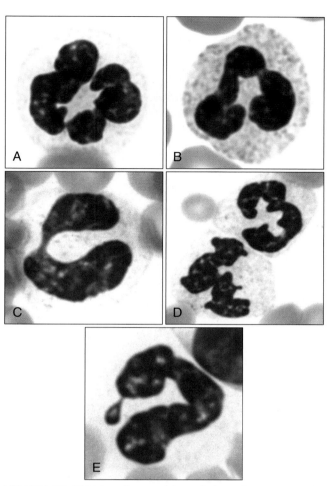

**FIGURE 12-17** Normal neutrophil morphology. (From Harvey JW: Veterinary hematology: A diagnostic guide and color atlas, St Louis, 2012, Saunders.)

## CLINICAL APPLICATION

### Neutrophilia and Leukocytosis

If there is an increased demand for neutrophils in tissue, bone marrow will release its reserve stores of mature—and, if necessary, immature—neutrophils into blood, so they can be transported to the site where neutrophils are needed. If a blood sample is drawn while these neutrophils are in transit, there will be a higher than normal number of neutrophils in the sample. This is called *neutrophilia*, and it is usually detected on a differential cell count.

The increased number of neutrophils will also increase the total number of white blood cells in the sample. This is called *leukocytosis* and usually is detected using an automated blood analyzer or by looking at the thickness of the buffy coat in a hematocrit tube. Leukocytosis with accompanying neutrophilia can indicate an infection somewhere in the body.

## CLINICAL APPLICATION

### Neutropenia and Leukocytopenia

If an infection is out of control, all the reserves of neutrophils can be used up faster than the bone marrow can replace them. If this happens, the number of neutrophils in circulation decreases, because the neutrophils are leaving the bloodstream and entering tissue, and there are no cells in the bone marrow to replace them. This condition is called *neutropenia*. The total white blood cell count will also decrease. This is *leukocytopenia*. The prognosis is poor for an animal that is clinically ill with accompanying neutropenia and leukocytopenia. It means the body is losing the war against the invading microorganisms.

## NEUTROPHILS

Neutrophils account for 40% to 75% of circulating leukocytes and are the most abundant white blood cell type in the blood of dogs, cats, and horses. Neutrophils are larger than red blood cells and smaller than monocytes. Mature neutrophils are also known as **polymorphonuclear** leukocytes (PMNs) because, when mature, their nuclei become lobulated or segmented and take on many different shapes. A mature neutrophil can have from two to five nuclear segments (Figure 12-17).

Normally a neutrophil will spend an average of 10 hours in circulation before it enters the tissue. This circulation time is shorter when there is an increased demand for neutrophils in the tissue. Once a neutrophil enters tissue it doesn't return to the blood, so all circulating neutrophils need to be replaced about two and a half times a day. Under normal conditions, they are replaced by mature neutrophils held in reserve in the bone marrow.

In peripheral blood there are two pools of mature neutrophils. The *circulating pool* represents the blood as it flows through the blood vessels. It is found toward the center of the lumen of the vessel. Blood samples obtained for laboratory analysis contain the neutrophils from this pool. The

normal range of neutrophil numbers in peripheral blood is based on the neutrophils contained in the circulating pool.

The *marginal pool* represents neutrophils that line the walls of small blood vessels, mainly in the spleen, lungs, and abdominal organs. These neutrophils are not circulating and are not contained in blood samples obtained for laboratory analysis.

Neutrophils stay in tissue until they die of old age or are destroyed by the microorganisms they are trying to destroy. Dead or abnormal neutrophils are picked up and destroyed by tissue macrophages.

If a neutrophil is released from the bone marrow before it is mature, it will have a horseshoe-shaped nucleus without any segmentation. This is called a *band neutrophil*. When band neutrophils are seen in peripheral blood, it is an indication that there is an increased demand for neutrophils beyond what the bone marrow can supply in mature neutrophils. If the bone marrow runs out of band neutrophils and still hasn't met the body's demand, it will start releasing progressively more immature cells. If band neutrophils or other immature neutrophils are seen in peripheral blood the condition is called a *left shift*.

## Hypersegmented Neutrophils

If a neutrophil nucleus in peripheral blood has more than five segments, it is called a *hypersegmented nucleus*. This indicates that the neutrophil has stayed in peripheral blood longer than normal, because hypersegmentation usually takes place in tissue as part of the normal aging process. The presence of hypersegmented neutrophils on a stained blood smear can be indicative of a pathologic condition that has prevented neutrophils from leaving the circulation, or it can mean the smear was made from old blood. Remember, blood is still living when it is removed from the animal, and it will continue the aging process as long as it can. Therefore, hypersegmented neutrophils may be just aging normally in the tube.

Hypersegmented neutrophils are seen within a day after the blood sample was drawn. For this reason, it is important that a smear be made as soon as possible after the blood sample is drawn.

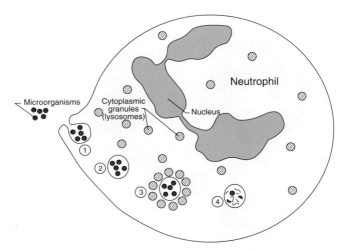

**FIGURE 12-18** Phagocytosis and destruction of microorganisms. **1,** Neutrophil membrane engulfs microorganisms. **2,** Phagocytic vacuole is formed. **3,** Cytoplasmic granules (lysosomes) line up around phagocytic vacuole and empty their digestive enzymes into vacuole. **4,** Microorganisms are destroyed.

**FUNCTION.** Neutrophils are involved in the early stages of the inflammatory response. Some neutrophils can always be found in tissues that are constantly exposed to microorganism invasion, such as the lungs and gastrointestinal tract. When microorganisms try to enter the body, the skin and mucous membranes mount the first attack. Next, neutrophils quickly respond by traveling in the blood to the site of inflamed tissue to mount a second attack. Neutrophils leave the blood vessel by squeezing between the cells of the endothelium in a process called **diapedesis.** They are attracted to a site of infection by **chemotaxis,** a process by which neutrophils and other cells are attracted by inflammatory chemicals produced by the interaction between microorganisms and the tissues they are invading. This allows the neutrophil to recognize what to ingest.

Sometimes microorganisms try to "hide" inside capsules that make them difficult for neutrophils to recognize. To help make the microorganism become more recognizable, the encapsulated microorganism is coated with a plasma protein, usually a specific antibody, called an **opsonin.** The coating process is called **opsonization** and allows the neutrophil to begin **phagocytosis.**

Neutrophils can phagocytize, or engulf, microorganisms such as bacteria and other microscopic debris in tissues (Figure 12-18). Their granules contain digestive enzymes that are capable of destroying bacteria and viruses that have been engulfed. During ingestion, the cell membrane of the neutrophil will enclose the bacteria to create a pouch called a **phagosome.** Although it sounds like it, the bacteria aren't really inside the neutrophil. Next the cytoplasmic granules will move closer to the edge of the phagosome and fuse with its membrane. These granules release *lysosomal enzymes,* which will help kill the bacteria.

Neutrophils increase their metabolism of oxygen during ingestion of microorganisms to produce substances that are toxic to ingested bacteria. *Hydrogen peroxide* is the product

of oxygen metabolism that is most important for the killing activity of neutrophils. Hydrogen peroxide is capable of killing bacteria *(bactericidal effect)* all by itself, but its action is enhanced by the enzyme *myeloperoxidase,* which is released from neutrophil granules. Lysozyme from the granules also enhances the bactericidal action of hydrogen peroxide and is capable of destroying the cell walls of microorganisms.

## Neutrophils and the Stress Response

Neutrophils can move freely between the circulating and marginal pools. At any given time, in dogs, cattle, and horses, there is about a 50:50 ratio between the number of neutrophils in the circulating pool and the marginal pool. In cats, the ratio is about 30:70.

Cells can detach from the marginal pool and enter the circulating pool when an animal is experiencing some sort of physical or mental stress. Trauma, fear, and exercise are a few of the stresses that may lead to a temporary transfer of neutrophils from the marginal pool to the circulating pool. This predictable neutrophil response is part of a larger physiologic reaction called the *stress response.*

Splenic contraction also plays an important role in this movement of cells out of the marginal pool. The temporary movement of neutrophils into the circulating pool can artificially elevate the total neutrophil count (neutrophilia) and the total white blood cell count (leukocytosis) because the normal values are based only on the number of cells normally found in the circulating pool. These artificially elevated results can lead to a possible misdiagnosis. Remember this when you have to chase a horse around a pasture or wrestle with a cat to get a blood sample.

The administration of corticosteroid drugs, which are similar to glucocorticoid hormones (see Chapter 11) will cause the same response. This is one good reason for drawing a blood sample before medications are administered.

## EOSINOPHILS

Eosinophils are named for the red granules in the cytoplasm of mature cells when the cells are viewed on a stained blood smear. They make up 1% to 6% of the total circulating white blood cells. Most cells have a bilobed, or two-lobed, nucleus with red granules in the cytoplasm (Figure 12-19). The appearance of the granules varies among species of animals. In the dog, the granules appear as dark reddish irregularly sized structures, whereas in the cat they appear rod shaped. In the horse, they appear as large round brightly eosinophilic granules. In cattle, sheep and pigs, eosinophils contain smaller, bright pink-stained granules.

Eosinophils are slightly larger than neutrophils. After eosinophils have been produced in the bone marrow, they stay there for several days before they go out into circulation. They stay in circulation about 3 to 8 hours before they migrate into tissues, where they live out the rest of their lives. An increased number of eosinophils in peripheral blood is called **eosinophilia**. A decreased number of eosinophils in peripheral blood is difficult to quantitate because there are normally so few in circulation. The correct term for a decrease in number in peripheral blood is **eosinopenia**.

**FUNCTION.** The functions of eosinophils are similar to those of the neutrophils and include phagocytosis and bactericidal properties, but to a lesser extent. Eosinophils are phagocytic cells, especially of antigen–antibody complexes (see Chapter 13). Large numbers of eosinophils are normally found in certain tissues in the body such as the gastrointestinal tract, skin, and lungs.

There are three key functions that are most often associated with eosinophils.

- Inflammatory response. Eosinophils are attracted to and inhibit local allergic and anaphylactic reactions. Their granules contain anti-inflammatory substances that are released at the site of an allergic reaction.
- Immunity. Eosinophils can ingest substances associated with the humoral immune response (e.g., antigen–antibody complexes).
- Phagocytosis. Eosinophils have minimal phagocytic and bactericidal functions. The contents of eosinophil granules are especially toxic to large pathogenic organisms, such as protozoa and some parasitic worms.

## BASOPHILS

Basophils are the least common leukocyte and constitute less than 1% of circulating white blood cells. It is therefore difficult to quantitate a **basophilia** or a **basopenia**. Basophils are recognized by of their large intensely staining basophilic or blue cytoplasmic granules (Figure 12-20). The basophil granules are water soluble and are frequently washed out during the staining procedure, so they are not always readily visible on a stained smear.

Basophils have multilobulated nuclei and are similar in size to neutrophils. They share some characteristics with tissue **mast cells** in that both contain immunoglobulin E, but some controversy exists over the relationship between these two cells.

**FUNCTION.** Not much is known about the function of basophils. They are the least phagocytic of the granulocytes. Their granules contain histamine and heparin. Histamine helps initiate inflammation and acute allergic reactions. Eosinophils are attracted to the site of an allergic reaction by

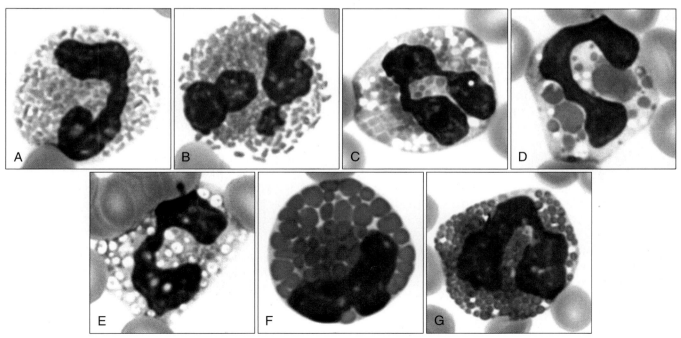

**FIGURE 12-19** Morphology of eosinophils. A, Cat. B, Cat. C, Dog. D, Dog. E, Dog. F, Horse. G, Cow. (From Harvey JW: Veterinary hematology: A diagnostic guide and color atlas, St Louis, 2012, Saunders.)

eosinophilic chemotactic factor released from the basophil or mast cell granules. Heparin acts as a localized anticoagulant to keep blood flowing to an injured or damaged area.

## AGRANULOCYTES

Agranulocytes are mature white blood cells that do not contain specific staining granules in their cytoplasm. They include lymphocytes and monocytes.

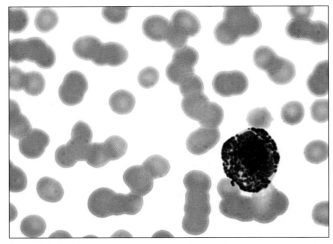

**FIGURE 12-20** Blood film from a horse. A basophil with purple granules is present in the bottom right of the image. (From Harvey JW: Veterinary hematology: A diagnostic guide and color atlas, St Louis, 2012, Saunders.)

## LYMPHOCYTES

Most of the lymphocytes seen in blood are small lymphocytes that can be recognized by their round or oval nucleus and minimal amount of clear, almost colorless cytoplasm (Figure 12-21). Small lymphocytes are smaller than neutrophils when viewed on a stained blood smear. Medium and large lymphocytes are sometimes seen in peripheral blood.

Most of the lymphocytes in the body actually live in what are called *lymphoid tissues* and constantly circulate between these tissues and blood. **Lymphocytosis** and **lymphocytopenia** refer to an increase and a decrease in the number of circulating lymphocytes, respectively.

**FUNCTION.** There are four main types of lymphocyte: T cells, B cells (which transform into plasma cells), and natural killer (NK) cells. They have individual functions that regulate an animal's immune system. These functions are discussed in depth in Chapter 13.

- **T lymphocytes (T cells).** T cells are processed in the thymus before going to peripheral lymphoid tissue. T cells are responsible for *cell-mediated immunity* (no antibody production involved) and for activating B cells. Most of the lymphocytes in peripheral blood are T cells.
- **B lymphocytes (B cells).** Inactive B cells travel through lymph nodes, the spleen, and other lymphoid structures, but rarely circulate in peripheral blood. B cells are ultimately responsible for *humoral immunity* (antibody production is involved). Each B cell is preprogrammed to produce only one specific **antibody** type against one

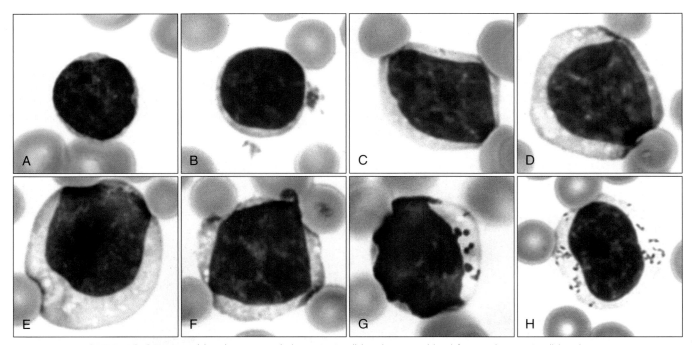

**FIGURE 12-21** Normal lymphocyte morphology. **A,** Small lymphocyte in blood from a dog. **B,** Small lymphocyte in blood from a cow. **C,** Medium-sized lymphocyte in blood from a horse. **D,** Medium to large lymphocyte in blood from a cow. **E,** Large lymphocyte in blood from a cow. **F,** Medium to large lymphocyte in blood from a cow. **G,** Granular lymphocyte in blood from a cow. **H,** Granular lymphocyte in blood from a cat. (From Harvey JW: Veterinary hematology: A diagnostic guide and color atlas, St Louis, 2012, Saunders.)

specific **antigen**. On its cell surface, a B cell has thousands of receptors shaped to fit only one antigen shape. Every antigen has a unique shape made up of amino acids on its cell surface. This area is called the *epitope*. The sequence of amino acids determines the shape of the epitope. There is a B cell that has a complementary combining site or receptor that fits the shape of the epitope. When the B cell and antigen are joined, an *antigen–antibody complex* is formed. All the other B cells will be unaffected. The amazing thing is that the B cells are preprogrammed to produce antibodies against antigens to which they have never been exposed. When B cells recognize an antigen, they transform into plasma cells that release antibodies. This is called humoral immunity.

- **Plasma cells** are derived from B cells in response to an antigenic stimulus. The B cells that are activated by their unique antigen multiply by mitosis in a process called *blastic transformation* to become plasma cells. Plasma cells produce, store, and release antibodies that are also known as *immunoglobulins*. Plasma cells can be found in any tissue in the body, but are most numerous in tissues engaged in antibody formation (e.g., lymph nodes, spleen). Plasma cells are rarely found in peripheral blood.

- **Natural killer (NK) cells** are found in the blood and lymph. These granular lymphocytes are able to identify and kill virus-infected cells, stressed cells, and tumor cells. They differ from phagocytes in that they do not ingest the target cell. Instead, they bind to the cell and induce cellular changes that lead to *apoptosis* (programmed cell death) or lysis of the cell. It is important to note that NK cells do not cause lysis of virus-infected cells, because this would release *virions* (virus particles) instead of controlling infection. Instead, apoptosis is triggered in virus-infected cells, to ensure death of the virus, which lysis does not. NK cells have two types of receptor to help determine which cells to kill: the killer-activating receptor (KAR) and the killer inhibitory receptor (KIR). The KIR binds with specific molecules on a cell's surface. This binding demonstrates that the cell is healthy and inhibits the NK cell from killing it. If the KIR does not bind to the cell, the NK cell will kill the cell. When there is decreased expression of the specific molecules on the cell's surface, the KAR is triggered, causing apoptosis of the cells. Cells with decreased numbers of molecules or damaged/altered molecules are destroyed because they are likely to be unhealthy. NK cells kill by binding to suspected cells. Once the KIR verifies a harmful cell, the NK cell with the KAR releases *perforins* (proteins that form pores in cell membranes) and *proteolytic enzymes* such as *granzymes*. Granzymes move into the target cell via the newly formed pores and cause apoptosis by breaking down the cell structure and its contents. NK cells are stimulated by *cytokines*, including *interleukins* and *interferons*. Tumor cells, damaged cells, and infected cells release cytokines as stress signals. This stimulates NK cell action and ultimate destruction of harmful cells.

Both T cells and B cells can become *memory cells*. These cells are clones of an original lymphocyte. They don't participate in an initial immune response to a specific antigen but survive in lymphoid tissue waiting for a second exposure to that same antigen. When the animal is exposed to the antigen for a second time, the memory cells are ready to respond. This response is much quicker and of greater magnitude than the initial immune response.

## MONOCYTES

Monocytes make up 5% to 6% of the circulating white blood cells in all common domestic species. Monocytes are the largest white blood cells in circulation. Their nuclei can be many shapes, from round to pseudolobulated. This means that monocyte nuclei can have similar shapes to those of neutrophils. Monocytes have abundant cytoplasm that stains gray and may contain **vacuoles** of varying sizes (Figure 12-22). **Monocytosis** and **monocytopenia** refer to an increase and decrease in the number of circulating monocytes, respectively.

*FUNCTION.* Monocytes participate in inflammatory responses. They do not spend much time in bone marrow or the circulation before they enter into tissues where they can live for up to 100 days. When monocytes enter tissues, they become **macrophages**. Collectively, the tissue macrophages and monocytes are known as the **mononuclear phagocyte system (MPS)**.

Both macrophages and monocytes clean up cellular debris that remains after an infection/inflammation clears up. Also, they process certain antigens, making them more antigenic. In addition, they can ingest antigens and present them on their cell membranes to the lymphocytes that will then destroy them.

> ✓ *TEST YOURSELF 12-5*
> 1. List the five types of white blood cell and indicate whether each one is a granulocyte or an agranulocyte.
> 2. What is the common function of all white blood cells?
> 3. Which cell is the only white blood cell not capable of phagocytosis?
> 4. Which white blood cell is known as a *PMN*?
> 5. Which white blood cell is known as "the second line of defense" after a microorganism has entered the body?
> 6. Which white blood cell would you likely see increased in peripheral blood during an allergic response?
> 7. Which white blood cell is least commonly seen in peripheral blood?
> 8. Which white blood cell is the largest cell normally seen in peripheral blood?
> 9. What are the four types of lymphocyte?

## THE LYMPHATIC SYSTEM

The lymphatic system can be viewed as two separate parts working together to contribute to an animal's immune system, which helps to keep the animal healthy. The first part

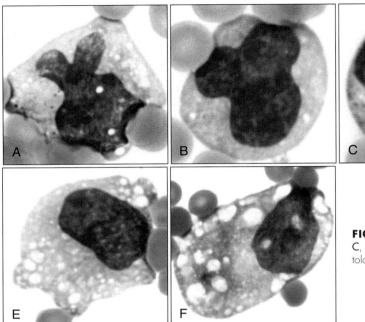

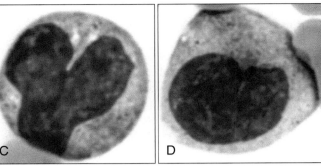

**FIGURE 12-22** Normal monocyte morphology. **A,** Horse. **B,** Cow. **C,** Dog. **D,** Horse. **E,** Horse. **F,** Cat. (From Harvey JW: Veterinary hematology: A diagnostic guide and color atlas, St Louis, 2012, Saunders.)

is composed of a system of ducts and fluid **lymph**. The second part of the system is composed of lymphoid organs and tissues.

The system of ducts picks up some of the fluid leaked from capillaries into interstitial tissue. When the fluid is in a lymph duct it is called lymph. The lymph ducts carry lymph to blood vessels near the heart, where it is processed and returned to systemic blood. Lymph contains very few blood cells other than lymphocytes. It contains nutrients, hormones, and other substances that have entered tissue fluid from the capillaries.

The lymphoid organs and tissues are scattered throughout the body and are involved in the immune response to help fight foreign invaders in the animal's body.

## FUNCTION

The lymphatic system has four primary functions:
- Removal of excess tissue fluid. Cells receive some of the nutrients carried by plasma through diffusion. The fluid that enters the interstitial (tissue) spaces will eventually be put back into the circulation. Part of the fluid will be picked up directly by the capillaries in the tissues and enter the venous part of the systemic circulation. Some of the fluid will enter lymphatic capillaries. If there is inadequate lymph drainage to an area, the interstitial fluid can build up, causing **edema** (excess fluid accumulation) of the tissues of the area. There are other causes of edema, but they all relate to inadequate fluid drainage from tissue.
- Waste material transport. The interstitial fluid that enters lymphatic capillaries will contain some of the waste materials from the tissue cell metabolism and will be carried to the systemic circulation by lymph and eventually eliminated.

- Filtration of lymph. Interstitial fluid that enters the lymphatic capillaries will also contain microorganisms, cellular debris, and other foreign matter that must be removed from lymph before it enters the bloodstream. This will occur as the lymph passes through the lymph nodes.
- Protein transport. Some large proteins, especially enzymes, are transported in lymph to the systemic circulation from their cells of origin. These proteins are too large to enter the venous circulation directly. Lymph has the ability to pick up larger protein molecules than the capillaries and deposit them into the systemic circulation.

## LYMPH FORMATION

Lymph starts out as excess tissue fluid that is picked up by small lymph capillaries found in the interstitial spaces of soft tissue. The excess tissue fluid accumulates when more fluid leaves blood capillaries than re-enters them. If it were not for the lymph vessels, the tissues of the body would all swell with the excess fluid.

Blood capillaries are very porous. Fluid can easily enter and leave them. At the arterial ends of capillaries, there is still enough blood pressure to force some of the plasma out into the tissues. The plasma carries substances such as nutrients, oxygen, and hormones out with it to bathe the cells and tissues. The blood pressure quickly drops in the tiny capillaries until there is no pressure at the venous end of a capillary bed. Rather, osmotic pressure due to proteins and other dissolved substances in blood in the capillaries draws fluid back in. Fluids will naturally flow from areas of low concentration (interstitial spaces) to areas of high concentration (blood vessels) to try to establish equilibrium. The problem is that the osmotic force drawing in fluid on the venous side is not as strong as the blood pressure force pushing it out on

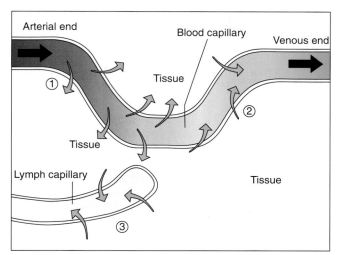

**FIGURE 12-23** Formation of lymph. **1**, Blood pressure forces plasma out into tissues. **2**, Osmotic pressure draws some of tissue fluid back into the capillary, but not all of it. **3**, A blind-ended lymph capillary picks up excess tissue fluid and carries it off into progressively larger lymph vessels that eventually return it to bloodstream.

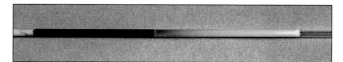

**FIGURE 12-24** Lipemic serum sample. (Courtesy of Heather Wamsley. In Harvey JW: Veterinary hematology: A diagnostic guide and color atlas, St Louis, 2012, Saunders.)

### 🔍 CLINICAL APPLICATION

#### Postprandial Lipemia

If an animal has eaten just prior to a blood sample being drawn, the plasma may appear cloudy owing to fat from the digested food suspended in the plasma. This condition is referred to as postprandial lipemia (*postprandial* means after eating, and *lipemia* means fat in the blood), and it can make the plasma or serum unsuitable for laboratory analysis, depending on the analytic method used. For this reason, blood samples for laboratory analysis should be drawn before an animal is fed or a couple of hours after feeding.

the arterial side. This could result in an accumulation of fluid in the tissues, known as edema. Fortunately, tiny lymph vessels gather up the excess fluid and carry it away (Figure 12-23).

The tiny lymph capillaries in tissue join together to form larger and larger lymph vessels, many of which contain one-way valves that prevent the lymph from flowing backward. These valves allow body movements to propel lymph toward the heart. Because lymph vessels don't have any muscles in their walls, they can't contract and force the lymph along, so they have to rely on body movement. The lymph vessels eventually join to form the *thoracic duct,* which empties lymph into the vena cava just before this large vein enters the heart. By this means, the lymph comes full circle: from its origin in plasma, back into plasma.

On its way to the thoracic duct, a lymph vessel passes through at least one *lymph node,* where it picks up lymphocytes. If the tissue fluid contained any microorganisms when it entered the lymph vessels, they will be removed from lymph by macrophages in the lymph nodes.

By the time the lymph reaches the thoracic duct, it is a transparent or translucent liquid containing varying numbers of cells, primarily lymphocytes. The fluid is different from plasma in that it is made up of more water, sugar, and electrolytes and fewer of the larger proteins (e.g., albumin, globulin, and fibrinogen) found in plasma that were too large to leave in the first place.

Lymph from the digestive system is called *chyle.* After a meal, the chyle contains microscopic particles of fat known as chylomicrons that cause the lymph to appear white or pale yellow and cloudy. The chylomicrons enter the systemic circulation with the rest of the lymph and cause plasma to also appear white or pale yellow and cloudy (**postprandial lipemia**) (Figure 12-24).

## LYMPHOID ORGANS AND TISSUES

Lymphoid organs and tissues are classified as primary and secondary. The primary organs function to regulate the lymphocyte maturation as the animal develops. These organs and tissues include the **thymus**, *bursa of Fabricius,* and *Peyer's patches.*

T cells mature in the thymus. B cells mature in other lymphoid organs. In birds, this lymphoid organ is the bursa of Fabricius; in rabbits, ruminants and pigs, this tissue is **gut-associated lymphoid tissue** (GALT).

### PRIMARY LYMPHOID ORGANS

***THYMUS.*** The thymus is located in the cranial thorax. It is largest in size when an animal is young, but shrinks and is replaced by fat as the animal matures, making it difficult to locate in adult animals. The thymus is made up of many lobules contained in a connective tissue capsule. The outer portion of the lobules contains a large number of lymphocytes.

The thymus is responsible for most of the production of mature T cells (thymus-derived lymphocytes) from precursors sent from the bone marrow. Once in the thymus they are called thymocytes. Here they divide rapidly and leave the thymus and travel to the secondary lymphoid organs. T cells are important in stimulating a cell-mediated immune response. Young animals do not have a fully developed immune system, which means that they rely heavily on the thymus to fight infections and ultimately survive.

### BURSA OF FABRICIUS

The bursa of Fabricius is found only in birds and is similar in structure and function to the thymus. It is a round sac that sits right above the cloaca.

### PEYER'S PATCHES

Peyer's patches are located in the wall of the small intestine. They have various structures and functions depending on the species. However, their common function is the activation of B cells to produce antibodies against antigens in the small intestines. Peyer's patches are just one type of gut-associated lymphoid tissue (GALT) located throughout various areas of intestinal mucosa and submucosa.

## SECONDARY LYMPHOID ORGANS

The secondary lymphoid organs are developed later in fetal development and persist in adult animals. They include the spleen, lymph nodes, and tonsils. Their main function is to trap and process antigens and mature lymphocytes that mediate immune responses. Unlike the primary lymphoid organs these organs will enlarge in response to antigenic stimulation.

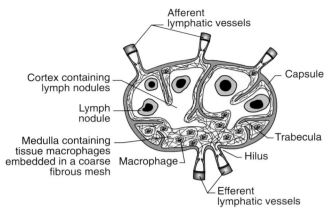

**FIGURE 12-25** Structure of a lymph node.

## CLINICAL APPLICATION

### Swollen Lymph Nodes

If there is an infection in some part of the body, the microorganism to blame may be picked up by a lymph vessel and carried to a lymph node. As the lymph passes through the lymph node, the tissue macrophages will attempt to remove the microorganisms. As the macrophages get more active, the lymph node becomes larger as a result of the multiplication of lymphocytes and the arrival of more macrophages. Some lymph nodes are located close to the surface of the body and can be palpated (felt) through the skin. If they are responding to an infection in their drainage area, they will become larger and be more readily palpated.

If enlarged, lymph nodes can be used as a clue to the location of an infection. You may be familiar with the mandibular lymph nodes located just behind each side of your jaw in your neck region. These are the "glands" that swell when you have a cold. This is because the mandibular lymph nodes (they are not true glands) drain the nasal cavity, mouth, and pharynx.

**LYMPH NODES.** Lymph nodes are small, kidney bean–shaped filters located at various points along lymphatic vessels. They trap antigens and other foreign material carried in lymph. A lymph node is divided into a cortex and a medulla, which have lymphatic sinuses running through them (Figure 12-25). Lymph flows from the tissues into the node in afferent vessels that empty just beneath the capsule, which lies outside the cortex. It leaves the lymph node in efferent vessels that exit the lymph node through the indented *hilus* area. The nodules located in the cortex are made up of predominantly B cells, although T cells and macrophages are also found in smaller numbers in lymph nodes.

In clinical practice, lymph nodes can give us clues to the health of an animal. Lymph nodes are found throughout the body, both superficially and deep, and drain the organs in their associated locations. If there is an infection in a particular area of the body, the activated superficial lymph nodes in that area will enlarge in response to antigenic stimulation, making them more easily palpated or visible to the

eye. They also may feel firmer in consistency. A diagnostic test called fine-needle aspiration (FNA) and cytology can be used to collect a microscopic sample of the enlarged lymph node and to evaluate for abnormalities such as infectious microorganisms or cancer cells.

**SPLEEN.** The spleen is a tongue-shaped organ located on the left side of the abdomen. It is near the stomach in simple-stomached animals and near the rumen in ruminants. Not only does the spleen store red blood cells and produce red blood cells during fetal development, but it also filters the blood and lymph.

The spleen is covered with a capsule made up of fibrous connective tissue and smooth muscle. The capsule sends branches called trabeculae into the soft tissue of the spleen. These trabeculae contain blood vessels, nerves, lymph vessels, and smooth muscle cells. In carnivores, the trabeculae are very muscular, whereas ruminants have trabeculae that are less muscular. When the smooth muscle cells contract, they squeeze stored blood cells out of the spleen and back into circulation. Because carnivores have more muscular branches, they are able to squeeze more blood out of the spleen.

The soft tissue interior of the spleen is divided into two areas, **white pulp** and **red pulp**, each with a distinct function (Figure 12-26). The white pulp is formed of localized areas of lymphoid tissue containing lymphocytes that can clone themselves during an immune response. The red pulp consists of blood vessels, tissue macrophages, and blood cell storage spaces called sinuses. The tissue macrophages filter out antigens and other foreign material from lymph and remove dead, dying, and abnormal red blood cells.

Remember, the spleen acts as a reservoir for blood when the animal is at rest and doesn't need large amounts of oxygen and other substances going to its muscles. When the storage spaces are filled with blood, the splenic reservoir is full and the spleen gets larger. When the body needs those "excess" blood cells, say for physical activity, the trabeculae contract, the blood is squeezed back into the circulation, and the spleen gets smaller. The spleen is not essential for the life of an animal and can be surgically removed if necessary. Splenic ruptures occurring from trauma such as being hit by

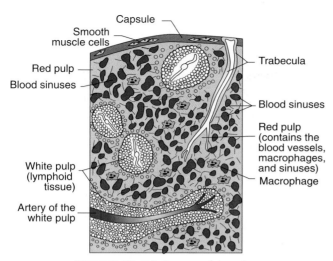

FIGURE 12-26 Structure of the spleen.

Labels: Capsule, Smooth muscle cells, Red pulp, Blood sinuses, White pulp (lymphoid tissue), Artery of the white pulp, Trabecula, Blood sinuses, Red pulp (contains the blood vessels, macrophages, and sinuses), Macrophage

a car and splenic tumors are the most common reasons for performing a splenectomy. An animal's immune system is still active because there are other lymphoid organs throughout the rest of the body.

## CLINICAL APPLICATION

### Autoimmune Diseases

In some instances, the immune system malfunctions and starts seeing "self" as "not self." In other words, part of the animal's own body becomes recognized as foreign. This results in a classification of diseases known as *autoimmune diseases.* For example, *autoimmune hemolytic anemia (AIHA)* is a disease in which the animal starts producing antibodies against its own red blood cells. The antibodies cling to the red blood cell membranes and cause the cells to clump together *(agglutination).* These clumps of cells are detected by the tissue macrophages in the spleen, removed by them, and destroyed. If enough red blood cells are removed this way, the animal will become anemic.

**TONSILS.** Tonsils are nodules of lymphoid tissue that are not covered with a capsule. They are found in epithelial surfaces all over the body, but we are most familiar with the ones in the pharyngeal (throat) region. Here, they function to prevent the spread of infection into the respiratory and digestive systems. Tonsils are classified as secondary lymphoid tissue where mature lymphocytes live. They are most prominent in young animals as they are developing their immune systems. Tonsils differ from lymph nodes in three significant ways: (1) tonsils are found close to moist epithelial (mucosal) surfaces, (2) tonsils don't have a capsule, (3) tonsils are found at the beginning of the lymph drainage system, not along the lymph vessels like lymph nodes. Other tonsils are found in the larynx, intestine, prepuce, and vagina.

## TEST YOURSELF 12-6

1. How does lymph differ from plasma?
2. Where is lymph formed?
3. What is the function of a lymph node?
4. Which lymphatic organ is composed of white pulp and red pulp?
5. Which lymphatic organ is large at birth and gradually gets smaller as the animal matures?
6. Where is the GALT located?

## TRANSFUSION THERAPY

Transfusion therapy is used to replace fluid or blood that has been lost or destroyed. Transfusion involves taking blood or a blood component from a donor animal and injecting it into a recipient animal. Keep in mind that the transfused blood does not treat disease, but supplements an absent or deficient component of blood while an underlying disease is being treated. The indications for blood transfusion include rapid blood loss, severe anemia, coagulation factor deficiency, a lower than normal plasma protein count, and thrombocytopenia.

## CLINICAL APPLICATION

### Blood Volume

Here's the question. How do you know if you can draw 200 ml of blood from an animal to use in a blood transfusion without causing serious problems? Our limit will be 25% of the total blood volume, which is more blood than you would routinely draw from an animal, because an animal that loses 25% of its total blood volume has about a 50:50 chance of survival, but let us examine a worst-case scenario.

First, you need to know how much blood an animal has. The total blood volume for any animal can be estimated using the animal's lean body weight. *Lean* is the operative word here. A 13.5 kg (30 lb) house cat is not lean. Therefore if you want to figure the total blood volume for this cat, think of it as a 3.5 to 4.5 kg (8 to 12 lb) cat. As a broad rule of thumb, figure 50 to 100 ml (average 75 ml) of blood/kg lean body weight. Highly strung animals tend to have more blood volume because they are always active—pacing, bouncing, and running—so they need more oxygen in their muscles.

Using these guidelines, a 454 kg (1000 lb) horse will have a total blood volume of about 34,000 ml or 34 L (454 kg × 75 ml of blood/kg = 34,050 ml total blood volume). Taking 200 ml of blood from this horse would result in a blood loss of 0.5% of the total blood volume (200 ml divided by 34,000 ml and multiplied by 100 to get a percentage). Not a problem.

Now let's consider a 16 kg (35 lb) dog with a total blood volume of 1193 ml. Drawing 200 ml from this dog would result in a blood loss of 16%. This is still not a problem, but we're getting closer to trouble.

### A Pint's a Pound the World Around

Another way to determine the total blood volume is to figure that blood makes up an average of 6% to 8% (average 7%) of an animal's lean body weight. Of course, that will give you

## CLINICAL APPLICATION—cont'd

the *weight* of total blood volume, so you need to convert that to a liquid measure. A pint of water weighs a pound. Therefore, because blood is mostly water, we'll use that conversion rate. From here we need to convert it into metric measurements because that's how syringes are calibrated. There are 2 pints in a quart, and a quart is approximately equivalent to a liter. There are 1000 ml in a liter. So now it becomes a simple math problem.

Using these guidelines, a dog weighing 75 lb (34 kg) will have a total blood volume of approximately 5.25 lb (75 pounds × 7%). That's 5.25 pints of blood. If 2 pints are 1 quart, 5.25 pints are 2.625 quarts, or approximately 2.625 liters. Move the decimal point to the right three places and the total blood volume of this dog is 2625 ml. A 200 ml blood loss for this animal would amount to about a 10% loss of total blood volume. This would not be a significant loss for the dog.

However, a cat weighing 10 lb (4.5 kg) will have a blood volume of 0.7 lb, or 0.7 pint. This converts to 350 ml. A blood loss of 200 ml would result in a loss of 57% of its total blood volume. The cat would probably die of shock before you could get that much blood out of it.

The three goals of transfusion therapy are to increase the oxygen-carrying capacity of blood, to replace coagulation factors or other proteins, and to replace blood volume. There are various veterinary blood banks that supply blood products such as whole blood, frozen plasma, frozen platelets, and many others. The blood product is chosen based on what component the recipient animal needs.

Prior to transfusing an animal, its blood group or type must be identified and matched against the donor's blood type. This process is called *blood typing* and *crossmatching* and is done to decrease any transfusion reactions in the recipient. All species have their own blood types.

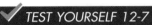

### TEST YOURSELF 12-7
1. What are the goals of transfusion therapy?

# 13 Immunity and Defense

*Christina M. Jeffries, AAS, CVT and
Morgan Rodgers, BS, AAS, CVT*

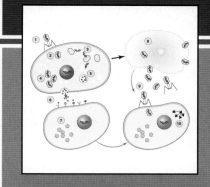

## OUTLINE

## LEARNING OBJECTIVES

*When you have completed this chapter you will be able to:*

1. List the organization and functions of the immune system.
2. Describe the structures and functions of the immune system, including the white blood cells, lymph nodes, spleen, thymus, tonsils, and GALT.
3. Differentiate between internal and external innate immune functions.
4. Understand complement proteins, cytokines, and interleukins along with their functions.
5. Differentiate between specific and nonspecific immune reactions.
6. Describe various nonspecific immune activities.
7. Differentiate between and understand the components of cell-mediated versus humoral immunity.
8. Describe the classes of immunoglobulin.
9. Differentiate between active and passive immunity.
10. Understand what can occur when the immune system doesn't function properly.

## VOCABULARY FUNDAMENTALS

*Active immunity* **ahck**-tihv ihm-**myoo**-nih-tē
*Adaptive immunity* ah-**dahp**-tihv ihm-**myoo**-nih-tē
*Antibody* **ahn**-tē-boh-dē
*Antigen* **ahn**-teh-jehn
*Apoptosis* ahp-ohp-**tō**-sihs
*Complement* **kohm**-pleh-mehnt
*Cytokine* **sī**-tō-kīn
*Disease* dihz-**ēz**
*Fever* **fē**-vər
*Infection* ihn-**fehck**-shuhn
*Inflammation* ihn-fluh-**mā**-shuhn
*Innate immunity* ihn-**āt** ihm-**myoo**-nih-tē

*Interferon* ihn-tər-**feer**-ohn
*Macrophage* **mah**-krō-fāj
*Memory cell* **mehm**-ohr-ē sehl
*Microbe* **mī**-krōb
*Passive immunity* **pah**-sihv ihm-**myoo**-nih-tē
*Pathogen* **pahth**-ō-jehn
*Pathogenicity* pahth-ō-jeh-**nihs**-ih-tē
*Phagocyte* **fahg**-ō-sīt
*Phagocytosis* fahg-ō-sī-**tō**-sihs
*Virulence* **vihr**-ū-luhnz
*Virulence factor* **vihr**-ū-luhnz **fahck**-tər

Every day an animal's body encounters millions of microorganisms. They are looking for food and a warm place to live and breed. Although many are harmless, others are capable of causing illness or even death. Thankfully, the body has the ability through its immune system to defend itself against **pathogens** (organisms capable of causing disease). The immune system has evolved to act as the security system of the body responsible for recognizing foreign material and protecting the body from anything that is not part of the animal. Its major function is distinguishing "self" from "nonself" cells, allowing easy identification and destruction of potential pathogens. Without the immune system, animals would be in a constant state of disease, if they survived at all. The first line of defense of the immune system is made of external barriers. The second line of defense includes cellular and chemical components. Together they make up the **innate immune system**. If a pathogen evades the first and second lines of defense, the third line of defense, also known as the **adaptive immune system**, will be activated (Figure 13-1).

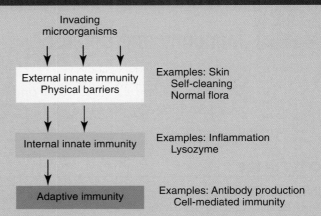

**FIGURE 13-1** The three major barriers that protect an animal's body against microbial invasion. Each barrier provides a more effective defense than the previous one. (Redrawn from Tizard I: Veterinary immunology, ed 9, St Louis, 2013, Saunders.)

## ANATOMIC ORGANIZATION OF THE IMMUNE SYSTEM

### SKIN AND MUCOUS MEMBRANES— THE FIRST LINE OF DEFENSE

The body's first line of defense against potential pathogens consists of physical barriers that prevent the pathogens from entering the body. By limiting pathogen entry, the body minimizes the effort required to defend the animal. If pathogens cannot enter, they cannot cause disease.

The first, and in many ways, most important defense mechanism is the skin. Covering the entire body surface, the skin serves as a physical barrier that protects the vital organs inside. In addition to serving as a physical barrier, the surface of the skin supports a variety of resident microorganisms (normal flora) that recognize and destroy potential invaders. Unless there is a break in the skin, most pathogens are destroyed before they can enter the body. Additionally, the acidic pH and fatty acid content of sweat inhibit bacterial growth.

Of course, if the animal's body were completely sealed off from the environment, it would be unable to acquire food, oxygen, and water—all requirements for life. It would also be unable to remove the waste products of metabolism. One or the other would eventually kill the animal. To sustain life, there must be pathways through the protective layer of the skin. The largest of these pathways include the respiratory, gastrointestinal, and urinary tracts. Although these openings are required, to leave them completely open would be just as dangerous as having no protective barrier. Thus, the body has several protective mechanisms that allow the materials entry into these pathways while still protecting the animal. For example, the respiratory system uses a combination of cilia and mucus to trap and remove potential pathogens away from the lower respiratory tract. The digestive system uses the acidity of the stomach to kill many **microbes** that gain entry through ingestion. In addition, fluids such as tears, saliva, nasal discharges, and urine flush pathogens from the body.

### ORGANS AND TISSUES— INTERNAL PROTECTION
#### SPLEEN

If a microbe is able to penetrate these physical and chemical barriers, there are internal organs with immunologic functions. The largest of these organs is the spleen, which is composed of white pulp and red pulp. White pulp is made of lymphoid tissue and is the portion of the spleen with immunologic functions. It surrounds blood vessels and contains phagocytic cells that react to **antigens** in the bloodstream. One of the functions of these cells is removing the antigens from the blood via **phagocytosis**, and initiating an immune response to produce antibodies against the antigen. Recall from Chapter 12 that the spleen acts as a reservoir for additional blood supply in the red pulp. Specialized blood-filled sinuses make up the red pulp, which is also responsible for removing worn, damaged, or aged blood cells by the action of tissue **macrophages**. Animals are capable of living without the spleen, and after a splenectomy, macrophages and lymphoid tissue in other areas of the body are able to compensate for the loss.

## LYMPHATIC SYSTEM

The next largest component of the immune system is the lymphatic system. The lymphatic system is responsible for collecting and returning excess interstitial tissue fluid to the cardiovascular system. Lymph vessels parallel the vessels of the circulatory system. As blood flows through arteries and capillaries, some of this fluid seeps into the interstitial tissue space. Lymphatic capillaries drain any excess fluid, as **lymph**, into lymphatic vessels (see Figure 12-23). As lymph travels through lymphatic vessels, it picks up water, electrolytes, sugar, and lymphocytes. Lymph collected from the digestive system is called **chyle**, which often contains small fat molecules called chylomicrons (which are responsible for the postprandial lipemia found in blood samples drawn just after an animal has eaten). Lymph travels through the vessels of the lymphatic system to the thoracic duct, which empties into the systemic circulation in the area of the right atrium of the heart. This mixes the lymph with blood returning to the heart. In this way the lymphatic system also helps maintain osmotic pressure and fluid balance.

## LYMPH NODES

Located throughout the body are lymph nodes, small structures that are responsible for lymph filtration as it travels back to the systemic circulation. Lymph enters the cortex of the lymph node via afferent vessels in most species (except pigs). This is where clusters of lymphocyte nodules exist. The lymph then passes into the medulla of the lymph node, which contains macrophages that remove potential pathogens such as microorganisms, cancer cells, or foreign debris. After passing through the medulla, the lymph exits the lymph node via the efferent vessels. As it moves through the lymph node, some of the lymphocytes enter the lymph and travel to other areas of the body, where they are capable of mounting an immune response (Figure 13-2).

As lymph returns from the periphery (e.g., the limbs), it has to flow through at least one lymph node. Although there are lymph nodes dispersed throughout the body, the peripheral lymph nodes can easily be palpated, and thus are easiest to assess. The peripheral nodes include the submandibular (caudal to the mandible), prescapular (cranial to the shoulder), axillary (where the front limb joins the trunk), inguinal (near the groin), and popliteal (distal/caudal aspect of the hamstring muscles) (Figure 13-3). As lymph fluid passes through successive nodes, the likelihood that any potential pathogen will survive decreases significantly.

Lymph from specific areas of the body will always pass through the same lymph node(s), which may aid in determining the location of an inflammatory response, **infection**, or tumor. A lymph node near an affected area becomes enlarged because of increased lymphocyte action (multiplication) and macrophage accumulation in response to the presence of an antigen. For this reason, in cases of suspected cancer it is common to biopsy the lymph nodes that filter lymph from an area where the tumors are present. Evaluation of the biopsy can help determine whether the cancer has begun to metastasize (spread) and assist in planning treatment protocols. If the cancer has metastasized to regional lymph nodes, they may need to be removed along with the original tumor.

## MALT

In addition to the peripheral lymph nodes, there are clusters of lymphoid tissue in various areas throughout the animal's body (Figure 13-4). Referred to as mucosa-associated lymphatic tissue (MALT), these small lymphatic nodules are located near mucosal surfaces but are not encapsulated like a lymph node. The function of MALT is to identify antigens and mount an immune response against them. There are subcategories of MALT that include conjunctiva-associated lymphoid tissue (CALT), nose or nasopharynx-associated lymphoid tissue (NALT), and gut-associated lymphoid tissue (GALT). The function of GALT is to ensure that pathogens that survive the acidic environment of the stomach cannot infect the animal via the gastrointestinal (GI) tract.

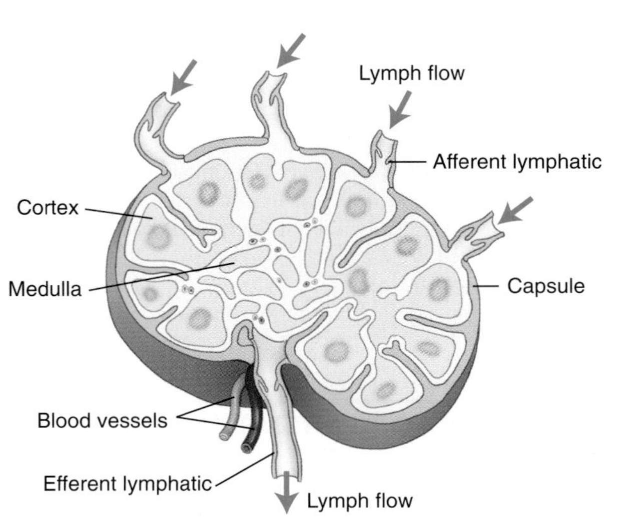

**FIGURE 13-2** The major structural features of a typical lymph node.

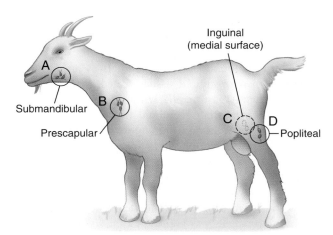

**FIGURE 13-3** Locations of common palpable lymph nodes in a goat. A, Submandibular lymph node; B, prescapular lymph node; C, Inguinal lymph node (in the groin area); D, popliteal lymph node.

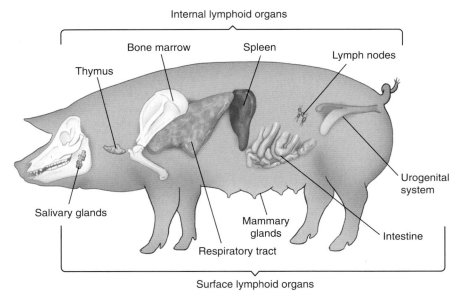

**FIGURE 13-4** The major lymphoid tissues of the pig, a typical mammal.

## TONSILS

Tonsils are found in the epithelial tissue in the pharynx, larynx, and urinary and reproductive tracts. They are part of the MALT system. Tonsils house lymphocytes to destroy foreign material before it is able to cause disease. Tonsils found in the posterior nasal cavity are called adenoid (pharyngeal) tonsils, whereas tonsils found in the posterior oral cavity are called palatine tonsils. Unlike lymph nodes, which are located along lymph vessels, tonsils are present at the beginning of the lymph drainage system and lack a capsule. Tonsils are also found in the prepuce and vagina where they perform a similar function.

## PEYER'S PATCHES

Peyer's patches are aggregations of lymphoid tissue in the small intestine of animals such as cattle, sheep, pigs, horses, and dogs. The majority of Peyer's patches are found in the lining of the ileum, the final section of the small intestine. A smaller percentage of Peyer's patches are found in the jejunum (the middle section of the small intestine).

## THYMUS

The **thymus** is found in young animals as an additional concentration of lymphoid tissue located in the mediastinum. The thymus is where T lymphocytes mature before they migrate into other lymphoid tissues and blood, and where T cells are programmed to fight specific antigens. The cell lines for the T lymphocytes are established while the animal is a juvenile. As the animal matures, the thymus atrophies and it is usually undetectable in an adult animal. However, microscopic clusters of cells in the area continue to produce T cells throughout the life of the animal.

## RED BONE MARROW

Red bone marrow, although not strictly an immune organ, is responsible for the production of all white blood cells, the

soldiers of the immune response. Look at Figure 13-5. Notice that the pluripotent stem cell will become either a common lymphoid progenitor or a common myeloid progenitor. The common lymphoid progenitor leaves the bone marrow and matures to one of the various types of lymphocyte in lymph tissue in other parts of the body. The common myeloid progenitor stays in the bone marrow and the cells that develop from it will mature in the bone marrow.

When the monocyte is called into tissue it becomes a macrophage. Depending on the location in which it is found, it can have a specific name. For example, a macrophage in the liver is called a Kupffer cell, in the central nervous system it is a microglial cell, in bone and bone marrow it is an osteoclast, and in the epidermis and lymph nodes it is a dendritic cell. The dendritic cell is a sentinel macrophage that can capture invading pathogens and take them to a lymph node for destruction. We'll discuss the importance of dendritic cells later in the chapter. See Chapter 12 for more detailed descriptions of the different types of white blood cell.

### ✓ TEST YOURSELF 13-1

1. What is the main function of the immune system?
2. What organs are involved in immunity?
3. Describe how the lymphatic system protects the body from disease.
4. Where is MALT found?
5. What is the significance of the thymus?

## FUNCTIONAL ORGANIZATION OF THE IMMUNE SYSTEM

The immune system is functionally divided into two categories: innate and adaptive immunity (Figure 13-6). The **innate**

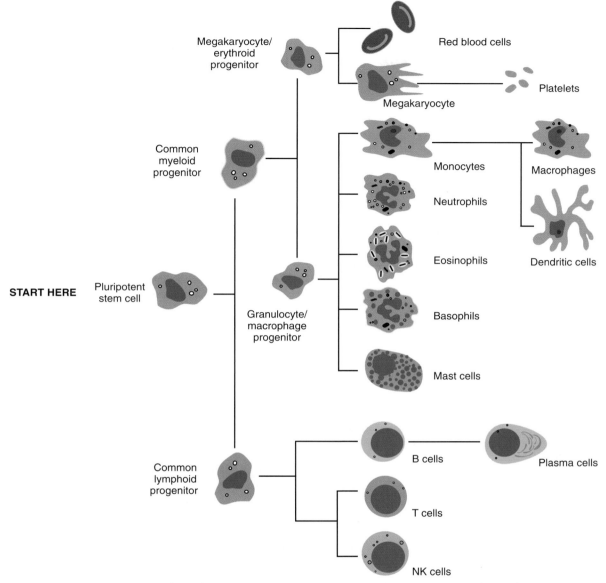

**FIGURE 13-5** The origin of cells from the red bone marrow. (From Tizard I: Veterinary immunology, ed 9, St Louis, 2013, Saunders.)

immune system is rapid, nonspecific and destroys "nonself" invaders indiscriminately. It is present at birth and uses physical, chemical, and cellular components to protect the body from anything identified as "nonself." The innate immune system is unable to target specific organisms; instead, it destroys all "nonself" invading organisms by the same mechanisms.

The **adaptive immune system** targets specific organisms, but it is slower to respond to an invading organism. It is not present at birth but develops and adapts as the animal matures and is exposed to a variety of antigens. Once an animal is exposed to an antigen, the adaptive immune system uses antibodies, memory cells, plasma cells, B lymphocytes, and T lymphocytes provide immunity.

**TEST YOURSELF 13-2**
1. What are the two main subcategories of the immune system?
2. How does specific immunity differ from nonspecific immunity?
3. Adaptive immunity is nonspecific immunity. True or False?

## INNATE IMMUNE SYSTEM

The innate or nonspecific immune system works independently or in conjunction with the adaptive immune system to prevent disease by providing mechanical (anatomic) and cellular barriers (Figure 13-7). It is present at

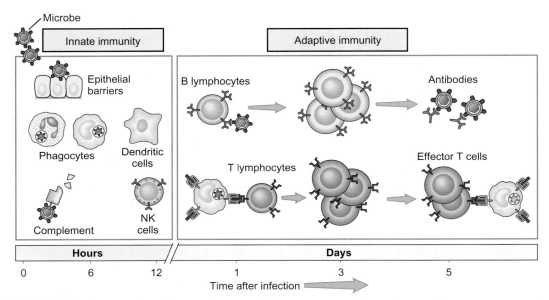

**FIGURE 13-6** The principal mechanisms of innate and adaptive immunity. The mechanisms of innate immunity provide the initial defense against infections. Some of the mechanisms prevent infections and others eliminate microbes. Adaptive immune responses develop later and are mediated by lymphocytes and their products. Antibodies block infections and eliminate microbes, and T lymphocytes eradicate intracellular microbes. *NK*, Natural killer cell. (From Abbas AK: Basic immunology updated edition: functions and disorders of the immune system, ed 3, St Louis, 2010, Saunders.)

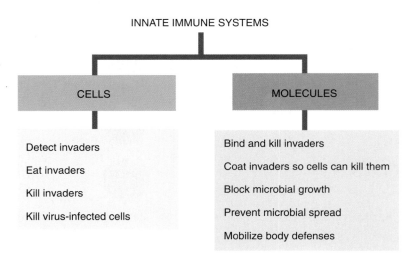

**FIGURE 13-7** The innate immune system consists of a collection of multiple subsystems. They can be divided into the cells that largely eat and kill invaders and the molecules that bind and kill the invaders. (From Tizard I: Veterinary immunology, ed 9, St Louis, 2013, Saunders.)

birth and remains virtually unchanged during the life of the animal.

Innate immunity acts as the animal's first and second lines of defense against pathogens that could cause disease in an animal. The innate immune system does not recognize specific pathogens, rather macrophages recognize common structures shared by large groups of pathogens. These *pathogen-associated molecular patterns (PAMPs)* are found on the membrane surface of invading pathogens. The membrane surface of a macrophage or dendritic cell has receptors called *pattern-recognition receptors (PRRs)* that fit the PAMP on the pathogen's cell membrane. This allows the macrophage to recognize and attach to the pathogen and trigger the innate immune system. Normal, nonpathogenic microbes (normal flora) are recognized as self and will not trigger the innate immune system.

## EXTERNAL INNATE IMMUNITY—THE FIRST LINE OF DEFENSE

Anatomic barriers that include structures on the surface of the body that prevent disease provide external innate immunity. The skin, the largest organ in the body, has a thick layer of keratinized epithelial tissue that is impermeable to a majority of pathogens. The keratinized epithelial cells have antimicrobial properties that inhibit bacterial growth. When the layer of dead keratinized cells is sloughed off the skin it takes with it any microorganisms that were clinging to the cells. In order for this to be an effective means of disease prevention, the skin must be intact to prevent pathogens from entering the body. When imperfections such as small cuts or lacerations are present on external barriers, pathogens can invade the body tissue and circulate to other areas of the body. Therefore, broken skin is always a weaker defense than intact tissue.

Mucous membranes of the epithelium that line the respiratory, digestive, urinary, and reproductive systems also have unique structures that provide innate immunity. Mucus produced by mucous membranes can trap pathogens. Cilia on the borders of epithelial cells move the pathogens away from entry into the body. For example, in the upper respiratory tract, mucus and cilia trap and propel foreign materials away from the lungs, preventing entrance into the lower respiratory tract. This is important because the lower respiratory tract is an ideal moist and warm location for bacterial growth.

Tears, saliva, and nasal discharge production create a flushing action that helps prevent infection in the eyes, mouth, and nose. Additionally, they contain lysozyme and phospholipase that break down bacterial cell walls and membranes, preventing microbial growth in these regions. The acidic environment in the stomach kills many of the microbes in the food that is ingested. If pathogens penetrate through these external barriers and into deeper tissues, the second line of defense is activated.

## INTERNAL INNATE DEFENSE—THE SECOND LINE OF DEFENSE

Once a pathogen has made its way past the physical barriers of the innate immune system, the body tries to control the spread of the infection through acute inflammation.

Phagocytes, natural killer cells, **interferons**, complement receptors, and PRRs play a key role in the inflammatory response.

***INFLAMMATION.*** **Inflammation** is the body's localized reaction created by the innate immune system in response to trauma, infection, chemical exposure, or excessive heat. The four cardinal signs of inflammation are: *redness, swelling, heat,* and *pain* (Figure 13-8). Loss of function is another attribute of inflammation that is sometimes considered the fifth sign.

During pathogen invasion, tissue cells are damaged. This triggers the release of various chemicals from specific cells, such as mast cells, that mediate the inflammatory response and result in the signs listed above. These chemicals include histamine, **prostaglandins**, **leukotrienes**, and **cytokines**.

During the inflammatory response arterioles dilate and venules constrict, which leads to increased blood flow and increased capillary permeability at the injured site. This allows large numbers of phagocytic white blood cells (WBCs) to enter the injured site and ingest foreign or cellular debris. Once the pathogens and/or foreign debris have been eliminated, the tissue begins to heal and inflammation is reduced.

Fever represents a systemic inflammatory response where the chemical mediators are carried throughout the body. An elevated body temperature can prevent proliferation of many microbes by creating an environment that exceeds their optimum temperature for growth. This prevents further pathogen growth and occasionally causes pathogen death. A fever can also result in increased cellular metabolism that in turn may cause more rapid phagocytosis, an acceleration of lymphocyte production, and increased antibody production.

Fever has many benefits to the immune system; however, a significant fever can be harmful to the body. An excessively high temperature (>~104° F (40° C)) may cause proteins to denature in the body and can lead to a number of problems,

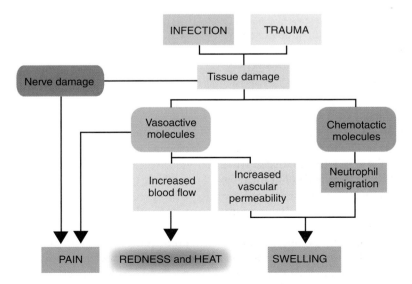

**FIGURE 13-8** The major signs of acute inflammation and how they are generated. (From Tizard I: Veterinary immunology, ed 9, St Louis, 2013, Saunders.)

## CLINICAL APPLICATION

### Disseminated Intravascular Coagulation (DIC)

Disseminated intravascular coagulation (DIC) is a condition that occurs as a complication of a variety of disorders, including hyperthermia. DIC is characterized by increased intravascular coagulation, worsened by the subsequent formation of microthromboses (clots) that lead to multiorgan failure. The result of DIC is either excessive bleeding or clotting which, without treatment, often leads to death. Animals with DIC typically show signs of bleeding, such as petechiae, ecchymoses, melena, and hematuria. Treatment involves remedying the initial cause of DIC by administering heparin, as well as blood product transfusion to replace consumed coagulation factors. Overall, the treatment or resolution of DIC is many times unsuccessful. DIC has also been called "Death Is Coming." The best way to prevent DIC is to treat the underlying cause rapidly before the sequence of DIC is initiated.

## CLINICAL APPLICATION

### Cat Bite Wound

Any animal bite wound has the likelihood of becoming infected. Cat bite wounds, whether on humans or other animals, are especially contaminated and infection is almost guaranteed. The cat's mouth has a large number of normal flora. Upon penetration of the its teeth through the skin of a person or another animal, those bacteria are deposited deep into the wound where they are no longer normal flora. This deep location often has a low oxygen concentration and becomes an ideal breeding ground for bacteria. The body responds to the presence of these bacteria by sending phagocytic white blood cells to the site to phagocytize the bacteria. This large accumulation of WBCs is known as pus, which often leads to the formation of an abscess (an accumulation of pus in a confined space). Treatment of an abscess typically consists of lancing, draining, and flushing out the wound. Sometimes a drain is placed to allow for further pus to exit the wound. Cat bite wounds, or any penetrating wound, should be addressed quickly to avoid abscess formation. Hint: In the case of bite wounds, look for four puncture sites—one for each of the cat's canine teeth.

including osmotic pressure changes, edema, and disseminated intravascular coagulation.

**PHAGOCYTOSIS.** Phagocytosis is one way the body can remove pathogens in the blood, fluids, and body tissues. There are several types of cell capable of phagocytosis but the most common phagocytic cells are the neutrophils, monocytes, macrophages, and dendritic cells. Phagocytes contain receptors on their outer membrane that help differentiate cells as being "self" versus "nonself." These receptors include PAMP receptors and complement receptors that recognize components of the **complement** system that enhance phagocytosis.

When tissues are injured or an infection is present, mast cells release histamine, which causes localized vasodilatation

and inflammation. Vasodilation creates increased permeability of the capillaries, allowing large numbers of phagocytic white blood cells to enter the injured site.

Typically, neutrophils are the first responders to the injured site, followed by macrophages. Phagocytosis includes five steps (Figure 13-9):

1. Activation and chemotaxis: Phagocytes are stimulated by inflammatory signals such as prostaglandins, cytokines, complement proteins, and bacterial components/products to begin moving toward the "nonself" cell (bacterium).
2. Attachment: Receptors on the phagocytes recognize the nonspecific components on the pathogen cell membrane and bind to them.
3. Ingestion or Endocytosis: The attached phagocyte extends projections from its plasma membrane, called pseudopods. Pseudopods engulf the microorganism into a vesicle called a *phagosome*.
4. Destruction: A lysosome (cellular organelle that contains digestive enzymes to help break down bacteria) fuses with the phagosome, creating a *phagolysosome*. The lysosome releases digestive enzymes into the phagolysosome. The enzymes break down the bacteria.
5. exocytosis The phagolysosome releases the indigestible material from the phagocyte.

**COMPLEMENT SYSTEM.** The **complement** system is a group of 30+ plasma proteins, mostly inactive proteolytic enzymes (break down peptide bonds that hold amino acids together), which are always present in plasma. They become active in the presence of an antigen or an antibody attached to an antigen. They are identified by the letter "C" followed by a number. For example C3 is complement 3. The number indicates the order in which it was discovered. So C3 was the third complement protein discovered.

Complement proteins are produced primarily in the liver and circulate in the blood in their inactive form. The two most important functions of the complement system are to trigger inflammation and to alter microbial cell membranes (Figure 13-10). To alter cell membranes the complement proteins can attach to the microbe's PAMPs and cause cell lysis. These complement proteins are part of the innate immune system because they don't need an antibody to be bound to the microbe first. The complement response to the PAMPs is rapid and provides nearly immediate protection against the antigen. The complement system can also alter microbe membranes through *opsonization* (coating the antigen with complement proteins to make it more visible to the phagocyte), for direct destruction by phagocytes (Figure 13-11).

There are also specific complement proteins that require a specific antibody to be bound to a specific antigen so that the specific complement protein can bind to it. This response is slower because it can take from 7 to 10 days for antibody production against an antigen to be effective.

In either case there are a series of complement protein reactions involved in a cascading process whereby when one complement protein is activated it activates the next complement protein in the series. This is called the *complement*

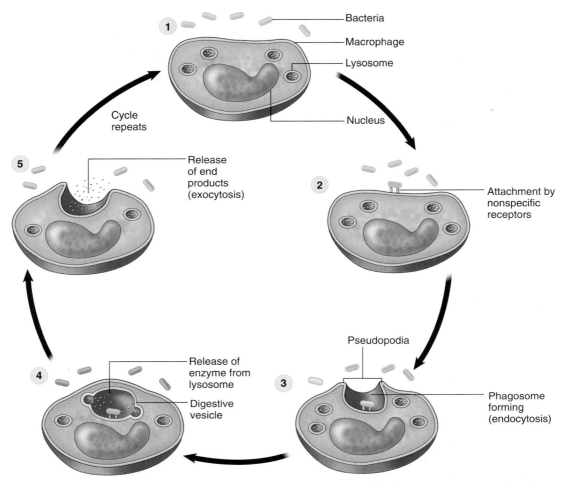

**FIGURE 13-9** Phagocytosis and destruction of bacteria. (From Patton KT, Thibodeau GA: Anatomy & physiology, ed 8, St Louis, 2013, Mosby.)

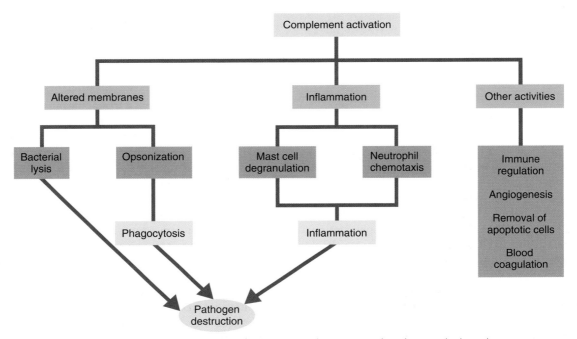

**FIGURE 13-10** The functions of the complement system. Complement may either alter microbial membranes or trigger inflammation. Either way, it hastens the elimination of microbial invaders and is thus a key component of the innate immune system. (From Tizard I: Veterinary immunology, ed 9, St Louis, 2013, Saunders.)

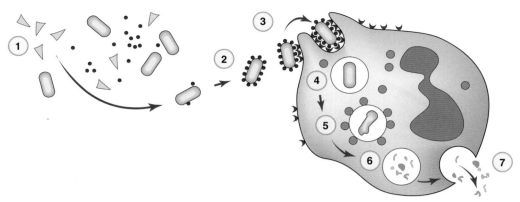

**FIGURE 13-11** Opsonization.
*1,* Macrophage with complement receptors ❤ on its cell membrane is attracted to the site of infection by chemotactic agents ◁.
*2,* Completment ● begins coating the microorganisms 🏷.
*3,* The complement-coated microorganism attaches to the complement receptors on the macrophage 🦠.
*4,* The complement-coated microorganism is engulfed into a phagosome ⬤.
*5,* Lysosomes surround the phagosome creating a phagolysosome and release substances that kill the microorganism 🦠.
*6,* The microorganism is digested in the phagolysosome ⬤.
*7,* The remnants of the microorganism are eliminated from the macrophage by exostosis 🦠.

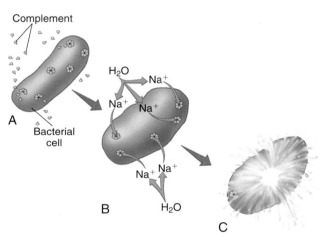

**FIGURE 13-12** Complement destruction of a bacterium. **A,** Activated complement molecules form doughnut-shaped complexes in a bacterium's cell membrane; **B,** Holes in the complement complexes allow sodium and then water to diffuse into the bacterium; **C,** After enough water has entered, the swollen bacterium bursts.

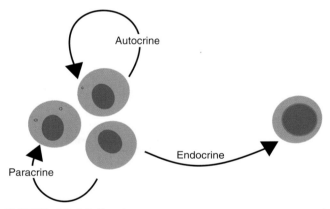

**FIGURE 13-13** The distinction among autocrine, paracrine, and endocrine effects. Cytokines differ from hormones in that most of their effects are autocrine or paracrine, whereas hormones usually act on distant cells in an endocrine fashion. (From Tizard I: Veterinary immunology, ed 9, St Louis, 2013, Saunders.)

*cascade.* The final step of the complement cascade is *complement fixation* where the molecules that are formed are gathered in clusters on the antigen's surface. Each cluster resembles a doughnut and in its center a hole is punched in the antigen cell wall. This results in antigen cell lysis or body cell **apoptosis** (Figure 13-12).

In addition to opsonization, activated complement proteins also play a part in chemotaxis of leukocytes to the site of tissue injury, regulating the inflammatory response and enhancing cell destruction.

**CYTOKINES.** **Cytokines** are part of the innate immune system. The term cytokine can be broken down into "cyto" meaning cell and "kinos" meaning movement. Cytokines are communicators. They provide communication between leukocytes and other cells and among leukocytes themselves. They are signaling proteins that are secreted by certain cells in the body. Cytokines can be autocrine (they act on the cell that secreted them), paracrine (they act on cells near the cell that secreted them), or endocrine (they travel to other parts of the body and act on cells in that location) (Figure 13-13). Often their role is to mediate the immune or inflammatory response by attracting immune cells to a specific site: the site of infection, inflammation, or trauma. They also play a major role in hematopoiesis.

There are many different cytokines but there are groups of cytokines that have similar effects on the cells they target. Some act as inhibitor molecules and others act to enhance immune processes. Many, but not all, cytokines are directly associated with immune activity. Currently nearly 50 cytokines have been described. **Interleukins**, **interferons**, and **chemokines** are types of cytokine.

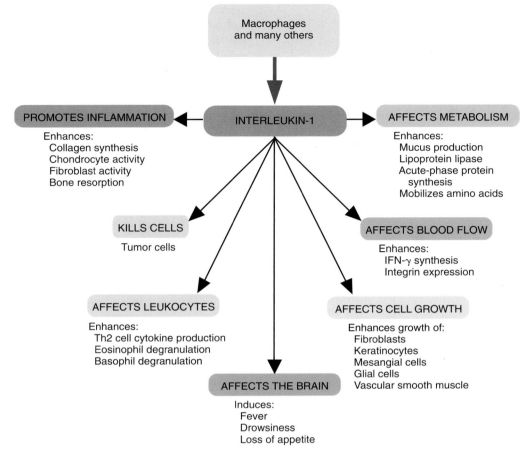

**FIGURE 13-14** The origins and some of the biological activites of interleukin (IL)-1. (From Tizard I: Veterinary immunology, ed 9, St Louis, 2013, Saunders.)

**INTERLEUKINS.** It was initially thought that interleukins were produced by leukocytes and acted on only leukocytes, which is how they got their name. Since that time other cells have been shown to produce interleukins. Interleukins are identified by "IL" followed by a number. Interleukins control leukocyte (especially T and B cells) growth, differentiation, and activation during an immune response. They have a variety of effects in the body. For example, T cells produce IL-2 during an immune response. This interleukin is necessary for the T cells to grow, proliferate, and differentiate into effector (cytotoxic) cells. The activities of IL-1 are shown in Figure 13-14.

**CHEMOKINES.** Chemokines are chemotactic cytokines. They stimulate the movement of leukocytes from blood into tissue and toward an injury/inflammatory site where there are high concentrations of the chemokines. This often causes an increased rate of clearance of pathogens at an injury site. They have many other effects in the body as well. Many injured or stressed cells will release chemokines, which leads to an influx of immune cells at the site.

**NATURAL KILLER (NK) CELLS.** Natural Killer (NK) cells are found in the blood and lymph and are part of both the innate immune system and the adaptive immune system.

These *granular lymphocytes* are able to identify and kill virus-infected cells, stressed cells, and tumor cells (Figure 13-15). They differ from phagocytes in that they do not ingest the target cell. Instead, they bind to the cell and induce cellular changes that lead to **apoptosis** (programmed cell death) before the virus can mature (Figure 13-16). It is important to note that NK cells do not cause lysis of virus-infected cells, as this would release virions (virus particles) instead of controlling infection. Instead, apoptosis is triggered for virus-infected cells; this ensures death of the virus whereas lysis does not.

All NK cells have two types of receptor on their cell membranes to help determine which cells to kill (abnormal, nonself) or not to kill (normal, self): the killer-activating receptor (KAR) and the killer inhibitory receptor (KIR).

All normal autogenous nucleated cells (self) have MHC-I (major histocompatibility complex class I) molecules on their surfaces that display a normal small protein fragment belonging to the cell (a "self" protein) to which a KIR receptor on an NK cell can bind. This binding demonstrates that the cell is expressing normal amounts of MHC-I and is healthy. This inhibits the NK cell from killing healthy cells (Figure 13-17).

Virus-infected cells or tumor cells in the body often have altered or missing MCH-I. The KIR receptor on the NK cell

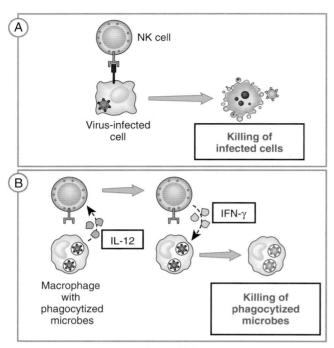

**FIGURE 13-15** Functions of natural killer (NK) cells. **A,** NK cells kill host cells infected by intracellular pathogens, thus eliminating reservoirs of infection. **B,** NK cells respond to IL-12 produced by macrophages and secrete interferon (INF)-gamma which activates the macrophages to kill phagocytized pathogens. (From Abbas AK: Basic immunology updated edition: functions and disorders of the immune system, ed 3, St Louis, 2010, Saunders.)

cannot bind to an altered or missing MHC-I molecule so it will not inhibit NK cell KAR action. The KAR receptor on the NK cell can still bind with other molecules on the cell membrane of the "nonself" cell, triggering apoptosis.

Once an infected or damaged cell is identified, the KAR of the NK cell binds with the cell. The NK cell then releases *perforins* (proteins that form pores in cell membranes), and proteolytic enzymes such as *granzymes* from their granules. Granzymes move into the target cell via the newly formed pores and cause apoptosis by breaking down the cell structure and its contents.

NK cells are stimulated by cytokines, including interleukins and interferons. Tumor cells, damaged cells, and virus-infected cells release cytokines as stress signals. NK cells respond, prompting the ultimate destruction of damaged or infected cells.

**INTERFERONS.** Interferons (IFNs) are proteins produced by an animal's immune system cells in response to the presence of viruses, bacteria, cancer, and other foreign invaders. IFNs are an especially effective mechanism to ward off viral invaders. Viruses lack the ability to replicate and survive on their own so they survive by invading the animal's cells (host cells). While in the host cell, they are able to utilize the cellular replicating machinery to produce adenosine triphosphate (ATP) for energy and proteins for viral replication. Viral infections are hard to treat, mainly because they are intracellular pathogens. In order to eradicate the virus, the host cell it inhabits must be damaged.

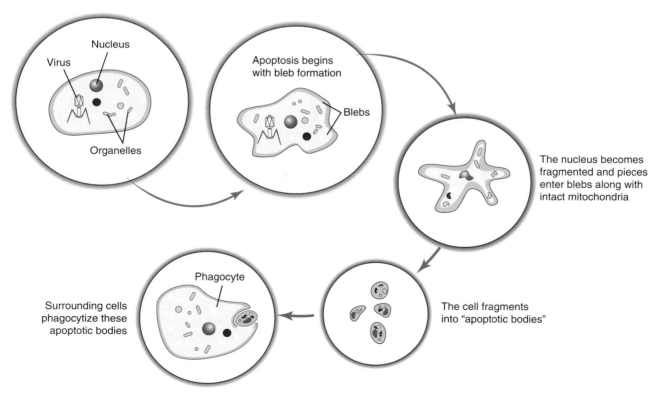

**FIGURE 13-16** Apoptosis of a virus-infected cell. (From Cunningham, JG: Textbook of veterinary physiology, ed 4, St Louis, 2007, Saunders.)

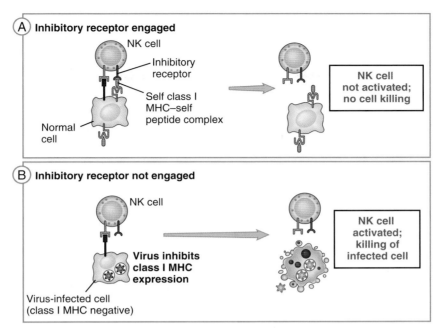

**FIGURE 13-17** Activating and inhibitory receptors of natural killer (NK) cells. **A,** Healthy host cells express self MHC-I molecules, which are recognized by inhibitory receptors (KIR), thus ensuring that NK cells do not attack normal host cells. **B,** NK cells are activated by infected cells when MHC-I is reduced so that the inhibitory receptors are not engaged. The result is that infected cells are killed. (Modified from Abbas AK, Lichtman AH: Basic immunology updated edition: Functions and disorders of the immune system, ed 3, St Louis, 2011, Saunders.)

Some virus-infected cells are able to secrete IFNs, which can be beneficial because they prevent the virus from spreading to healthy unaffected cells. Once produced in one cell, IFNs are able to diffuse to neighboring cells and promote the production of "interfering" proteins that help block protein synthesis and degrade viral RNA in the infected cell (Figure 13-18).

More specifically, IFNs are secreted from virus-infected cells and bind to the membrane-bound receptors on surrounding cells. Once the interferon is bound to the noninfected cell, second messengers relay a signal to the inner portion of the uninfected cell to produced inactive antiviral particles (AVP). When a virus enters the cell the inactive AVPs become activated and the overall effect is inhibition of virus replication within that cell.

IFNs stimulate an increase in expression of both MHC-I and MHC-II. MHC-II is found on the cell membranes of professional *antigen presenting cells (APCs)* (Figure 13-19). The APCs are cells whose "profession" it is to phagocytize antigens, process and destroy them, and present fragments of antigen protein attached to an MHC-II on the phagocytic cell membrane. APCs include phagocytes, macrophages, dendritic cells, and B cells. Increased MHC-II expression on antigen-presenting cells leads to recognition by helper T cells to stimulate the action of NK cells and cytotoxic cells.

There are several classes of IFN. Biologically engineered IFNs are now available and have some uses in veterinary medicine, for example in supportive treatment of feline leukemia (FeLV) and feline immunodeficiency virus (FIV).

**TEST YOURSELF 13-3**

1. What is the difference between the first and second lines of defense against invading pathogens?
2. The body's innate defense against viral pathogens is driven by the production of what?
3. What are the pros and cons of fever?
4. What cell type of innate defense targets tumor cells?
5. What types of cell are phagocytic?
6. What are the four cardinal signs of inflammation?

## ADAPTIVE (ACQUIRED) IMMUNE SYSTEM

In addition to the nonspecific innate immune system, an animal has a third line of defense that is able to target specific foreign invaders called pathogens or antigens. Unlike the innate immune system, which eliminates anything identified as nonself, the adaptive or acquired immune system is slower to respond, specific, and has memory (Figure 13-20). It targets pathogens with precision. Although the innate immune system protects the body from all pathogens using the same population of cells and chemicals, the cells of the adaptive immune system are programmed to respond only to specific pathogens. The adaptive immune system also has the ability to remember pathogens that have infected the organism and destroy them before they can cause disease in an animal a second time. The adaptive immune system has a systemic, rather than local, impact and is able to respond to pathogens throughout the entire body. Its response to a pathogen involves primarily B lymphocytes and T lymphocytes (Figure 13-21).

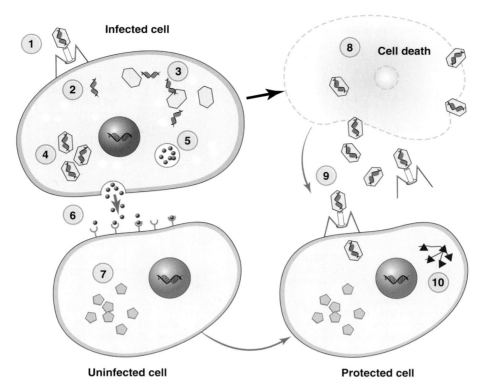

**FIGURE 13-18** Action of interferons.

*1,* Virus invades host cell.

*2,* Outer protein shell is removed to expose the genome (DNA or RNA).

*3,* Using the host cell's replicating machinery, the virus produces more genomes and proteins.

*4,* Virus genomes and proteins are reassembled into more viruses.

*5,* Virus replication in the host cell triggers production of interferons.

*6,* Interferon is released and diffuses to a nearby uninfected cell with receptors for the interferon on its cell wall.

*7,* Interferon binding triggers the production of inactive antiviral proteins (AVP).

*8,* The originally infected cell with eventually be killed by the virus causing virus particles to be released.

*9,* A virus may infect the original uninfected cell and release its genome into the cytoplasm.

*10,* This activates the AVP which degrade the genome and eventually stopping protein synthesis and virus replication.

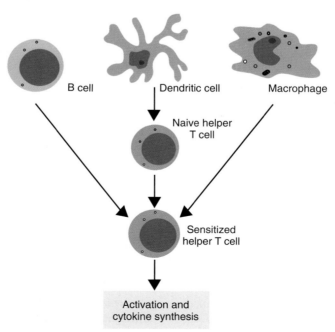

**FIGURE 13-19** Three major populations of antigen-presenting cells (APCs): B cells, dendritic cells, and macrophages. (From Tizard I: Veterinary immunology, ed 9, St Louis, 2013, Saunders.)

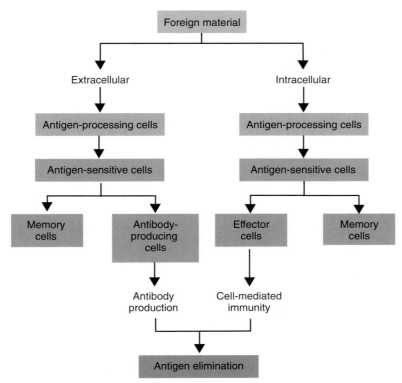

**FIGURE 13-20** A simple flow diagram showing the essential features of the adaptive immune responses. (From Tizard I: Veterinary immunology, ed 9, St Louis, 2013, Saunders.)

## B LYMPHOCYTES

Like all blood cells, B lymphocytes (B cells) originate in the red bone marrow. They then migrate to lymphoid tissues (e.g., lymph nodes, spleen) where they can initiate an immune response. B cells do not directly destroy pathogens. Each B cell is programmed to secrete a specific **antibody** (also known as **immunoglobulin** or Ig) that will lead to phagocytosis and destruction of the pathogen. Since the antibodies that are produced by the B cells are circulating in blood, lymph, and tissue fluid, they are most effective in providing immunity against extracellular pathogens.

(Historical note: The "B" refers to an organ found in birds called the *bursa of Fabricius*. When B cells were first distinguished from T cells in the 1960s, researchers were working with birds and the *bursa of Fabricius* was determined to be the site of development. Although mammals do not have this organ, think "B = bone marrow" to remember that B cells mature in the bone marrow.)

B cells are stimulated by the presence of a specific antigen and a signal from a helper T cell to differentiate into **plasma cells** that are responsible for the actual production, storage, and release of antibodies. Once created, plasma cells remain in the lymph nodes and spleen. Other B cells can differentiate into memory B cells. Should the original pathogen reappear, memory B cells are prepared to respond quickly to the same antigen.

## T LYMPHOCYTES

The precursor cells of T lymphocytes (T cells) are *thymocytes*. These cells originate in the red bone marrow and migrate to the thymus where they mature, multiply, and enter the bloodstream as T cells. They take up residence in the lymph nodes and the spleen, where they coordinate cell-mediated immunity (against intracellular pathogens) and activate B cells.

In an adult animal, B cells and T cells exist in at least three different stages of differentiation:

- Naive cells have entered the lymphatic system, but have not encountered an antigen.
- Cytotoxic or effector cells have been activated and are involved in eliminating a pathogenic antigen.
- **Memory cells** are the survivors of past infections, capable of providing long-term immunity.

When T cells and B cells are activated in an immune response, they produce clones, which are the memory cells. These clones stay in the lymph nodes or circulate in blood, looking for the same antigen that originally triggered the activation of their parent cell. Should that antigen enter the animal again, memory cells will initiate an immune response. This response is stronger and faster than the initial immune response, hopefully preventing the animal from getting sick.

The adaptive immune system can be divided into two distinct types of immunity, humoral and cell-mediated (Figure 13-22).

## HUMORAL IMMUNITY

The humoral immune response, part of adaptive immunity, is triggered by extracellular pathogens and results in antibody production. The antibodies produced by B cells/plasma

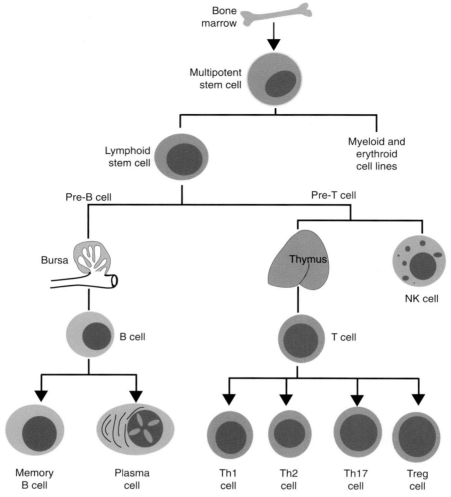

**FIGURE 13-21** Development of T and B lymphocytes, and natural killer (NK) cells. (From Tizard I: Veterinary immunology, ed 9, St Louis, 2013, Saunders.)

cells target specific antigens for destruction. Each pathogen has a unique series of amino acid antigen markers on its surface that form a unique shape called an *epitope*. On the surface of each B lymphocyte there is a corresponding shape that binds to the epitope like two pieces of a jigsaw puzzle. When the B lymphocyte and the antigen bind they wait for a signal from a helper T cell, and then an immune response is initiated. The B lymphocyte creates copies of itself, which will develop into plasma cells that produce an antibody unique to the antigen.

## IMMUNOGLOBINS

- **IgM** antibodies are produced when an animal is first exposed to an antigen (Figure 13-23, *A*).
  - IgM is a temporary antibody that disappears within 2 or 3 weeks after the initial infection and is replaced by the IgG antibody.
  - IgM antibodies are the largest antibody. They are found in blood and lymph fluid and are the first immunoglobulin made by newborn animals.

- **IgG** is the smallest but most common antibody (Figure 13-23, *B*). It is produced and released by plasma cells and found in blood and extracellular fluid when the animal has been exposed to an antigen for an extended time.
  - Elevated IgG levels can indicate a chronic infection in an animal.
  - IgG is the only antibody capable of crossing the placenta to provide **passive immunity** to the fetus.
  - IgG antibodies are involved in fighting bacterial and viral infections.
  - Production of IgG antibodies is relatively slow, so the animal may become sick from the initial exposure before the immune response can neutralize the antigen.

- **IgA** antibodies protect body surfaces from foreign substances. These antibodies play an important role in preventing diseases caused by antigens that may enter the body through mucosal surfaces (e.g., intestinal tract and lungs). Intranasal applications, such as those used in intranasal vaccination, create this type of antibody.

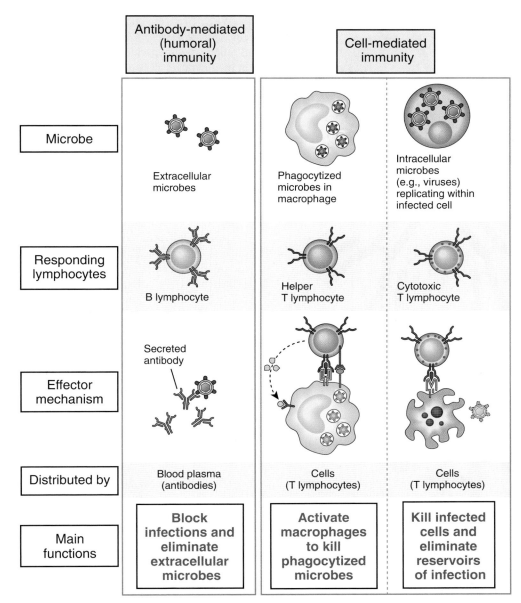

| | Antibody-mediated (humoral) immunity | Cell-mediated immunity | |
|---|---|---|---|
| **Microbe** | Extracellular microbes | Phagocytized microbes in macrophage | Intracellular microbes (e.g., viruses) replicating within infected cell |
| **Responding lymphocytes** | B lymphocyte | Helper T lymphocyte | Cytotoxic T lymphocyte |
| **Effector mechanism** | Secreted antibody | | |
| **Distributed by** | Blood plasma (antibodies) | Cells (T lymphocytes) | Cells (T lymphocytes) |
| **Main functions** | **Block infections and eliminate extracellular microbes** | **Activate macrophages to kill phagocytized microbes** | **Kill infected cells and eliminate reservoirs of infection** |

**FIGURE 13-22** Types of adaptive immunity. In humoral immunity, B cells secrete antibodies that eliminate extracellular pathogens. In cell-mediated immunity, T cells either activate machrophages to destroy phagocytosed pathogens or kill infected cells. (From Abbas AK, Lichtman AH: Basic immunology updated edition: Functions and disorders of the immune system, ed 3, St Louis, 2011, Saunders.)

- **IgE** binds to allergens and triggers histamine release from mast cells and basophils. It also protects against some parasitic helminth (worm) infections.
- **IgD** has been shown to activate basophils and mast cells but its exact mechanism is unknown.

B lymphocytes and plasma cells remain in lymphoid tissue. The antibodies released by plasma cells are secreted directly into blood, allowing them to find and bind to the invading antigens. When the antibody binds to the antigen an antigen–antibody complex is formed. The results can (1) render antigenic toxins incapable of destroying cells, (2) agglutinate antigens into large clumps that can be destroyed by macrophages, or (3) activate the **complement** system in plasma that in turn destroys the cell.

 **CLINICAL APPLICATION**

### Serologic Testing
Veterinarians often need to distinguish between acute and chronic infections in animals. To help do this, serum samples from a sick animal are sent to a reference laboratory where levels of IgG and IgM are measured. The results help the veterinarian determine whether the illness affecting the animal is recent or whether it has been around for a long time. IgM antibodies are produced early in illness and are usually detectable within 1 to 2 weeks after onset of symptoms. High serum levels of IgM indicate an acute disease. IgG antibodies generally appear 2 to 6 weeks after infection and high serum levels indicate a more chronic disease.

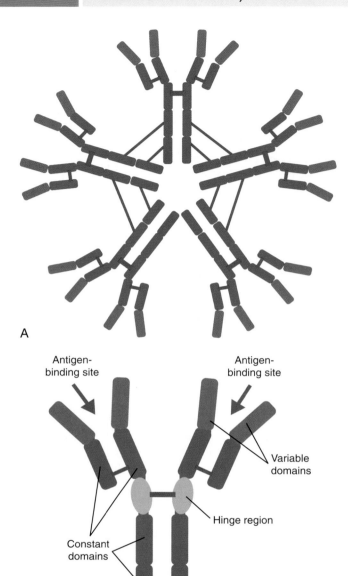

A

Antigen-
binding site                    Antigen-
                                binding site

Variable
domains

Hinge region

Constant
domains

B

**FIGURE 13-23** Immunoglobin structure. **A,** The structure of IgM. **B,** The structure of IgG. (From Tizard I: Veterinary immunology, ed 9, St Louis, 2013, Saunders.)

Remember, some B lymphocytes become memory cells after the initial exposure to a pathogen. These cells are capable of protecting the animal from this pathogen should a subsequent exposure occur. In this way, B lymphocytes can both destroy the invading pathogens and create a defense system to protect the body against future infections.

## CELL-MEDIATED IMMUNITY

Cell-mediated immunity is also part of the adaptive immune system. It is controlled by T cells, which do not depend on antibody production, but provide immunity against intracellular pathogens. T cells attach directly to antigen markers on the surfaces of phagocytes that have already processed the pathogen.

When T cells are maturing in the thymus, they develop specific antigen receptors on their cell membranes. Each receptor is unique to one specific antigen marker. After being processed in the thymus, T cells travel via the blood to lymph nodes and the spleen. Unlike B cells, T cells leave the lymphoid tissue and circulate throughout the blood and lymph. For this reason, most of the lymphocytes found in peripheral blood are T cells.

Unlike B cells, T cells fail to recognize antigens on their own. For a T cell to recognize an antigen, it must first be processed by an APC (usually a dendritic cell) (Figure 13-24). The antigen is phagocytized by the APC and broken down to its component parts. Antigenic protein fragments are bound to cellular proteins (MHC-II) in the cell and migrate to the surface of the APC. The T cell recognizes the combination of MHC-II and the antigenic marker on the macrophage surface as the antigen to which it was programmed in the thymus during development.

When the T cell encounters a corresponding antigenic marker on an APC, the antigenic marker and T cell bind, resulting in the T cell becoming activated, or sensitized. The sensitized T cell then divides, creating two populations of new cells. The first population contains multiple clones of the first cell, called memory T cells. The second population subdivides into three distinct populations:

- **Helper T cells** ($T_H$): These are the most numerous T cells. They help the immune response by secreting **cytokines** into the surrounding tissue. The effects of these signaling proteins include:
  - The cytokine that increases activation of B cells, cytotoxic T cells, and suppressor T cells
  - Interleukins, such as interleukin 2 (IL-2), a cytokine that stimulates the activity of other T cells
  - Macrophage migration inhibiting factor (MIF), a cytokine that attracts tissue macrophages to the affected area via chemotaxis. This activates the macrophages to accelerate the rate of phagocytosis that will result in more antigenic markers on the surface of the macrophage. MIF also inhibits the antigens from leaving the site of infection.
- **Cytotoxic T cells** ($T_C$): These cells are also known as effector cells, killer cells, or killer T cells. They attach to antigenic markers and destroy the cells to which they are attached. However, they are not damaged themselves. T cells that do not become cytotoxic cells can become helper T cells.
- **Regulatory T cells** ($T_S$): These cells inhibit helper T cell and cytotoxic T cell function by negative feedback. They also prevent B cells from transforming into plasma cells. These antagonistic actions provide a certain degree of control over the cell-mediated and humoral immune responses.

## ACTIVE IMMUNITY

**Active immunity** is, as the name implies, the result of an active immune process. During an initial exposure to an antigen, the immune response can be slow, allowing the disease to develop. During subsequent exposures to the same antigen, the immune system recognizes the antigen and can respond faster. Using memory T and B cells, the body

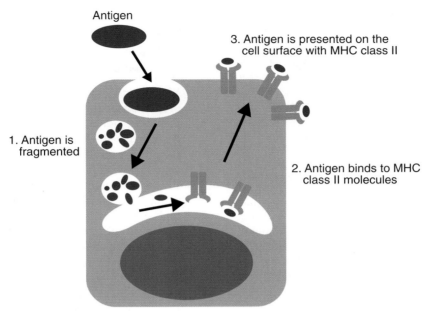

Antigen

3. Antigen is presented on the cell surface with MHC class II

1. Antigen is fragmented

2. Antigen binds to MHC class II molecules

**FIGURE 13-24** The processing of exogenous antigen by an antigen-presenting cell. (From Tizard I: Veterinary immunology, ed 9, St Louis, 2013, Saunders.)

produces antibodies, protecting the individual from developing the disease a second time.

In nature, animals are exposed to a variety of antigens in their environment and develop a natural immunity against these antigens without ever showing signs of disease. In a similar manner, using vaccines we can protect animals against certain diseases without ever exposing the animals to the actual disease.

There are two primary types of vaccine used in veterinary medicine today: modified live and killed virus. Modified live vaccines contain like-virus particles that have been weakened (attenuated) so they are nonpathogenic but still recognized by the animal as antigenic. These inactivated particles are unlikely to cause disease. A modified live vaccine produces a strong immune response because they mimic a natural infection.

Killed virus vaccines contain virus particles that have been treated with chemicals, heat, or radiation to render them inactive. Once killed, the viruses are unable to revert to their disease-causing state, but the immune system is still able to recognize the remnants of the virus and respond appropriately. This response is weaker than when modified live vaccines are used so multiple doses must be administered before immunity is achieved. Regardless of whether exposure is through the environment or vaccination, the body's immune system actively responds to the antigens, resulting in active immunity.

## PASSIVE IMMUNITY

Receiving antibodies from an external source can also protect the animal but its immune system is not actively involved. This is passive immunity. The most common method of providing passive immunity is through maternal antibodies

### CLINICAL APPLICATION

#### Vaccination Protocols 1

Occasionally a client will come into a veterinary clinic and ask to have a pet vaccinated so it can go to the groomer, boarding facility, or daycare facility. Or a client wants some livestock vaccinated so it can be shipped across a border that same day. It is important for clients to understand that although vaccines will protect their animals from disease, the protection is not immediate. Vaccines stimulate the immune system (active immunity), but it takes time, usually about 2 weeks. As veterinary technicians, we need to help educate clients so they can help keep the animals in their care healthy and up to date on vaccines.

that are passed from mother to the fetus through the placenta (transplacentally), or to the neonate via colostrum (the antibody-rich milk the mother produces right before and after birth). Although these antibodies will protect the newborn animal, they do not activate the immune system and memory cells are not produced. Once the antibodies against a specific disease are cleared from the newborn's system it is no longer protected from the disease.

## MECHANISMS OF DISEASE

In a healthy animal, once exposure to a pathogen has occurred, the innate immune system should immediately recognize the pathogen as nonself and begin its attack. Inflammation, phagocytosis, and fever should work together to destroy the pathogen, without regard to its type. Bacterial, viral, and fungal infections elicit similar initial responses from the innate immune system.

## CLINICAL APPLICATION

### Vaccination Protocols 2

Vaccination protocols in young animals are established using the characteristics of both passive and active immunity. The newborn animal likely has some passive immunity from its mother (transplacentally or through colostrum) that will protect it against commonly encountered antigens. As the newborn matures the passively received antibodies are lost and protection must be activated by vaccinations and the active immune system. There is no way to know when the passive immunity disappears so initial vaccinations usually require a series of injections.

For example, most puppies receive their initial vaccination somewhere around 4 to 6 weeks of age. Prior to this time we assume the puppy is protected by passive immunity. When it is about 6 weeks old the puppy must start providing its own antibodies through active immunity. To make sure we are protecting the puppy as best we can we will continue providing vaccines up to about 16 weeks of age.

Most vaccines do not provide lifetime immunity so the animal's immune system must be "boosted" at regular intervals, e.g. annually, every 2 years, or every 3 years.

---

### ✔ TEST YOURSELF 13-4

1. Where are B cells produced? Where do they mature?
2. Where are T cells produced? Where do they mature?
3. Which cell produces antibodies?
4. Describe the three stages of differentiation of lymphocytes.
5. Describe the function of each of the five immunoglobulins. When would the levels of each increase?
6. Describe the three types of T lymphocyte.
7. Describe how vaccines protect patients from disease. Is this an example of active or passive immunity?

---

The adaptive immune system also responds to the pathogen. Although its response is slightly delayed, it is specific to the invading pathogen and is able to target it more directly. Typically, this multifaceted defense system is sufficient to prevent an animal from becoming seriously ill. However, there are cases where the pathogen is too strong or the immune system is too weak and the animal succumbs to disease.

The following factors determine the likelihood of a pathogen causing disease in the animal:

- **Exposure:** The process of a pathogen infecting a host begins with exposure to the pathogen. In order to invade a host, the animal must be exposed to the pathogen. Exposure can occur via a variety of methods including contact with contaminated secretions (aerosolized or nonaerosolized), direct ingestion of the pathogen, or contact via a break in the skin (wound). In all of these cases, there has been a failure of the first and second lines of defense that are designed to prevent the pathogen from gaining entry into the body.
- **Mode of infection/transmission:** Pathogens that use aerosol transmission to move from one animal to another

have an easier time finding and invading the bodies of potential hosts. If, however, transmission requires direct contact with another infected animal, transmission is less likely and the pathogen may have a harder time infecting subsequent hosts.

- **Virulence:** The **virulence** of the pathogen and the degree of **pathogenicity** refer to the relative strength of the pathogen. Some pathogens are weak and are easily destroyed by the immune system. Others are able to resist the protective methods of the immune system and cause illness in the animal.
- **Immune system strength:** The immune systems of young, old, or immunosuppressed animals are usually not functioning at 100% capability. Also, animals fighting a concurrent disease are more susceptible to disease. If an animal's immune system is using its resources to fight one pathogen, there are fewer resources available to fight the second pathogen. This increases the chance that the second pathogen will cause disease.
- **Resistance:** There are various types of resistance that can help an animal remain protected from a particular pathogen. *Acquired resistance* is the most common. It is acquired over an animal's lifetime, either through natural exposure to the pathogen or via vaccination against the pathogen. In both cases, the immune system has been primed, through memory cell production, to fight the pathogen, making subsequent encounters less likely to result in disease. Some animals never develop a disease when exposed to a particular pathogen, even if they have never been vaccinated. These animals have resistance based on their DNA rather than their lifetime exposure. *Species resistance* protects all members of a species from some diseases. For example, dogs do not contract human measles and people do not get sick after exposure to canine parvovirus.

## HYPERSENSITIVITY REACTIONS

The immune system is critical to an animal's survival, but occasionally it malfunctions, resulting in mild health disturbances, major illnesses, or even death. What we recognize as an allergic reaction is actually an overreaction of the immune system. Instead of the usual controlled response, the immune system goes into overdrive. This results in the signs we commonly associate with allergies.

In sensitized animals, allergic reactions can become even more severe, resulting in hypersensitivity reactions, which are classified into four types.

- **Type I reactions** are generally severe and can include anaphylactic shock (urticaria or hives, edema, excess salivation, vomiting, dyspnea, diarrhea, cyanosis, shock, and death). Atopy (atopic dermatitis), flea allergy dermatitis, and food allergies in dogs and cats are examples of type I reactions. In type I reactions, antigens bind to the surface of IgE antibodies on the surfaces of basophils and mast cells rather than IgA, IgG, or IgM. This sensitizes the animal. Once sensitized, a second exposure to the same antigen results in the release of inflammatory chemicals into the bloodstream, which leads to the symptoms often associated with severe allergic reactions and anaphylactic shock. Without immediate medical intervention, these reactions can quickly become fatal.

- **Type II reactions** occur when infection is present, antibodies are being produced, and the complement system is activated. Cross-reactive antibodies form, leading to antibody-mediated cytotoxic reactions (AMCR). This reaction occurs when reactive antibodies bind antigens on the host cell surface and destroy the body's own cells. This leads to diseases where the immune system is the cause of disease rather than the cure. These reactions often involve red blood cells, leading to diseases such as immune mediated hemolytic anemia (IMHA) where the animal's immune system destroys its own red blood cells indiscriminately, causing a life-threatening anemia.
- **Type III reactions** occur when an antibody and an antigen bind and form an immune complex. These immune complexes are insoluble and become trapped in the basement membrane of small blood vessels in tissues, especially joints, kidneys, lungs, brain, and skin. Activation of the complement cascade leads to chemotaxis of a large number of neutrophils and other inflammatory cells and chemicals to the site. This typically produces acute inflammation and damage to affected tissues. Type III reactions are some of the most common immunologic diseases.

Examples include systemic lupus erythematosus, hypersensitivity pneumonitis, and vasculitis.

- **Type IV reactions.** Type IV or cell-mediated reactions occur when antigens trigger helper T cells ($T_H$), which in turn activate cytokines, macrophages, and cytotoxic T cells. Type IV reactions are often caused by intracellular pathogens and are accompanied by inflammation. An example of a Type IV reaction is systemic inflammatory response syndrome (SIRS). SIRS is a form of shock characterized by an exaggerated inflammatory response, usually due to a severe infection or extensive tissue damage. Although most commonly seen during bacterial infections, other pathogens (such as fungi, viruses, and parasites) can all cause SIRS.

---

### ✔ TEST YOURSELF 13-5

1. What three factors influence the ability of a pathogen to cause disease?
2. Describe the three types of resistance that prevent an animal from contracting a disease. Which type of resistance prevents humans from contracting canine distemper?
3. Which hypersensitivity reaction is likely involved in a vaccine reaction?

---

 **CLINICAL APPLICATION**

## Immune Mediated Hemolytic Anemia

Lucy, a 23 lb, 7-year-old female spayed Cocker Spaniel, presented with acute lethargy/weakness, anorexia, exercise intolerance, and hematuria. According to her owner, Lucy was vaccinated 3 weeks prior to the onset of clinical signs. Lucy appeared depressed in the exam room and was quiet, but alert and responsive.

Based on the diagnostic test results the veterinarian diagnosed Lucy with immune mediated hemolytic anemia (IMHA) and autoimmune thrombocytopenia (ITP), likely secondary to vaccination. Lucy was hospitalized and placed on intravenous (IV) fluids, glucocorticoids (to prevent destruction of red blood cells and suppress the overactive immune system), and was given a transfusion of whole blood to treat anemia.

Patients with IMHA and thrombocytopenia may have coagulopathies, which will interfere will blood clotting, so a large vessel like the jugular vein should not be used to draw blood samples. Caution stickers were also placed on Lucy's cage stating "NO JUGULAR BLOOD SAMPLES."

## What Are IMHA and ITP?

Immune mediated hemolytic anemia is a immune malfunction where the body destroys its own red blood cells (RBCs), either by creating antibodies directed at its own RBCs, or by IgG and complement binding to the RBCs marking them for destruction.

There are two types of IMHA, primary and secondary. Primary IMHA occurs when the body creates antibodies directed at its own RBCs. Secondary IMHA occurs when

foreign proteins bind to RBC membranes (e.g., FeLV in cats, vaccines, *Ehrlichia canis* infection, toxins, zinc toxicity, onion toxicity, or heartworm infection).

A diagnosis of IMHA is based on a combination of clinical signs and diagnostic test results. Patients typically present with lethargy, weakness, pale mucous membranes, icterus, hematuria, bruising/petechiae, and possibly vomiting and diarrhea. Examination often shows hepatosplenomegaly, due to removal of increased numbers of destroyed RBCs from circulation.

Icterus is caused by the excess destruction of RBCs, which releases more bilirubin into the bloodstream than the liver can conjugate. This results in the bilirubin being deposited in skin and mucous membranes and giving them a yellow tinge.

Blood tests will show hyperglobulinemia (excessive antibodies in the circulation, indicating an active immune system), hyperbilirubinemia, anemia, reticulocytosis (increase reticulocyte count, indicating regenerative anemia), and the presence of spherocytes (small RBCs lacking an area of central pallor).

Treatment consists of identifying the underlying cause of the IMHA (if any), and treatment with an immunosuppressant drug, such as prednisone, which acts to decrease the activity/sensitivity of the immune system and stop destruction of the RBCs.

ITP is a decreased thrombocyte (platelet) count, which often is seen concurrent with IMHA. The two conditions are often seen together because the same mechanism (destruction of self cells) causes both. When ITP is present, the animal may also have impaired clotting abilities that need to be taken into account when caring for the animal (blood draws, injections, and so on). Treatment for ITP is similar to the treatment for IMHA.

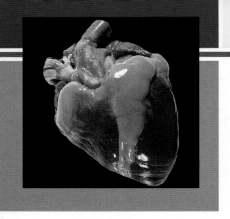

# The Cardiovascular System

*Joann Colville*

## OUTLINE

## LEARNING OBJECTIVES

*When you have completed this chapter you will be able to:*

1. Describe the external and internal anatomy of the heart.
2. Follow the flow of blood through the heart, pulmonary circulation, and systemic circulation.
3. Explain how the heart valves keep blood flowing in the proper direction through the heart.
4. Describe the components of the cardiac conduction system and explain how it works to keep the heart beating in an organized fashion.
5. Explain what happens during one cardiac cycle.

6. Understand cardiac output and what conditions can affect it.
7. Describe the anatomy of arteries, veins, and capillaries and understand the function of each type of blood vessel.
8. Understand the difference between fetal and newborn circulation.
9. Understand the different methods used to evaluate the cardiovascular system.
10. Know the common pulse points and venipuncture sites for common species of animal.

## VOCABULARY FUNDAMENTALS

*Afterload* **ahf**-tər-lōd
*Aorta* ā-**ohr**-tah
*Aortic valve* ā-**ohr**-tihck vahlv
*Apex of heart* ā-**pehcks** *of* hahrt
*Arteriole* ahr-**teer**-ē-ōl
*Artery* **ahr**-tər-ē
*Atrioventricular node* ā-trē-ō-vehn-**trihck**-ū-lahr nōd
*Atrioventricular septum* ā-trē-ō-vehn-**trihck**-ū-lahr **sehp**-tuhm
*Atrioventricular valve* ā-trē-ō-vehn-**trihck**-ū-lahr vahlv
*Atrium* ā-**trē**-uhm
*Auricle* **ohr**-eh-kuhl
*Auscultation* aws-kuhl-**tā**-shuhn

*Autorhythmic* aw-tō-**rihth**-mihck
*Base of heart* bās *of* hahrt
*Bicuspid valve* bī-**kuhs**-pihd vahlv
*Blood pressure* bluhd **prehsh**-ər
*Bundle of His* **buhn**-duhl *of* hihs
*Capillary* **kahp**-eh-lahr-ē
*Cardiac cycle* **kahr**-dē-ahck **sī**-kuhl
*Cardiac output* **kahr**-dē-ahck **out**-puht
*Cardiovascular system* kahr-dē-ō-**vahsk**-ū-lahr **sihs**-tehm
*Carotid artery* kahr-**oht**-ihd **ahr**-tər-ē
*Cephalic vein* seh-**fahl**-ihck vān
*Chordae tendonae* **kohr**-dā **tehn**-duhn-ā
*Coccygeal vein* **kohck**-sehj-ē-ahl vān

*Coronary artery* **kohr**-ah-nār-ē **ahr**-tər-ē
*Coronary sinus* **kohr**-ah-nār-ē **sī**-nuhs
*Coronary vein* **kohr**-ah-nār-ē vān
*Cusp* kuhsp
*Deoxygenated* dē-**ohck**-seh-jeh-**nā**-tehd
*Depolarization* dē-pō-lər-ih-**zā**-shuhn
*Diastole* dī-**ahs**-stō-lē
*Diastolic blood pressure* dī-ah-**stohl**-ihck bluhd **prehsh**-ər
*Doppler echocardiography* **dohp**-lər ehck-ō-kahr-dē-**ohg**-rah-fē
*Ductus arteriosus* **duhck**-tuhs ahr-**teer**-ē-ō-suhs
*ECHO* **ehck**-ō
*Echocardiography* ehck-ō-kahr-dē-**ohg**-rah-fē
*Elastic artery* eh-**lahs**-tihck **ahr**-tər-ē
*Electrocardiogram* ē-**lehck**-trō-**kahr**-dē-ō-grahm
*Electrocardiography* ē-**lehck**-trō-kahr-dē-**ohg**-rah-fē
*Endocardium* ehn-dō-**kahr**-dē-uhm
*Endothelium* ehn-dō-**thē**-lē-uhm
*Epicardium* ehp-ih-**kahr**-dē-uhm
*Femoral vein* fehm-**ohr**-ahl vān
*Foramen ovale* fohr-**ā**-mehn ō-**vah**-lē
*Heart rate* hahrt rāt
*Interatrial septum* ihn-tər-**ā**-trē-uhl **sehp**-tuhm
*Interventricular groove* ihn-tər-vehn-**trihck**-ū-lər groov
*Interventricular septum* ihn-tər-vehn-**trihck**-ū-lər **sehp**-tuhm
*Jugular vein* **juhg**-ū-lər vān
*Mean arterial pressure* mēn ahr-**teer**-ē-ahl **prehsh**-ər
*Mediastinum* mē-dē-ah-**stīn**-uhm
*Mitral valve* **mī**-trah vahlv
*Murmur* **mər**-mər
*Muscular artery* **muhs**-kyoo-lər **ahr**-tər-ē
*Myocardium* mī-ō-**kahr**-dē-uhm
*Oscillometric* aws-uh-lō-**meh**-trihck
*Oxygenated* **ohck**-suh-jehn-**ā**-tehd
*P wave* P wāv
*Papillary muscle* pah-pihl-**leər**-ē **muhs**-uhl
*Parietal layer of the serous pericardium* pah-**rī**-eh-tahl **lā**-ər *of the* **seer**-uhs peər-ih-**kahr**-dē-uhm

*Pericardial fluid* peər-ih-**kahr**-dē-ahl **floo**-ihd
*Pericardial sac* peər-ih-**kahr**-dē-ahl sahck
*Pericardial space* peər-ih-**kahr**-dē-ahl spās
*Pericardium* peər-ih-**kahr**-dē-uhm
*Polarization* pōl-ər-ih-**zā**-shuhn
*Preload* **prē**-lōd
*Pulmonary artery* puhl-muh-**neər**-ē **ahr**-tər-ē
*Pulmonary circulation* puhl-muh-**neər**-ē sər-kyoo-**lā**-shuhn
*Pulmonary valve* puhl-muh-**neər**-ē vahlv
*Pulse* puhls
*Pulse wave* puhls wāv
*Purkinje fiber system* pər-**kihn**-jē **fī**-bər **sihs**-tehm
*QRS complex* Q-R-S **kohm**-plehkx
*Repolarize* rē-**pō**-lər-īz
*Saphenous vein* **sahf**-uh-nuhs vān
*Semilunar valve* seh-mē-**lū**-nər vahlv
*Serous pericardium* **seer**-uhs peər-ih-**kahr**-dē-uhm
*Sinoatrial node* **sī**-nō-**ā**-trē-ahl nōd
*Sphygmomanometer* sfihg-mō-muh-**nohm**-uht-ər
*Starling's law* **stahr**-lihngz lahw
*Stroke volume* strōk **vohl**-ūm
*Systemic circulation* sihs-**tehm**-ihck sər-kyoo-**lā**-shuhn
*Systole* **sihs**-tuh-lē
*Systolic blood pressure* sih-**stohl**-ihck bluhd **prehsh**-ər
*Systolic discharge* sih-**stohl**-ihck dihs-**chahrj**
*T wave* T wāv
*Tricuspid valve* trī-**kuhs**-pihd valv
*Umbilical artery* uhm-**bihl**-ihck-ahl **ahr**-tər-ē
*Umbilical vein* uhm-**bihl**-ihck-ahl vān
*Valvular insufficiency* vahl-vyoo-lər ihn-suh-**fihsh**-ehn-sē
*Valvular stenosis* vahl-vyoo-lər steh-**nō**-sihs
*Vein* vān
*Vena cava* vē-nah **kā**-vah
*Ventricle* vehn-**trihck**-ehl
*Venule* **vehn**-yool
*Visceral layer of the serous pericardium* vih-sər-ahl **lā**-ər *of the* **seer**-uhs peər-ih-**kahr**-dē-uhm

## INTRODUCTION

Imagine the world blood lives in. Think of it as a water world. The plasma is the fluid all the elements live and swim in. The outer limits of this world are the walls of the blood vessels where blood resides. The **erythrocytes** (red blood cells) are the planes, trains, and automobiles that move oxygen and other substances from place to place. The **leukocytes** (white blood cells) are the military vehicles ready for battle at a moment's notice. The thrombocytes (platelets) are the EMTs, the first responders to the scene of a vessel wall injury.

So far this is a static world; nothing is moving. Enter the heart. Each time the heart beats blood is propelled through blood vessels throughout the animal's body. This is the world of the **cardiovascular system** (i.e., the circulatory system). It is responsible for the movement of blood and everything it carries throughout the animal's body. It is made up of the heart, all the blood vessels, and the blood itself. Normally there are no external openings to the cardiovascular system so it is considered a closed system. Electrolytes, waste materials, nutrients, hormones, antibodies, and drugs are carried by blood contained in the structures of the cardiovascular system to every living cell in the animal's body.

Blood is continuously flowing around the animal's body and through the heart in a circuit propelled by the beating (pumping) heart. **Arteries** carry blood away from the heart; **veins** carry blood toward the heart; and **capillaries** form the transition between arteries and veins.

The cardiovascular system is divided into two parts that all blood cycles through in a "figure 8" configuration: the **pulmonary (lung) circulation** and the **systemic (body) circulation**. One side of the heart controls each part. The right side of the heart controls the pulmonary circulation. It receives **deoxygenated** blood from throughout the animal's body (carried in veins) and pumps it into the lungs where it becomes oxygenated. The left side of the heart controls the systemic circulation. It receives **oxygenated** blood from the lungs and pumps it out to the rest of the animal's body. More on this later.

## THE HEART

### LOCATION

The heart is located in the middle of the thoracic cavity in the **mediastinum**, the space between the two lungs (Figure 14-1). The mediastinum in bounded by the thoracic inlet crainially, the diaphragm caudally, the sternum ventrally, and the spinal column dorsally. In addition to the heart, the mediastinum also contains blood vessels, the thoracic portion of the trachea, the esophagus, the thymus in young animals, lymph nodes, and nerves.

Generally speaking, when viewing a standing animal the heart is located between the elbows (Figure 14-2).

### SIZE AND SHAPE

The heart is sort of heart-shaped (Figure 14-3). It has a rounded cranial end called the **base of the heart**. The more pointed caudal end is the **apex of the heart**. This is just the opposite of what we normally think of base (wide bottom) and apex (narrow top) but if you go strictly by shape and forget orientation the wide end is the base and the narrow end is the apex.

The heart doesn't sit straight along the median plane in an animal. The base is shifted to the right and faces more dorsally. The apex is shifted to the left and sits more ventrally (Figure 14-4).

## COVERINGS OF THE HEART

The heart is contained in a fibrous sac called the **pericardium**. The pericardium is divided into two parts: the fibrous sac called the **pericardial sac** and the **serous pericardium**. The pericardial sac is a little loose so the heart can beat inside it but it is not elastic so it cannot stretch if the heart becomes abnormally enlarged.

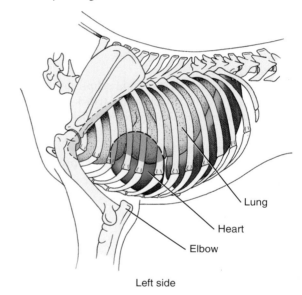

Lung

Heart

Elbow

Left side

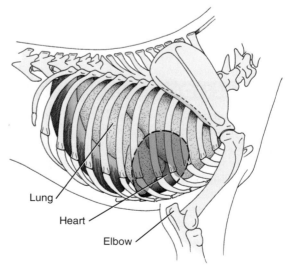

Lung

Heart

Elbow

Right side

**FIGURE 14-2** Location of the heart between the elbows in a standing animal. (Redrawn from Dyce KM, Sack WO, Wenseng CJG: Textbook of veterinary anatomy, ed 4, St Louis, 2010, Saunders.)

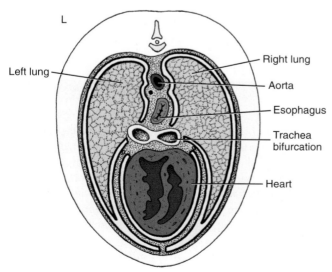

L

Left lung

Right lung

Aorta

Esophagus

Trachea bifurcation

Heart

**FIGURE 14-1** Transverse section through the thorax at the level of the heart showing structures in the mediastinum. (Redrawn from Dyce KM, Sack WO, Wenseng CJG: Textbook of veterinary anatomy, ed 4, St Louis, 2010, Saunders.)

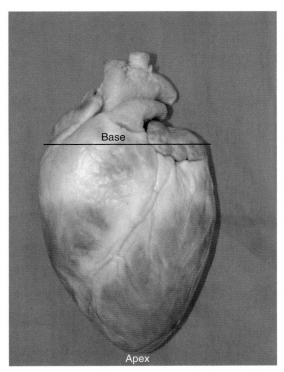

**FIGURE 14-3** Shape of the heart showing the base and the apex.

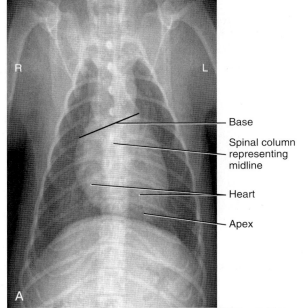

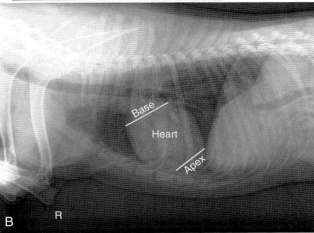

**FIGURE 14-4** Radiograph showing the position of the heart in the thoracic cavity. **A,** ventral view; **B,** lateral view. (**A,** From Evans H, Lahunta A: Miller's Anatomy of the Dog, ed 4, St Louis, Saunders. **B,** From Brown M, Brown: Lavin's Radiography for Veterinary Technicians, ed 5, St Louis, 2014, Saunders.)

The serous pericardium consists of two membranes. A smooth, moist serous membrane called the **parietal layer** of the serous pericardium lines the pericardial sac, and the **visceral layer** of the serous pericardium lies directly on the surface of the heart. The **pericardial space** is the area between the two serous membranes. It is filled with **pericardial fluid** that lubricates the two membranes and prevents friction as they rub together during contractions and relaxations of the heart muscle (Figure 14-5).

## WALL OF THE HEART

The wall of the heart has three layers (Figure 14-6). The middle and thickest layer is the muscular layer called the **myocardium** because it is made up of cardiac muscle. Remember that cardiac muscle fibers are joined side-to-side by multiple branches and end-to-end by intercalated discs. These two anatomic characteristics mean that the myocardium is made up of continuous muscle sheets that wrap around the chambers of the heart. These muscle sheets make a greater force of contraction possible.

Two other advantageous characteristics of cardiac muscle are that it is **autorhythmic** and it doesn't fatigue. This means that without outside stimulus it can start beating (contracting and relaxing) in a steady rhythm before an animal is born and continue beating through birth, adolescence, adulthood, middle age, and old age without taking a break. When the heart stops beating and it isn't restarted the animal dies.

The **epicardium** is the outermost layer of the heart wall. It is a membrane that lies on the external surface of the myocardium. Sound familiar? Another name for the epicardium is the visceral layer of the serous pericardium. Two names; same membrane.

The **endocardium** is the membrane that lies on the internal surface of the myocardium. It is composed of thin, flat simple squamous epithelium and forms the lining of the heart chambers. The endocardium is continuous with the endothelium that lines blood vessels. The endocardium also covers the valves that separate the chambers of the heart.

The inside surface of the myocardium is not smooth. It forms ridges and nipplelike projections called **papillary muscles** that are covered by the endocardium.

## CHAMBERS OF THE HEART

There are four chambers or cavities in the heart: two **atria** (singular: **atrium**) that receive blood into the heart, and two **ventricles** that pump blood out of the heart (Figure 14-7). The

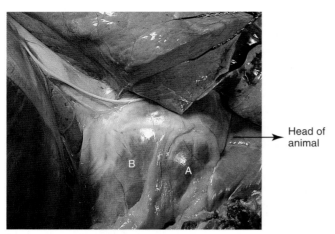

**FIGURE 14-5** The heart enclosed in the pericardium. **A,** The wall of the right ventricle visible through the pericardium; **B,** the wall of the left ventricle visible through the pericardium. The heart is sitting in the area of the mediastinum. (Modified from Clayton HM, Flood P, Rosenstein D: Clinical anatomy of the horse, London 2005, Mosby Ltd.)

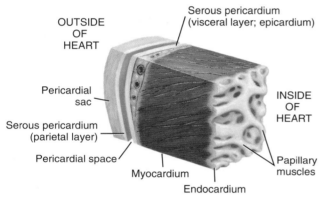

**FIGURE 14-6** Section of the wall of the heart showing the pericardial sac, the parietal and visceral layers of the serous pericardium, the pericardial space, the myocardium, and the endocardium. (Modified from Huether SE, McCance KL: Understanding pathophysiology, ed 4, St Louis, 2007, Mosby.)

---

✔ **TEST YOURSELF 14-1**

1. Which type of blood vessel carries blood away from the heart? Toward the heart?
2. What are the two parts of the cardiovascular system? Which part carries blood to and from the left rear leg of a pony?
3. List three structures found in the mediastinum.
4. Which is located more caudally in a standing pig, the apex or the base of the heart?
5. What is the difference between the endocardium and the pericardium?

---

two atria sit on top of the two ventricles and their walls form part of the base of the heart. The two ventricles sit below the two atria and the wall of the left ventricle forms the apex of the heart.

## ATRIA

The left atrium and the right atrium are separated by the **interatrial septum** that is a continuation of the myocardium. The atria receive blood from large veins that carry

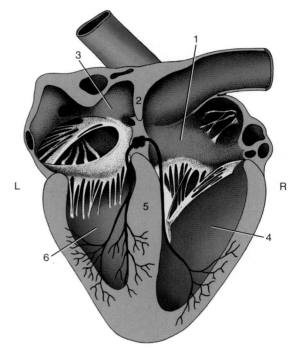

**FIGURE 14-7** Section of the heart exposing the four chambers. **1,** Right atrium; **2,** interatrial septum; **3,** left atrium; **4,** right ventricle; **5,** interventricular septum; **6,** left ventricle. (Modified from Dyce KM, Sack WO, Wenseng CJG: Textbook of veterinary anatomy, ed 4, St Louis, 2010, Saunders.)

blood to the heart. When the atria have filled with blood their walls (composed of myocardium) contract and force blood through one-way valves into the ventricles.

The atria are identified on the outside of the heart by their **auricles.** These are blind pouches that come off the main part of the atria and look like earflaps.

**_That's Interesting:_** Auricle means "ear flap" or "ear." In humans the auricle also refers to the external ear flap. Since the atrial auricle looks somewhat like an earflap it seems to make sense to name it accordingly.

The auricle is part of the atrium but is not the entire atrium so the two terms cannot be used interchangeably.

The myocardium of an atrium is not very thick because it only has to contract with enough force to move blood into a ventricle. The same is not true for the walls of the ventricles.

## VENTRICLES

The left and right ventricles are separated by the **interventricular septum**, which is a continuation of the interatrial septum. Together they form the **atrioventricular septum**. The area of the interventricular septum is visible on the outside of the heart as the **interventricular** groove (Figure 14-8). The groove contains **coronary** (heart) blood vessels and is frequently filled with fat. When the ventricles have received blood from the atria the myocardium of the ventricular walls contract and force blood through one-way valves into arteries. The right ventricle pumps blood to the pulmonary circulation through the **pulmonary artery;** the left ventricle pumps blood into the systemic circulation through the **aorta.** Since blood from the right ventricle doesn't have very far to go the right ventricular wall is thinner than the left ventricular wall. The left ventricular wall has the most work to do pumping blood to the rest of the animal's body so it has a thicker wall that will contract with greater force. In fact the left ventricular wall is so thick that it pushes the right ventricular wall to the right. Consequently the left ventricular wall makes up the apex of the heart (Figure 14-9).

## VALVES OF THE HEART

There are four one-way valves that control blood flow through the heart (Figure 14-10). Two of the valves are located between the right and left atria and their respective ventricles. The other two are located between the right and left ventricles and the arteries they eject blood into. The valves close at specific times to prevent backflow of blood into the chamber it just

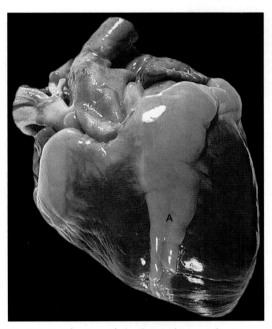

**FIGURE 14-8** Left view of the heart showing the interventricular groove filled with fat. (Modified from Clayton HM, Flood P, Rosenstein D: Clinical anatomy of the horse, London 2005, Mosby Ltd.)

came from. In order for the heart to function properly blood must flow through it in one direction only.

The **atrioventricular valves** (**AV valves**) are located between the atria and the ventricles. The right AV valve consists of three flaps or **cusps** of endothelium and is called the **tricuspid valve**. It opens when the pressure from the amount of blood in the right atrium forces it open and allows blood to flow into the right ventricle. When the pressure from the blood in the right ventricle exceeds the pressure of blood in the right atrium the tricuspid valve is forced to snap shut. The valve is prevented from opening backward into the atrium by collagen fiber cords that are attached to the edge of each cusp and to papillary muscles in the wall of the right ventricle. These cords are called the **chordae tendonae** (Figure 14-11).

The left AV valve has only two cusps and is called the **bicuspid valve**. It is also known as the **mitral valve** because of its resemblance to the headgear, called the miter, worn by Roman Catholic bishops. This valve also has attached chordae tendonae.

The two valves that control blood flow out of the ventricles and into arteries are the **semilunar valves**, so named because they have three cusps, each of which resembles a crescent moon. The right semilunar valve is the **pulmonary valve** because blood from the right ventricle flows through it into the pulmonary circulation. The left semilunar valve is the **aortic valve** because blood from the left ventricle flows through it into the aorta, which is the major artery that is the beginning of systemic circulation.

## SKELETON OF THE HEART

The skeleton of the heart is located between the atria and the ventricles (Figure 14-12). It is made up of four dense fibrous connective tissue rings and has four primary functions:
- It separates the atria and ventricles.
- It anchors the heart valves.
- It provides a point of attachment for the myocardium.
- It provides some electrical insulation between the atria and the ventricles.

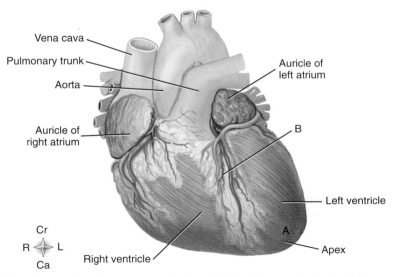

**FIGURE 14-9** Ventral view of the heart showing **A**, the wall of the left ventricle forming the apex of the heart and **B**, the interventricular groove. (Modified from Brown M, Brown L: Lavin's Radiography for veterinary technicians, ed 5, St Louis, 2014, Saunders.)

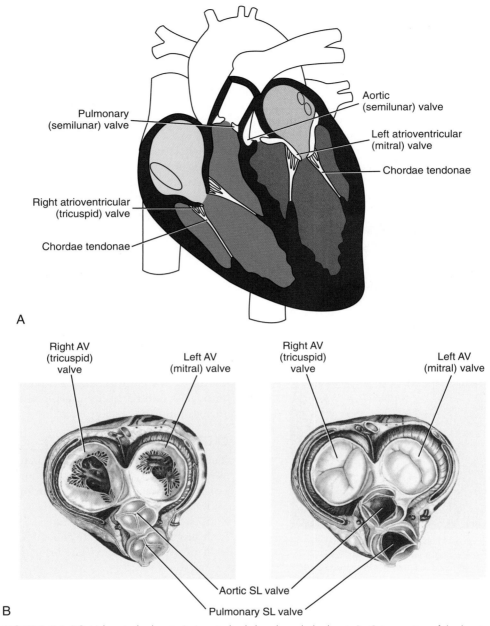

**FIGURE 14-10** Valves in the heart. **A,** Longitudinal slice through the heart. **B,** Cross section of the heart. *AV,* Atrioventricular; *SL,* semilunar. (**B,** From Thibodeau D: Structure and function of the body, ed 14, St Louis, 2012, Mosby.)

## BLOOD SUPPLY TO THE HEART

Like any living tissue, the cells of the heart need nourishment and oxygen brought to them and waste materials carried away. **Coronary arteries** and **coronary veins** are responsible for these functions (Figure 14-13). Coronary arteries branch off the aorta just past the aortic valve (left semilunar valve). They continue to branch around the heart until they completely encircle it. The left ventricle gets the largest blood supply because it has the most work to do pumping blood through the systemic circulation. After the blood from the coronary arteries has passed through the capillaries in the myocardium it enters the coronary veins. To return the

blood to the circulation the coronary veins join together near the right atrium and form a channel called the **coronary sinus** that drains directly into the right atrium.

## NERVE SUPPLY TO THE HEART

Cardiac muscle is autorythmic and can create its own contractions and relaxations through its internal conduction system. But there are times when the heart needs to beat faster to increase the oxygen supply to certain tissues. For example, an animal being exercised needs an increased oxygen supply to its muscles. To help accommodate this increased oxygen demand the heart receives some external

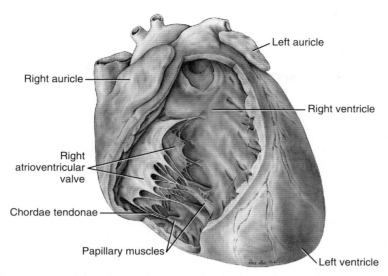

Left auricle

Right auricle

Right ventricle

Right atrioventricular valve

Chordae tendonae

Papillary muscles

Left ventricle

**FIGURE 14-11** Interior view of the right ventricle showing the chordae tendonae of the right AV (tricuspid) valve. Only two cusps of the valve are visible. (Modified from Evans H, Lahunta A: Miller's anatomy of the dog, ed 4, St Louis, 2013, Saunders.)

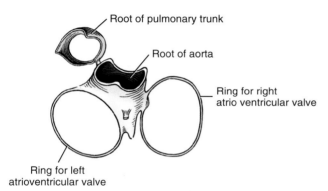

Root of pulmonary trunk

Root of aorta

Ring for right atrio ventricular valve

Ring for left atrioventricular valve

**FIGURE 14-12** Skeleton of the heart. (Modified from Evans H, Lahunta A: Miller's anatomy of the dog, ed 4, St Louis, 2013, Saunders.)

motor stimulation. The nerve fibers enter the heart and terminate primarily in the right atrium near the area of cardiac muscle cells that is the control center for the cardiac conduction system. Some nerve fibers will stimulate an increased heart rate and others will stimulate a decreased heart rate. The nervous system is discussed in detail in Chapter 9. The nerve supply to the heart serves a purpose, but is not essential. Transplanted hearts lose their nerve supply and usually continue to function well.

 **TEST YOURSELF 14-2**

1. Which sits closer to the base of the heart, the left atrium or the right ventricle?
2. What is the name of the structure that is a continuation of the myocardium that forms a wall between the two atria? The two ventricles?
3. Why is the wall of the right ventricle thinner than the wall of the left ventricle?
4. What is another name for each of these valves: right AV valve, semilunar valve in the right ventricle, left AV valve, semilunar valve in the left ventricle?
5. What is the function of the chordae tendonae?

## CLINICAL APPLICATION

### Hardware Disease

In cattle, the **reticulum** (the most cranial stomach compartment) rests directly behind the heart, and the two organs are separated by the muscular diaphragm. Cattle are not very selective when eating, and it is not uncommon for them to ingest wires, nails, and other foreign metallic objects along with their feed. These bits of "hardware" are ingested into the rumen, from which digestive contractions move them forward into the reticulum. Continued ruminal contractions, particularly when combined with factors that increase abdominal pressure, such as pregnancy and parturition, may push pieces of wire through the cranial wall of the reticulum. Puncture of the reticulum wall by a foreign object often results in traumatic **reticuloperitonitis**, also called **hardware disease**, which is an inflammation and infection of the reticulum and abdominal cavity. More severe disease occurs when a wire is pushed even farther cranially, through the diaphragm and into the pericardium. This can result in **septic pericarditis**, which is an infection of the pericardium that usually progresses to heart failure and death.

Hardware disease can be prevented by the oral administration of a magnet about the size of a 5 ml blood tube. The magnet stays in the rumen or reticulum, usually for the rest of the animal's life. Wire or other metal objects ingested by the animal stick to the magnet instead of being pushed cranially through the wall of the reticulum and beyond.

## BLOOD FLOW THROUGH THE HEART

You've read about heart chambers, one-way valves, and unidirectional blood flow so now it's time to follow the blood as it moves through the heart. The entire purpose of the heart is to receive deoxygenated blood from the systemic circulation (right atrium), send it out to the pulmonary circulation for oxygenation (right ventricle), receive the freshly oxygenated blood back from the pulmonary

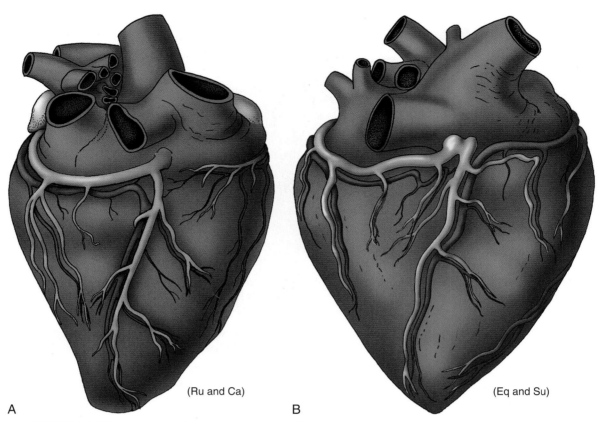

**FIGURE 14-13** Coronary circulation of the heart viewed from the right. **A,** Ruminants and carnivores, **B,** horse and pig. *Ru,* Ruminants; *Ca,* cat; *Eq,* equine; *Su,* pig. Red blood vessels, coronary arteries; blue blood vessels, coronary veins. (Modified from Dyce KM, Sack WO, Wenseng CJG: Textbook of veterinary anatomy, ed 4, St Louis, 2010, Saunders.)

 **CLINICAL APPLICATION**

### Pericardial Effusion and Cardiac Tamponade

The heart is able to expand and contract in the chest thanks to the layer of fluid that provides lubrication between layers of the serous pericardium. Normally, only a small amount of fluid is contained within the pericardial sac. A number of conditions such as infection, inflammation, or hemorrhage may cause excess fluid to accumulate in the pericardial sac. This condition is called *pericardial effusion.* Sometimes pericardial effusion is idiopathic, meaning it may occur spontaneously with no known cause.

The outer layer of the heart, called the *fibrous pericardium,* is not elastic, so when the pericardial space is overfilled with fluid, the heart becomes unable to expand normally between contractions. This condition, called **cardiac tamponade,** leads to less complete cardiac filling, decreased stroke volume, and decreased cardiac output. Pericardial effusion, with or without cardiac tamponade, may be treated by inserting a needle into the pericardial sac (usually through the chest wall) and withdrawing the excess fluid.

heart sits in the middle pumping blood through both loops (Figure 14-15).

We'll arbitrarily start our journey through the heart in the **vena cava,** the large vein that brings deoxygenated blood from the systemic circulation (but not the pulmonary circulation) to the heart. The vena cava enters the right atrium of the heart. The deoxygenated blood passes from the right atrium through the tricuspid valve into the right ventricle. At this point the pulmonary valve in the right ventricle is closed. When the right ventricle is full the tricuspid valve is forced closed and the pulmonary valve is forced open. The right ventricle contracts and the deoxygenated blood leaves the right ventricle through the pulmonary valve and enters the pulmonary circulation via the pulmonary artery. After the deoxygenated blood has been oxygenated in the pulmonary circulation it comes back to the heart via the pulmonary vein that empties into the left atrium. The mitral valve opens and the blood from the left atrium enters the left ventricle. When the ventricle is full the mitral valve is forced closed and the aortic valve is forced open. The left ventricle contracts and oxygenated blood leaves through the aortic valve and enters the systemic circulation via the aorta, the largest artery in the body. Once in the systemic circulation the blood is distributed throughout the animal's body through arteries that become progressively smaller until they transition to become capillaries. At the tissue capillary level, blood gives up its oxygen in exchange for carbon dioxide and

circulation (left atrium), and put it into systemic circulation (left ventricle) (Figure 14-14). Note that each chamber has its own specific function. Think of blood flow as a figure 8. One loop represents the pulmonary circulation, the other loop represents the systemic circulation, and the

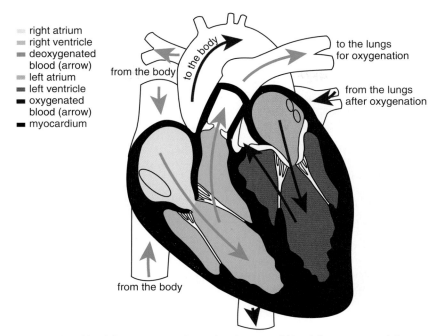

right atrium
right ventricle
deoxygenated blood (arrow)
left atrium
left ventricle
oxygenated blood (arrow)
myocardium

to the body

from the body

to the lungs for oxygenation

from the lungs after oxygenation

from the body

**FIGURE 14-14** Cardiac blood flow. Arrows indicate the direction of blood flow. (From Colvile J, Oien S: Clinical veterinary language, St Louis, 2014, Mosby.)

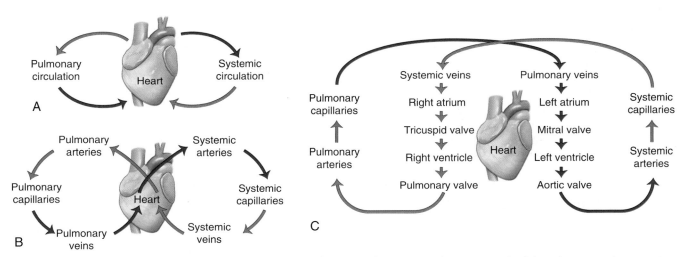

Pulmonary circulation      Heart      Systemic circulation

**A**

Pulmonary arteries      Systemic arteries

Pulmonary capillaries      Heart      Systemic capillaries

Pulmonary veins      Systemic veins

**B**

Pulmonary capillaries

Pulmonary arteries

Systemic veins      Pulmonary veins

Right atrium      Left atrium

Tricuspid valve      Mitral valve

Right ventricle      Heart      Left ventricle

Pulmonary valve      Aortic valve

Systemic capillaries

Systemic arteries

**C**

**FIGURE 14-15** Schematics of the circulation. **A,** Pulmonary and systemic circulation, **B,** vessels of the pulmonary and systemic circulation, **C,** blood flow through the heart plus the pulmonary and systemic circulation.

other waste materials in tissue fluid. From this tissue level the capillaries converge to form small veins that become progressively larger as the deoxygenated blood is carried back to the heart. The veins eventually join the vena cava and the deoxygenated blood flows into the right atrium. The cycle is complete.

To make sure blood is entering and leaving the heart in an orderly, coordinated fashion, the heart has to have rhythmic, coordinated contractions. The actual rhythm pattern is simple. Even though the two sides of the heart pump blood to different areas they do so at the same time: deoxygenated blood enters the right atrium and oxygenated blood enters the left atrium at the same time; the tricuspid and mitral

valves open and close at the same time; the right and left ventricles contract at the same time, and so forth. When the ventricles are full the pressure from the blood in them forces the AV valves closed and the semilunar valves open. When the pressure in the pulmonary artery (right side) and aorta (left side) exceeds the pressure in the right and left ventricles the semilunar valves are forced close. At this point the pressure in the atria exceeds the pressure in the ventricles so the AV valves open and ventricular filling begins again. To keep blood flowing, the ventricles are emptying while the atria are filling and the atria are emptying while the ventricles are filling. The valves closing produce sounds that can be heard with a stethoscope: the heartbeat.

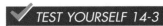

1. List, in order, the structures an erythrocyte will pass through (including valves) to move in a complete circuit from the left ventricle back to the left ventricle.

## CLINICAL APPLICATION

### Defibrillation

If you've watched a few hospital shows on television, chances are you've seen someone grab a couple of paddles, yell "clear" or something like it, place the paddles on the patient's chest, and "shock" them to restart the heart. In real life, this process is called **defibrillation**, and it has to do with the electrical conduction system of the heart.

Sometimes a diseased heart will develop one or more *ectopic pacemakers*. The word *ectopic* means *out of place*, and an ectopic pacemaker is located outside the heart's normal pacemaker, which is the sinoatrial (SA) node in the right atrium. Despite the presence of any ectopic pacemakers, the SA node continues to fire, meaning that the cardiac muscle cells receive electric currents from more than one direction. The synchronized contraction of the heart, which begins in the atria and flows through the ventricles, is lost. If there is enough ectopic pacemaker activity, a condition called *ventricular fibrillation* may develop, in which heart muscle cells in different areas contract independently of one another. In ventricular fibrillation, all coordinated pumping activity of the ventricles is lost.

The defibrillator sends a large electric current of short duration through the heart, with the objective of repolarizing all of the cells at the same time. If defibrillation is successful, the SA node and the heart's normal conduction system will resume control over depolarization of the heart after the cells have been "reset" by defibrillation.

## CARDIAC CONDUCTION SYSTEM

Even though cardiac muscle is autorhythmic it does need some sort of control to keep it beating at a steady rate. Areas of cardiac muscle cells have developed that initiate an impulse that moves through the myocardium, stimulating first the muscle cells in the walls of the atria to contract, then moving through the walls of the ventricles to cause them to contract. After each contraction the muscle cells relax. One cycle of atrial and ventricular contraction and relaxation is a **cardiac cycle**. The cardiac cycle produces one heartbeat.

The impulse for each heartbeat comes from the **sinoatrial node** (**SA node**) located in the wall of the right atrium. It is the pacemaker of the heart. The SA node is an area of cardiac muscle cells that automatically generate the impulses that trigger each heartbeat.

At rest, a cardiac muscle cell is polarized. Sodium and calcium ions are located on the outer membrane of the cell and potassium ions are located inside the cell. In order for the cell to contract it must depolarize. During cardiac muscle cell **depolarization** (Figure 14-16) two sets of events occur.

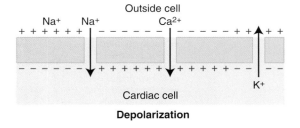

**Depolarization**

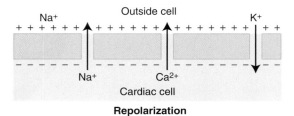

**Repolarization**

**FIGURE 14-16** Depolarization and repolarization of a cardiac muscle cell. (From Wanamaker BP: Applied pharmacology for veterinary techinicians, ed 4, St Louis, 2008, Saunders.)

First, sodium ($Na^+$) and calcium ($Ca^{2+}$) ions move through channels in the cell membrane from the exterior to the interior of the cell. This reverses the polarity of the cell membrane. Second, potassium ($K^+$) ions move through channels in the cell membrane from the interior of the cell to the exterior. This restores the original polarity, but now the $Na^+$, $Ca^{2+}$, and $K^+$ ions are on the wrong sides of the cell membrane. During **repolarization** the ions are pumped back to their original locations and the cell is ready to depolarize again. In this way, the heart automatically keeps going through the cardiac cycle of cellular depolarization (contraction) and repolarization (relaxation).

The impulse generated by the SA node travels from the base of the heart to the apex and back to the base of the heart. The impulse passes through the muscle fibers of the wall of the atria. When the impulse passes through these cardiac muscles, the muscles contract. Remember, unlike other muscle fibers, cardiac muscle can transmit an impulse from one muscle cell to another, so impulses and the resulting muscle contractions spread across the atria in a wavelike fashion.

The structures that make up the primary cardiac conduction system are the SA node, the **atrioventricular node** (**AV node**), the **bundle of His**, and the **Purkinje fiber system** (Figure 14-17).

As stated above, after the impulse is initiated in the SA node in the right atrium, it spreads in a wave across both atria, causing them to contract and push blood through the AV valves into the ventricles, which are still relaxed. The impulse generated by the SA node travels through the walls of the atria to the atrioventricular node located in the atrioventricular septum that separates the left and right sides of the heart. The only route of conduction the impulse can take from the atria to the ventricles is through the AV node. When the impulse from the SA node reaches the AV node it delays

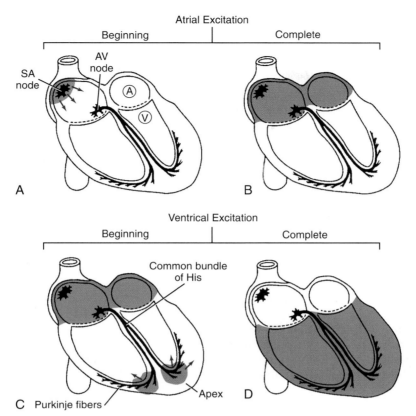

**FIGURE 14-17** Cardiac conduction system. **A,** The SA node has initiated an impulse; **B,** the impulse has spread through the walls of both atria and reached the AV node (atrial depolarization); **C,** the impulse has traveled down the interventricular septum through the bundle of His, and the Purkinje fiber system has initiated ventricular contraction beginning at the apex, **D,** the impulse has spread through the walls of both ventricles (ventricular depolarization). (From Cunningham JG: Textbook of veterinary physiology, ed 4, St Louis, 2007, Saunders.)

for a fraction of a second. The delay permits the atria to complete their contraction before ventricular contraction begins. If atrial and ventricular contraction took place at the same time, the pressure in the contracting ventricles would be so high that the weaker, thin-muscled atria could not push blood into the ventricles.

After the delay at the AV node, the impulse resumes its speedy journey, this time through the bundle of His and the Purkinje fiber system. The fibers of the bundle of His travel down the interventricular septum to the apex of the heart. Here the Purkinje fiber system picks up the impulses, makes a U-turn, and carries them from the bundle of His up into the right and left ventricular myocardium. Because the impulse is delivered to the apex more quickly than it can spread from cell to cell in the ventricular myocardium, the ventricles actually contract starting from the apex and moving toward the base of the heart. This apex-to-base direction of ventricular contraction facilitates ejection of blood into the aorta and pulmonary arteries, which are located at the base of the heart (Box 14-1).

Just as the atria begin their contractions while the ventricles are relaxed, the atria also enter their relaxation phase while the ventricles are contracting. When the ventricles are contracting but the atria are relaxed, the pressure in the ventricles is much higher than the pressure in the atria, so

**BOX 14-1 | Try This At Home**

As mentioned in the text the two atria contract while the two ventricles relax and vice versa. To get a better sense of how this works make a fist with both hands. Put your right fist representing the atria on top of your left fist representing the two ventricles. First squeeze your right fist in a rolling movement starting with your thumb and forefinger and going down. This represents the systolic wave of the atria, which begins at the cardiac base and moves to the atrioventricular septum. Now as you relax your right fist (atrial diastole) squeeze your left fist (ventricular systole) in a rolling movement starting with your little finger and moving up. The systolic wave through the ventricle starts at the cardiac apex with the Purkinje fiber system (i.e., your pinkie finger), and moves toward the base (i.e., your thumb). Relax your left fist and squeeze your right fist again. Each time you go through one squeeze and relaxation of each fist you have completed a cardiac cycle. Once you have mastered the squeezing and relaxing sequence, try and set up a rhythm of contractions of one "cardiac cycle" per second. This represents a heart rate of 60 beats per minute (bpm).

the AV valves are forced shut. With the AV valves closed, the relaxed and expanding atria can fill with blood again. At about the time the atria are becoming completely full, contraction comes to an end in the ventricles, and they begin to relax. This results in the pressure in the ventricles dropping lower than the pressure in the arteries they supply, so the aortic and pulmonary valves are forced shut. Pressure in the ventricles also falls below the pressure in the full atria, so the AV valves are pushed open.

After the AV valves open, the ventricles again fill with blood from the atria. The negative pressure caused by ventricular relaxation pulling blood in from the atria generates most ventricular filling. Just as the pressure in the atria and the ventricles begins to reach equilibrium, the SA node "fires," causing the atria to contract and forcibly push the rest of their blood into the ventricles, and the cardiac cycle begins again.

There are two clinical terms associated with contraction and relaxation of cardiac muscles. **Systole** is the myocardium contracting, causing a chamber to empty itself of blood. This is the working phase of the cardiac cycle when the cardiac muscle cells are depolarized. **Diastole** is the myocardium relaxing and repolarizing after a contraction, allowing the chambers to fill with blood again. This is the resting phase of the cardiac cycle.

Each chamber goes through systole and diastole, but not all at the same time. In one cardiac cycle first the atria contract (atrial systole) while the ventricles are relaxed (ventricular diastole). This allows blood to flow from the atria into the ventricles. Next the ventricles contract (ventricular

systole) while the atria are relaxed (atrial diastole). This allows the ventricles to eject blood from the heart and for the atria to fill with blood again.

## NORMAL HEART SOUNDS

If you've had a chance to listen to a heart with a stethoscope you know it makes sounds as it beats. The heart valves snapping shut produce these sounds. One cardiac cycle produces two distinct heart sounds (Box 14-2). The sounds are often described as "lub" and "dub." The first sound, "lub," is produced when the tricuspid and mitral valves snap shut after atrial systole. The pressure in the ventricles is greater than the pressure in the atria at this point so the AV valves are forced closed. Remember these are one-way valves so blood cannot backflow into the atria.

The second heart sound, "dub," is produced after ventricular systole when the pulmonary and aortic valves (semilunar valves) snap shut. The pressure in the pulmonary artery and aorta exceeds that in the ventricles at this point so the valves are forced closed. These are also one-way valves so blood cannot backflow into the ventricles. Most heart sounds are best heard on the left side of the standing animal by placing the stethoscope on the chest wall at about the point of the elbow. From this point, by moving slightly forward and backward, the pulmonary, aortic, and mitral valve sounds are heard. The tricuspid valve sound is best heard on the left side of the standing animal at approximately the same level (Figure 14-18).

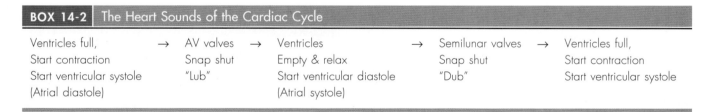

| BOX 14-2 | The Heart Sounds of the Cardiac Cycle | | | |
|---|---|---|---|---|
| Ventricles full, Start contraction Start ventricular systole (Atrial diastole) | → | AV valves Snap shut "Lub" | → | Ventricles Empty & relax Start ventricular diastole (Atrial systole) | → | Semilunar valves Snap shut "Dub" | → | Ventricles full, Start contraction Start ventricular systole |

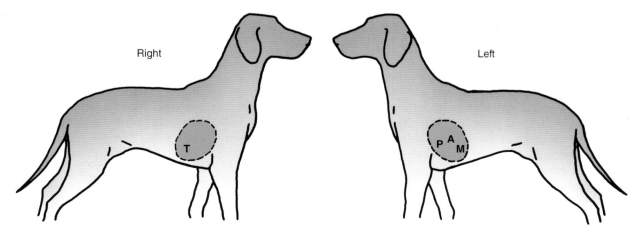

**FIGURE 14-18** Approximate locations for auscultation of the cardiac valves on the thoracic wall. *T*, Tricuspid valve; *P*, pulmonary valve; *A*, aortic valve; *M*, mitral valve. (From Nelson RC: *Small animal internal medicine*, ed 4, St Louis, 2009, Mosby.)

## ABNORMAL HEART SOUNDS

If the two AV valves or the two semilunar valves are not closing simultaneously you may hear extra heart sounds.

**Valvular insufficiency** is a heart condition where one or more of the cardiac valves don't close all the way. When this happens a **murmur** is produced. The murmur sound is produced by turbulence in the blood flow and sounds like a swishing or whooshing sound rather than a lub or dub. In the case of valvular insufficiency the murmur is caused by blood backflowing abnormally into a chamber. For example, a murmur caused by *mitral valve insufficiency* results when the mitral valve doesn't close all the way when the left ventricle begins systole. Instead of all the blood being ejected through the aortic valve into the aorta, some of the blood backflows into the left atrium. This results in less blood entering the systemic circulation.

**Valvular stenosis** is a heart condition where any one or more of the cardiac valves don't open all the way. Again a murmur is produced by turbulent blood flow. In the case of valvular stenosis the murmur is caused by blood flowing through a partially open valve and producing the same whooshing or swishing sound. For example, a murmur caused by *mitral valve stenosis* results when the mitral valve doesn't open entirely during left atrial systole. Instead of all the blood from the left atrium being ejected into the left ventricle, some of the blood remains in the left atrium. This results in less blood in the left ventricle to be ejected into the systemic circulation. It also results in less blood being able to enter the left atrium from the pulmonary circulation because the left atrium doesn't empty completely.

---

### ✓ TEST YOURSELF 14-4

1. What is the pacemaker of the heart and where is it located?
2. List the four conductors that make up the rapid conduction system for an impulse created by the heart's pacemaker.
3. The working phase of a cardiac cycle is ___. It involves ___ that generates an impulse that results in muscle contraction.
4. What is happening in the other three heart chambers during left atrial diastole?
5. When the mitral valve is forced closed it produces part of which heart sound, the first or the second?

---

## CARDIAC OUTPUT

The **cardiac output** (CO) is the volume of blood that is ejected out of the left ventricle over a unit of time, usually 1 minute. In a healthy animal the cardiac output has to be sufficient to supply oxygen and nutrients throughout the animal's body. Two factors determine the cardiac output (1) stroke volume and (2) heart rate.

### CLINICAL APPLICATION

#### Congestive Heart Failure

In older dogs, **congestive heart failure (CHF)** is a fairly common problem. CHF occurs when the pumping ability of the heart decreases, usually due to disease of the heart muscle or a valve malfunction that restricts the forward flow of blood through a valve or allows a backward flow. CHF may be predominantly right-sided or left-sided. When the right side of the heart begins to fail, blood returning from the systemic circulation is no longer able to move through the right heart as quickly. This causes increased blood pressure in the systemic circulation, which results in fluid accumulation in the form of **ascites** (fluid in the abdomen) and **edema** (fluid in the tissues).

When the left side of the heart fails, venous return from the lungs is decreased, resulting in pulmonary edema, which interferes with respiratory function. The decrease in cardiac output associated with heart failure may also reduce perfusion of important organs, such as the kidneys, to dangerously low levels.

Medications used to treat CHF include cardiac glycosides to increase the strength of cardiac contractions, diuretics to promote elimination of extra fluid to relieve edema, and vasodilators to enhance blood flow to the organs and decrease vascular resistance to outflow from the heart. CHF in pets cannot be cured, but it can often be medically managed to improve the animal's quality of life.

---

The **stroke volume (SV)** is the volume of blood ejected from the left ventricle during one contraction or systole. Another name for the stroke volume is **systolic discharge**. The **heart rate (HR)** is the number of times the ventricle contracts or beats in 1 minute. For an individual animal the HR is based in part on the rate at which the SA node spontaneously depolarizes:

$$\text{cardiac output (CO)} = \text{stroke volume (SV)} \times \text{heart rate (HR)}$$

For example if we know that a dog's heart ejects 100 milliliters (ml) of blood into the aorta with each systolic contraction, and its heart rate is 100 beats per minute, the animal's cardiac output can be calculated using our formula:

$$CO = 100 \text{ ml/min (SV)} \times 100 \text{ beats/min (HR)} = 10,000 \text{ ml/min}$$

Cardiac output for this dog would be 10,000 ml of blood per minute. This equation can help explain why cows and horses survive with much slower heart rates than cats and dogs. A horse or cow needs more cardiac output than a dog or cat because it has much greater tissue mass, yet it normally has a slower heart rate. How can that be? Well, if

$$CO = SV \times HR$$

and CO goes up but HR goes down, we can write the equation as:

$$CO = ?SV \times \downarrow HR$$

In order to balance the equation the stoke volume has to increase. Horses and cows have much larger hearts than dogs and cats; this allows them to have such a large stroke volume that they can generate sufficient cardiac output, even with a slower heart rate than smaller animals.

The stroke volume represents the strength of the heartbeat. It is determined by two factors: preload and afterload. **Preload** is the volume of blood the ventricle receives from the atrium. Eighty percent of ventricular filling occurs passively by gravity; the remaining 20% happens during atrial systole when the atrium contracts. When the atrium doesn't contract sufficiently the preload will decrease and the ventricle receives less blood.

**Afterload** is the physical resistance presented by the artery the ventricle is ejecting blood into. If there is resistance in the artery (e.g., partial blockage) the ventricle will not be able to contract all the way and the amount of blood ejected into the artery will be decreased.

Another factor that can affect the stroke volume is the length of the cardiac muscle cells. The longer the cells the more force they produce when they contract. The myocardial cells can be stretched to a certain degree by introducing an increased amount of blood into the ventricle during ventricular diastole. In this way myocardial cells are somewhat elastic. So if the ventricular wall is stretched the ventricle chamber increases in size and holds more blood. In order to get rid of the increased amount of blood the ventricular wall has to contract with increased force. The result is an increased stroke volume.

The normal heart rate for each species of animal is set internally by the rate of spontaneous SA node depolarization (Box 14-3). External control of the heart rate comes through the autonomic nervous system (discussed in Chapter 9).

---

### ✔ TEST YOURSELF 14-5

1. Stroke volume (SV) is a measurement of what?
2. If the cardiac output and stroke volume both decrease what has to happen to the heart rate to achieve equilibrium?
3. What is the difference between the preload and the afterload in reference to the stroke volume?
4. How could mitral valve stenosis affect the stroke volume?

---

| BOX 14-3 | Normal Heart Rate (and Pulse Rate) for Common Animal Species (*bpm) | | |
|---|---|---|---|
| Cat | 120-140 | Goat | 70-80 |
| Dog | 70-120 | Pig | 70-120 |
| Cow | 36-60 | Chicken | 250-300 |
| Dairy cow | 48-84 | Guinea Pig | 200-300 |
| Horse | 28-40 | Rabbit | 180-350 |
| Sheep | 70-80 | Rat | 250-400 |

*Beats per minute.

## BLOOD VESSELS

Blood vessels in the pulmonary and systemic circulations make continuous loops to and from the heart. In the pulmonary circulation this means the blood vessels are branches from the pulmonary artery and vein. In the systemic circulation the blood vessels are branches from the aorta and vena cava. All blood vessels are arteries, veins, or capillaries. They are hollow tubes with similar but not identical anatomy and function.

The walls of arteries and veins have three layers (Figure 14-19). The inner layer that lines the lumen of the vessel is the **endothelium**. It is composed of thin, smooth simple squamous epithelium and is continuous with the endocardium that lines the chambers of the heart. The endothelium provides a smooth surface for the vessel lumen so blood flows easily through the vessel with little or no friction.

The middle layer of a blood vessel wall is made up of smooth muscle, elastic fibers, or both. The smooth muscles contract and relax to change the diameter of the vessel. They are controlled by the autonomic nervous system. The elastic fibers provide stretchability to the vessel wall. They allow the blood vessel to stretch and recoil without outside control.

The outer layer of a blood vessel is composed of fibrous connective tissue and collagen fibers. The connective tissue is strong and flexible which prevents vessel walls from tearing. The collagen fibers extend outward from the connective tissue and anchor the vessels so they can't move around too much. They also help keep the lumen of the vessel pulled open.

### ARTERIES

Arteries carry blood away from the heart. In the pulmonary circulation they carry deoxygenated blood to the lungs for oxygenation. In systemic circulation they carry oxygenated blood throughout the animal's body. There are two types of artery: **elastic arteries** and **muscular arteries**. Elastic arteries have the greatest ability to stretch when blood passes through them because they have a large number of elastic fibers in the middle layers of their walls. These arteries are found closest to the heart because they have to be able to stretch and recoil without damage each time a surge of blood is ejected from a ventricle during ventricular systole.

The aorta is the largest elastic artery in the body. It has the largest layer of elastic fibers in its wall because it must be able to withstand the entire surge of blood ejected from the left ventricle. Other elastic arteries branch off the aorta. They have smaller diameters than the aorta but still have more elastic fibers than smooth muscle fibers in their wall.

Muscular arteries have more smooth muscle fibers than elastic fibers in their walls. They are found farther away from the heart than elastic arteries and usually direct blood to specific organs and tissues. Muscular arteries branch off the smallest elastic arteries and therefore have a smaller diameter. They are located far enough away from the heart that the blood surge is not severe enough to cause damage. Muscular arteries branch into arterioles.

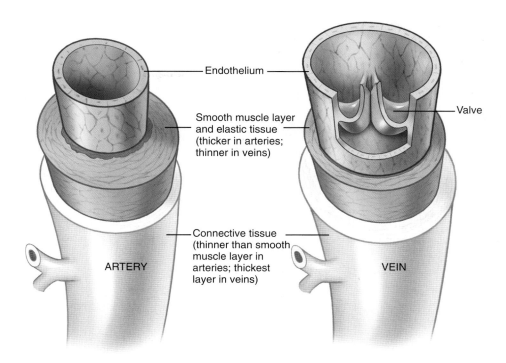

Endothelium

Smooth muscle layer
and elastic tissue
(thicker in arteries;
thinner in veins)

Valve

Connective tissue
(thinner than smooth
muscle layer in
arteries; thickest
layer in veins)

ARTERY

VEIN

**FIGURE 14-19** Anatomy of arteries and veins. (From Colvile J, Oien S: Clinical veterinary language, St Louis, 2014, Mosby.)

**Arterioles** are the smallest branches of the arterial tree. They are in effect small muscular arteries and have the narrowest diameter. Blood flow to areas of the animal's body is controlled through contraction of the smooth muscles in their walls under autonomic nervous system control. Their smaller diameter produces blood flow resistance, which in turn helps maintain blood pressure.

Muscular arteries and some elastic arteries are frequently named for the organ or tissue they are carrying blood to (e.g., the renal artery carries blood to a kidney). An animal's body is pretty much bilaterally symmetric so arteries usually come in pairs (e.g., the right and left ovarian arteries supply blood to the right and left ovary respectively) (Figure 14-20).

## CAPILLARIES

Arterioles branch into many microscopic blood vessels called capillaries. Capillaries do not occur singly but in groups called capillary beds or capillary networks. One arteriole will give rise to an entire capillary bed. The wall of a capillary is one endothelial cell thick. It has no middle or outer layer. For this reason the exchange of gases and nutrients takes place at this level. No cell in an animal's body is far from a capillary bed so the waste products of cellular metabolism are easily exchanged for the oxygen and nutrients necessary for cellular metabolism.

## VEINS

In order to get the blood back to the heart the capillaries join together to form tiny veins called **venules**. In the pulmonary

circulation the venules carry oxygenated blood; in the systemic circulation they carry deoxygenated blood and waste materials. Venules have thin enough walls that some fluid exchange between interstitial fluid and plasma can take place. Their walls consist of endothelium, a thin muscle layer, and a few fibrous connective tissue cells. White blood cells leave the circulation at the venule level to enter tissues at a site of inflammation.

Venules join together to form veins. Veins and arteries in a specific area run close to each other so veins are named for their corresponding arteries. For example, the femoral veins that drain blood from the hind legs accompany the femoral arteries that supply blood to the hind legs.

As veins approach the heart they become larger in diameter as more veins draining other areas of the body join together. The largest vein in the animal's body is the vena cava, and all other systemic veins eventually drain into it. Figure 14-21 shows the major veins in a cat's body.

Many veins are working against gravity to get the blood back to the heart and they don't have the force of ventricular contraction to propel blood flow. For this reason small and medium veins have one-way valves in their lumens. The valves allow blood to flow only in the direction of the heart. When blood tries to flow backward, the valves close. These valves are similar to the semilunar valves in the heart, but they each have only two cusps. Muscular movements in the body compress small veins and the one-way valves allow blood to move only toward the heart. This is the only mechanism that propels blood back to the heart.

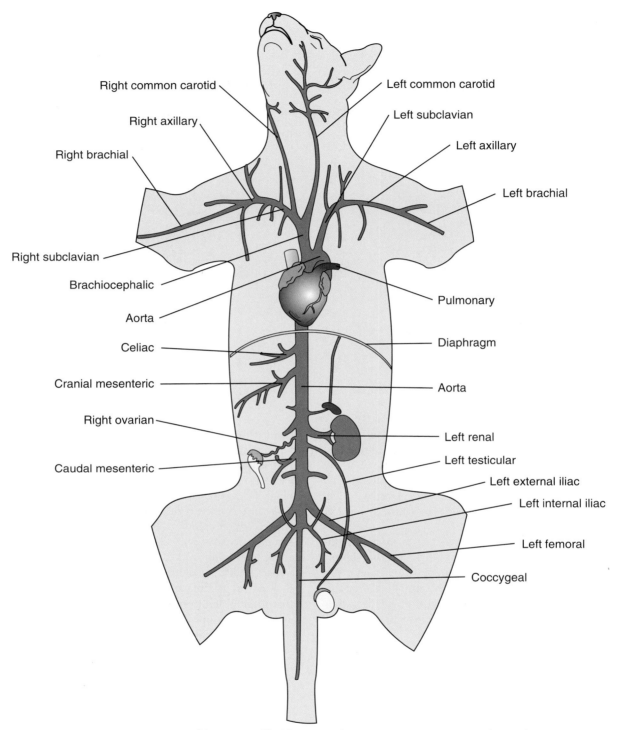

**FIGURE 14-20** Major arteries of the cat. (Modified from McBride DF: *Learning Veterinary terminology*, ed 2, St Louis, 2002, Mosby.)

## BLOOD CIRCULATION IN THE FETUS

Now that you are familiar with how blood moves through an animal, we'll look at some differences in blood flow in a developing fetus. The major difference between a fetus and a newborn is that the newborn receives oxygen through its own lungs, and a fetus receives oxygen from the blood of its mother. Because fetal lungs are not used for oxygen/carbon dioxide exchange, they need only enough blood to keep the growing lung tissues alive. Consequently, in the fetus there are bypasses that allow most of the blood in the fetal circulation to go around the lungs instead of through them.

The fetus receives oxygen through the placenta, an organ containing a network of tiny blood vessels that allows oxygen exchange between fetal and maternal circulation (Figure 14-22). The oxygenated blood from the mother flows from

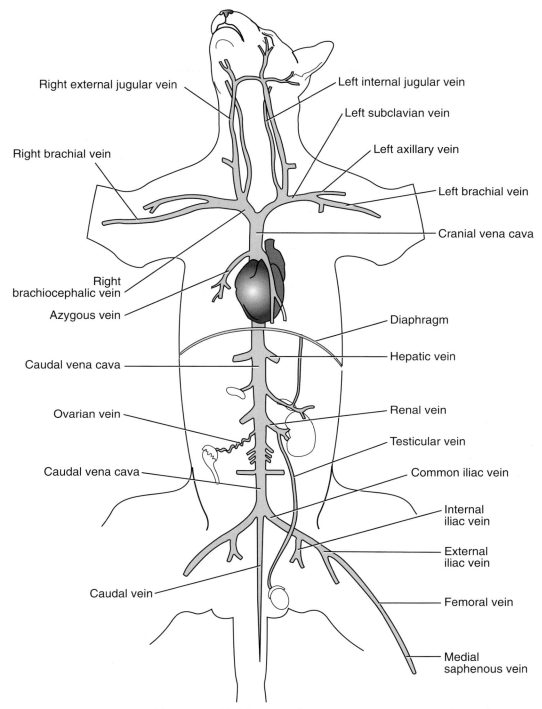

**FIGURE 14-21** Major veins of the cat. (Modified from McBride DF: Learning Veterinary terminology, ed 2, St Louis, 2002, Mosby.)

the placenta into the fetus through the **umbilical vein**. The vessel that carries oxygenated blood to the fetus is called a *vein* because it flows toward the heart of the fetus.

The oxygenated blood in the umbilical vein flows through the fetal liver and into the caudal vena cava, where it mixes with deoxygenated blood from the fetal systemic circulation. Just as in the newborn animal, blood from the vena cava fills the right atrium. However, in the fetus two structures allow

most of the fetal blood to bypass the lung tissue, because the blood in the right atrium has already been oxygenated from the maternal blood, and the lungs of the fetus do not perform oxygen exchange. The first bypass is the **foramen ovale** between the right and left atria (*foramen* means "opening," and *ovale* means "oval"). Much of the blood from the right atrium flows directly into the left atrium, but some does flow through the tricuspid valve into the right ventricle and then

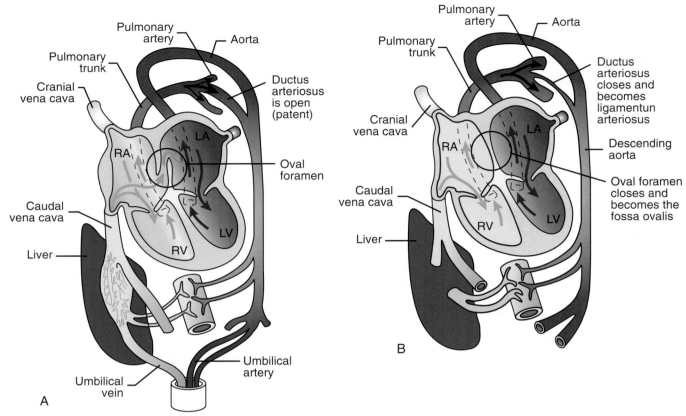

**FIGURE 14-22** Circulation in the fetus and the newborn. A, Fetal circulation, B, newborn circulation. *LA,* Left atrium; *LV,* left ventricle; *RA,* right atrium; *RV,* right ventricle.

into the pulmonary artery. Blood from the pulmonary artery may flow into the lungs or through another bypass, the **ductus arteriosus**, directly into the aorta. Remember that this blood was oxygenated when it passed through the placenta. Blood travels through the fetal aorta to the fetal systemic circulation, where it supplies oxygen and collects waste products from the tissues. The deoxygenated blood is then sent back to the placenta for oxygenation through the umbilical arteries.

With the first breath after birth, the lungs inflate, and the newborn begins to oxygenate its own blood. In a normal newborn, the foramen ovale and ductus arteriosus close at that time so that blood can no longer bypass the lungs.

---

### TEST YOURSELF 14-6

1. From the aortic valve in the left ventricle to the right atrium, list, in order, the types of blood vessel a drop of blood will pass through.
2. The coronary artery is the first branch off the aorta. Is it a muscular or elastic artery? Why?
3. In a pregnant ewe, which are the only two *veins* that are carrying *oxygenated* blood?
4. What two bypass structures are found in the fetus that allow most of its blood to bypass the pulmonary circulation?

---

### 🔍 CLINICAL APPLICATION

#### Patent Ductus Arteriosus

During gestation, the fetal circulation does not carry much blood through the lungs; instead, there is an opening between the left pulmonary artery and the aorta that allows much of the blood that leaves the right ventricle to bypass the lungs on the way to the aorta and systemic circulation. Because the fetus does not breathe air—oxygen is provided to the fetus from the blood of the dam—there is only enough pulmonary circulation to nourish the tissues of the growing lungs. Following the rupture of the umbilical cord at birth, the fetus must generate its own oxygenated blood, so circulation through the lungs must be increased to include all of the blood that leaves the right ventricle.

Normally, the shortcut opening between the pulmonary artery and aorta, known as the *ductus arteriosus,* closes soon after birth. Occasionally, the opening fails to close in the newborn, a condition called **patent ductus arteriosus** (**PDA**). Young animals with PDA suffer from inadequate oxygenation of their blood; in the long term, the condition is incompatible with life. PDA may be treated with drug therapy to promote closure, or surgical closure of the ductus arteriosus may be an option.

# PULSE

The **pulse** is the rate of alternating stretching and recoiling of the elastic fibers in an artery as blood passes through it with each heartbeat. The artery has to stretch and recoil because the left ventricle doesn't eject blood in a continuous flow. Every time the left ventricle contracts (systole) it ejects a bolus of blood into the aorta. When the left ventricle relaxes (diastole) blood flow into the aorta stops. This sets up a **pulse wave** of stretching and recoiling that travels through all the arteries and arterioles and dissipates in the capillaries. In most animals the pulse is felt on superficial arteries lying against firm surfaces such as bones.

Clinically the pulse is used to evaluate the regularity of the pulsations and the strength of the pulsations. The pulse and the heartbeat in an animal are not the same thing. The pulse is felt on a superficial artery; the heartbeat is counted using a stethoscope to listen to the animal's chest (**auscultation**) to hear the heart sounds. In some animals the heartbeat can be felt through the chest wall. This is still not a true pulse because it is not felt over an artery.

## PULSE POINTS

The pulse is best felt on different arteries in different species of animal (Box 14-4). It is most commonly evaluated over a medium-sized artery. In a healthy animal the pulse rate and the heart rate should be equal. When feeling for a pulse, use the tips of your index and middle fingers, not your thumb because the thumb has its own pulse (Figure 14-23). The pulse wave that passes through your thumb may be confused

with the animal's pulse. As a general rule, larger animals have slower pulse rates and smaller animals have faster pulse rates. The pulse cannot be taken over a vein because the pulse wave dissipates in the capillaries and none of it is passed into the veins.

# BLOOD PRESSURE

As the name implies **blood pressure** is a measure of the amount of pressure flowing blood exerts on arterial walls. It is dependent on the interaction between the heart rate, stroke volume, the diameter and elasticity of the artery, and the total blood volume. Any condition or medication that affects any one or more of these factors will also affect the blood pressure.

| BOX 14-4 | Common Pulse Points in Common Animal Species |
|---|---|
| Cat | Femoral artery—medial surface of the thigh near the belly |
| Dog | Femoral artery—medial surface of the thigh near the belly |
| Cow | Coccygeal artery—ventral midline of the tail near the base<br>Facial artery—passes over the mandible near the angle of the jaw |
| Horse | Mandibular artery—passes over the mandible near the angle of the jaw<br>Posterior digital artery—on the pastern between the coronary band and the fetlock |
| Sheep | Femoral artery—medial surface of the thigh near the belly |
| Goat | Femoral artery—medial surface of the thigh near the belly |
| Piglet | Femoral artery—medial surface of the thigh near the belly |
| Pig | Coccygeal artery—ventral midline of the tail near the base |

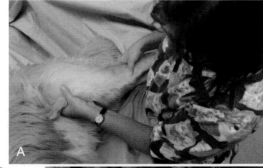
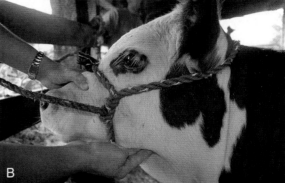
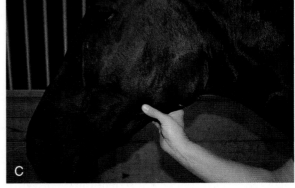

**FIGURE 14-23** Finding the pulse on **A,** a dog or cat, **B,** a cow, **C,** a horse. (**A,** From Thomas J, Lerche, P: Anesthesia and analgesia for veterinary technicians, ed 4, St Louis, 2011, Mosby; **B** and **C,** From Bassert J, McCurnin D: McCurnin's clinical textbook for veterinary technicians, ed 8, St Louis, 2014, Saunders.)

Blood pressure varies during the cardiac cycle. If you've ever had your blood pressure measured you know that two numbers are recorded. One number, the highest number, is the **systolic blood pressure**. It is produced by ejection of blood from the left ventricle into the systemic circulation by way of the aorta. The second number, the lowest number, is the **diastolic blood pressure**. It measures the pressure remaining in the artery during left ventricular diastole when the ventricle is relaxing and refilling with blood. A third value, the **mean arterial pressure** (MAP), is sometimes measured. This is the average pressure during one cardiac cycle. The MAP can be used when monitoring an anesthetized animal as an indication of tissue perfusion.

Blood pressure is most commonly measured using one of two methods. The **oscillometric** method is the method often used in your doctor's office. A cuff is placed over the area of an artery and inflated until blood flow either stops or nearly stops. The air is gradually released from the cuff and an instrument attached to the cuff measures the magnitude and frequency of pulsations. The instrument automatically determines the systolic and diastolic blood pressures. Many instruments will also determine heart rate.

The second method used to determine blood pressure is Doppler ultrasound. The ultrasound instrument measures arterial blood flow as air is released from an inflated cuff attached to a **sphygmomanometer**. The cuff is proximal to the position of the Doppler transducer that is placed over an artery. This method accurately measures systolic blood pressure only.

## CARDIOVASCULAR MONITORING

Given that the heart is not visible by direct observation, a number of direct and indirect tests have been developed to monitor it and the entire cardiovascular system. These tests include:

- **Auscultation** of the thorax to determine heart rate and rhythm, and to detect heart murmurs
- Peripheral artery palpation to evaluate the rate, regularity, and strength of the pulse
- Measurement of arterial blood pressure to evaluate cardiac output
- Thoracic radiography to evaluate the size and position of the heart
- Electrocardiography to evaluate the electrical activity of the heart
- Echocardiography to evaluate the size, shape, and movement of heart structures

## ELECTROCARDIOGRAPHY

**Electrocardiography** produces an **electrocardiogram** (ECG or EKG) based on the electrical activity of the heart. The electrical impulse that originates in the SA node and spreads through the cardiac conduction system can be detected on the surface of the animal's body. Leads are placed at specific locations on the animal's body and attached to an ECG machine. When the ECG machine is turned on, the electric impulses generated in the heart muscle are picked up at the

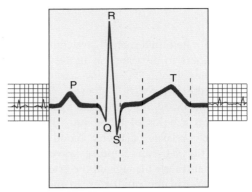

**FIGURE 14-24** The electrocardiogram (ECG) of normal heartbeats. The enlarged area represents one cardiac cycle or heartbeat. (Adapted from Koeppen BM, Stanton BA: Berne & Levy physiology, ed 6, St Louis, 2010, Mosby.)

various locations on the body surface where the leads were placed, and are recorded. A series of heartbeats are followed for a specified period of time, recording them at a standardized rate on a strip of graph paper moving through the instrument.

Figure 14-24 shows the ECG of one cardiac cycle. An explanation of the various components in Figure 14-24 follows:

- **P wave**
  - Is the time it takes the wave of depolarization (contractions) to travel from the SA node through the atria
  - It corresponds to the mechanical activity of atrial contractions in a normal animal
- **QRS complex**
  - Is the time of ventricular depolarization (contraction)
  - It corresponds to the mechanical activity of ventricular contraction
  - It is composed of three different waves
    - Q wave corresponds to depolarization of the interventricular septum.
    - R wave corresponds to depolarization of the main mass of the ventricles so it is the largest wave
    - S wave corresponds to the final part depolarization of the ventricles near the base of the heart
- **T wave**
  - Is the time of ventricular relaxation (repolarization)
  - It corresponds to the time taken by the ventricles to get ready for the next contraction by refilling with blood from the atria

## ECHOCARDIOGRAPHY

Another way to evaluate the heart is through **echocardiography** (**ECHO** or cardiac ultrasound). This procedure uses ultrasound to bounce sound waves off parts of the heart to watch the heart beating. ECHO can be used to evaluate the size, shape, and movement of the heart and its parts.

Two-dimensional echocardiography produces an overall 2-D cross-sectional image of the heart (Figure 14-25). (The image is much like the image produced of a fetus when ultrasound is used on a pregnant woman.) Two-dimensional echocardiography is a trans-thoracic procedure where the

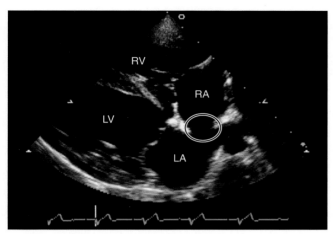

**FIGURE 14-25** Two-dimensional echocardiography (ECHO) of a heart with an interatrial septal defect (**A**). All four chambers of the heart are visible. (Modified from Ettinger SJ, Feldman E: Textbook of veterinary internal medicine, ed 7, St Louis, 2010, Saunders.)

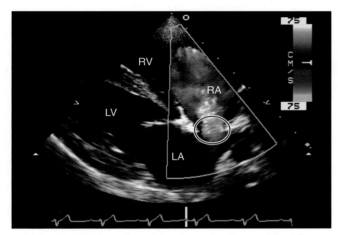

**FIGURE 14-26** Doppler echocardiography showing blood flowing between the two atria (**B**) of the same heart as in Figure 14-25. (Modified from Ettinger SJ, Feldman E: Textbook of veterinary internal medicine, ed 7, St Louis, 2010, Saunders.)

transducer that emits ultrasound waves is moved over the thorax in the area of the heart. The sound waves bounce or "echo" off the heart and are sent to a computer that produces an animated image of the heart. Two-dimensional echocardiography is especially useful for evaluating the relative size of the heart chambers, the thickness of the myocardium, and the functioning of the valves. With this method you are able to see the heart working in real time.

**Doppler echocardiography** (Figure 14-26) is a more sophisticated ultrasound procedure that measures blood flow through the heart and adds color to the image. It is usually done in conjunction with two-dimensional echocardiography and is especially useful for evaluating valvular stenosis and insufficiency.

## VENIPUNCTURE

Most blood vessels are buried deep within an animal's body, but some are superficial and can be seen or felt just under

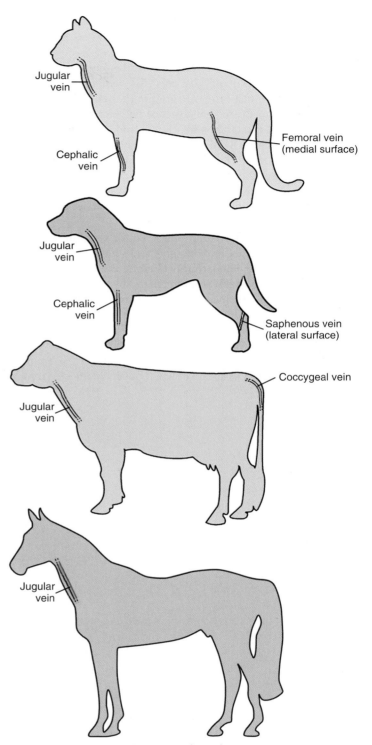

**FIGURE 14-27** Commonly used venipuncture sites.

the skin. These superficial blood vessels are used to collect blood samples, administer medications intravenously, and place venous or arterial catheters. It is important to become familiar with the names and locations of these superficial blood vessels (Figure 14-27).

In dogs and cats, the **cephalic vein** of the thoracic limb is commonly used for venipuncture. It runs between the elbow and the carpus on the cranio-medial aspect of the forearm. The cephalic vein carries blood from the distal extremity to the jugular vein.

In the pelvic limb of dogs and cats, the **femoral vein** or the **saphenous vein** may be used for venipuncture. The femoral vein, which is more commonly used in cats than dogs, runs along the medial aspect of the hind limb between the groin and the tarsal joint (hock) and carries blood to the iliac vein, which joins the vena cava. The saphenous vein, which is more commonly used in dogs, runs along the lateral aspect of the hind limb from the cranial aspect of the leg just above the hock (tarsus) to the caudal aspect just below the knee (stifle). The saphenous vein carries blood to the femoral vein.

The **jugular vein** is commonly used for venipuncture in nearly all animal species, both large and small. Jugular veins travel in muscular jugular grooves along the ventral aspect of each side of the neck, from the mandible to the shoulder. The jugular veins are located near the **carotid arteries**. In all species, but especially in the horse, care must be taken to avoid accidental injection into the carotid artery of substances that are meant to be injected into the jugular vein. The carotid artery carries blood very quickly to the brain; substances that act as sedatives when normally injected into the jugular vein may actually cause seizures and/or death if accidentally injected into the carotid artery.

In lactating dairy cattle, the superficial caudal epigastric vein, commonly called the *milk vein,* is easily seen as it travels along the ventral aspect of each side of the abdomen from the udder to about the level of the sternum. This vein is not to be used for routine venipuncture, because its thin-walled, superficial character makes it prone to excessive bleeding and hematoma formation, which may lead to the development of an abscess.

In ruminants and rodents, the **coccygeal vein** may be used for venipuncture. The coccygeal vein carries blood from the tail to the vena cava. It runs along the ventral midline of the tail.

---

✔ **TEST YOURSELF 14-7**

1. What is the difference between a heart rate and a pulse?
2. What does systolic blood pressure measure?
3. What is the difference between an ECG and an ECHO?
4. Which vein can be used in most common animal species for venipuncture? Where is it located?

# 15 The Respiratory System

*Thomas Colville*

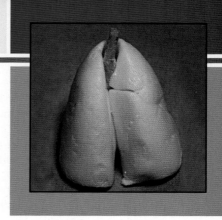

## OUTLINE

## LEARNING OBJECTIVES

*When you have completed this chapter you will be able to:*

- Differentiate between internal and external respiration.
- List the secondary functions of the respiratory system.
- List the components of the upper respiratory tract and describe their structure and functions.
- List the components of the lower respiratory tract and describe their structure and functions.
- Describe the events that occur during inspiration and expiration.
- List the muscles involved in inspiration and expiration.
- Define the terms *tidal volume, minute volume,* and *residual volume.*
- Describe the processes of oxygen and carbon dioxide exchange between the alveoli and the blood.

## VOCABULARY FUNDAMENTALS

*Alveolar duct* ahl-**vē**-ō-lahr duhckt
*Alveolar sac* ahl-**vē**-ō-lahr sahck
*Alveolus* ahl-**vē**-ō-luhs
*Arytenoid cartilage* eǝr-eh-**tih**-noyd **kahr**-tih-lihj
*Bifurcation of the trachea* bī-fǝr-**kā**-shuhn *of the* trā-kē-ah
*Breathing* **brē**-thihng
*Bronchial tree* **brohn**-kē-ahl trē
*Bronchiole* **brohn**-kē-ōl
*Bronchitis* brohn-**kīt**-ihs
*Bronchoconstriction* brohn-kō-kuhn-**strihck**-shuhn
*Bronchus* **brohn**-kuhs
*Chemical control system* **kehm**-ih-kuhl **kohn**-trōl **sihs**-tehm
*Congenital* kohn-**jehn**-ih-tahl
*Cough* kawf
*Cricoid cartilage* **krī**-koyd **kahr**-tih-lihj
*Diaphragm* **dī**-ah-frahm

*Endotracheal intubation* ehn-dō-**trā**-kē-ahl **ihn**-too-bā-shuhn
*Endotracheal (ET) tube* ehn-dō-**trā**-kē-ahl toob
*Epiglottis* ehp-ih-**gloht**-ihs
*Expiration* ehcks-puh-**rā**-shuhn
*External respiration* ehcks-tǝr-nahl rehs-puh-**rā**-shuhn
*False vocal cord* fahls **vō**-kahl kohrd
*Glottis* **gloh**-tihs
*Hiccup* **hihck**-uhp
*Hilus* **hī**-luhs
*Inspiration* ihn-spuh-**rā**-shuhn
*Intercostal space* ihn-tǝr-**kohst**-ahl spās
*Internal respiration* ihn-tǝr-nahl rehs-puh-**rā**-shuhn
*Laryngeal hemiplegia* **lahr**-ehn-jē-ahl hehm-ih-**plē**-jē-ah
*Laryngoscope* lah-**rihn**-jeh-skōp
*Laryngospasm* lah-**rihn**-gō-spahzm
*Larynx* **leǝr**-ihngks
*Lateral ventricle* **laht**-ǝr-ahl **vehn**-trihck-ehl

*Lobe* lōb

*Lower respiratory tract* lō-ər **rehs**-pər-uh-tohr-ē trahkt

*Mechanical control system* meh-**kahn**-ih-kahl kohn-**trōl** sihs-tehm

*Mediastinum* mē-dē-ah-**stīn**-uhm

*Minute volume* **mihn**-iht **vohl**-ūm

*Nares* **neər**-rēs

*Nasal meatus* **nāz**-ahl mē-**āt**-uhs

*Nasal passage* **nāz**-ahl **pahs**-ihj

*Nasal septum* **nāz**-ahl **sehp**-tuhm

*Olfactory sense* ohl-**fahck**-tuh-rē sehnz

*Paranasal sinus* peər-ah-**nā**-sahl **sī**-nuhs

*Partial pressure* **pahr**-shahl **prehsh**-ər

*pH* **pē**-H

*Pharynx* **feər**-ihnks

*Phonation* fō-**nā**-shuhn

*Pleura* **ploor**-ah

*Pneumonia* nū-**mōn**-yah

*Pneumothorax* nū-mō-**thōr**-ahx

*Pulmonary* puhl-muh-**neər**-ē

*Residual volume* rih-**zihj**-yoo-ahl **vohl**-ūm

*Respiration* rehs-puh-**rā**-shuhn

*Respiratory center* **rehs**-pər-uh-tohr-ē **sehn**-tər

*Roaring* **rohr**-ihng

*Sigh* **sī**

*Sinus* **sī**-nuhs

*Sinusitis* sī-nuhs-**ī**-tihs

*Sneeze* snēz

*Surfactant* sər-**fahck**-tahnt

*Thoracic cavity* thohr-**ah**-sihck **kahv**-ih-tē

*Thorax* **thohr**-ahx

*Thyroid cartilage* **thī**-royd **kahr**-tih-lihj

*Tidal volume* **tī**-dahl **vohl**-ūm

*Trachea* **trā**-kē-uh

*Turbinate* **tər**-buh-nāt

*Upper respiratory tract* **uhp**-ər **rehs**-pər-uh-tohr-ē trahkt

*Ventilation* vehn-tih-**lā**-shuhn

*Vestibular fold* vehs-**tihb**-yoo-lahr fōld

*Vocal cord* **vō**-kahl kohrd

*Vocal fold* **vō**-kahl fōld

*Yawn* yahn

---

## INTRODUCTION

What do you think of when you read the term *respiration?* Do you imagine the process of breathing—drawing air into the lungs and blowing it back out? That is certainly an important part of respiration, but it is only one part of the whole, complex process. In simplest terms **respiration** is the process of bringing oxygen ($O_2$) from the outside air in to all of the body's cells, and carrying carbon dioxide ($CO_2$) out in the opposite direction. The body's cells need a constant supply of oxygen to burn nutrients to produce energy. Carbon dioxide is a waste product of these energy-producing reactions and must be eliminated. In a simple, single-celled animal, these gases are exchanged between the interior of the cell and the outside environment directly through the cell membrane by simple diffusion (movement of molecules from an area of high concentration to an area of lower concentration). In a complex animal such as a horse or dog, most of the body's cells are located too far from the outside world for that simple system to work. Regardless, oxygen somehow has to reach *all* of the body's cells, and carbon dioxide has to be transported away from them. These vital processes are carried out by the respiratory system working together with the cardiovascular system.

Two steps are needed for respiration to take place in an animal's body—**external respiration** and **internal respiration**. External respiration occurs in the lungs. It is the exchange of oxygen and carbon dioxide between the *air* inhaled into the lungs and the *blood* flowing through the **pulmonary** (lung) capillaries. Internal respiration, on the other hand, occurs all over the body. It is the exchange of oxygen and carbon dioxide between the *blood* in the capillaries all over the body (the *systemic capillaries*), and all of the *cells and tissues* of the body.

Internal respiration is the real "business end" of respiration. It is the means by which the body's cells receive the oxygen they need and get rid of the waste carbon dioxide they produce. Without external respiration, however, there would be no oxygen in the blood for the cells to absorb, and no way for the cells to get rid of their carbon dioxide.

In this chapter, we concentrate on the organs and structures that contribute to external respiration. These are parts of what we call the *respiratory system*—the lungs and the complex system of tubes that connect them with the outside world. Box 15-1 lists the main components of the respiratory system in order, from outside in.

In addition to its primary function of swapping oxygen for carbon dioxide, the respiratory system has some

---

| **BOX 15-1** | Main Structures of the Respiratory System |
|---|---|

In order, from outside in, the main structures of the respiratory system are as follows:

**Upper Respiratory Tract**
- Nostrils
- Nasal passages
- Pharynx
- Larynx
- Trachea

**Lower Respiratory Tract**
- Bronchi
- Bronchioles
- Alveolar ducts
- Alveoli

secondary functions that are also important to an animal's well-being. These include voice production, body temperature regulation, acid–base balance regulation, and the sense of smell.

Voice production is also called **phonation**. The process usually begins in the **larynx**, or *voice box*, as it is commonly called. Two fibrous connective tissue bands called the **vocal cords** (also known as the **vocal folds**) stretch across the lumen of the larynx and vibrate as air passes over them. This produces the basic sound of the animal's voice. Other structures, such as the **thorax** (chest cavity), nose, mouth, **pharynx** (throat), and sinuses contribute resonance and other characteristics to the vocal sounds.

Body temperature regulation involves many body systems, including the respiratory system. Under cold environmental conditions, the network of superficial blood vessels just under the epithelium of the nasal passages helps warm inhaled air before it reaches the lungs. (The location of these blood vessels is illustrated in Figure 15-2.) This helps prevent hypothermia (low body temperature) by avoiding chilling of the blood circulating through the lungs. Under hot environmental conditions, the respiratory system aids cooling in many animals by the mechanism of panting. The rapid respiratory movements of panting cause increased evaporation of fluid from the lining of the respiratory passages and mouth, which helps cool the blood circulating just beneath the epithelium.

Acid–base balance is an important homeostatic mechanism in the body. For normal chemical reactions to occur in the cells, the relative acidity or alkalinity of their environment must be controlled carefully. The unit used to express relative acidity or alkalinity is **pH**. Literally, pH is a mathematical value representing the negative logarithm of the hydrogen ion concentration. In simpler terms, pH is a number that tells us the relative acidity or alkalinity of something.

The pH ranges from 0 to 14. The lower the pH, the more acidic the environment, and the higher the pH, the more alkaline the environment. A pH of 7 is neutral, that is, neither acidic nor alkaline. The normal pH of the blood in most animals is 7.4, with an acceptable range of 7.35 to 7.45. A blood pH outside that narrow range spells danger for the animal's health.

The respiratory system contributes to the process of acid–base control by its ability to influence the amount of $CO_2$ in the blood. The more $CO_2$ there is in the blood, the lower the blood pH and the more acidic the blood ($CO_2$ dissolves in the plasma to form carbonic acid [$H_2CO_3$]). The respiratory system can alter the $CO_2$ content of the blood by adjusting the volume and rate of breathing. We describe this process more completely in the section on the control of breathing.

The sense of smell, also called the **olfactory sense**, is very important to many animals. The receptors for the sense of smell are contained in patches of sensory epithelium located high in the nasal passages. More information on the olfactory sense can be found in Chapter 10.

> ✓ **TEST YOURSELF 15-1**
> 1. What is the primary function of the respiratory system?
> 2. What are secondary functions of the respiratory system?
> 3. What is the difference between breathing and respiration?
> 4. What is the difference between internal respiration and external respiration? Which one occurs in the lungs?

## STRUCTURE

Structurally, the respiratory system consists of the lungs and a system of tubes that connects them with the world outside the animal's body. For this discussion, we classify all the respiratory structures outside the lungs as parts of the **upper respiratory tract** and all the structures within the lungs as parts of the **lower respiratory tract**.

### UPPER RESPIRATORY TRACT

The upper portion of the respiratory tract includes the nose, the nasal passages, the *pharynx* (throat), the *larynx* (voice box), and the **trachea** (wind pipe) (Figure 15-1). All of the air that enters and leaves the lungs does so through the upper respiratory structures.

### NOSE

If we were air molecules being inhaled into the respiratory system of an animal, the nose would be the first structure we would encounter. It begins with the nostrils, which are also

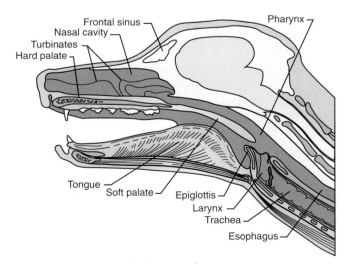

**FIGURE 15-1** Longitudinal section of canine upper respiratory tract.

known as the **nares**. The nostrils are the external openings of the respiratory tube, and they lead into the **nasal passages**.

**NASAL PASSAGES.** The nasal passages are located between the nares (nostrils) and the pharynx (throat). A midline divider called the **nasal septum** separates the left nasal passage from the right, and the hard and soft palates separate the (dorsal) nasal passages from the (ventral) mouth.

The nasal passages are not just simple tubes. Their linings are convoluted and full of twists and turns because of the presence of the **turbinates** (also called the *nasal conchae*). Turbinates are thin, scroll-like bones covered with nasal epithelium that occupy most of the lumen of the nasal passages (see Figure 7-14).

Two sets of scroll-like turbinates are found in each nasal passage: a *dorsal turbinate* and a *ventral turbinate*. They divide each nasal passage into three main passageways, each called a **nasal meatus** (*meatus* means "passageway"). The *ventral nasal meatus* is located between the ventral turbinate and the floor of the nasal passage, the *middle nasal meatus* is located between the two sets of turbinates, and the *dorsal nasal meatus* is located between the dorsal turbinate and the roof of the nasal passage. A small fourth meatus, called the *common nasal meatus,* is located on either side of the nasal septum. It is continuous with the other three main nasal meatuses. See Chapter 7 for a more complete description of the turbinates.

The lining of the nasal passages is critical to their function and is illustrated in Figure 15-2. It consists of pseudostratified columnar epithelium with cilia projecting from the cell surfaces up into a layer of mucus that is secreted by many mucous glands and goblet cells. The cilia beat back toward the pharynx (throat). An extensive complex of large blood vessels lies just beneath the nasal epithelium.

Aside from housing the receptors for the sense of smell, the main function of the nasal passages is to "condition" the inhaled air that passes through them. The three main conditioning roles performed by the nasal lining are *warming, humidifying,* and *filtering* the inhaled air. The scroll-like twists and turns of the turbinates increase the surface area of the nasal lining tremendously. They allow it to function as a combination radiator and humidifier. The air is warmed by the blood flowing through the complex of blood vessels just beneath the nasal epithelium, and it is humidified by the mucus and other fluids that lie on the epithelial surface.

The filtering function of the nasal passages helps remove particulate matter, such as dust and pollen, from the inhaled air before it reaches the lungs. The filtering mechanism relies on the many twists and turns of the nasal passages produced by the turbinates, the mucus layer on the surface of the nasal epithelium, and the cilia that project up into it. Given that air is a gas, it easily passes along the tortuous path of the nasal lining as it is inhaled, but particles of dust and other debris do not negotiate the twists and turns as readily and become trapped in the mucous layer. The beating of the cilia sweeps the mucus and the trapped foreign material back to the pharynx, where it is swallowed. One of the damaging effects of respiratory infections is that the swelling and thick inflammatory secretions "gum up" the cilia and prevent them from doing their sweeping job. Excess secretions can then build up on the epithelial surfaces, obstruct airflow, and stimulate coughing and sneezing.

**PARANASAL SINUSES.** The **paranasal sinuses** are usually just called the **sinuses**. They are outpouchings of the nasal passages that are contained within spaces in certain skull bones. Each sinus is named for the skull bone that houses it. Most animals have two *frontal sinuses* and two *maxillary sinuses*, within the frontal and maxillary bones, respectively. Figure 15-3 shows the locations of the frontal

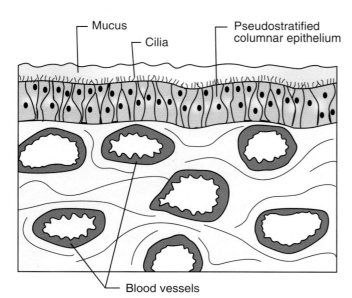

**FIGURE 15-2** Lining of nasal cavity. Note cilia protruding up into the overlying mucous layer and numerous large blood vessels immediately below the epithelium.

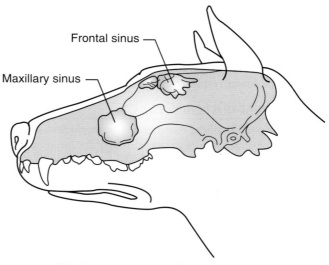

**FIGURE 15-3** Paranasal sinuses of the dog.

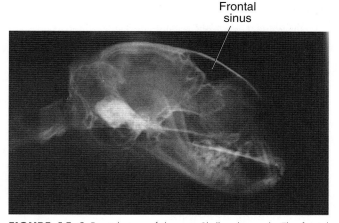

Frontal
sinus

**FIGURE 15-4** Frontal sinus of the cat. Skull radiograph. The frontal sinus appears dark because it contains air, which is very transparent to x-rays. Note the lighter appearance of the surrounding skull bones.

and maxillary sinuses of the dog. Figure 15-4 shows the location of the frontal sinus of the cat on a skull radiograph (x-ray). (See also Figure 7-15.) Some animals, including humans, have two more sinuses—the *sphenoidal sinus* and the *ethmoidal sinus*—located in the sphenoid and ethmoid bones. See Chapter 7 for more information on the skull bones that house paranasal sinuses.

The sinuses have the same kind of ciliated lining as the nasal passages. The cilia constantly sweep mucus produced in the sinuses down into the nasal passages. This sweeping action helps prevent fluid and debris from accumulating in the sinuses and obstructing the openings into the nasal passages.

 **CLINICAL APPLICATION**

### Sinusitis

The sinuses can be clinically significant if they become inflamed and swollen as a result of allergies, infections, tumors, and so on. If the openings into the nasal passages swell shut or become plugged with inflammatory debris, fluids in the sinus have nowhere to go, and the resulting buildup of pressure can be very painful for the animal. This condition is known as **sinusitis**. Sinusitis can often be treated effectively with drugs such as antibiotics to combat disease-causing microorganisms and decongestants to reduce the swelling in the lining of the sinus. However, in some severe cases, a hole must be surgically drilled into an inflamed sinus to allow fluid to drain from it.

### PHARYNX

The nasal passages lead back to the pharynx, or what we commonly call the "throat." It is a common passageway for both the respiratory and digestive systems. At its rostral (front) end, the soft palate divides the pharynx into the dorsal *nasopharynx* (respiratory passageway) and the ventral *oropharynx* (digestive passageway). These lead back to the main part of the pharynx, which is common to both systems.

At its caudal end, the pharynx opens dorsally into the esophagus (digestive passageway) and ventrally into the larynx (respiratory passageway). Take a look at Figure 15-1 and note that the respiratory and digestive passageways switch places at the pharynx. The respiratory passageway (nasal passage) starts out *dorsal* to the digestive passageway (the mouth) but, further caudally, the respiratory passageway (larynx) is *ventral* to the digestive passageway (esophagus). If you have ever wondered why it is so easy to choke if you try to swallow and breathe or laugh at the same time, this is the reason.

Because it is a common passageway that must allow both breathing and swallowing, some delicate reflexes control the actions of the muscles around the pharynx. Breathing is easy. The pharynx just has to stay open to allow airflow. Swallowing is the tricky part. As discussed next, the larynx and the pharynx work together to prevent swallowing from interfering with breathing and vice versa. This is one of those spots in the body where timing is everything. The seemingly simple act of swallowing actually involves a complex series of actions that stop the process of breathing, cover the opening into the larynx, move the material to be swallowed to the rear of the pharynx, open the esophagus, and move the material into it. Once swallowing is complete, the opening of the larynx is uncovered and breathing resumes. It is no wonder that things occasionally don't work quite right and choking results.

### LARYNX

The larynx is what we commonly refer to as the "voice box." It is a short, irregular tube that connects the pharynx with the trachea. It is made up mainly of segments of cartilage that are connected to each other and the surrounding tissues by muscles. The larynx is supported in place by the hyoid bone.

The pattern of the cartilage components of the larynx, as well as their number, varies among species. The major cartilages in the common animal species are the single **epiglottis**, the paired **arytenoid cartilages**, the single **thyroid cartilage**, and the single **cricoid cartilage**. Of these, the epiglottis and the arytenoid cartilages are most commonly of clinical importance.

The somewhat leaf-shaped epiglottis is the most rostral of the laryngeal cartilages. It projects forward from the ventral portion of the larynx, and its bluntly pointed tip is usually tucked up behind the caudal edge of the soft palate when the animal is breathing. When the animal swallows, however, the epiglottis covers the opening of the larynx, much like a trapdoor. This keeps the swallowed material out of the larynx and helps direct it dorsally into the opening of the esophagus.

The vocal cords are attached to the two arytenoid cartilages. Muscles adjust the tension of the vocal cords by moving the cartilages. The arytenoid cartilages and the vocal cords form the boundaries of the **glottis**—the opening into the larynx.

In nonruminant animals, a second set of connective tissue bands, called the **false vocal cords**, or **vestibular folds**, is present in the larynx in addition to the vocal cords. They are not involved in voice production. On each side of the larynx of these animals, blind pouches called the **lateral ventricles** project laterally into the space between the vocal cords and the vestibular folds. These lateral ventricles are often involved in the treatment of a condition in horses called **roaring** (see the Clinical Application on roaring).

Aside from its role as part of the upper airway, the larynx has three main functions: voice production, prevention of foreign material being inhaled, and control of airflow to and from the lungs.

As described earlier, the basic sound of an animal's voice originates from the vocal cords in the larynx. These two fibrous connective tissue bands are attached to the arytenoid cartilages and stretch across the lumen of the larynx parallel to each another. As air passes over the taut vocal cords, they vibrate and produce sounds. The muscles that attach to the arytenoid cartilages control the tension of the vocal cords. They can adjust the tension from a state of complete relaxation, which opens the glottis wide and produces no sound, to a very tight condition that can completely close off the glottis and prevent airflow. Voice production requires a tension somewhere between these two extremes. In general, by lessening the tension of the vocal cords, lower-pitched sounds are made, and by tightening them, higher-pitched sounds result.

The larynx also helps keep foreign material from entering the trachea and passing down into the lungs. This is accomplished mainly by the trapdoor action of the epiglottis. Part of the process of swallowing consists of muscle contractions that pull the entire larynx forward and fold the epiglottis back over its opening. You can feel part of this process by putting your fingertips on your "Adam's apple" (the thyroid cartilage of your larynx) and swallowing. You can feel your Adam's apple move up as you swallow. This extremely effective process helps protect the delicate tissues of the trachea and lungs from trauma due to inhaled foreign material.

The larynx controls airflow to and from the lungs partially through the trapdoor action of the epiglottis when swallowing occurs, but also through adjustments in the size of the glottis. Small adjustments aid the movement of air as the animal draws air into its lungs and blows it out. At times, complete closure of the glottis is helpful. For example, the process of coughing starts with a closed glottis. To generate a cough, the glottis closes and the respiratory muscles contract, compressing the thorax. This builds pressure behind the closed glottis. When the glottis suddenly opens, the forceful release of air that results is what we call a **cough**. The purpose of coughing is usually to clear mucus and other matter from the lower respiratory passages.

Closure of the glottis even aids nonrespiratory functions that involve straining, such as urination, defecation, and parturition (the birth process). Straining begins with the animal holding the glottis closed while applying pressure to the thorax with the breathing muscles. This stabilizes the thorax and allows the abdominal muscles to compress the abdominal organs effectively when they contract. Without the closed glottis, contraction of the abdominal muscles merely forces air out of the lungs (exhalation).

 **TEST YOURSELF 15-2**

1. By what mechanisms is inhaled air warmed, humidified, and filtered as it passes through the nasal passages? How do the turbinates aid these processes?
2. Describe how the respiratory and digestive passageways "switch places" in the pharynx.
3. How do the pharynx and larynx work together to keep swallowed material from entering the trachea? What role does the epiglottis play in that process?
4. How is the larynx involved in the straining process that aids functions such as defecation?

## CLINICAL APPLICATION

### Endotracheal Intubation

**Endotracheal intubation** is a common clinical procedure in which a soft rubber or plastic tube, called an **endotracheal (ET) tube**, is inserted through the glottis and advanced down into the trachea. Its purpose is to provide an open airway, usually for the administration of an inhalant anesthetic, or to allow effective artificial ventilation.

Techniques for passing ET tubes vary among species. In horses and cattle, species with long heads and soft palates, endotracheal intubation is often done blindly. The unconscious animal's head and neck are extended to give a straighter path into the larynx, and the ET tube is lubricated and gently inserted into the animal's mouth. It is then slowly advanced until it passes through the glottis and into the trachea. The long, soft palate forces the tip of the tube ventrally, so it usually enters the glottis on the first try.

The soft palates of dogs and cats are generally too short for the blind technique to work. They are usually intubated with the help of an instrument called a **laryngoscope**. A laryngoscope consists of a battery-containing handle to which is attached a long, narrow blade with a small light source near the end. With the animal's head and neck extended, the laryngoscope blade is introduced into the mouth and advanced caudally until the epiglottis is identified. The tip of the laryngoscope blade is used gently to press the tip of the epiglottis ventrally. Once the epiglottis is out of the way, the arytenoid cartilages can be seen forming the entrance into the glottis. The tip of the lubricated ET tube is directed between the cartilages and down into the trachea.

If the ET tube has an inflatable cuff (to provide a leak-proof seal), the cuff is positioned just beyond the larynx to avoid passing the tube too far down into the trachea. If an ET tube is inserted too far, its tip can enter one of the two main bronchi. This can cause the other lung to collapse because it does not receive any air.

In dogs, endotracheal intubation is usually just that simple. They generally have a large larynx that is easy to pass an ET tube into. A cat, however, usually has a more sensitive larynx. As soon as an ET tube touches any part of the glottis, it typically slams shut—a condition called **laryngospasm**. The purpose of this reflex is to prevent anything but air from entering the larynx. The way to get the tube through the sensitive opening is either to time the insertion of the tube for when the opening is of maximum size, during expiration, or to apply a small amount of local anesthetic to the glottis. This numbs the surface and temporarily eliminates the protective laryngospasm reflex.

## Roaring in Horses

An abnormal respiratory condition that is sometimes seen in horses is called *roaring,* which is the common name for **laryngeal hemiplegia**. *Hemi* means "half," and *plegia* means "paralysis"; therefore, *laryngeal hemiplegia* literally means "paralysis of half of the larynx." Actually, it is a paralysis of the muscles that tighten the arytenoid cartilage and vocal cord on one side (usually the left) of the larynx. The result is that the affected vocal cord just "flaps in the wind" as the animal breathes. It usually does not cause a problem when the animal is at rest, but when the animal exercises and breathes heavily, the paralyzed vocal cord partially obstructs the glottis each time the animal inhales. This produces the characteristic "roaring" sound as the animal breathes and makes it difficult for the animal to get enough air. The lack of air causes the animal to tire quickly, thereby producing what is known as *exercise intolerance.*

The cause of roaring is a **congenital** (present at birth) degeneration of the left recurrent laryngeal nerve that supplies the muscles that tighten the left arytenoid cartilage. The cause of this degeneration is not known, but it may be an inheritable genetic defect. In other words, it may be a trait that can be passed on to offspring by affected parents.

The treatment of roaring usually requires surgery to stabilize the "loose" side of the larynx. The most common procedure is *laryngeal ventriculectomy* (removal of the lateral ventricle on the affected side). The purpose of the procedure is to produce enough scar tissue as the area heals to tighten the affected cartilage and vocal cord and hold it out of the airstream. It does not cure the condition, but it may lessen the severity of the clinical signs. More extensive (and expensive) surgical procedures are sometimes performed on affected high-value animals, such as racehorses.

## Aspiration Pneumonia

Aspiration pneumonia is an inflammatory condition of the lungs produced by inhalation of foreign material. Common causes include oral liquids administered too rapidly for an animal to swallow and inhalation of regurgitated material by an anesthetized animal. It is a much easier condition to prevent than to treat.

When large quantities of oral liquids are to be administered to an animal, care must be taken not to administer them faster than the animal can swallow. If the delivery rate is too rapid, the animal may inhale some of the fluid down into the lungs. The amount of damage caused depends on the quantity and composition of the inhaled material. If the quantity is large or the material is irritating, the damage to the lungs can be considerable—even fatal.

An anesthetized animal must be protected from aspiration of foreign material, because its swallowing reflex disappears as it becomes anesthetized. Anesthetized animals are often positioned horizontally with their heads at the same level as their stomachs, so it is easy for small amounts of stomach contents to be regurgitated up the esophagus into the pharynx. Without the protective swallowing reflex, the regurgitated material can be inhaled easily down into the lungs. The stomach contents are very acidic because of secretions from the stomach wall, so you can imagine how irritating that material can be to the delicate structures of the lungs.

The biggest risk of aspiration in anesthetized animals is in those that do not have an ET tube in place. A properly sized ET tube effectively blocks foreign material from entering the larynx and trachea because it fills the lumen of the airway. Placement of ET tubes in anesthetized animals is always desirable to ensure an open airway and to prevent aspiration pneumonia. However, danger periods still arise even in animals that are intubated. Just before the ET tube is inserted and just after it is removed, the animal is potentially vulnerable to aspiration of liquids from the mouth, throat, or stomach. We must monitor animals closely during these periods.

## TRACHEA

The *trachea,* or windpipe, is a short, wide tube that extends from the larynx down through the neck region into the thorax, where it divides into the two main bronchi that enter the lungs. This division, called the **bifurcation of the trachea**, occurs at about the level of the base of the heart. Structurally, the trachea is a tube of fibrous tissue and smooth muscle held open by hyaline cartilage rings and lined by the same kind of ciliated epithelium that is present in the nasal passages. It is shaped like an upside-down Y. The main part of the trachea forms the base of the Y, and the bifurcation forms the arms of the arms of the Y (the left and right main bronchi that enter the lungs).

If nothing held the trachea open, it would collapse each time the animal inhaled as a result of the partial vacuum created by the inhalation process. Incomplete rings of hyaline cartilage spaced along the length of the trachea prevent this collapse. Each tracheal ring is C-shaped with the open part of the C facing dorsally. The gap between the ends of each ring is bridged by smooth muscle (Figure 15-5).

The ciliated lining of the trachea is similar to that of the nasal passages. The mucous layer on its surface traps tiny particles of debris that have made it down this far into the respiratory tube. The cilia that project up into the mucous layer move the trapped material up toward the larynx. It eventually reaches the pharynx and is swallowed. If large amounts of debris are inhaled, such as might occur in a dusty environment, an increased amount of mucus is produced to help trap the foreign particles. The increased mucus accumulation irritates the lining of the trachea and stimulates coughing to help clear the passageway.

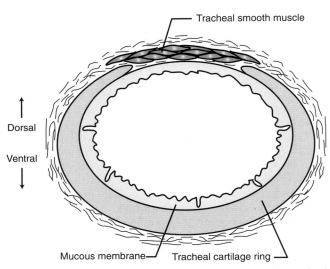

FIGURE 15-5 Cross section of canine trachea. Note that tracheal cartilage ring is incomplete dorsally.

 **CLINICAL APPLICATION**

## Tracheal Collapse

Tracheal collapse is a condition seen most commonly in toy and miniature breeds of dog. The cause is unknown, but what happens is that the usually narrow space between the ends of several of the C-shaped tracheal rings is wider than normal. When the animal inhales, the widened area of smooth muscle gets sucked down into the lumen of the trachea and partially blocks it. This can cause a dry, honking cough and difficulty breathing (dyspnea). Because the soft tissue gets sucked down into the tracheal lumen mainly during inspiration, the breathing difficulty can be described as an *inspiratory dyspnea* (the animal has difficulty inhaling air). The clinical signs are often most severe when the animal is breathing hard from excitement or exercise. Affected animals are commonly overweight.

Therapy for tracheal collapse includes weight loss in obese animals, exercise restriction, reduction of excitement and stress, medical therapy to help control clinical signs, and surgical procedures that help hold the affected area of the trachea open.

## LOWER RESPIRATORY TRACT

The lower respiratory tract starts with the **bronchi**, ends with the **alveoli,** and includes all the air passageways in between. Except for the two main bronchi that are formed by the bifurcation of the trachea, all the structures of the lower portion of the respiratory tract are located within the lungs.

### BRONCHIAL TREE

The air passageways that lead from the bronchi to the alveoli are often called the **bronchial tree,** because they divide into smaller and smaller passageways much like the branching of a tree. Figure 15-6 gives an impression of the branching of

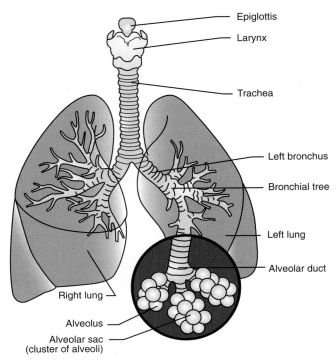

FIGURE 15-6 Lower respiratory tract. (Modified from McBride DF: *Learning veterinary terminology,* St Louis, 1996, Mosby.)

the bronchial tree. If you imagine a bushy tree, the trunk represents the main bronchus that enters each lung. It divides into some fairly large branches, which divide into smaller and smaller branches that finally terminate in leaves. The leaves are the equivalent of the alveoli at the ends of the many branches of the bronchial tree.

After it enters the lung, each main bronchus divides into smaller bronchi, which divide into even smaller bronchi and, finally, into tiny **bronchioles.** The bronchioles continue to subdivide down to the smallest air passageways—the microscopic **alveolar ducts.** The alveolar ducts end in groups of alveoli arranged like bunches of grapes. These groups of alveoli are called **alveolar sacs** (Figures 15-6 and 15-7).

The air passageways that make up the bronchial tree are not just rigid tubes. The diameter of each one can be adjusted by smooth muscle fibers in its wall. The *autonomic* (unconscious) portion of the nervous system controls this smooth muscle. During times of intense physical activity, the bronchial smooth muscle relaxes, allowing the air passageways to dilate to their full maximum diameters in a process (*bronchodilation*) that helps the respiratory effort move the greatest amount of air back and forth to the alveoli with each breath. At more relaxed times, fully dilated air passageways would actually create more work for the respiratory muscles to move air through gently. So, at rest, the bronchial smooth muscle partially contracts, reducing the size of the air passageways (partial **bronchoconstriction**) to a more appropriate size. Sometimes irritants in inhaled air can stimulate severe bronchoconstriction. This can make it difficult for an animal to breathe (see the Clinical Application on asthma).

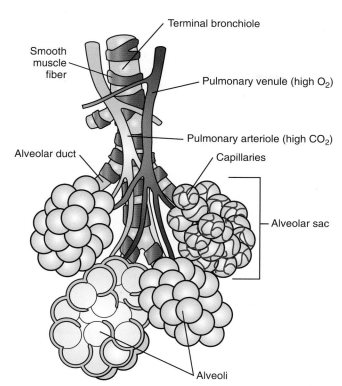

**FIGURE 15-7** Alveoli and alveolar sacs. The smallest terminal bronchioles divide into alveolar ducts that lead to clusters of alveoli called *alveolar sacs*.

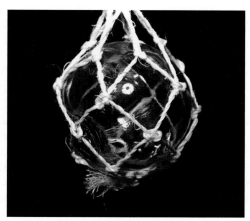

**FIGURE 15-8** Representation of an alveolus and alveolar capillaries, consisting of a glass fishing-net float surrounded by netting. Imagine that the blue glass ball is an alveolus and the net is the network of alveolar capillaries surrounding it. The capillary network around an actual alveolus is denser than this, but this gives an impression of the intimate relationship between an alveolus and the capillary network that surrounds it.

## ALVEOLI

External respiration takes place in the alveoli, where oxygen and carbon dioxide are exchanged between the blood and the air. The rest of the respiratory structures exist just to move air in and out of the alveoli.

Structurally, the alveoli are tiny, thin-walled sacs that are surrounded by networks of capillaries. Figure 15-8 gives an impression of the netlike arrangement of capillaries around an individual alveolus. The wall of each alveolus is composed of the thinnest epithelium in the body—simple squamous epithelium. The capillaries that surround the alveoli are also composed of simple squamous epithelium. Therefore, the main physical barriers between the air in the alveoli and the blood in the capillaries are the thin epithelium of the alveolus and the adjacent, equally thin epithelium of the capillaries. These two thin layers allow oxygen and carbon dioxide to diffuse freely back and forth between the air and the blood. We will discuss how the movement of gases takes place shortly.

Each alveolus is lined with a thin layer of fluid that contains a substance called **surfactant**. Surfactant helps reduce the *surface tension* (the attraction of water molecules to each other) of the fluid. This prevents the alveoli from collapsing as air moves in and out during breathing.

### 🔍 CLINICAL APPLICATION

#### Asthma

Asthma is a disease that causes the bronchial tree to become overly sensitive to certain irritants. Exposure causes inflammation with resulting thickening of the lining of the air passageways, excess mucus production, and bronchoconstriction that can range from mild and annoying to severe and life threatening.

Asthma is seen less commonly in domestic animals than in humans. It occurs most often as an allergic condition in cats that is usually chronic and progressive, and for which there is, as yet, no cure. Mild attacks can cause signs such as wheezing and coughing. More severely affected animals may show severe dyspnea (difficulty breathing), cyanosis (bluish color of the gums and lining of the eyelids), and frantic attempts to get air. Preventing asthma attacks usually involves trying to minimize the cat's exposure to potential allergens and irritants such as litter box dust, cigarette smoke, perfumes, pollen, air fresheners, molds, and hair sprays. Treatments range from emergency treatments with inhaled medications to long-term treatments with bronchodilators and anti-inflammatory drugs to help prevent attacks.

## LUNGS

The two lungs together form a shape that is somewhat like a cone. Each lung is described as having a base, an apex, and a convex lateral surface. The base of each lung is in the caudal part of the thoracic cavity and lies directly on the cranial surface of the **diaphragm** (the thin, domelike sheet of muscle that separates the thoracic cavity from the abdominal cavity). The apex of each lung is much narrower than the base and lies in the cranial portion of the thoracic cavity. Figures 15-9 through 15-12 show this conelike shape. The convex lateral surface lies against the inner surface of the thoracic wall. The area between the lungs is called the **mediastinum**. It contains most of the rest of the thoracic contents, such as the heart, large blood vessels, nerves, trachea, esophagus, lymphatic vessels, and lymph nodes.

← Cranial          Caudal →

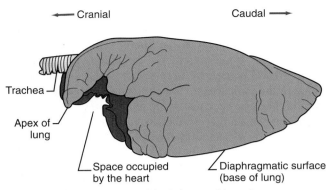

**FIGURE 15-9** Left lateral view of horse lungs.

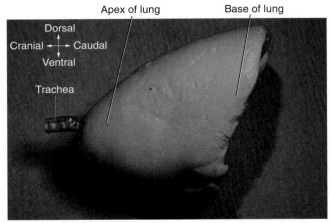

**FIGURE 15-10** Left lateral view of rat lungs. Freeze-dried specimen.

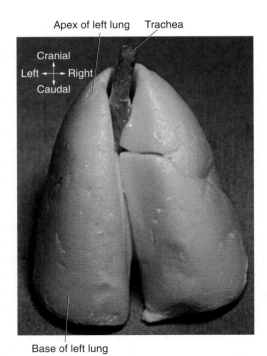

**FIGURE 15-11** Dorsal view of rat lungs. Freeze-dried specimen.

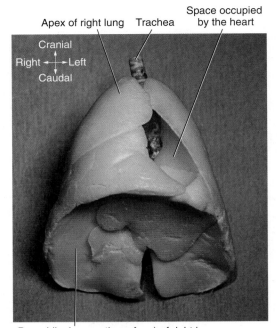

**FIGURE 15-12** Ventral view of rat lungs. Freeze-dried specimen.

| TABLE 15-1 | Lung Lobes | |
| --- | --- | --- |
| **SPECIES** | **LEFT LUNG** | **RIGHT LUNG** |
| Cat, cow, dog, goat, pig, sheep | Cranial lobe | Cranial lobe |
| | Middle lobe | Middle lobe |
| | Caudal lobe | Caudal lobe |
| | | Accessory lobe |
| Horse | Cranial lobe | Cranial lobe |
| | Caudal lobe | Caudal lobe |
| | | Accessory lobe |

The lungs are subdivided into sections called **lobes**. There are two ways to distinguish the lobes: (1) by externally visible grooves and clefts and (2) by the internal major branches of the bronchi. The external divisions are easiest to see with the naked eye, so we will use them as our examples. In some species the clefts between the lobes are pronounced and easy to see. In others they are more subtle. The pattern of lung lobes is fairly consistent among most of the common domestic species. Cats, cattle, dogs, goats, pigs, and sheep all have the same basic arrangement of lung lobes. The left lung has three lobes: *cranial, middle,* and *caudal.* The right lung is divided into four lobes: *cranial, middle, caudal,* and a small *accessory* lobe. The horse is somewhat unique in that it has two poorly defined lobes in its left lung, the *cranial* and *caudal* lobes, and three in its right lung, the *cranial, caudal,* and *accessory* lobes (Table 15-1 and Figure 15-9).

Each lung has a small, well-defined area on its medial side called the **hilus**. This is where air, blood, lymph, and nerves enter and leave the lung, and it is the only area of the lung that is "fastened in place." The rest of the lung is free within the thorax. This physical arrangement is important to lung function. (We will discuss this in more detail shortly.)

The blood supply to and from the lungs is called the *pulmonary circulation.* (The term **pulmonary** refers to the lungs.) Blood enters the lungs through the pulmonary artery. The blood in this large blood vessel is dark red because it contains very little oxygen but a lot of carbon dioxide. It has returned to the heart in the large systemic veins after delivering oxygen to the body's cells and picking up the carbon dioxide that was produced. This $CO_2$-rich blood enters the right side of the heart and is pumped out into the pulmonary artery by the right ventricle. The pulmonary artery splits into left and right pulmonary arteries that enter the two lungs.

Within the lungs, the blood vessels basically follow and subdivide along with the bronchial tree. Figure 15-7 shows the smallest pulmonary blood vessels as blood from pulmonary arterioles enters capillary networks around the alveoli. This is where the blood gets rid of its $CO_2$ and picks up $O_2$. Next it enters the pulmonary venules. The blood in the venules is bright red because of its high $O_2$ content and low $CO_2$ content. The venules join together into increasingly larger veins, eventually forming the large pulmonary veins that leave each lung and enter the left side of the heart. From there, this $O_2$-rich blood is pumped back out into the systemic circulation to supply the body's cells with oxygen and carry away their carbon dioxide.

Physically the lungs are very light and have a spongy consistency. Before birth the lungs of a fetus are nonfunctional because the fetus floats in fluid as it develops. The structures of the lungs develop along with the rest of the fetus, but until birth, the alveoli do not expand into their saclike shapes. The fetal lungs have a solid consistency, much like liver. If a piece of lung from a fetus that has never breathed air is dropped into water, it will sink. Once an animal is born and takes its first breaths, the lungs expand, and surfactant in the alveolar fluid prevents the expanded alveoli from collapsing again. In those first few moments after birth, the lungs of the breathing newborn change from a dense, solid consistency to the light, spongy consistency we usually associate with the lungs. If a piece of lung from an animal that has taken even one breath is dropped into water, it will float. This technique is sometimes used to determine whether a dead newborn animal was born alive and subsequently died or was born dead.

## THORAX

The *thorax,* also known as the **thoracic cavity,** is the chest cavity. It is bounded by the thoracic vertebrae dorsally, the ribs and intercostal muscles laterally, and the sternum ventrally. Its main contents include the lungs, heart, large blood vessels, nerves, trachea, esophagus, lymphatic vessels, and lymph nodes. A thin membrane called the **pleura** covers the organs and structures in the thorax and lines the inside of the thoracic cavity. The membrane that covers the thoracic organs and structures is called the *visceral layer* of pleura,

## CLINICAL APPLICATION

### Respiratory Tract Infections
Respiratory tract infections are common in all animals. However, a significant difference is noted between infections of the upper respiratory tract and infections of the lower respiratory tract. An upper respiratory tract infection (URI) affects some combination of the nasal passages, pharynx, larynx, and trachea. Although they can be severe, URIs are generally less likely to be life threatening than infections of the lower respiratory tract. The main reason is the body's ability to drain excess mucus and inflammatory fluids away from infected areas in the upper respiratory tract. The body can cough up the fluids, which are either expelled through the nose or mouth or swallowed. This kind of moist cough actually accomplishes something beneficial and is referred to as a *"productive" cough.* We usually don't want to suppress a productive cough, because it helps the animal.

A lower respiratory tract infection is usually called **bronchitis** or **pneumonia.** As its name implies, bronchitis affects the lining of the bronchial tree. Pneumonia involves the tiny bronchioles and alveoli. In either case, the animal's condition is often more severe than with a URI because inflammatory fluids tend to accumulate deep in the lungs in the small, dead-end air passageways. The fluids are more difficult to cough up, and so they can accumulate and obstruct airflow. Lower respiratory tract infections can be very serious and sometimes life threatening.

and the portion that lines the cavity is called the *parietal layer* of pleura. Between the two layers is a potential space that is filled with a small amount of lubricating fluid. The smooth surfaces of the pleural membranes lubricated with the pleural fluid ensure that the surfaces of the organs, particularly the lungs, slide along the lining of the thorax smoothly during breathing.

The *mediastinum* is the portion of the thorax between the lungs. It contains the heart and most of the other thoracic structures, including the trachea, esophagus, blood vessels, nerves, and lymphatic structures. Figure 15-13 shows the position of the heart in the thorax relative to the lungs. Figure 15-14 shows the main thoracic structures on a radiograph (x-ray) of a dog's thorax. Figure 15-15 shows the contents of the thorax at three different cross-sectional levels. Note the relationship of the visceral and parietal layers of pleura and the differing contents of the mediastinum in different parts of the thorax.

The diaphragm is a thin sheet of skeletal muscle that forms the caudal boundary of the thorax and acts as an important respiratory muscle. In its relaxed state, the diaphragm assumes a dome shape with its convex surface facing in a cranial direction. The bases of the lungs lie directly on the cranial surface of the diaphragmatic dome, and the liver and stomach lie just behind it. When the diaphragm contracts, its dome shape flattens out somewhat. This enlarges the volume of the thorax and helps accomplish the process of inspiration (inhalation). It also pushes the abdominal

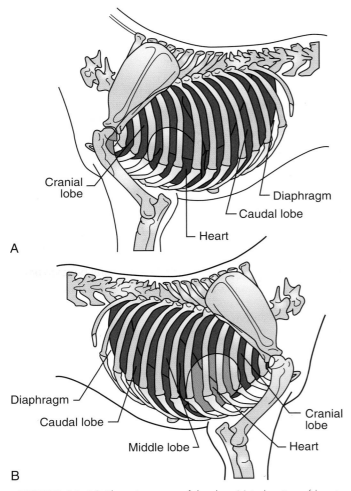

**FIGURE 15-13** Thoracic organs of the dog. Note location of heart at the level of the elbow joint. **A,** Left side. **B,** Right side.

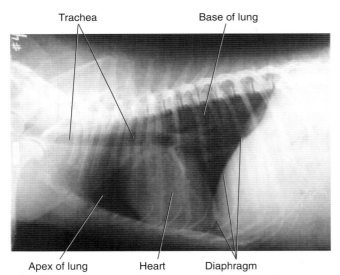

**FIGURE 15-14** Thoracic organs of the dog. Lateral thoracic radiograph. Compare with Figure 15-13, A. The lungs and the air in the trachea appear dark, because they are very transparent to x-rays. Note that the heart is a little lighter in shade and the bones are even lighter. The heart and the bones stop some of the x-rays from reaching the film, and so they appear lighter than the air-containing lungs and trachea.

organs caudally. Try an experiment: Raise your hands over your head. This raises your ribcage. Now, keep your ribcage elevated, lower your hands, and place one hand on your abdomen. Take a deep breath. Did your abdomen push your hand out? This is called a diaphragmatic breath, since it is produced solely by contraction of the diaphragm, which pushed on your abdominal organs. Actors and singers are often urged to "breathe from the diaphragm" in order to have more control over airflow through the larynx. This allows more consistent notes or tones of voice than when the chest muscles are involved. Cool, huh?

---

✓ *TEST YOURSELF 15-3*

1. Why are the hyaline cartilage rings important to the function of the trachea?
2. Describe the basic structure of the bronchial tree in the lung.
3. How do the physical characteristics of the alveoli and the capillaries that surround them facilitate the exchange of gases between the air in the alveoli and the blood in the capillaries?
4. What is the hilus of the lung and why is it important?
5. What is the mediastinum and what organs and structures are located there?
6. Which main pulmonary blood vessel contains bright red, high-oxygen blood: the pulmonary artery or the pulmonary vein? Why?
7. When a piece of lung from a dead newborn animal is dropped into water, it sinks. What conclusion can be drawn about whether the newborn animal was born dead and never breathed or took some breaths before dying?
8. Why are the smooth pleural surfaces important to the process of breathing?

---

## FUNCTION

The process of respiration requires effective movement of air into and out of the lungs at an appropriate rate and in a sufficient volume to meet the body's needs at any particular time. Once fresh air has been drawn into the lungs, oxygen has to be moved into the bloodstream and carbon dioxide must be extracted from it. The "old" air must then be blown out and the whole process repeated as long as the animal lives. The balance of this chapter is devoted to the mechanisms and controls that allow all of this to happen—the physiology of respiration.

### NEGATIVE INTRATHORACIC PRESSURE

The pressure within the thorax is negative with respect to atmospheric pressure. This is a fancy way of saying that a partial vacuum exists within the thorax. That partial vacuum pulls the lungs tightly out against the thoracic wall. The soft, flexible nature of the lungs allows them to conform closely to the shape of the inside of the thoracic wall. Pleural fluid between the lungs and the thoracic wall provides lubrication. As the thoracic wall moves, so do the lungs. The lungs follow

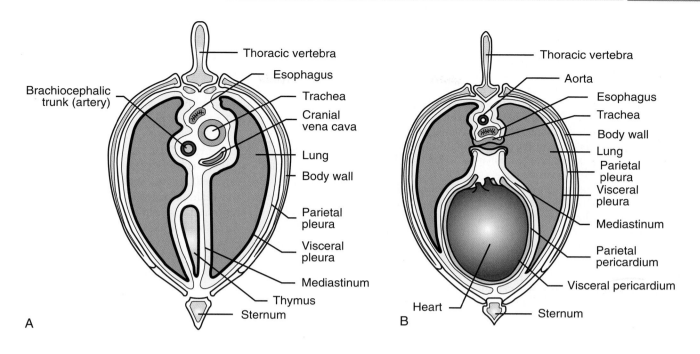

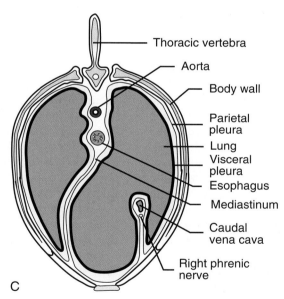

**FIGURE 15-15** Cross sections of thorax showing contents. **A,** Section cranial to heart. **B,** Section through heart. **C,** Section caudal to heart.

passively as movements of the thoracic wall and diaphragm alternately enlarge and diminish the volume of the thorax. The whole system functions like a bellows, pulling air into the lungs (**inspiration**) and blowing it back out (**expiration**).

The negative pressure in the thorax also aids the return of blood to the heart. It helps pull blood into the large veins in the mediastinum, such as the cranial vena cava, the caudal vena cava, and the pulmonary veins. These veins return large volumes of blood to the heart but have no muscular pump to facilitate the process. The negative intrathoracic pressure

helps draw blood from the midsize veins into these large veins, which then dump the blood into the right and left atria (receiving chambers) of the heart.

## INSPIRATION

**Inspiration** is the process of drawing air into the lungs—what we commonly call *inhalation.* The basic mechanism for inspiration is enlargement of the volume of the thoracic cavity by the inspiratory muscles. The lungs follow the enlargement passively, and air is drawn into them through the respiratory passageways.

### Pneumothorax and Lung Collapse

Without negative intrathoracic pressure, normal breathing cannot take place. If air leaks into the pleural space (the space between the lungs and the thoracic wall), the partial vacuum is lost. The presence of free air in the thorax is called **pneumothorax**. It results in the lung in that area falling away from the thoracic wall because nothing is holding it in place any longer. This causes the lung to collapse, which can be a serious, life-threatening situation.

The possible causes of pneumothorax and lung collapse are numerous. Generally, the air comes either from the outside, as in the case of a penetrating wound into the thorax, or from the lung itself, due to the rupture of some air-containing structure as a result of lung disease or injury.

Regardless of the cause, the treatment for a collapsed lung consists of re-establishing the partial vacuum within the pleural space. This can be done in an emergency situation either by sucking the air out with a needle and syringe or by placing a chest tube that is connected to some sort of suction device into the thorax. The cause of the original air leak must be identified and corrected.

The main inspiratory muscles are the *diaphragm* and the *external intercostal muscles.* As discussed earlier, the diaphragm is dome shaped when relaxed, with its convex surface projecting cranially into the thorax. It enlarges the thoracic cavity by flattening out its dome shape. As their name implies, the external intercostal muscles are located in the external portion of the spaces between the ribs—the **intercostal spaces**. Their fibers are oriented in an oblique direction so that, when they contract, they increase the size of the thoracic cavity by rotating the ribs upward and forward. The lifting of the ribs is also aided by some of the muscles of the shoulder, neck, and chest that attach to the rib cage.

### EXPIRATION

*Expiration* is the process of pushing air out of the lungs—what we commonly call *exhalation.* The basic mechanism is the opposite of inspiration in that the size of the thoracic cavity is decreased. This compresses the lungs and pushes air out through the respiratory passageways.

The main expiratory muscles are the *internal intercostal muscles* and the *abdominal muscles.* The internal intercostal muscles are located between the ribs. Their fibers run at right angles to those of the external intercostals. When the internal intercostal muscles contract, they rotate the ribs backward, which decreases the size of the thorax and helps push air out of the lungs. When abdominal muscles contract, they push the abdominal organs against the caudal surface of the diaphragm. This pushes the diaphragm forward into its full dome shape, which decreases the size of the thorax.

Other external muscles can also contribute to the expiratory effort. Actually, expiration usually does not require as much work as inspiration because gravity pulls the ribs down, helping to decrease the thoracic cavity volume. Expiration becomes more work when breathing is fast and labored, such as when an animal is exerting itself. Then the lungs must be filled deeply and emptied quickly. Think about how different your breathing is when you are at rest and when you are exerting yourself physically.

### RESPIRATORY VOLUMES

The quantity of air involved in respiration can be described with some standardized terms, such as **tidal volume, minute volume**, and **residual volume**. The *tidal volume* is the volume of air inspired and expired during one breath. The tidal volume varies according to the body's needs. It is smaller when an animal is at rest and larger when it is excited or active.

The *minute volume* is the volume of air inspired and expired during 1 minute. It is calculated by multiplying the tidal volume by the number of breaths per minute. For example, an animal with a tidal volume of 450 milliliters (ml) that is taking 12 breaths per minute has a minute volume of 5400 ml ($450 \times 12 = 5400$), or 5.4 L.

The *residual volume* is the volume of air remaining in the lungs after maximum expiration. No matter how hard an animal tries, the lungs cannot be completely emptied of air. The residual volume always remains.

### EXCHANGE OF GASES IN ALVEOLI

Getting a fresh breath of air down into the alveoli of the lungs is a complex process, but the actual exchange of gases that occurs once it is down there is elegantly simple. The basic force behind the exchange is simple diffusion of gas molecules from areas of high concentration to areas of low concentration. It's as easy as rolling a ball down a hill (Figure 15-16).

Atmospheric air contains a high level of oxygen (about 21%) and very little carbon dioxide (about 0.03%). When that air is inhaled down into the alveoli of the lungs, it is only a couple of thin epithelial layers away from the blood in the surrounding capillaries. The alveolar capillary blood contains very little oxygen but a high level of carbon dioxide. Remember that it gave up its oxygen to the body's cells and picked up their carbon dioxide as it flowed through the systemic circulation.

So, as this low-oxygen, high-carbon dioxide blood circulates right next to an alveolus containing high-oxygen, low-carbon dioxide air, something amazing happens: Oxygen diffuses from the alveolar air (an area of high concentration) into the blood of the alveolar capillary (an area of low concentration). At the same time, carbon dioxide diffuses from the blood (area of high concentration) into the alveolus (area of low concentration). The differences in the concentrations of the gases (the *concentration gradient*) stay fairly constant because as the blood picks up oxygen and dumps carbon dioxide, it flows away and is replaced by more low-oxygen, high-carbon dioxide blood. At the same time, the air in the alveoli is refreshed with each breath.

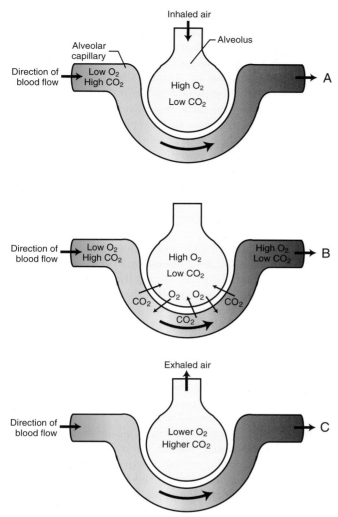

**FIGURE 15-16** Gas exchange in alveoli of the lung. **A,** Inspiration. Inhaled air contains a high level of oxygen and a low level of carbon dioxide. Blood entering the alveolar capillary contains a low level of oxygen and a high level of carbon dioxide. **B,** Gas exchange. Oxygen diffuses from the air in the alveolus, where its level is high, into the blood in the alveolar capillary, where its level is low. Carbon dioxide does the reverse, diffusing from the alveolar capillary into the alveolus. **C,** Expiration. Exhaled air contains less oxygen and more carbon dioxide than is present in room air. The next breath brings in a fresh supply of high-oxygen air.

## PARTIAL PRESSURES OF GASES

How and why respiratory gases diffuse as they do becomes clearer if we understand a physical concept called the *partial pressures* of gases. It really is not as complicated as it sounds. John Dalton, a British scientist, formulated the law of partial pressures of gases a couple hundred years ago. Dalton's law states that *the total pressure of a mixture of gases is the sum of the pressures of each individual gas.*

The pressure of each individual gas is known as its **partial pressure**. Partial pressure is abbreviated by placing a capital letter *P* before the chemical symbol for the gas. For example, atmospheric air contains about 21% $O_2$. At a total atmospheric pressure of 760 mm of mercury (mm Hg), the

partial pressure of oxygen (the $PO_2$) is equal to 21% × 760 mm Hg, or 159.6 mm Hg.

The concept of partial pressures holds true even for gases that dissolve in liquids such as blood. The amount of a particular gas that dissolves in liquid exposed to a gaseous environment is determined by the partial pressure of the gas in the gaseous environment. So the partial pressure of $O_2$ and $CO_2$ in the blood moving through the alveolar capillaries (the liquid) is affected by the partial pressures of $O_2$ and $CO_2$ in the alveolar air (the gaseous environment). If the $PO_2$ in the alveolar *air* is about 100 mm Hg, and the $PO_2$ in the *blood* of the alveolar capillaries is about 40 mm Hg. Doesn't it make sense, then, that $O_2$ would diffuse from the alveolar air into the blood of the alveolar capillaries? It is moving from an area of high concentration (100 mm Hg in the alveolar air) to an area of low concentration (40 mm Hg in the capillary blood). The $CO_2$ diffuses in the other direction because its partial pressure is higher in the blood (46 mm Hg) than in the alveolar air (40 mm Hg). So the $CO_2$ diffuses from the alveolar capillary blood into the alveolar air.

After circulating around the alveoli and swapping gases with the alveolar air, the blood in the pulmonary veins now contains a high level of oxygen and a low level of carbon dioxide. It flows back to the heart and is ready to be pumped back out into the systemic circulation to deliver its oxygen to the cells in exchange for their carbon dioxide. And so it goes on. The respiratory system takes care of the air movement, and the cardiovascular system manages the blood movement.

As long as everything goes as planned, the net effect is that all of the body's cells are constantly supplied with the vital oxygen they need and relieved of the waste carbon dioxide they produce. However, as you can imagine, this system is rather delicate. Anything that interferes significantly with either the flow of air in the respiratory system or the flow of blood in the cardiovascular system can throw off the whole balance and endanger the health and well-being of the animal.

> ### TEST YOURSELF 15-4
> 1. Why is negative intrathoracic pressure important to breathing? What happens if it is lost?
> 2. What are the main muscles of inspiration? How do they cause air to be drawn into the lungs?
> 3. What are the main muscles of expiration? How do they push air out of the lungs?
> 4. Describe the basic processes by which oxygen moves from the air in the alveoli into the blood in the alveolar capillaries and how carbon dioxide moves in the other direction.

## CONTROL OF BREATHING

Even though all of the inspiratory and expiratory muscles are skeletal muscles, and therefore under voluntary control, breathing does not require conscious effort. An animal does not have to think consciously about how much and how often to inhale and exhale. It just seems to happen. Just for grins, try an experiment to put this into context. For the next few breaths, try to control consciously how often you breathe, how much air you inhale with each breath, and how much air you blow out when you exhale. After a short time, your breathing will probably become a real chore. Fortunately, by ignoring your breathing and turning your attention back to reading about it, your breathing will once again return to its normal, rhythmic pattern. So how do the voluntary respiratory muscles carry out the seemingly automatic activity of breathing?

Breathing is controlled by an area in the medulla oblongata of the brainstem known as the **respiratory center**. Within the respiratory center are individual control centers for functions such as inspiration, expiration, and breath-holding. These centers send nerve impulses out to the respiratory muscles at a subconscious level, telling them when and how much to contract. Therefore the voluntary respiratory muscles are controlled by nerve impulses from a subconscious part of the brain.

Of course, this automatic system can be overridden by voluntary control from the conscious part of the brain (which is what you did if you tried the experiment of consciously controlling your breathing). Conscious control usually only lasts for a short time, however, before the automatic system kicks back in. The conscious mind just has too many other things to think about and control. (So when young children threaten to hold their breath to get their way about something, never fear. They cannot consciously suffocate themselves. Their automatic respiratory control system will start up after they've made a dramatic show of holding their breath for a while!)

The body has two main systems that control breathing: (1) a **mechanical system** that sets *routine* inspiration and expiration limits and (2) a **chemical system** that monitors the levels of certain substances in the blood and directs *adjustments* in breathing if they get out of balance.

## MECHANICAL CONTROL

The mechanical control system operates through stretch receptors in the lungs that set limits on routine, resting, inspiration and expiration. When the lungs inflate to a certain preset point during inspiration, a nerve impulse is sent to the respiratory center, indicating that the lungs are full. The respiratory center sends out nerve impulses to stop the muscle contractions that have been producing inspiration, and to start the muscle contractions that will produce expiration. When the lungs deflate to another preset point during expiration, another nerve impulse is sent to the respiratory center, indicating that the lungs are sufficiently empty. The respiratory center sends out the appropriate nerve impulses to stop expiration and start the process of inspiration again. The whole process repeats itself unless some modification of the breathing process is necessary. The net effect of the mechanical control system is to maintain a normal, rhythmic, resting breathing pattern.

## CHEMICAL CONTROL

The mechanical breathing control system is pretty much preset and automatic, whereas the chemical control system monitors the blood and only affects the breathing pattern if something gets out of balance. Chemical receptors in the blood vessels (the carotid and aortic bodies located in the carotid artery and aorta, respectively) and in the brainstem constantly monitor various physical and chemical characteristics of the blood. Three characteristics important to the control of the breathing process are (1) the $CO_2$ *content,* (2) the *pH,* and (3) the $O_2$ *content* of the arterial blood. If any of these varies outside preset limits, the chemical control system signals the respiratory center to modify the breathing process to bring the errant level back into balance.

The blood level of $CO_2$ and the blood pH are usually linked. Earlier, in our brief discussion of acid–base balance, we explained that as the $CO_2$ level in the blood rises, the pH of the blood goes down, indicating that the blood is becoming more acidic. Therefore, if the chemical control system detects a rise in the blood level of $CO_2$ and a decrease in the blood pH, it signals the respiratory center to increase the rate and depth of respiration so that more $CO_2$ can be eliminated from the lungs. If the $CO_2$ level falls too low, which is usually accompanied by a rise in the blood pH level, the opposite occurs; that is, respiration is decreased to allow the $CO_2$ level to rise back into the normal range.

We sometimes see this effect clinically in anesthetized patients that have been "bagged" for a time. *Bagging* is the term used to describe manual control of an anesthetized patient's breathing by squeezing and releasing the rebreathing bag of an inhalant anesthesia machine. Bagging often hyperventilates the patient somewhat, causing more $CO_2$ than normal to be eliminated via the lungs. The decreased blood $CO_2$ level often causes the patient to stop breathing for a while when the bagging stops, until the $CO_2$ level rises back into the normal range. At that point, normal breathing generally resumes. Unless you know to expect this effect, it can be quite scary when it happens. (Do you see how important this anatomy and physiology stuff is?)

The effects of variations in the blood $O_2$ level are not as clear-cut as the $CO_2$ effects. If a slight decrease in the blood $O_2$ level occurs (hypoxia), the chemical control system signals the respiratory center to increase the rate and depth of breathing so that more $O_2$ will be taken in. If, however, the blood $O_2$ level drops below a critical level, the neurons of the respiratory center can become so depressed from the hypoxia that they cannot send adequate nerve impulses to the respiratory muscles. This can cause breathing to decrease or stop completely.

The net effect of the chemical control system is to adjust the normal, rhythmic breathing pattern produced by the mechanical control system when the $CO_2$ content, pH, or $O_2$ content of the blood varies outside preset limits. In other words, ***the mechanical control system sets a baseline respiratory rate and depth,*** and ***the chemical control system makes adjustments as needed*** to maintain homeostasis.

## CLINICAL APPLICATION

### Coughs, Sneezes, Yawns, Sighs, and Hiccups

Coughs, sneezes, yawns, sighs, and hiccups are temporary interruptions in the normal breathing pattern. They can be responses to irritation (coughs and sneezes) or attempts to correct imbalances (yawns and sighs), or they may occur for unknown reasons (hiccups).

A *cough* is a protective reflex that is stimulated by irritation or foreign matter in the trachea or bronchi. It consists of a sudden, forceful expiration of air. Moist coughs, also known as *productive coughs*, help an animal clear mucus and other matter from the lower respiratory passages. They are generally beneficial to the animal, and we usually do not try to eliminate them with medications. Dry coughs, also known as *nonproductive coughs*, are generally not beneficial and are often treated with cough-suppressant (**antitussive**) medications.

A **sneeze** is similar to a cough, but the irritation originates in the nasal passages. The burst of air is directed through the nose and mouth in an effort to eliminate the irritant.

A **yawn** is a slow, deep breath taken through a wide-open mouth. It may be stimulated by a slight decrease in the oxygen level of the blood, or it may just be due to boredom, drowsiness, or fatigue. Yawns can even occur in humans by the power of suggestion, such as seeing someone else yawn or even thinking about yawning. (Did you just yawn?)

A **sigh** is a slightly deeper than normal breath. It is not accompanied by a wide-open mouth, like a yawn. A sigh may be a mild corrective action when the blood level of oxygen gets a little low or the carbon dioxide level gets a little high. It may also serve to expand the lungs more than the normal breathing pattern does. Anesthetized animals are often manually given deep sigh breaths periodically to keep their lungs well-expanded. This is done to prevent the partial collapse of the lungs, which can occur in anesthetized animals as a result of respiratory system depression produced by general anesthetic drugs.

**Hiccups** are spasmodic contractions of the diaphragm accompanied by sudden closure of the glottis, causing the characteristic "hiccup" sound. Although hiccups can result from serious conditions, such as nerve irritation, indigestion, and central nervous system damage, most of the time they are harmless and temporary. Many folk remedies have been suggested for hiccups, but because they are usually self-limiting, the best approach is to just let them run their course. However, prolonged or recurrent hiccups may require medical attention.

### TEST YOURSELF 15-5

1. Describe how the mechanical respiratory control system maintains a normal, rhythmic, resting breathing pattern.
2. What is the basic difference between the functions of the mechanical and chemical respiratory control systems?
3. When does the chemical respiratory control system kick in and override the mechanical control system?
4. Why do animals cough, sneeze, yawn, sigh, and hiccup?

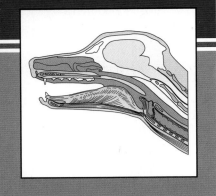

# Digestive System  16

*Sabrina M. Timperman, DVM*

## LEARNING OBJECTIVES

*When you have completed this chapter you will be able to:*

1. List the functions of the digestive system.
2. Describe the epithelial and muscle layers of the gastrointestinal tract.
3. Explain the process of peristalsis and segmentation.
4. List the structures of the oral cavity.
5. Name the types of tooth found in carnivores and herbivores.
6. Describe the structure of teeth.
7. Differentiate between mechanical and chemical digestion.

8. List the structures of the monogastric stomach and describe the function of each area.
9. Explain the effects of amylase, lipase, gastrin, pepsin, pepsinogen, prostaglandins, mucin, bicarbonate, secretin, cholecystokinin, proteases, and hydrogen and chloride ions on the gastrointestinal system.
10. Describe the structure and functions of the rumen, reticulum, omasum, and abomasums.
11. Differentiate between fermentative and nonfermentative digestion.

12. List the segments of the small intestine and describe the structure of the small intestinal mucosa.

13. List the segments of the large intestine and describe the general functions of each segment.

14. Describe carbohydrate, protein, and fat digestion.

## VOCABULARY FUNDAMENTALS

*Aborally* ahb-**ohr**-ahl-ē

*Acetylcholine* ah-sēt-ehl-**kō**-lēn

*Amino acid* ah-**mē**-nō **ah**-sihd

*Amylolytic bacteria* ahm-ah-lō-**liht**-ihck bahck-**teer**-ē-ah

*Apical* **ā**-pihck-ahl

*Aradicular hypsodont* ā-rah-**dihck**-yoo-lər **hihp**-suh-dohnt

*Bilirubin glucuronide* bihl-ē-rū-bihn gloo-**kyuhr**-uh-nīd

*Brachyodont* **brah**-kē-ō-dohnt

*Brush border* bruhsh **bohr**-dər

*Buccal cavity* **buhck**-ahl **kahv**-ih-tē

*Canine* **kā**-nīn

*Cardia* **kahr**-dē-ah

*Carnassial teeth* karh-**nās**-ē-ahl tēth

*Carnivore* **kahr**-nah-vohr

*Cecum* **sēk**-uhm

*Cellulolytic* sehl-ū-lō-liht-ihck

*Chemical* **kehm**-ih-kuhl

*Chief cell* chēf sehl

*Cholecystokinin* kō-leh-sihs-tuh-**kī**-nihn

*Chyme* kīm

*Chymotrypsinogen* kī-mō-trihp-**sihn**-ō-jen

*Colon* **kō**-luhn

*Coronal* kuh-**rō**-nahl

*Crown* kroun

*Deciduous teeth (baby or milk teeth)* dē-**sihd**-ū-uhs tēth (**bā**-bē or mihlk tēth)

*Deglutition (swallowing)* dē-**gloo**-tihsh-uhn (**swahl**-lō-ihng)

*Dental formula* dehn-tahl **fohr**-myoo-lah

*Dentin* **dehn**-tihn

*Duodenum* doo-ō-**dēn**-uhm

*Emesis* **ehm**-eh-sihs

*Enamel* ē-**nahm**-ahl

*Endocrine* **ehn**-dō-krihn

*Endopeptidase* ehn-dō-**pehp**-teh-dāz

*Enteric* ehn-**teər**-ihck

*Enteric nervous system* ehn-**teər**-ihck **nər**-vuhs **sihs**-tehm

*Enterochromaffin-like cell (ECL-cell)* ehn-teh-rō-**krō**-mah-fihn-līk sehl (ECL-sehl)

*Enterohepatic circulation* ehn-teh-rō-heh-**paht**-ihck sər-kyoo-**lā**-shuhn

*Enteropeptidase* ehn-teh-rō-**pehp**-teh-dāz

*Eructation* ē-ruhck-**tā**-shuhn

*Eustachian tube (auditory tube)* yoo-**stā**-shehn toob (**ahw**-dih-tohr-ē toob)

*Exocrine* **ehcks**-ō-krihn

*Exopeptidase* ehcks-ō-**pehp**-teh-dāz

*Fermentation* fər-mehn-**tā**-shuhn

*Forestomach* fohr-**stuhm**-uhck

*Fundus* **fuhn**-duhs

*G cell* jee sehl

*Gastric* **gahs**-trihck

*Gastrin* **gahs**-trihn

*Gluconeogenesis* gloo-kō-nē-ō-**jehn**-eh-sihs

*Glycogenolysis* glī-kō-jehn-**ohl**-eh-sihs

*Hepatocyte* heh-**paht**-ō-sīt

*Herbivore* **hər**-bah-vohr

*Heterodont teeth* **heht**-ər-ō-dohnt tēth

*Hydrolysis* hī-**drohl**-uh-sihs

*Hypsodont* **hihp**-s-ō-dohnt

*Ileum* **ihl**-ē-uhm

*Incisor* ihn-**sī**-zər

*Jejunum* jeh-**joo**-nuhm

*Labial surface* **lā**-bē-ahl **suhr**-fihs

*Lactase* **lahck**-tāz

*Maltase* **mahl**-tāz

*Mastication* mahst-eh-**kā**-shuhn

*Mechanical digestion* meh-**kahn**-ih-kahl dī-**jehst**-shuhn

*Mesentery* **mehs**-ehn-teər-ē

*Microvilli* mī-krō-**vihl**-lī

*Molar* **mō**-lər

*Monogastric animal* mohn-ō-**gahs**-trihck **ahn**-uh-muhl

*Monoglyceride* mohn-ō-**glihs**-ər-rīd

*Monosaccharide* mohn-ō-**sahck**-ah-rīd

*Mucosa* myoo-**kō**-sah

*Mucus neck cell* **myoo**-kuhs nehck sehl

*Myenteric plexus (Auerbach's plexus)* mī-ehn-**teər**-ihck **plehck**-suhs (**awb**-ər-bohckz **plehck**-suhs)

*Neck* nehck

*Nonprotein nitrogen compound (NPN compound)* nohn—**prō**-tēn **nī**-truh-*jehn* kohm-*pohwnd* (NPN **kohm**-pohwnd)

*Omnivore* **ohm**-nah-vohr

*Palate* **pahl**-iht

*Parietal cell* pah-**rī**-eh-tahl sehl

*Pepsin* **pehp**-sihn

*Peptidase* **pehp**-teh-dāz

*Peristalsis* peər-ih-**stahl**-sihs

*Plication* plī-**kā**-shuhn

*Polysaccharide* pohl-ē-**sahck**-uh-rīd

*Prehension* prē-**hehn**-shuhn

*Premolar* prē-**mō**-lər

*Procarboxypeptidase* prō-kahrb-**ohck**-sē-**pehp**-tīd-āz

*Proelastase* prō-ē-**lahs**-tāz

*Proenzyme (zymogen)* prō-**ehn**-zīm (**zī**-mō-jen)

*Proteolytic enzyme* **prō**-tē-ō-liht-ihck **ehn**-zīm

*Pyloric antrum* pī-**lohr**-ihck **ahn**-truhm

*Pyloric sphincter* pī-**lohr**-ihck **sfihnk**-tər

*Radicular hypsodont* rah-**dihck**-yuh-lər **hihp**-ō-dohnt

*Reticulorumen* reh-**tihck**-ū-lō-r ū -mehn

*Reticulum* reh-**tihck**-ū-luhm

*Root* root

379

*Rumen* **rū**-mehn
*Ruminant* **rū**-mehn-ahnt
*Rumination* rū-meh-**nā**-shuhn
*Saliva* sah-**lī**-vah
*Salivary gland* **sahl**-eh-veɘr-ē glahnd
*Secretin* seh-**krēt**-ihn
*Segmentation* sehg-mehn-**tā**-shuhn
*Submucosa* suhb-myoo-**kō**-sah
*Submucosal plexus (Meissner's plexus)* suhb-myoo-**kō**-sahl **plehck**-suhs (**mīz**-nɘrz **plehck**-suhs)

*Sucrase* **soo**-krās
*Temporomandibular joint* **tehm**-pohr-ō-mahn-**dihb**-ū-lahr joynt
*Triadan system* **trī**-ah-dehn **sihs**-tehm
*Trypsin* **trihp**-sehn
*Urobilinogen* yɘr-ō-bih-**lihn**-ō-jehn
*Villi* **vihl**-lī
*Volatile fatty acid (short chain fatty acid)* **vohl**-uh-tihl **faht**-ē **ah**-sihd (shohrt chān **faht**-ē **ah**-sihd)

## INTRODUCTION

All animals need to provide energy and nutrients to their body's cells and tissues to perform daily activities, ensure the cells' ability to do work, and promote growth and normal development. In the animal kingdom, often these needs are met by breaking down and absorbing nutrients that the animal has consumed. The process of extracting nutrients and creating energy from food begins when an animal consumes a meal.

What an animal eats, however, varies among species. **Herbivores** eat plants. In herbivores, such as horses and cattle, the process of converting consumed plant material into usable nutrients and energy is heavily dependent on microbial fermentation chambers within the animals' **gastrointestinal** (GI) tract. **Carnivores** eat meat. In carnivores, such as the cat, the gastrointestinal tract itself is responsible for converting consumed meals into nutrients and energy without the aid of a microbial fermentation chamber. Dogs have similar dental anatomy to cats. Both have sharp, pointed **canine** teeth for tearing flesh and sharp **premolars** and **molars**, which can be used for cutting meat, but dogs are no longer strictly carnivores. They are now omnivores because they have evolved to utilize both plant material and meat. **Omnivores**, such as humans and pigs, eat a combination of plant materials and meats.

Although domestic animals share many similarities, there are distinct anatomic differences depending on what they consume. **Ruminants** such as cattle, sheep, and goats are herbivores. They have large microbial **fermentation** chambers where the plant materials are partially broken down before the food reaches the true stomach. Nonruminant herbivores, such as horses, are called *hindgut fermenters*. They have an extremely well developed and expansive fermentation chamber (the **cecum**) at the junction of the small and large intestines that allows microbes to help break down plant materials (Figure 16-1). In contrast, carnivores have an inconspicuous and small cecum because microbes play an insignificant role in breaking down their food.

Digestion is a process that begins inside the gastrointestinal tract but, interestingly, anything within the gastrointestinal tract can be considered still outside the body. During embryonic development, the animal starts off as a flat sheet of cells that folds in and forms a tube. The lumen of the tube is what will become the lumen of the gastrointestinal tract.

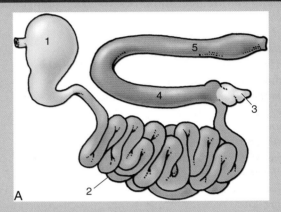

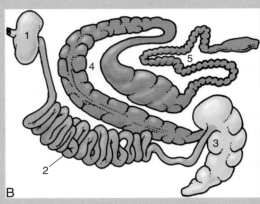

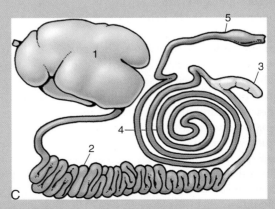

**FIGURE 16-1** Gastrointestinal tracts **A**, of the dog, **B**, of the horse, and **C**, of cattle laid out in one plane. *1*, Stomach; *2*, small intestine; *3*, cecum; *4*, ascending colon; *5*, descending colon. (From Dyce KM, Sack WO, Wenseng CJG: Textbook of veterinary anatomy, ed 4, St Louis, 2010, Saunders.)

Initially the tube is closed at both ends but soon the oral and anal openings will develop so that the gastrointestinal tract essentially becomes a continuous tube with openings at either end. The breakdown of nutrient macromolecules into their more basic parts occurs within the lumen of this tube. Even after they have been broken down into basic parts, the smaller nutrients do not enter into the body until they are absorbed across the intestinal tract wall.

**Digestion** refers to the part of the process in which larger molecules are broken down into their smaller component parts. This breakdown process occurs in two very different ways, **mechanical digestion** and **chemical digestion**. Mechanical digestion refers to the gastrointestinal tract movements, which physically break food up into its smaller parts. In chemical digestion, a chemical reaction breaks the bonds holding macromolecules together, resulting in the production of smaller molecules. When they are small enough, molecules are able to be absorbed across the intestinal membrane and enter the body.

## BASIC STRUCTURE OF THE GASTROINTESTINAL TRACT

The gastrointestinal (GI) tract runs from the oral cavity to the anus and includes structures such as the oral cavity, esophagus, stomach, small intestine, and large intestine. When referring to the stomach, the term **gastric** is used and when referring to the intestines, the term **enteric** is used.

Most of the GI tract wall consists of four layers of tissue, from the lumen outward the **mucosa**, the **submucosa**, the muscular layers (circular and longitudinal), and the **serosa** (Figure 16-2). Within these layers there are some variations, depending on which part of the GI tract you are looking at.

The mucosa or innermost layer consists of its own three parts, the epithelium, the **lamina propria**, and the **muscularis mucosae**. The epithelium, which lines the lumen, is made up of different types of epithelial tissue based on its location. The epithelial tissues near the mouth and anus consist of layers of *stratified squamous epithelium*. The stratified cells make up many layers, which enable them to provide protection. The rest of the epithelium of the gastrointestinal tract consists of *simple columnar epithelium*. These epithelial cells are connected to one another with tight junctions, helping to protect the animal by creating a barrier that prevents harmful or unwanted substances from entering the body.

The second layer of the mucosa, the lamina propria, is made up of *loose areolar connective tissue*. This layer contains blood and lymph vessel, and glands. The third layer of the mucosa is the muscularis mucosae, a thin layer of smooth muscle, which helps form the mucosa into folds that help to increase the surface area of the lining of the stomach and intestines. The increased surface area provides a larger area for absorption of nutrients into the body.

The submucosa, which is not part of the mucosa but lies underneath it, consists of *dense connective tissue*.

The muscular layer is the third layer and in most parts of GI tract consists of two smooth muscle layers, an inner circular and an outer longitudinal one. In the oral cavity, pharynx, and in some species the esophagus, skeletal muscle is also present. There is also an external anal sphincter that is made of skeletal muscle, which assists animals in controlling the timing of their defecation.

The last layer making up the gastrointestinal tract wall is the serosa or adventitia, depending on whether that part of the GI tract is suspended from the body cavity (serosa) or surrounded by other tissue (adventitia). This layer is made up of *loose connective tissue*.

## REGULATION OF GASTROINTESTINAL FUNCTION

The gastrointestinal tract is regulated by two different control systems. The first system involves a combination of the central nervous system and the endocrine system. The second system is unique to the gastrointestinal tract and consists of an *enteric* or *intrinsic nervous system* with an *intrinsic endocrine/paracrine* component. The enteric nervous system is commonly known as the "brain of the gut" and consists of different receptors, sensory neurons, interneurons, and motor neurons. The enteric nervous system controls both motor and secretory functions of the gastrointestinal tract and contains its own "pacemaker" cells. It is influenced by the autonomic nervous system, which can alter its degree of activity. The parasympathetic branch of the autonomic nervous system usually enhances digestive processes, whereas the sympathetic branch usually inhibits digestion. Afferent neurons travel to the central nervous system (CNS) from different types of receptor in the gut that monitor changes in GI tract tension as well as monitoring the chemical conditions of the GI tract. These neurons are associated with the autonomic nervous system and provide this sensory information to the CNS.

Two plexuses make up the enteric nervous system, the **submucosal plexus** (*Meissner's plexus*) and the **myenteric plexus** (*Auerbach's plexus*). The nerve fibers of both plexuses run the length of the GI tract. The submucosal plexus is located in the submucosa and controls secretions and blood flow in the GI tract. The myenteric plexus runs between the circular and longitudinal layers of smooth muscle, and is important in controlling movements of the GI tract through local reflexes.

The GI tract also contains intrinsic endocrine and paracrine systems, which have a regulatory function rather than a digestive one. For example, the endocrine hormone **cholecystokinin** inhibits gastric emptying and the endocrine hormone **gastrin** stimulates stomach motility. Endocrine

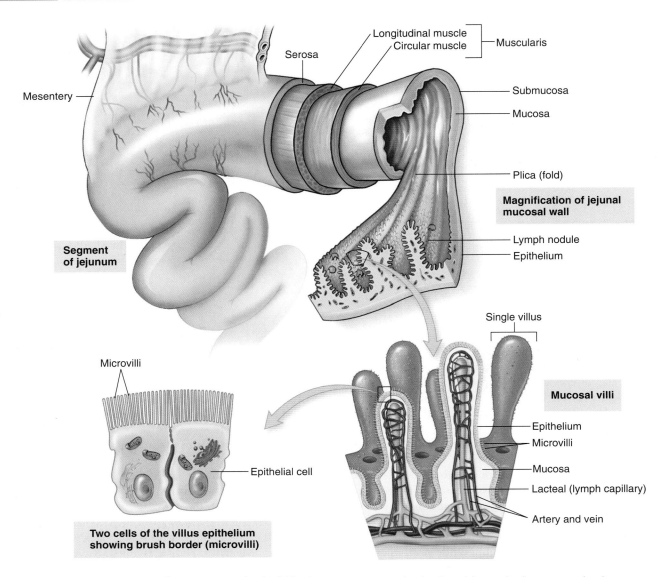

**FIGURE 16-2** Small intestine. Note that the folds of mucosa are covered with villi and that each villus is covered with epithelium, which increases the surface area for absorption of food. (From Thibodeau G, Patton KT: Structure and function of the body, ed 14, St Louis, 2012 Mosby.)

cells secrete hormones directly into the bloodstream and have their effect at a distant site. Paracrine cells secrete substances into the interstitial fluid, which then travel by diffusion and affect nearby cells.

> ### ✓ TEST YOURSELF 16-1
> 1. What is the primary diet of a carnivore, an omnivore, and an herbivore?
> 2. What are two species of animal that require microbial fermentation to digest their food?
> 3. What is the purpose of the stratified squamous epithelium that lines much of the GI tract?
> 4. How many layers of muscle make up the muscular layer of the wall of the intestines?
> 5. What are the two nerve plexuses that make up the intrinsic enteric nervous system?

## ORAL CAVITY, PHARYNX, AND ESOPHAGUS

The entrance to the gastrointestinal tract is the mouth or oral cavity, also known as the **buccal cavity**. It contains the teeth, tongue, and everything else required to ingest food (Figure 16-3). The oral cavity consist of two parts: (1) the *vestibule* is the space between the outer surface of the teeth and the surrounding lips and cheeks and (2) the *oral cavity* proper is the space bordered by the inner surface of the teeth laterally and rostrally and by the hard and soft **palate** dorsally.

The *oral fissure* is the opening into the oral cavity. The lips mark the boundary of the oral fissure. There are both long, tactile hairs and regular hairs at the margins of the lips. Depending on the species, the lips can be very maneuverable

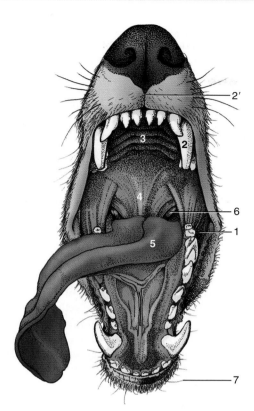

**FIGURE 16-3** General view of the oral cavity of the dog. **1**, Vestibule; **2**, canine tooth; **2′**, philtrum; **3**, hard palate; **4**, soft palate; **5**, tongue; **6**, palatine tonsil; **7**, tactile hairs. (From Dyce KM, Sack WO, Wensing CJG: Textbook of veterinary anatomy, ed 4, St Louis, 2010, Saunders.)

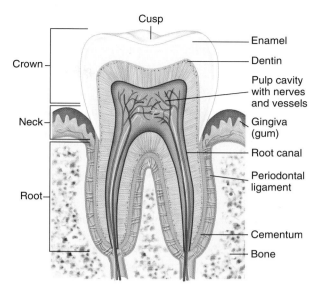

**FIGURE 16-4** Longitudinal section through a tooth. A molar is sectioned to show its bony socket and details of its three main parts: crown, neck, and root. Enamel (over the crown) and cementum (over the neck and root) surround the dentin layer. The pulp contains nerves and blood vessels. (From Thibodeau G, Patton K: Structure and function of the body, ed 14, St Louis, 2012, Mosby.)

and be used to assist the animal in **prehension**, which is the process of bringing food into the oral cavity. The cheeks form the lateral walls of the vestibule. The lips and cheeks are made up of an outer layer of haired skin, a middle layer of muscles and fibroelastic tissue, and an inner layer of mucosa that lines the vestibule and oral cavity. The middle muscular layer consists of the muscles of **mastication** (chewing), which contribute to the biting strength of the mouth. The **philtrum** is the cleft that divides the two halves of the upper lip. In some species the philtrum is deeper and more prominent, such as in carnivores, whereas other animals have a shallow inconspicuous philtrum that is hard to see, such as in horses.

The **palate**, which acts as the dorsal border of the oral cavity (roof of the mouth), consists of two distinct parts, the *hard palate* and the *soft palate.* The more rostral part is the hard palate, which is made up of the palatine, maxillary, and incisive bones that are covered by a mucous membrane. Several elevations cross the hard palate transversely, creating ridges. The soft palate is the caudal part of the palate. It is made up of muscle and connective tissue and divides the pharynx (throat) into an *oropharynx,* the lower area that connects with the mouth, and the *nasopharynx,* the upper area that leads into the nasal passageway. The soft palate is raised to close off the nasal

passage, preventing food from entering the nasal passageway, during swallowing.

## TEETH

Within the oral cavity you will find the teeth and tongue. The teeth are embedded in the upper maxilla bone and lower mandible bone. They are found in sockets or cavities called *alveoli* and are held in place by the *periodontal ligament.* Teeth are important in assisting the animal with the mechanical breakdown of food. Food is broken into smaller pieces by the tearing, cutting, and crushing action of the teeth that occurs during the process of mastication (chewing).

The **crown** is the part of the tooth that projects above the **gingiva** (gums). The **root** is embedded in the alveoli below

---

 **CLINICAL APPLICATION**

### Tooth Resorption

Feline odontoclastic resorptive lesions were first discovered in the necks of teeth, which explains why these lesions were initially known as "neck lesions." Other species can also acquire similar lesions, so the name has been changed from feline odontoclastic resorptive lesion to tooth resorption. In this condition, tooth resorption occurs to form erosions, which are then covered with calculus or gingival tissue. Some affected animals will show signs of pain and discomfort, resulting in changes in behavior or appetite, whereas others show few symptoms. The level of treatment ranges from monitoring with minimal treatment to multiple tooth extractions.

the gingiva. The tip of the root of a tooth is called the **apex** (plural: apices) where the blood vessels and nerves enter the tooth. The area where the crown and the root meet is called the **neck** (Figure 16-4).

## TOOTH SURFACES

When performing a dental cleaning it is important to know what the different surfaces of the teeth are called in order to document properly where a lesion has occurred on the tooth. The outer surfaces, facing toward the cheeks and lips, are *buccal* and *labial* respectively. The inner surfaces, facing the tongue and soft palate, are *lingual* and *palatal* (Figure 16-5). In the space between the teeth, the edge of the tooth facing the midline or center of the dental arch is the *mesial* surface. The edge facing away from the center of the dental arch is called the *distal* surface. Both the mesial and distal surfaces refer to the part of the tooth that is touching or nearly touching an adjacent tooth. The *occlusal* or *masticatory* surfaces are the surfaces on the upper and lower teeth that come together when the mouth is closed. When referring to something toward the crown of a tooth the term **coronal** is used, whereas something toward the root is *apical*.

## TOOTH STRUCTURE

An understanding of the anatomy of the tooth is also crucial in any dental procedure. The crown is covered by a thin layer of white hard material called **enamel**. Enamel is the hardest substance in the body. Under the enamel is the **dentin**. Dentin forms the bulk of the tooth and is as hard as bone,

but not nearly as hard as enamel. The dentin surrounds an inner area called the **pulp cavity** that contains the blood supply and nerves which supply the tooth (see Figure 16-4).

The type or classification of teeth an animal has varies depending on its species. Carnivores, humans, and pigs (except for their tusks) have teeth that are classified as **brachyodont** teeth. They have relatively small crowns and well developed roots. Ruminant **incisors** are also brachyodont teeth. These teeth do not continually grow because the apices of their roots are open for only a finite period of time.

A horse's incisors and cheek teeth, a boar's canine teeth (tusks), ruminant cheek teeth, and some of the teeth of rodents and lagomorphs are classified as **hypsodont** teeth (Figure 16-6). These teeth grow continuously during most of the life of the animal because of a large reserve of crown beneath the gingiva. Hypsodont teeth can be further divided into two different types of tooth, **radicular hypsodont** and **aradicular hypsodont**. All the cheek teeth of the horse are radicular hypsodont, meaning that the apices of their roots remain open for a significant part of the horse's life, leading to continued growth. They do eventually close and stop growing. The wear on the teeth is offset by their continued eruption until growth ceases. In horses, points and hooks can develop on the teeth owing to uneven wear on the occlusal or masticatory surfaces. These sharp elongated ridges must then be filed down through a process called *floating the teeth* to create a level occlusal surface.

Lagomorphs and some rodents have incisor and cheek teeth that are classified as aradicular hypsodont teeth. These

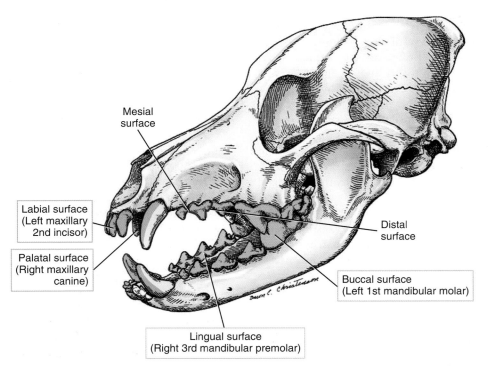

Mesial surface

Labial surface
(Left maxillary
2nd incisor)

Palatal surface
(Right maxillary
canine)

Distal surface

Buccal surface
(Left 1st mandibular molar)

Lingual surface
(Right 3rd mandibular premolar)

**FIGURE 16-5** Tooth surfaces. (Redrawn from Christenson DE: Veterinary medical terminology, ed 2, St Louis, 2008, Saunders.)

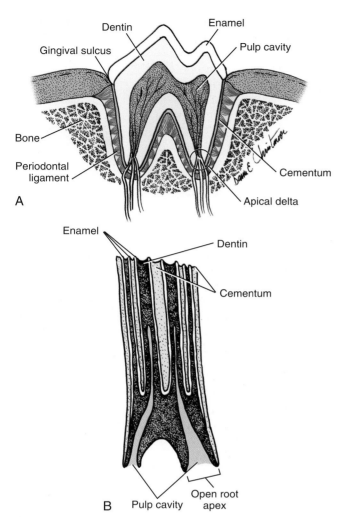

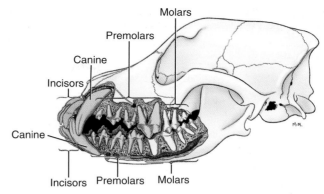

**FIGURE 16-7** Jaws and teeth of an adult dog. Lateral view of the jaws, sculpted to show tooth roots. (From Evans H, de Lahunta A: Miller's anatomy of the dog, ed 4, St Louis, 2013, Saunders.)

**FIGURE 16-6** Comparative tooth anatomy. **A,** Carnivorous tooth (premolar; brachyodont tooth). **B,** Herbivorous tooth (premolar; hypsodont tooth). (From Christenson DE: Veterinary medical terminology, ed 2, St Louis, 2008, Saunders.)

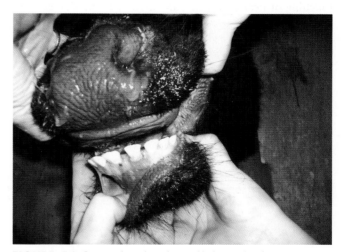

**FIGURE 16-8** Dental pad and mandibular teeth of a cow. (From Holtgrew-Bohling K: Large animal clinical procedures for veterinary technicians, ed 2, St Louis, 2012, Mosby.)

teeth lack a true root and grow continuously throughout the life of the animal. The continued growth compensates for the wear on the teeth. A pet rabbit's or rodent's diet is different from what it would be in the wild. This prevents normal wear, but the teeth continue growing. These animals also may develop points or overgrowths on their teeth, which will require floating or *odontoplasty* (the process of recontouring a tooth surface).

The **cementum** is a thin bonelike covering over the roots of brachyodont teeth and most of the entire tooth superficial to the enamel in hyposodont teeth. The **periodontal membrane** is made of dense fibrous connective tissue that links the cementum with the alveolar wall, anchoring the tooth into the jaw.

## DECIDUOUS TEETH (BABY TEETH)

All domestic species have two sets of teeth, **deciduous dentition**, also called the *milk teeth* or *baby teeth*, and **permanent dentition**, also called the adult teeth. The deciduous

teeth tend to be smaller and whiter. They are present in the jaw at birth but erupt through the gums at different times in different species. For example, in the cat the deciduous teeth erupt starting at around 3 weeks and continue to erupt for about 6 weeks. The permanent set of teeth erupts at around 12 to 24 weeks (3 to 6 months) (Table 16-1). Some animals, especially horses, can have their age determined from their dentition. This skill requires a lot of practice to be accurate.

## HETERODONT DENTITION

**Heterodont dentition** refers to teeth of differing shapes and sizes. Domestic animals have heterodont dentition. There are four different types of teeth and each has a different function (Figure 16-7). **Incisors** are found in the premaxilla or incisive bone. They are small and are often used to cut and nibble on food. In some species, such as in ruminants, the upper front incisors are missing. Instead they have a thickened region called the **dental pad** that

| TABLE 16-1 | Eruption of Teeth in Domestic Animals | | | |
|---|---|---|---|---|
| | | **ERUPTION** | | |
| **ANIMAL** | | **DECIDUOUS** | **PERMANENT** | |
| Cat | Incisors | 3-4 weeks | Incisors | 3.5-5.5 months |
| | Canines | 3-4 weeks | Canines | 5.5-6.5 months |
| | Premolars | 5-6 weeks | Premolars | 4-5 months |
| | | | Molars | 5-6 months |
| Dog | Incisors | 4-6 weeks | Incisors | 3-5 months |
| | Canines | 3-5 weeks | Canines | 5-7 months |
| | Premolars | 5-6 weeks | Premolars | 4-6 months |
| | | | Molar | 4-7 months |
| Ox | Incisors before birth to ≤2-14 days postnatally | | Incisor 1 | 1.5-2 years |
| | | | Incisor 2 | 2-2.5 years |
| | | | Incisor 3 | 3 years |
| | | | Incisor 4 | 3.5-4 years |
| | Premolars before birth to ≤2-3 weeks | | Premolars | 2-3 years |
| | | | Molar 1 | 5-6 months |
| | | | Molar 2 | 15-18 months |
| | | | Molar 3 | 24-28 months |
| Horse | Incisor 1 | 1 week | Incisor 1 | 2.5 years |
| | Incisor 2 | 1 month | Incisor 2 | 3.5 years |
| | Incisor 3 | 5-9 months | Incisor 3 | 4.5 years |
| | Canines | Never erupt | Canines | 4-5 years |
| | Premolars | Before birth or 1st week postnatally | Premolar 1 | 5-6 months |
| | | | Premolar 2 | 2.5 years |
| | | | Premolar 3 | 3 years |
| | | | Premolar 4 | 4 years |
| | | | Molar 1 | 1 year |
| | | | Molar 2 | 2 years |
| | | | Molar 3 | 3.5-4.0 years |

From Studdert V: Saunders comprehensive veterinary dictionary, ed 4, Philadelphia, 2012, Saunders, VitalBook file.

the lower incisors can grind and crush food upon (Figure 16-8). Other animals, such as the elephant, have tusks, which are modified first incisors. The bulk of the incisor is composed of very hard dentin, which is more commonly called ivory in the tusks of the elephant, walrus, and hippopotamus.

The **canine teeth** are located in the maxilla bone and the mandible. They are single teeth on each side of the jaw caudal to the incisors. These teeth are sharp and pointed and are used to tear flesh and hold prey. Ruminants do not have canine teeth. In horses, both mares and geldings may have canine teeth, but they are usually small if they are present at all. A stallion, on the other hand, can have well-developed canine teeth. In pigs, the canine teeth of a boar are exaggerated and open rooted, allowing continued growth. These teeth are also known as tusks.

The **premolars** and **molars** are called the *cheek teeth* and are also found in the maxilla bone and the mandible. The premolars act like shears, cutting and slicing meat from bones and grinding the food into smaller pieces. The premolars of the dog have sharp points. The horse's rudimentary upper first premolar is called the *wolf tooth* and is often missing or vestigial. Molars, which are only found in adult dentition, also assist in grinding and shearing. The largest

cutting teeth in the jaw of the carnivore are the **carnassial teeth**, premolar 4 on the upper jaw and molar 1 on the mandible.

## DENTAL FORMULA

Although the types of tooth are similar, the number of each type of tooth differs with each species. The **dental formula** indicates how many of each type of tooth are present. The types of tooth are abbreviated as incisors (I), canines (C), premolars (P), and molars (M), and each abbreviation is followed by a number representing the number of the teeth of that type on one side of the upper and lower jaw. The dental formulas for several species are shown in (Table 16-2). Upper case letters represent the adult set of dentition; lower case letters denote the deciduous or baby set of teeth. The dental formula lists only half of the teeth, or one side of the oral cavity. In order to get the total number of teeth you would need to add all the numbers up from the maxilla and the mandible and then multiply by two.

Often it is necessary to document in a chart or make a record of a damaged or missing tooth. It is therefore crucial to also have a numeric system that can be used during charting to locate a specific tooth. The most commonly used

| TABLE 16-2 | Comparative Dental Formulas | |
| --- | --- | --- |
| **COMPARATIVE DENTAL FORMULAS** | **DECIDUOUS (BABY) TEETH** | **PERMANENT (ADULT) TEETH** |
| Cat | $2\left(I\frac{3}{3}C\frac{1}{1}P\frac{3}{2}\right)$ | $2\left[I\frac{3}{3}C\frac{1}{1}P\frac{3}{2}M\frac{1}{1}\right]$ |
| Dog | $2\left(I\frac{3}{3}C\frac{1}{1}P\frac{3}{3}\right)$ | $2\left[I\frac{3}{3}C\frac{1}{1}P\frac{4}{4}M\frac{2}{3}\right]$ |
| Horse | $2\left(I\frac{3}{3}C\frac{1}{1}P\frac{3}{3}\right)$ | $2\left[I\frac{3}{3}C\frac{1(0)}{1(0)}P\frac{3(4)}{3}M\frac{3}{3}\right]$ |
| Pig | $2\left(I\frac{3}{3}C\frac{1}{1}P\frac{3}{3}\right)$ | $2\left[I\frac{3}{3}C\frac{1}{1}P\frac{4}{4}M\frac{3}{3}\right]$ |
| Ruminant | $2\left(I\frac{0}{4}C\frac{0}{0}P\frac{3}{3}\right)$ | $2\left[I\frac{0}{3}C\frac{0}{1}P\frac{3}{3}M\frac{3}{3}\right]$ |

Adapted from Christenson DE: Veterinary medical terminology, ed 2, Philadelphia, 2008, WB Saunders Company; Noden DM, Delahunta AD: Embryology of domestic animals, Baltimore, 1985, Williams & Wilkins; Studdert V: Saunders comprehensive veterinary dictionary e-book, ed 4, St Louis, 2015, Saunders.

*I*, Incisor; *C*, canine; *P*, premolar; *M*, molar.

system is the **Triadan System** (Figure 16-9). Using this system, tooth numbering begins at the midline of the upper arch and is numbered as follows: right maxillary arch (100 series), left maxillary arch (200 series), left mandibular arch (300 series), and right mandibular arch (400 series). The first right maxillary incisor starting at the midline therefore is numbered 101 and the numbering continues caudally. The second incisor going away from the midline is 102, the third incisor is 103, and the canine is 104 and so forth. The deciduous teeth are numbered in the same fashion but starting in the right maxillary arch as the 500 series and moving in the same direction. Some teeth are missing in different species but the numbering continues in the same way and the number corresponding to the missing tooth is skipped. For example, right maxillary premolar 1 is missing in the cat so the numbering goes from right maxillary canine (104) to premolar 2 (106). Cats are also missing their first and second premolars on the lower mandible and the

### ✓ TEST YOURSELF 16-2

1. What are the two parts of the roof of the mouth?
2. The part of the tooth that sticks above the gum line is the __. It is covered with __.
3. What substance makes up the bulk of a tooth?
4. The inside surface of a tooth that faces the tongue is the __ surface.
5. Where is the occlusal surface of a tooth?
6. What type of tooth will continue to grow throughout the life of an animal?
7. What are the four types of tooth that make up heterodont dentition?
8. What numeric system is used to assign a specific number to each tooth in the mouth?

numbering continues in the same way. Regardless of species, the numbering in the Triadan system is consistent so if you know that the left maxillary canine in the dog is 204, you know that the same tooth in a cat or a pig is also 204.

## TONGUE

The tongue is also located in the oral cavity. It consist of both extrinsic muscles that anchor it in place and the intrinsic muscles that originate and insert on the tongue itself and make up the majority of the mass of the tongue. The fibers of the intrinsic muscles cross in multiple directions across the tongue making it flexible and maneuverable, which accounts for its fine and delicate movements. The ruminant tongue is especially flexible and is used to assist in prehension.

The tongue normally lies on the ventral surface of the oral cavity and consist of three parts, an *apex*, *body*, and *root*. The free unattached mobile tip of the tongue is called the apex; the body is the long and slender part that links the apex with the root. The root anchors the tongue to the hyoid bone and the sides of the mandible. The exterior of the tongue is covered by cornified stratified squamous epithelium.

Located on the dorsal surface of the tongue are different types of papilla. Some papillae have a mechanical function and assist in the grooming process and in moving the food bolus down into the pharynx. Specialized papillae contain taste buds, which allow the animal to experience a variety of different taste sensations.

The tongue not only senses taste but also has a nerve supply, which allows for sensations of pain, temperature, and touch. In addition to innervation the tongue is well supplied with blood. The superficial positioning of some of these blood vessels, especially in the dog, reflects an additional function of the tongue: thermoregulation through panting.

## SALIVARY GLANDS

**Salivary glands** deposit **saliva** into the oral cavity via ducts. Saliva is extremely important in the process of digestion. It is composed mainly of water but also contains protein, electrolytes, antibodies (immunoglobulin [Ig]A), glycoproteins, other organic molecules, salivary bicarbonate and enzymes. **Lysozyme**, an enzyme found in the saliva, along with immunoglobulins, helps control the bacterial population in the oral cavity. Some species, mainly omnivores, as well as some avian species, have the starch-digesting enzyme **amylase** in their saliva. Amylase assists in the breakdown of starchy carbohydrates. Although it is secreted in the oral cavity, minimal digestion occurs there because of the short time food stays in the mouth. In pigs, rats, and humans, salivary amylase contributes significantly to the breakdown of starchy carbohydrates in the proximal stomach before the amylase is inactivated by hydrochloric acid in the stomach. Among the domestic animals, dogs, cats, and ruminants lack salivary amylase, horses produce a limited amount, whereas pigs produce the most.

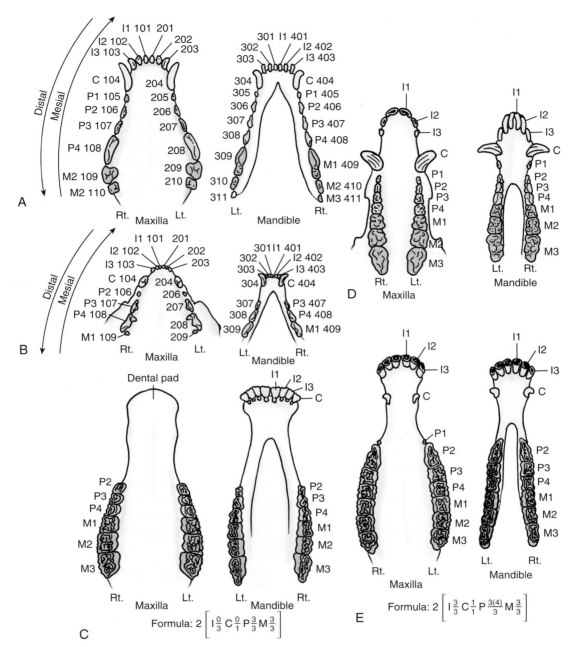

**FIGURE 16-9** Comparative dental arcades. **A,** Canine. **B,** Feline. **C,** Bovine, ovine, and caprine. **D,** Porcine. **E,** Equine. (From Christenson DE: Veterinary medical terminology, ed 2, St Louis, 2008, Saunders.)

Saliva production varies depending on species and diet. Cattle can secrete up to 200 L of saliva per day. Ruminant saliva has a high pH (alkaline) and a high concentration of bicarbonate and other bases that are important for neutralizing the acids produced in the fermentation chambers of the forestomach.

Saliva has many functions including lubrication, antibacterial action, pH regulation, thermoregulation, and enzymatic digestion. The salivary glands are usually paired and located near the oral cavity. There are three main salivary glands, the *parotid, mandibular,* and *sublingual* glands, along with multiple smaller minor glands, such as the *zygomatic*

(Figure 16-10). Depending on the gland, the secretion can be serous (watery), mucous (viscous), or mixed.

The parotid gland is located ventral to the ear and has a long duct extending to the oral cavity. Its secretion is serous in most species and accounts for approximately half of the total volume of saliva produced. The sublingual and the mandibular glands are located under the tongue and caudal to the angle of the jaw respectively, and both secret a mixed secretion in most species. The sublingual gland is divided into two parts in some species. In the dog there is a polystomatic part, which is more rostral and located on either side of the tongue, and a monostomatic part which is more caudal, but rostral to the mandibular salivary gland. The horse on the other hand has only the polystomatic part, whereas the ruminant has both parts, but they are in the opposite position to those of the dog, with the polystomatic part coming after the more rostral monostomatic part (Figure 16-11).

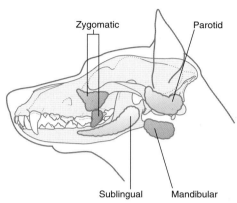

**FIGURE 16-10** Salivary glands of the dog. (Adapted from Aspinall V, O'Reilly M: Introduction to veterinary anatomy and physiology, Oxford, 2004, Butterworth Heinemann. In Studdert V: Saunders comprehensive veterinary dictionary e-book, ed 4, St Louis, 2015, Saunders.)

## TEMPOROMANDIBULAR JOINT

The **temporomandibular joint** (TMJ) is a condylar joint that forms the connection between the condylar process of the mandible (lower jaw) and the mandibular fossa of the temporal bone, which is part of the cranium. This connection occurs on both sides of the head, so there are two temporomandibular joints. The area where the two bones, the mandible and the temporal, articulate is enclosed in a joint capsule, and a thin fibrocartilagenous disc, or *meniscus,* divides the joint cavity into two compartments. The movements allowed by the TMJ include extension, flexion, and translation. The movement of the mandible to the side (laterally) and forward (rostrally) is called *translation.*

The dietary preferences of different species influence how much translation can occur. The cat, a carnivore, has a very different degree of translation from a cow, an herbivore. Many carnivores barely chew their food and instead use their teeth to rip off small chucks, which they swallow whole. Herbivores, such as a cow, have a greater degree of lateral translation. Moving the lower jaw in a rostral or lateral

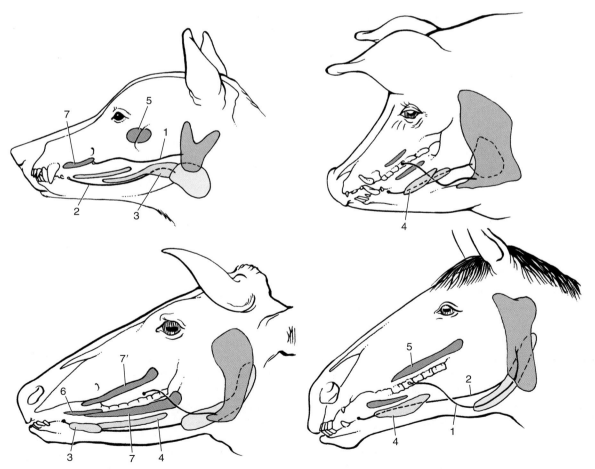

**FIGURE 16-11** The major salivary glands of the dog, pig, cattle, and horse. Orange, parotid gland; blue, mandibular gland; yellow, sublingual glands; red, buccal glands. 1, Parotid duct; 2, mandibular duct; 3, compact (monostomatic) part of sublingual gland; 4, diffuse (polystomatic) part of sublingual gland; 5, dorsal buccal glands (zygomatic gland in the dog); 6, middle buccal glands; 7, ventral buccal glands; 7', middle buccal gland. (From Dyce KM, Sack WO, Wenseng CJG: Textbook of veterinary anatomy, ed 4, St Louis, 2010, Saunders.)

direction increases the grinding effect of the molars. This lateral movement can be clearly appreciated when examining a cow chewing its cud. Chewing cannot take place on both sides of the mouth at the same time because herbivores have a wider maxilla than their mandible. Because of their coarse plant-based diet, herbivores also require more extensive mastication, to mash and grind their food into smaller particles so they can be properly digested.

---

✓ *TEST YOURSELF 16-3*

1. The majority of the tongue is made up of what type of tissue?
2. Besides water, list three substances found in saliva.
3. What are three primary salivary glands in a dog?
4. What does TMJ mean?
5. When speaking of the movement of the mandible, what is translation?

---

## PHARYNX

From the oral cavity food enters the **pharynx** (throat), which is part of both the gastrointestinal tract and the respiratory tract (Figure 16-12). It is here that food is directed into the esophagus through the act of swallowing. The pharyngeal structures are crucial in directing food into the esophagus while at the same time preventing food from entering the larynx and trachea. The **epiglottis** is the part of the laryngeal cartilage that covers the glottis during the act of swallowing, thus preventing the food from being aspirated into the trachea. The opening of the **Eustachian tube** is located in the pharynx. The Eustachian tube travels between the nasopharynx and the middle ear. It helps equalize the atmospheric pressure with the pressure in the middle ear. Diffuse areas of lymphoid tissue called **tonsils** that protect the animal against some diseases are also located in the pharynx.

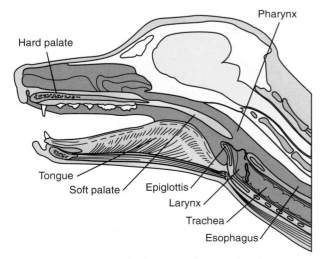

**FIGURE 16-12** Longitudinal section of canine head showing the pharynx.

Labels: Hard palate, Pharynx, Tongue, Soft palate, Epiglottis, Larynx, Trachea, Esophagus

## ESOPHAGUS

The **esophagus** is a muscular tube that connects the pharynx to the stomach. It travels dorsal to the trachea at first, but then moves more to the left as it travels down the neck. After passing through the thoracic cavity it passes through the diaphragm and enters the stomach. The inside of the esophagus is lined by a mucosa that is formed into folds, allowing for the expansion or dilation necessary when food passes through it.

The tunica muscularis consist of two layers of muscle, the inner circular layer and the outer longitudinal layer. Whether the muscle is smooth or skeletal, however, depends on the species. In dogs, horses, and ruminants, the muscle is skeletal throughout the entire length of the esophagus. In cats and primates the distal esophagus changes from skeletal to smooth muscle. Both the circular and longitudinal muscle layers are needed to move food down the esophagus.

---

 **CLINICAL APPLICATION**

### Myasthenia Gravis

Myasthenia gravis interferes with normal skeletal muscle function and movement. It is an autoimmune disease in which antibodies target the receptors for acetylcholine, preventing the transmission of nerve impulses to the skeletal muscle, thereby preventing contraction. Given that the dog's esophagus consists of skeletal muscle throughout, myasthenia gravis causes a loss of muscle tone in the esophagus, resulting in an esophageal dilation termed megaesophagus. Food is not properly moved down the esophagus and the dog presents with a history of regurgitation of undigested food. Owners often mistake regurgitation for vomiting. Regurgitation does not involve the profound muscular contractions associated with vomiting. With regurgitation, the food coming up is not digested because it has not yet reached the stomach. Animals with megaesophagus are fed in a position where the head is elevated to allow gravity to assist movement of food into the stomach. Animals with megaesophagus are more prone to aspirating food into the lungs so they must be monitored for signs of aspiration pneumonia.

---

There is a thickening at the gastric end of the esophagus called the **cardiac sphincter** that functions to prevent the highly acidic contents of the stomach from backflowing or refluxing into the esophagus and damaging its mucosa.

## DIGESTION IN THE ORAL CAVITY AND PHARYNX

In order to begin the process of digestion food must be brought into the mouth. This is **prehension**. Different species rely on different anatomic structures such as the teeth, tongue, and lips, as well as movement of their head and jaws, for prehension. Horses have extremely flexible lips, cows have very mobile tongues, whereas pigs use their noses to root.

After getting the food into the mouth, the animal needs to break down the food into smaller pieces that can be easily swallowed. This is accomplished by mastication, or chewing, that involves the lips, cheeks, tongue, teeth, and jaw. In addition to breaking down macromolecules, mastication serves to mix food with saliva, which acts to lubricate and soften the food.

Salivary secretion is regulated primarily by the nervous system. Afferent neurons carry nerve impulses from sensory cells within various parts of the gastrointestinal tract to the salivary center in the medulla oblongata, located in the brainstem. The brainstem then regulates the parasympathetic and sympathetic activity of the salivary glands. Both branches of the autonomic nervous system enhance the secretion of saliva. In many species parasympathetic stimulation produces more watery saliva whereas sympathetic stimulation produces a smaller amount of thick, mucoid saliva. The parasympathetic and sympathetic responses work in combination to produce the consistency and volume of saliva needed. When the animal is consuming a meal, parasympathetic stimulation predominates.

In addition to the sight and smell of food and the presence of food in the oral cavity, saliva secretion can be triggered by a variety of different stimuli, including conditioned responses. Conditioned responses are learned responses in which salivation is initiated by associating a certain unrelated factor or stimulus with the feeding process. Over time, this association strengthens until eventually the unrelated stimulus alone without the presence of food initiates an increase in salivary secretions. This is the learned response that was studied by Dr. Pavlov in his classic experiments in which he conditioned dogs to salivate at the sound of a bell.

## SWALLOWING/DEGLUTITION

Once the food is sufficiently macerated and mixed with saliva it forms a **bolus** that must now be transported from the oral cavity into the esophagus and ultimately to the stomach. Swallowing or **deglutition** is the process by which food from the oral cavity is transported to the stomach (in simple-stomached animals) or reticulorumen (in ruminants).

The swallowing reflex occurs in three different phases. The first phase is voluntary, which is why animals require some degree of consciousness to swallow. In an animal with decreased consciousness, the swallowing reflex center is depressed and these animals do not respond well to stimulation of receptors in the mouth and pharynx. This is important in anesthetized animals because it makes them more prone to aspirating saliva into the trachea. In stage one, the voluntary stage, the tongue pushes the bolus toward the pharynx.

Stage two, the pharyngeal stage, is an involuntary reflex that is controlled by the swallowing center in the brainstem. The food bolus stimulates pressure receptors in the pharyngeal wall, causing all openings into the pharynx, except for the esophagus, to close. Once the swallowing reflex begins it cannot be stopped. During this phase breathing stops momentarily and the epiglottis covers the glottis, preventing food from entering the trachea. A wave of muscle contraction moves across the pharynx, pushing the food bolus into the esophagus.

Stage three, the esophageal stage, is also an involuntary reflex. The presence of food in the esophagus stimulates the swallowing center to initiate **peristalsis** (Figure 16-13A).

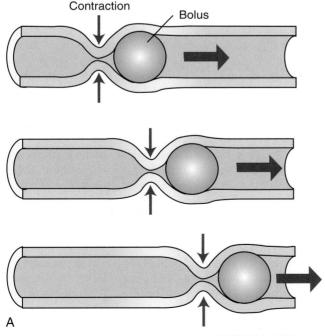

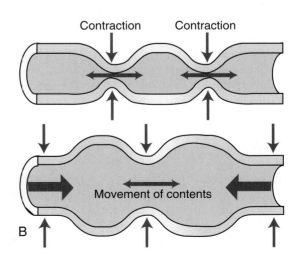

**FIGURE 16-13** A, Peristalsis. B, Segmentation.

Peristalsis is the pattern of muscle contraction, involving the circular muscle layer in the esophagus (and other parts of the GI tract), that propels food through the GI tract. In the esophagus, peristaltic contractions travel caudally, pushing the food toward the stomach. Peristaltic contractions consist of a moving wave of luminal constriction cranial to the food bolus. Contraction of the circular smooth muscle causes constriction of the lumen, whereas relaxation of the circular smooth muscle allows the food to pass through the lumen.

The esophagus travels through the thoracic cavity and diaphragm, then connects with the stomach after entering the abdominal cavity. When the food bolus enters the stomach, digestion continues.

---

### ✓ TEST YOURSELF 16-4

1. What is the structure that covers the opening of the trachea when an animal is swallowing food?
2. How many muscle layers are found in the esophagus? Which direction do the fibers run in each layer?
3. What is the proper medical term for the throat?
4. What happens during prehension? During deglutination? During mastication?
5. Which of the three phase of swallowing is under conscious control?
6. What is the name of the pattern of muscular contractions and dilations that moves food forward through the esophagus and other parts of the digestive system?

---

## ABDOMINAL CAVITY

Within the abdominal cavity, the surfaces of the organs are covered by a serous membrane called the **visceral peritoneum**; the abdominal body wall is lined by the **parietal peritoneum**. *Connecting peritoneum* forms folds that connect the organs to the parietal peritoneum and to one another. **Mesentery, omentum**, and ligaments are types of connecting peritoneum. The mesentery suspends the intestines from the abdominal wall (see Figure 16-2). Many blood vessels and nerves run through the mesentery to supply different sections of the intestinal tract. The mesentery is named according to the organs it suspends. That is, the prefix "meso" is added to the organ name. For example, mesoduodenum is the mesentery that suspends the **duodenum** and the mesocolon is the mesentery that suspends the **colon**. The omentum is a double-layered connecting peritoneum that links the stomach to the abdominal wall or other organs. The smaller inner curve of the stomach is called the lesser curvature and it is connected to the first part of the duodenum and the liver by the *lesser omentum*. The greater curvature is the larger outer curve of the stomach and it is connected to the dorsal abdominal wall by the *greater omentum* (Figure 16-14). The omentum contains a large amount of fat and it is clearly seen covering the loops and coils of the rest of the intestinal tract when the abdomen is opened. The purpose of the omentum is to store fat, and assist in insulating the abdomen.

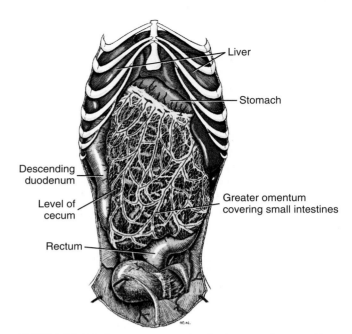

**FIGURE 16-14** Greater omentum of male dog, ventral aspect. (From Evans H, de Lahunta A: Miller's anatomy of the dog, ed 4, St Louis, 2013, Saunders>)

---

## STOMACH

### BASIC STRUCTURE AND OVERALL FUNCTION

The functions of the stomach are the storage of ingested food, mechanical and chemical breakdown of food, and production of intrinsic factor, which is required for vitamin B12 absorption in the small intestine. Given that the stomach acts as a storage compartment, animals such as dogs can consume a large meal quickly and then digest the food over a more prolonged time frame. Food that enters the stomach is subject to mechanical digestion that mixes and kneads the food, as well as to chemical digestion, which results in the disruption of chemical bonds by the action of the enzymes and acids secreted in the stomach. Mechanical digestion acts to reduce the size of the ingested particles, which increases the surface area that is available for the enzymes to do their work.

When the food is in a semiliquid state it leaves the stomach and enters the duodenum, where it is called **chyme**. Chyme is usually hypertonic and has a low pH due to the acidity of the stomach contents. Small amounts of chyme need to be released into the duodenum in a slow and controlled fashion to prevent large fluid shifts from occurring. The hypertonic chyme draws fluids from outside the GI tract into the lumen of the intestine by osmotic forces. If a significant volume of water moved from the vasculature into the GI tract, it could lead to a dangerous drop in blood pressure. In addition, because the chyme is acidic, it requires proper buffering to prevent damage to the duodenal mucosa.

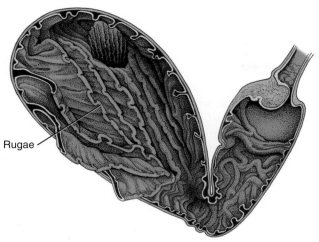

**FIGURE 16-15** Gastric rugae in the abomasum. (From Dyce KM, Sack WO, Wensing CJG: Textbook of veterinary anatomy, ed 4, St Louis, 2010, Saunders.)

## MONOGASTRIC STOMACH AND DIGESTION

Animals can be divided into two main groups based upon their stomach anatomy. **Monogastric** animals, including the dog, cat, and horse, have a single or simple stomach with one chamber. Ruminants, such as cows, goats, and sheep, have a complex stomach consisting of four chambers. The monogastric stomach is a C-shaped organ located just behind the diaphragm in the left cranial abdomen. The stomach's main blood supply is from the *celiac artery,* which is the first branch of the abdominal aorta. Veins leaving the stomach join the *portal vein* that travels to the liver. The size or volume of the stomach varies depending on how full or empty it is. **Rugae** are transient folds of gastric mucosa, which allow the stomach to expand when it is filled with food and increase the surface area for absorption (Figure 16-15). The gastric mucosa is made up of simple columnar epithelium containing surface mucous cells that produce a layer of mucus that helps protect the stomach from the acidity of the gastric secretions. If the surface mucous cells are not producing adequate mucus, this can lead to the development of *gastric ulcers.*

Depending on the species, the luminal surface of the gastric mucosa can be either glandular, nonglandular, or both. Monogastric animals such as the horse and pig have a *composite stomach,* which means the stomach wall contains both glandular and nonglandular tissue. The carnivore's monogastric stomach contains only glandular tissue. The equine stomach has a clear line of demarcation, called the *margo plicatus,* dividing the upper nonglandular half and the lower glandular portion. The pig's nonglandular region is much smaller and located where the esophagus enters the stomach.

The glandular portion of the stomach can be divided into three basic regions, called the **cardia**, **fundus**, and **pylorus** (Figure 16-16). In all three glandular regions *gastric pits* or shallow depressions dot the mucosal surface of the stomach. The gastric pits are the openings of ducts that are lined by glandular cells. The type of glandular cell depends on the region of the stomach. The secretions produced by the

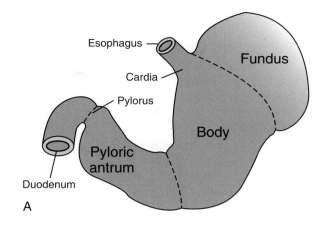

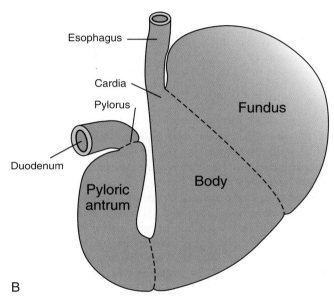

**FIGURE 16-16** Gastric anatomy. **A,** The empty and **B,** the full monogastric stomach. (From Washabau RJ, Day MJ: Canine & feline gastroenterology, St Louis, 2013, Saunders.)

glandular cells move into the ducts and empty into the gastric lumen.

The cardia is the part of the stomach where the esophagus enters and is so named because of its close proximity to the heart. In this region of the stomach, mucous glands secrete a thick layer of alkaline mucus to protect the mucosa against damage from the gastric acids.

The expanded, dome-shaped, blind-ended sac that is adjacent to the cardia is called the fundus. This is the section where the rugae are prominent so the fundus can expand to store the food after a large meal is consumed. The fundus leads into the body, or *corpus,* which is the largest section of the stomach. It links the fundus with the distal part of the stomach, called the pylorus.

The gastric pits in the glandular regions of the fundus and the body of the stomach contain different types of glandular cell, including **mucous neck cells**, **parietal cells**, and **chief cells**, each producing different secretions (Figure 16-17). The parietal cells are gastric glands that secrete hydrogen and

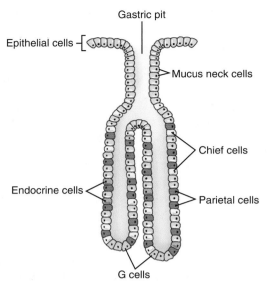

**FIGURE 16-17** The gastric pit—the anatomic unit of gastric secretion. (From Washabau RJ, Day MJ: Canine & feline gastroenterology, St Louis, 2013, Saunders.)

chloride, which form hydrochloric acid (HCl) in the lumen of the stomach. Parietal cells also secrete intrinsic factor, which is necessary for absorption of vitamin B12 in the small intestine. In the cat, the pancreas, not the parietal cells of the stomach, secretes intrinsic factor.

Cells close to the opening of the duct, called mucous neck cells, secrete a thinner, less viscous, mucus than the surface mucous cells and are considered *progenitor cells.* This means they are capable of dividing and creating new cells. The new cells can migrate either up into the mucosal surface or further down into the gastric glands, where they can remain mucous cells or become parietal or chief cells.

The third cell type located in the fundic glandular region is the chief cell, which secretes *pepsinogen.* Pepsinogen is an inactive precursor form of the enzyme pepsin. It is converted into pepsin by the acidic environment of the stomach created by hydrochloric acid (HCl). **Pepsin** is a **proteolytic** enzyme that begins the chemical digestion of proteins. Once pepsinogen is activated to pepsin it can also activate other pepsinogen molecules. Secretion of proteolytic proenzymes such as pepsinogen is essential in the digestive process because the constant presence of the active enzyme pepsin would lead to the breakdown of the very cell that is making it.

The last glandular portion of the stomach is called the pyloric gland region. This region consists of the **pyloric antrum,** which is the area continuous with the body of the stomach. The stomach then narrows into the *pyloric canal,* terminating at the *pylorus,* which opens into the duodenum through a circular muscle called the **pyloric sphincter.** The sphincter helps determine the *rate of gastric emptying,* which is the rate at which the stomach empties chyme into the duodenum. The glands found in the pyloric region include mucus secreting cells and **G cells.** G cells are endocrine cells that secrete the hormone *gastrin* into the bloodstream.

## STIMULATION OF SECRETIONS

Three substances, **acetylcholine**, gastrin, and histamine, stimulate secretions by glandular cells in the stomach. Histamine is secreted by **enterochromaffin-like cells** (ECL cells) in the gastric mucosa, acetylcholine comes from cholinergic neurons, and gastrin is released by G cells. Acetylcholine stimulates both chief cells and parietal cells; gastrin and histamine mainly stimulate the parietal cells. Both acetylcholine and histamine act directly on the parietal cells to increase hydrogen and chloride ion production, whereas gastrin acts indirectly by causing the ECL cells to release histamine.

The *cephalic phase of secretion* begins when an animal anticipates or is preparing to eat a meal. The enteric nervous system is stimulated by a parasympathetic response, leading to the release of acetylcholine. When acetylcholine binds to its receptors, it directly causes the parietal cells to secrete hydrogen and chloride ions and the chief cells to secrete pepsinogen into the stomach and the G cells to secret gastrin into the bloodstream. Gastrin eventually travels to the parietal and ECL cells; it stimulates the ECL cells to release histamine. Acetylcholine can also trigger histamine release by ECL cells. Histamine further stimulates the parietal cells to produce more hydrogen and chloride ions.

The *gastric phase of secretion* begins when food enters the stomach. Glandular cells are further stimulated by the stomach wall stretching. Formation of peptides by protein breakdown triggers long vagal reflexes to and from the brain, as well as local enteric reflexes. In addition, the acetylcholine released stimulates the secretion of histamine from the ECL cells and gastrin from the G cells. Gastrin goes on to stimulate even more histamine release from the ECL cells, which in turn increases HCl production. Peptides that are present from the breakdown of proteins have a direct effect on the release of gastrin from the G cells, ultimately leading to even more histamine release, with the same overall result of increasing HCl production. As a result, the pH of the stomach can be as low as 2.0.

> ✓ **TEST YOURSELF 16-5**
> 1. The serous membrane that covers the organs of the abdominal cavity is the __.
> 2. The connecting peritoneum that links the stomach to the abdominal wall is the __.
> 3. Semiliquid, partially digested food that leaves the stomach and enters the duodenum is __.
> 4. What are the four sections of a monogastric stomach?
> 5. What proteolytic enzyme in the stomach begins protein digestion?
> 6. What three actions result from acetylcholine release during the cephalic phase of gastric secretion?

## MONOGASTRIC STOMACH MOTILITY

The muscle contractions of the monogastric stomach wall contribute to the mechanical breakdown of food particles that will be further digested in the small intestine. The stomach releases gastric contents into the small intestine at a controlled rate. The smooth muscle that makes up the muscle layer of the stomach is an excitable tissue. Specialized smooth muscle cells located within the stomach and intestine act as pacemaker cells regulating the contraction of the gastric and intestinal smooth muscle, similar to cardiac sinoatrial (SA) node cells that control heart muscle contractions. These pacemaker cells lie at the junctions between the submucosa and the circular muscle and between the longitudinal and circular muscle extending the length of the gut. They do not have constant resting membrane potentials but instead have repetitive, spontaneous, slow fluctuations in their resting membrane potentials. When the changing resting membrane potentials of the pacemaker cells reach threshold they initiate action potentials that result in synchronized smooth muscle contractions. These slow fluctuations in resting potential vary among different parts of the gastrointestinal tract and, although they are spontaneous, they can be regulated by the autonomic nervous system.

The fluctuations in resting membrane potential do not always initiate an action potential. Only when the peak of a slow wave crosses threshold and leads to an action potential does a muscle contract. The slow waves therefore cannot cause contractions unless they reach threshold. Acetylcholine from parasympathetic neurons elevates the baseline resting membrane potential, resulting in the slow waves approaching threshold more often. This stimulates an increase in action potentials and consequently more smooth muscle contractions. Norepinephrine released by sympathetic neurons does the opposite and lowers the baseline resting membrane potential, making it less likely to cross threshold and therefore reducing the frequency of smooth muscle contractions.

When threshold is reached, the opening of voltage-gated $Ca^{2+}$ channels and entry of calcium into the muscle cell initiates the contraction process. A greater frequency of action potentials means more calcium enters the muscle cell, resulting in a greater force of muscle contraction.

Each part of the stomach differs in its degree of movement based on the function it is designed to perform. When an animal eats a meal, the fundus expands and adapts to accommodate large volumes of food without significantly increasing intraluminal gastric pressure. The corpus (body) is a large mixing chamber, whereas the pyloric antrum acts like a pump, regulating the movement of food toward the pyloric sphincter.

The peristaltic contractions that occur in the fundus and corpus are weak but get progressively stronger as food moves toward the pylorus. The peristaltic movements fragment the food into smaller particles, while also influencing the rate of gastric emptying into the small intestine. As the peristaltic wave gets closer to the pylorus, the pressure in the pyloric lumen rises forcing a small amount of chyme to exit the stomach. When the peristaltic contraction reaches the pyloric sphincter, the sphincter narrows and prevents larger particles of food from leaving the stomach. Instead, they are forced back into the corpus, in a process called *retropulsion*. This allows for more remixing and grinding into small enough particles that will allow them to pass through the pyloric sphincter.

## CONTROL OF GASTRIC MOTILITY

The motility of the stomach is under neurohumeral control, meaning that both neurotransmitters and hormones can affect the motility of the stomach and the rate of gastric emptying. In the neural component, the nerve fibers of the vagus nerve synapse on nerve cell bodies of the gastric myenteric plexus. This has a profound effect on the control of gastric motility. The motility of the stomach decreases when food enters it. The motility increases as the food approaches the pyloric region. These opposing responses are both the result of vagal (vagus nerve) stimulation. The vagal nerve fibers release a neurotransmitter other than acetylcholine that suppresses movement. Some sources identify this neurotransmitter as vasoactive intestinal peptide (VIP). In the pyloric region the vagal nerve fibers release acetylcholine, which is excitatory and increases peristaltic contractions. The distention that accompanies ingestion of a large meal triggers both adaptive relaxation of the fundus and corpus and peristalsis in the pylorus.

The hormonal control of gastric motility by gastrin is excitatory, but its effect on motility is not nearly as pronounced as its effect on secretion of gastric juices.

## GASTRIC EMPTYING

The rate of gastric emptying is primarily controlled by the strength of the pyloric antral muscle contractions and to a lesser extent the degree of contraction of the pyloric sphincter. The strength of the pyloric antral muscle contractions is a result of interplay between the stimulatory effect of gastrin, secreted by G cells, and the inhibitory effect of the duodenum. When a meal is consumed and the stomach stretches, both local and central reflexes are stimulated, leading to the release of acetylcholine and causing an increase in pyloric antral muscle contractions and more rapid emptying of the stomach. Gastrin stimulates contraction of the pyloric antral smooth muscle and dilates the pyloric sphincter, thus increasing the rate of gastric emptying.

The neurohumeral stimulatory effects of the stomach are balanced by the neurohumeral inhibitory effects of the small intestine. When food enters the duodenum, multiple neural reflexes are initiated that slow the rate of gastric emptying by inhibiting the strong contractions of the stomach and increasing the tone of the pyloric sphincter. These neural reflexes involve both short (local, through the enteric nervous system) and long reflex arcs. The long reflex arc consists of a signal sent to the central nervous system, and a response that results in increased sympathetic stimulation and decreased parasympathetic stimulation to the stomach. This results in decreased gastric smooth muscle contractions.

The neuronal reflexes are initiated when sensory nerve endings in the duodenal mucosa perceive duodenal distention in the presence of chyme, high concentrations of peptides or fat breakdown products, osmolarity of chyme (hyper- or hypo-osmotic chyme empties slower than iso-osmotic chyme), and/or low chyme pH. Not only nervous reflexes, but also hormones, such as **secretin, cholecystokinin** (CCK) and *gastric inhibitory peptide* (GIP), released by the small intestine, play a role in delaying gastric emptying by inhibiting pyloric antral contractions and further constricting the pyloric sphincter. Release of these hormones is most strongly associated with an increase in fatty or acidic chyme entering the duodenum.

 **CLINICAL APPLICATION**

### Emesis

**Emesis** is a protective mechanism that provides animals with the ability to remove harmful or toxic substances from the stomach or upper intestine. Some species, such as swine, dogs, and cats, vomit easily. The vomiting reflex is controlled by the vomiting center in the medulla. The reflex begins with the animal taking a deep inspiration, followed by closure of the glottis and contraction of the abdominal muscles, but not the gastric muscles. The combination of abdominal muscle contraction and inspiration results in an increase pressure in the abdomen. This force is transferred to the contents of the stomach. The cardiac sphincter relaxes and food is forced into the esophagus. *Antiperistalsis* moves the food up the esophagus and into the oral cavity. Antiperistalsis is reverse peristalsis where the peristalsic wave moves partially digested food toward the oral cavity, as opposed to peristalsis that moves chyme toward the anus.

Horses rarely vomit because their cardiac sphincter is so strong and because the angle at which the esophagus enters the stomach causes the stomach wall to push against the sphincter. The cardiac sphincter closes tightly when the stomach is full, making it difficult for it to open from a reverse direction. In the horse, attempting to vomit can increase the pressure in the stomach considerably, resulting in dilation and rupture of the stomach.

## DIGESTION IN THE STOMACH

Mechanical digestion in the oral cavity and in the stomach is essential to increase the amount of food surface area that can be exposed to the digestive enzymes. Digestive enzymes are responsible for the second phase of digestion, chemical digestion. Chemical digestion is divided into two phases: *luminal and membranous chemical digestion.*

Luminal chemical digestion results in large macromolecules being broken down into short chain polymers through the process of **hydrolysis.** Hydrolysis is a chemical reaction in which a bond is broken by the insertion of a water molecule. Hydrolysis is then repeated in membranous chemical digestion, where the short chain polymers are completely broken down into their most basic component parts.

A meal may include carbohydrates, proteins, and lipids as energy sources as well as other nutrients, such as vitamins and minerals. Carbohydrates are made up of repeating units called **monosaccharides**, such as glucose, galactose, and fructose. *Starches* are large carbohydrates made up of repeating glucose monosaccharide units and may be branched or unbranched. *Sugars* can be simple monosaccharides (such as glucose) or made up of two or more monosaccharide units linked together (such as the disaccharides sucrose and lactose). *Cellulose* is a complex carbohydrate, which makes up the structural part of a plant. Mammalian digestive enzymes cannot break down cellulose.

Proteins are made up of repeating **amino acid** units. A protein is defined as a chain of more than 50 amino acids, held together by peptide linkages. Peptides are chains of fewer than 50 amino acids linked together. For example, dipeptides consist of two amino acids, tripeptides consist of three amino acids, and so forth.

Lipids, such as triglycerides, are made up of a glycerol backbone and three fatty acids. Although other lipids are found in food, the majority of the fat found in an animal's diet consists of triglycerides.

In some animals, such as omnivores, chemical digestion begins with amylase in the saliva. *Amylase* is an enzyme that breaks down starch carbohydrates. Because food is held in the oral cavity for such a short period of time, starch digestion by salivary amylase takes place primarily in the stomach. Starch digestion is continued in the small intestine by pancreatic amylase. In animals that do not have amylase in their saliva, the digestion of starch does not begin until the food has reached the small intestine and pancreatic amylase is released. Both luminal and membranous chemical carbohydrate digestion then continue within the small intestine.

Protein digestion, on the other hand, begins in the stomach. Pepsinogen released by the chief cells is activated to pepsin by the acidic environment produced by HCl in the stomach. This begins luminal chemical protein digestion, which will continue in the small intestine. In luminal protein digestion, larger proteins are broken into smaller peptide chains.

✓ **TEST YOURSELF 16-6**

1. Which neurotransmitter, released by sympathetic neurons, causes a reduction in the frequency of smooth muscle contractions in the stomach?
2. What part of the monogastric stomach increases in size to accommodate a large meal?
3. What nerve can elicit opposite types of gastric movement through the release of different neurotransmitters in the myenteric plexus?
4. List three conditions in the duodenum that can decrease the rate of gastric emptying.
5. What are the two types of digestion that take place in the stomach?
6. Repeating units of monosaccharides make up ___.

## RUMINANT STOMACH AND DIGESTION

The ruminant stomach consists of four chambers. It is important to note that the ruminant has only one stomach, even though it is made up of four chambers. The first three chambers are known as the **forestomach** or **forestomachs**.

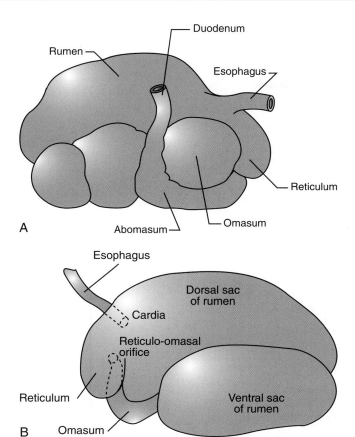

A

B

**FIGURE 16-18 A,** Stomach and forestomachs of a cow as seen from the right side of the cow. **B,** Rumen topographic anatomy as seen from the left side of the cow.

Some references refer to all three chambers as one forestomach, whereas other references refer to the three chambers as three separate forestomachs. These three chambers, the **reticulum**, **rumen**, and **omasum**, are nonglandular. As food leaves the forestomachs, is enters the fourth chamber or the "true" stomach, the **abomasum**, which is glandular (Figure 16-18).

Ruminants are herbivores, and their highly fibrous and less nutritive diet requires that they consume greater quantities of food than carnivores. To digest this food properly, ruminants also require a more complex and involved digestion process than carnivores. The forestomachs are lined by stratified squamous epithelium and are nonglandular, meaning they do not produce digestive enzymes. The rumen and reticulum are where the majority of cellulose is degraded, yet because they lack the enzymes necessary to break down the complex carbohydrates (cellulose) that make up the bulk of their diet they need another way to begin the digestive process. The rumen and reticulum contain a large number of microorganisms (bacteria, protozoa, and fungi) that are responsible for a fermentation process that yields adequate nutrition for the ruminant. During fermentation, complex carbohydrates such as cellulose and hemicellulose are broken down into a variety of different end products such as volatile fatty acids that the ruminant absorbs and uses for energy.

The abomasum functions in the same way as the monogastric simple stomach in carnivores. As mentioned previously, the forestomachs in ruminants such as the cow, sheep, goat, deer, reindeer, and moose consists of three chambers: the reticulum, rumen and omasum. There are other ruminants, however such as camels and llamas, that have only the reticulum and the rumen and lack the omasum.

To enter the forestomachs the food must pass through a powerful sphincter that is found at the junction of the esophagus and the reticulum and rumen.

## FORESTOMACHS AND ABOMASUM

Each of the forestomachs performs a different digestive function, so their anatomic features are different. The rumen is a large expansible chamber where fermentation occurs. It contains many microorganisms that assist in breaking down the carbohydrate substances that make up the structural parts of plants: cellulose, hemicellulose and pectin. The rumen occupies most of the left side of the abdominal cavity and extends from the diaphragm to the pelvis when it is full. This means that the other abdominal organs are located to the right (Figure 16-19). The rumen is commonly referred to as the "paunch" because of its large volume, which in an adult cow can reach 100 L. The ruminal mucosa contains numerous papillae, which help to increase the surface area available for absorption. Pillars (muscular folds) divide the rumen into the *dorsal sac, ventral sac,* and *two caudal sacs.*

The reticulum is located cranial to the rumen and is on the median plane, lying against the diaphragm. The reticulum is also called the "honeycomb" because its mucosa resembles a honeycomb, with its crisscross pattern (Figure 16-20). The contents of the reticulum can enter and exit the rumen fairly easily, meaning that the rumen and reticulum essentially act like one unit in which fermentation occurs. The reticulum and the rumen are indeed frequently referred to as one unit, the **reticulorumen**.

The reticular or **esophageal groove** (Figure 16-21) links the esophagus with the omasum and plays a crucial role in the young ruminant. When a young ruminant nurses, the groove folds in and essentially turns into a tube for milk to travel directly into the omasum and abomasum, bypassing the reticulum and rumen. If the groove did not close, the milk could spill into the reticulorumen, and the bacteria present could ferment the milk, producing lactic acid. This would decrease the rumen pH, causing acidosis, and inhibiting normal microbial development in the reticulorumen.

The next chamber, the omasum, is also called the *many plies* or *book stomach* because of its many leaves, which resemble pages (plies) in a book (Figure 16-22). The leaves are actually folds of mucosa that have many papillae on their surfaces. This increases the absorptive surface area in the omasum, where absorption of water and salts takes place. The omasum is a spherical compartment located on the right side of the abdominal cavity. It connects the reticulorumen to the abomasum.

The abomasum is the elongated "true stomach," lined with glandular tissue (see Figure 16-15). It is located on the

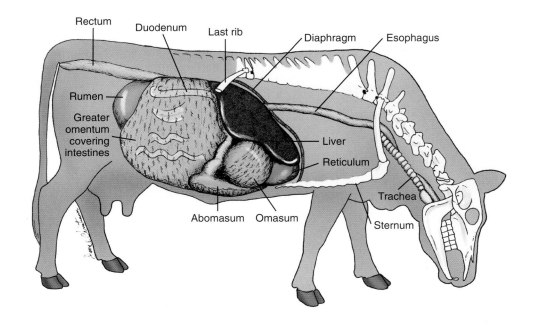

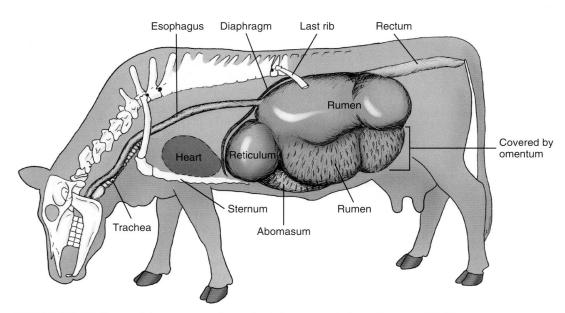

**FIGURE 16-19** Bovine abdominal viscera (left and right lateral views). (From Christenson DE: Veterinary medical terminology, ed 2, St Louis, 2008, Saunders.)

right side of the abdomen, in contact with the ventral abdominal wall. The abomasum functions much like the simple stomach in the monogastric animal, except that in ruminants the abomasum does not act like a storage compartment. The flow of **ingesta** into the abomasum is continuous. As the abomasum expands it inhibits contractions of the reticulorumen, limiting the amount of ingesta that can enter the abomasum and keeping the abomasum's volume relatively constant.

Abomasal emptying is controlled in a similar fashion to the monogastric stomach. The abomasum contains numerous glands, which secrete substances such as pepsinogen, and

hydrogen and chloride ions, just like the monogastric stomach. In the young ruminant the enzyme **rennin** that causes milk protein coagulation is also released. Milk coagulation prolongs the amount of time milk proteins stay in the abomasum, allowing more time for pepsin to break down the proteins.

## MOTILITY OF THE RUMINANT STOMACH

Digestion in the ruminant begins like that in a nonruminant. Food is consumed and the process of mastication breaks larger food particles up into smaller parts, mixing them with saliva to create a rounded mass called a bolus that the

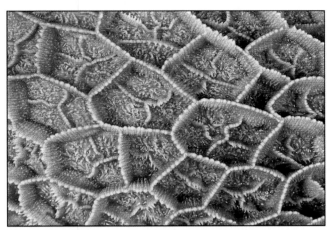

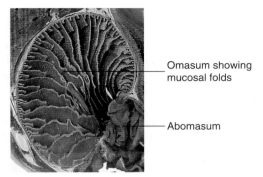

FIGURE 16-22 The mucous membrane lining of the omasum. (From Dyce KM, Sack WO, Wenseng CJG: Textbook of veterinary anatomy, ed 4, St Louis, 2010, Saunders.)

**FIGURE 16-20** The mucous membrane lining of the reticulum. Note the honeycomb appearance. (From Dyce KM, Sack WO, Wenseng CJG: Textbook of veterinary anatomy, ed 4, St Louis, 2010, Saunders.)

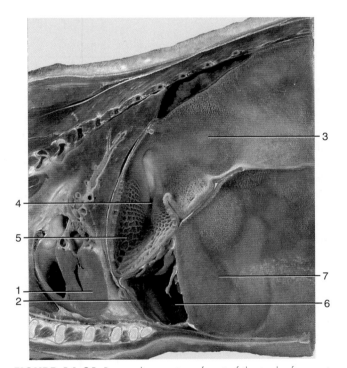

**FIGURE 16-21** Paramedian section of part of the trunk of a goat. 1, heart; 2, diaphragm; 3, dorsal sac of rumen; 4, esophageal groove; 5, reticulum; 6, abomasum; 7, ventral sac of rumen. (From Dyce KM, Sack WO, Wensing CJG: Textbook of veterinary anatomy, ed 4, St Louis, 2010, Saunders.)

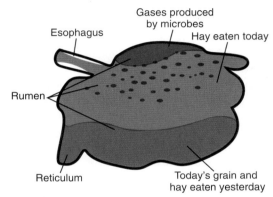

**FIGURE 16-23** Layers of material in the rumen. Grain and yesterday's hay are the heaviest materials, so they have fallen to the bottom of the rumen and into the reticulum. (From Colvile J, Oien S: Clinical veterinary language, St Louis, 2014, Mosby.)

ruminant swallows. An adult cow can secrete as much as 200 L of saliva per day (the adult human that produces only 1 to 2 L per day). Ruminant saliva is alkaline and contains bicarbonate and phosphate. The bicarbonate helps to neutralize the acids produced by fermentation in the reticulorumen; the high phosphate content is necessary for both buffering and microbial growth.

The reticulorumen undergoes three types of contraction. The *primary contractions* or mixing contractions help ensure adequate movement of the contents back and forth between

the reticulum and the rumen. This serves to separate particles on the basis of size: the heavier, larger particles will fall into the lower portions of the reticulorumen and the smaller, lighter particles move to the top of the rumen to be carried into the omasum (Figure 16-23). The primary contractions also provide the force necessary to move the liquid contents from the reticulorumen into the omasum.

The second type of contraction in the reticulorumen is associated with the process of **rumination** or *chewing the cud*. During rumination, the ingesta moves up from the reticulorumen into the oral cavity, where additional saliva and continued chewing help to break down the coarse plant materials further.

The rumination process involves four steps. The first step is *regurgitation*. During regurgitation the reticulum contracts, bringing material from the dorsal reticulum to the cardiac sphincter. Next the cardiac sphincter relaxes, followed immediately by the animal taking a breath against a closed glottis. This causes negative pressure in the thorax, which pulls open the esophagus and the cardiac sphincter. At the same time, the rumen contracts, increasing pressure within the rumen. Pressure in the rumen is now higher than in the esophagus so the food bolus passes into the esophagus. The bolus is then moved toward the oral cavity by an antiperistaltic wave of contraction (reverse peristalsis) of the esophageal smooth muscle.

The process of rumination then proceeds with the next three steps: *re-insalivation, re-mastication,* and *re-swallowing.* During re-insalivation and re-mastication the ruminant adds more saliva and chews the regurgitated bolus much more thoroughly and completely than the first time it was in its mouth. The number of chews is based on the diet; ruminants that eat fiber-rich forage ruminate over a longer period of time than those fed a low fiber diet.

Rumination is completed when the animal re-swallows the bolus. The entire time spent ruminating also varies with the type of diet that is consumed. For example, animals consuming a mostly hay diet ruminate for approximately 8 hours per day. Rumination occurs in a number of distinct periods spread out over the entire day.

The third type of reticulorumen contraction is responsible for the release of gases, such as carbon dioxide and methane, produced during fermentation. This process is called **eructation** and is how ruminants belch. These contractions are known as *secondary contractions.* Carbon dioxide is produced as the microorganisms break down carbohydrates and amino acids. Methane-producing bacteria then use the carbon dioxide to produce methane. Both gases start to accumulate in the reticulorumen during the fermentation process and need to be released, or the ruminant could develop a condition known as **bloat** (*acute rumenal tympani*). When bloat occurs the accumulating gases build up, causing the reticulorumen to expand. The expansion compresses the thoracic and abdominal organs and compromises blood flow to abdominal organs. It also interferes with lung function by putting pressure on the diaphragm. Tissue hypoxia (inadequate tissue oxygenation) and death of the ruminant can follow if the bloat is not treated.

The amount of gas produced by fermentation in a high yielding dairy cow over a 24-hour period can be as high as 4000 L. These gases must be removed through eructation before they can build up. Eructation occurs about once a minute.

Eructation begins with secondary contractions in the caudal blind sac of the rumen. The contractions move cranially along the dorsal sac. They force air forward toward the cranial part of the reticulorumen. As this is occurring, the folds of the rumen wall keep the contents away from the opening of the esophagus. The cardiac sphincter and lower esophagus relax and air is able to enter the relaxed esophagus. The gas is then propelled up the esophagus by antiperistaltic contractions. Rather than producing a burp, most of the gas is directed into the lungs during inspiration and then expelled through expiration.

Although the enteric nervous system plays a part in regulating the motility of the ruminant digestive system, longer reflexes from the central nervous system play an even more important role in coordination of normal motility. There is an area in the brainstem that is responsible for control of reticuloruminal motility. The area is innervated by vagal afferent nerve fibers that receive input from intraluminal

sensors located in the reticulorumen. These sensors monitor conditions such as pH, osmolarity, and expansion of the walls within the reticulorumen. The brainstem sends efferent signals through the vagus nerve to the smooth muscle of the reticulorumen, controlling its contractions. Because the vagus nerve carries both afferent and efferent fibers, these reflexes are often referred to as *vagovagal reflexes.* The brainstem also receives nerve impulses from other parts of the body, such as the olfactory organ and taste buds in the oral cavity, that can also affect the reflex.

✓ **TEST YOURSELF 16-7**

1. List the four chambers that make up the ruminant stomach.
2. Which of the four chambers is the largest fermentation chamber and on which side of the animal would you look to see whether it was bloated?
3. Which chamber is known as the *many plies?*
4. What is the importance of the esophageal groove?
5. Explain the difference between eructation and rumination.
6. What does a cow do when she chews her cud?

## RETICULORUMEN ECOSYSTEM

The microbial species that inhabit the reticulorumen consist of a wide variety of bacteria, protozoa, and fungi that help create a complex ecosystem within the reticulorumen. The reticulorumen must maintain the proper balance among the different types of bacteria, protozoa, and fungi to promote the fermentation process. This delicate balance is largely controlled by diet and how much food the ruminant consumes. For example, when there is an increase in grain content of the diet, an imbalance is created in the reticulorumen. The microbes that break down starch flourish whereas microbes that break down the complex carbohydrates are diminished.

When the ruminant consumes its food, a small amount of oxygen is ingested. This oxygen is quickly used up by some of the microorganisms, creating a low oxygen environment in the reticulorumen. This low oxygen environment allows facultative anaerobic bacteria and protozoa, which are crucial players in the fermentation process, to thrive.

The number of microorganisms inhabiting the reticulorumen is large and the interaction among them is complex, but a ruminant is not born with this ecosystem already established. When a ruminant is born, its gastrointestinal tract is usually sterile. The microorganisms that will one day be so crucial to its survival must be acquired. The young ruminant attains these different microbes by ingesting them from the environment. The interactions that occur between mother and young, such as during grooming, nursing, or cleaning, help facilitate this transfer of microorganisms. By the time the young animal is weaned, its microbial environment is established and contains a large variety of bacteria, protozoa, and fungi.

The different types of bacterium are classified on the basis of what nutrients they metabolize and the substances they produce. For example, **amylolytic** bacteria break down starch and soluble carbohydrates into **volatile fatty acids** (VFA). **Cellulolytic** bacteria break down components of cell walls, including cellulose, hemicelluloses, and pectin, into VFA. The protozoa in the reticulorumen are unicellular, anaerobic, and mostly ciliates. In terms of size, ciliates are much larger than most bacteria. The importance of ciliates in the digestion process of the ruminant is unclear but they do produce volatile fatty acids, carbon dioxide, lactate, and hydrogen from different varieties of plant. The ruminant can live without protozoa in its gastrointestinal tract but protozoa are thought to play a role in slowing down the digestion starches and proteins that are rapidly fermented. The number of fungi that make up the final portion of the microbial population is small but they are thought to play a crucial role in the breakdown of the plant cell wall.

## CARBOHYDRATE DIGESTION IN RUMINANTS

The ruminant's natural diet consists mostly of grasses or roughage and some grains. The grasses or roughage are composed of complex carbohydrates such as cellulose, hemicelluloses, and pectin, which makeup the structural components of the plant and provide the main nutrients for the ruminant. Grains, also known as concentrates, are primarily composed of carbohydrates that are nonstructural. These nonstructural carbohydrates include energy stored in the form of starches, fructosans (hydrolyzed to fructose), and simple sugars. Although most mammals produce enzymes that are capable of breaking down starches and soluble sugars, there are no known mammalian enzymes that can break down complex carbohydrates. In order to survive on their fibrous diet, ruminants have evolved a symbiotic relationship with the microorganisms living in their digestive systems. The microorganisms use the nutrients the ruminant consumes for their own growth and development. The microorganisms then produce their own end or waste products that ruminants can use for their own growth and development. In addition the ruminant can digest the microorganisms themselves as a source of protein.

In the reticulorumen, cellulase enzymes bound to the surfaces of cellulolytic bacteria break down complex carbohydrates through hydrolysis, releasing specific monosaccharides (simple sugars) such as glucose and less complex **polysaccharides** (multiple sugars linked together). Starches and soluble sugars are also broken down into monosaccharides and polysaccharides through hydrolysis by the amylolytic bacteria. These initial steps do not take place in the microorganisms and the saccharides released are not immediately available to the ruminant. Instead, the saccharides are absorbed by the microorganisms and further metabolized to pyruvate. As this process is occurring nicotinamide adenine dinucleotide (NAD) is reduced to NAD hydrogen (NADH) and two molecules of adenosine triphosphate (ATP) are produced. Because the reticulorumen has an anaerobic environment, the pyruvate is converted into volatile fatty acids

(VFAs) such as *acetic acid (acetate), propionic acid (propionate),* and *butyric acid (butyrate).*

When an animal consumes a diet high in starch, the total production of VFAs is increased, the proportion of propionate is increased, and the VFAs are produced faster than when a diet is high in fiber. This illustrates what a profound effect feed composition has on VFA production.

The VFAs that are produced in the forestomachs are absorbed into the blood. Most of the VFAs are absorbed from the reticulorumen, some from the omasum and abomasum, and the last small bit of absorption is completed in the small intestine. The VFAs are the main source of energy for the ruminant, functioning in the same role as glucose for monogastric animals.

## LIPID DIGESTION IN RUMINANTS

Lipids constitute a small portion of the diet of ruminants. Diets with too many lipids result in decreased appetite, reduced motility of the reticulorumen, and decreased fermentation of cellulose. Lipids can be found in grasses and plants in the form of triglycerides, glycolipids, and a small amount of free fatty acids.

Microorganisms in the reticulorumen rapidly hydrolyze triglycerides. During this process free fatty acids are separated from the glycerol backbone of the triglyceride. The glycerol then goes through the process of fermentation, producing VFAs, whereas most of the fatty acids go through the process of hydrogenation. The hydrogenated fatty acids leave the stomach and are absorbed in the small intestine. The absorbed fatty acids are ultimately used by the ruminant to produce energy or are stored.

## PROTEIN DIGESTION IN RUMINANTS

In the ruminant, ingested food travels through the reticulorumen and then moves into the omasum and abomasum. This means the fermentation process occurs before enzymatic digestion and that the nutrients in the food are first available to the microbes living in the reticulorumen. A majority of the protein in the ruminant's diet is actually degraded and used by the microorganisms to meet their own metabolic needs. **Peptidases** released by rumen bacteria break down proteins to form small peptide chains. These small peptide chains are then absorbed by the microorganisms and further hydrolyzed inside the cell, culminating in the production of amino acids. Some of the amino acids are used by the bacteria to create microbial proteins. If the amino acids are not used to make microbial proteins, they can be further broken by the microbes, which deaminate the amino acids into ammonium. Ammonium is ultimately used to produce VFAs, which are required by some microbes as growth factors.

Breakdown of peptides by extracellular peptidase is only one way in which microbial amino acids are produced, however. Microbes can make amino acids from ammonium. In turn, ammonium can be produced by microbes not only through deamination of amino acids, but also by conversion of **non-protein nitrogen (NPN) compounds.** These NPN compounds may be endogenous, such as urea, or found in the diet as nitrates. Ruminants ingest nitrates because they are used as plant fertilizers. In fact, NPN compounds are sometimes added to a ruminant diet because this is cheaper than adding more expensive dietary protein. The microorganisms in the reticulorumen are then required to synthesize the protein needed.

In the ruminant, proteins synthesized by microbes are transported to the small intestine where they are broken down by proteolytic enzymes in a similar fashion to that in the carnivore small intestine. Bypass proteins, which are proteins that pass through the forestomachs unaltered, are also degraded enzymatically in the small intestine. The end products of protein breakdown are amino acids, which are absorbed across the intestinal mucosa into the bloodstream and transported to the liver. In the liver, the absorbed amino acids can be metabolized to make proteins. As the amino acids are metabolized, urea is produced as a waste product. The liver also produces urea from endogenous proteins as well as from ammonium absorbed from the rumen. In monogastric animals the kidneys are responsible for excreting urea but in the ruminant the urea travels back to the rumen and ultimately the saliva, where it is available to be used by the microbes once again to make microbial proteins.

## GLUCOSE PRODUCTION IN RUMINANTS

In the ruminant, fermentation in the reticulorumen occurs before enzymatic digestion in the small intestine. The ruminal microbes process most carbohydrates and proteins before they are exposed to the intestinal digestive enzymes. In fact, almost no ingested carbohydrates make it to the small intestine. This prevents their exposure to intestinal digestive enzymes and subsequent breakdown into monosaccharides. As a result, the ruminant is constantly faced with a potential glucose deficiency.

Although the ruminant receives most of its energy from metabolizing the VFAs produced by microbes, a source of glucose is still required by some tissues. To meet this need, the ruminant has developed a very effective method of producing and conserving glucose. Almost all of the glucose the ruminant needs is made through **gluconeogenesis**, production of glucose by the liver from noncarbohydrate sources. In the case of the ruminant, the noncarbohydrate source is the VFA propionate.

Propionate, a waste product of microbial metabolism, is absorbed from the rumen into the blood and travels directly to the liver where it is used to make glucose. Propionate never enters the systemic circulation. Most butyric acid, another VFA, is absorbed and metabolized by the liver into beta-hydroxybutyrate, a ketone. This molecule is easily metabolized by most tissues in the body but cannot be used to make glucose. Acetate, which is the most abundant VFA in the circulation, is absorbed and passes through the liver mostly unchanged, but it also cannot be used to make glucose. Both acetate and butyric acid are used in the mammary gland to synthesize fatty acids.

Propionate is not the only substance to undergo gluconeogenesis. Amino acids that are absorbed from the intestinal tract can also be used to make glucose through gluconeogenesis.

Producing glucose more efficiently is only one of the strategies that the ruminant uses to ensure adequate glucose levels. The other strategy involves conserving glucose more effectively. In the ruminant, glucose is not used to make fatty acids. Fatty acids are made in adipose tissue from acetate rather than in the liver as in other species. In the ruminant this frees up glucose to ensure a supply of glucose will be available for those tissues that require it.

> ✔ **TEST YOURSELF 16-8**
> 1. The main source of energy in ruminants is the production of __.
> 2. In the reticulorumen complex carbohydrates are broken down to __ or __.
> 3. What are the three most important volatile fatty acids produced by conversion from pyruvate?
> 4. Lipids are found in grasses and plants in the form of (three compounds)?
> 5. Proteins in ruminant diets are broken down extracellularly by peptidase into __.
> 6. Urea produced as a by-product of amino acid metabolism in the ruminant liver goes to the __ for reuse.
> 7. What is gluconeogenesis and where in the ruminant does it mostly take place?

## SMALL INTESTINE AND ASSOCIATED STRUCTURES

### BASIC STRUCTURE AND FUNCTION

The small intestine extends from the pyloric sphincter of the stomach to the beginning of the large intestine. It is essentially a tube that carries the chyme away from the stomach and deposits it in the large intestine. The small intestine consists of three distinct parts: **duodenum**, **jejunum**, and **ileum**. In those animals that do not rely on large amounts of fermentation to supply their need for energy and nutrients, the small intestine is the principal site for digestion and absorption.

The intestines are suspended from the body wall by the mesentery. The duodenum is the first portion of the small intestine. It receives the chyme as it exits the stomach through the pyloric sphincter. From the pyloric sphincter, the duodenum extends in a somewhat cranial direction for a short distance before turning caudally and descending on the right side of the abdomen (descending duodenum) toward the right kidney. The duodenum then turns medially and moves in a cranial direction again for a short distance (ascending duodenum), before ending at the duodenojejunal flexure where it attaches to the jejunum (Figure 16-24).

The **pancreas** runs right alongside the descending duodenum and next to the greater curvature of the stomach (Figure 16-25). It consists of an **endocrine** portion, which

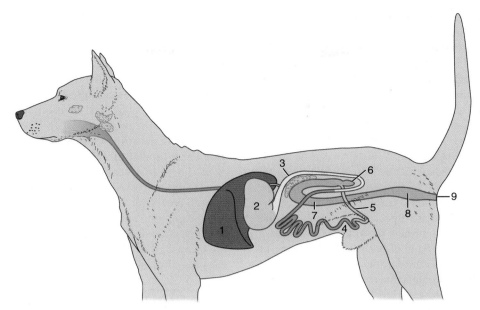

**FIGURE 16-24** Schematic representation of the intestines in a dog. **1**, Liver; **2**, stomach; **3**, duodenum; **4**, jejunum; **5**, ileum; **6**, cecum; **7**, colon; **8**, rectum; **9**, anus.

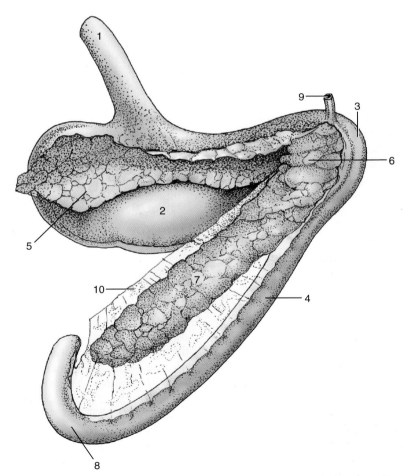

**FIGURE 16-25** The pancreas of the dog (caudal view). **1**, Esophagus; **2**, stomach; **3**, cranial flexure of duodenum; **4**, descending duodenum; **5**, left lobe of pancreas; **6**, body of pancreas; **7**, right lobe of pancreas; **8**, caudal flexure of duodenum; **9**, bile duct; **10**, mesoduodenum. (From Dyce KM, Sack WO, Wenseng CJG: Textbook of veterinary anatomy, ed 4, St Louis, 2010, Saunders.)

produces various hormones and deposits them directly into the bloodstream, and an **exocrine** portion, which produces digestive proenzymes that are deposited through a duct into the duodenum. More on this organ later.

The jejunum continues the intestinal tract and is the longest part of the small intestine, forming a mass of many coils and loops that occupy the ventral abdominal cavity. The bulk of chemical digestion and absorption occurs in the jejunum. Its mesentery is long and allows the jejunum to have a great range of motion.

The small intestine ends with the ileum, which is indistinguishable grossly from the jejunum. **Peyer's patches**, which are aggregates of lymphoid tissue, are found throughout the small intestine and are especially prominent in the ileum. These structures help protect the animal from disease by controlling local populations of bacteria, functioning in antibody production, and aiding in filtration of fluids. The ileum empties into the large intestine at the cecum (*ileocecal junction*) in the horse, at the colon (*ileocolic junction*) in the dog and cat, and at the cecum and colon (*ileocecocolic junction*) in the ruminant and pig.

To assist the small intestine in digestion and absorption, several features help increase its surface area. First, the small intestine is long and consists of many loops and coils. Second, the mucosa lining the small intestine is thrown into folds or **plications**. These plicae are permanent structures of the small intestine, in contrast to gastric rugae (the folds of the gastric mucosa), which disappear when the stomach fills. Third, the intestinal mucosa is made of simple columnar epithelial cells that have fingerlike projections called **villi**, which in turn contain smaller projections called **microvilli** (Figure 16-26). The villi move back and forth, helping move liquid contents into close contact with the mucosa. The microvilli form what is called the **brush border** (see Figure 16-2) that provides the majority of the surface area of the small intestine. Embedded in this brush border are brush-border enzymes that are responsible for membranous

digestion. Membranous digestion in the small intestine plays the ultimate role in the digestion of carbohydrates, proteins, and nucleotides.

Between adjacent villi are found groups of undifferentiated cells, in an area called the *intestinal crypts* (or crypts of Langerhans). These undifferentiated cells are the only intestinal cells undergoing cell division and they replace those further up on the tips of the villi as they are lost due to wear. An extensive network of blood capillaries is found inside the villi. These capillaries collect some of the nutrients absorbed from the gastrointestinal tract and transport them to the liver. Lymphatic capillaries called **lacteals** also are found in the villi (see Figure 16-26). Lipids are too large to enter the blood capillaries and must be transported in the lacteal. The lacteal carries absorbed lipids and fat-soluble substances to the thoracic duct, which empties into the venous blood of the vena cava.

## SECRETIONS OF THE SMALL INTESTINE

Many secretions are released from the small intestine that contribute to the digestive process. The duodenal mucosa, for example, secretes two very important hormones, *cholecystokinin (CCK)* and *secretin*. The stimulus for secretion of CCK is the presence of chyme with a high amino acid concentration, high fatty acid concentration, or a low pH entering the small intestine. The role of CCK is multifaceted. First, it inhibits gastric emptying. This allows the chyme to exit the stomach at a controlled rate, allowing more time to neutralize the acidic chyme, which in turn protects the small intestine. Second, CCK causes increased secretion of pancreatic digestive proenzymes as well as bicarbonate ($HCO_3^-$) secretion. Third, it is the main trigger for gallbladder contraction. Finally, CCK stimulates the secretion of **enteropeptidase** from the duodenal mucosa. Enteropeptidase is responsible for converting one of the pancreatic proenzymes, trypsinogen, into its active form, trypsin.

Secretin, another hormone released by the duodenal mucosa, decreases the HCl production in the stomach, and increases pancreatic and biliary bicarbonate secretions. The stimulus for secretin release is the presence of chyme with a low pH or high fatty acid concentration. The digestive enzymes, which are released from the pancreas, function optimally when the pH is more alkaline than the acidic chyme as it exits the stomach. The release of bicarbonate from the pancreas and liver helps neutralize the acids leaving the stomach, ensuring that the pancreatic digestive enzymes are most effective.

## PANCREAS

The pancreas, as mentioned earlier, has both endocrine and exocrine functions. The endocrine part of the pancreas consists of the *pancreatic islets* (formally known as islets of Langerhans). These pancreatic islets contain several different cell types and each cell type produces its own hormone. For example, beta cells secret insulin, which is needed to

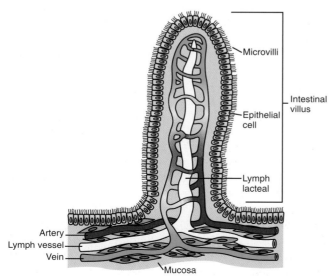

**FIGURE 16-26** Microanatomy of intestinal villus.

Labels: Microvilli; Intestinal villus; Epithelial cell; Lymph lacteal; Artery; Lymph vessel; Vein; Mucosa

transport glucose into most cells, thereby lowering the glucose levels in the blood. Alpha cells produce glucagon, which has the opposite effect, raising blood glucose levels by stimulating processes such as gluconeogenesis.

The exocrine portion of the pancreas consists of groups of acini. An *acinus* is made up of a single layer of columnar epithelial cells, resembling a cluster of grapes, surrounding a lumen. The cells of the acini release their secretions into the lumen, which merge with other lumina to form ducts that eventually converge into the *pancreatic duct.* The pancreatic duct empties into the duodenum. Some species have one pancreatic duct whereas others have two. In humans, sheep, and goats, the pancreatic duct combines with the common bile duct just before it enters the duodenum.

The secretions of the exocrine pancreas contain bicarbonate and pancreatic digestive enzymes. Pancreatic cells have surface receptors that are stimulated by acetylcholine, cholecystokinin, and secretin. During the cephalic and gastric phases of digestion, anticipation of food and food stretching the stomach causes an increase in pancreatic secretions. This is brought about mainly by an increase in vagal activity (acetylcholine release). During the intestinal phase of digestion, both a neural and an endocrine stimulus increase pancreatic secretions. Distention of the duodenum results in vagal stimulation of the pancreatic cells *(neural stimulation),* whereas chyme entering into the duodenum stimulates the release of secretin and cholecystokinin (CCK) *(hormonal stimulation).*

Enzymes derived from the exocrine pancreas are vital to the digestion of proteins, carbohydrates, lipids, and nucleic acids. **Lipases** break down lipids into two free fatty acids and a **monoglyceride.** Pancreatic **amylase** breaks down starches primarily into maltose (two glucose molecules linked together). Nucleases break down nucleic acids into nucleotides. Finally, proteolytic enzymes, also called **proteases,** break down proteins into amino acids.

All of the proteolytic enzymes are secreted by the pancreas in an inactive form called a **proenzyme** (or zymogen). These proenzymes need to be activated in the lumen of the intestine, just like pepsinogen, the proenzyme released by the chief cells in the stomach. The pancreatic proenzymes are **trypsinogen, chymotrypsinogen, proelastase,** and **procarboxypeptidase** *A* and *B.* They are activated as follows: CCK stimulates duodenal mucosal cells to secrete enteropeptidase. In the duodenal lumen, enteropeptidase then activates trypsinogen into trypsin, its active form. Trypsin is then responsible for activating the other proenzymes released by the pancreas. For example, chymotrysinogen is activated into chymotrypsin, proelastase is activated into elastase, and procarboxypeptidases A and B are activated into carboxypeptidases A and B. Trypsin can also activate additional trypsinogen to trypsin.

## LIVER, BILE DUCT, AND GALLBLADDER

The liver is located near the stomach, immediately caudal to the diaphragm (see Figure 16-24). Its secretions are essential

**TEST YOURSELF 16-9**

1. List, in order as they leave the stomach, the three sections of the small intestine.
2. What is the brush border in relation to the small intestine, and what is its function?
3. What characteristics of chyme are necessary to stimulate the release of cholecystokinin (CCK)?
4. Which hormone, released in the duodenum, is responsible for decreased hydrochloric acid production in the stomach?
5. What substance, released by the pancreas and liver into the duodenum, helps neutralize the acidic chyme leaving the stomach?
6. What are two substances secreted by the exocrine portion of the pancreas?

for digestion and absorption of nutrients. The liver has a multitude of other functions not directly related to digestion. These functions include synthesizing nutrients and regulating their release into the bloodstream, excreting toxic substances, both those originating within the body and those that have been brought into the body, and producing most of the plasma proteins, cholesterol, and many of the blood coagulation factors.

The liver is the largest digestive gland in the body and, like the pancreas, is considered an extramural gland, meaning it is outside the lumen of the gastrointestinal tract. It has two surfaces, a diaphragmatic surface that is the convex surface in contact with the diaphragm, and a visceral surface in contact with the abdominal organs. The *falciform ligament* attaches the liver to the diaphragm, whereas the right kidney, stomach, duodenum, colon, and jejunum leave impressions on the visceral surface. The mammalian liver consists of lobes. For example, carnivore livers have six lobes: left lateral, left medial, quadrate, right medial, right lateral, and caudate lobes. The caudate lobe has two parts: a papillary process which is on the left of the median plane lying in the lesser curvature of the stomach and a caudate process, which is more caudal on the right side of the liver, enclosing the cranial pole of the right kidney in the right dorsal abdomen. The **gallbladder** is located between the quadrate and the right medial lobe. Microscopically each lobe of the liver is made up of many *hepatic lobules.*

The liver is strategically placed between the vessels draining the intestine, and associated structures, and the general circulation. This means that the liver is able to process the blood leaving the gastrointestinal tract, preventing harmful substances, such as toxins, from entering the general circulation. The liver receives blood from two sources, the **hepatic portal vein** from the gastrointestinal tract and the **hepatic artery**, a branch of the celiac artery. The celiac artery branches directly off the abdominal aorta and supplies oxygenated blood to the liver tissue. Both the hepatic artery and the hepatic portal vein enter the liver near the periphery of the lobules, in areas known as *triads,* so called because the bile ducts also are found there in addition to the hepatic artery and hepatic portal vein. The hepatic artery and the hepatic portal vein travel from the periphery of the lobule toward its interior, coming together and emptying their blood into sinusoids, which are the large capillaries of the liver. The endothelial cells making up the walls of the sinusoids have large fenestrations or pores in them so that they are much more "leaky" then normal blood capillaries.

Adjacent to the sinusoids are **hepatocytes**, which come into close contact with the blood. The pores in the walls of the sinusoid endothelial cells allow large molecules, such as proteins, made by the hepatocytes to enter the blood easily.

Attached to the inner surface of the sinusoids are macrophages called **Kupffer cells**, which engulf foreign substances. The blood from the sinusoids enters the central vein, which is located at the center of each lobule, and ultimately exits the liver, returning back to the general circulation via the **hepatic vein**. Located between the individual hepatocytes are bile ductules called bile **canaliculi**. Bile is excreted from the hepatocytes into these canaliculi and travels in the opposite direction from the blood, away from the central vein, emptying into larger bile ductules, and ultimately into the bile duct at the triad. Bile is necessary for lipid digestion in the intestines (Figure 16-27).

Bile exits the liver and travels through the **hepatic ducts**, emptying into the **common bile duct**. The *cystic duct* also comes off the common bile duct. It connects the gallbladder, if the species has one, to the common bile duct. The common bile duct can empty directly into the duodenum, but in some species it combines with the pancreatic duct before entering the duodenum at the **major papillae**. There is a sphincter, called the *sphincter of Oddi,* which controls the entrance of the bile duct into the duodenum. When the sphincter of Oddi is closed, bile backs up into the gallbladder (Figure 16-28).

The gallbladder concentrates and stores bile until it is needed. The cat and dog usually eat meals once or twice a day so fat digestion does not occur continuously. In these animals, the gallbladder stores bile until the animal eats a meal. When fats are consumed, a large quantity of bile enters the duodenum. The gallbladder also provides the liver with a storage container so it can continue to excrete waste products through bile production even during periods when the animal isn't eating.

When chyme with a high fat or peptide concentration enters the small intestine, cholecystokinin (CCK) is released from the duodenal mucosa. CCK is the major stimulus for contraction of the gallbladder and relaxation of the sphincter of Oddi. This allows bile to enter the duodenum.

Given that ruminants have a more continuous digestive process, their gallbladders have a short retention time and do not concentrate the bile as much as that of carnivores. Horses do not have gallbladders. Because they also have a more continuous digestive process that requires a more continuous secretion of bile into the duodenum, bile storage isn't needed.

Bile is composed primarily of bile salts, phospholipids, cholesterol, and bile pigments. Hepatocytes form bile acids from cholesterol. Bile acids contain a water-soluble (hydrophilic) side and a lipid-soluble (hydrophobic) side. Bile acids tend to aggregate and position themselves with their hydrophobic parts facing inward, away from water, and their hydrophilic parts pointing out, toward water. This configuration is called a *micelle*. In the digestive process, these micelles in the intestine are important because they emulsify lipids, allowing the lipids to come close to the intestinal mucosa so they can be absorbed.

## BILE FORMATION AND BILIRUBIN EXCRETION

Bile production begins with bile salts (conjugated bile acids) being secreted into the bile canaliculi. The bile salts draw water out of the hepatocytes by osmosis, making bile a liquid. The composition of the bile is altered as it passes through the canaliculi by both absorptive and secretory processes; that is, water and ions are moved into and out of the canaliculi. One of the secretory processes involves secretin, which stimulates duct cells to secrete bicarbonate, which is added to the bile. The hepatic bicarbonate, along with the pancreatic bicarbonate, helps to neutralize the acid chyme entering into the duodenum from the stomach.

When the bile is released into the intestine, it emulsifies fats. The bile salts themselves are not reabsorbed until they reach the ileum. After they are reabsorbed in the ileum, they enter the hepatic portal vein and travel back up to the liver. The liver is responsible for reabsorbing almost all of the bile salts out of the hepatic portal vein and recycling them back into the bile. If the liver is functioning properly, only insignificant amounts of bile salts will bypass the liver and end up in the systemic circulation. This pathway for bile, from the liver to the intestine to the hepatic portal vein back to the liver, is called **enterohepatic circulation**.

The amount of bile salts that recirculates from the intestine to the liver influences how much bile is synthesized by the hepatocytes. As long as enterohepatic circulation of bile continues, bile synthesis will continue. When the stimulus for CCK secretion is gone, CCK secretion ceases and the sphincter of Oddi closes, diverting the bile back into the gallbladder. This means that the reabsorption of bile salts from the ileum back to the liver will diminish. Because the return of bile salts to the liver is the stimulus for continued bile acid production, this results in diminished bile acid synthesis.

In addition to their role in digestion and absorption of fats, bile acids are important in the excretion of organic compounds. Bilirubin, one of the breakdown products of hemoglobin, is an organic compound that is eliminated through the bile. Red blood cells, like all cells, have a finite life span and must be removed from circulation when that life span comes to an end. The majority of senescent (dead or dying) red blood cells are broken down through *extravascular hemolysis* (outside the vascular system). They are removed from circulation by the mononuclear phagocytic system. The mononuclear phagocytic system consists of macrophages found in the liver, spleen, bone marrow, lungs,

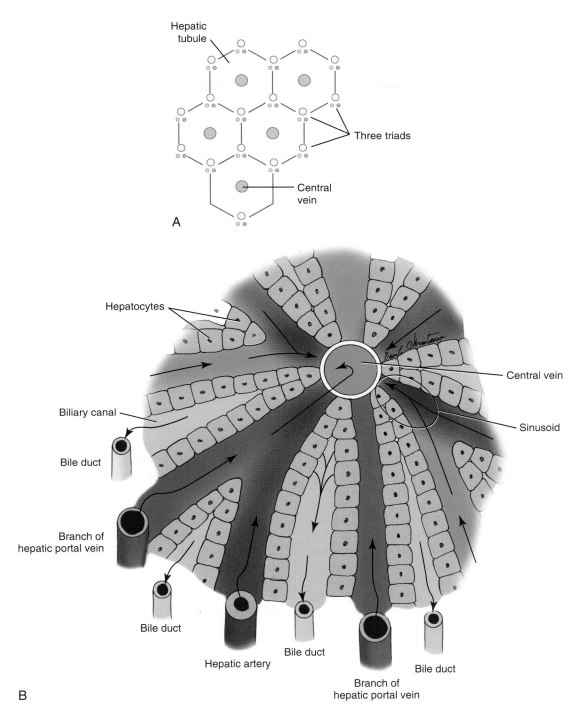

**FIGURE 16-27** A, Anatomy of a hepatic lobe. B, Anatomy of a hepatic lobule. (B, From Christenson DE: Veterinary medical terminology, ed 2, St Louis, 2008, Saunders.)

and lymph nodes. These macrophages phagocytize or engulf senescent red blood cells, rupturing them and releasing hemoglobin. This process is called hemolysis.

In the macrophage, hemoglobin is broken down into its component parts, globin and heme. Globin is degraded into amino acids that are reutilized by the animal. The iron is separated from heme and is either stored in macrophages or transferred into plasma, where it combines with plasma proteins, becoming transferrin. Transferrin circulates to the

bone marrow and the iron is reused to make new hemoglobin.

Heme, which is a red pigment, is converted to **biliverdin**, a green pigment. Biliverdin is then converted into **free** or **unconjugated bilirubin**, a yellow to orange pigment. Unconjugated bilirubin is released into the bloodstream, where it combines with the plasma protein albumin and travels to the liver. At this point the unconjugated bilirubin is not water soluble. The liver absorbs the unconjugated bilirubin. In the

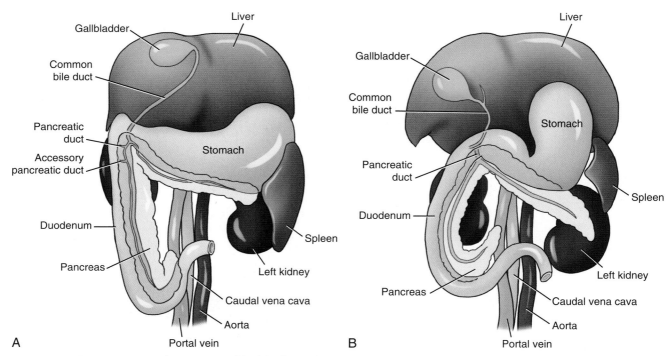

**FIGURE 16-28** Schematic view of the bile duct and pancreatic duct emptying into the duodenum of **A**, the dog and **B**, the cat. (From Washabau RJ, Day MJ: Canine & feline gastroenterology, St Louis, 2013, Saunders.)

hepatocyte, bilirubin is conjugated (joined) to **glucuronic acid** to form **bilirubin glucuronide** or **conjugated bilirubin**, which is water soluble. The hepatocyte releases the conjugated bilirubin into the bile, and when bile enters the small intestine conjugated bilirubin is transported along with it. In the small intestine, glucuronide is removed from conjugated bilirubin by bacterial enzymes. Fecal bacteria reduce the bilirubin to **urobilinogen**. Several different things can then happen to urobilinogen. Most urobilinogen is oxidized to *urobilin* and *stercobilin* and excreted from the body in feces. Urobilin is a yellow to orange pigment, depending on its degree of oxidation, whereas stercobilin is a brownish pigment. Together they give feces its characteristic color. The rest of the urobilinogen is reabsorbed into the enterohepatic circulation. From there it has two possible fates. Most of the urobilinogen is taken up by the liver and re-excreted into the bile, ultimately re-entering the enterohepatic circulation. Some of the urobilinogen in the hepatic portal vein bypasses the liver and enters the general circulation. The urobilinogen then travels to the kidney, where it is converted into **urobilin** and excreted from the body in urine, giving urine its characteristic color.

If this process is disrupted at any point, the level of bilirubin in the blood becomes elevated. As a result, the animal may become icteric (jaundiced), a condition in which the tissues turn a yellow or orange color. Disruptions can occur anywhere in the pathway, including before the liver (prehepatic), within the liver (hepatic), and after the liver (posthepatic) (Figure 16-29). If too many red blood cells are hemolyzed in the circulation, the amount of bilirubin can overwhelm the normally functioning liver and lead to

*prehepatic bilirubinemia.* Bilirubinemia is an abnormal increase of bilirubin in the blood. If the liver is not functioning normally and the ability of hepatocytes to conjugated bilirubin is reduced, this can result in *hepatic bilirubinemia.* Cholestasis refers to a condition that prevents or slows the flow of bile through the bile ducts, causing a buildup of substances that would normally be excreted through the bile. If there is an obstruction of the bile duct (extraheptic cholestasis) or some impairment of bile flow within the canaliculi (intrahepatic cholestasis), this would results in *posthepatic bilirubinemia.*

> ✓ **TEST YOURSELF 16-10**
>
> 1. What three structures are found in the triad located at the periphery of a hepatic lobule?
> 2. What is the function of Kupffer cells?
> 3. Where does the common bile duct enter the small intestine?
> 4. What common species of domestic animal does not have a gallbladder?
> 5. What is enterohepatic circulation?
> 6. Unconjugated bilirubin in blood is not water soluble. How does it become water soluble?

## NUTRIENT PROCESSING IN THE LIVER

The liver plays a vital role in keeping blood glucose levels normal. In the nonruminant animal, carbohydrate digestion results in the production of monosaccharides, such as glucose, fructose, and galactose. Glucose is the primary monosaccharide absorbed from the small intestine, entering the hepatic

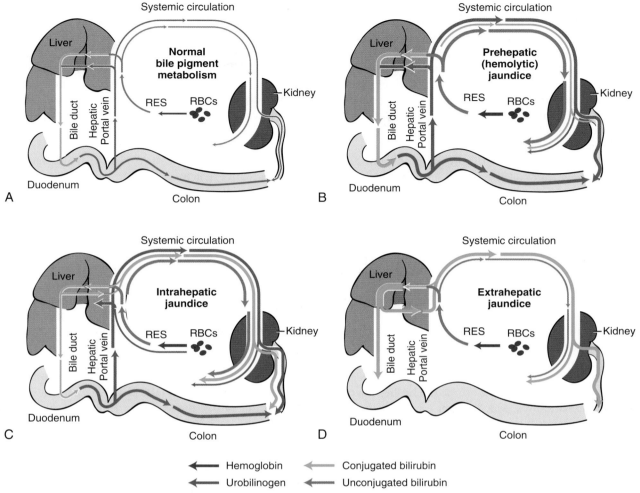

**FIGURE 16-29** Diagrams comparing the formation, excretion, and enterohepatic circulation of bilirubin and other bile pigments. **A,** The normal animal; **B,** *prehepatic* jaundice associated with hemolysis and overproduction of bilirubin; **C,** *intrahepatic* jaundice associated with hepatocellular disease; **D,** *posthepatic* jaundice associated with extrahepatic bile duct obstruction. *RBCs,* Red blood cells; *RES,* reticuloendothelial or mononuclear phagocytic system. (Courtesy Dr. Susan Johnson, The Ohio State University. In Washabau RJ, Day M: Canine & feline gastroenterology, St Louis, 2013, Saunders.)

portal vein and arriving at the liver. In the liver, glucose can be metabolized to produce energy in a number of forms, including ATP. Conversion of glucose to energy occurs through the process of glycolysis. In addition to glucose, two other monosaccharides that are absorbed in the nonruminant (fructose and galactose) can be converted to glucose by the liver and, therefore, can be used as energy sources.

In the liver, as well as in skeletal muscle, if there is an excess amount of glucose, it can be stored as **glycogen**. When blood glucose levels are high, some excess glucose can be taken up by adipose cells and converted to triglycerides. In the nonruminant the liver can turn glucose into triglycerides when glucose levels remain high, even after glucose has been stored by the skeletal muscle and adipose tissue. In the ruminant, there is less glucose available so this does not occur.

Glycogen, the major storage form of glucose, can be broken down to glucose monomers through a process called **glycogenolysis** when the animal needs to use glucose as an energy source. The process of glycogenolysis can occur when

the animal is in the postabsorptive state (after absorption has occurred, between meals) and glucose is no longer so readily available.

During the postabsorptive state, when the availability of glucose is reduced, *gluconeogenesis* can also occur in the liver and sometimes the kidney. Gluconeogenesis is the synthesis of glucose from noncarbohydrate sources, providing the animal with a source of glucose when glucose levels decline. The substrates used in this glucose-making process are pyruvate (formed from amino acids during protein breakdown), lactate, and glycerol.

When glucose is scarce, tissues can utilize lipids as an energy source. Triglycerides in adipose tissue can be broken down into glycerol and fatty acids by the enzyme lipase. Glycerol can then be converted into glucose in the liver by gluconeogenesis, whereas the fatty acids are oxidized in various tissues as a source of energy. This process can be helpful when the animal's glucose level is low between meals. In severe starvation, however, fatty acid mobilization from adipose tissue can increase tremendously, overwhelming the oxidative capability of the liver to convert fatty acids to energy. Instead the fatty acids are converted into **ketones**. Some tissues can use ketones as an alternative energy source, but too many ketones can ultimately cause a metabolic acidosis, called *ketosis*. It is important to note that, in nonruminants, ketones come only from the liver, as a consequence of the mobilization of fats, but in ruminants the ketone betahydroxybutyrate is also produced during normal digestion from butyrate, one of the VFAs.

Another function of the liver is protein production. The liver synthesizes nearly all the plasma proteins, including albumin and blood clotting proteins. Albumin is a blood protein that plays a vital role in keeping fluids in the vascular system. Because of its large size, albumin does not easily pass through most capillary walls. It exerts osmotic pressure, preventing water from moving out of the capillaries into the extravascular space. As a result, it helps to maintain the balance of fluids between the blood, interstitial spaces, and cells. If that balance is upset, abnormal fluid accumulations in body tissues can occur.

The liver also can convert amino acids into ketoacids. Ketoacids can be used by the liver for energy production, or they can be converted to glucose or fatty acids, which can be used in lipid synthesis. When amino acids are degraded in the liver, ammonia, a toxin, is formed. The hepatocytes convert ammonia to urea, which is later excreted primarily by the kidney in nonruminants. In ruminants, some urea re-enters the salivary glands and the rumen. Once it is in the rumen, microorganisms can use it again to synthesize proteins.

## SMALL INTESTINAL MOTILITY

The two primary movements in the small intestine are peristalsis and **segmentation**. As described in the section on esophageal motility, peristalsis is a moving wave of luminal constriction preceded by an area of luminal distention (see Figure 16-13A). Peristalsis in the small intestine propels the intestinal contents toward the large intestine. Segmentation is a different type of movement carried out in the small intestine (see Figure 16-13B). The presence of chyme stretches the intestinal wall, triggering the ring of circular muscle to contract; as one set of contractions relaxes, another area of circular muscle contracts in a different area. These random, localized contractions of the circular muscle layer help mix the digestive contents and move the digestive fluid closer to the epithelial surface of the intestine, increasing its contact with the mucosal enzymes and absorptive surfaces. Segmentation is a mixing action only and does not move the chyme toward the large intestine.

## REGULATION OF SMALL INTESTINAL MOTILITY

The pacemaker cells within the small intestinal wall are similar to those in the stomach and function as described in the section on gastric motility.

## DIGESTION IN THE SMALL INTESTINE

### CARBOHYDRATE DIGESTION

The small intestine is where the majority of carbohydrate chemical digestion occurs. Starches are one of the few carbohydrates broken down in the *luminal phase*. In luminal carbohydrate digestion, the enzyme alpha-amylase, which is secreted by the pancreas, breaks starch down into smaller chains of glucose molecules. These include the disaccharide maltose (two glucose molecules), trisaccharides (three glucose molecules), and oligosaccharides (three to ten glucose molecules).

The second phase of chemical digestion is the *membranous phase*. Embedded in the brush border are the specific enzymes for each type of polysaccharide. The polysaccharides must therefore come into contact with the intestinal epithelium to be broken down by the brush border enzymes. The enzymes are named according to the polysaccharides they break down. For example, the enzyme **maltase** breaks down the disaccharide maltose. The enzyme isomaltase breaks down the disaccharide isomaltose. Remember that starch is made up solely of repeating glucose units; luminal digestion of starch will yield only glucose molecules.

Sugars, such as sucrose and lactose, are not broken down in the luminal phase and instead are degraded in the membranous phase by the enzymes embedded in the brush border. The membranous enzyme **sucrase** breaks down sucrose into a glucose molecule and a fructose molecule, whereas **lactase** breaks down lactose into a glucose molecule and galactose molecule. Some adult mammals do not produce the enzyme lactase and therefore cannot digest lactose. Ultimately, enzymatic digestion of carbohydrates yields monosaccharides, which are small enough to be absorbed through the intestinal wall (Figure 16-30).

### PROTEIN DIGESTION

Luminal protein digestion, which began in the stomach with pepsin, must be completed in the small intestine. The pancreas releases proenzymes that are activated in the lumen of the small intestine. Two types of enzyme participate in luminal digestion, the **endopeptidases** and the **exopeptidases**. Endopeptidases include pepsin as well as the pancreatic enzymes **trypsin**, chymotrypsin, and elastase. These enzymes break proteins at internal points along the polypeptide chains, resulting in smaller peptide chains. They do not release free amino acids. Exopeptidases, on the other hand, break proteins at the ends of the polypeptide chains, releasing free amino acids. Carboxypeptidases A and B are examples of exopeptidases. Protein luminal digestion by exopeptidases yields free amino acids.

The enzymes responsible for membranous protein digestion are also embedded in the brush border, and the peptides must come into contact with the epithelial surface for membranous digestion to occur. Peptide-digesting enzymes, or *peptidases,* hydrolyze the small peptide products of luminal phase protein digestion, yielding free amino acids. Some

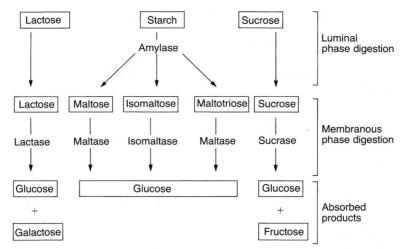

**FIGURE 16-30** Carbohydrate digestion. (From Cunningham JG: Textbook of veterinary physiology, ed 4, St Louis, 2007, Saunders.)

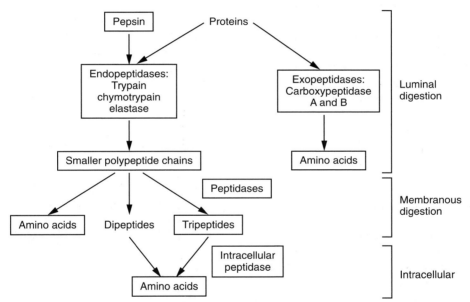

**FIGURE 16-31** Protein digestion. (From Cunningham JG: Textbook of veterinary physiology, ed 4, St Louis, 2007, Saunders.)

peptide chains are incompletely hydrolyzed and form dipeptides and tripeptides. These dipeptides and tripeptides are small enough to be absorbed into enterocytes (intestinal wall cells). Within the enterocytes are intracellular peptidases that complete hydrolysis, producing free amino acids that are available for passage into the blood. Only free amino acids are small enough to be absorbed into the blood (Figure 16-31).

## ABSORPTION OF MONOSACCHARIDES, DIPEPTIDES, TRIPEPTIDES, AND AMINO ACIDS

Absorption across the intestinal mucosa can occur in a multitude of ways, including both passive and active processes.

Although some molecules are transported passively by diffusion down their concentration gradients, others must use an active transport process, using energy to enter the body. Some substances rely on multiple methods. For example, electrolytes are absorbed by attaching to one of several transport molecules and use a variety of mechanisms responsible for completing their absorption. Other molecules are transported by *antiports* that allow one molecule to be exchanged for another, such as the sodium/hydrogen exchange. Glucose and amino acids often have to rely on secondary active transport for absorption. Glucose relies on the establishment of a sodium gradient to help move it into the enterocyte against its concentration gradient. When glucose levels are high within the enterocyte and lower in the lumen of the GI tract, an unfavorable concentration gradient is formed preventing glucose from passively entering into the enterocyte. The body cannot allow this glucose to be lost in the feces. A sodium–potassium pump found on the enterocyte near the blood side of the cell pumps three sodium atoms out and two potassium atoms in, helping to create a lower concentration of sodium inside the cell. This creates a concentration gradient that favors the movement of sodium from the lumen of the gastrointestinal tract into the enterocyte. As the sodium is moving into the cell, glucose moves by cotransport into the cell along with the sodium, against the glucose concentration gradient. This is an example of *secondary active transport* and both glucose and amino acids can be brought into the enterocyte through this process. To complete the process, glucose must then move through the cell wall into interstitial space by facilitated diffusion. *Facilitated diffusion* is a passive transport process, meaning it does not require ATP, but uses a carrier molecule to move glucose out of the cell. The glucose completes its absorption process by entering the capillaries from the lateral space by *simple diffusion.*

## LIPID DIGESTION AND ABSORPTION

Fats and fat-soluble vitamins are also digested in and absorbed from the small intestine. Triglycerides are the primary dietary lipids; other lipids include cholesterols, phospholipids, and esters. Lipids are not water soluble and cannot dissolve in the watery medium of the gastrointestinal fluids. In order to digest and absorb fats, a four-step process must occur, comprising emulsification, hydrolysis, micelle formation, and absorption.

The first step, emulsification, begins in the stomach, where lipids are warmed to body temperature and thoroughly mixed. This process helps break lipids into smaller droplets. Emulsification is then completed in the small intestine by the detergent action of bile salts and phospholipids. If bile salts were not available, the smaller fat droplets would coalesce back into larger fat droplets in the intestine, which does not have the intense mixing action of the stomach. Bile salts coat the lipid droplets, causing them to repel one another and remain as small individual droplets. Decreasing the size of lipid droplets increases the surface area available for the hydrolytic pancreatic enzymes, lipase and colipase, to break down each triglyceride into a monoglyceride and two fatty acids. The monoglyceride and the two fatty acids are not yet soluble in water, which again would cause a problem if it were not for the bile salts forming *micelles.* The monoglycerides and fatty acids form a union with the bile salts and phospholipids in a mass, where the water-soluble bile salts and phospholipids are on the outside and the water-insoluble monoglyceride and fatty acids are on the inside, completely surrounded by the bile salts and phospholipids. It looks as though the entire molecule is water-soluble, not just the outside surface. The micelles essentially act like tiny ferries, transporting the fatty acids and monoglyceride to the enterocyte surface. At this point the monoglyceride and fatty acids diffuse into the cell and the bile salts do not. This keeps the bile salts available to transfer other monogylcerides and

fatty acids. Inside the enterocyte, the monoglyceride and the two fatty acids are reassembled into a triglyceride and packaged into **chylomicrons**. Chylomicrons are spherical structures that are made up of triglycerides, cholesterol, phospholipids, and proteins. The Golgi apparatus packages the chylomicrons into vesicles, which are transported to the cell membrane, from which they are released into the interstitial fluid by exocytosis. Chylomicrons cannot enter the capillaries because of their large size; instead they are picked up by the lymphatic system and transported to the systemic circulation without passing through the liver.

---

✓ *TEST YOURSELF 16-11*

1. The major storage form of glucose is __.
2. How are triglycerides in adipose tissue converted into glucose for energy?
3. Which plasma protein produced in the liver plays a crucial role in fluid movement between plasma and interstitial fluid?
4. Which movement in the small intestine propels intestinal content toward the rectum?
5. In the luminal phase of the chemical digestion of starches, which enzyme, secreted by the pancreas, is needed?
6. In the membranous phase of chemical digestion of sugars, where are the necessary enzymes located?
7. What is an exopeptidase?
8. Both glucose and amino acids are brought into a cell through secondary active transport? What does this mean?

---

## THE LARGE INTESTINE

### BASIC STRUCTURE AND FUNCTION

The end of the small intestine, the ileum, leads into the large intestine, which consists of the **cecum, colon, rectum,** and **anus.** The large intestine overall has a wider diameter then the small intestine, hence the name. The amount of microbial fermentation that occurs within the large intestine contributes to how extensive and complex its anatomy is. Whether the ileum opens into the colon, cecum, or both depends on the species.

The cecum is a blind diverticulum at the beginning of the colon. It varies from being small and inconspicuous in the carnivore, where little fermentation is required, to a voluminous and expansive cecum in equine species that rely heavily on hindgut microbial fermentation. In the horse, the comma-shaped cecum is so expansive that it takes up a large portion of the abdomen on the right side of the animal (Figure 16-32). It consists of a base, the main body, and an apex (point of the blind diverticulum). The cecum in the ruminant is a large blind tube that extends caudally.

The colon can be divided into three parts, ascending, transverse and descending, with the most variation between species appearing in the ascending colon (Figure 16-33). In the carnivore, the ascending colon is short and straight,

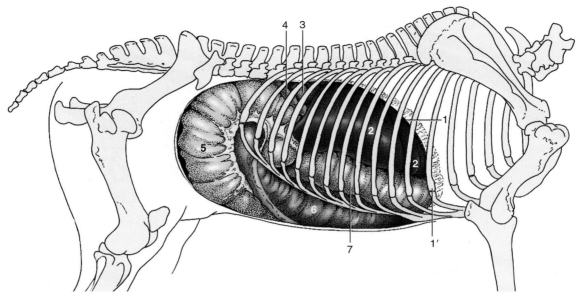

**FIGURE 16-32** Visceral projections on the right abdominal wall (including the diaphragm) of a horse. **1**, Cut edge of the diaphragm; **1′**, rib #6; **2**, liver; **3**, right kidney; **4**, descending duodenum; **5**, body of cecum; **6**, right ventral colon; **7**, right dorsal colon. (From Dyce KM, Sack WO, Wensing CJG: Textbook of veterinary anatomy, ed 4, St Louis, 2010, Saunders, VitalBook file.)

extending cranially and leading into the transverse colon. The transverse colon goes from the right side of the abdomen to the left, often running between the stomach and the small intestine, and terminates at the longest part of the colon, the descending colon. The descending colon follows the left side of the abdomen before going medially to the rectum.

The colon in the pig and ruminant consists of the same three parts. However, the ascending colon forms a coil or spiral, which is quite different from the carnivore's short and straight ascending colon. The ruminant's ascending colon in fact can be further subdivided into a proximal loop, forming an S shape; a spiral loop, which coils toward the center of the mesentery and then coils back up in the reverse direction; and a distal loop, which connects the ascending with the transverse colon. In the pig, the ascending colon also forms a spiral arrangement but instead of being in a flat plane, it is shaped more like a cone. In both animals, the ascending colon then leads into the transverse colon, which crosses from right to left, similar to that of the carnivore, leading into the descending colon.

The horse has the largest and most complicated colon of the domestic species and it is often referred to as the great colon. The horse's ascending colon actually forms a double horseshoe-shaped loop, with one loop (the dorsal colon) lying on top of the other (the ventral colon). The bottom of the horseshoe is toward the front of the animal and the turn between the two occurs at the pelvic inlet. The colon narrows significantly at the transition from ventral to dorsal colon, and therefore transport can be delayed in this area.

During segmentation in the colon and cecum of the horse and pig, both the longitudinal muscle, which runs in bands called *teniae*, and the circular muscle contract, forming bulging saclike structures called *sacculations*. These sacculations are also called haustra. Certain areas contract then relax, then different areas contract and relax in another location. The sacculations are semipermanent and may even be visible post mortem. Sacculations prolong the time during which the contents stay in the large intestine by creating extra volume. This allows more time for absorption and microbial digestion.

## MOTILITY OF THE LARGE INTESTINE

The intestinal contents (ingesta) travel slowly in the large intestine, especially in animals such as the horse and the rabbit that require extensive hindgut fermentation to provide energy. In the large intestine, the ingesta must be thoroughly mixed to allow contact with the absorptive surface of the colon, where absorption of water and ions occurs. Different types of motility pattern occur within the large intestine with the function of mixing, retaining, and propelling ingesta toward the anus. Although they vary among species, the motility patterns in general consist of four different types: segmentation, peristalsis, antiperistalsis, and mass movement.

Segmentation is the most common type of movement in the cecum and colon. Segmental contractions move the ingesta in a slow back and forth movement, increasing the contact between the ingesta and the epithelial surface. Peristalsis in the large intestine is similar to peristalsis in other parts of the GI tract, moving ingesta toward the anus.

Antiperistalsis occurs in the opposite direction, toward the stomach. The movement helps slow down the transit

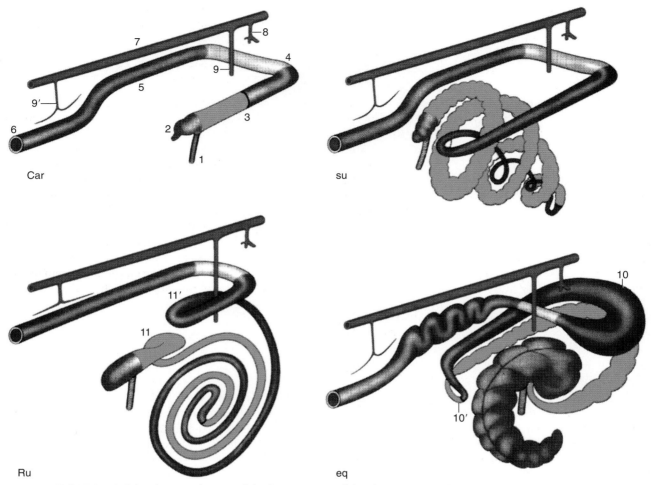

**FIGURE 16-33** Schematic drawing of the large intestine of the domestic mammals: carnivores (Car), the pig (su), ruminants (Ru), and the horse (eq). Cranial is to the upper right. **1**, Ileum; **2**, cecum; **3**, ascending colon; **4**, transverse colon; **5**, descending colon; **6**, rectum and anus; **7**, aorta; **8**, celiac artery; **9**, **9'**, cranial and caudal mesenteric arteries; **10**, **10'**, dorsal diaphragmatic and pelvic flexures of ascending colon; **11**, **11'**, proximal and distal loops of ascending colon. (From Dyce KM, Sack WO, Wenseng CJG: Textbook of veterinary anatomy, ed 4, St Louis, 2010, Saunders.)

of the ingesta, allowing more time for reabsorption to occur. The hairpin turn between the ventral colon and the dorsal colon is narrow, and functions in a very similar way to the pylorus of the stomach. In the horse, this area is often where the antiperistalsis movements originate. Antiperistalsis in this area also prevents larger food molecules that require further digestion from passing through, allowing smaller, more liquid, ingesta to continue its journey into the dorsal colon.

The last type of movement seen in the large intestine is called mass movement. It consists of a period of intense propulsive activity, moving the contents of the large intestine toward the rectum. Mass movement contractions occur within both the colon and the cecum.

## REGULATION OF LARGE INTESTINE MOTILITY

Slow waves are initiated by large intestinal pacemaker cells that have the same fluctuating membrane potential as seen in

other parts of the gastrointestinal tract. The pacemaker cells can be found throughout the large intestine; they have alternating periods of activity and rest, allowing different areas of the large intestine to be the active pacemakers. Depolarizing waves from the various pacemaker cells can be sent toward the stomach, creating antiperistaltic movements, or toward the rectum, resulting in peristaltic movements. The autonomic nervous system influences the activity of the pacemaker cells in the large intestine, just as in the small intestine.

## DIGESTION AND ABSORPTION IN THE LARGE INTESTINE

Two very important functions of the large intestine are absorption of water and ions, and completion of carbohydrate or protein microbial digestion and absorption. The forestomachs in the ruminant are the primary location of microbial digestion, whereas in nonruminant hindgut fermenting herbivores, such as horses and rabbits, microbial digestion occurs mainly in the cecum and colon. Although the physical location of fermentation is different, the substrates being broken down in the cecum are similar to those fermented in the rumen. These substrates are mainly the structural and nonstructural carbohydrates found in plants, as well as some proteins.

The horse's fermentation center, being positioned after the stomach where enzymatic digestion occurs, influences how food is processed in the cecum and colon. Carbohydrates are exposed to enzymes in the small intestine, making them more susceptible to breakdown by microbes in the cecum and colon. Some simple carbohydrates may be broken down by the enzymes and acids in the stomach, but in comparison to the carnivore, the enzymatic digestion process that occurs in the horse is far less efficient. Additionally, the high concentration of cell wall or structural elements found in plant food may act to protect the simple nonstructural components from exposure to digestive enzyme, thus preventing their degradation.

Similar to the ruminant, the horse, through the process of fermentation, produces VFAs that are absorbed from the cecum and colon and used as an energy source. There also are local glands in the wall of the large intestine that produce bicarbonate that helps to neutralize acids produced during the fermentation process.

Proteins from the food the microbes would have used for their growth and metabolism have already been broken down and absorbed by the horse during enzymatic digestion, prior to the ingesta entering the cecum and colon. This presents the microbes in the cecum and colon with a potential nitrogen deficiency. To solve this problem, extensive amounts of urea are transferred from the blood to the large intestine.

The microbes use the urea, along with the small amount of protein that has escaped enzymatic digestion, to make amino acids and proteins.

## EMPTYING OF THE RECTUM

When chyme (ingesta) passes through the large intestine much of the water is absorbed, leaving a semisolid material called feces. The consistency of normal feces varies among species from semiliquid "cow pies" to small, hard sheep pellets. When **feces** are transported to the rectum sensory receptors are stimulated. This initiates the *defecation reflex* that causes the colon and rectum to contract, and relaxes the *inner anal sphincter muscle,* a smooth muscle. The animal then perceives the need to defecate. Some species such as the cat and the dog can be trained to close the voluntary *outer anal sphincter,* a skeletal muscle, and delay defecation. Other animals such as ruminants, horses, and birds seem unable to learn how to control this sphincter voluntarily.

### ✔ TEST YOURSELF 16-12

1. List the four parts of the large intestine.
2. Which species of large animal is a hindgut fermenter?
3. Name a common species of animal that has a short ascending colon?
4. Name a common species of animal that has a spiral ascending colon shaped like a cone?
5. What is the purpose of the sacculations?
6. What are the four movements associated with the large intestine?
7. How are feces formed?

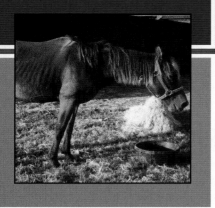

# Nutrients and Metabolism

*Joanna M. Bassert*

## OUTLINE

## LEARNING OBJECTIVES

*When you have completed this chapter you will be able to:*

1. List the six categories of nutrient.
2. List and describe the three categories of carbohydrate.
3. List and describe the four categories of lipid.
4. Give the general structure of proteins.
5. Differentiate between water-soluble vitamins and fat-soluble vitamins and list their dietary sources and functions.
6. List the common macrominerals, microminerals, and trace elements found in the body.
7. Describe the processes of catabolism and anabolism.
8. List the events that occur in each stage of cellular metabolism.
9. Describe the process of glycolysis, the Krebs cycle, and the electron transport system.
10. Describe the general structure of enzymes and explain the role of enzymes in initiation and control of metabolic reactions.

## VOCABULARY FUNDAMENTALS

*Adenosine diphosphate (ADP)* ah-**dehn**-ō-sēn dī-**fohs**-făt
*Adenosine triphosphate (ATP)* ah-**dehn**-ō-sēn trī-**fohs**-făt
*Anaerobic glycolysis* ahn-ər-**rō**-bihck glī-**kohl**-ih-sihs
*Anaerobic respiration* ahn-ər-**rō**-bihck res-puh-**rā**-shuhn
*Biologic value* bī-ah-**lohj**-ihck **vahl**-yoo
*Cell metabolism* sehl meh-**tahb**-uh-lihz-ehm
*Cellular respiration* sehl-ū-lər res-puh-**rā**-shuhn
*Cellulose* **sehl**-ū-lōs
*Citric acid cycle* **siht**-rihck **ah**-sihd **sī**-kuhl
*Coenzyme* kō-**ehn**-zīm
*Cofactor* kō-**fahck**-tər
*Contractile protein* kohn-**trahck**-tehl **prō**-tēn
*Crude protein* krood **prō**-tēn
*Cytochrome* **sī**-tō-krōm
*Deamination* dē-**ahm**-ih-ā-shuhn
*Electron transport system* ē-**lehck**-trohn **trahnz**-pohrt **sihs**-tehm
*Essential amino acid* eh-**sehn**-shuhl ah-**mē**-nō **ah**-sihd
*Essential fatty acid* eh-**sehn**-shuhl **faht**-ē **ah**-sihd
*Essential nutrient* eh-**sehn**-shuhl **noo**-trē-ehnt

*Fat soluble* faht **sohl**-yuh-buhl
*Functional group* **fuhngk**-shuh-nuhl groop
*Glycolysis* glī-**kohl**-ih-sihs
*Ketone body* kē-tōn **boh**-dē
*Krebs cycle* krehbz **sī**-kuhl
*Lipolysis* lī-**pohl**-ih-sihs
*Macromineral* mah-krō-**mihn**-ər-ahl
*Membrane protein* **mehm**-brān **prō**-tēn
*Metabolic turnover* meh-tah-**bawl**-ihck **tərn**-ō-vər
*Micromineral* mī-krō-**mihn**-ər-ahl
*Mitochondrial matrix* mī-tō-**kohn**-drē-ahl **mā**-trihks
*Monounsaturated fat* mohn-ō-uhn-**sahch**-ər-rā-tihd faht
*Monounsaturated fatty acid* mohn-ō-uhn-**sahch**-ər-rā-tihd **faht**-ē **ah**-sihd
*Myositis* mī-ō-**sīt**-uhs
*NADH* N-A-D-H
*Negative balance* **nehg**-uh-tihv **bahl**-ehnz
*Nicotinamide adenine dinucleotide (NAD)* nihck-uh-**tihn**-ah-mīd **ahd**-eh-nīn dī-**noo**-klē-ō-tīd
*Nitrogen balance* nī-**truh**-jehn **bahl**-ehnz

*Nonessential amino acid* nohn-eh-**sehn**-shuhl ah-**mē**-nō **ah**-sihd

*Osmoregulator* aws-mō-**rehg**-ū-lā-tǝr

*Peptide bond* **pehp**-tīd bohnd

*Phosphorylation* fohs-fohr-eh-**lā**-shuhn

*Polypeptide* pohl-ē-**pehp**-tīd

*Polyunsaturated fat* pohl-ē-uhn-**sahch**-ǝr-rā-tihd faht

*Polyunsaturated fatty acid* pohl-ē-uhn-**sahch**-ǝr-rā-tihd **faht**-ē **ah**-sihd

*Positive balance* **pawz**-eh-tihv **bahl**-ehnz

*Product molecule* **prohd**-uhckt **mohl**-uhl-kyool

*Protective protein* prō-**tehck**-tihv **prō**-tēn

*Provitamin* prō-**vī**-tah-mihn

*Regulatory protein* rehg-ū-lah-**tohr**-ē **prō**-tēn

*Saturated fatty acid* sahch-ǝr-rā-tihd **faht**-ē **ah**-sihd

*Short-chain fatty acid* shohrt – chān **faht**-ē **ah**-sihd

*Simple sugar* **sihmp**-ehl **shoog**-ǝr

*Starch* stahrch

*Storage protein* **stohr**-ihj **prō**-tēn

*Structural protein* **struhck**-shǝr-uhl **prō**-tēn

*Sugar* **shoog**-ǝr

*Trace element* trās **ehl**-eh-mehnt

*Transamination* trahnz-ahm-ih-**nā**-shuhn

*Transport protein* **trahnz**-pohrt **prō**-tēn

*Triacylglycerol* trī-**ah**-sihl-**glihs**-ǝr-ahl

*Triglyceride* trī-**glihs**-ǝr-rīd

*Unsaturated fatty acid* uhn-**sahch**-ǝr-rā-tihd **faht**-ē **ah**-sihd

*Water soluble* **wah**-tǝr **sohl**-yuh-buhl

## INTRODUCTION

Anyone who has ever watched a Labrador Retriever gulp down his dinner in 2 seconds, or someone else's dinner, for that matter, knows how glorious food is to most dogs. If you have had the experience of feeding cattle or horses at mealtime, you know the level of excitement that the herds express as they bellow and whinny or "sing" for their supper. And alas, for some overweight pets on restricted diets, those pets that sit patiently and plaintively by their masters during dinner, food is just a bit too wonderful. All living things, plants and animals, need to take in nutrients to stay alive. Because food is required for survival, the nervous and endocrine systems of healthy living creatures not only generate the desire to eat but also instill the pleasure of eating to make food a glorious thing!

Most food consumed by animals is used for metabolic fuel. This means that the nutrients derived from eating are broken down into smaller molecules and, along with oxygen, are used to make **adenosine triphosphate (ATP)**, which is the chemical energy used by cells. The amount of energy that can be acquired from these nutrient molecules is measured in kilocalories (kcal). Kilocalories are also called Calories (with a capital C). A kilocalorie is the amount of energy needed to raise the temperature of a kilogram of water by 1 degree.

In the previous chapter, we explored the structure and function of each part of the digestive system, and we learned how food is digested into fundamental nutrient molecules, which are then absorbed into the bloodstream. But what happens after these molecules are transported throughout the body via blood and lymph? How do the cells that make up tissues and organs absorb the nutrients and use them to stay alive? And how is the energy that is stored in the nutrient molecules converted to the usable form, ATP? How does the cell use ATP to make new molecules needed for repair and maintenance? In this chapter, we will answer these and other questions.

## NUTRIENTS

A nutrient is a substance derived from food that is used by the body to carry out all of its normal functions. Nutrients are divided into six categories:

- Water
- Carbohydrates
- Lipids
- Proteins
- Vitamins
- Minerals

Water, carbohydrates, lipids, and protein are consumed in large quantities relative to vitamins and minerals, which are consumed in very small quantities (Figure 17-1). In addition, carbohydrates, fats, and proteins produce energy when consumed, but water, vitamins, and minerals do not. Box 17-1 offers a summary of the energy-producing nutrients and gives examples of their sources in the diet.

Cells, especially those found in the liver, have a remarkable ability to convert one type of molecule into another. This ability enables the body to break apart large molecules and use the "building blocks" to make new and completely different molecules. The body knows what molecules it needs to stay alive, so it will build the necessary molecules and transport them to where they are needed. This process is analogous to dismantling an old bank building that is not needed anymore and using the old bricks to build a new school or post office. In this way, the body is able to use a wide range of nutrient molecules found in food, dismantle them into their fundamental units, and build new molecules. This process enables animals to adjust to variations in diet.

However, there are limits. Creating new molecules from old ones cannot be done for all needed molecules. Each animal species has a select group of **essential nutrients** that it cannot manufacture from building blocks; therefore, the animal must obtain these essential nutrients from its diet.

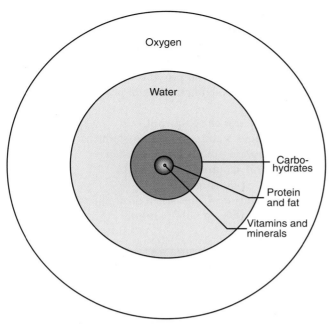

**FIGURE 17-1** A nutrient target. Oxygen and six classes of nutrient are essential for life. The amount of water needed daily by an animal (in milliliters) is equal to the amount of its daily energy requirement (in Calories). Notice that vitamins and minerals are consumed in minute amounts relative to the other nutrients.

For example, many animals are able to make vitamin C from the nutrients they ingest, but guinea pigs cannot; to get vitamin C, guinea pigs must eat foods rich in vitamin C, such as fruits and vegetables or vitamin C-fortified pelleted feed. Cats cannot make the essential amino acid taurine, but dogs can, therefore cat food is fortified with taurine, but dog food is not. For this reason, you should not feed dog food to cats or, with time, they will develop disorders such as blindness and cardiac disease as a result of the taurine deficiency.

When animals are fed diets that contain both the essential and nonessential nutrients required for their species, they are able to synthesize all of the other additional molecules required for a healthy life. Keep in mind that the terms *essential* and *nonessential* are misleading, because both are required for life. Perhaps more accurate descriptions would be *manufacturable* and *not manufacturable*.

## OXYGEN AND WATER

Oxygen is the most vital requirement for survival. Without oxygen, animal life would cease in an extraordinarily short period of time. I would last about 3 minutes without taking a breath, but a whale might last over an hour. Without the ability to take oxygen into our bodies, we would quickly die.

In the priority of life's essential requirements, water would be second only to oxygen. However, in terms of the diet, water is the most important nutrient. Most animals cannot survive longer than a few days without it, but there are some adapted to desert conditions that can survive for several weeks. Water is obtained not only by ingesting food and drink but also by oxidizing proteins, fats, and

carbohydrates. This metabolic source of water accounts for about 10% of the daily water requirement, though this is higher in desert animals and birds.

Mammals consist of about 70% water: newborns have somewhat more (75% to 80%), and adults have somewhat less (50% to 60%). Remarkably, even though an animal can survive the loss of almost all of its body fat and half of its protein, a loss of as little as 10% of its water can cause serious illness in most animals, and a 15% loss would be fatal without immediate treatment. The amount of water that is needed daily by an animal (in milliliters) is equal to the amount of its daily energy requirement (in Calories). Refer to the clinical application box to learn more about treating sick and dehydrated animals.

Water is involved in almost all of the metabolic processes of the body. It is the major component of blood and is found inside all cells (intracellular) as well as outside the cell (extracellular). Water serves many functions in the body. It is a lubricant for body tissues, a circulatory and transport medium, and a chemical reactant in digestion (hydrolysis). In addition, water is excreted as sweat and evaporated during panting to assist in temperature regulation. Finally, it is the medium in which the biochemical reactions of metabolism

## CLINICAL APPLICATION

### Taurine Deficiency in Cats

Taurine is an essential amino acid in cats and is found in high quantities in meat and fish, but it is virtually nonexistent in plant-based foods, including dog food. Therefore cats that are fed dog food or home-cooked vegetarian diets develop taurine deficiency after several months. The result is a progressive, irreversible **retinal degeneration** that ultimately leads to blindness. In addition, taurine deficiency has been associated with **dilated cardiomyopathy**, a condition in which the heart enlarges because of dilation of the cardiac chambers. In some cases, the walls of the ventricles become very thin and the ability of the heart to pump blood efficiently is altered. Cats may exhibit signs of heart failure, such as depression, shortness of breath, decreased exercise tolerance, and coughing. Fortunately, cardiomyopathy caused by taurine deficiency is reversible, and affected cats recover with nutritional supplementation.

    **Queens** that are taurine deficient may appear clinically normal but may have diminished reproductive success, including problems with abortion, early embryonic death, and malformations of neonates. An examination of the eyes of these cats usually reveals some degree of retinal degeneration.

    Kittens that are born to taurine-deficient queens and fed deficient diets often die. Those that do survive exhibit neurologic signs, including **cerebellar dysfunction** and **paresis** in the hind legs, which frequently splay outward.

    Occasionally, even cats that are fed diets adequate in taurine develop clinical signs of deficiency. In these cases, a biochemical disturbance in the retinal cells is thought to prevent normal taurine uptake and use.

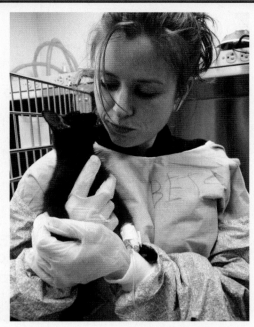

Kittens fed diets deficient in taurine are particularly vulnerable to serious illness or death. (Courtesy Joanna Bassert.)

---

occur, such as those involved in the growth, repair, and maintenance of cells.

## CARBOHYDRATES

With the exception of lactose, which is the sugar found in milk, and a small amount of glycogen from meat, all dietary carbohydrates come from plants. Carbohydrates are divided into three categories:

- **Sugars**—monosaccharides and disaccharides that come from fruits, sugar cane, honey, milk, and sugar beets
- **Starches**—polysaccharides that come from grains, root vegetables, and legumes
- **Cellulose**—polysaccharides that are found in most vegetables

Glucose is the fundamental building-block molecule that results from breaking down large molecules of carbohydrates. It is used by the cell to make other molecules. Glucose is a *monosaccharide,* which is the simplest and smallest form of dietary carbohydrate (Figure 17-2). Fructose and galactose are also derived from the digestion of carbohydrates, but these monosaccharides are converted by the liver into glucose before they enter the general circulation.

    Remember from the previous chapter that many nutrient molecules are absorbed in the small intestine and transported to the liver via the hepatic portal system. Once in the liver, they are often converted to other molecules, before they are either used by the liver itself or released into the general circulatory system for the benefit of other organs and tissues.

    Glucose is readily used to make ATP through a process called **glycolysis**. ATP is the major fuel for the body. Although there are several types of cell that use fat as a primary source of energy, red blood cells and neurons rely almost exclusively on glucose for their energy needs. Perhaps this explains why brain-drained students crave candy bars and other high-sugar foods while studying for long periods of time. (I like espresso chocolate chip ice cream when I'm doing a lot of brain work. It has sugar *and* caffeine!)

    The brain is exquisitely sensitive to decreases in blood glucose levels, and even temporary decreases in glucose can severely depress brain function and lead to the death of neurons. For this reason, the endocrine system keeps a vigilant watch over blood glucose levels by releasing glucose-controlling hormones from the pancreas (refer to our discussion of the endocrine system in Chapter 11). These hormones help to provide the brain and other tissues with a relatively steady level of glucose. However, as mentioned, even slight decreases in glucose can affect brain function, so if you find it difficult to make a decision at the end of the day, when you are tired and hungry, it is not your imagination. Glucose that is not immediately used by cells

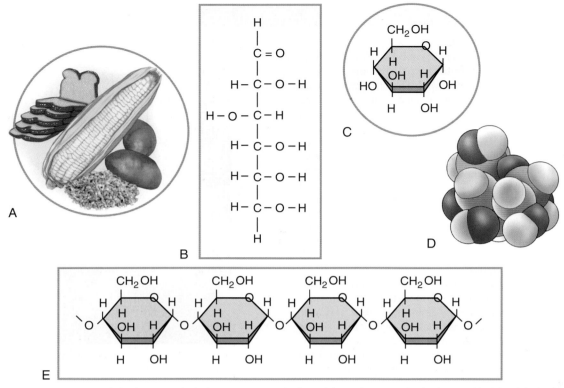

**FIGURE 17-2** Carbohydrates. Carbohydrates are primarily derived from plants. **A**, The fundamental building block of carbohydrates is the monosaccharide. Glucose is the most important monosaccharide in the body. It may be composed of a straight chain of carbon atoms (**B**), or it may bend into a more stable ring (**C**), which in three dimensions (3-D) appears as a tight cluster of atoms (**D**). **E**, Monosaccharides link together to form disaccharides (*di* means "two") or polysaccharides (*poly* means "many").

is converted to glycogen and stored in the liver, or it is converted to fat and stored in adipose tissue throughout the body.

## FATS AND LIPIDS

Lipids are organic molecules that are soluble in other lipids and in organic solvents, such as alcohol and ether, but are not soluble in water. Lipids are divided into four major categories:

- Neutral fats
- Phospholipids
- Steroids
- Other lipoid substances

### NEUTRAL FATS

Neutral fats are commonly known as *fats* when they are solid and *oils* when they are liquid. It is important to keep in mind that fats are a kind of lipid, but not all lipids are fats. The building blocks of neutral fats are *fatty acids* and *glycerol.* Fatty acids are linear molecules classified as *long-chain, medium-chain,* or **short-chain fatty acids** depending upon the number of carbon atoms in the backbone of the molecule. Glycerol is a modified **simple sugar**. When fat is made in the body, three chains of fatty acid molecules are attached to a single molecule of glycerol, resulting in a molecule that looks like the letter E. Because there are three fatty acids in

each molecule of fat, neutral fats are also called **triglycerides** or **triacylglycerols**. Although the glycerol component is the same in all neutral fats, the fatty acid chains vary, resulting in different types of neutral fat.

Whether a neutral fat is solid or liquid at room temperature depends upon two factors: the length of the fatty acid chains and the degree of saturation with hydrogen atoms within the chains. Fatty acids with single bonds between the carbon atoms can accommodate the greatest number of hydrogen atoms and are said to be **saturated fatty acids**, because the maximum number of hydrogen atoms is attached to the chain of carbon atoms. Saturated fatty acids tend to have long chains and are primarily found in meat and dairy foods, such as milk, cream, cheese, lard, and butter (Figure 17-3). Coconuts are one of the few plant sources of saturated fats.

On the other hand, fatty acids with one or more double bonds between the carbon atoms can accommodate fewer hydrogen atoms and are said to be **unsaturated fatty acids**, which includes **monounsaturated** and **polyunsaturated** *fats.* Fatty acids with short chains and those that are unsaturated are found in seeds, nuts, and most vegetables. Olive and peanut oils are rich in **monounsaturated fats,** and corn, soybean, and safflower oils contain a high percentage of **polyunsaturated fats** (Figure 17-4). Neutral fats with short-chain fatty acids and unsaturated fats are liquid at room

## Ketosis and Eclampsia: The Importance of Carbohydrates

We know how important carbohydrates are in providing animals with adequate energy levels. We also know how profoundly sensitive the brain is to even small decreases in blood glucose levels. For herbivores, the consumption of sufficient amounts of starch and cellulose from plants plays a vital role in their management, particularly if they are pregnant. The nutritional requirements in the first two trimesters of pregnancy are close to those needed for maintenance during the nonpregnant state. However, in the last trimester and during lactation, nutritional demands increase dramatically. Energy requirements are proportional to the number of fetuses and are highest during lactation. Thus, cows carrying twins and ewes carrying twins or triplets have the highest nutritional needs. Serious metabolic disease can occur if the nutrition to these pregnant or lactating animals is interrupted.

When pregnant ewes and cows receive inadequate nutrition, their bodies will compensate for the caloric deficiency by metabolizing their own tissues, primarily their fat reserves. Ketones are formed from the breakdown of the tissue and are released into the bloodstream, called *ketonemia,* and into the urine, called *ketonuria.* Even the breath of the animal contains ketones, and it therefore smells like acetone or nail polish remover. This condition is called *ketosis.* Ketosis is considered *primary* if the animal is fed an insufficient or unpalatable diet. It is called *secondary* ketosis if the animal is provided adequate nutrition but stops eating because of an illness, such as mastitis or metritis. Left abomasum displacement is the primary cause of secondary ketosis in cows. In both primary and secondary ketosis, the cow or ewe is not able to supply enough glucose from the digestion of food or from the catabolism of tissues to meet the needs of the developing fetuses or lactation and her own needs.

When ketosis occurs in preparturient, or pregnant, cows and ewes, it may precipitate a dangerous and often fatal metabolic disorder known as **eclampsia**. The primary sign is hypoglycemic encephalopathy, because the brain is adversely affected by the extremely low glucose level. The illness lasts 2 to 5 days. Affected animals are usually fat, as a result of overfeeding in the early part of gestation, but subsequently consume inadequate nutrition during the last trimester. Initially they are often restless and uncoordinated, as though drunk; later, they become listless, anorexic, and they walk aimlessly, sometimes bumping into things because of a condition known as *cortical blindness.* They may grind their teeth, develop unusual postures, and may exhibit muscle twitching on the face and ears. Finally, the animals become sternally recumbent, develop rapid, weak pulses; and do not get up. Coma and death often follow, and mortality is about 80%. Not surprisingly, blood tests show high ketone and low glucose levels. Guinea pigs, ferrets, and rabbits are also predisposed to developing eclampsia.

Postparturient ketosis usually appears a few days to weeks after giving birth, when milk production is high. Lactation requires huge amounts of glucose to make lactose for milk. When inadequate carbohydrates are consumed, glycogen stores in the liver are used first. The metabolism of tissues, which promotes ketogenesis, soon follows once the glycogen stores have been depleted. Clinical signs of postparturient ketosis include depression, lethargy, a staring expression, decreased milk production, weight loss, and a humped-back appearance consistent with abdominal pain. Occasionally, postparturient ketosis will cause frenzied behavior, such as circling, staggering, bellowing, head pressing, and compulsive walking, which occurs for about an hour. As with all ketotic states, ketones are present in the blood, urine, and breath, and there is a marked decrease in blood glucose levels. Unlike eclampsia, however, postparturient ketosis is self-limiting, because the reduction of food intake eventually causes milk production and the corresponding glucose drain to stop.

By far the best and least expensive treatment for ketosis is prevention. Providing fresh, palatable feed in appropriate quantities at the appropriate times is the key to a successful breeding program.

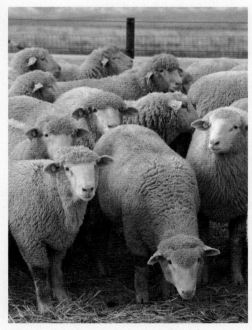

(From McCurnin DM, Bassert JM: Clinical textbook for veterinary technicians, ed 6, St Louis, 2006, Saunders.)

temperature (oils). In ruminants, short-chain fatty acids are found in the gas and liquid contents of the rumen and reticulum. In species such as cattle, sheep, and goats, these *volatile* short-chain fatty acids, derived from the microbial breakdown of ingested plant matter, are a vital source of energy.

The liver is adept at converting one fatty acid to another, but some fatty acids, such as linoleic acid, cannot be synthesized. Linoleic acid is a fatty acid component of lecithin. Thus, in all domestic species and in humans, linoleic acid is an **essential fatty acid** that must be available in the diet.

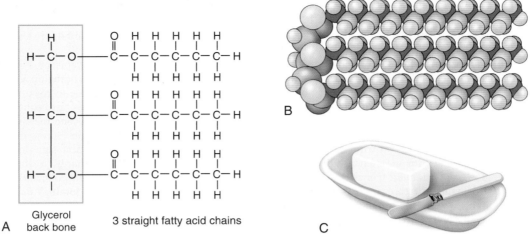

**FIGURE 17-3** Neutral fats. **A,** Neutral fats are composed of triglycerides. Each triglyceride molecule includes a glycerol backbone and three fatty acid chains. These molecules together create an E shape. **B,** The saturated triglyceride does not have any double bonds in the molecule and can therefore hold the maximum number of hydrogen atoms, making the chains very straight. **C,** Saturated fats tend to come from animal fat and are found in butter, lard, and meat.

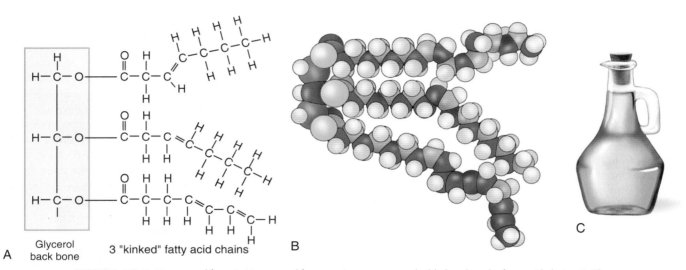

**FIGURE 17-4** Unsaturated fats. **A,** Unsaturated fats contain one or more double bonds in the fatty acid chains. **B,** These double bonds cause the chains to bend and kink. **C,** Unsaturated fats tend to be liquid at room temperature and are derived from plants and vegetable oils.

Fortunately, it is found in most vegetable oils. Lino*lenic* and arachidonic acids are also considered to be essential fatty acids. Though it is possible for the body to convert linoleic acid into arachidonic acid, the process is extremely inefficient and does not yield adequate results for many species. Thus arachidonic acid is also considered to be an essential fatty acid.

Neutral fats are amazing. They contain over twice as much potential energy by weight as proteins or carbohydrates. Fat is easily digestible, makes food taste good, staves off hunger for long periods of time, and helps the body absorb the fat-soluble vitamins A, D, E, and K. Stored, subcutaneous fat is an important insulator, and fat also surrounds and cushions vital organs, such as the heart, kidneys,

and eyes. In the digestive tract, neutral fats are broken down into their fatty acid and glycerol components before being absorbed by the intestine and sent into the hepatic portal system. The liver rebuilds neutral fats, forming many different kinds of E-shaped triglycerides before they are sent off to other parts of the body. Not surprisingly, triglycerides are the major energy source for hepatocytes (liver cells) and skeletal muscle cells, which are some of the most active cells in the body.

## PHOSPHOLIPIDS

Phospholipids are modified triglycerides derived primarily from the cell membranes of plant and animal cells. Like the triglycerides, phospholipids have a glycerol core but contain two, rather than three, fatty acid chains; therefore you could call them *diglycerides.* In addition, phospholipids have a phosphorus group attached to the glycerol molecule—the infamous *polar head,* for which the phospholipids are so well known. The polar head and the two fatty acid chains make the phospholipid molecule look like the head, shoulders, and dropped arms of a stick person (see Chapter 3).

## STEROIDS

Steroids are lipids that are dramatically different from neutral fats. Unlike the E-shaped molecule typical of fats or the "head, shoulders, and arms" of phospholipids, steroids are made of four flat interlocking rings of hydrocarbons. Steroids include cholesterol, bile salts, sex hormones, and hormones released from the cortex of the adrenal gland. Of these, **cholesterol** is the most vital nutritionally, because all of the other steroid molecules can be made from cholesterol: it is the essential precursor. Like phospholipids, cholesterol is found in the plasma membrane and is nutritionally derived from animal products such as egg yolks, meat, and cheese. In addition, the liver is able to manufacture cholesterol; without it, animals would not be able to carry out many vital biochemical processes.

## OTHER LIPOID SUBSTANCES

A diverse range of other lipoid substances, such as fat-soluble vitamins, eicosanoids, and lipoproteins, are vital for an animal's survival. Eicosanoids are regulatory molecules derived from arachidonic acid, which is a 20-carbon fatty acid found in the plasma membrane. These substances include prostaglandins, leukotrienes, and thromboxanes, which are hormones that play an important role in the inflammatory process, blood clotting, and labor contractions. Prostaglandins are also important in smooth muscle contraction and in controlling blood pressure.

---

### ✔ TEST YOURSELF 17-1

1. What is a Calorie?
2. What are the six fundamental nutrients? Which ones generate energy when consumed?
3. Why is water so vital to the survival of an animal?
4. What are the three categories of carbohydrate?
5. What are the four major categories of lipid?
6. What is the difference between a *saturated* and an *unsaturated* fat? Why is this difference important nutritionally?
7. What is an essential fatty acid?
8. Give a specific example of a steroid.

---

## PROTEINS

Proteins make up 10% to 30% of a cell's mass and are therefore the dominant structural material of the animal body. Proteins are used for building critical structural materials, such as keratin, collagen, and elastin for the skin; connective tissues; and muscle proteins. But not all proteins are construction materials. Many play vital and diverse roles in cell function: enzymes and hormones regulate an incredible variety of body functions; hemoglobin carries oxygen in red blood cells; and contractile proteins in muscle cells enable the body to move.

Though the roles of proteins vary, all proteins are composed of amino acids. There are 22 different types of amino acid, but they are all composed of three important **functional groups**: a *basic amine group* ($-NH_2$), an *organic acid group* ($-COOH$), and an *R group*. Differences in the *R* group make each amino acid unique, but the acidic and basic groups are identical among all amino acids. Proteins are created when the amino acids link together, like pearls on a string (Figure 17-5). The acid group from one amino acid links to the basic group on the next, forming a **peptide bond**. When two amino acids link together, the resulting molecule is called a *dipeptide.* Three amino acids together form a *tripeptide,* and more than 10 amino acids link to form a **polypeptide**.

Proteins are huge molecules, called *macromolecules.* They are commonly composed of 100 to 10,000 amino acids, though any polypeptide with 50 or more amino acids is considered a protein. The type and order of the amino acids determine the structure and function of the protein. Each of the 22 amino acids is analogous to a letter in an alphabet. The letters used and the order in which letters are arranged determine a particular action or meaning. For example, if the chain reads "Have a nice day," and only one amino acid is altered in the chain to make it read "Have a *mice* day," the meaning becomes very different and possibly nonsensical.

There are 10 essential and 12 **nonessential amino acids** in most species. **Essential amino acids** must be present in the diet because the animal either cannot make them at all or cannot make them fast enough to meet the body's needs for tissue maintenance and growth. For the body to make new proteins, all of the needed amino acids—essential and nonessential—must be present in the cell in *sufficient quantity* and *all at the same time.* This is called the *all or none rule.* If one amino acid is missing, the protein cannot be manufactured.

Animal products, such as meat, eggs, and dairy products, contain proteins that include the largest number of essential amino acids. In fact, meat products contain all of the essential amino acids for many species and are therefore called *complete proteins.* However, animal-based protein is more expensive than plant-based protein, so many pet foods contain primarily plant-based proteins, such as soy. Cereals, rice, nuts, and legumes, such as beans, are protein rich, but their proteins are nutritionally incomplete, because they are low in one or more of the essential amino acids. Leafy green vegetables are also rich in essential amino acids, but have little methionine and tryptophan. When ingested together, legumes, grains, and cereals provide all of the essential amino acids for many species, including humans; these foods are therefore said to be *complements* of one another (Figure 17-6).

Amino acids cannot be stored. Those not immediately used to make protein are oxidized by the cell to make energy or are

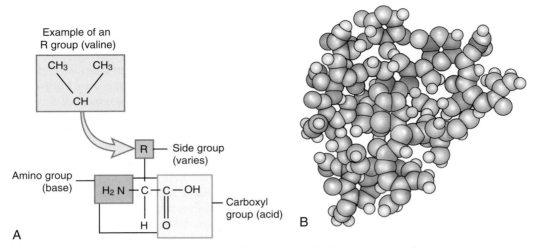

**FIGURE 17-5** Proteins. **A,** Proteins are composed of amino acids, which are composed of an amino group, a carboxyl group, and a variety of side chains (*R* groups). Amino acids link together to form long chains. **B,** When the protein becomes particularly large, it coils to increase its molecular stability. Meat is an excellent source of protein, because it contains the complete assortment of amino acids needed for the body to make all of the proteins required for maintenance and growth.

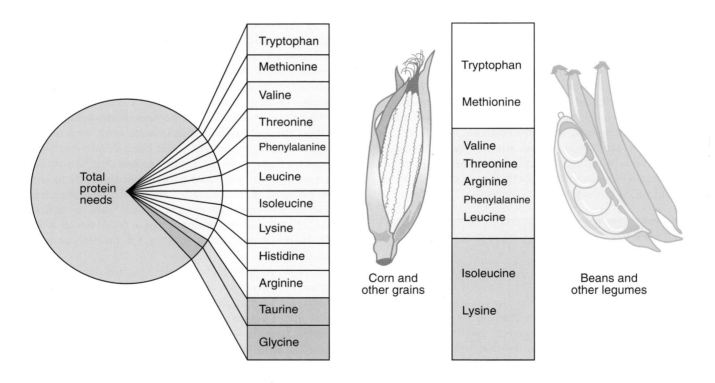

**FIGURE 17-6** Protein synthesis. **A,** Protein synthesis depends upon all of the essential amino acids being present in sufficient amounts simultaneously. The *essential amino acids* make up a relatively small portion of the total protein needs of animals. Notice that the amino acids considered essential vary from species to species. The amino acids in yellow are essential for the dog. Taurine *(pink)* is essential for cats and is found in meat. Glycine *(blue)* is essential for poultry. **B,** Foods such as corn and grains are rich in certain essential amino acids, such as tryptophan and methionine, but lack other amino acids, such as isoleucine and lysine, which are found in legumes. When consumed together, a diet of corn, grain, and legumes contains all of the essential amino acids needed by many species, including dogs. Thus, dogs can do well on home-cooked vegetarian diets, as well as on meat-based diets, if adequate complement foods are present, but cats are strict carnivores and must consume animal proteins (because taurine is found naturally only in animal tissue). Therefore, cats should not be fed a home-cooked vegetarian diet.

converted to carbohydrates or fats. If the body does not have enough carbohydrate or fat calories in the diet to make ATP, the cell will use proteins from the diet or will catalyze tissue to make ATP. In the healthy animal, the rate of protein synthesis equals the rate of protein breakdown and loss. This is called the **nitrogen balance**. When the amount of nitrogen ingested in the form of protein equals the amount of nitrogen that is excreted, the body is said to be in nitrogen balance. Nitrogen from protein is packaged by the liver into a molecule called urea, which can be measured by a *blood urea nitrogen (BUN)* test, before it is excreted by the kidney.

A **positive balance** occurs when the body is incorporating more protein into tissues than it is breaking down to make energy (ATP). This happens normally during healing, and during pregnancy because of the growing fetus. It also occurs in growing animals. Certain hormones, called *anabolic hormones,* accelerate protein synthesis and growth. For example, pituitary growth hormone stimulates tissue growth in young animals and conserves protein in mature animals. Sex hormones trigger growth spurts. Growth and lactation increase the protein requirements of animals above what is needed for body maintenance and exertion (work or exercise). The metabolism of excess amino acids increases the workload of the liver and kidney because of the processing and excretory requirements for the urea and organic acid waste by-products. In other words, eating too much protein causes the liver and kidneys to work harder. This is why animals with kidney disease are fed a low-protein diet.

A **negative balance** occurs when protein breakdown exceeds the amount of protein being incorporated into tissues. This occurs during physical and emotional stress—infection, injury, debilitation—and during starvation, or when the quality of the dietary protein is poor. Glucocorticoids released during stress enhance protein breakdown and the conversion of amino acids to glucose. Cats are the consummate carnivore and are specifically adapted to a high-protein diet. They commonly manufacture proteins from the amino acids released from gluconeogenesis.

Pet foods often identify the **crude protein** content on the label of the can or bag of food. Most people assume that the best food for their pet contains the highest percentage of crude protein. This, however, is not necessarily true. Crude protein content gives no indication of the quality or utilization potential of the protein. A dog food, for example, may have a high protein content, but the *biologic value* of the protein may be low. The **biologic value** is the percentage of absorbable protein that is available for productive body functions. It defines the amount of amino acids available for metabolic processes.

The ideal protein content in food includes all of the essential amino acids needed to meet the specific metabolic requirements of a particular species. For example, if a protein has a missing essential amino acid, its quality may be low. However, by adding the missing amino acid, the full potential of the biologic value of the protein can be restored. This is one reason why mixed animal and plant protein sources are often complementary to each other in food formulations.

In addition, the quality of proteins is improved if feeds are not overprocessed or overheated in storage, because heating can denature proteins.

In ruminants, the digestion of protein is facilitated by microbes, which break down protein derived from the grasses and grains consumed in the diet. The amino acids generated from this process are further degraded into ammonia, organic acids, and carbon dioxide. The ammonia is either absorbed through the wall of the rumen or is used by the microorganisms to make new proteins. Interestingly, the microbial-made protein has a consistent quality regardless of the quality of the nutrient source. Thus, protein in lower-quality feeds is improved by microbial metabolism. On the other hand, the usefulness of high-quality protein from feed may be lowered by microbial metabolism, so feeding high-quality protein to a ruminant may give the same results nutritionally as feeding low-quality protein. Amazingly, the rumen also has the ability to convert non-protein sources of nitrogen, such as urea and ammonium salts, into protein. These nitrogen sources, however, must be used judiciously in feeds, because an excess or an imbalance can be toxic to the herbivore.

## VITAMINS

Although consumed in minute amounts, vitamins are essential for life. Not surprisingly, the Latin word *vita* means *life*. Unlike nutrient molecules, such as carbohydrates, proteins, and fats, vitamins do not produce energy when metabolized, nor are they broken down into building-block units. Rather vitamins are, for the most part, coenzymes or parts of coenzymes. Their molecular structure is the "key" that activates an enzyme and enables it to carry out its diverse metabolic reactions. For example, during the biochemical breakdown of glucose, the B vitamins riboflavin and niacin are required. Without them, the reaction cannot be completed and glucose cannot be used to generate energy. Thus, the full use of nutrient proteins, carbohydrates, and fats is dependent upon the presence of coenzymes. However, not all vitamins are coenzymes. Vitamins A, D, and E have important and varied roles in the body. Vitamin D, for example, is converted to calcitriol, which regulates calcium levels in the body, and a form of vitamin A, retinal, helps sensory cells in the retina of the eye to detect light.

Plants can manufacture the vitamins they require, but animals cannot. Therefore, most vitamins are not made in the body and must be consumed in the diet, but there are exceptions. Vitamin D, for example, is made in the skin, and vitamin K and biotin are made in the intestine by bacteria. In addition, the body can convert beta carotene, which is an orange pigment found in carrots and deep green leafy vegetables, into vitamin A. For this reason, beta carotene is called a **provitamin** and is essential for many species.

Vitamins were assigned their letters in the order that they were discovered. In addition, they also have been given a descriptive title that indicates their function in the body and have been classified as either **fat soluble** or **water soluble** (Table 17-1).

## CLINICAL APPLICATION

### Starvation: A Life and Death Issue

We have all marveled at the fortitude of wild animals that survive severe winters, drought, and food deprivation. Neglected domestic animals may also endure inadequate shelter, food supplies, and access to water. For them, food deprivation and subsequent starvation are a threat to their lives. Fortunately, evolution has dictated physiologic adaptations that extend the time animals can live without food. Except for the terminal phase, starvation is reversible, and the reproductive capacity of the animal is preserved for as long as possible. How does the body do this?

The process of starvation can be organized into three stages.

### Stage I

Initially, the body tries to balance the animal's energy expenditure with energy intake by lowering the basal metabolic rate. In this way, the animal needs less food for maintenance but may feel weak, dizzy, and tired. Although many tissues can use nutrients other than glucose, certain tissues—such as blood cells, the kidney, and nervous tissue (brain and spinal cord)—are normally glucose dependent. The body, therefore, uses glycogen stores in the liver to provide glucose to these important tissues. However, the glycogen stores are depleted after several hours, and the body must turn to other sources of energy. Glycerol and fatty acid stores from fat and amino acids from body proteins are catabolized next to produce glucose. Ketone bodies are released as a product of fatty acid metabolism, causing the blood levels of ketone bodies and glucose to rise.

### Stage II

After 1 to 2 weeks, depending on the species, a change occurs in the body that allows the brain and other tissues to use ketones and glucose for energy. Stored body fat becomes the primary source of energy as the body breaks down fatty acids into ketone bodies. This process continues until fat reserves are depleted. The length of this stage varies among individual animals, depending on the amount of body fat that is available for catabolism. Generally, this stage lasts for several weeks.

Because body fat serves primarily as an energy storage tissue, an insulator, and protector of internal organs, progressive loss of adipose tissue does not threaten normal body functions or survivability until the stores are nearly depleted.

### Stage III

Once fat reserves are used up, protein becomes the principal metabolic fuel. Even during the first stages of starvation, the body catabolizes protein to produce glucose. However, the level of protein catabolism remains high after the fat reserves are depleted. Initially, liver and plasma proteins are used, followed by protein from the gastrointestinal tract, heart, and skeletal muscle. These structures decrease dramatically in size, and critical body functions are lost. Decreases in plasma proteins, for example, lead to changes in oncotic pressure, and fluid subsequently leaks into the abdominal cavity, causing abnormal distention called *ascites*. Loss of muscle between ribs and in the diaphragm may lead to respiratory failure. The heart, which can lose 50% of its mass, may simply stop beating. Gastric emptying and intestinal transit times are prolonged, and the absorption of fat and protein is impaired as the inner layers of the intestine degenerate. Diarrhea and nausea may result. In addition, malnourished animals are immunocompromised and often develop pneumonia and other infections. Only the skeletal system seems remarkably unaffected by starvation.

### Treatment

Warm, intravenous fluids in conjunction with antibiotics and parenteral nutrition are important in the treatment of end-stage starvation. In addition, malnourished animals are less able to maintain adequate body temperature and should be given a warm environment in which to recover. Good nursing care is important in these cases, because animals will need thick, soft bedding and care for any decubital ulcers or sores that may have developed from prolonged recumbency. After the animal has been stabilized through the use of parenteral nutrition, high-protein liquid diets should be given by mouth initially until semisolid foods can be tolerated.

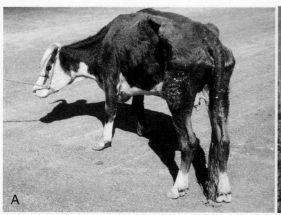
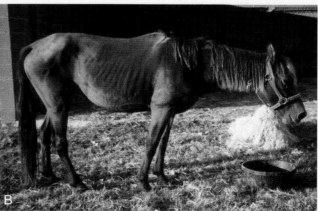

The emaciated cow **(A)** and horse **(B)** seen here stand with lowered heads, characteristic of depression and lethargy. Malnourished animals, such as these, are experiencing a negative nitrogen balance and have already metabolized all of their fat stores and much of their muscle tissue to generate the energy needed for vital metabolic functions. These animals are vulnerable to infection, particularly parasitism and bacterial pneumonias, owing to immunosuppression. (**A** from Hendrix CM, Robinson E: Diagnostic parasitology for veterinary technicians, ed 3, St Louis, 2006, Mosby. **B** from McCurnin DM, Bassert JM: Clinical textbook for veterinary technicians, ed 6, St Louis, 2006, Saunders.)

| TABLE 17-1 | Summary of Vitamins, Dietary Sources and Importance | |
|---|---|---|
| **VITAMIN** | **DIETARY SOURCE** | **IMPORTANCE IN THE BODY** |
| *WATER-SOLUBLE VITAMINS* | *EXCESS IS EXCRETED IN URINE SO TOXICITIES ARE RARE* | |

**B Complex Vitamins:**

| | | |
|---|---|---|
| Vitamin B1 (thiamine) | Meat, fish, eggs, leafy green vegetables, legumes, liver | Limited amount stored in the body |
| Required for the transformation of pyruvic acid to acetyl coenzyme A (CoA) in carbohydrate metabolism. Needed in the synthesis of some neurotransmitters (acetylcholine). Rapidly destroyed by heat | | |
| Vitamin B2 (riboflavin) | Milk, meat (fish, poultry, and red meats), liver, eggs, grains, legumes | Found in the body as flavin mononucleotides (FAD and FMN), which serve as hydrogen acceptors. Also needed for oxidation of amino acids |
| Vitamin B3 (niacin or nicotinamide) | Milk, meat (fish, poultry, and red meats), liver, eggs, grains, potatoes, peanuts, leafy green vegetables, yeast, liver | The amino acid tryptophan, which is found in many food groups, is easily converted to niacin. Niacin is part of nicotinamide adenine dinucleotide (NAD⁺), which is important in glycolysis, and in the catabolism of fats. |
| Vitamin B5 (pantothenic acid) | Found in large quantities in internal organs such as brain, kidney, liver, adrenal, and heart. Also found in grains, legumes, eggs, and yeast. Name refers to the Greek word *panthos*, meaning *everywhere*, and referring to the diverse dietary sources | Stable when heated. Is a major component of coenzyme A. Important in the oxidation of fatty acids and in the synthesis of steroids and hemoglobin |
| Vitamin B9 (folacin or folic acid) | Lean beef, eggs, veal, whole grains, liver, orange juice, deep green vegetables, yeast. A crystalline vitamin that is bright yellow | Essential for the formation of red blood cells. Is one of many coenzymes that are part of methionine, choline, and DNA synthesis |
| Vitamin B12 (cyanocobalamin) | Found in liver, meat (poultry, fish, and red meat), dairy (but not eggs), and butter. Not found in plants. *Intrinsic factor* is required for absorption in the intestine. | Stored in the liver in quantities that meet bodily needs for 3 to 5 years. Essential for the synthesis of methionine and choline. Is a coenzyme in all cells in the body, particularly in the nervous system, bone marrow, and gastrointestinal tract |

**Others:**

| | | |
|---|---|---|
| Biotin (vitamin H) | Liver, eggs, nuts, and legumes. In some species, it is generated by enteric bacteria in the gut. | Essential for reactions in the Krebs cycle. Functions as a coenzyme in a number of reactions, including carboxylation, decarboxylation, deamination, and anabolism of purines and nonessential amino acids |
| Vitamin C (ascorbic acid) | Found in fruits and vegetables, especially large quantities in citrus fruits, leafy green vegetables, tomatoes, cantaloupe, and strawberries | Important antioxidant. Needed for the formation of collagen fibers in connective tissue and the conversion of tryptophan to serotonin. Aids absorption of iron. Activates folicin (a B vitamin) |
| **Fat-Soluble Vitamins:** | Fat-soluble vitamins are stored for long periods of time in tissues. Excess is not excreted, making toxicity a possibility if high levels are consumed | |
| Vitamin A (retinol) | Can be formed in the body from ingested beta-carotene, which is found in dark green leafy and dark yellow vegetables. Vitamin A is found in fish oils, milk, eggs, and liver. | 90% is stored in the liver, so feeding liver routinely to dogs or cats can cause toxicity. Enough is stored to meet the body's needs for one year |
| Vitamin D (antirachitic factor or calciferol) | Formed in the skin when ultraviolet (UV) light converts 7-dehydrocholesterol. Modified to the active form in the liver and kidneys. Also found in liver oil, eggs, and fortified milk | Essential for blood clotting and bone and tooth formation. Acts as a hormone that regulates calcium levels in the blood by increasing absorption from the gut and mobilizing calcium from bone |
| Vitamin E (antisterility factor or tocopherols) | Found in wheat germ, nuts, whole grains, vegetable oils, and green leafy vegetables. Stored in muscle and fat tissue; chemically similar to sex hormones | An important antioxidant. Prevents oxidation of unsaturated fatty acids and cholesterol. Helps prevent oxidative damage to cell membranes |
| Vitamin K (coagulation factor or quinones) | Found in leafy green vegetables, cauliflower, broccoli, pork liver, and cabbage. Also synthesized by bacteria in the large intestines of some species | Essential for the generation of clotting factors and many proteins made by the liver. Contributes to the process of oxidative phosphorylation in cells |

Water-soluble vitamins are absorbed through the gut wall when water is absorbed in the gastrointestinal tract. The water-soluble vitamins include vitamin C and eight of the B-complex vitamins. An exception is vitamin B12, however, which must bind to gastric intrinsic factor before it can be absorbed. Very small amounts of water-soluble vitamins are stored in the body, and excesses not used within an hour are excreted in the urine. Hypervitaminosis conditions involving water-soluble vitamins are therefore extremely rare.

Fat-soluble vitamins include A, D, E, and K. These bind to ingested lipids before they are absorbed with the ingesta. Thus, if fat absorption is impaired, so too is the absorption of fat-soluble vitamins. Except for vitamin K, fat-soluble vitamins are stored in the body; therefore, if an excessive amount of a fat-soluble vitamin is consumed, vitamin toxicity due to hypervitaminosis may result. For example, liver is high in vitamin A, and owners who frequently feed liver to their dogs or cats may unknowingly induce a toxic condition in their pets.

Proteins, carbohydrates, and lipids are oxidized as part of the normal metabolic processing of food. This process uses oxygen and generates some potentially harmful **free radicals**. Vitamins A, C, and E are potent antioxidants that disarm dangerous free radicals. Certain foods such as broccoli, cauliflower, cabbage, and Brussels sprouts are all good sources of vitamins A and C.

Antioxidants are thought to act like a bucket brigade, passing dangerous free radicals from one molecule to another until they can be excreted. For example, vitamin E returns a free radical to a less harmful state but, in doing so, vitamin E itself becomes a free radical. It is subsequently inactivated by carotenoids, and the carotenoid free radicals that are produced are then inactivated by vitamin C. Water-soluble free radicals are subsequently formed, which can be flushed from the body in urine.

## MINERALS

Minerals are inorganic substances that are essential for life, though they make up less than 4% of an animal's body by weight. Like vitamins, minerals do not generate energy, but they work with other nutrients to ensure that the body functions normally. Minerals are classified as **macrominerals**, **microminerals**, and **trace elements**, depending upon how much is required by the body; however, the amount of a particular mineral in the body does not tell you how important that mineral is. Iodine, for example, is needed in extremely small quantities, yet it is vital for normal thyroid function, which controls metabolic rate.

Macrominerals include calcium, chlorine, magnesium, phosphorus, potassium, and sodium. Calcium and phosphorus are the most abundant minerals in the body and together compose three quarters of the minerals by weight. These, together with magnesium salts, harden the teeth and form the rigid, hard material that gives bone its strength. Sodium and chlorine are the primary electrolytes found in blood. They are vital for maintaining normal oncotic pressures in the body and for assisting in water absorption in the kidney. Macrominerals are expressed in parts per hundred (1 pph = 10 g per kg of food).

| BOX 17-2 | Summary of the Minerals Found in the Body |
| --- | --- |

| MACROMINERALS | MICROMINERALS | TRACE MINERALS |
| --- | --- | --- |
| *Calcium (Ca) | Copper (Cu) | Chromium (Cr) |
| Chlorine (Cl) | Iodine (I) | Cobalt (Co) |
| Magnesium (Mg) | Iron (Fe) | Fluorine (F) |
| *Phosphorus (P) | Manganese (Mn) | Molybdenum (Mo) |
| Potassium (K) | Selenium (Se) | Nickel (Ni) |
| Sodium (Na) | Zinc (Zn) | Silicon (Si) |
| | | Sulfur (S) |
| | | Vanadium (V) |

*By far the most abundant minerals in the body.

Microminerals include copper, iodine, iron, manganese, selenium, and zinc. These are expressed in parts per million (1 ppm = 1 mg per kg of food). Iron is one of the most vital microminerals, because it is the core of the hemoglobin molecule that carries oxygen in red blood cells. Without iron, cells could not receive the oxygen needed to make ATP, and the animal would die.

Trace elements include chromium, cobalt, fluorine, molybdenum, nickel, silicon, sulfur, and vanadium. Of these, fluorine is perhaps the most well known, because of its importance in healthy teeth. Refer to Box 17-2 for a complete listing of all of the minerals.

### ✓ TEST YOURSELF 17-2

1. What is the principal building-block unit of proteins? How are these units arranged?
2. What are the four basic components of an amino acid molecule? Which parts of the molecule change to create the different kinds of amino acids?
3. Some amino acids cannot be synthesized in the body and must be provided in the diet. What are these amino acids called? Can you give an example of one in cats? Can you give an example of one in birds?

## METABOLISM

The cell is a dynamic, living powerhouse. It undergoes hundreds of metabolic reactions in its lifetime, building molecules and breaking down nutrients, manufacturing, packaging, and excreting. All of these biochemical events are part of the cell's metabolism. **Cell metabolism** is divided into two categories: *catabolism* and *anabolism*.

Catabolism is a process that involves *breaking down* nutrients into smaller molecules to produce energy. Energy is stored in the bonds of the ATP molecule, which can be transported to other parts of the cell where it is needed. Anabolism is a process in which the stored energy is used to *assemble* new molecules from the small components that are produced from catabolism. Catabolic and anabolic reactions occur simultaneously, and each must be in exquisite balance with the other so that adequate levels of energy are maintained.

## CATABOLIC METABOLISM

The breakdown of large molecules into small ones is the basis of catabolism. Catabolism occurs in three stages. The first stage occurs in the lumen of the gastrointestinal tract, and stages two and three occur inside the cells of tissues; stage two occurs in the cytoplasm and stage three occurs in the mitochondria.

### STAGE ONE: THE GASTROINTESTINAL TRACT

As you know, the chewed food that animals swallow is too big to pass through the wall of the intestine, and therefore it must be digested and broken down into tiny units so that it can enter the absorptive cells that line the intestinal tract. Digestion of food occurs in the stomach and in the first part of the small intestine, the duodenum, where acids and emulsifiers work together to break down the nutrient molecules into fundamental nutritional units. Water, vitamins, and minerals are also derived from food. Potatoes, for example, may be broken down into molecules of carbohydrate, and a steak may be broken down into protein and fat molecules.

Carbohydrates, proteins, and fats are further broken down, or catabolized, before being absorbed. This part of the catabolic process is called *hydrolysis*—*hydro* means *water* and *lysis* means *to break down*—because at least one molecule of water is used up each time a nutrient molecule is broken down. Hydrolysis is the first stage of catabolism. A large sugar molecule, such as a polysaccharide, can be broken down into disaccharides, for example, and disaccharides, in turn, can be hydrolyzed into two smaller sugar molecules, called *monosaccharides:*

$$1\,Disaccharide + Water \rightarrow 1\,Monosaccharide + 1\,Monosaccharide$$

Through the process of hydrolysis, protein is broken down into *amino acids;* carbohydrates into monosaccharides; *nucleic acids* into nucleotides; and fats into fatty acids and glycerol (Figure 17-7). Once hydrolysis is complete, the smaller nutrient molecules are taken up by absorptive cells that line the small intestine and are transported through the cell away from the lumen of the intestine. On the basal surface of the cell, the nutrient molecules are expelled and transferred to capillaries and extracellular spaces deeper in the wall of the intestine. Here they are picked up by blood

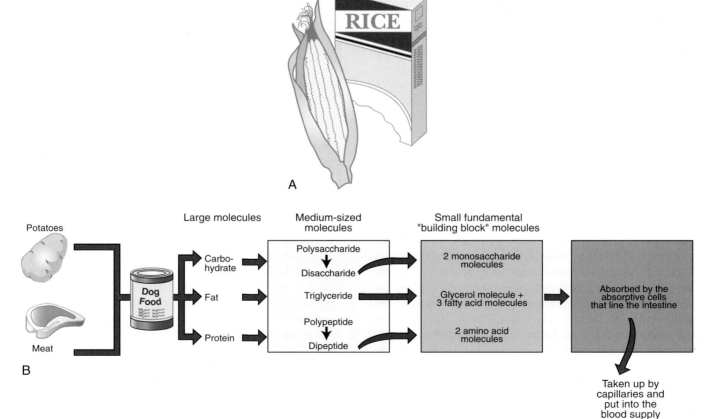

**FIGURE 17-7** Building blocks. Large molecules that make up carbohydrates, fats, and proteins are broken down into fundamental building blocks to make new and different molecules. This process is the foundation of nutrition and cell metabolism.

and lymph and carried to the hungry cells that make up the organs and tissues found throughout the body. Many nutrients are carried to the liver, where the nutrient molecules are either assembled into larger molecules or are further metabolized before being used by the body (Figure 17-8).

## STAGE TWO: THE CYTOSOL

The second stage of catabolism occurs inside the cell's cytosol. Amino acids, monosaccharides, fatty acids, and glycerol enter cells and are further catabolized in the cytoplasm through a process called **anaerobic respiration**. Because *an* means *not,* and *aerobic* means *using oxygen,* **anaerobic** respiration therefore is simply a metabolic process that does not use oxygen. An important molecular product of anaerobic respiration is acetyl coenzyme A (CoA), which carries a lot of the energy derived from food; acetyl CoA is transported through the cytosol to the mitochondria, where it is used in **aerobic respiration**, which is the third and final stage of catabolism.

## STAGE THREE: THE MITOCHONDRIA

As its name implies, aerobic respiration requires oxygen; it involves the attachment of an inorganic phosphate group ($PO_4$) to a molecule of **adenosine diphosphate (ADP)**. The result is the formation of **adenosine triphosphate (ATP)**, which is a critical molecule used in the cell to carry much of the energy that is derived from food; this energy is essential for making new molecules.

The mitochondrion can be viewed as an energy-producing factory; much of the energy that is derived from food is stored in the bonds of the ATP molecule. The catabolic pathways of proteins, carbohydrates, and fats are vital to the survival of the cell and therefore to the animal as a whole, because the pathways transfer the energy stored in the nutrient molecules to a small, transportable unit—ATP—which can then be used by the cell to grow, divide, heal, and maintain itself.

## ANABOLIC METABOLISM

The cell uses energy in the form of ATP to manufacture a wide range of substances and to perform many vital functions. These *constructive* duties define anabolism, and the ATP that powers them is supplied by catabolism. Anabolic events are also called *biosynthetic processes,* because a biochemical substance is manufactured. Examples of anabolism are evident in many aspects of cellular life. When cells grow, for example, additional proteins are needed for the expanded cell membrane. The cytoskeleton and additional organelles are manufactured. Cell locomotion, the production and secretion of hormones, the movement of materials from one place to another inside the cell, active membrane processes, and preparation for cell division are all examples of cellular activities that require the production of biochemical substances via anabolism. With the exception of deoxyribonucleic acid (DNA), molecular substances are routinely broken down, and replacement molecules are manufactured continuously. This process is called **metabolic turnover**, and it

represents the largest demand for protein and enzymes in the cell.

An important part of anabolism is *dehydration synthesis,* the effect of which is the opposite of hydrolysis. Monosaccharides, for example, are assembled—not broken down—to form chains of polysaccharides. A disaccharide, which is a chain of two monosaccharides, can be constructed as follows:

$$1\,Monosaccharide + 1\,Monosaccharide \rightarrow 1\,Disaccharide + Water$$

Glycerol and fatty acid molecules are connected to form fat molecules, and proteins are created from chains of amino acids. All of these anabolic processes begin with dehydration synthesis.

Many of the anabolic cellular processes occur in the cytosol during stage two of metabolism. Here, the building blocks glucose, glycerol, fatty acids, and amino acids are incorporated into larger molecules, which may be used by the cell itself or exported and used elsewhere in the body. The liver in particular is an important organ because of its active anabolic efforts; it manufactures proteins such as albumin and clotting factors, and it manufactures and stores glycogen and fat.

Refer to Figure 17-9 for a summary of both catabolic and anabolic metabolism. Here, glycolysis is represented in blue, the Krebs cycle is in orange, and the electron transport chain appears in yellow.

---

✓ **TEST YOURSELF 17-3**

1. What is cellular metabolism? Can you think of routine cellular processes that represent specific examples of cell metabolism?
2. Cellular metabolism is divided into two categories. What are they?
3. What is the first stage of cellular catabolism called? Is energy produced or consumed?
4. Is energy produced or consumed during an anabolic process? What is an example of anabolism?
5. What cellular process represents the largest demand for protein and enzymes?

---

## CONTROL OF METABOLIC REACTIONS

Living cells are composed of and contain thousands of molecules. How is it possible for all of these molecules to interact in a structured and orderly fashion that maintains life for the cell? As discussed in the previous chapter, compartments are created within or on the surface of organelles, such as the mitochondria, endoplasmic reticulum, or ribosome. These "work areas" help to isolate molecules and allow chemical reactions to take place without interference. The organelles not only create separate environments for the different metabolic pathways, but also assist in storing the enzymes and cofactors required for various biochemical processes. However, grouping molecules together does not guarantee that they will react with one another. Molecules must collide with sufficient force to initiate a

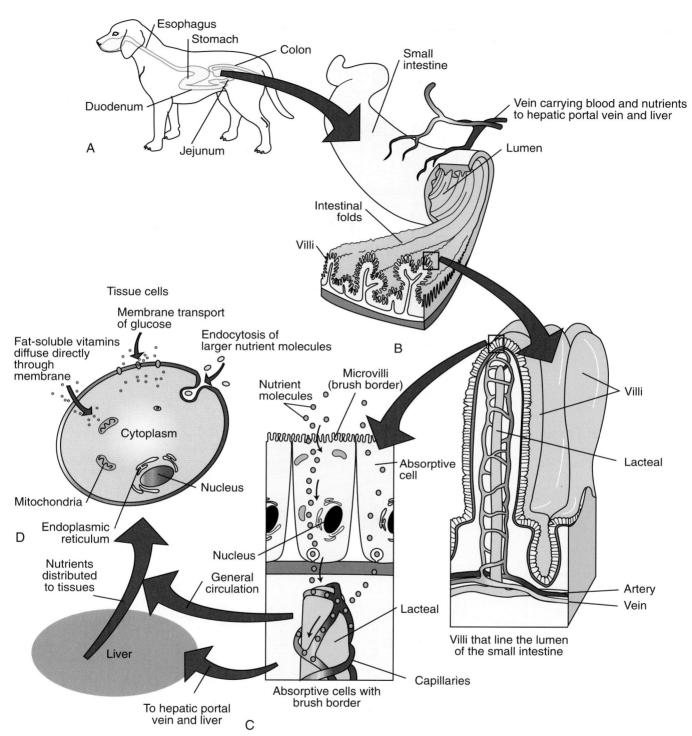

**FIGURE 17-8** Summary of stage one of metabolism. **A**, Food is broken down in the stomach, and the digested stomach contents (chyme) pass into the small intestine. Here the food is broken down further by enzymes in the lumen of the intestine. **B**, In addition, the cell membranes in the microvilli brush border produce more enzymes, which further catabolize the nutrient molecules into their building-block units. Monosaccharides, fatty acids, glycerol, and amino acids are taken up by the absorptive cells. **C**, The nutrient molecules are then transported through the absorptive cell and are taken up by capillaries (amino acids and sugars) or lacteals (fatty acids) in the villi. Once in the blood or lymph, nutrient molecules are carried quickly away from the gastrointestinal tract. Most of the nutrient-rich blood flows directly to the liver via the hepatic portal vein. In the liver, the nutrient molecules are either incorporated into the production of larger molecules or are further broken down. From the liver, nutrients continue to travel through the general circulation to other body tissues. **D**, Cells throughout the body absorb the nutrient molecules from blood and lymph. Once in the cytoplasm, the molecules can undergo the second stage of metabolism.

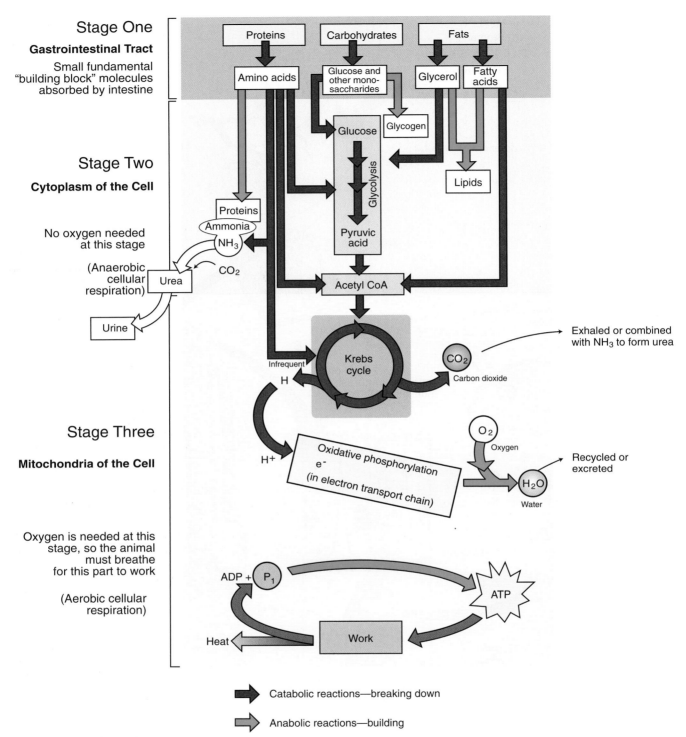

**FIGURE 17-9** Summary of metabolism. Cell metabolism occurs in three stages. In the first stage, large nutrient molecules from food are degraded by enzymes and emulsifiers in the lumen of the stomach and intestine. Much smaller molecules are formed, which are absorbed through the intestine and transferred to blood and lymph. They are transported to various parts of the body. In the second stage, tissue cells absorb the small building-block molecules from the bloodstream. In the cytoplasm of the cell, the small molecules may be either used to make larger molecules (anabolism) or broken down into even smaller molecules, such as pyruvic acid and acetyl CoA (catabolism). Stage three is entirely catabolic: acetyl CoA is transported to the mitochondria of the cell, where it is broken down in the Krebs cycle. The hydrogen atoms that result are channeled into the electron transport chain, where ATP is produced via oxidative phosphorylation.

reaction. The moderate temperatures of the intracellular environment and the relative stability of intracellular organic molecules preclude forceful collisions. How, then, are molecular reactions initiated and controlled? The answer is simple: through the formation and use of specialized proteins called *enzymes.*

## ENZYMES

Each enzyme reacts with a particular molecule called a *substrate* to produce a new molecule called a *product.* Because one enzyme reacts only with one substrate or combination of substrates, enzymatic reactions are considered highly specific. Hundreds of different biochemical reactions take place within the cell, so there must be hundreds of different enzymes available, each with the ability to locate and bond to its own special substrate. The DNA contained within the nucleus of the cell carries instructions for manufacturing all of the enzymes needed to drive these vital metabolic pathways. Metabolism therefore is a multi-enzyme sequence of events in which the product of one step is the substrate of the next. Some metabolic pathways include as many as 20 enzyme-driven steps. Although many of these pathways are linear, some are circular and all have branches leading into or out of them.

Most chemical reactions require an input of energy to get started. The energy needed to initiate a biochemical reaction is called the *energy of activation.* In the laboratory, the energy of activation is often supplied by heat. Heat causes molecules to become more active and to bang into one another. When molecules collide, existing bonds can be broken and new bonds can be formed. In this way, new substances are created. However, increased temperatures would be destructive to organelles and other structures within the cell. In addition, temperature changes would affect *all* of the chemical reactions at once and would not be selective for a particular type of reaction. The cell therefore relies on enzymes to initiate and control metabolic reactions.

An enzyme's ability to locate and bond to a particular substrate depends on the molecular *shape* of the enzyme. Enzymes are globular proteins that consist of one or more flexible polypeptide chains. These chains twist and coil to form a unique, three-dimensional shape that fits the special shape of the substrate molecules. When the enzyme and substrate bind together, they form a temporary enzyme–substrate complex.

The region of the enzyme molecule that binds to the substrate is called the *active site.* Like other portions of the enzyme, the active site is flexible and can exert pressure on the substrate that, in turn, weakens the bonds that keep the substrate molecule intact. In this way, one or more **product molecules** are formed, which subsequently separate from the enzyme. In biosynthetic reactions, enzymes unite smaller molecules to form one large molecule. These enzymes therefore require more than one active site, as shown in Figure 17-10. The enzyme is not altered by the reactions that it initiates and is able to move on to other substrate molecules to complete more of the same kind of reaction.

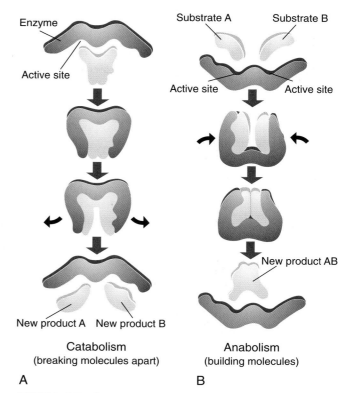

**FIGURE 17-10** Enzyme activity. **A,** Enzymes are flexible molecules with dynamic active binding sites; they are able to bond to one substrate to produce two product molecules via catabolism. **B,** They can also bind to two substrates to form a single product molecule via anabolism.

Because enzymes bring reactant substrate molecules into close proximity and form temporary associations with them, they are able to speed up the rate of molecular reactions. For this reason, enzymes are also called *catalysts,* which are substances that speed up reactions by lowering the activation energy. Heat and various elements, ions, and chemicals can also act as catalysts. In the cell, enzymes speed up molecular reactions by a factor of a million or more. The rate at which a catalyzed reaction occurs is related to the amount of substrate and enzyme present. In general, an increase in the amount of an enzyme or a substrate causes an increase in the rate of the reaction. In addition, different enzymes have varying innate rates; that is, one type of enzyme might perform fewer reactions per second than another type of enzyme.

As mentioned earlier, each enzyme is specific for a particular reaction; for example, hexokinase is an enzyme that converts glucose to glucose-6-phosphate (G6P), and this is the *only* reaction that hexokinase initiates and controls. It binds with glucose and ATP to create G6P and ADP, and it repeats this reaction over and over again. The amount of enzymes needed by the cell to carry out thousands of reactions is therefore relatively small, because the enzymes are not used up during the reactions but are used multiple times to complete more reactions.

When studying cell metabolism, you can easily pick out the enzyme, because its name ends in the suffix *-ase.* In addition, the enzyme is usually named for the substrate on which it acts. For example, *proteinases* are enzymes that break down protein, *lipase* breaks down lipid, *lactase* breaks down lactose, and so on. The name of the enzyme may also indicate the kind of reaction that the enzyme initiates. For example, *synthetases* are enzymes that *synthesize* or make new substances, and *transferases* are enzymes that move one part of a molecule to another molecule. Phosphotransferase, for example, is an enzyme that transfers a phosphate group from one molecule to another molecule. For these reasons, enzymes may have long names, such as glucose-1-phosphate uridylyltransferase and phosphoglucomutase. Although they may be a linguistic challenge at times, the names of enzymes are very useful and may indicate the biochemical reactions that are taking place.

## COENZYMES AND COFACTORS

Some enzymes are not able to complete a reaction without the assistance of another substance. Elements such as iron, zinc, or copper, for instance, are needed to complete the shape of a binding site. These nonprotein substances are called **cofactors**. Certain ions, such as magnesium, are cofactors in reactions that involve the transfer of a phosphate group and are therefore found in virtually all cells. The negative charges on the phosphate group are attracted to the positive charges on the magnesium cation. The attraction of these opposite charges helps to stabilize the enzyme–substrate complex. $K^+$ and $Ca^{2+}$ play a similar role in other molecular reactions.

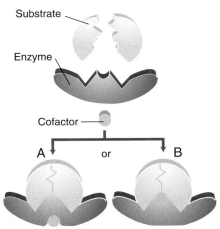

**FIGURE 17-11** Cofactors and coenzymes assist in the activity of enzymes in one of two ways. **A**, A cofactor is added to the structure of a molecule in such a way that it indirectly changes the shape of the active site to enable a better fit between substrate and enzyme. **B**, A cofactor is part of the active site and plays a direct role in creating the correct shape of the active site.

Nonprotein organic substances may also act as cofactors. These substances are called **coenzymes** and often are, or are derived from, vitamins. They may be bound temporarily or permanently to the enzyme and are usually located near the active site (Figure 17-11). **Nicotinamide adenine dinucleotide (NAD)** and flavin adenine dinucleotide (FAD), for example, are commonly encountered cellular coenzymes and are critical in powering important cellular functions.

 **CLINICAL APPLICATION**

### Thermolabile Enzymes

Because enzymes are protein molecules with complicated three-dimensional structures, they are able to bend and move to accommodate bonding activities. Their shape is critical in enabling the enzyme to bond with the correct substrate. However, the shape of the binding site in some enzymes is affected by changes in the surrounding temperature. These enzymes are called **thermolabile enzymes**, because changes in temperature bring about changes in the structure and shape of the enzyme molecule.

For example, in the Siamese cat, a thermolabile enzyme that affects coat color functions well at cooler temperatures but is rendered nonfunctional at higher temperatures; therefore, a dark brown or black pigment is produced in the cooler regions of the body, such as the tips of the ears and the tail, face, and paws, but not in warmer areas, such as the torso, neck, and thighs. Himalayan rabbits also carry thermolabile enzymes that affect coat color. For example, Himalayan rabbits raised at temperatures of around 5° C are entirely black; those raised at moderate temperatures are white with black ears, tail, and paws; and those raised at temperatures above 35° C are completely white.

### An Easy Diagnosis

It is not uncommon for cats or dogs to develop Horner's syndrome, a condition caused by damage to a chain of nerves

that extends from the chest, up the neck, and into the head and face. Possible causes include ear infections, particularly those caused secondarily by ear mites; trauma to the neck, often from misuse of choke chains; tumors in the chest; and trauma to the nerves in the armpit region. Usually only one side of the face is affected, and the most pronounced clinical signs include abnormal changes to the affected eye.

Horner's syndrome also causes profound dilation of blood vessels in the muscles and skin of the face, an abnormality that is obvious in horses because they sweat profusely on the affected side. However, in domestic dogs and cats that do not sweat this change is usually not clinically apparent. In Siamese cats, the increased blood flow and the increased temperature in their faces change the shape of thermolabile enzymes, making them unable to function normally. The production of pigment in the hair is halted, and in cases of long-term Horner's syndrome, the characteristic dark brown or black color of the Siamese face fades to a light tan or buff. Keep in mind that the appearance can look comical, because this condition usually affects only one side of the face. Fortunately, for most cats, Horner's syndrome is a short-term disorder.

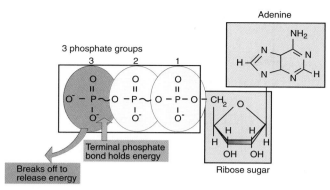

**FIGURE 17-12** Conversion of ATP to ADP. When the terminal phosphate bond in an ATP molecule is broken, it releases stored energy that can be used by the cell to make other molecules. The remaining molecule, ADP, has two phosphate groups.

## ENERGY FOR METABOLIC REACTIONS

Energy is required for the survival of all living cells. In mammals, energy is supplied to cells by the breakdown of nutrients, and energy is transferred to various energy-holding molecules such as ATP, NADH, and $FADH_2$. In these convenient molecular packages, energy can be stored for extended periods and easily transported to regions of the cell where energy is in demand. Energy is captured and stored in the formation of atomic bonds but is released when these bonds are broken. ATP, for example, stores energy in the terminal phosphate bond. When the phosphate group is broken off, energy is released and the molecule is transformed into ADP (Figure 17-12). The released energy is used during subsequent biochemical reactions.

The molecules that make up animal cells are adept at transforming themselves, from nutrient molecules to molecular energy stores and from substrate to product, cleaving off portions here and adding extensions there. Thus it is the molecule that stores, transforms, and uses energy in the cell through the formation and breakage of its molecular bonds.

### TEST YOURSELF 17-4

1. Why are enzymatic reactions considered highly specific?
2. What is a substrate? What is a product?
3. Why is the total number of enzymes present in the body relatively low, when compared with the number of metabolic reactions?
4. What is the energy of activation in a biochemical reaction?
5. What is a catalyst? Why are enzymes considered catalysts?
6. How can you tell that a molecule is an enzyme? List three characteristics of enzymes.
7. What are some specific examples of cofactors?
8. How might vitamins play a role in enzyme-driven reactions?
9. How is energy stored in molecules? When is it released?
10. Give three examples of energy-holding molecules.

## METABOLIC PATHWAYS

The goal of metabolizing nutrients derived from food is to generate the energy needed to keep the body going. The breakdown of carbohydrates, proteins, and fats each follows a different metabolic pathway, and each pathway generates different amounts of energy. As mentioned, some phases of the pathways occur in the cytoplasm and do not require oxygen (anaerobic), whereas other parts occur in the mitochondria and do require oxygen (aerobic). These pathways represent a complex series of biochemical steps that must occur in a particular sequence, and each step involves an enzyme specific for that particular step.

## CARBOHYDRATE METABOLISM

**Carbohydrate metabolism** occurs in virtually all living cells and includes all of the catabolic and anabolic processes involving carbohydrates. In mammals, carbohydrates may be supplied either through the diet or from the breakdown of glycogen, glycerol, or, in the case of ruminants, propionate stored in the liver. In most mammals, carbohydrates provide well over half the energy required to fuel metabolic functions, such as absorption, secretion, excretion, mechanical work, growth, and repair. Refer to Figure 17-13 for an overview of carbohydrate metabolism.

Glucose is the primary carbohydrate found in blood. It is absorbed by all cells and is used to produce energy in the form of ATP. Certain types of cell, such as red blood cells and brain cells, are exquisitely sensitive to fluctuations in blood glucose levels, because they cannot derive energy from other sources. Other cells, however, such as skeletal muscle cells, can derive energy from ketones and fatty acids and therefore are not as affected by falls in blood glucose supplies. Nevertheless, when glucose is urgently needed and in short supply, the body is able to provide it quickly by mobilizing stores of glycogenic molecules in the liver.

Glucose may enter a cell either by *facilitated diffusion* or via *active transport*. Once inside the cell, glucose is further broken down to form pyruvate, or pyruvic acid. This process is called *glycolysis* (*lysis* means "break apart") and occurs in the cytoplasm. Because glycolysis does not require oxygen, it is referred to in some texts as *anaerobic respiration*.

After pyruvate is formed from glycolysis, one of several pathways may follow. Most of the time, cells are fed with good quantities of oxygen via circulating red blood cells. In an oxygen-rich environment, pyruvate is transported from the cytosol to the mitochondria, where it undergoes further degradation as part of aerobic respiration. The Krebs cycle and the electron transport chain are two important components of aerobic respiration. **Anaerobic glycolysis** and aerobic respiration (the Krebs cycle and the electron transport chain) are collectively known as **cellular respiration**.

Some cells, such as skeletal muscle cells, may take a different pathway than aerobic respiration if their oxygen supply has become depleted. During vigorous exercise, for example, skeletal muscle cells rapidly consume oxygen. Once the oxygen is depleted, the cells take a different metabolic

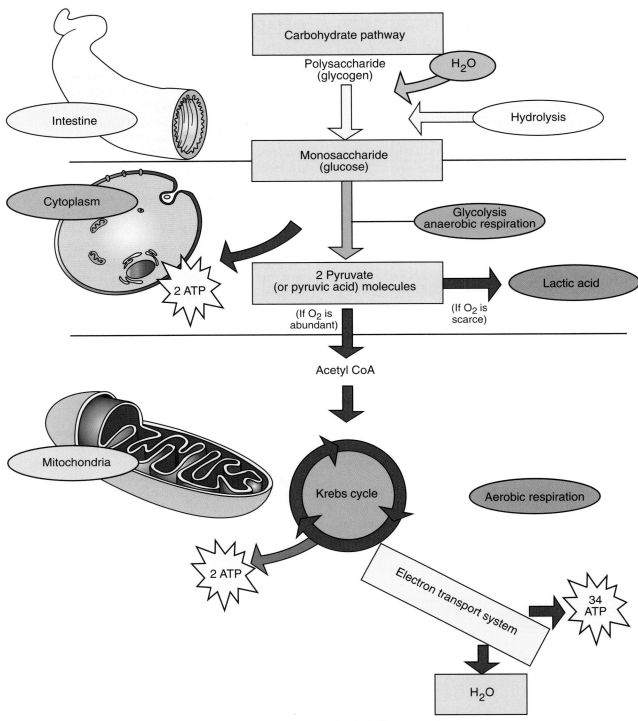

**FIGURE 17-13** Overview of carbohydrate metabolism.

pathway and convert pyruvate to *lactic acid.* We have all experienced the effects of lactic acid production in our own muscles at one time or another, particularly after performing strenuous work that we do not normally do. Lactic acid builds up in muscles during and after exercise and causes a stiff feeling the next day. In horses, this stiffness can be severe and can cause a condition called **myositis** or *"tying up."* It is not uncommon for horses ridden for pleasure to "tie up" on Mondays, because many owners only ride them on weekends. For this reason, myositis in horses is sometimes called *"Monday morning syndrome."*

The biochemical pathways of cellular respiration have been studied extensively by biochemists and therefore are discussed in detail. However, keep in mind that the principles involved in their function and regulation are common to all pathways of cell metabolism.

### ANAEROBIC RESPIRATION: GLYCOLYSIS.

Glycolysis, or "sugar splitting," occurs in all animals and includes 10 biochemical steps, each of which relies on a specific enzyme found in the cytoplasm. As mentioned, it does not require oxygen. For every molecule of glucose metabolized, the cell must use two molecules of ATP and two molecules of NAD to initiate the process. Two molecules of pyruvic acid, four molecules of ATP, and two molecules of **NADH** are produced. Thus, the net energy yield from glycolysis is two molecules of NADH and two molecules of ATP.

The chemical reactions of glycolysis can be summarized in three phases. Refer to Figure 17-14. In the initial phase, energy—one ATP molecule—is invested in the process of adding a phosphate molecule to glucose, which results in the formation of glucose-6-phosphate (G6P). This process is called **phosphorylation**, and although it costs the cell energy, it is important in preventing the glucose molecule from leaving the cell; this is because phosphorylated glucose cannot cross the cell membrane. Phosphorylation also prepares the glucose molecule for further manipulations, either in a catabolic or anabolic pathway. Subsequently, G6P is rearranged to form fructose-6-phosphate. From here, phosphorylation occurs again, using one more ATP molecule to form fructose-1,6-diphosphate.

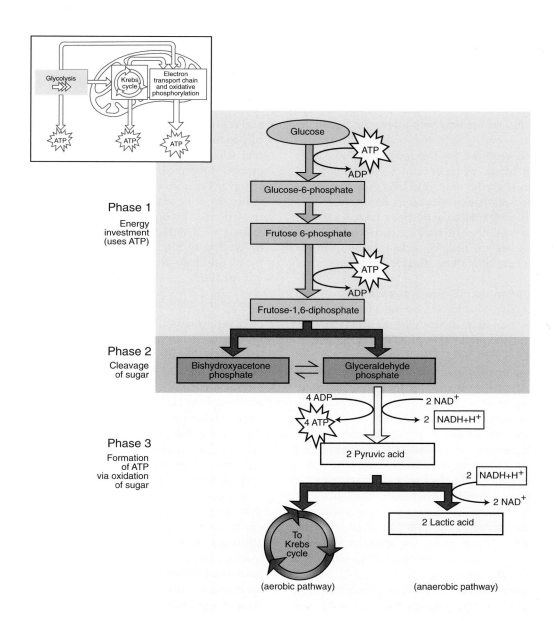

**FIGURE 17-14** Glycolysis. In glycolysis, a six-carbon glucose molecule is split into a pair of three-carbon molecules of pyruvic acid (pyruvate). This process includes 10 steps and produces six energy-holding molecules: two molecules of NADH and four molecules of ATP. Given that two molecules of ATP were used in phase one, the net production of energy is two molecules of NADH and two of ATP.

During phase two, fructose-1,6-diphosphate is cleaved. A pair of three-carbon molecules is formed, but they can be one of two reversible isomers: *bishydroxyacetone phosphate* and *glyceraldehyde phosphate.* The molecules change back and forth between these two forms.

Phase three includes six steps, which result in the formation of four ATP molecules and two molecules of pyruvic acid. The net energy production by glycolysis, however, is two ATP, because two ATP molecules were used in phase one to "prime the pathway."

Although its contribution of energy to animal cells is important, glycolysis is *not* the cell's primary source of ATP. A great deal of potential energy from the original glucose molecule still remains in pyruvic acid. This molecule can be further broken down in the mitochondria to form larger quantities of energy for the cell through an aerobic sequence of biochemical events.

**AEROBIC RESPIRATION.**  When animals breathe in air, they are performing a vital function. Everyone knows that when animals *stop* breathing, they die. Like humans, animals can only survive for a short time without oxygen before the cells in the body—particularly the brain—start to die, because oxygen is required for the production of energy (ATP) by the cell. Many cell types cannot live without ATP for very long. Blood carries oxygen to cells throughout our bodies. After blood releases oxygen molecules to the cells, it picks up carbon dioxide molecules that have been discharged by the cell. These molecules are then circulated back to our lungs, where they are exhaled. We exhale carbon dioxide because our cells give off carbon dioxide in the process of making ATP.

Aerobic respiration occurs in the mitochondria in two stages: the *Krebs cycle,* also known as the *citric acid cycle,* and the *electron transport chain.* The mitochondrion is uniquely suited for the production of ATP; it is the powerhouse of the cell.

The smooth outer membrane of the mitochondrion is permeable to most small molecules, but the undulating inner membrane is more selective and permits the passage of only certain molecules, such as pyruvic acid and ATP. The folds of the inner membrane are called *cristae,* and they contain within their walls some of the enzymes and cofactors needed in the Krebs cycle. Other enzymes are found in the **mitochondrial matrix**, which is the thick solution that bathes the cristae within the mitochondria. Enzymes in the mitochondria responsible for aerobic respiration have positioned themselves on the cristae in the order in which they are needed for oxidation. This assembly-line approach is an efficient way to carry out molecular alterations and minimizes the potential for errors.

The inner membrane of the mitochondrion houses a series of cytochrome molecules, which make up the electron transport system. As electrons are passed from one cytochrome molecule to another, energy is released that is used to transport protons from the mitochondrial matrix across the inner membrane to the intermembrane space. Because protons are positive, this establishes a positive charge on the outside of the inner membrane relative to the matrix side. The electrical gradient that is established is a form of stored energy. Energy is released when protons rush back into mitochondrial matrix; this release of energy is the ultimate power source that converts ADP into ATP. Refer to Figure 17-15 for a summary of cellular respiration.

**KREBS CYCLE.**  Pyruvic acid enters the mitochondria from the cytoplasm by passing through both the outer and inner membranes. Before it enters the **Krebs cycle**, it is transformed from a three-carbon molecule of pyruvic acid into a two-carbon acetyl group; this, in turn, binds to a compound known as *coenzyme A* to form *acetyl CoA,* the molecule that represents the link between glycolysis and the Krebs cycle. During this process, one molecule of carbon dioxide and one of NADH are also generated for every molecule of pyruvic acid.

Acetyl CoA enters the Krebs cycle and reacts with oxaloacetic acid to form citric acid; therefore, the Krebs cycle is also known as the **citric acid cycle** (Figure 17-16). As citric acid is produced, coenzyme A is released and is used repeatedly to make acetyl CoA. After seven additional steps, citric acid is converted back to oxaloacetic acid, and the entire process is repeated. Each turn of the Krebs cycle generates energy in the form of one ATP, one FADH$_2$, and three NADH molecules. For every molecule of glucose, the Krebs cycle can run twice and produce two molecules of ATP, two of FADH$_2$, and six of NADH. Carbon dioxide, which is formed as a by-product of respiration, diffuses out of the cell and into the bloodstream as waste and is carried to the lungs, where it is exhaled.

**ELECTRON TRANSPORT SYSTEM.**  The final stage of cellular respiration, which produces the majority of ATP for the cell, occurs in the inner wall of the mitochondrion and is known as the **electron transport system**. NAD and FAD molecules released from the conversion of pyruvic acid to acetyl CoA, glycolysis, and the Krebs cycle bind to hydrogen atoms to form NADH and FADH$_2$. The electrons in NADH and FADH$_2$ are at a very high energy level, because they hold most of the energy once held by the original glucose molecule. In a sense, they are at the top of an energy "hill" and are carried down a chain of electron carrier molecules, collectively known as the **cytochromes**.

Each cytochrome molecule contains a central core of iron that accepts electrons and then releases them at a lower energy level. At each step, large amounts of free energy are released and used to pump protons from the mitochondrial matrix through the inner membrane to the intermembranous space, which is the space between the inner and outer membranes of the mitochondrion. This establishes a difference in electrical charge, because more positive hydrogen ions are pumped to the outside than remain on the inside of the inner mitochondrial membrane. Thus, the outside has a positive charge relative to the matrix side of the membrane. The result is the formation of potential energy that is

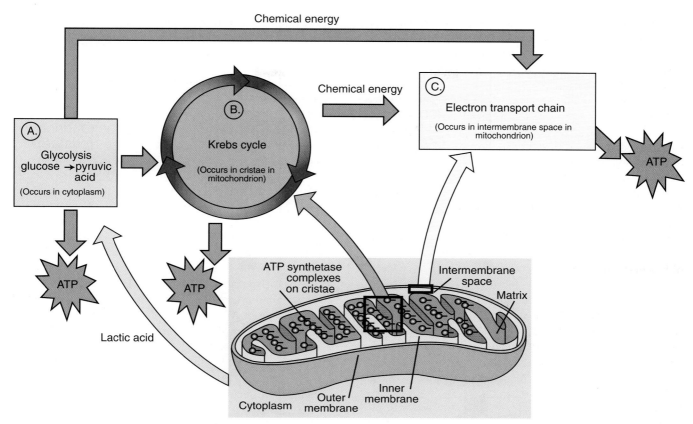

**FIGURE 17-15** Summary of cellular respiration. **A,** Glycolysis occurs in the cytoplasm, where glucose is converted to two molecules of pyruvic acid. A net production of two ATP molecules occurs. Other chemical energy in the form of two NADH molecules is produced, which is converted to ATP in the electron transport system. **B,** Krebs cycle. The inner membrane of the mitochondrion has infoldings and outpouchings, called *cristae,* which form separate "work spaces" for the Krebs cycle. Many of the enzymes involved in ATP production, such as ATP synthetase, are built into the wall of the inner membrane. These molecules form an assembly line, which improves efficiency and helps to prevent errors. The matrix that fills the internal spaces of the cristae is rich with electron carriers, phosphates, coenzymes, and other solutes necessary for ATP production. **C,** The electron transport chain. The inner membrane of the mitochondrion houses a series of cytochrome molecules, which make up the electron transport system. As electrons are passed from one cytochrome molecule to another, energy is released that is used to transport protons from the mitochondrial matrix across the inner membrane to the intermembrane space. Because protons are positive, this establishes a positive charge on the outside of the inner membrane relative to the matrix side. The electrical gradient that is established is a form of stored, potential energy. Energy is released when protons rush back into the mitochondrial matrix. This release of energy is the ultimate power source that converts ADP into ATP.

available when the protons flow back to the matrix side of the inner mitochondrial membrane (Figure 17-17). The energy released during this downhill pathway is captured in the formation of ATP from ADP. At the end of the electron transport chain, oxygen accepts the low-energy electrons, joins with hydrogen ions, and forms water ($H_2O$). Thus oxygen is the final acceptor of the electrons.

### SUMMARY OF ATP SYNTHESIS. The biochemistry of glucose catabolism is complicated, so let us take a step back and look at the overall picture of what the cell is doing.

Through the breakdown of glucose, the cell produces units of usable energy called *ATP.* For every molecule of glucose metabolized by an animal, a maximum of 38 ATP molecules are formed, although in some cells only 36 ATP molecules are formed. Two ATP molecules are made in the cytoplasm, and the rest are made in the mitochondria.

In the cytoplasm, glycolysis gives rise to two molecules of ATP directly and two molecules of NADH. The NADH molecules are shuttled to the electron transport system in the mitochondria, where they produce six ATP molecules (three for every molecule of NADH). Thus, the total gain from glycolysis is eight ATP molecules. However, in certain cells, such as brain and skeletal muscle cells, there is an energy cost for transporting NADH into the mitochondria. In these cells, each NADH molecule produces only two ATP, rather than three; therefore, in some cells, glycolysis produces only six ATP, not eight.

Inside the mitochondria, pyruvic acid is converted to acetyl CoA before it enters the Krebs cycle. During this process, two molecules of NADH are formed, one from each of the two molecules of pyruvic acid. Each of these NADH molecules forms three molecules of ATP, so a total of six ATP molecules are derived from the conversion of pyruvic acid to acetyl CoA.

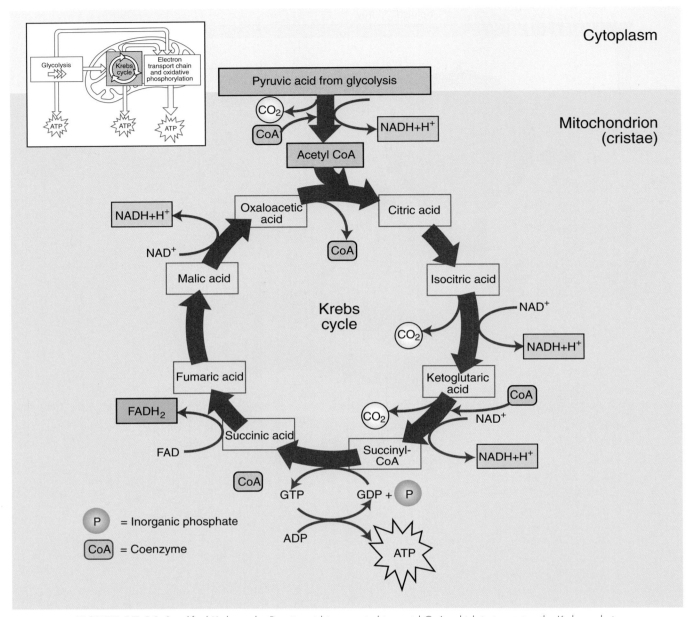

**FIGURE 17-16** Simplified Krebs cycle. Pyruvic acid is converted to acetyl CoA, which in turn enters the Krebs cycle in the matrix of the mitochondrion. Carbon and oxygen are released from the cycle as waste and are ultimately exhaled by the animal in the form of carbon dioxide. For every molecule of glucose, the Krebs cycle can run twice and in doing so produces two molecules of ATP, two of $FADH_2$, and six of NADH. From these energy-carrying molecules, hydrogen atoms are released and used in the electron transport system to produce ATP.

Also in the mitochondria, the Krebs cycle yields two molecules of ATP, two of $FADH_2$, and six of NADH. The electron transport system converts the NADH and $FADH_2$ molecules into 22 ATP; so the Krebs cycle produces a total of 24 ATP.

Table 17-2 provides a summary of ATP production in the cell. Notice that all but two of the 38 ATP molecules are produced in the mitochondria and that all but four ATP result from the passage down the electron transport chain of electrons carried by NADH and $FADH_2$. Once formed, the energy-carrying ATP molecules are exported across the mitochondrial membrane, and a molecule of ADP is brought into the mitochondrion for each ATP exported.

## LIPID METABOLISM

Lipids are molecules composed of carbon, hydrogen, and oxygen, which are insoluble in water but dissolve easily in other lipids or organic solvents. One common type of lipid is the *triglyceride* or *neutral fat.*

Triglycerides contain a higher number of carbon–hydrogen bonds than other nutrient molecules and therefore contain more chemical energy than either carbohydrates or proteins,

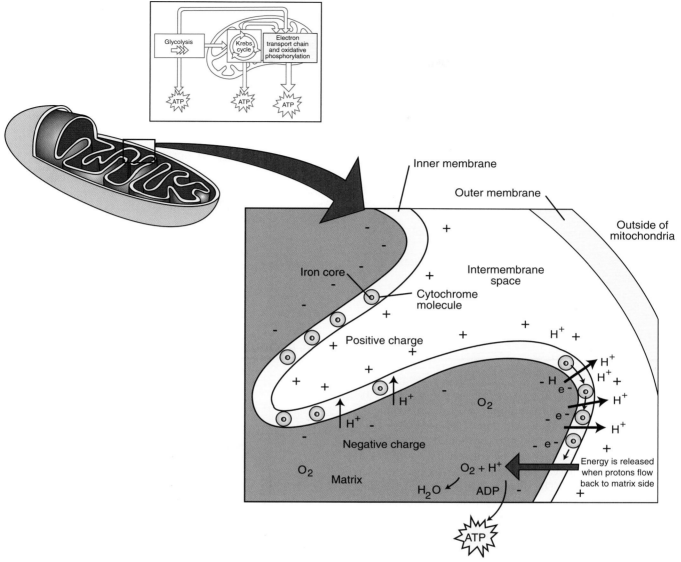

**FIGURE 17-17** The electron transport system. Cytochrome molecules are located in the inner membrane of the mitochondrion. Each cytochrome molecule contains a central iron core that accepts electrons and then releases them to another cytochrome molecule at a lower energy level. At each step, a large amount of free energy is used to pump protons from the matrix through the inner membrane to the intermembrane space. This establishes an electrical charge difference (potential energy) between the matrix and the intermembrane space, because more protons are pumped to the outside than remain on the inside of the inner membrane. Energy is released when the protons flow back to the matrix side. This energy is used to convert ADP to ATP. The low-energy electrons left at the end of the cytochrome chain and the hydrogen atoms in the matrix bind to oxygen and form water ($H_2O$).

because energy is stored in the bonds between atoms. Gram for gram, fat contains over *twice* as much chemical energy as carbohydrate and stores *six* times as much energy as glycogen. This fact is important, particularly in birds, because it illustrates that fat concentrates energy in a form that is relatively lightweight—an essential requirement for flight. Herbivores do not consume the large amount of fat that is prevalent in the diet of meat eaters. For them, the formation of fat is derived primarily from the conversion of carbohydrates in excess of what can be stored as glycogen.

The liver is the primary controller of lipid metabolism. Triglycerides can be removed from circulating blood by the liver and structurally altered. For example, lipids may be broken into smaller fragments that enable them to enter the glycolytic pathway to form pyruvic acid, or they may be fed directly into the Krebs cycle. This process is called **lipolysis**.

Triglycerides, specifically, are hydrolyzed into one molecule of glycerol and three fatty acid chains. The glycerol head is further catabolized in the cytoplasm to acetyl CoA and subsequently enters the Krebs cycle; or it may be used to synthesize glucose. The fatty acid tails, on the other hand, are long chains of 18 carbon atoms or more and are handled by enzymes found in the mitochondria.

| **TABLE 17-2** | Summary of Energy Production from One Glucose Molecule | | |
|---|---|---|---|

## CYTOSOL

*Anaerobic Cellular Respiration (Glycolysis—no oxygen needed)*

| | PRODUCTS | ATP PRODUCTION FROM ELECTRON TRANSPORT SYSTEM (OXIDATIVE PHOSPHORYLATION) | TOTAL PRODUCTION |
|---|---|---|---|
| | 2 molecules of **pyruvic acid** (goes to mitochondria) 2 ATP 2 NADH | 6 ATP | 2 ATP 6 ATP |

## MITOCHONDRIA

*Aerobic Respiration (Oxygen Required from Inhalation)*

| | | | |
|---|---|---|---|
| Intermediate stage: conversion of pyruvic acid (from cytosol) to acetyl CoA | 2 NADH $CO_2$ (exhaled) | 6 ATP | 6 ATP |
| Krebs cycle (citric acid cycle) | Two turn of Krebs cycle produce: 2 ATP 2 $FADH_2$ 6 NADH $CO_2$ (exhaled) | 4 ATP 18 ATP | 2 ATP 4 ATP 18 ATP |
| | | **FINAL PRODUCTION** | **38 ATP** |

Through a process known as *beta oxidation,* each fatty acid chain is broken into multiple two-carbon fragments. Some of these fragments are converted to acetyl CoA, whereas others are converted into compounds called **ketone bodies**. Later, the ketones can be converted to acetyl CoA, which can be further catabolized in the Krebs cycle to form ATP (Figure 17-18). The energy gain from the complete oxidation of an 18-carbon fatty acid chain is substantial—about 148 ATP, which is about 4 times more energy than that generated from the catabolism of one molecule of glucose. Because fat, for the most part, is not soluble in water and is therefore difficult to mobilize, it serves primarily as a reserve energy source, rather than a supply to meet immediate energy demands.

If not immediately used to produce energy, glycerol and fatty acid chains may be reconstructed into lipids and stored in fatty tissue. This is nature's way of protecting the health of animals and humans when food supplies become low.

## PROTEIN METABOLISM

Proteins are found in great abundance in animals. The body of a cow, for instance, may contain several thousand different proteins, each with a unique function and a unique structure to fit its function. Proteins include **structural proteins**, such as hair, microtubules, and collagen; **regulatory proteins**, such as insulin and other hormones; **contractile proteins**, such as actin and myosin in muscle tissue; **transport proteins**, such as hemoglobin and myoglobin; **storage proteins**, such as those found in egg whites; **protective proteins**, such as antibodies; **membrane proteins**, such as cell receptors and membrane transport molecules; and **osmoregulators**, such as albumin and enzymes. Clearly

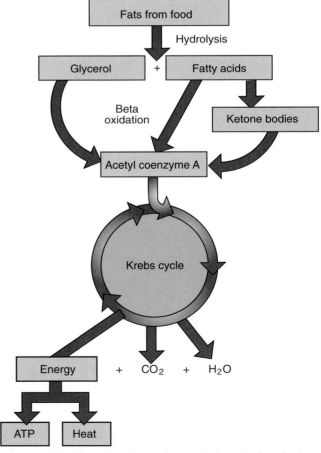

**FIGURE 17-18** Triglyceride metabolism. Triglycerides from food are digested into glycerol and fatty acids. These can be further broken down to form acetyl CoA, which enters the Krebs cycle to form ATP. Excess nutritional triglycerides not immediately catabolized for energy are stored in tissue as fat.

the diversity of proteins and the functions they perform are extensive.

**PROTEIN CATABOLISM.** In addition to the multiple roles that proteins play in the structural and functional maintenance of the body, proteins may also be catabolized and used to make energy (ATP) (Figure 17-19). Although amino acid catabolism occurs in most tissues, it is of particular importance in the intestinal mucosa, kidney, brain, liver, and skeletal muscle, where the amino acid molecules may undergo one of two processes: **deamination** or **transamination**. These processes occur in the mitochondria (Figure 17-20).

In transamination, the amine group ($-NH_2$) is transferred to another carbon chain to form a different amino acid. These newly constructed amino acids then diffuse across the mitochondrial membranes into the surrounding cytosol, where they become the building blocks for other proteins.

In deamination, the amine is removed from the carbon chain and becomes an ammonia molecule. Because ammonia is toxic, even in small quantities, most deamination reactions occur in the liver, where specialized enzymes are present to convert ammonia to *urea,* a nontoxic water-soluble molecule that is excreted in urine. After the amine has been removed by deamination, the remaining carbon chain may enter the Krebs cycle at one of several locations, resulting in the formation of ATP. Some of the pathways, for example, enter the Krebs cycle from the formation of acetyl CoA; others enter much later. As a result, deamination may give rise to a variable amount of ATP, depending on where the cycle was entered. If energy is not immediately required, the carbon chains may not enter the Krebs cycle but instead will be converted to glucose or fat.

**PROTEIN ANABOLISM.** The manufacture of new protein from nutrient building blocks is an important function for cells. The genetic material housed in the nucleus contains the instructions for the manufacture of thousands of different types of protein. Refer to Chapter 4 for a detailed description of the processes by which proteins are made.

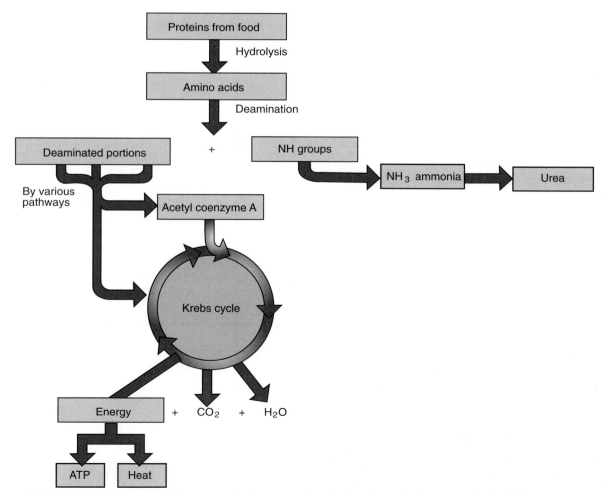

**FIGURE 17-19** Overview of protein metabolism. Protein from food is digested into amino acids, but before they are completely catabolized, the amine group ($NH_2$) is removed and converted to ammonia, which is later excreted in urine. The remainder of the deaminated portion is then converted to acetyl CoA and subsequently is used to generate ATP.

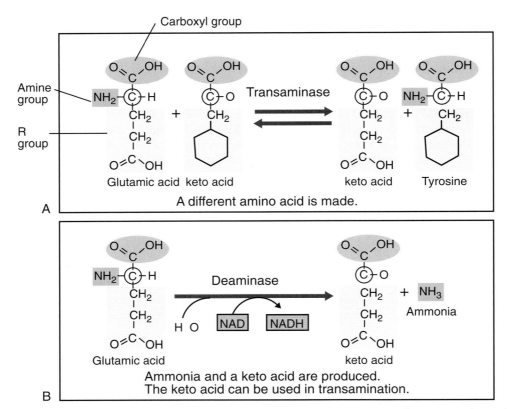

**FIGURE 17-20** Transamination and deamination. **A**, During transamination, an amine group of an amino acid is transferred to another molecule by the enzyme transaminase, and a different amino acid is subsequently formed. When stripped of its amine group, an amino acid becomes a keto acid. **B**, During deamination, an amine group is removed from an amino acid by the enzyme deaminase. The amino acid then becomes a keto acid, which can be reused in transamination reactions. The amine group is converted to ammonia, a toxin; the liver subsequently converts ammonia to a nontoxic molecule called *urea*.

 **CLINICAL APPLICATION**

### Liver and Kidney Failure

During protein catabolism, ammonia is produced. Because ammonia is toxic, it is converted by the liver to a nontoxic molecule called *urea*.

$$\text{Protein} \rightarrow \text{(liver)} \rightarrow \text{ammonia} \rightarrow \text{(kidney)} \rightarrow \text{urea} \rightarrow \text{urine}$$

Urea is a type of nitrogenous waste; it is a compound that contains nitrogen and is excreted. Nitrogenous waste is normally pulled out of the bloodstream by the kidneys and put into urine. When the kidney becomes diseased, however, it is sometimes unable to excrete urea effectively. The urea therefore builds up in the bloodstream, causing a condition called *uremia*. Uremia can be detected by a blood test that evaluates the blood urea nitrogen (BUN) level of the patient. Veterinarians look for this in the blood chemistry profiles of sick animals. Similarly, if the BUN is abnormally low, the veterinarian might suspect liver disease, because the liver is responsible for converting ammonia to urea. If the liver is not functioning normally, it cannot carry out this conversion. Can you guess what might happen to the ammonia level in an animal with liver disease?

### TEST YOURSELF 17-5

1. What is the most common carbohydrate found in blood?
2. Where does carbohydrate metabolism begin in nonruminant animals?
3. What part of carbohydrate metabolism occurs in the cytoplasm?
4. Under what conditions is lactic acid formed in muscle cells?
5. How many biochemical steps are involved in glycolysis? Does glycolysis require oxygen?
6. Cellular respiration is composed of what two parts?
7. How does the membrane structure of the mitochondrion assist in the process of cellular respiration?
8. What role does oxygen play in the electron transport system?
9. What is oxidative phosphorylation?
10. What is the maximum number of ATP molecules that can be formed from the catabolism of one molecule of glucose?
11. What are transamination and deamination?

# 18 The Urinary System

*Angela Beal*

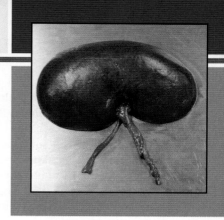

## OUTLINE

## LEARNING OBJECTIVES

*When you have completed this chapter you will be able to:*

1. List and describe the functions of the kidneys.
2. Describe the gross and microscopic anatomy of the kidneys.
3. List the main blood vessels associated with the kidneys.
4. Define the terms *glomerular filtration, renal threshold, polyuria, polydipsia, urolithiasis,* and *uremia.*
5. Describe the production of urine.
6. Describe the mechanisms that affect urine volume.
7. Explain the renal mechanisms that help regulate blood pressure.
8. Describe the structures and functions of the ureters and urinary bladder.
9. Describe the processes involved in urination.
10. Describe the structure and functions of the urethra.

## VOCABULARY FUNDAMENTALS

*Afferent glomerular arteriole* ā-fər-ehnt glō-**meər**-ū-lahr ahr-**teer**-ē-ōl
*Aldosterone* ahl-**dohs**-tuhr-ōn
*Antidiuretic hormone (ADH)* **ahn**-tē-dī-ū-**reht**-ihck **hohr**-mōn
*Anuria* ahn-**yər**-ē-ah
*Azotemia* ā-zō-**tē**-mē-ah
*Bowman's capsule* **bō**-mahnz **kahp**-sehl
*Capsular space* **kahp**-sehl-ahr spās
*Collecting duct* kah-**lehck**-tihng duhckt
*Cortex* **kohr**-tehx
*Distal convoluted tubule (DCT)* **dihs**-tahl kohn-vah-**lū**-tehd **too**-būl
*Diuresis* dī-ū-**rē**-sihs
*Efferent glomerular arteriole* ē-fər-ehnt glō-**meər**-ū-lahr ahr-**teer**-ē-ōl
*Erythropoietin* ē-rihth-rō-**poy**-eh-tihn
*Fenestration* fehn-ih-**strā**-shuhn

*Glomerular filtrate* glō-**meər**-ū-lahr fihl-**trāt**
*Glomerular filtration rate (GFR)* glō-**meər**-ū-lahr fihl-**trā**-shuhn rāt
*Glomerulus* glō-**meər**-ū-luhs
*Glycosuria* glī-kōs-**yər**-ē-ah
*Hilus* **hī**-luhs
*Homeostasis* hō-mē-ō-**stā**-sihs
*Loop of Henle* loop of **hehn**-lē
*Medulla* meh-**duhl**-uh
*Micturition* mihck-tuhr-**ihsh**-shuhn
*Nephron* **nehf**-rohn
*Oliguria* awl-ihg-**yər**-ē-ah
*Osmotic diuresis* ohs-**moh**-tihck dī-ū-**rē**-sihs
*Peritubular capillary* peər-ih-**too**-būl-ahr **kahp**-eh-leər-ē
*Podocyte* **pōd**-ō-sīt
*Polydipsia* pohl-ē-**dihp**-sē-ah
*Polyuria* pohl-ē-**yər**-ē-ah
*Postrenal uremia* pōst-**rē**-nuhl yər-ē-**mē**-ah

*Prerenal uremia* prē-**rē**-nuhl yər-**ē**-mē-ah
*Prostaglandin* prohs-tuh-**glahn**-duhn
*Proximal convoluted tubule (PCT)* **prohck**-sih-mahl
  kohn-vah-**lū**-tehd **too**-būl
*Reabsorption* rē-ahb-**sohrp**-shuhn
*Renal artery* **rē**-nuhl **ahr**-tər-ē
*Renal corpuscle* **rē**-nuhl **kohr**-puhs-ehl
*Renal pelvis* **rē**-nuhl **pehl**-vihs
*Renal uremia* **rē**-nuhl yər-**ē**-mē-ah
*Renal vein* **rē**-nuhl vān
*Renin* **reh**-nihn
*Renin–angiotensin–aldosterone system* **reh**-nihn
  ahn-jē-ō-**tehn**-sihn ahl-**dohs**-tuhr-ōn **sihs**-tehm

*Retroperitoneal* reh-trō-peər-ih-tō-**nē**-ahl
*Secretion* seh-**krē**-shuhn
*Glomerular capillary* thuh glō-**meər**-ū-lahr
  **kahp**-eh-leər-ē
*Trigone* **trī**-gōn
*Tubular filtrate* **too**-būl-ahr fihl-**trāt**
*Uremia* yər-**ē**-mē-ah
*Uresis* yər-**ē**-sihs
*Ureter* **yər**-eh-tər
*Urinary calculi* **yər**-ih-neər-ē **kahl**-kyoo-lī
*Urinary stone* **yər**-ih-neər-ē stōn
*Urination* yər-ih-**nā**-shuhn
*Urolith* **yər**-ō-lihth

## INTRODUCTION

An animal's body is a finely tuned machine that relies on numerous metabolic reactions to keep it alive and healthy. These chemical reactions are of great benefit to the body but also result in the production of many by-products, some of which are useful to the body and are recycled. Other by-products, on the other hand, are of no further use to the body and can be harmful if allowed to accumulate. These potentially harmful substances are called *waste products* and must be eliminated from the body (Box 18-1). Some examples of metabolic waste products are:

- Carbon dioxide and water from carbohydrate and fat metabolism
- Nitrogenous wastes, primarily urea, from protein metabolism
- Bile salts and pigments from red blood cell breakdown
- Various salts from tissue breakdown and excessive consumption

The body has several routes by which waste products are eliminated:

- The respiratory system removes carbon dioxide and water vapor.
- The sweat glands eliminate water, salts, and a small amount of urea.
- The digestive system removes bile salts and bile pigments.
- The urinary system removes urea, salts, water, and other soluble waste products.

The urinary system is the single most important route of waste-product removal in the body. It removes nearly all the soluble waste from blood and transports it out of the body. The urinary system is also a major route for the elimination of excess water from the body.

| BOX 18-1 | Summary of Waste Removal |

### Excretion

The urinary system's chief function is to regulate the volume and composition of body fluids and excrete unwanted material, but it is not the only system in the body that is able to excrete unnneded substances. The table below compares the excretory functions of several systems. Although all of these systems contribute to the body's effort to remove wastes, only the urinary system can finely adjust the water and electrolyte balance to the degree required for normal homeostasis of body fluids.

| SYSTEM | ORGAN | EXCRETION |
|---|---|---|
| Urinary | Kidney | Nitrogen compounds |
| | | Toxins |
| | | Water |
| | | Electrolytes |
| Integumentary | Skin-sweat glands | Nitrogen compounds |
| | | Electrolytes |
| | | Water |
| Respiratory | Lung | Carbon dioxide |
| | | Water |
| Digestive | Intestine | Digestive wastes |
| | | Bile pigments |
| | | Salts of heavy metals |

From Patton KT, Thibodeau GA: Anatomy & physiology, ed 8, St Louis, 2013, Mosby.

## Urinalysis

A urinalysis ("UA") is the laboratory analysis of a urine sample. It can be performed by a commercial laboratory or by veterinary personnel within a veterinary clinic. Performing a complete urinalysis involves three major steps:

1. A gross examination of the physical properties of the sample.
2. A chemical analysis of substances dissolved in the urine.
3. A microscopic examination of the solid components in the urine.

Before beginning a urinalysis, a urine sample must be obtained from the patient. There are several options for urine collection. Ideally, the sample should be collected in a sterile manner so that any bacteria observed in the sample are derived from the urinary tract and not from contamination of the sample during collection. Sterile collection methods include urinary catheterization or cystocentesis. To perform cystocentesis (A), a sterile needle is inserted through the skin of the lower abdomen and into the bladder. Urine is drawn directly from the bladder through the needle and into the sterile syringe. Nonsterile methods of sample collection include "catching" the urine in a container as it is voided (free catch method) and collecting the sample in a container as the bladder is compressed manually.

After collection, the physical properties of the urine are evaluated. The volume, color, odor, transparency, and specific gravity of the sample are observed and recorded (B). Normal urine is light yellow to amber in color, depending on the amount of water it contains. The odor of normal urine varies between species. The urine of most animals is clear or transparent; however, equine urine normally contains mucus, which gives it a cloudy appearance. Specific gravity (SG) is a reflection of the concentration of the urine and is measured using an instrument called a refractometer. Normal specific gravity measurements vary among species.

Chemical analysis of the urine sample is performed using a reagent strip (C). Each strip contains a series of pads, and each pad is impregnated with a chemical that causes a color change to indicate the presence of a particular substance in the urine. Urine is placed on the reagent strip using a pipette or syringe. The color change of the various reagent pads is observed at specific times and compared to a reference chart provided by the manufacturer. Chemical analysis reagent strips commonly provide information about urine pH and the presence of protein, glucose, ketones, bile pigments (bilirubin and urobilinogen), red blood cells, and white blood cells in the sample.

Lastly, a microscopic examination of the solid components (sediment) of the urine sample is performed. To prepare the sample, urine is placed in a test tube and centrifuged to concentrate the sediment into a pellet at the bottom of the tube. The sediment is then examined microscopically for the presence of various microscopic elements such as red blood cells, white blood cells, epithelial cells, tubular casts, crystals (D), and microorganisms such as bacteria, fungi, and parasites.

A thorough urinalysis is essential to identify conditions affecting the urinary system such as infections, crystalluria and urinary calculi, diabetes mellitus, and many others. Being proficient in performing a urinalysis is an important component of becoming an invaluable veterinary technician.

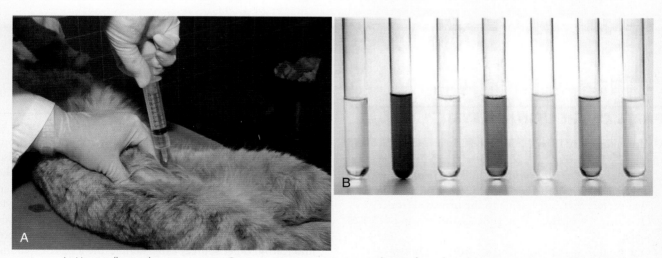

A, Urine collection by cystocentesis. Cystocentesis is a common procedure performed to obtain an uncontaminated urine sample. B, An array of urine specimens with variations in color. In veterinary hospitals where there are healthy and sick animal patients, urine samples are found with a variety of colors and levels of clarity depending upon the species and relative health of the patient.

*Continued*

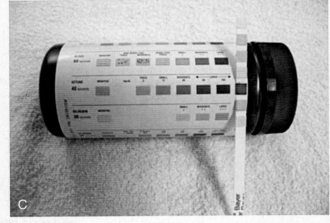

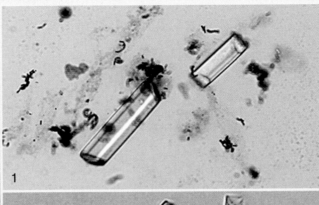

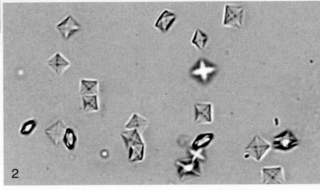

**C,** Commercial urine dipstick testing. A reagent strip is used to measure multiple substances (glucose, blood cells) that may be present in urine. **D,** Examples of crystals that may be observed during microscopic evaluation of urine. Microscopic view of struvite *(D1)* and calcium oxalate *(D2)* crystals in urine sediment from a dog. (**A,** From Taylor SM: Small animal clinical techniques, St Louis, 2010, Elsevier Saunders; **B,** from Little S: The cat, clinical medicine and management, ed 1, St Louis, 2011, Elsevier Saunders; **C,** from Pugh AN, Baird DG: Sheep and goat medicine, ed 2, St Louis, 2012, Elsevier Saunders; **D,** from Bassert JM, Thomas J: McCurnin's clinical textbook for veterinary technicians, ed 8, St Louis, 2014, Elsevier Saunders.)

## PARTS OF THE URINARY SYSTEM

As shown in Figure 18-1, *A* and *B*, the urinary system is made up of:

- Two kidneys that make urine and carry out other vital functions
- Two ureters that carry urine to the urinary bladder
- One urinary bladder that collects, stores, and releases urine
- One urethra that conducts urine from the body

## KIDNEYS

In medical terminology, the combining word forms for kidney are *nephro* (Greek) and *reno* (Latin). For example, *nephrology* is the study of the kidney, and the artery and vein that supply and drain blood from the kidney are the ***renal artery*** and *renal vein*.

## FUNCTION

The kidney's most obvious role is the production of urine to facilitate the elimination of metabolic waste materials from the body. In the process of making urine, the kidney also helps maintain **homeostasis** in the body by manipulating the composition of blood plasma. In this way, the kidney can regulate such things as body acid–base and fluid–electrolyte balances. The kidney must filter enough water and electrolytes out of the blood to equal the amount that is being put into it from other sources. For example, the levels of sodium, potassium, chloride, and nitrogenous waste (primarily urea from protein breakdown) in plasma must be maintained within specific, narrow concentration limits for health and life to continue. If the kidney fails to remove these substances from plasma adequately, their concentrations can rise to toxic levels, leading to illness and potentially death.

Maintaining homeostasis in the body is the most important overall function of the kidneys. The main processes by which the kidneys help maintain homeostasis include:

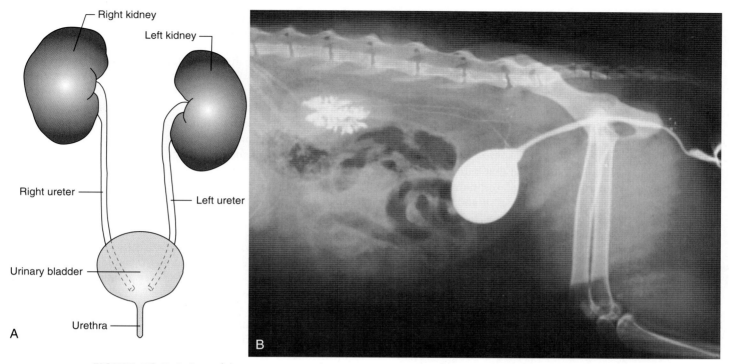

**FIGURE 18-1 A,** Parts of the urinary system. The urinary system is made up of two kidneys, two ureters, one urinary bladder, and one urethra. **B,** Cystogram. Lateral view of the urinary system distended by contrast medium. (From Lavin L: *Radiography for veterinary technicians, ed 4,* St Louis, 2007, Elsevier Saunders.)

- *Blood filtration, reabsorption, and secretion.* The blood is filtered, useful substances are returned to the circulation, and waste products are secreted from the bloodstream into the fluid that eventually becomes urine. More on these processes later in the chapter.
- *Fluid balance regulation.* The amount of urine produced depends on the amount of water it contains, which helps ensure that the body contains the right amount of water to maintain a healthy internal environment. If the body has excess water and needs to get rid of it, more urine is formed (**diuresis**). If the body needs to conserve water, less urine will be produced, and the animal will pass little urine (**oliguria**) or no urine at all (**anuria**). The amount of water contained in the urine is under the control of the hormones **antidiuretic hormone (ADH)** and **aldosterone**.
- *Acid–base balance regulation.* The kidneys help maintain acid–base homeostasis by their ability to remove acidic hydrogen and basic bicarbonate ions from the blood and excrete them in urine. By eliminating these ions in the appropriate amounts, blood pH can be maintained in the proper range.
- *Hormone production.* The kidneys have close associations with the endocrine system—the hormones that help regulate body functions. The kidneys produce hormones, regulate the release of hormones from other organs, and are themselves influenced by hormones. For example, the kidney can influence the rate of release of **ADH** from the posterior pituitary gland and **aldosterone**, the mineralocorticoid secreted by the cortex of the adrenal gland. The kidneys are also influenced by both of these hormones.

Specialized cells in the kidneys produce **erythropoietin**, the hormone necessary for red blood cell production, and some **prostaglandins**. (Consult Chapter 11 for more information about these and other hormones.)
- *Blood pressure regulation.* The kidneys contain internal receptors that monitor blood pressure. When blood pressure falls, the kidneys secrete a hormone called renin. The release of renin will start a cascade of reactions that will result in vasoconstriction and the retention of sodium and water. By increasing the fluid volume of the blood, blood pressure will also be increased.

## LOCATION

The kidneys are located in the dorsal part of the abdomen, just ventral to and on either side of the first few lumbar vertebrae. In common domestic animals, except the pig, the right kidney is more cranial than the left. A thick layer of fat (*perirenal fat*) usually surrounds the kidneys and helps protect them from pressure exerted by surrounding organs.

The kidneys are located **retroperitoneal** to the abdominal cavity; that is, they are outside the parietal peritoneum (between the peritoneum and the dorsal abdominal muscles) and are therefore considered officially *outside* the abdominal cavity. To a limited extent, the kidneys move with movements of the diaphragm. As the diaphragm contracts, the kidneys are pushed caudally, sometimes by nearly half the length of a vertebra. This is one of the reasons abdominal radiographs should be taken when the patient has exhaled completely. In many species, the right kidney is less mobile, because it fits into a depression in the liver that helps stabilize it. The left kidney doesn't have this stabilization, so it is more mobile. The positions of the kidneys and abdominal organs are more standardized that way.

## GROSS ANATOMY

The kidneys are bean-shaped in most animals and are covered by a fibrous connective tissue capsule (Figure 18-2). Look at a kidney bean and you'll have a good idea of the origin of its name. The right kidney in horses appears compressed end to end, so it becomes somewhat heart-shaped. Kidneys are reddish brown. Look at that kidney bean again. The color is about right. With the exception of cattle, the kidneys of domestic animals have a smooth surface. The surface of cattle kidneys is divided into about 12 lobes that give it a lumpy appearance.

The indented area on the medial side of the kidney is called the **hilus**. This is the area where blood and lymph vessels, nerves, and the **ureters** enter and leave the kidney. If

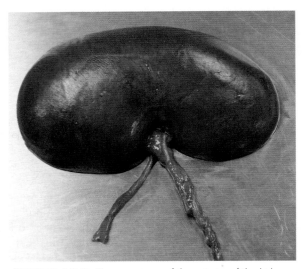

**FIGURE 18-2** Gross anatomy of the exterior of the kidney.

you cut the kidneys of most animals in half longitudinally through the hilus, you'll find a funnel-shaped area inside the hilus (Figure 18-3). This area is the **renal pelvis**. It is a urine collection chamber that forms the beginning of the ureter. The renal pelvis is lined with transitional epithelium, the type of epithelium that is capable of considerable stretching without being damaged. Cattle don't have a distinct collection chamber that can be called a renal pelvis.

The outer portion of the kidney is called the renal **cortex**. It is reddish brown and has a rough granular appearance. The inner portion around the renal pelvis is the renal **medulla**. It has a smooth appearance with a dark purple outer area that sends rays up into the cortex and a pale, gray–red inner area that extends down to the renal pelvis. The shapes of the cortex and medulla and how they relate to each other vary among species (Figure 18-4). In some species, such as cattle and pigs, the medulla is made up of numerous, pyramid-shaped areas (they look like candy corn) with the apex pointing to the renal pelvis (pigs) or directly to the ureter (cattle). This gives the medulla a scalloped appearance. The cortex fills in around the scallops. Kidneys with this structure are called *multipyramidal* or *multilobar*. In other species, such as dogs, horses, and cats, the medullary pyramids fuse to occupy the entire inner area, and the cortex is pushed to the outside area only. These kidneys are called *unipyramidal* or *unilobar*.

Each medullary pyramid fits into a cuplike extension of the renal pelvis called a calyx. These funnel-shaped calyces direct urine into the renal pelvis. From there the urine will move into the ureter. In cattle, the calyces empty directly into the ureter.

## MICROSCOPIC ANATOMY

Within the cortex and medulla of the kidney are packed hundreds of thousands of microscopic filtering, reabsorbing, and secreting units called *nephrons*. The **nephron** is the basic functional unit of the kidney. It is the smallest part of the kidney that can carry out its basic functions. The number of

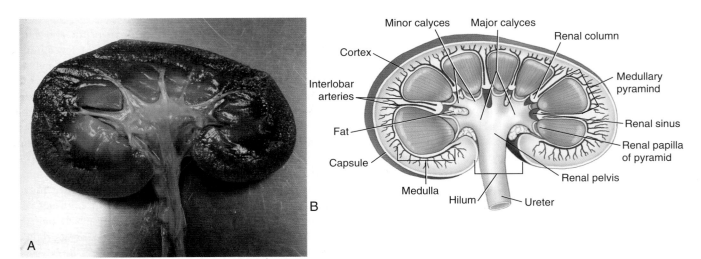

**FIGURE 18-3** Canine kidney. **A,** Gross anatomy of the interior of the kidney, transected through the renal pelvis. **B,** Artist's rendering of the transected kidney of a dog.

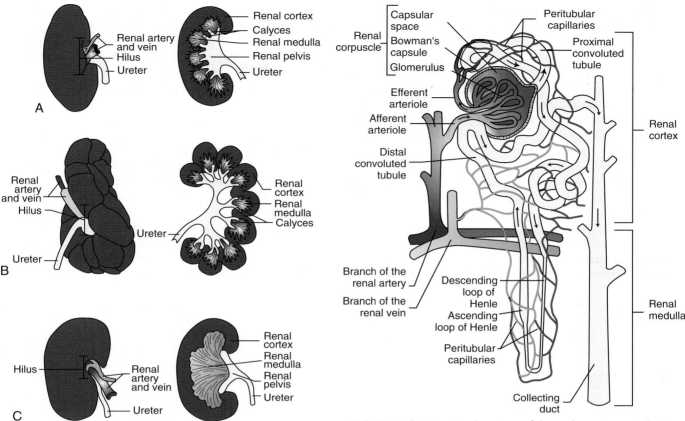

**FIGURE 18-4** Renal morphology varies with species. **A,** Pig and **B,** cattle kidneys are multipyramidal (multilobar). **C,** Cat and dog kidneys are unipyramidal (unilobar).

**FIGURE 18-5** Functional anatomy of the nephron. Arrows indicate the direction of fluid flow through the nephron.

nephrons per kidney varies with the size of the animal. For example, a medium-sized cat will have about 200,000 nephrons per kidney and a medium-sized dog will have about 700,000. Sheep, pigs, and humans have about 1,000,000 nephrons per kidney, and cattle have about 4,000,000. Each nephron is composed of a *renal corpuscle,* a *proximal convoluted tubule,* a *loop of Henle,* and a *distal convoluted tubule* (Figure 18-5).

The **renal corpuscle** is located in the cortex of the kidney. It is made up of the *glomerulus* and *Bowman's capsule.* The **glomerulus** is a tuft of glomerular capillaries. **Bowman's capsule** is a double-walled capsule that surrounds the glomerulus (see Figure 18-5). The inner layer of Bowman's capsule is the *visceral layer,* and it adheres closely to the surfaces of all glomerular capillaries. The outer layer is called the *parietal layer.* The visceral layer of Bowman's capsule is made up of **podocytes** ("foot cells") that have footlike extensions that cover the glomerular capillaries. The podocytes covering the capillaries have spaces between them, creating a permeable layer through which fluid and dissolved substances can pass during filtration. The space between the visceral and parietal layers is the **capsular space**. The capsular space is continuous with the proximal convoluted tubule. The function of the renal corpuscle is to filter blood in the first stage of urine production. The fluid that is filtered out of blood is called the **glomerular filtrate**.

The **proximal convoluted tubule (PCT)** is a continuation of the capsular space of Bowman's capsule. It is the longest part of the tubular system of the nephron. The epithelial cells that line the PCT are cuboidal and have a brush border (thousands of tiny projections of the cell membrane) on their lumen side. The brush border increases the cellular surface area exposed to the fluid in the tubule by a factor of about 20. This is especially important to the PCT's reabsorption and secretion functions. The PCT follows a twisting (hence the name *convoluted*) path through the cortex. The glomerular filtrate, now called the **tubular filtrate** (sometimes referred to as *primitive urine*) begins its journey through the tubular part of the nephron in the PCT.

The **loop of Henle** continues from the PCT, descends into the medulla of the kidney, makes a U-turn, and heads back up into the cortex. The descending part of the loop of Henle has cuboidal epithelial cells similar to the cells of the PCT, including the brush border. As the loop of Henle makes its U-turn, the wall becomes thinner and the epithelial cells flatten to simple squamous epithelial cells and lose their brush border. The lumen gets narrower here, too. As the loop of Henle ascends back up into the cortex, its wall becomes thicker again, but the cells don't regain the brush border. The lumen also expands as the loop of Henle ascends towards the cortex.

The **distal convoluted tubule (DCT)** is a continuation of the ascending part of the loop of Henle. The DCT follows a twisting path through the cortex. Even though it is also called a *convoluted tubule,* the DCT is not as twisted as the PCT.

The distal convoluted tubules from all the nephrons in the kidney empty into a series of tubules called **collecting ducts.** The collecting ducts carry tubular filtrate through the medulla into the calyces, which lead to the renal pelvis. The collecting ducts also play an important role in urine volume, because they are the primary site of action of antidiuretic hormone (ADH). Potassium regulation and acid–base balance control are two other important functions that take place in the collecting ducts.

## NERVE SUPPLY

The nerve supply to the kidney is primarily from the sympathetic portion of the autonomic nervous system. Sympathetic stimulation causes vasoconstriction of renal vessels and temporarily decreases urine formation. Although this controls the blood flow through the glomerular capillaries, it is not essential for the kidney to function. A transplanted kidney will work well even though its sympathetic nerve supply has been disrupted.

## BLOOD SUPPLY

Each kidney has a very large blood supply (Figure 18-6). This makes sense when you realize that the function of the kidney

is to clear waste products from the blood. Up to 25% of the blood pumped by the heart goes to the kidneys. In fact, every 4 or 5 minutes, all the circulating blood in the body passes through the kidneys. The main blood vessels responsible for this journey through the kidneys each have unique functions.

- The **renal artery** branches off the abdominal portion of the aorta. It enters the kidney at the hilus. It then divides and subdivides into smaller arteries and arterioles until it becomes a series of afferent glomerular arterioles.
- The **afferent glomerular arterioles** carry blood into the glomerular capillaries of the renal corpuscle.
- **The glomerular capillaries** are a continuation of the afferent arterioles. They filter some of the plasma out of blood, which enters the capsular space of Bowman's capsule, where is it known as the *glomerular filtrate.* Not all the plasma is filtered out; if it were, blood flow would come to a screeching halt. The blood in the glomerular capillaries leaves the glomerulus and enters the efferent glomerular arterioles. Notice that the blood is still arterial blood at this point, because oxygen exchange hasn't taken place yet. This is the only place in the body where blood entering *and* leaving the capillaries is oxygenated blood.
- The **efferent glomerular arterioles** divide into a network of capillaries that surround the rest of the nephron. These capillaries are known as the *peritubular capillaries* (see Figure 18-5). Oxygen transfer to the cells of the nephron takes place here. Also at this level, substances are taken

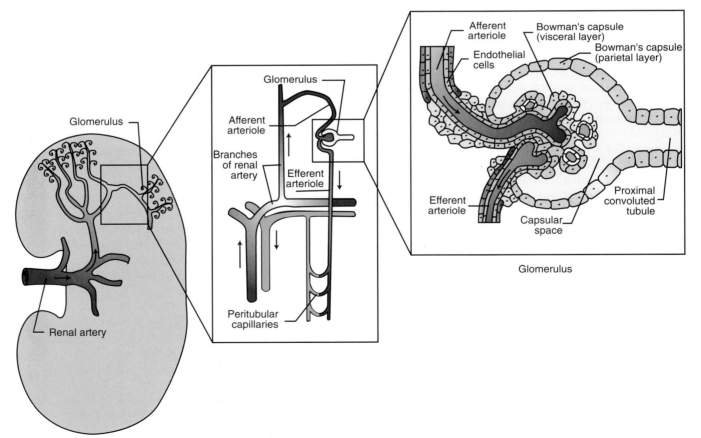

**FIGURE 18-6** Arterial blood supply to renal corpuscle. Arrows show the direction of blood flow.

out of the tubular filtrate and put back into blood. This is known as *tubular reabsorption.* Other substances are secreted from the blood into the tubules at this level. This is called *tubular secretion.* More on these actions later.

- The **peritubular capillaries** that surround the nephron converge to form venules that in turn converge to form larger veins that eventually become the renal vein.
- The **renal vein** leaves the kidney at the hilus and joins the abdominal portion of the caudal vena cava. With regard to waste content, the blood in the renal veins is the purest in the body.

### ✓ TEST YOURSELF 18-1

1. List the three steps involved in performing a urinalysis.
2. What are the six structures that make up the urinary system?
3. Nitrogenous waste materials from protein breakdown are eliminated from the body primarily as what?
4. Name one hormone whose release is regulated by the kidney, one hormone that directly affects kidney function, and one hormone produced by the kidney.
5. What is the difference between the hilus of the kidney and the renal pelvis?
6. What is meant by the term *retroperitoneal?*
7. List, in order, the parts of the nephron. Indicate whether each specific part is found in the cortex or the medulla of the kidney.

## MECHANISMS OF RENAL ACTION

The three main mechanisms by which the kidneys carry out their waste elimination role are *filtration* of the blood, *reabsorption* of useful substances back into the bloodstream, and *secretion* of waste products from the blood into the tubules of the nephron.

### FILTRATION OF BLOOD

Filtration of blood occurs in the renal corpuscle. Normally, capillaries are found between arterioles and venules and have very low blood pressure. The glomerular capillaries are different in that they are found between two arterioles and have a high blood pressure that is only about 30% lower than the blood pressure in the aorta. This high blood pressure is created by a difference in size between the afferent and efferent glomerular arterioles. The diameter of the efferent glomerular arteriole is smaller than that of the afferent arteriole, causing blood (and therefore pressure) to build up within the glomerular capillaries. The high blood pressure in the glomerular capillaries forces some of the plasma out of the capillaries and into the capsular space of Bowman's capsule. The transfer of plasma out of the glomerular capillaries is helped by the presence of many **fenestrations**, or pores, in the capillary endothelium. These fenestrations are larger than the fenestrations found in the endothelium of other capillaries, and they allow more fluid to leave the bloodstream. This fluid is known as the *glomerular filtrate* when it enters

the capsular space and is similar to plasma except that it contains virtually no proteins. The filtration of blood in the glomerulus is mainly a size-regulated process. Molecules within the blood that fit through the fenestrations will move through with the plasma and end up as part of the glomerular filtrate. Larger molecules that cannot fit through the fenestrations will stay in the bloodstream. Most of the plasma protein molecules are too large to pass through the glomerular capillary fenestrations. Blood cells are also too large to fit through the fenestrations. If the endothelium of the glomerulus is damaged, proteins and blood cells can leak into the glomerular filtrate. Because there is no mechanism to get the proteins back into the bloodstream through tubular reabsorption, they will show up as abnormal constituents of urine. The presence of abnormal amounts of proteins in urine can be used as an indicator of glomerular damage.

The **glomerular filtration rate (GFR)** is the term used to describe how fast plasma is filtered as it passes through the glomerulus. The GFR depends on the rate of blood flow (and therefore plasma flow) to the kidney. It is expressed in milliliters per minute. In a 25-lb dog, approximately 180 ml of plasma (that's about 300 ml of blood by the time you factor in the cells) flows to the kidney every minute. As blood passes through the kidney, about 45 ml of glomerular filtrate is formed every minute. In other words, about 25% of the plasma (45 ml/180 ml) is removed from the circulation each minute. Over a 24-hour period, that amounts to about 64 L of glomerular filtrate being formed. That's more than 16 gallons. If all that glomerular filtrate became urine that had to be eliminated from the body, imagine how often this poor dog would have to urinate (and he would shrivel up with dehydration within an hour)! Luckily, there is another mechanism (*reabsorption*) used by the kidney to reduce the volume of glomerular filtrate to about 680 ml of urine produced over a 24-hour period.

### REABSORPTION

Once plasma leaves the circulation and passes into the capsular space to become the glomerular filtrate, it is considered to be outside the body proper, even though physically it is still contained within the boundaries of the body. Remember, the glomerular filtrate is composed of fluid containing the small molecules that fit through the glomerular fenestrations. Some of these molecules are waste products that need to be cleared from the body. This is a good thing. Unfortunately, some of the molecules found in the glomerular filtrate the body doesn't want to lose, because it needs them to maintain homeostasis. Some of the most important of these substances are *sodium, potassium, calcium, magnesium, glucose, amino acids, chloride, bicarbonate,* and *water.* So there has to be a mechanism to get these useful substances back into the body by way of the blood. This mechanism is **reabsorption** of useful substances from the tubules of the nephron into the blood of the peritubular capillaries.

The glomerular filtrate enters the PCT and becomes tubular filtrate. Changes in its composition begin immediately. Some of those changes involve removal of some of the

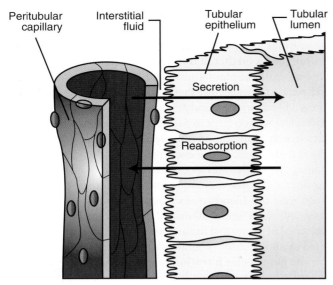

Peritubular capillary    Interstitial fluid    Tubular epithelium    Tubular lumen

Secretion

Reabsorption

**FIGURE 18-7** Reabsorption and secretion. Reabsorption involves movement of substances out of the tubular lumen, through the tubular epithelium and interstitial fluid, and into the peritubular capillary. Secretion involves movement of substances in the opposite direction—from the peritubular capillary, through the interstitial space, tubular epithelium, and tubular lumen.

constituents of the tubular filtrate through reabsorption back into the bloodstream. For any substance to be reabsorbed back into the body, it must pass out of the tubular lumen, through or between the tubular epithelial cells, into the interstitial fluid, and through the endothelium into the peritubular capillaries (Figure 18-7). Some substances make this movement passively through osmosis or diffusion. Others have to be actively transported across cell membranes.

As the glomerular filtrate enters the lumen of the PCT, sodium is actively "pumped" out of the fluid and back into the bloodstream. Sodium in the tubular filtrate attaches to a carrier protein that carries it into the cytoplasm of the PCT epithelial cell. The transfer of sodium from the tubular lumen into the epithelial cell requires energy. At the same time, glucose and amino acids attach to the same protein as the sodium ions and follow the sodium into the epithelial cell by passive transport. This process is called **sodium cotransport**. No extra energy is expended, because the glucose and amino acids are hitching a ride with the sodium by attaching to the same protein. Once the sodium is in the epithelial cell, it must be actively pumped out of the cell into the interstitial fluid, where it will move into the peritubular capillaries. Glucose and amino acids passively diffuse out of the tubular epithelial cell into the interstitial fluid and then into the peritubular capillaries. Sodium ions are also reabsorbed in the ascending part of the loop of Henle and the DCT, where they are usually exchanged for hydrogen, ammonium, or potassium ions that are secreted into the tubular filtrate. This exchange is under the influence of aldosterone—the mineralocorticoid hormone produced in the cortex of the adrenal gland.

Potassium diffuses out of the tubular filtrate by moving between the epithelial cells into the interstitial fluid and then into the peritubular capillaries. Potassium reabsorption takes

place in the PCT, the ascending part of the loop of Henle, and the DCT. Calcium moves through the epithelial cells under the influence of vitamin D, parathyroid hormone (PTH), and calcitonin, a hormone produced by the thyroid gland. Calcium reabsorption takes place in the PCT, the ascending loop of Henle, and the DCT. Magnesium is reabsorbed from the PCT, the ascending loop of Henle, and the collecting duct. PTH release increases the reabsorption of magnesium.

When sodium ($Na^+$) has been pumped out of the epithelial cell into the interstitial fluid, an electrical imbalance is created between the tubular lumen, which becomes negatively charged, and the interstitial space, which becomes positively charged. Chloride ($Cl^-$), which readily diffuses through cell membranes, moves from the tubular filtrate into the epithelial cells and interstitial space to restore electrical neutrality. When sodium, glucose, amino acids, and chloride have left the tubular filtrate, some of the water left behind in the filtrate moves into the interstitial space and peritubular capillaries by osmosis. Once some of the water has left the tubular filtrate, the concentration of other substances in the filtrate increases beyond their concentration in the blood of the peritubular capillaries. This concentration gradient results in these substances passively diffusing through cell membranes, moving through the epithelial cells into the interstitial fluid, and passing into the peritubular capillaries. One of the substances passively reabsorbed is urea. Even though urea is one of the waste products the body wants to get rid of, not all of the urea that is filtered through the glomerulus is eliminated in urine. The body maintains a normal level of urea in the blood that can be measured as the blood urea nitrogen, or BUN.

About 65% of all tubular reabsorption takes place in the PCT, where about 80% of the water, sodium, chloride, and bicarbonate and 100% of the glucose and amino acids in the tubular filtrate are reabsorbed. Additional reabsorption also takes place in the loop of Henle, DCT, and collecting ducts.

## SECRETION

Many waste products and foreign substances are not filtered from the blood in sufficient amounts from the glomerular capillaries. The body still needs to get rid of these substances, so it transfers them from the peritubular capillaries to the interstitial fluid to the tubular epithelial cells and into the tubular filtrate in the tubules. This is called tubular **secretion** (see Figure 18-7). Most tubular secretion takes place in the DCT. Hydrogen, potassium, and ammonia are some of the more important substances eliminated by secretion. Antibiotic drugs such as penicillin and some of the sulfonamides are also eliminated from the body by secretion. This can be useful if an animal has a urinary tract infection with microorganisms sensitive to one of these drugs.

## URINE VOLUME REGULATION

Urine volume is determined by the amount of water contained in the tubular filtrate when it reaches the renal pelvis. Two hormones, *antidiuretic hormone (ADH)* released from the posterior pituitary gland and *aldosterone* secreted by the adrenal cortex, are responsible for the majority of urine volume regulation.

ADH plays the most important role in regulating urine volume. It acts on the DCT and collecting ducts to promote water reabsorption and thereby prevent water loss from the body. If ADH control is absent, water will not be reabsorbed and will be lost in the urine. This results in increased urine volume (**polyuria**).

Aldosterone increases reabsorption of sodium into the bloodstream in the DCT and the collecting duct. This causes an osmotic imbalance that encourages water to follow the sodium out of the tubular filtrate and into the blood. The

---

 **CLINICAL APPLICATION**

### Renal Threshold of Glucose

There is a limit to the amount of glucose that can be reabsorbed by the proximal convoluted tubules. This limit is known as the *renal threshold of glucose*. If the blood glucose level gets too high, the amount of glucose filtered through the glomerulus exceeds the amount that can be reabsorbed (the renal threshold), and the excess is lost in urine.

In dogs, the renal threshold for glucose is approximately 180 mg/dl (deciliter). This means that if the blood glucose level exceeds 180 mg/dl (normal blood glucose = 62–108 mg/dl) the PCT cannot reabsorb any more than 180 mg/dl back into the body. So if a dog has a blood glucose level of 500 mg/dl, only 180 mg/dl will be reabsorbed and 320 mg/dl will be lost in the urine.

In cats, the renal threshold for glucose is 240 mg/dl (normal blood glucose = 60–124 mg/dl). Fortunately, the renal threshold exceeds the *normal* amount of glucose found in blood,

so 100% of the glucose filtered through the glomerulus is reabsorbed back into the body, and no glucose is lost in the urine.

However, in pathologic conditions such as uncontrolled diabetes mellitus, where blood glucose levels can be extremely high because of insufficient insulin production, the amount of glucose filtered through the glomerulus exceeds the limit that can be reabsorbed by the PCT. When this occurs, glucose appears in the urine (**glycosuria**). The glucose in urine pulls water out with it, which results in an abnormally high urine volume production (polyuria) due to osmosis (**osmotic diuresis**). The loss of water will cause a water imbalance in the body that the animal will try to correct by drinking increased amounts of water (**polydipsia**). Although polyuria and polydipsia (PU/PD) are nonspecific clinical signs associated with many pathologic conditions, PU/PD with an accompanying glucosuria can help pinpoint diabetes mellitus.

---

 **CLINICAL APPLICATION**

### Renal Failure

Like any functional organ of the body, the kidneys can deteriorate and fail to work properly. Renal failure can be acute (sudden), and these cases are often caused by toxicity (exposure to toxins such as antifreeze or some pharmaceutical drugs) or decreased renal perfusion due to low a blood pressure event or systemic disease. Acute renal failure is caused by necrosis of the renal tubules resulting either from exposure to the toxic substance or from lack of blood flow.

More commonly, however, renal failure is chronic, characterized by a progressive and irreversible destruction of nephrons over months to years causing a gradual loss of renal function. Chronic renal failure is a common disease condition of both cats and dogs.

In the early stages of chronic renal failure, the glomerular fenestrations become larger than normal and allow larger molecules such as proteins to pass into the tubular filtrate. One of the earliest signs of chronic renal failure is proteinuria, or the presence of protein in the urine. Unfortunately, at this stage, there are no clinical signs that we can observe. This proteinuria can only be detected by urinalysis (see Clinical Application on urinalysis), which is often not performed in the absence of clinical signs. As the renal failure progresses, complete destruction of nephrons follows. The kidneys do an amazing job of compensating for this loss until enough nephrons are lost that those left can no longer filter the blood sufficiently and remove unwanted toxins. It is not until two thirds of the nephrons have been lost that clinical signs of renal

failure start to appear! This is a double-edged sword. On the one hand, the kidneys are able to compensate and continue adequately to remove enough waste products from the blood, even working at decreased capacity. On the other hand, however, it is not until renal failure reaches the end stages, when little can be done to improve the quality or length of life, that we often diagnose its presence.

When nephron destruction reaches this critical point, the kidneys lose their ability to perform their basic duties: filtration, reabsorption, and secretion. With glomerular damage, important blood proteins are lost into the urine because of impaired filtration. In addition, an increased amount of water is lost in the urine instead of being reabsorbed, causing dilute urine and dehydration of the patient. Also, waste materials that the kidneys normally eliminate through secretion accumulate in the body and cause many of the clinical signs of renal failure. Two of the main nitrogenous waste products that the kidneys normally eliminate are urea and creatinine, both by-products of protein metabolism. The accumulation of urea in the blood is called uremia, whereas the buildup of creatinine is called **azotemia**. Levels of these substances can be measured by performing blood chemistry analysis (see figure). The buildup of these toxins is mainly responsible for the nausea and vomiting that often characterize advanced renal failure.

The goals of treating chronic renal failure are to slow the progression of the disease and improve the quality of life of the patient by treating the clinical signs. Fluid therapy is the

*Continued*

## CLINICAL APPLICATION—cont'd

mainstay of treatment for renal failure. Increasing the flow of fluid through the kidneys facilitates removal of urea and creatinine and improves hydration. If the animal is being kept in the hospital, fluids will likely be administered intravenously. If the patient is being treated by the owner at home, the owner can often be trained to administer fluids subcutaneously on a daily basis. Renal patients are often fed a diet that contains lowered levels of protein, as well as low levels of several minerals (such as phosphorus) that the kidneys are no longer able to remove sufficiently.

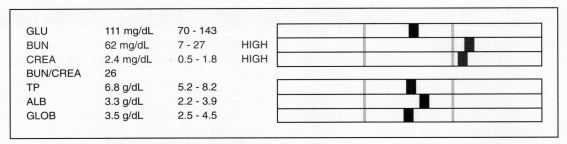

| | | | |
|---|---|---|---|
| GLU | 111 mg/dL | 70 - 143 | |
| BUN | 62 mg/dL | 7 - 27 | HIGH |
| CREA | 2.4 mg/dL | 0.5 - 1.8 | HIGH |
| BUN/CREA | 26 | | |
| TP | 6.8 g/dL | 5.2 - 8.2 | |
| ALB | 3.3 g/dL | 2.2 - 3.9 | |
| GLOB | 3.5 g/dL | 2.5 - 4.5 | |

Example of blood work results indicating renal failure, with elevations in BUN and creatinine.

## CLINICAL APPLICATION

### Diabetes Insipidus
Antidiuretic hormone (ADH) released by the posterior pituitary gland plays a major role in controlling urine volume by regulating water reabsorption from the collecting ducts. If the pituitary is not releasing adequate amounts of ADH, the collecting ducts will not reabsorb adequate amounts of water, and polyuria develops, along with a compensatory polydipsia. This condition is known as *diabetes insipidus,* and it has to be distinguished from diabetes mellitus. Both diseases are associated with polyuria and polydipsia, as are many other diseases. The urine produced in diabetes mellitus contains large amounts of glucose and therefore would taste sweet (if you were inclined to taste it to find out). The word *insipid* means *tasteless.* The disease *diabetes insipidus* was given its name because clinically it looked similar to diabetes mellitus; but the urine was tasteless, rather than sweet, because it didn't contain glucose.

Another form of diabetes insipidus results from an inability of the collecting ducts to respond to the presence of adequate amounts of ADH. The clinical signs are the same. Further diagnostic testing would have to be done to reach a definitive diagnosis of diabetes insipidus. Like diabetes mellitus, diabetes insipidus occurs most often in dogs and cats among domestic species.

## CLINICAL APPLICATION

### Urine Production Review
Urine is constantly being produced by the kidneys and sent down through the ureters into the urinary bladder for storage until it is eliminated. As plasma containing metabolic wastes passes through a nephron, the kidney converts it into urine that can be eliminated from the body. It accomplishes this through a series of processes designed to eliminate waste materials and preserve substances needed by the body to maintain homeostasis. Refer to Figure 18-5 Urine production can be broken down into six basic steps:

1. Blood enters the glomerulus via the afferent glomerular arteriole.
2. High blood pressure in the glomerular capillaries forces some plasma (minus large proteins and the blood cells) out of the capillaries and into the capsular space of Bowman's capsule. At this point, the fluid is known as the *glomerular filtrate.* From there, it moves into the proximal convoluted tubule and is then called *tubular filtrate.*

3. The balance of the plasma not forced out of the glomerular capillaries leaves the glomerulus via the efferent glomerular capillaries and enters a peritubular capillary network around the rest of the nephron.
4. While the tubular filtrate travels through the tubules of the nephron, some of its constituents, or useful substances, are reabsorbed back into the peritubular capillaries *(A).*
5. Waste products are secreted from the peritubular capillaries into the tubular filtrate as it travels through the tubules *(B).*
6. By the time the tubular filtrate reaches the collecting ducts, it has decreased in volume, has changed chemical composition many times, and is now ready to leave the kidney on its way to being eliminated. When the tubular filtrate enters the renal pelvis, it is *urine,* and nothing more will be done to alter its composition. (One exception here is that mucus may be added to equine urine after it reaches the renal pelvis. See also Figure 18-5.)

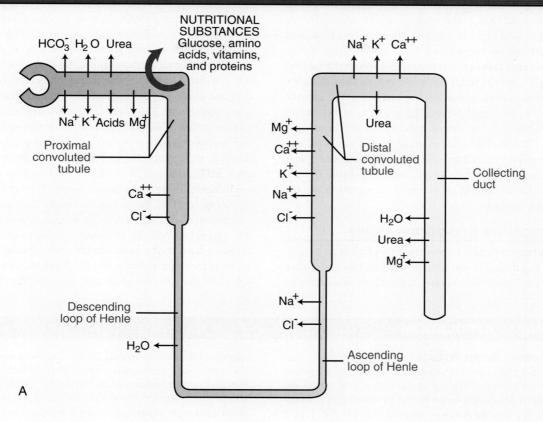

A

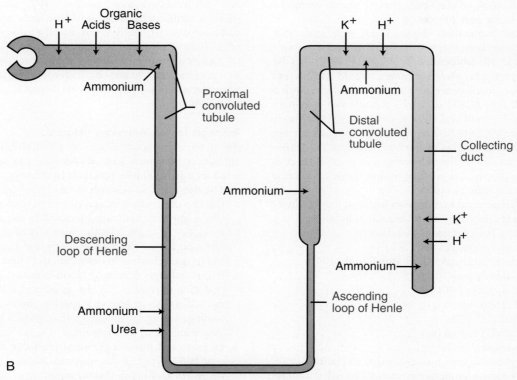

B

Substances involved in reabsorption and secretion. **A,** Substances that are recovered from the tubular filtrate through reabsorption into peritubular capillaries. **B,** Substances that are eliminated from the body as necessary through secretion into the tubular filtrate from peritubular capillaries.

hitch is that the water cannot move out of the DCT and collecting duct unless sufficient ADH control is present. This is one of those situations in the body in which several things have to happen just right in order for normal function (and thereby health) to be maintained.

The glomerular tubular filtrate moves through the tubules and eventually into the renal pelvis because of the difference in pressure that exists between the fluid in Bowman's capsule and the fluid in the renal pelvis. The pressure in Bowman's capsule is higher than the almost nonexistent pressure in the renal pelvis. Like the difference in pressure that forces plasma to leave the afferent capillary and enter the capsular space, the difference in pressure between Bowman's capsule and the renal pelvis forces the fluid to move along through the tubules of the nephron.

## REGULATION OF BLOOD PRESSURE

The kidneys help maintain homeostasis by playing an important role in regulating blood pressure. When blood pressure falls, a system called the **renin–angiotensin–aldosterone system** responds to bring it back up to a normal level. Within the afferent glomerular arterioles are specialized *juxtaglomerular cells* that constantly monitor blood pressure within the arterioles. In addition, there is a group of densely packed cells within the ascending limb of the loop of Henle, called the *macula densa,* that monitors the NaCl concentration of the tubular filtrate. If the juxtaglomerular cells detect a decrease in blood pressure or if the macula densa cells come into contact with less NaCl (either because of a lower NaCl concentration or sluggish flow of filtrate through the tubules) the juxtaglomerular cells will respond by releasing **renin**. Renin is an enzyme that facilitates the splitting of angiotensin I from angiotensin. Angiotensin I is then converted to angiotensin II by angiotensin-converting enzyme (ACE). Angiotensin II is the active molecule that causes arterial constriction and stimulates the release of aldosterone from the adrenal glands. By increasing sodium and water reabsorption back to the bloodstream, aldosterone will cause an increase in blood volume. As blood volume increases, it will better fill the vascular space and increase blood pressure.

 **CLINICAL APPLICATION**

### Feline Chronic Renal Failure

A 12-year-old male castrated, domestic shorthair cat named "Magic" is presented for lethargy, anorexia, and vomiting. After taking a thorough history, the veterinary technician learns that the cat has had a decreased appetite for 1 to 2 months and has been uncharacteristically reclusive and hides under the bed much of the time. The cat has also vomited several times in the past 2 weeks.

On physical examination, the veterinary technician finds Magic to be quiet, alert, and responsive (QAR) with multiple mats in his coat. His temperature is 100.2°F (37.89°C), pulse 180 beats per minute, and respiratory rate 38 breaths per minute. Mucous membranes are pale pink and tacky, with a capillary refill time (CRT) of 2 to 3 seconds. The veterinary technician finds a small oral ulcer and estimates Magic's body condition score (BCS) to be 2 out of 5. When Magic's current weight is compared with his weight 8 months ago, it is discovered that he has lost 1.2 lb. When the skin over the neck is tented, the tent persists longer than normal. Little to no urine is palpable in the urinary bladder.

Based on her physical examination findings, the veterinary technician makes the following technician evaluations:
- Hypovolemia (tacky mucous membranes)
- Decreased perfusion (delayed CRT)
- Inappropriate elimination (little urine production)
- Vomiting and nausea
- Exercise intolerance (lethargy)
- Abnormal eating behavior (anorexia)
- Underweight (2/5 BCS)
- Self-care deficit (matted fur)
- Altered mentation (reclusive)
- Altered oral health (mucous membrane ulceration)

The veterinary technician alerts the veterinarian to her findings and readies the materials needed for venipuncture and urine collection. After examining the cat, the veterinarian orders a complete blood count (CBC), blood chemistry, and urinalysis. The veterinary technician draws blood from the jugular vein and obtains urine via cystocentesis. Using the in-clinic laboratory equipment, the veterinary technician completes the blood tests and urinalysis ordered by the veterinarian. The CBC results reveal a decreased packed cell volume (PCV) and an increased total protein (TP). Blood chemistry shows a significantly increased blood urea nitrogen (BUN) and creatinine. Urinalysis results reveal a urine specific gravity of 1.010 and proteinuria. The lab results, along with a 1- to 2-month history of clinical signs, lead the veterinarian to conclude that Magic is in chronic renal failure, and promptly meets with the owner to discuss the seriousness of his condition.

#### Rationale for the Veterinary Diagnosis

All of the abnormalities seen on physical examination and analyses of the patient's blood and urine can be attributed to a lack of normal kidney function. Here's why....
1. The decreased production of red blood cells, which gives rise to a diminished PCV, is due to the lack of erythropoietin, a hormone normally produced by the kidney.
2. As kidney function fails, the mechanisms that concentrate urine no longer function properly and excessive water is lost in urine, leading to dehydration. Dehydration is manifest as lethargy, decreased blood pressure, and decreased perfusion of tissues. It is also associated with an elevation in PCV and an isosthenuric specific gravity of urine. Both findings are strong indicators that Magic's kidneys are no longer able to concentrate urine.
3. Elevations of physiologic waste products, both BUN and creatinine, occur as the weakened kidneys fail to remove them. The buildup of these compounds in blood is responsible for the symptoms of nausea, vomiting, and anorexia seen commonly in cases of renal failure.

4. The presence of large molecules, such as protein, in the urine is a result of damage to the delicate filtration membranes in the glomerulus.

### Questions to Consider Before Treatment is Started

- What are the goals of treating a patient with chronic renal failure?
- How will Magic's dehydration be addressed, both in the hospital and potentially at home?
- How can urine output be monitored while Magic is hospitalized?
- How will the clinical signs of renal failure be managed (vomiting, lethargy, anorexia) to improve Magic's quality of life?

### Treatment

Magic is admitted to the hospital in an effort to slow the progression of his renal failure and to control the clinical signs of the disease. An intravenous catheter is placed in his cephalic vein and intravenous fluids are administered to replace Magic's fluid losses and to meet his ongoing needs for fluids (see figure). A urinary catheter is placed and is connected to a urine collection system so that urine production can be monitored. Medications are also administered to help control the clinical signs of renal failure such as anorexia, vomiting, and anemia.

Magic will be hospitalized for several days with the goals of rehydrating him, flushing some of the built-up waste products from his body, and controlling his clinical signs. If blood work results show an improvement in his condition, Magic may be able to continue treatment at home. With home care, he may have several more months of quality time with his owner.

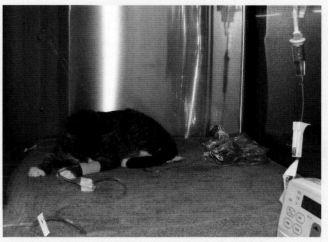

Treatment for renal failure often includes intravenous fluid administration. A urinary collection system is also used to monitor and evaluate urine production and output.

---

### TEST YOURSELF 18-2

1. What is the difference between *glomerular* filtrate and *tubular* filtrate?
2. What is the function of the brush border on the epithelial cells of the proximal convoluted tubule?
3. How does the blood in the *efferent* glomerular arteriole differ from the blood in the *afferent* glomerular arteriole?
4. What is the difference between tubular *reabsorption* and tubular *secretion?*
5. How does ADH deficiency affect urine volume? What is the mechanism?
6. What is the mechanism by which glucose and amino acids are reabsorbed out of the proximal convoluted tubule and back into the body?
7. Explain the concept of the renal threshold of glucose.
8. Explain why proteinuria occurs with renal failure.
9. Why are clinical signs of renal failure not observed until the disease process is advanced?
10. Diabetes insipidus gets its name from what physical characteristic of urine produced by patients with this disease?
11. How do the kidneys respond to a decrease in blood pressure?

## URETERS

The **ureter** is a tube that exits the kidney at the hilus and connects to the urinary bladder near the neck of the bladder at its caudal end. The two openings from the ureters into the bladder and the opening from the bladder into the urethra, if connected, form an upside-down triangle. This arrangement is referred to as the **trigone** of the bladder (Figure 18-8).

### ANATOMY

The ureters are tubes composed of three layers: an outer, *fibrous layer;* a middle, *muscular layer* made up of smooth muscle; and an inner, *epithelial layer* lined with transitional epithelium. The transitional epithelium allows the ureters to stretch as urine is passed through them on its way to the urinary bladder. The ureters are a continuation of the renal pelvis, and each ureter leaves its kidney at the hilus.

### FUNCTION

The ureters continuously move urine from the kidneys to the urinary bladder. The smooth muscle layer propels the urine through the ureter by peristaltic contractions, much like the contractions of the intestines. This enables urine to move to the urinary bladder regardless of the position of the animal's body.

The ureters enter the urinary bladder at such an oblique angle that, when the bladder is full, it collapses the opening of the ureter, preventing urine from backing up into the ureter (Figure 18-9). It doesn't prevent more urine from entering the bladder, though, because the strength of the peristaltic contractions is enough to force the urine through the collapsed opening into the urinary bladder.

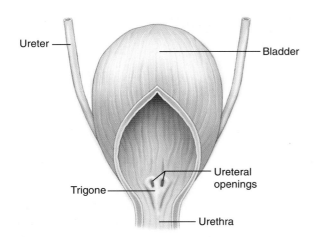

**FIGURE 18-8** Trigone of the bladder.

> ✓ *TEST YOURSELF 18-3*
> 1. Why is it important that the ureters have an inner lining of transitional epithelium?
> 2. What prevents urine from backing up into the ureters when the bladder wall contracts to expel urine?
> 3. The ureter is continuous with what structure in the kidney (except in cattle)?

## URINARY BLADDER

The urinary bladder stores urine as it is produced and releases it periodically from the body.

### ANATOMY

The urinary bladder has two parts: a muscular *sac* and a *neck*. The bladder looks and acts a lot like a balloon. The size and position of the bladder sac vary depending on the amount of urine it contains. The bladder is lined with transitional epithelium that stretches as the bladder becomes filled with urine. Have you ever made a water balloon? The principle is the same. The wall of the urinary bladder contains smooth muscle bundles that run lengthwise, obliquely, and in a circular direction. These bundles of smooth muscle are collectively called the *detrusor muscle*. When these muscles contract, the bladder is squeezed and urine is expelled—like forcing the water out of the water balloon. The neck of the bladder extends caudally from the sac into the pelvic canal, and joins the urethra. Around the neck of the urinary bladder are circular sphincter muscles composed of skeletal muscle fibers. The contraction and relaxation of these sphincter muscles, which are under voluntary control, open and close the passageway for urine to leave the bladder and enter the urethra. This provides voluntary control over the process of urination.

When the urinary bladder is empty, it is round and rests on the pubic bones. Structurally it has a thick wall, is lined with many thick folds of transitional epithelium, and has virtually no lumen. In large animals the empty bladder is confined to the pelvic cavity, but in carnivores it extends into the abdominal cavity. As the bladder fills with urine, it

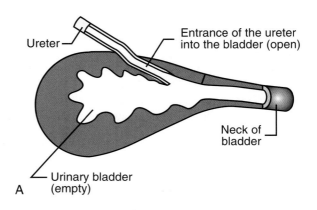

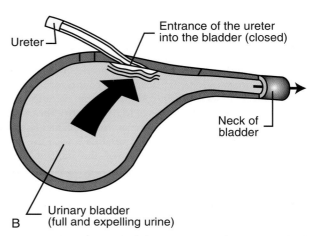

**FIGURE 18-9** Entrance of the ureters into the urinary bladder. **A,** When the bladder is empty and while it is filling, its entrances remain open and urine flows freely into bladder. **B,** When bladder is full, the pressure of the urine present collapses the entrances so that when urine is expelled it does not flow back into the ureters.

becomes pear-shaped, it extends cranially into the abdominal cavity, the folds smooth out, and the wall becomes thinner (see Figure 18-9).

### FUNCTION

The function of the urinary bladder is to collect, store, and release urine. The kidneys constantly produce urine, so if it weren't for the storage function of the urinary bladder, animals would constantly drip urine as it was being produced.

### CONTROL OF URINATION

**Urination** (also known as **micturition** or **uresis**) is the expulsion of urine from the urinary bladder into the urethra for elimination from the body. The process involves two to three steps.

### URINE ACCUMULATION

The urinary bladder constantly accumulates urine, until the pressure of the filling bladder reaches a certain trigger point that activates stretch receptors in the bladder wall.

## MUSCLE CONTRACTION

When the trigger point is reached, a spinal reflex is activated that returns a motor impulse to the detrusor muscle and the smooth muscle of the bladder wall contracts. These contractions are responsible for the sensation of having to urinate. In animals that are not housebroken, emptying of the bladder will occur at this point.

## SPHINCTER MUSCLE CONTROL

Animals that have been trained can control the reflex release of urine by voluntary control of the muscular sphincter around the neck of the bladder. This results in temporary control of urination. There is a limit, however, to how long an animal can hold urine in its bladder. Remember, urine is constantly being produced, so the bladder just keeps getting fuller if the animal has not urinated. The fuller the bladder gets, the more pressure is applied to the muscular sphincter, until it eventually relaxes, and urine is released. Something to consider when an animal has an "accident" is how long that animal had been expected to hold its urine.

As the bladder fills with urine, its walls become thinner as the transitional epithelium becomes thinner. This makes the bladder more susceptible to rupture. Remember the water balloon? If you fill the balloon to its stretched capacity and then squeeze it too hard, you can guess what will happen. The same thing happens if a urinary bladder is traumatized when it is too full. A common consequence of blunt trauma to the abdomen, such as when an animal is hit by a car, is a ruptured bladder. Manual palpation of an overextended bladder has also been known to cause it to rupture.

> ✓ **TEST YOURSELF 18-4**
> 1. How does the bladder know when to empty itself?
> 2. What part of the urinary bladder is under voluntary control and allows an animal to be housebroken?
> 3. Does urine production stop when the urinary bladder is full?

## URETHRA

### ANATOMY

The urethra is a continuation of the neck of the urinary bladder that runs through the pelvic canal. Like the ureters and urinary bladder, it is lined with transitional epithelium that allows it to expand. The female urethra is shorter and straighter than the long, curved male urethra (Figure 18-10). In the female, the urethra opens on the floor (ventral portion) of the vestibule of the vulva. In the male, the urethra runs along the ventral aspect of the penis (see Chapter 19).

### FUNCTION

In both females and males, the urethra carries urine from the urinary bladder to the external environment.

In the female, the urethra has a strictly urinary function; it carries only urine. In males, the urethra also has a reproductive function. The vas deferens and accessory reproductive glands enter the urethra as it passes through the pelvic canal. Here, spermatozoa and seminal fluid are discharged into the urethra during ejaculation and are pumped out as semen. At the beginning of ejaculation, the sphincter at the neck of the urinary bladder closes to prevent semen from entering the bladder and mixing with urine (see Chapter 19).

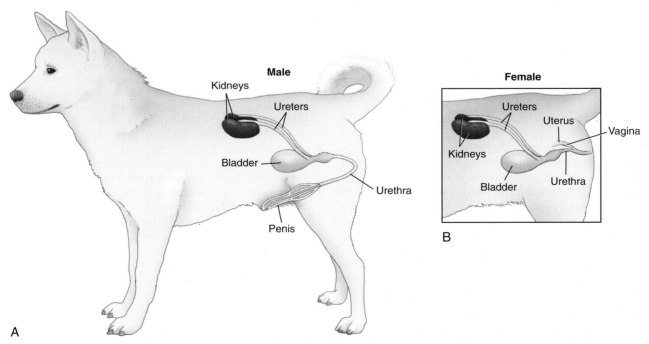

**FIGURE 18-10** The canine urinary tract. **A,** The urethra of the male dog is curved and longer because it travels the length of the penis; **B,** the urethra of the bitch is short and straight.

## CLINICAL APPLICATION

### Renal Dysfunction and Uremia

Renal dysfunction is the term used to describe any pathologic condition that results in inability of the urinary system to remove waste materials adequately from the blood. When this happens, the waste materials, especially nitrogenous wastes from protein breakdown (e.g., BUN), build up in the blood and become toxic to the animal. The resulting condition is called **uremia** (literally "urine in the blood"). Uremia can be *prerenal, renal,* or *postrenal.*

**Prerenal uremia** is associated with decreased blood flow to the kidneys and may be caused by conditions such as dehydration, congestive heart failure, or shock, if these conditions are left untreated. In these cases, the kidneys are functioning normally, but not enough blood is reaching them, so waste materials can't be adequately removed.

**Renal uremia** is associated with an inability of the kidney to regulate urine production adequately because of damage to the nephrons (refer to the Clinical Application on feline chronic renal failure). Toxins, inflammation, or infections that localize in the kidneys and destroy nephrons are some of the causes of uremia due to kidney dysfunction. Even though there may be adequate blood flow to the kidneys, there are not enough functional nephrons present to regulate normal urine production, so waste materials can't be removed from the

blood. The kidneys have far more nephrons than they need to function properly under normal conditions, so there is a large reserve of nephrons to take over if some of the nephrons are damaged or destroyed. Two thirds of the total nephrons in both kidneys must be nonfunctional before clinical signs of renal dysfunction start to become evident.

**Postrenal uremia** is usually associated with an obstruction that prevents urine from being expelled from the body. Tumors, blood clots, or uroliths (stones) can cause the obstruction. Remember that urine is constantly being produced, even if it is prevented from being expelled from the body by the obstruction. Eventually urine will back up into the renal pelvis and then into the nephrons. This will result in increased pressure in the nephrons and kidney damage. Now it becomes a case of renal dysfunction, but the underlying cause was a postrenal obstruction.

Uremia is diagnosed by evaluating a blood sample for the presence of increased amounts of waste materials. The easiest waste material to evaluate is urea, the nitrogenous waste product of protein breakdown. The amount of blood urea nitrogen (BUN) in plasma is an indication of how well the blood is being cleaned. Elevated BUN levels indicate a problem but will not distinguish among prerenal, renal, and postrenal uremia. Further diagnostic testing will be necessary to make that distinction.

## CLINICAL APPLICATION

### Uroliths and Urolithiasis

Urine normally contains waste products dissolved in water. Some of these waste products are just barely soluble and, under certain conditions, they will precipitate out of solution to form crystals. This may not cause problems if the crystals move through the urinary system rapidly. If their transit time through the urinary system is prolonged, they may interact with each other and form aggregates known as **uroliths**, **urinary stones**, or **urinary calculi**. Uroliths are commonly seen in dogs, cattle, sheep, and goats *(A)* but are uncommon in horses. They take on a slightly different morphology in cats. (Refer to the Clinical Application on feline urolithiasis.)

All uroliths have an organic matrix that stays fairly constant and makes up about 2% to 10% of its structure. The remaining 90% to 98% of the urolith structure is made up of one or more of about 20 different minerals. Some of the more common mineral compounds involved are *magnesium ammonium phosphate hexahydrate (struvite), calcium oxalate, calcium phosphate, urate, ammonium urate,* and *cystine.* Struvite stones are the most common stones found in dogs. Calcium carbonate, struvite, and calcium oxalate stones are some of the more common stones found in ruminants. The mechanism of urolith formation is not understood. We know that uroliths form when there are adequate amounts of the minerals present in the urine, the transit time of crystals through the urinary system is lengthened, and the pH of the urine favors precipitation. Some crystals stay in solution in acidic urine but precipitate out of solution in alkaline urine (e.g., struvite crystals), and other crystals stay in solution in alkaline urine but precipitate out of solution in acid urine (e.g., urate crystals). Diet,

frequency of urination, urinary tract infection, and urine volume can influence these factors. For example, diet and the presence of certain bacteria associated with urinary tract infections can influence the pH of the urine. In addition, a housebroken animal that must consistently hold its urine for long periods of time will have a decreased crystal transit time through the lower urinary tract (bladder and urethra).

**Urolithiasis** (the presence of *urinary stones*) can occur anywhere in the urinary system (the kidneys, ureters, urinary bladder, or urethra). Clinical signs associated with uroliths depend on where the stones are located. Some stones may cause no noticeable signs. Others may cause inflammation of the bladder (cystitis) or urethra (urethritis) or an obstruction anywhere along the urinary tract *(B).* Urethral obstruction is more common in males in general; in male ruminants, it occurs most often at the urethral sigmoid flexure (see Chapter 19). If the stone is obstructing the renal pelvis or ureter of one kidney, urine is prevented from leaving the kidney, and the pressure in the nephrons from fluid backup will eventually destroy that kidney. As long as the other kidney is functioning normally, no clinical signs may be evident. Remember that two thirds of the nephrons in both kidneys must be nonfunctional before clinical signs of renal dysfunction start to become evident.

Treatment of urolithiasis is aimed at removing the stones and preventing them from forming again. There are commercially available diets for dogs and cats that dissolve and prevent some types of stones. Some stones will have to be surgically removed. In ruminants, surgical removal of the stones is often necessary. Diets and urinary tract infections have to be controlled to prevent urolith recurrence.

## CLINICAL APPLICATION—cont'd

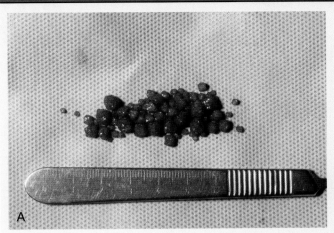

A, A cluster of calcium carbonate uroliths from the bladder of a 2-year-old goat. (From Pugh AN, Baird DG: Sheep and goat medicine, ed 2, St Louis, 2012, Elsevier Saunders.)

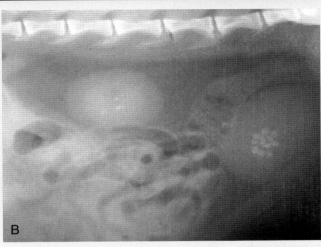

B, Numerous opacities in the kidney and bladder indicating the presence of uroliths. (From Pugh AN, Baird DG: Sheep and goat medicine, ed 2, St Louis, 2012, Elsevier Saunders.)

## CLINICAL APPLICATION

### Feline Urolithiasis

Feline uroliths differ from uroliths in other species in that they are much smaller and resemble sand rather than large stones (see figure). Feline urolithiasis can be very irritating—like having sandpaper in the urine. If the sand contains a lot of the organic matrix, it clumps together to become a gelatinous plug with a gritty, toothpaste consistency. This plug can cause an obstruction, most often at or near the urethral orifice and most often in male cats. These are the "plugged tomcats" that are seen so often in emergency situations. Struvite and calcium oxalate uroliths are the most common types of urolith in cats.

As with uroliths in other species, urine pH, diet, and the presence of a urinary tract infection play important roles in urolith formation. Keeping the urine acidic, sometimes with a special diet or medications, will keep the struvite in solution. Struvite crystals are composed of magnesium, ammonium, and phosphate, so a diet low in these substances may play some part in reducing the chance of crystals forming.

If a plug has formed, it will have to be manually removed to prevent urinary bladder rupture or postrenal uremia from developing. One method of removal involves passing a catheter into the urethra and flushing the plug back into the urinary bladder. Manipulating the urine pH to make it more acidic can dissolve the plug. If back-flushing doesn't work, the plug may have to be surgically removed.

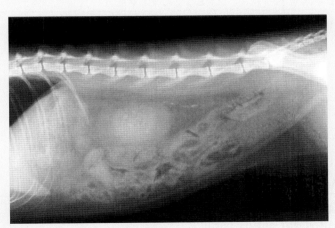

Cystogram of feline patient showing urolithiasis in bladder and ureter. (From Little S: The cat, clinical medicine and management, ed 1, St Louis, 2011, Elsevier Saunders.)

---

### ✓ TEST YOURSELF 18-5

1. Besides its urinary function, what other function does the urethra play in a male animal?
2. How much kidney function must be destroyed before clinical signs of renal dysfunction become evident?
3. Explain the difference between *prerenal* uremia and *postrenal* uremia.
4. What is a urolith?
5. Name two conditions that can predispose an animal to urolith production.
6. How do uroliths in cats differ from uroliths in other species?
7. What is the chemical composition of a struvite crystal?

### REFERENCES AND FURTHER READING

Hendrix CM, Sirois M: Laboratory procedures for veterinary technicians, ed 5, St Louis, 2007, Mosby/Elsevier.

Marieb EN, Hoehn K: Human anatomy & physiology, ed 9, Glenview, IL, 2013, Benjamin Cummings.

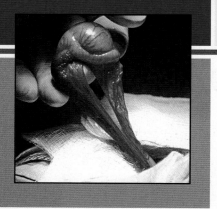

# The Reproductive System  19

*Thomas Colville*

## LEARNING OBJECTIVES

*When you have completed this chapter you will be able to:*
1. Differentiate between meiosis and mitosis.
2. Describe the process of spermatogenesis.
3. Describe the process of oogenesis.
4. Describe the structure of spermatozoa.
5. List the components of the male reproductive system and describe the functions of each.
6. List the characteristics and functions of the accessory structures of the male reproductive system.
7. List the components of the female reproductive system and describe the functions of each.
8. Describe the events that occur during the ovarian cycle.
9. List the stages of the estrous cycle and describe the events that occur during each stage.
10. Differentiate among monoestrous, diestrous, polyestrous, and seasonally polyestrous cycles.

## VOCABULARY FUNDAMENTALS

*Acrosome* **ahck**-rō-sōm
*Afterbirth* **ahf**-tər-bərth
*Ampulla* ahm-**pyool**-uh
*Androgen* **ahn**-drō-jehn
*Anestrus* ahn-**ehs**-truhs
*Antrum* **ahn**-truhm
*Body of the penis* **boh**-dē *of the* **pē**-nihs
*Broad ligament* brawd **lihg**-ah-mehnt
*Bulb of the glans* buhlb *of the* glahnz
*Bulbourethral gland* buhl-bō-ū-**rē**-thruhl glahnd
*Cervix* **sər**-vihx
*Chromosome* **krō**-muh-sōm
*Clitoris* **klih**-tohr-ihs
*Common vaginal tunic* kohm-uhn **vahj**-ihn-ahl **too**-nihck
*Cornification* kohr-nih-fih-**kā**-shuhn
*Corona glandis* kuh-**rō**-nuh **glahn**-dihs
*Corona radiata* kuh-**rō**-nuh ād-ē-**aht**-ah

*Corpus cavernosum penis* **kohr**-puhs kahv-ər-**nō**-suhm **pē**-nihs
*Corpus cavernosum urethrae* **kohr**-puhs kahv-ər-**nō**-suhm ū-**rē**-thrē
*Corpus hemorrhagicum* **kohr**-puhs hehm-uh-**rahj**-uh-kuhm
*Corpus luteum* **kohr**-puhs **lū**-tē-uhm
*Cremaster muscle* krē-**mahs**-tər **muhs**-uhl
*Crura* **krər**-uh
*Cryptorchidism* krihpt-**ohr**-kihd-ihsm
*Cumulus oophorus* kyoo-myuh-luhs ō-**ō**-fər-uhs
*Diestrous* dī-**ehs**-truhs
*Diestrus* dī-**ehs**-truhs
*Diploid chromosome number* **dihp**-loyd **krō**-muh-sōm **nuhm**-bər
*Efferent ducts of the testes* ē-**fər**-ehnt duhcktz *of the* **tehs**-tēs

*Ejaculation* eh-jahck-ū-**lā**-shuhn

*Epididymis* ehp-ih-**dihd**-eh-mihs

*Erectile tissue* eh-**rehck**-tihl **tihsh**-yoo

*Erection* eh-**rehck**-shuhn

*Estrogen* **ehs**-trō-jehn

*Estrous* **ehs**-truhs

*Estrous cycle* **ehs**-truhs **sī**-kuhl

*Estrus* **ehs**-truhs

*Fimbriae* **fihm**-brē-ē

*Follicle* **fohl**-ih-kuhl

*Follicular atresia* fuh-**lihck**-yuh-lər ā-**trē**-zhuh

*Follicular cell* fuh-**lihck**-yuh-lər sehl

*Fossa glandis* **fohs**-ah **glahn**-dihs

*Gamete* **gahm**-ēt

*Glans of the penis* glahnz *of the* **pē**-nihs

*Glycoprotein* glī-kō-**prō**-tēn

*Gonad* **gō**-nahd

*Granulosa cell* **grahn**-ū-lō-sah sehl

*Gubernaculum* goo-bər-**nahck**-yuh-luhm

*Haploid chromosome number* **hahp**-loyd **krō**-muh-sōm **nuhm**-bər

*Homologous* hō-**mohl**-ō-guhs

*Hydraulic pressure* hī-**draw**-lihck **prehsh**-ər

*Infundibulum* ihn-fuhn-**dihb**-yuh-luhm

*Inguinal ring* **ihn**-gwih-nahl rihng

*Interstitial cell* ihn-tər-**stihsh**-ahl sehl

*Labia* **lā**-bē-uh

*Ligate* **lī**-gāt

*Mature follicle* **maht**-chər **fohl**-ih-kuhl

*Meiosis* mī-ō-sihs

*Metestrus* meht-**ehs**-truhs

*Mitosis* mī-**tō**-sihs

*Monoestrous* mohn-ō-**ehs**-truhs

*Multiparous* muhl-**tihp**-er-uhs

*Oocyte* **ō**-ō-sīt

*Oogenesis* ō-ō-**jehn**-eh-sihs

*Orchiectomy* ohr-kihd-**ehck**-tō-mē

*Os penis* ohs **pē**-nihs

*Ovarian follicle* ō-**veer**-ē-uhn **fohl**-ih-kuhl

*Ovary* **ō**-vər-ē

*Oviduct* **ō**-vih-duhckt

*Ovulation* ohv-yoo-**lā**-shuhn

*Ovum* **ō**-vuhm

*Pampiniform plexus* pahm-**pihn**-eh-fohrm **plehck**-suhs

*Parietal vaginal tunic* pah-**rī**-eh-tahl **vahj**-ihn-ahl **too**-nihck

*Penis* **pē**-nihs

*Placenta* plah-**sehn**-tah

*Polar body* **pō**-lər boh-dē

*Polyestrous* pohl-ē-**ehs**-truhs

*Prepuce* **prē**-pyoos

*Proestrus* prō-**ehs**-truhs

*Progestin* prō-**jehs**-tihn

*Proper vaginal tunic* **praw**-pər **vahj**-ihn-ahl **too**-nihck

*Prostate gland* **prah**-stāt glahnd

*Pseudocyesis* soo-dō-sī-**ē**-sihs

*Pseudopregnancy* soo-dō-**prehg**-nuhn-sē

*Retractor penis muscle* rih-trahck-tər **pē**-nihs **muhs**-uhl

*Roots of the penis* rootz *of the* **pē**-nihs

*Round ligament of the uterus* round **lihg**-ah-mehnt *of the* **ū**-tər-uhs

*Scrotum* **skrō**-tuhm

*Seasonally polyestrous* sē-zuhn-**ahl**-ē pohl-ē-**ehs**-truhs

*Seminal vesicle* **sehm**-ihn-uhl **vehs**-ih-kuhl

*Seminiferous tubule* sehm-uh-**nihf**-ər-uhs **too**-būl

*Sertoli cell* sər-**tō**-lē sehl

*Sex chromosome* sehx **krō**-muh-sōm

*Sigmoid flexure* **sihg**-moyd **flehck**-shər

*Spermatic cord* spər-**maht**-ihck kohrd

*Spermatogenesis* spər-**mah**-tō-**jehn**-eh-sihs

*Spermatozoon* spər-maht-uh-**zō**-uhn

*Sphincter* **sfihnk**-tər

*Suspensory ligament of the ovary* suh-**spehn**-suh-rē **lihg**-ah-mehnt *of the* **ō**-vər-ē

*Testes* **tehs**-tēs

*Tie* tī

*Uniparous* ū-**nihp**-er-uhs

*Urethra* ū-**rē**-thrah

*Urethral process* ū-**rē**-thruhl **proh**-sehs

*Uterus* **ū**-tər-uhs

*Vagina* vah-**jī**-nah

*Vaginal tunic* **vahj**-ihn-ahl **too**-nihck

*Vas deferens* vahs **dehf**-ər-ehns

*Vestibule of the vulva* **vehs**-tuh-byool *of the* **vuhl**-vah

*Visceral vaginal tunic* **vih**-sər-ahl **vahj**-ihn-ahl **too**-nihck

*Vulva* **vuhl**-vah

## INTRODUCTION

To say the least, the reproductive system is unusual. The rest of the body's systems work to ensure the survival of the individual animal they are part of, whereas the reproductive system works to ensure the survival of the *species* of animal. The reproductive system does interact with other body systems, but purely reproductive structures are not essential to the life of an animal. Think about it: The testes, ovaries, and other reproductive organs of male and female animals are commonly removed surgically to prevent reproduction and influence behavior. If no complications result from the surgery, the rest of the body systems continue to go merrily on their way, and the animal is none the worse for its loss. It simply cannot reproduce. Of course it is a different story with structures that the reproductive system shares with other systems. For example, the urethra in the male has both urinary and reproductive functions. It *is* essential to life and must not be damaged or removed.

Something else unique about the reproductive system is that it requires a *second* animal (of the opposite sex) to fully carry out its function, which is to produce a brand new animal (the offspring). What we refer to as the *reproductive system* in an individual animal is really only half a system. A complete reproductive system is made up of all the male reproductive organs and structures in one animal *and* all the female reproductive organs and structures in another. Both are necessary for an offspring to be produced.

The basic reproductive process starts with fertilization: the head of a **spermatozoon** must penetrate into the cytoplasm of an **ovum**. The fertilized ovum must then be provided with a hospitable place to grow and develop until the offspring is born. After birth, the offspring must be fed and cared for until it can fend for itself. For these basic processes to occur, the physical characteristics and behavior of two different animals must be synchronized and coordinated with delicate precision. This elegant process of developing and bringing together a male animal and a female animal at the appropriate time and in appropriate states of readiness to produce a viable offspring is the amazing role of the reproductive system.

For simplicity's sake, we discuss the male and female reproductive systems as separate physical entities. Remember, though, that a whole reproductive *system* is made up of both the male and female systems working in concert with each other.

## MEIOSIS

Our discussion of reproduction begins at the most basic, cellular level. **Gametes** (reproductive cells—ova and spermatozoa) are produced by the unique process of cell division called **meiosis**. This is the first step in the process by which nature "shuffles the genetic cards" each time a new animal is conceived. Meiosis ensures that the genetic makeup of each new animal is unique. Each animal that enters the world has characteristics similar to others of its species and breed, but its precise genetic makeup is unique. Except for identical twins or clones, it is virtually impossible for two animals to have exactly the same genetic makeup.

### CLINICAL APPLICATION

#### Unique Patients

The fact that each animal has an individual, unique genetic composition is not just hypothetical or interesting in an abstract sense. This uniqueness is an important concept for us to keep in mind as we examine and treat patients. It can significantly affect things such as behavior, clinical signs of disease, doses of drugs, and response to treatments. Even though all Golden Retrievers look a lot alike, a particular Golden Retriever we are working with may respond differently to our drugs and treatments than others of its breed we have worked with before. This is an important concept to grasp if we are to be effective in our work in clinical veterinary medicine. Each of our patients is an absolutely unique, original individual. It is reasonable to expect more similarities than differences among animals of a particular species and breed, but always keep in the back of your mind the possibility that this animal may not react exactly the same as others you have worked with in the past.

## CHROMOSOMES

### DIPLOID CHROMOSOME NUMBER

The genetic material in the body's cells is contained in the nuclei in the form of coiled masses of DNA called **chromosomes**. This genetic material contains a complete "blueprint" for all of the structures and functions in the animal's body. For the body to function efficiently, each cell must contain the same genetic information. So each of the cells in an animal's body, with the exception of the gametes (spermatozoa or ova), contains identical chromosomes.

Another member of the same species has a slightly different genetic code in its chromosomes (the cause of that uniqueness business), but the total *number* of chromosomes in the nucleus of each of its body cells (except for the gametes) is the same. The total number of chromosomes in the nucleus of each cell is called the **diploid chromosome number**, which is always an even number, because the chromosomes occur in pairs (*di* means "double," and *ploid* refers to chromosomes). Therefore all cattle have the same number of chromosomes in the nuclei of their cells. The same goes for all dogs, horses, humans, and even corn and tomato plants. Table 19-1 contains the diploid chromosome numbers of some selected species. The diploid chromosome number is sometimes expressed generically with the abbreviation *2n*. The *n* is a mathematical expression that represents a number, and the *2* indicates that the number is doubled (diploid).

### SEX CHROMOSOMES

One of the pairs of chromosomes that make up the diploid chromosome number are the **sex chromosomes**. They determine the genetic gender (male or female) of the animal. They are designated as being either *X* chromosomes or *Y* chromosomes. If both of the sex chromosomes are *X* chromosomes (*XX*), the individual is genetically female. If one is an *X* and the other is a *Y* (*XY*), the individual is genetically male. The *YY* combination is not possible, for reasons that we will discuss. Many other factors, including the influence of hormones, help determine the overall maleness or femaleness of an individual, but the makeup of the sex chromosomes is a basic determining factor. (Table 19-2 lists common female and male gender terms.) So the full diploid chromosome makeup of a female animal is often abbreviated as *2n,XX* and that of a male animal as *2n,XY*.

| TABLE 19-1 | Diploid Chromosome Numbers of Some Selected Species |
|---|---|
| **SPECIES** | **DIPLOID CHROMOSOME NUMBER** |
| African Hedgehog | 90 |
| Cat | 38 |
| Cattle | 60 |
| Corn | 20 |
| Dog | 78 |
| Donkey | 62 |
| Fox | 34 |
| Goat | 60 |
| Gray Fox | 66 |
| Horse | 64 |
| Human | 46 |
| Mosquito | 6 |
| Mouse | 40 |
| Pig | 38 |
| Rabbit | 44 |
| Rat | 42 |
| Red Panda | 36 |
| Sheep | 54 |
| Tomato | 24 |

| TABLE 19-2 | Selected Common Gender Terms | |
|---|---|---|
| **SPECIES** | **FEMALE** | **MALE** |
| Ass/Donkey | Jenny | Jack |
| Bison | Cow | Bull |
| Camel | Cow | Bull |
| Cat | Queen | Tom |
| Cattle | Cow | Bull |
| Chicken | Hen | Rooster |
| Deer | Doe | Buck |
| Dinosaur | Cow | Bull |
| Dog | Bitch | Dog |
| Dolphin | Cow | Bull |
| Elephant | Cow | Bull |
| Ferret | Jill | Hob |
| Fox | Vixen | Dog |
| Gerbil | Doe | Buck |
| Guinea Pig | Sow | Boar |
| Goat | Doe | Buck |
| Hamster | Doe | Buck |
| Hedgehog | Sow | Boar |
| Horse | Mare | Stallion |
| Jellyfish | Sow | Boar |
| Leopard | Leopardess | Leopard |
| Llama | Cow | Bull |
| Mouse | Doe | Buck |
| Mule | Molly | John |
| Otter | Sow | Boar |
| Parrot | Hen | Cock |
| Pig | Sow | Boar |
| Porcupine | Sow | Boar |
| Porpoise | Cow | Bull |
| Rabbit | Doe | Buck |
| Rat | Doe | Buck |
| Red Panda | Sow | Boar |
| Sheep | Ewe | Ram |
| Squid | Hen | Cock |
| Tiger | Tigress | Tiger |
| Turkey | Hen | Tom |
| Whale | Cow | Bull |
| Wolf | Bitch | Dog |
| Zebra | Mare | Stallion |

## HAPLOID CHROMOSOME NUMBER

Some basic mathematics reveals why the gametes cannot have the diploid number of chromosomes. If the ovum of a goat and the spermatozoon that fertilizes it each contained the full caprine diploid chromosome number of 60, the fertilized ovum would contain a total of 120 chromosomes! That is way too many. The number of chromosomes in the reproductive cells must be reduced to half of the diploid number for things to work out, so when the spermatozoon and the ovum come together, the total number of chromosomes in the fertilized ovum equals the diploid number.

The reduced number of chromosomes in the gametes is called the **haploid chromosome number** (*hapl-* means "single") and is abbreviated *n,X* or *n,Y*, depending on which sex chromosome is present. The haploid chromosome number in the reproductive cells results from a "reduction division" of cells called *meiosis*. Meiosis is referred to as a *reduction division* because as a cell *divides* by this process, the total number of chromosomes in each of the daughter cells is *reduced* to one half the number in the parent cell. One of each pair of diploid chromosomes from the parent cell goes to each of the daughter cells. Each daughter cell then has the haploid chromosome number.

## MEIOSIS VERSUS MITOSIS

You recall that when most of the body's cells divide, they do it through a process called **mitosis**. When a cell divides by mitosis, each of its chromosomes first produces a duplicate copy of itself. When the two daughter cells pull apart, half the chromosomes go to one cell and half go to the other. Each cell ends up with an identical, full diploid set of chromosomes. The genetic makeup of the two daughter cells is exactly the same, and identical to that of the parent cell. This ensures that the genetic information in all of the body's cells, except for the gametes, stays exactly the same.

When the gametes are produced by meiosis, the chromosomes do not produce duplicate copies of themselves before the daughter cells pull apart. Half of the total number of chromosomes (one from each diploid chromosome pair), including one sex chromosome, goes to each daughter cell. Which chromosomes go to which daughter cell is entirely random. The chromosomes merely pull apart into their new cells. In this way, the genetic material of the reproductive cells gets "shuffled," resulting in genetically unique offspring.

## CLINICAL APPLICATION

### Chromosome Combinations

If you want to do some interesting mathematical calculations, determine how many different combinations of chromosomes could result for different species by randomly assigning one of each pair of diploid chromosomes to each reproductive cell. *Hint:* Because the diploid chromosomes occur in pairs, you can start with the number 2 and multiply it times itself as many times as there are *pairs* of chromosomes. For example, a diploid chromosome number of 8 would have four pairs of chromosomes, so the number of possible haploid chromosome combinations would be $2^4$, or 16 possible combinations. Try using that calculation for some of the diploid chromosome numbers listed in Table 19-1. (Divide the diploid chromosome number in half and multiply 2 by itself that many times.) You are going to get some very large numbers. Those large numbers represent the number of possible combinations

of chromosomes that could occur in each spermatozoon *or* ovum from an animal of that species.

If you want to calculate the number of chromosome combinations possible in an *offspring* of that species, you need to take the number of possible chromosome combinations for a spermatozoon and multiply it by the number of possible chromosome combinations for an ovum: you are going to come up with some *ginormous* numbers.

In a human, for example, the diploid chromosome number is 46, so the number of possible combinations of chromosomes in each spermatozoon or ovum is $2^{23}$, or 8,388,608. The number of possible combinations of chromosomes in a human infant would then be $2^{23} \times 2^{23}$, or 70,368,744,177,664. Barring an identical twin, the chance of your parents producing a brother or sister with the exact same chromosome combination as you is 1 in 70,368,744,177,664!

## SPERMATOGENESIS

Spermatozoa, the male gametes, are produced in the seminiferous tubules of the testes through a process called **spermatogenesis** (*genesis* means "creation"). Spermatozoa are produced continuously and in very large numbers in an effort to ensure that one spermatozoon will successfully reach and fertilize the ovum when breeding occurs. So the process of spermatogenesis is designed to produce huge numbers of spermatozoa continuously (Figure 19-1).

Spermatogenesis begins at the periphery of the **seminiferous tubule** with a cell called a *primary spermatocyte*. This cell has the normal diploid chromosome number for the species. The chromosome complement of the cell is abbreviated as *2n,XY.* Keep in mind that the *XY* refers to the sex chromosomes, which in a male are always an *X* and a *Y.* The primary spermatocyte divides by meiosis into two secondary spermatocytes, which are pushed inward toward the tubule lumen. These now have haploid chromosome numbers. One

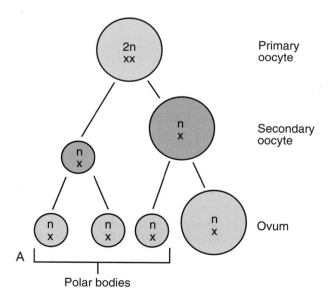

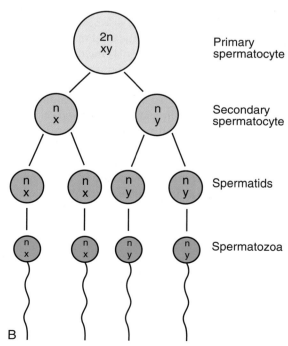

**FIGURE 19-1** Meiosis. This process reduces the diploid chromosome number to the haploid number in reproductive cells. **A,** Oogenesis. Note that only one functional ovum is produced from the original primary oocyte. **B,** Spermatogenesis. Note that four spermatozoa are produced from the original primary spermatocyte.

has an *n,X* chromosome complement, and the other has an *n,Y* complement. The two secondary spermatocytes divide by *mitosis* (so that the chromosome number does not get reduced further) into four spermatids. Two of the spermatids have *n,X* chromosome complements, and two have *n,Y.* As a result of the cell divisions that produced them, the spermatids are now located near the center of the tubule lumen. They do not undergo any further cell divisions, but they grow tails and undergo other physical changes that convert them to spermatozoa. When the spermatozoa are fully developed, they detach and are carried to an organ called the *epididymis* for storage before ejaculation. This is discussed in more detail below.

Half of the spermatozoa produced have an *X* sex chromosome, and half have a *Y* sex chromosome. This is the means by which the genetic sex of the offspring will be determined. If an *X*-bearing spermatozoon fertilizes the ovum (which always contains an *X* sex chromosome), the offspring will have *XX* sex chromosomes and be genetically female. If a *Y*-bearing spermatozoon is successful, the offspring will have *XY* sex chromosomes and will be genetically male. This ensures sexual equality of numbers in that about the same number of females and males will be conceived.

## OOGENESIS

Ova, the female gametes, are produced in follicles in the ovaries through a process called **oogenesis**. They are not produced continuously, unlike spermatozoa. At or soon after birth, a female has a fixed number of primary **oocytes** (which are the precursor cells to ova) already formed in her ovaries. That is the total number available in her lifetime. They remain in a quiet, immature state until they are recruited as part of an ovarian cycle. Each ovarian cycle produces one or more mature ova, depending on the species. Because spermatozoa come to the ovum to fertilize it, large numbers of ova are not needed. Therefore the process of oogenesis is designed to produce small numbers of ova at one time (see Figure 19-1).

Oogenesis takes place in the developing **ovarian follicle**. The primary oocyte is the immature cell that waits quietly in the ovary for the signal to start developing. It has the normal diploid chromosome number for the species. The chromosome complement of the cell is abbreviated as *2n,XX*. When it becomes activated, the primary oocyte divides by meiosis into a large, secondary oocyte and a small **polar body**. Each has the haploid chromosome number *n,X*. Polar bodies are essentially garbage cans for excess chromosomes. They will not develop into ova. The secondary oocyte and the first polar body divide *by mitosis* (to preserve the haploid chromosome number) into an ovum and three polar bodies. So from one primary oocyte, one mature ovum will result.

## MALE REPRODUCTIVE SYSTEM

The tasks for the male component of the reproductive system sound pretty simple: produce male sex hormones, develop male gametes (spermatozoa), and deliver the spermatozoa to the female system at the appropriate time. However, a rather complicated system of organs, glands, structures, and tubes is required to carry out these tasks. Figure 19-2 illustrates the reproductive system of the bull, and Figure 19-3 illustrates that of the dog. Let us start our examination of the male reproductive system with the basic organs of male reproduction: the testes.

## TESTES
### CHARACTERISTICS

The **testes** are the male **gonads**—the organs where the male reproductive cells are formed (Figures 19-4 and 19-5). They are generally oval, and their size varies considerably among species. In common domestic animals, they are located outside the abdomen in the inguinal (groin) region, housed in a sac of skin called the **scrotum**.

### FUNCTIONS

The testes have two main functions: *spermatogenesis* and *hormone production*. Spermatogenesis is the process by which spermatozoa, the male gametes, are produced in the seminiferous tubules of the testes. Between the seminiferous tubules, cells called **interstitial cells** (*interstitial* means *between*) produce male sex hormones, or **androgens**. The principal androgen they produce is *testosterone,* which is responsible for the development of male secondary sex characteristics (such as the male body shape) and the male libido (sex drive). It also has a general anabolic (protein-building) effect on the body, which results in the enhanced muscle and bone development that gives male animals their size and bulk.

### SPERMATOZOA

Spermatozoa are long, thin cells with three main parts: an enlarged *head,* a *midpiece,* and a long, narrow *tail* (Figure 19-6). The head contains the payload of the cell, the nucleus, and is covered by a caplike structure called the **acrosome**. The acrosome contains digestive enzymes that are released once the spermatozoon is inside the female reproductive tract. It helps the spermatozoon penetrate through the layers surrounding the ovum to accomplish fertilization. The midpiece is the "power plant" of the cell. It contains a large concentration of energy-producing mitochondria arranged

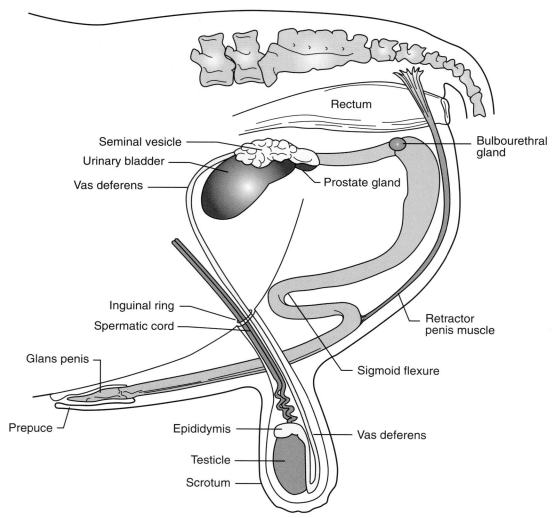

**FIGURE 19-2** Reproductive system of the bull. Lateral view.

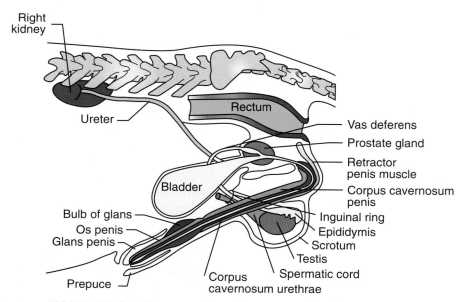

**FIGURE 19-3** Male urinary and reproductive organs of the dog. Lateral view.

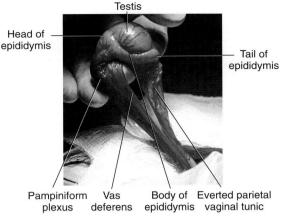

**FIGURE 19-4** *Canine testis. Lateral view.*

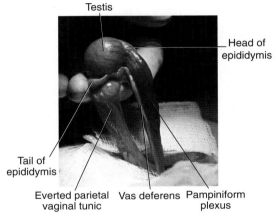

**FIGURE 19-5** *Canine testis. Medial view.*

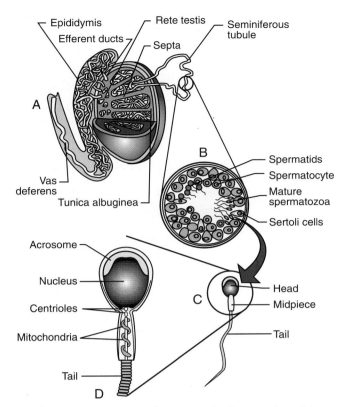

**FIGURE 19-6** Structure of a testis. **A,** Testis and epididymis. **B,** Enlarged cross section of seminiferous tubule. **C,** Mature spermatozoon. **D,** Head area detail of mature spermatozoon.

in a spiral pattern. The long, thin tail resembles the flagellum that many single-celled organisms use for propulsion. It contains musclelike contractile fibrils that produce a whip-like movement of the tail and propel the cell forward once it is activated.

## DEVELOPMENT AND LOCATION

Before birth, the testes begin development in the abdominal cavity near the kidneys. They are attached to their eventual permanent home in the scrotum by a band of connective tissue called the **gubernaculum**. As the tiny embryo grows, the gubernaculum remains fairly constant in length. This results in the testes gradually being pulled caudally and ventrally. What is actually happening is that the fetus is growing longer and larger while the testes are being held in place. At or soon after birth, the testes are normally pulled down through the **inguinal rings** into the scrotum. The inguinal rings, located in the groin region, are two slitlike openings in the abdominal muscles. This process is referred to as the *descent of the testes* and is illustrated in Figure 19-7.

## SCROTUM

The **scrotum** is the sac of skin that houses the testes. Besides providing a home for the testes, the scrotum also helps

regulate their temperature. The testes have to be kept slightly cooler than body temperature to produce spermatozoa. A bandlike muscle, the **cremaster muscle**, passes down through the inguinal ring and attaches to the scrotum. It can adjust the position of the testes relative to the body. In warm conditions, the cremaster muscle relaxes, and the testes hang down away from the warm body. This position helps to reduce their temperature. In cold conditions, however, the cremaster muscle pulls the testes up tight against the body wall, which helps warm them.

## SPERMATIC CORD

The **spermatic cords** link the testes with the rest of the body. They are tubelike, connective tissue structures that contain blood vessels, nerves, lymphatic vessels, and the *vas deferens*. The arrangement of blood vessels in the spermatic cord is particularly interesting. They form a heat-exchange mechanism that helps keep the temperature of the testes slightly lower than that of the rest of the body. As Figures 19-8 and 19-9 show, the single testicular artery carries blood down to the testis. Surrounding the artery is a structure called the **pampiniform plexus**, which is an intricate meshwork of tiny veins derived from the testicular veins. As body-temperature blood passes down to the testis through the testicular artery, it is cooled by the blood returning from the testis in the pampiniform plexus. At the same time, the blood in the pampiniform plexus is warmed by the blood in the testicular

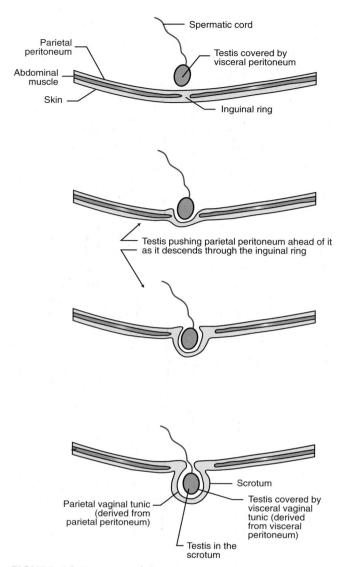

**FIGURE 19-7** Descent of the testes and derivation of the vaginal tunics.

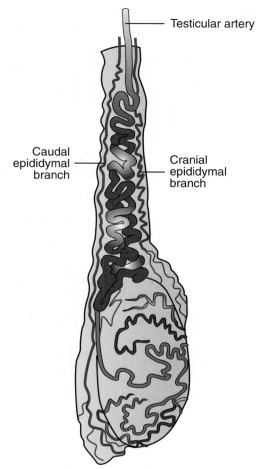

**FIGURE 19-8** Arterial blood supply to testis and epididymis of a bull. The testicular artery passes down the center of the spermatic cord.

artery. This heat-exchange mechanism helps maintain the testes at a temperature slightly lower than body temperature but keeps the body as a whole from losing heat by warming the blood from the testes back to body temperature before it returns to the abdomen.

## STRUCTURE

**TUNICS.** Two layers of connective tissue called the **vaginal tunics** surround the testes in the scrotum and the spermatic cord. The "vaginal" part of the name refers to the fact that the tunics form sheathlike covering layers. They are derived from layers of peritoneum that were pushed ahead of the testes as they descended through the inguinal rings (see Figure 19-7). The thin, inner layer, the **visceral vaginal tunic** (also known as the **proper vaginal tunic**), is derived from the visceral layer of peritoneum that coated the testes as they developed in the abdomen. It is tightly adherent to the surface of the testes and the structures of the spermatic

cords. It is so thin and transparent that it is invisible to the naked eye. The thick, outer layer, the **parietal vaginal tunic** (also known as the **common vaginal tunic**), is derived from the parietal layer of peritoneum that lines the abdominal cavity. It forms a visible fibrous sac around each testis and spermatic cord.

The tunics become significant when an animal is to undergo a castration (**orchiectomy**). An incision into the scrotum will reveal the tunic-covered testis. In one common method of castration, an incision is made in the outer, parietal vaginal tunic, and the testis is then everted through the incision in the tunic, thereby exposing the blood vessels in the spermatic cord. The blood vessels can then be **ligated** (tied off) or clamped for a time before the testis is removed. Figure 19-10 shows the initial incision through the parietal vaginal tunic during a dog castration. Note the testis, covered in the visceral vaginal tunic, bulging up through the incision in the parietal tunic.

**CAPSULE.** Beneath the tunics, each testis is enclosed by a heavy, fibrous connective tissue capsule called the **tunica albuginea** (see Figure 19-6). This capsule protects and supports the soft contents of the testis. Many small partitions,

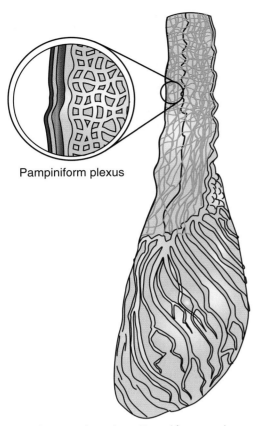

Pampiniform plexus

**FIGURE 19-9** Pampiniform plexus. Formed from testicular veins visible on the surface of the testis, it surrounds the testicular artery and helps cool the blood passing down to the testis.

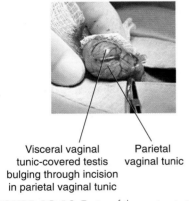

Visceral vaginal tunic-covered testis bulging through incision in parietal vaginal tunic

Parietal vaginal tunic

**FIGURE 19-10** Tunics of the canine testis.

called *septa*, extend into the testis from the capsule. The septa divide each testis into tiny lobules that contain the seminiferous tubules, as well as other cells and structures.

**SEMINIFEROUS TUBULES.** The seminiferous tubules are where spermatogenesis takes place. Each tubule is shaped like a long, convoluted "U" that is attached at both ends to a complex system of ducts called the *rete testis* (a *rete* is a complex *network* of something in the body). Between the seminiferous tubules are the endocrine cells of the testis known as the **interstitial cells**. The interstitial cells produce

androgens, the male sex hormones, under the influence of luteinizing hormone (LH) from the anterior pituitary gland. LH is sometimes referred to as *interstitial cell-stimulating hormone (ICSH)* in the male.

Inside the seminiferous tubules (see Figure 19-6), spermatozoa are produced by the process of meiosis (see Figure 19-1). The "parent" cells stay out toward the periphery of the tubule and push the "daughter" cells toward the center of the tubule as they divide. Primary spermatocytes divide to produce secondary spermatocytes, which divide to produce spermatids. The spermatids undergo physical changes to become spermatozoa. While they are undergoing these transformations, the spermatids are attached to large "nurse" cells called **Sertoli cells**.

In addition to providing mechanical and nutritional support, the Sertoli cells also help shield the developing spermatozoa from the body's immune system. Proteins on the surfaces of the genetically unique spermatozoa would stimulate the immune system to produce antibodies against them if they were not shielded. This would cause an autoimmune reaction, meaning the immune system would attack part of its own body—the spermatozoa. The Sertoli cells are also known to produce small amounts of estrogens under the stimulation of follicle-stimulating hormone (FSH) from the anterior pituitary gland.

 **CLINICAL APPLICATION**

### Cryptorchidism

Sometimes one or both of the testes do not descend into the scrotum. This is referred to as **cryptorchidism**. This condition can be either unilateral, when one testis has failed to descend, or bilateral, when both testes have failed to descend. An undescended testis can be located anywhere along the normal path of descent, from the region of the kidney to an area just outside the inguinal ring but not completely down in the scrotum (called a "high flanker"). Testes retained in the abdominal cavity are usually sterile (cannot produce spermatozoa) because spermatogenesis requires a temperature slightly lower than body temperature. The interior of the abdomen is too hot for spermatozoa to be produced. However, testosterone continues to be produced, so a bilaterally cryptorchid animal has all the characteristics of a male animal but typically cannot reproduce.

**DUCT SYSTEM.** When spermatozoa complete their physical development in the seminiferous tubules, they are transported to a storage site where they will be prepared for ejaculation. After they detach from their protective Sertoli cells, the spermatozoa enter the complex of ducts that make up the rete testis. From there, they flow through the **efferent ducts of the testes** to their storage site—the epididymis.

Grossly, the **epididymis** is a flat, ribbonlike structure that lies along the surface of the testis (see Figures 19-4 and 19-5). It is actually a single, long, very convoluted tube that connects the efferent ducts of the testis with the vas deferens. If the tube that makes up the human epididymis were stretched out, it would be about 6 m (20 feet) in length. The epididymis is divided into three regions: (1) the *head* of the epididymis is where the spermatozoa enter from the efferent ducts, (2) the *body* is the main portion that lies along the surface of the testis, and (3) the *tail* continues on as the vas deferens.

The epididymis functions as a storage site for spermatozoa and a place for them to mature before they are expelled by ejaculation. Spermatozoa are immature when they leave the seminiferous tubules. They must mature in the epididymis for a week or more before they can fertilize ova. If the spermatozoa are never ejaculated (e.g., in an individual who has had a vasectomy), they live out their lives in the epididymis, die, and are broken down and absorbed by the tubular lining cells.

## CLINICAL APPLICATION

### Sertoli Cell Tumor

On occasion, Sertoli cells can multiply out of control, particularly in dogs. This produces what is termed a *Sertoli cell tumor* in the testis. Because normal Sertoli cells produce small amounts of estrogens, this action can become exaggerated as the cells multiply out of control. The level of estrogens in the animal's bloodstream rises rapidly, producing feminization of the male dog. The prepuce often becomes pendulous, and the mammary glands may become enlarged (gynecomastia) and can even produce milk. The penis and the opposite testis atrophy, and other male dogs may be attracted to the affected animal as if he were a female in heat. The signs of feminization are often the primary complaints when affected animals are presented to the veterinary clinic. The primary treatment for a Sertoli cell tumor is usually castration of the animal.

---

 **TEST YOURSELF 19-3**

1. What are the two main functions of the testis? Where in the organ does each take place?
2. What are the three main parts of a spermatozoon? What is the main purpose or function of each?
3. Why is a bilaterally cryptorchid animal usually sterile?
4. Would a bilaterally cryptorchid animal exhibit normal male behavior? Why or why not?
5. What is important about the scrotum's ability to adjust the position of the testes relative to the body?
6. What are the main components of the spermatic cord?
7. From what are the visceral and parietal vaginal tunics that cover the testes derived?
8. Where are spermatozoa stored before ejaculation?

## VAS DEFERENS

Something has to move the spermatozoa from the epididymis (located way down in the scrotum) up to the urethra (within the pelvic cavity) when ejaculation occurs. This is the job of the **vas deferens**. Also known as the *ductus*

*deferens,* the vas deferens is a muscular tube that connects the tail of the epididymis with the pelvic portion of the urethra. Thick layers of smooth muscle in its wall give it a very solid, cordlike texture. The vas deferens passes up through the inguinal ring as a part of the spermatic cord. Once inside the abdomen, each vas deferens separates from the rest of the spermatic cord, loops back caudally, and connects with the urethra just caudal to the neck of the urinary bladder (see Figures 19-2 through 19-5, and Figure 19-11). In many species, the vas deferens enlarges just before joining the urethra. This enlargement, if present, is called the **ampulla**, which may contain glands that contribute material to semen.

The job of the vas deferens is to propel spermatozoa and the fluid they are suspended in quickly from the epididymis to the urethra when ejaculation occurs. Once they are in the urethra, the spermatozoa are mixed with secretions from accessory reproductive glands to form *semen,* which is pumped out into the female reproductive tract.

## URETHRA

The **urethra** of the male has two functions. Most of the time it carries urine from the urinary bladder out of the body. This is its *urinary* function. However, when ejaculation occurs, urine flow is temporarily blocked. Spermatozoa from the vas deferens and secretions from the accessory reproductive glands enter the urethra and are pumped out as semen. **Ejaculation** is its reproductive function.

The urethra is spoken of as having two portions. The *pelvic portion,* within the pelvic cavity, is where the vas deferens and accessory reproductive glands enter. The remainder of the urethra, which runs down the length of the penis, is known as the *penile portion* of the urethra.

## ACCESSORY REPRODUCTIVE GLANDS

Spermatozoa make up only a small portion of the total volume of semen. The majority is made up of secretions from the various accessory reproductive glands. The ducts of all the accessory reproductive glands enter the pelvic portion of the urethra (see Figure 19-11). Different species have different combinations of accessory reproductive glands. Table 19-3 provides a summary of which common animals have which glands.

The accessory reproductive glands produce alkaline fluid containing substances such as electrolytes, fructose, and prostaglandins. The alkalinity of the fluid helps counteract the acidity of the female reproductive tract. This helps more spermatozoa survive to reach the oviducts, where they hope to meet up with an ovum. Fructose is a simple sugar that acts as an energy source for the very active spermatozoa. Some of the prostaglandins are thought to stimulate the contractions of the female reproductive tract which help move the spermatozoa up to the oviducts.

## SEMINAL VESICLES

Ducts from the two **seminal vesicles**, sometimes called *vesicular glands,* enter the pelvic urethra in the same area as the

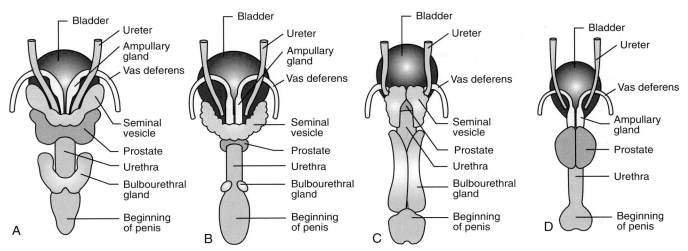

**FIGURE 19-11** Accessory reproductive glands. Comparisons among some common domestic species (dorsal views). A, Stallion. B, Bull. C, Boar. D, Dog.

| TABLE 19-3 | Male Accessory Reproductive Glands | | |
|---|---|---|---|
| **ANIMAL** | **SEMINAL VESICLES** | **PROSTATE GLAND** | **BULBOURETHRAL GLANDS** |
| Boar | + | + | + |
| Bull | + | + | + |
| Cat | − | + | + |
| Dog | − | + | − |
| Human | + | + | + |
| Ram | + | + | + |
| Stallion | + | + | + |

+, Indicates the presence of a gland; −, indicates the gland is absent.

### CLINICAL APPLICATION

#### Vasectomy

If a section of each vas deferens is removed surgically from an animal, the animal is rendered sterile (it cannot reproduce). This procedure is known as a *vasectomy*. It prevents spermatozoa from reaching the urethra during ejaculation. The other components of semen are ejaculated, but no spermatozoa are included. The individual is "firing blanks," so to speak. The spermatozoa live out their lives in the epididymis, die, and are absorbed by the lining cells.

Vasectomy is a common contraceptive surgery to prevent pregnancy in humans. It is performed less commonly for that reason in nonhuman animals but is sometimes performed on bulls to create "teaser" animals. Teaser bulls are used to help identify cows in heat so that they can be bred, often by artificial insemination, to other males.

vas deferens. They are present in all common domestic animals except for cats and dogs.

## PROSTATE GLAND

The **prostate gland** is a single structure that more or less completely surrounds the urethra. Multiple ducts carry its secretions into the urethra. It is present in all common domestic animals. In dogs, it is particularly large because it is the only accessory reproductive gland they have.

## BULBOURETHRAL GLANDS

The two **bulbourethral glands**, also known as the *Cowper's glands*, are located further caudally than the other accessory reproductive glands. Their ducts enter the urethra back near the caudal border of the pelvis. They secrete a mucinous (mucus-containing) fluid just before ejaculation that clears and lubricates the urethra for the passage of semen. All common domestic animals have bulbourethral glands except for the dog.

## PENIS

The **penis** is the male breeding organ. It is made up mainly of muscle, erectile tissue, and connective tissue, with the urethra running down its center. It has a very large blood supply and many sensory nerve endings. When the male is sufficiently aroused and stimulated, the erectile tissue becomes engorged with blood, causing the penis to enlarge and stiffen. This allows it to be inserted into the vagina of the female for breeding.

The three main parts of the penis are the *roots*, the *body*, and the *glans*.

### ROOTS

The **roots of the penis** attach it to the brim of the pelvis. They consist primarily of two bands of connective tissue, called the **crura**, covered by the ischiocavernosus muscles.

### BODY

The **body of the penis** is its largest part. It is mainly made up of two bundles of **erectile tissue**. Erectile tissue is composed of a spongy network of fibrous connective tissue and many tiny, blood-filled spaces called *sinuses*. In the nonerect state, the amount of blood flowing into the erectile tissue is the same as the amount flowing out. When more blood flows into erectile tissue than leaves it, however, the sinuses engorge with blood and try to enlarge. The network of connective tissue surrounding the engorged sinuses prevents them from swelling up like a bunch of water balloons. Instead, the relatively inelastic connective tissue around the blood sinuses generates enough **hydraulic pressure** in the engorged erectile tissue to cause the penis to become a little larger and a lot stiffer. This is called **erection** of the penis.

The two erectile tissue structures that make up the body of the penis are the smaller **corpus cavernosum urethrae** and the larger **corpus cavernosum penis**. The corpus cavernosum urethrae, also called the *corpus spongiosum,* forms a sleeve around the urethra as it passes through the body of the penis. The larger body of erectile tissue dorsal to the urethra is the corpus cavernosum penis.

## CLINICAL APPLICATION

### Canine Prostate Problems

The prostate gland in dogs is large—about the size of a walnut in a medium-size dog. Many conditions can cause it to become even larger, such as infection, tumors, or just normal aging. Because the urethra runs through the center of the gland, significant enlargement of the prostate squeezes the urethra. This can partially or completely block the passage of urine, leading to difficulty urinating. Instead of urine passing in a large stream, it dribbles out or may stop entirely. The cause of prostate gland enlargement must be determined to formulate an effective treatment strategy. Some conditions can be managed with medication, but others require surgery.

### GLANS

The **glans of the penis** is its tip, or the distal, free end of the organ. Its structure and appearance vary considerably among species. Horses have a well-defined glans that contains a considerable amount of erectile tissue. In ruminants, the glans is small and not well defined. Cats have short spines covering their glans. The penis of the dog is a special case that is described more completely below. Regardless of the species, the surface of the glans has a rich supply of sensory nerve endings that make it very sensitive to physical stimulation.

### PREPUCE

The **prepuce** is the sheath of skin that encloses the penis when it is not erect. The outer part of the prepuce is normal skin, but the inner portion that is in contact with the penis is a smooth, moist, mucous membrane. The prepuce of the boar also contains a small preputial pouch in which urine and cellular debris accumulate. Decomposition of the material in this pouch gives boars their typical ripe odor. (This is considered very sexy to sows—a clear case of different strokes for different folks!)

### PENIS OF THE DOG

The penis of the dog and other canine species is unusual (see Figure 19-3). It includes a bone and an erectile structure that

causes the male and female to remain stuck together after breeding is completed. The bone in the penis of the dog is called the **os penis** (see Figure 7-37). The urethra runs through a groove in the ventral surface of this bone. No other domestic animals have a similar bone, but several wildlife species do, including raccoons, beaver, and walruses. It is rarely of clinical significance unless it is fractured (very rare) or unless urinary stones (calculi) lodge in the urethra, where it enters the groove in the os penis, and obstruct urine flow.

The other unique structure in the penis of the dog is an enlargement toward the rear of the glans called the **bulb of the glans**. It is made up of erectile tissue that is derived from the corpus cavernosum urethrae. During breeding, the bulb becomes engorged with blood more slowly than the other erectile structures. It usually does not reach full size until after ejaculation has taken place. Once it enlarges, however, the swollen bulb is tightly clamped in place by contractions of the muscles surrounding the vagina and vulva of the female. This makes it impossible for the male to withdraw the penis. The male then typically dismounts from the female and turns so that he faces the opposite direction from her. The two stand in a tail-to-tail position looking for all the world like the fictional "Pushme-Pullyou" from the Dr. Doolittle story. This is known as the **tie** and seems to be important for conception to occur in the dog. The tie typically lasts 15 to 20 minutes and does not seem uncomfortable for either animal. Once the erection of the bulb subsides, the animals can separate. Forcing the animals apart prematurely can cause injury. So tell well-meaning people *not* to throw cold water on a pair of tied dogs in an effort to separate them. Just let nature take its course. The positions of dogs during copulation are shown in Figure 19-12.

### PENIS OF THE HORSE

The penis of the horse contains a large component of erectile tissue, and the glans at the distal end flairs into a distinctive mushroom shape, the widest part of which is called the **corona glandis** (Figure 19-13). The distal end of the urethra, the **urethral process**, extends from a central depression, the **fossa glandis**, at the tip of the penis. Because of the large amount of erectile tissue it contains, the penis of the horse enlarges considerably in both length and circumference when erect.

### SIGMOID FLEXURE

The nonerect penis of the bull, ram, and boar is normally bent into an "S" shape. This is called the **sigmoid flexure** (see Figure 19-2); *sigmoid* means S-*shaped*. The penises of these animals also have a higher proportion of connective tissue to erectile tissue than other species, and so the penis does not enlarge much when erection occurs. Rather, the main mechanism of erection in these species is a straightening of the sigmoid flexure resulting from internal hydraulic pressure. The basic principle is the same as in a garden hose that wants to straighten out when the water is turned on. This causes the penis to protrude from the prepuce for breeding. A long, thin, cordlike muscle, the **retractor penis muscle**,

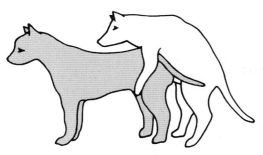

First stage coitus

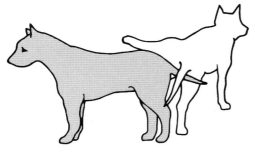

The turn

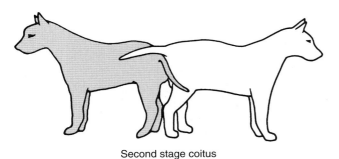

Second stage coitus

**FIGURE 19-12** Illustration of the three most obvious stages of breeding in dogs. (From Feldman E, Nelson R: Canine and feline endocrinology & reproduction, ed 3, Philadelphia, 2004, WB Saunders Company.)

originates near the base of the tail and attaches to the bend of the sigmoid flexure. It functions like a small bungee cord: When erection straightens out the sigmoid flexure, the retractor penis muscle stretches. When the erection subsides, the retractor penis muscle pulls the penis back into its nonerect, S shape.

## REPRODUCTIVE FUNCTIONS

**ERECTION.** Erection enlarges and stiffens the penis to prepare it for breeding. See Chapter 20 for information about the processes of erection.

**EJACULATION.** *Ejaculation* is the process by which semen is expelled from the penis. See Chapter 20 for more information about ejaculation.

## FEMALE REPRODUCTIVE SYSTEM

The female part of the reproductive system is a bit more complex than the male part, because it has more jobs to do.

Some are similar to those of the male, such as the production of sex hormones and development of gametes. But, in addition, the female system receives the male gametes, furnishes a site for them to fertilize the ovum (the oviduct), provides a hospitable environment for the embryo to grow and develop, carries it for the entire period of pregnancy, and then pushes the offspring out into the world when it is fully developed. All these jobs do not stop at birth: In the period immediately after, the mammary glands provide nutrition to the newborn. This is a lot of work for one system to do.

Nearly all of the female reproductive system is internal and is located within the abdominal and pelvic cavities. Figures 19-14 and 19-15 illustrate the female reproductive system of the bitch, and Figure 19-16 compares the female reproductive systems of several species; Figures 19-17 and 19-18 show reproductive structures of the cat.

## LIGAMENTS

The main reproductive organs—the *ovaries, oviducts,* and *uterus*—hang by broad sheets of peritoneum from the dorsal part of the abdominal cavity. The sheets of peritoneum are collectively called the left and right **broad ligaments** (see Figure 19-17). Each broad ligament has segments that are named according to the organ they directly support, although the divisions are not clearly apparent at a quick glance. The *mesovarium* supports the ovary, the *mesosalpinx* supports the oviduct, and the *mesometrium* supports the uterus. (The term *meso* refers to a sheet of tissue that attaches an organ to the body wall.) The broad ligaments contain blood vessels and nerve fibers that supply the ovaries, oviducts, and uterus; they also contain fat.

The ovarian end of the broad ligament extends cranially and attaches to the body wall in the area of the last rib. This forms the **suspensory ligament of the ovary** (see Figure 19-18). During surgical removal of the ovaries and uterus (ovariohysterectomy) in dogs and cats, the suspensory ligament must often be stretched or divided to allow the ovary to be elevated into the incision, so the ovarian blood vessels can be tied off.

A cord of fibrous tissue and smooth muscle called the **round ligament of the uterus** is contained in the free edge of a lateral fold of the broad ligament on each side

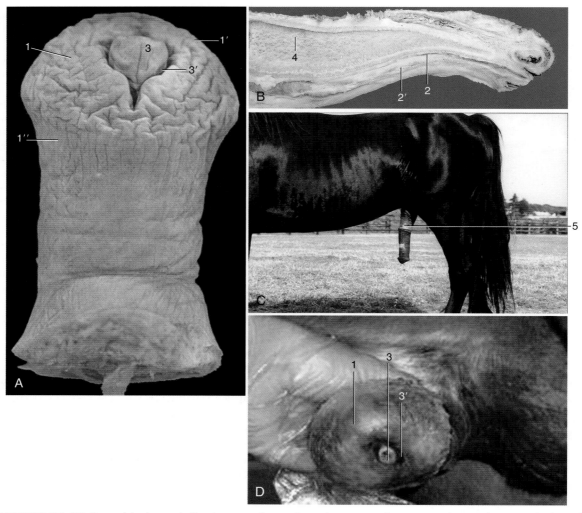

**FIGURE 19-13** Penis of the horse. **A,** Distal portion of penis; **B,** median section; **C,** penis just after copulation; **D,** distal tip of glans. *1,* Glans; *1',* corona; *2,* urethra; *2'* corpus cavernosum urethrae; *3,* urethral process within *3'* fossa glandis; *4,* corpus cavernosum penis; *5,* prepuce. (From Dyce KM, Sack WO, Wensing CJG: Textbook of veterinary anatomy, ed 4, St Louis, 2010, W.B. Saunders Company.)

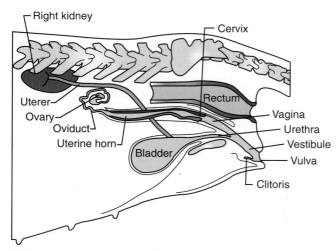

**FIGURE 19-14** Urinary and reproductive organs of bitch. Lateral view.

(see Figure 19-17). The round ligament extends from the tip of the uterine horn caudally and to the inguinal ring area ventrally. During ovariohysterectomy in dogs and cats, the round ligament is transected (cut) along with the broad ligament to allow the uterine horns to be removed.

## OVARIES
### CHARACTERISTICS

The **ovaries** are the female gonads; they are the female equivalent of the male testes. They are located in the dorsal part of the abdominal cavity near the kidneys. Their shape varies among species; in most, they are somewhat almond shaped, but the ovaries of the horse are indented, making them bean-like in appearance. The ovaries of sows, because their large litter sizes require large numbers of follicles, often look like clusters of grapes.

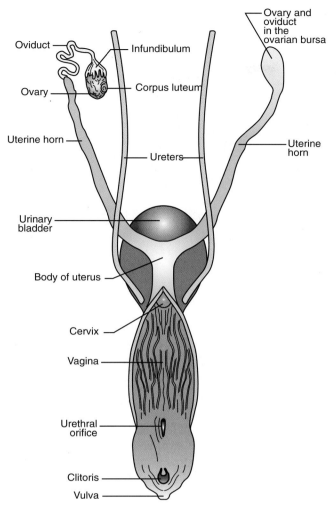

FIGURE 19-15 Reproductive system of bitch. Dorsal view.

**CLINICAL APPLICATION**

## Ovariohysterectomy

Ovariohysterectomy is a surgical procedure in which the ovaries, oviducts, and uterus are removed from an animal. It is commonly known as *spaying* an animal. Despite the frequency with which it is performed, ovariohysterectomy is a major surgical procedure that involves opening the abdominal cavity. To remove the reproductive organs safely, the blood vessels supplying them must first be tied off (ligated). The blood vessels to each ovary are usually ligated along with the portion of the broad ligament *(mesovarium)* that contains them. This portion is referred to surgically as the *ovarian pedicle* or *ovarian stump*. The ovaries then can be severed safely from their ligated blood vessels. The remainder of the broad ligament is usually either ligated en masse or cut back toward the body of the uterus. The blood vessels in this part of the broad ligament are usually small. The body of the uterus and its accompanying blood vessels are ligated and transected (cut). The reproductive organs then can be removed safely from the abdominal cavity and the incision sutured closed.

## FUNCTIONS

Like the testes, the ovaries have two main functions: producing gametes and producing hormones. **Oogenesis** is the process by which *ova* (the female gametes) are produced in **follicles** in the ovaries. Unlike spermatozoa, ova are not constantly produced during the reproductive life of the animal. At or soon after birth, the ovaries are seeded with tens of thousands of immature reproductive cells called **oocytes**. Some of these oocytes will mature into ova, the mature female reproductive cells, through the activities of the ovarian cycle. The rest will either degenerate or never begin development. No more oocytes are produced during the

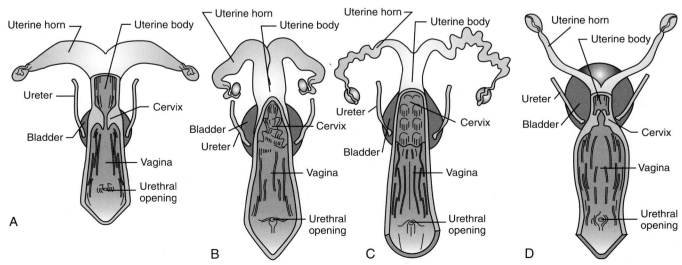

FIGURE 19-16 Female reproductive tract. Comparisons among some common domestic species (dorsal views). A, Mare. B, Cow. C, Sow. D, Bitch.

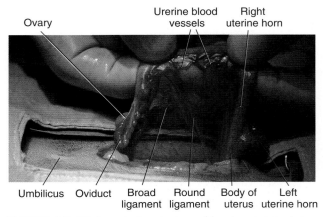

FIGURE 19-17 Reproductive structures of female cat. Lateral view.

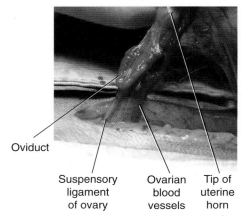

**FIGURE 19-18** Reproductive structures of female cat. Lateral view.

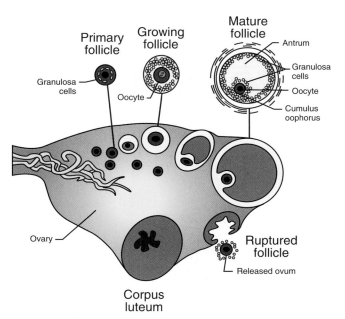

**FIGURE 19-19** Ovarian cycle. Schematic representation of the sequence of events in the ovarian cycle, starting with the primary follicle and proceeding (clockwise) to the mature follicle, ovulation, and formation of the corpus luteum. These stages would not all be present at one time in an ovary.

animal's life, however. The number of oocytes in the ovaries soon after birth is the maximum number that will be available to that animal during her lifetime.

The hormones produced in the ovaries fall into two categories: *estrogens* and *progestins*. **Estrogens** are produced by the cells of the developing ovarian follicles and are responsible for the physical and behavioral changes that prepare the animal for breeding and pregnancy. **Progestins**, principally progesterone, are produced by the **corpus luteum** that develops from the empty follicle after ovulation. Progestins help prepare the uterus for implantation of a fertilized ovum. They are also necessary for pregnancy to be maintained once implantation occurs.

## OVARIAN CYCLE

Ova are not constantly produced in the ovaries. Their production involves a complex sequence of events carried out in a cyclic (repeating) fashion under the influence of two hormones from the anterior pituitary gland: *follicle-stimulating hormone (FSH)* and *luteinizing hormone (LH)*. Each cycle includes the development of an ovum within a follicle, its release from the follicle (called **ovulation**), formation of a corpus luteum, and the degeneration of unripened follicles and, eventually, the corpus luteum. Figure 19-19

illustrates the main sequence of events in this process, and Figure 19-20 shows steps in follicular development in cattle.

The number of follicles involved in each cycle depends on the species. **Uniparous** species, such as horses, cattle, and humans, normally give birth to only one offspring at a time. Their ovaries produce one mature ovum per cycle. **Multiparous** species, such as cats, dogs, and sows, give birth to *litters* of young. Their ovaries produce multiple ova per cycle.

The beginning stage of follicle development in the ovary is the primordial, sometimes called the *primary*, follicle. The thousands of immature oocytes in the ovaries of newborn animals reside in this stage until they become activated later in life and begin to develop further. The primordial follicle consists of the immature gamete (the oocyte) surrounded by a single layer of flattened **follicular cells**. When FSH is released from the anterior pituitary, the whole ovary is bathed in it. Something, however, causes just a few of the thousands of primordial follicles to begin developing. This is known as *follicular recruitment* or *follicular activation*.

Once a primordial follicle has become activated, it is referred to as a *growing follicle*. The oocyte starts to grow in size, the **glycoprotein zona pellucida** layer forms just outside the cell membrane, and the follicular cells enlarge into cuboidal shapes and begin to multiply. Multiple layers of follicular cells form around the zona pellucida of the developing oocyte. At this stage, the follicular cells are called **granulosa cells**. As the granulosa cells multiply, the follicle starts to grow rapidly in size. The granulosa cells do more than just physically surround the developing oocyte. They also produce estrogen hormones that begin preparing the animal for breeding and pregnancy. The larger the follicle

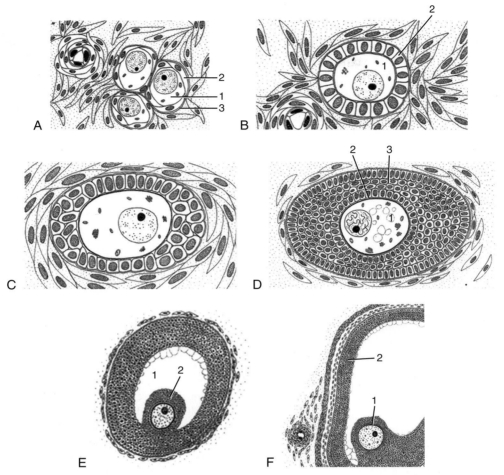

**FIGURE 19-20** Follicular development in cattle. (Not to scale.) **A,** Primordial follicle. The oocyte (1) is surrounded by flat follicular cells (2) resting on a basement membrane (3). **B,** Primary follicle. The oocyte (1) is surrounded by cuboidal granulosa cells (2). **C,** Early growing follicle. **D,** Slightly larger early growing follicle. The oocyte (1) is surrounded by the developing zona pellucida (2) and a multilayered granulosa cell compartment (3). **E,** Larger growing follicle showing the antrum (1) and the oocyte located in the cumulus oophorus (2). **F,** Large growing follicle presenting the oocyte in the cumulus oophorus (1) and the granulosa cell layer (2) surrounding the antrum. (Courtesy Sinowatz and Rüsse (2007). From Hyttel P, Sinowatz, F, Vejlsted M: Essentials of domestic animal embryology, St Louis, 2010, Saunders.)

becomes, the greater the amount of estrogens produced. As the follicle continues to grow, fluid-filled spaces begin to form between the granulosa cells. The spaces gradually become confluent (they join together), forming one large, fluid-filled space called the **antrum.**

When the follicle has reached its maximum size, it looks like a large, blisterlike structure on the surface of the ovary. At this stage, it is called a **mature follicle.** Alternative names for the mature follicle include *Graafian follicle* and *vesicular ovarian follicle.* Inside the mature follicle, the oocyte sits on a little mound of granulosa cells called the **cumulus oophorus,** and its zona pellucida is surrounded by a thin layer of granulosa cells called the **corona radiata.** Most of the volume of the mature follicle is made up of the fluid-filled antrum. At this stage, estrogen production from the follicle is at a peak level, and the animal is ready for breeding to take place. In most animal species, **ovulation** (rupture of the mature follicle with release of the reproductive cell into the **oviduct**)

occurs spontaneously as a result of the rising level of LH. This generally occurs regardless of whether breeding has taken place. In some species, however, such as cats, camels, rabbits, and ferrets, breeding must take place before ovulation can occur. For this reason, cats, camels, rabbits, and ferrets are called *induced ovulators.* (This is also why the heat periods of cats can be so prolonged if they are not bred.) Once the mature gamete is released from the follicle, its name changes. It is now called an **ovum.**

Ovulation is a traumatic and somewhat explosive event. The surface of the mature follicle weakens and physically ruptures, suddenly releasing the fluid from the antrum. The rush of fluid out of the follicle carries the ovum with it, still surrounded by its halo of granulosa cells, the corona radiata. The empty follicle fills with blood that rapidly clots, forming the **corpus hemorrhagicum.**

Under continued stimulation by the high LH level, the granulosa cells that line the corpus hemorrhagicum begin to multiply again. This time they form a solid structure, the corpus luteum, that gets about as large as the mature follicle was just before ovulation. The term *corpus luteum* literally means "yellow body," because it has a pale yellow color grossly (without magnification). The corpus luteum produces hormones called *progestins*. The principal progestin is *progesterone*, which is necessary for pregnancy to be maintained if the ovum is fertilized. If the ovum has been fertilized and implants in the uterus, it sends an endocrine signal to the ovary that causes the corpus luteum to be maintained. If the ovum has not been fertilized, no "we are pregnant" endocrine signal is sent and the corpus luteum degenerates after a short period.

Not all follicles that were activated in a particular ovarian cycle fully develop and ovulate. It is as if the ovary "auditions" follicles and chooses particular ones to fully develop. The rest may degenerate at any stage of their development. This is called **follicular atresia** and is a normal part of each ovarian cycle.

---

✓ **TEST YOURSELF 19-5**
1. What two main types of hormone are produced in the ovary? Where is each produced?
2. What changes does an ovarian follicle undergo as it develops from a primordial follicle to a mature follicle?
3. After ovulation has occurred, what cells in the ovary multiply to form the corpus luteum?

---

## OVIDUCTS

The two **oviducts** also are known as the *Fallopian tubes* and *uterine tubes;* they are small, convoluted tubes that extend from the tips of the uterine horns (see Figures 19-17 and 19-18). Their roles are to guide ova from the ovary to the uterus and to serve as the usual site for fertilization of ova by spermatozoa. The oviducts are not attached to the ovaries at all; when ovulation takes place, they have to "catch" the ova in the funnel-like **infundibulum**, which is the enlarged opening at the ovarian end of each oviduct. At the time of ovulation, it more or less surrounds the area of the ovary where follicles have formed. Muscular, fingerlike projections called **fimbriae** form the margin of the infundibulum. They "feel" along the surface of the ovary and position the infundibulum where the follicles are located. This helps ensure that the infundibulum is properly positioned to catch the ova when ovulation occurs. If ova miss the opening of the oviduct, they fall into the abdominal cavity, where they usually just disintegrate after a time.

When examined closely, the complex physical structure of the oviducts becomes apparent. They contain many smooth muscle fibers in their walls. Their linings are very intricate and folded, and the lining cells are covered with countless, movable cilia. When an ovum enters the oviduct after ovulation, delicate muscle contractions and gentle movements of the cilia begin slowly and gently moving it toward the uterus. The greatly folded lining of the oviduct keeps it in continuous, gentle contact with the ovum. If breeding has taken place, spermatozoa are already up in the oviducts when ovulation occurs. The oviducts are the usual place where the ovum and some lucky spermatozoon come together. This is called *fertilization* of the ovum. Once fertilization has taken place, the oviducts gently conduct the fertilized ovum down to the uterus for implantation.

## UTERUS

The **uterus** is the womb, where the fertilized ovum implants and lives while it grows and develops into a new animal. When the fetus is fully developed, the uterus helps push it through the birth canal out into the world. Although it seems like a simple receptacle in which the fetus can develop, the roles of the uterus are actually quite complex. It has to grow along with the developing offspring and then return to its original size after birth. It forms part of the **placenta**, which is the life-support system that keeps the fetus alive while it develops during pregnancy. The uterus must remain quiet during pregnancy, and it must contract powerfully at the time of birth. After it has delivered the newborn and the placenta (the **afterbirth**), it has to contract quickly to stop bleeding from the sites where the placenta was attached to its lining. It does not have the complex, cyclic functions of the ovaries or the intricate structure of the oviducts, but the uterus is vital to the success of reproduction.

Physically, the uterus is a hollow muscular organ. In common domestic animals, it is somewhat Y-shaped, with the uterine body forming the base of the Y and the two uterine horns forming the arms. The body of the uterus extends in a caudal direction, eventually joining with the cervix at its caudal end. The two uterine horns project cranially (see Figure 19-16). The oviducts extend from the tips of the uterine horns. The whole organ is suspended from the dorsal part of the abdomen by the mesometrium portion of the broad ligament.

The thick wall of the uterus is made up of three layers. The *endometrium* is composed mainly of simple columnar epithelium and simple tubular glands that secrete mucus and other substances. The thickest layer of the wall is the *myometrium*, which is made up of layers of smooth muscle that give the uterus the strength to push the fetus out at parturition. The outermost layer is the *perimetrium*, which is covered by the visceral layer of peritoneum.

The fertilized ovum implants in the uterus and begins to grow. As the offspring develops, the placenta forms around it and attaches to the lining of the uterus so that nutrients, wastes, and respiratory gases can be exchanged between the fetal bloodstream and the maternal bloodstream. (This is explained more fully in Chapter 20.) When the time comes for the offspring to be delivered, the muscular uterus provides most of the force necessary to open (dilate) the cervix so the fetus can pass through it on its way to the outside world.

## CERVIX

The **cervix** is a muscular "valve" that seals off the uterus from the outside most of the time. It is a powerful, smooth muscle **sphincter** located between the body of the uterus and the vagina. It functions to control access to the lumen of the uterus from the vagina. The cervix is normally tightly closed, except at the two ends of pregnancy: *estrus* (the heat period) and *parturition* (the birth process). The cervix relaxes at estrus to admit spermatozoa during breeding. It then tightly closes again during pregnancy and does not relax again until birthing time. Uterine contractions during the first stage of labor push the newborn against the relaxed cervix and gradually pry it open (called *dilation* of the cervix) so that "junior" can slide down the birth canal and out into the world.

## VAGINA

The **vagina** is the tube that receives the penis at breeding time and acts as the birth canal at parturition. It is a muscular tube that extends caudally from the cervix and connects it with the vulva. Although the lumen of the vagina is a "potential" space and is collapsed most of the time, it can stretch considerably to accommodate the penis at breeding and the newborn during the birth process. Mucous glands lining the vagina lubricate it at the time of breeding.

## VULVA

The **vulva** is the only portion of the female reproductive system that is visible from the outside. Its main parts are the *vestibule,* the *clitoris,* and the *labia.* The word *vestibule,* in anatomic terms, means the entrance into a canal of some sort. In this case, the **vestibule of the vulva** is the entrance into the vagina from the outside world. It is the short space between the **labia** and the opening of the vagina. The urethra, the tube that carries urine out from the urinary bladder, opens on the floor (ventral portion) of the vestibule. The **clitoris** is also located on the floor of the vestibule a little nearer to the exterior than the urethral opening. The clitoris is the female equivalent of the penis of the male. It is **homologous** (equivalent in embryologic origin) to the penis and has a similar basic structure. It is attached by two roots and has a body composed of erectile tissue and a glans that is extensively supplied with sensory nerve endings. The **labia** (lips) form the external boundary of the vulva.

---

### ✔ TEST YOURSELF 19-6

1. When ovulation occurs, what causes the ovum to enter the oviduct?
2. Describe the functions of the uterus relating to pregnancy and parturition.
3. Where is the urethral opening located in the female?

---

## THE ESTROUS CYCLE

To get the ovum and some lucky spermatozoon together at the right time (when both are mature) in the right place (the oviduct), some intricate coordination has to take place between two different animals. The situation in the male is pretty straightforward. Spermatozoa are constantly produced in the testes, and the testosterone level stays fairly constant. So the male is basically always ready for breeding.

---

**BOX 19-1** | Estrous versus Estrus

**Estrous** is an adjective used with the noun "cycle" to refer to the entire reproductive cycle in females.

**Estrus** is a noun that is the name of the stage of the estrous cycle that is commonly referred to as the "heat period" when the female is sexually receptive to the male.

---

He just needs the appropriate signals from the female to get the process underway. Because ovum production in the ovary of the female is not continuous but occurs in a cyclic manner, the timing of breeding is controlled by the ovarian cycle of the female.

In all common domestic animals, breeding takes place only during a definite period in each reproductive cycle, when the chance of a successful pregnancy is the highest. This period when the female is receptive to the advances of the male is known as the *heat period,* or **estrus.** (Box 19-1 explains the difference between the words "estrous" and "estrus.") It is characterized by physical and behavioral changes that communicate the "window of opportunity" for breeding to the male. The timing of breeding is critical if pregnancy is going to result. The spermatozoa and the ovum must enter the oviduct at just the right times with respect to each other.

The **estrous cycle** is defined as the time from the beginning of one heat period to the beginning of the next. It is controlled by the anterior pituitary hormones, FSH and LH. FSH and LH stimulate activity in the ovaries that causes one or more reproductive cells (ova) to mature and be released. They also stimulate the production of hormones by the developing follicle (estrogens) and the corpus luteum (progestins) after ovulation. The estrogens and progestins are directly responsible for the physical and behavioral changes in the female that are associated with the estrous cycle. Different animal species have different patterns of estrous cycles, although all go through the same basic stages.

### ESTROUS CYCLE INTERVALS

Animals can be classified according to how and when their estrous cycles occur during the year. **Polyestrous** animals, such as cattle and swine, cycle continuously throughout the year if they are not pregnant. As soon as one cycle ends, another begins. Some polyestrous animals show seasonal variations in their estrous cycles. They cycle continuously at certain times of the year and not at all at others. These animals, such as horses, sheep, and cats, are called **seasonally polyestrous. Diestrous** animals, such as dogs, have two cycles per year, usually in the spring and fall. **Monoestrous** animals, such as foxes and mink, usually have only one cycle each year.

### STAGES OF THE ESTROUS CYCLE

Although it is a continuous process, the estrous cycle can be divided into a series of characteristic stages. These stages reflect what is going on in the ovary as follicles develop, mature, rupture, and are replaced by corpora lutea. Keeping the events of the ovarian cycle in mind makes it easier to correlate what is going on in the ovary with the stages of the estrous cycle. The estrous cycle stages are *proestrus, estrus, metestrus,* and *diestrus.* (Another stage, **anestrus,** occurs in some animals between breeding seasons.)

**Proestrus** is the period of follicular development in the ovary. During this stage, follicles begin developing and growing. As they increase in size, the follicles' output of estrogen increases accordingly, causing many physical changes that prepare the rest of the reproductive tract for ovulation and breeding. These include thickening and development of the linings of the oviduct, uterus, and vagina. The epithelial lining of the vagina also begins undergoing **cornification;** that is, forming a layer of tough keratin on its surface, to help protect against the physical trauma of breeding that is about to occur. These changes in the epithelial lining of the vagina can be conveniently used to detect the stage of the estrous cycle, particularly in dogs. See the Clinical Application on Vaginal Cytology.

**Estrus** is the heat period, or the period of sexual receptivity in the female. It occurs when the estrogen level from the mature follicles reaches its peak. This high estrogen level causes physical and behavioral changes that signal the female's willingness to breed to the male. In most species, ovulation occurs near the end of estrus. In some species, however, such as camels, cats, ferrets, and rabbits, ovulation does not occur until the animal is bred. These species, called *induced ovulators,* remain in a prolonged state of estrus if they are not bred. The behavioral signs of estrus in the cat— particularly the vocalizing, rolling, and rubbing—can be very annoying to owners; they may even be misinterpreted as signs of illness by novice owners.

**Metestrus** is the period after ovulation, when the corpus luteum develops. The granulosa cells left in the now-empty follicle begin to multiply under continued stimulation from LH. They soon produce a solid structure, the corpus luteum (yellow body), which is about the same size as the former mature follicle. The hormone progesterone, which is produced by the corpus luteum, temporarily inhibits follicular development in the ovary, causes the lining of the uterus to get very thick and "juicy" in preparation for implantation of a fertilized ovum, and causes loss of the cornified epithelial lining that developed in the vagina during proestrus and estrus. In the dog and cat there is little distinction between the metestrus and diestrus stages, so the metestrus stage is usually excluded for these species. Their estrous cycles go directly from the estrus stage to the diestrus stage.

**Diestrus** is the active luteal stage, when the corpus luteum has reached maximum size and exerts its maximum effect. If the animal is bred and becomes pregnant, the corpus luteum receives an endocrine signal from the developing embryo and is retained well into the pregnancy. If the animal is not pregnant, the corpus luteum degenerates at the end of diestrus. Depending on the species and the type of estrous cycle it has, the animal then either goes straight back into proestrus, or the ovary shuts down and the animal goes into anestrus. Some animals, particularly bitches, can have an exaggerated diestrous period, resulting in **pseudocyesis,** or what is commonly called **pseudopregnancy** (false pregnancy). Affected animals may act and look pregnant. The mammary glands often enlarge, the pelvis may relax, and the animal often shows maternal behavior patterns, such as nest building. In extreme cases, lactation and signs of labor may occur. Most cases of pseudopregnancy resolve spontaneously, but hormonal therapy may be required in some severe cases.

**Anestrus** is a period of temporary ovarian inactivity seen in seasonally polyestrous, diestrous, and monoestrous animals. It is the period between breeding cycles, when the ovary essentially shuts down temporarily. The anestrous period can be cited to dog and cat owners who are reluctant to have their animals spayed because they are afraid the animals will become fat and lazy after the procedure. In reality, dogs and cats are functionally "spayed" for a good portion of each year while they are in anestrus. Animals become fat and lazy if they are fed too much and exercised too little, regardless of whether or not they have been spayed.

---

✔ **TEST YOURSELF 19-7**

1. What is the difference in the estrous cycle intervals of polyestrous, seasonally polyestrous, diestrous, and monoestrous animals?
2. How do the stages of the estrous cycle relate to the physical events of the ovarian cycle?

---

 **CLINICAL APPLICATION**

## Vaginal Cytology in the Dog

Changes in the epithelial lining of the vagina during proestrus and estrus can be utilized to determine the most effective time to breed a bitch, or the most likely time she must be kept away from males to prevent unplanned breeding. The basic principle is that the vaginal lining becomes progressively thicker and the surface epithelial cells become increasingly cornified (keratinized) during the proestrus period, and this reaches a peak when the animal is in estrus and most likely to conceive if bred.

The most common technique is to insert a saline-moistened cotton swab into the vagina while avoiding contact with the lining of the vulva. The swab is gently twirled or moved back and forth, removed, and rolled onto a glass microscope slide in several rows. Then any of several different stains are applied to make the epithelial cells more visible under the microscope.

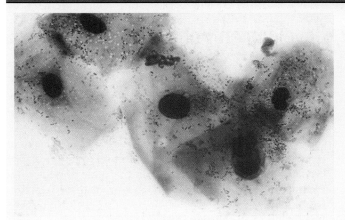

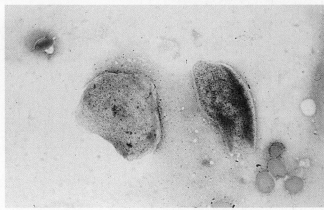

Vaginal cytology in the bitch. **A,** Proestrus. The large cells are vaginal epithelial cells with large purple and blue nuclei. The small scattered dots are normal bacteria. The prominent nuclei indicate that this dog has not reached the estrous stage yet. (Sample provided by Rolf Larsen, University of Florida. From Raskin R, Meyer D: Canine and feline cytology, ed 2, St Louis, 2010, Saunders.)

Vaginal cytology in the bitch. **B,** Estrus. Note that no nuclei are visible in the large epithelial cells. They are cornified, indicating that the bitch is in estrus and ready for breeding. (Sample provided by Rolf Larsen, University of Florida. From Raskin R, Meyer D: Canine and feline cytology, ed 2, St Louis, 2010, Saunders.)

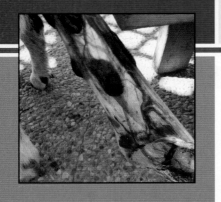

# Pregnancy, Development, and Lactation

*Thomas Colville*

## OUTLINE

## LEARNING OBJECTIVES

*When you have completed this chapter you will be able to:*

1. Describe the processes by which spermatozoa move from the male reproductive tract to the oviduct of the female at breeding.
2. Describe the processes of capacitation of spermatozoa and fertilization of the ovum.
3. Describe the events that occur between fertilization of the ovum and implantation of the blastocyst.
4. Describe the structure and functions of the placenta and explain the relationship between the fetus and the amniotic and allantoic sacs of the placenta.
5. Describe the structures and functions of the components of the umbilical cord.

6. Differentiate between *diffuse, cotyledonary, zonary,* and *discoid* placental attachments.
7. Describe the events that occur in each stage of gestation.
8. Describe the structure and development of the mammary glands.
9. Describe the general composition of colostrum and explain its importance to the health of the neonate.
10. Describe the process of lactation and milk let-down.
11. Describe the key hormones in the female that are involved in the processes of breeding, gestation, parturition, and lactation.

## VOCABULARY FUNDAMENTALS

*Acrosome* **ahck**-rō-sōm
*Afterbirth* **ahf**-tər-bərth
*Allantoic sac* ahl-ahn-**tō**-ihck sahck
*Allantois* ah-lahn-**tō**-ihs
*Alveolar duct* ahl-**vē**-ō-lahr duhckt
*Alveoli* ahl-**vē**-ō-lī
*Amnion* **ahm**-nē-ahn
*Amniotic sac* **ahm**-nē-aw-tihck sahck
*Antibody* **ahn**-tē-boh-dē
*Blastocyst* **blahs**-tō-sihst
*Capacitation* kah-**pahs**-uh-tā-shuhn
*Caruncle* **kahr**-uhn-kuhl

*Chorion* **kohr**-ē-ohn
*Cleavage* **klē**-vihj
*Colostrum* kō-**loh**-struhm
*Copulation* kohp-ū-**lā**-shuhn
*Corona radiata* kuh-**rō**-nah rād-ē-**oht**-ah
*Cotyledon* kohd-eh-**lē**-duhn
*Cotyledonary placental attachment* kohd-eh-**lē**-duh-neər-ē plah-**sehn**-tahl ah-**tahch**-mehnt
*Delivery of the newborn* dih-**lihv**-ər-ē *of the* **nū**-bohrn
*Delivery of the placenta* dih-**lihv**-ər-ē *of the* plah-**sehn**-tah

*Diffuse placental attachment* dih-**fyoos** plah-**sehn**-tahl ah-**tahch**-mehnt

*Diploid chromosome number* **dihp**-loyd **krō**-muh-sōm **nuhm**-bər

*Discoid placental attachment* **dihs**-koyd plah-**sehn**-tahl ah-**tahch**-mehnt

*Dystocia* dihs-**tō**-shuh

*Ejaculation* eh-jahck-ū-**lā**-shuhn

*Erection* eh-**rehck**-shuhn

*Embryo* **ehm**-brē-ō

*Female pronucleus* **fē**-māl prō-**noo**-klē-uhs

*Fertilization* fər-tihl-ih-**zā**-shuhn

*Fetal development* **fē**-tahl dih-**vehl**-ehp-mehnt

*Fetal growth* **fē**-tahl grōth

*Fetus* **fē**-tuhs

*Gamete* **gahm**-ēt

*Gestation* jeh-**stā**-shuhn

*Gland sinus* glahnd **sī**-nuhs

*Haploid chromosome number* **hahp**-loyd **krō**-muh-sōm **nuhm**-bər

*Implantation* ihm-plahn-**tā**-shuhn

*Intromission* ihn-trōh-**mihsh**-uhn

*Involution of the mammary gland* ihn-vō-**loo**-shuhn *of the* **mahm**-uh-rē glahnd

*Involution of the uterus* ihn-**vōuh**-**loo**-shuhn *of the* **ū**-tər-uhs

*Lactation* lahck-**tā**-shuhn

*Male pronucleus* māl prō-**noo**-klē-uhs

*Mastitis* mahs-**tī**-tihs

*Meconium* meh-**kō**-nē-uhm

*Milk let-down* mihlk **leht**-doun

*Morula* **mohr**-yoo-lah

*Multiparous* muhl-**tihp**-eər-uhs

*Myoepithelial cell* **mī**-ō-ehp-eh-**thē**-lē-ahl sehl

*Neonatal period* nē-ō-**nā**-tahl **pihr**-ē-uhd

*Parturition* pahr-chuhr-**ih**-shuhn

*Passive immunity* **pah**-sihv ihm-**myoo**-nih-tē

*Placenta* plah-**sehn**-tah

*Placentome* **plah**-sehn-tōm

*Quarter* **kwahr**-tər

*Streak canal* strēk kuh-**nahl**

*Stages of labor* **stā**-jehz *of* **lā**-bər

*Teat sinus* tēt **sī**-nuhs

*Trimester* trī-**mehs**-tər

*Udder* **uhd**-ər

*Umbilical artery* uhm-**bihl**-ihck-ahl **ahr**-tər-ē

*Umbilical cord* uhm-**bihl**-ihck-ahl kohrd

*Umbilical vein* uhm-**bihl**-ihck-ahl vān

*Urachus* yər-ā-kuhs

*Uterine contraction* **ū**-tər-ihn kohn-**trahck**-shuhn

*Zona pellucida* zō-nuh puh-**loo**-sih-duh

*Zonary placental attachment* zō-nuh-rē plah-**sehn**-tahl ah-**tahch**-mehnt

*Zygote* **zī**-gōt

## INTRODUCTION

The processes that lead to a new animal being born are almost impossibly intricate, unforgivingly sequential, and amazingly elegant. A multitude of events has to happen at just the right times, and in just the right order, in, and between, two separate animals for breeding and fertilization of an ovum to take place. Then if that minor miracle occurs, a whole new collection of events has to proceed in just the right manner for the fertilized ovum (the zygote) to implant in the uterus, undergo all the stages of growth and development during pregnancy (gestation), and survive the birth process (parturition) that pushes it out of the dark, quiet, moist environment in which it has developed, into the bright, noisy, comparatively dry environment in which it will spend the rest of its life. It has to inflate its lungs for the first time and begin breathing, alter blood flow through its heart and lungs, and make its way to a teat or nipple to begin receiving nourishment via its newly functioning digestive tract.

While all this is happening to junior, mom's uterus has to stay quiet as it expands during pregnancy, supply all of junior's needs for growth and development via the placenta, and, at just the right time, contract to start the birth process. Her mammary glands have to develop and be ready to produce their first secretion, colostrum, at just the right time so junior will receive what s/he needs soon after birth. She then has to maintain milk production (lactation) for as long as junior needs it before being weaned onto solid food.

Did you notice how many "and then(s) ..." there were in these introductory paragraphs? They give an impression of how complex the processes of breeding, fertilization of the ovum, pregnancy, zygote/embryo/fetal development, birth, and lactation/nursing are. That is what we explore in this chapter.

## BREEDING AND FERTILIZATION OF THE OVUM

### ERECTION

**Erection** is the enlargement and stiffening of the penis that prepares it for breeding. It results from a parasympathetic reflex triggered by sexual stimuli. In most species, the important stimuli are olfactory cues (smells) and behavioral changes from the female that signal to the male that she is receptive to breeding. These cues from the female, and her willingness to participate in breeding, are primarily due to the high level of estrogen hormones in her system. Table 20-1 shows the predominant female hormones at the times of

| TABLE 20-1 | Key Female Hormones of Breeding, Gestation, Parturition, and Lactation | |
| --- | --- | --- |
| | HORMONE | SOURCE |
| **Breeding** | Estrogens | Ovary |
| | Oxytocin | Posterior pituitary |
| **Gestation** | Progestins (Progesterone) | Ovary (and placenta in some species) |
| **Parturition** | Relaxin | Placenta |
| | ACTH | Anterior pituitary (fetus) |
| | Glucocorticoids | Adrenal glands (fetus) |
| | Estrogens | Placenta |
| | Prostaglandin F$_2$alpha | Placenta and uterine wall (dam) |
| | Oxytocin | Posterior pituitary (dam) |
| **Lactation** | Growth hormone | Anterior pituitary |
| | Prolactin | Anterior pituitary |
| | Oxytocin | Posterior pituitary |

breeding, gestation (pregnancy), parturition (birth), and lactation (milk production).

Erection occurs when more blood enters the penis via the arteries than leaves it via the veins. The connective tissue-enclosed erectile tissue becomes engorged with blood, causing the penis to become enlarged and rigid. Mechanically, what happens is that the arteries supplying blood to the penis dilate, increasing the blood flow into the organ. At the same time, the veins carrying blood away from the penis are compressed against the cranial brim of the pelvis by contractions of the ischiocavernosus muscles (part of the roots of the penis). This acts like a tourniquet and decreases the flow of blood out of the penis. The net effect is that more blood enters the penis than leaves it. This generates hydraulic pressure within the erectile tissue, producing the enlargement and stiffening of the penis that we call *erection*. In species with a sigmoid flexure in the penis, such as ruminants and the boar, the primary erection mechanism is lengthening of the penis by straightening of the sigmoid flexure. In species with a high proportion of erectile tissue in the penis, such as dogs and stallions, engorgement of the erectile tissue with blood results in increases in both length and diameter.

## COPULATION

Copulation, or the act of breeding, is allowed by the female during the estrus (heat) period. In most animals, it is done in a standing position with the male mounting the female from behind (Figure 20-1). Exceptions to this include the camelids (camels, llamas and alpacas) which breed in a kneeling (cushed) position (Figure 20-2). Mounting is followed by **intromission** (insertion of the penis into the vagina), thrusting, and ejaculation.

## EJACULATION

**Ejaculation** is the reflex expulsion of semen from the penis. It is produced by a continuation of the stimuli that produced erection, plus the physical actions and sensations of breeding. The process has two stages. The first involves the movement of spermatozoa from the epididymis, and fluids from the accessory reproductive glands, into the pelvic portion of the urethra. At the same time, the sphincter muscle around the neck of the urinary bladder closes tightly to prevent the movement of semen into the bladder. This is quickly followed by the second stage of ejaculation: rhythmic contractions of smooth muscle around the urethra that pump the semen out into the female reproductive tract.

In most animals, ejaculation deposits semen in the upper portion of the vagina. Exceptions to this include the horse and pig, in which semen is usually deposited through the open cervix directly into the uterus.

## TRANSPORT OF SPERMATOZOA

The spermatozoa have to cover a lot of territory to travel from where they are deposited up to the oviducts, where their mission is to seek out the ovum. The distance is huge on the microscopic scale of these tiny cells. They start actively swimming as soon as they are deposited in the female reproductive tract, but if they were to cover the whole distance under their own power, it would take over an hour for them to arrive in the oviducts. In actuality, they begin arriving within a few minutes after ejaculation. How do they make the trip so quickly? The answer is that they are transported mainly by contractions of the uterus and oviducts and the action of cilia in the oviducts. Copulation causes the hormone oxytocin to be released from the posterior pituitary gland of the female. Oxytocin causes the smooth muscle of the estrogen-primed female reproductive tract to contract, giving the spermatozoa a free ride.

The reason for the rush to get the spermatozoa up to the oviducts so quickly is that timing is everything at this point. The spermatozoa must arrive at the oviducts before the ovum does so they have time to undergo a process (**capacitation**) that will enhance their fertility.

Nature has an exquisite method for arranging the proper timing. Breeding is only allowed by the female during the estrous, or heat, period. So spermatozoa enter the female reproductive tract when the oocyte in the follicle is fully developed but has not yet been released. Release of the ovum (ovulation) is delayed until near the end of the estrous period in most species. This nifty bit of traffic control helps ensure that the spermatozoa arrive at the oviducts first and have time to undergo the process of capacitation before the ovum shows up ready to be fertilized.

## CAPACITATION

**Capacitation** describes a series of changes that spermatozoa undergo in the female reproductive tract that collectively serve to increase their chances of successfully fertilizing an ovum. Many of the changes are subtle, involving adjustments in ion movement through the cell membranes, increases in the cells' metabolic rates, and increases in the rates at which simple sugars are used for energy production. A more dramatic change is in the **acrosome**, the digestive enzyme-containing caplike structure that covers the head of the spermatozoa. Capacitation causes exposure of the enzymes that, up until now, have been sealed off. These digestive

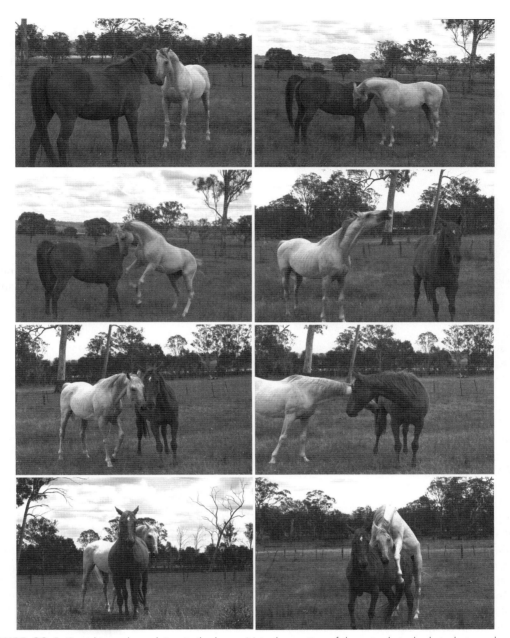

**FIGURE 20-1** Courtship and copulation in the horse. Note the position of the animals in the last photograph when copulation is occurring. (From McGreevy P: Equine behavior: a guide for veterinarians and equine scientists, ed 2, St Louis, 2013, Elsevier Health Sciences.)

enzymes will help the spermatozoa penetrate through the layers surrounding the ovum to accomplish fertilization.

## FERTILIZATION OF THE OVUM

Spermatozoa are preprogrammed to seek out anything large and round and attempt to penetrate it. Many go astray and attempt to fertilize things other than ova, such as epithelial cells in the oviducts. This is one of the reasons why such a large number of spermatozoa must be introduced into the female reproductive tract in the first place: to increase the odds that one will successfully reach and fertilize (penetrate into) the ovum. A significant number of spermatozoa find

and swarm around the ovum once it moves down into the oviduct. Many begin tunneling through the **corona radiata** (layers of cumulus cells from the follicle) and **zona pellucida** (thick, gel-like membrane that surrounds the ovum's cell membrane) surrounding the ovum, aided by the digestive enzymes of their acrosomes. Only one spermatozoon, however, will achieve **fertilization**—physical penetration through the cell membrane of the ovum, delivering its genetic material into the ovum's cytoplasm. Once the head of a single spermatozoon has entered the ovum, a change takes place in the cell membrane that blocks other spermatozoa from entering.

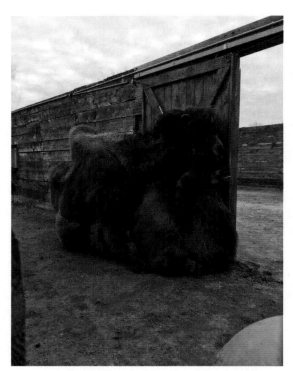

**FIGURE 20-2** Camelid copulation position—Bactrian Camels. Note that the female is kneeling in a sternal (cushed) position and the male is kneeling over her. (Photograph by the author and used with permission from the Red River Zoo, Fargo, ND; www.redriverzoo.org)

## PREGNANCY AND DEVELOPMENT

### THE ZYGOTE

Once an ovum is fertilized, it gets a name change and becomes known as a **zygote**. Immediately after fertilization, the nucleus of the spermatozoon is called the **male pronucleus**, and the nucleus of the ovum is called the **female pronucleus**. Each carries the haploid chromosome number, that is, one half the number in the rest of the body's cells. The male and female pronuclei quickly join together to restore the diploid chromosome number and determine the unique genetic makeup of the offspring. The full genetic map for the new animal has now been established.

### CLEAVAGE

As soon as the two pronuclei join to form a single nucleus, each chromosome makes a copy of itself, and the zygote begins to divide rapidly by the normal process of mitosis. This rapid division is called **cleavage**. Figure 20-3 shows what happens to the genetic material from the ovum and the sperm from just after fertilization up to the first cleavage division. The single cell divides into two cells, which quickly divide into four, then eight, then 16, and so forth. Cleavage occurs so rapidly that the cells of the zygote do not have time to grow between divisions. The number of cells making up the zygote is increasing dramatically, but its overall size is still about the same as the original ovum, even after several days.

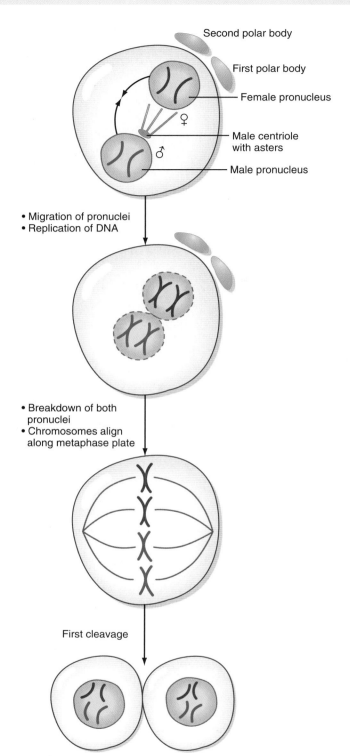

Second polar body

First polar body

Female pronucleus

♀

Male centriole with asters

♂

Male pronucleus

- Migration of pronuclei
- Replication of DNA

- Breakdown of both pronuclei
- Chromosomes align along metaphase plate

First cleavage

**FIGURE 20-3** Overview of events in a zygote from just after fertilization up to the first cleavage division. (Modified from Porterfield SP, White BA: Endocrine physiology, ed 3, Philadelphia, 2007, Mosby. In Koeppen B, Stanton B: Berne & Levy physiology [updated], ed 6, St Louis, 2010, Mosby.)

While cleavage is taking place, the zygote is slowly moving down the oviduct toward the uterus (Figure 20-4). Delicate muscular contractions and the movements of cilia are gently propelling it along. After a few days the zygote is a solid mass of cells that looks like a tiny raspberry; this is known as the

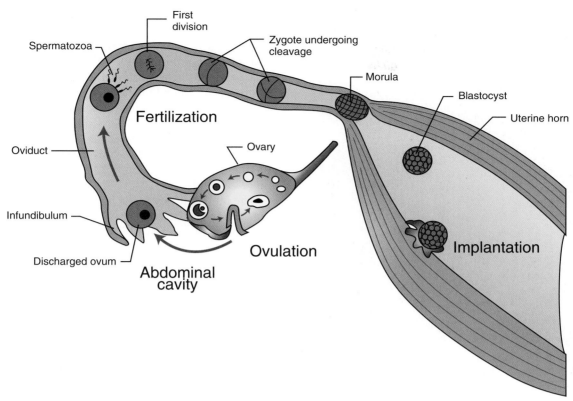

**FIGURE 20-4** Fertilization and implantation. After ovulation, the ovum starts moving slowly down the oviduct toward the uterus. A spermatozoon in the oviduct fertilizes the ovum, forming the single-celled *zygote*. Cleavage of the zygote begins almost immediately as the single cell divides into two cells, two cells divide into four, and so on. After a day or two, the zygote has formed into a solid mass of cells called the *morula*. The morula continues to develop into a hollow ball of cells, the *blastocyst*, which enters the uterus and implants in its wall.

**morula** stage. The cells of the morula continue to divide and gradually form a hollow cavity in the center. By the time it reaches the uterus a few days later, it is formed into a hollow ball of cells with a "bump" on one side that eventually forms into the **embryo** (Figure 20-5). It is now called a **blastocyst**, and it is ready to implant itself in the lining of the uterus.

## IMPLANTATION

**Implantation** is the means by which the blastocyst makes itself a home by embedding itself in the endometrium (lining) of the uterus. When it comes to rest against the endometrium, enzymes from the blastocyst dissolve away a small pit. The blastocyst implants itself in the pit. In **multiparous** species (those that normally give birth to multiple offspring), such as swine, the multiple blastocysts randomly space themselves along the horns and body of the uterus as they implant.

During the early part of pregnancy, the developing offspring is called an **embryo**. Later it is referred to as a **fetus**. We discuss this further later in the chapter.

Up until now, the dividing zygote has obtained its nourishment by diffusion from the fluid of the oviduct and uterus. By the time of implantation, it has become too large and metabolically active for its needs to be met by this mechanism. A more effective method of supplying oxygen and

nutrients and carrying wastes away must be developed. This role is carried out by the **placenta**, a complex structure that begins to form as soon as the blastocyst implants in the uterus.

> ✓ *TEST YOURSELF 20-1*
> 1. Why is the timing of copulation so important? How is the precise timing accomplished?
> 2. Describe what happens to a zygote between fertilization and implantation.

## THE PLACENTA

The placenta is a life-support system for the developing offspring that surrounds it and connects it with the uterus. During gestation (pregnancy), the offspring leads a parasitic existence as it grows and develops; that is, it receives all the nutrients and other substances it needs to grow and develop from its mother. It also depends on her to dispose of the waste products it produces. Remember that, during the period of pregnancy, the offspring is undergoing incredibly rapid growth, and its cells are differentiating into all of the tissues, organs, and systems needed to support independent life after it is born. Its need for nutrients and waste elimination is huge and grows minute by minute along with its body.

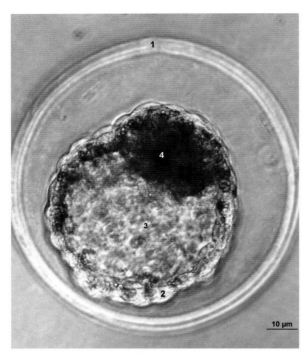

**FIGURE 20-5** Pig blastocyst at day 6 of development, as seen through a microscope. *1*, Zona pellucida; *2*, Trophoblast (future placenta); *3*, Blastocyst cavity; *4*, Inner cell mass (future embryo). (From Hyttel P: Essentials of domestic animal embryology, St Louis, 2010, Saunders.)

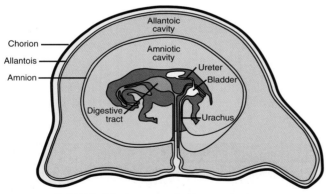

**FIGURE 20-6** Fetus and placenta of a horse.

Fortunately, the placenta grows right along with the fetus and meets its needs every step of the way.

## STRUCTURE

The placenta is a multilayered, fluid-filled, membranous sac that develops around the embryo and is connected to it by the **umbilical cord** (Figures 20-6 and 20-7). In some areas the outermost layer of the placenta attaches to the lining of the uterus. It is at these areas of attachment that the actual exchange of nutrients and wastes takes place between the fetal circulation and the maternal circulation. The fetal and maternal blood vessels are separate but in close proximity to each other in this area. Normally, no direct mixing of fetal and maternal blood occurs. The nutrients and wastes are

exchanged across the very thin layers that separate the two sets of blood vessels.

Grossly, the placenta consists of layers of soft membranes that form two fluid-filled sacs around the developing fetus. The layer immediately around the fetus is called the **amnion**. It forms a sac around the fetus called the **amniotic sac**. The fetus floats in amniotic fluid inside this sac. Surrounding the amniotic sac is another layer called the **allantois**, which forms the fluid-filled **allantoic sac**. The outside of the allantoic sac is covered by the **chorion**, which attaches to the uterine lining. The chorion is linked to the fetus by the umbilical cord.

The umbilical cord is the link between the fetus and the nutrient and waste exchange structures of the placenta. As its name implies, it is a cordlike structure that contains blood vessels (the *umbilical arteries* and *umbilical vein*) and a drainage tube from the fetus' urinary bladder (the *urachus*). The two **umbilical arteries** carry unoxygenated, waste-filled blood from the fetus to the placenta. The single **umbilical vein** carries nutrient- and oxygen-rich blood back from the placenta to the fetus. The **urachus** is a tube that runs from the cranial tip of the fetus' urinary bladder through the umbilical cord to the allantoic sac. The kidneys of the developing fetus are not fully functional through most of the pregnancy, therefore they do not produce urine as we know it. They do, however, produce a watery fluid that must be removed from the urinary bladder. The urachus drains this fluid out into the allantoic sac. It normally closes at birth.

### CLINICAL APPLICATION

#### The Afterbirth

At birth, the placenta is often referred to as the **afterbirth** because it is delivered *after* the offspring. What actually happens is that the fetus is delivered *through* the placenta. The powerful contractions of uterine and abdominal muscles during labor cause the membranes of the placenta to rupture and release their fluid. This is called the *water breaking*. Often the amnion still partially covers the newborn after it is delivered. The dam will usually lick this off, starting at the face so that the newborn can draw those important first breaths. If the mother does not perform this important duty, humans must intervene if they are present. The membrane is very soft and is easily broken and pulled away from the newborn's face. Few things in veterinary medicine are more rewarding than removing the membrane from the face of a newborn animal and watching it take its first breaths!

## ATTACHMENT TO THE UTERUS

The area where the chorion attaches to the lining of the uterus is where the fetal and maternal blood vessels intertwine with each other. The exchange of nutrients and wastes between the fetal and maternal bloodstreams takes place here. The type of attachment varies among species but can be categorized into one of four general types: *diffuse, cotyledonary, zonary,* and *discoid*.

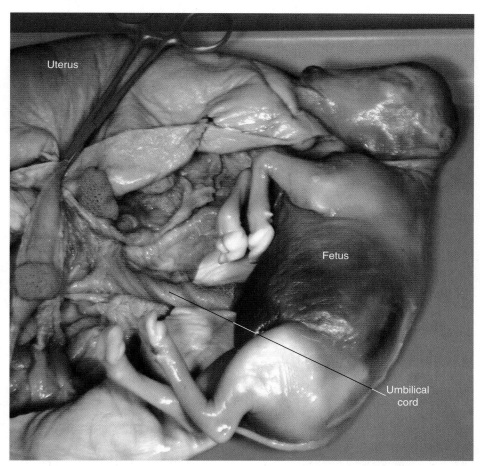

**FIGURE 20-7** Umbilical cord in preserved pregnant cow uterus. The umbilical cord links the fetus with the placenta. It contains arteries that bring waste-filled blood from the fetus to the placenta, a vein that brings nutrient and oxygen-rich blood back to the fetus from the placenta, and the urachus, a tube that runs from the urinary bladder of the fetus to one of the placental sacs around the fetus (the allantoic sac). (From Colville T, Bassert J: Clinical anatomy and physiology laboratory manual for veterinary technicians, St Louis, 2009, Mosby.)

**DIFFUSE PLACENTAL ATTACHMENT.** Diffuse placental attachment means that the attachment sites are spread diffusely over the whole surface of the placenta and the whole lining of the uterus. There are no small, focal areas of attachment. Species with this type of placenta include pigs, horses, and camelids (Figure 20-8). Because the attachment sites are so diffuse and loosely attached, this type of placenta usually detaches easily from the uterine lining and is readily passed after the **delivery of the newborn.**

**COTYLEDONARY PLACENTAL ATTACHMENT.** Cotyledonary placental attachment is the most complicated type and is somewhat the opposite of the diffuse placental attachment. The areas of attachment are small, discrete, and numerous. Each of the many separate attachment sites is called a **placentome.** Each placentome consists of an area on the surface of the placenta called a **cotyledon** that joins with a mushroomlike **caruncle** in the lining of the uterus. The cotyledon and caruncle interdigitate tightly with each other. This type of placenta is found in ruminants, such as cattle, sheep, and goats. See Figure 20-9.

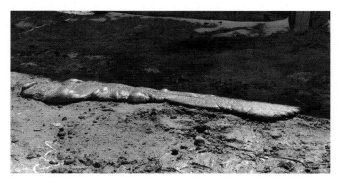

**FIGURE 20-8** Diffuse placentation. Afterbirth from a Bactrian Camel. Like those of horses and swine, the attachment of the placenta of the camel to the lining of the uterus is diffuse. This afterbirth is about 6 feet long by about 12 to 18 inches wide. Note the relatively smooth surface. (Photograph by the author and used with permission from the Red River Zoo, Fargo, ND; www.redriverzoo.org)

For a cotyledonary placenta to pass after the birth of the offspring, each of the individual placentomes must separate completely. Sometimes this does not occur, and part or all of the placenta is retained in the uterus after the birth process. This retained portion of placenta dies and

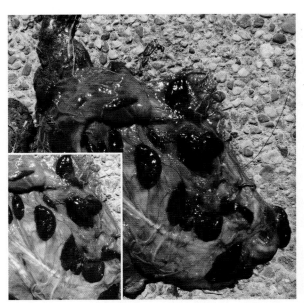

**FIGURE 20-9** Cotyledonary placentation. Afterbirth from an African Pygmy Goat with detail. Note the dark cotyledons, the former attachment sites of the placenta with the caruncles in the lining of the uterus during gestation. (Photograph by the author and used with permission from the Red River Zoo, Fargo, ND; www.redriverzoo.org)

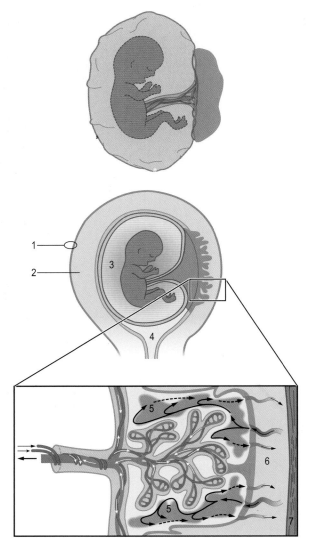

**FIGURE 20-11** The discoid primate placenta. (From Hyttel P: Essentials of domestic animal embryology, St Louis, 2010, Saunders.)

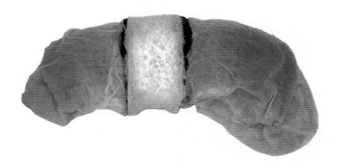

**FIGURE 20-10** Zonary placentation. Note the pale area of attachment encircling the placenta like a belt. (From Dyce KM, Sack WO, Wensing CJG: Textbook of veterinary anatomy, ed 4, St Louis, 2010, Saunders.)

degenerates within the uterus, creating a potentially dangerous situation for the already stressed dam. It can lead to a serious postpartum (after birth) metritis (infection of the uterus) because bacteria can live and multiply in the dead placental tissue. Ensuring that the placenta is delivered by ruminant animals is important, and appropriate treatment must be given if it is not.

### ZONARY PLACENTAL ATTACHMENT. With **zonary placental attachment**, the placenta attaches to the uterus in a belt-shaped zone that encircles the placenta. See Figure 20-10. Found in dogs and cats, this type of attachment also detaches fairly easily after delivery of the newborn. Retained placentas are not common in dogs and cats.

### DISCOID PLACENTAL ATTACHMENT. The pattern of **discoid placental attachment** is fairly self-descriptive. The area of attachment between the placenta and uterus is a single, discrete, disc-shaped area. This type of attachment is found in humans and other primates, as well as in rabbits and many rodents. See Figure 20-11.

---

✓ **TEST YOURSELF 20-2**

1. Why is the placenta so important to a successful pregnancy?
2. Describe the relationship between the fetus and the amniotic and allantoic sacs of the placenta.
3. Describe the main structures that make up the umbilical cord and the function of each.
4. Which type of placental attachment to the uterus is the simplest and detaches most easily after parturition? Which is most complicated and most often results in retention of the placenta?

## GESTATION

The period of pregnancy is called **gestation**, or the **gestation period.** It is the time from fertilization of the ovum to delivery of the newborn. It is convenient to divide it into three, often unequal, segments, called **trimesters**. The first trimester is the period of the embryo, when the newly implanted zygote is getting itself organized and developing its life-supporting placenta. During this period, the developing offspring is often referred to as an *embryo*. Starting with the second trimester, the developing offspring is usually called a *fetus*. The second trimester is the **fetal development** period, when all the various parts of the fetus are taking shape and differentiating from each other. All the body tissues, organs, and systems develop during this period. The third trimester is the period of **fetal growth**. All parts of the fetus grow dramatically during this last period of development, preparing it to transition from a parasitic to a free-living existence after birth. The lengths of the gestation period in some common species are listed in Table 20-2.

## PARTURITION

The whole, grand purpose of the male and female reproductive systems is fulfilled when **parturition**, the birth process, successfully takes place. At birth the fetus, which has led a parasitic existence up until now, is pushed out of the warm, dark, moist environment of the uterus into the cold, bright, outside world as a free-living, independent animal. In a very short time the body of the fetus has to undergo some dramatic changes. Its lungs, which have been nonfunctional until now, must suddenly expand with air and immediately start supplying the newborn with the oxygen it needs and eliminating the carbon dioxide its cells are producing as a waste product. Contributing to this process are some

dramatic changes in blood flow in and around the heart and lungs. The foramen ovale and ductus arteriosus, which shunted most of the blood from the right side of the fetal heart around, rather than through, the lungs, must both close fairly quickly. (See Chapter 14 for a complete description of these two fetal structures.) The lungs now need their full blood supply to oxygenate the blood properly and eliminate carbon dioxide.

Precisely what triggers parturition is not known. Many factors seem to be involved, including the size and weight of the uterus and fetus, and changing hormone levels in the fetus and the dam. The hormonal changes form a chain of events that leads to the onset of labor. Late in pregnancy the placenta of some species produces the hormone relaxin which helps relax ligaments between the bones around the birth canal, to ease the passage of the newborn. When it is time for parturition to get started, things start happening quickly, both in mom and in the fetus. The progesterone level in the bloodstream of the dam plummets (decreases rapidly) owing to the luteolytic effect of prostaglandin $F_2$alpha. This causes the corpus luteum of the ovary to regress quickly and stop producing progesterone. Up until now, the high progesterone level from the corpus luteum, and other sources, has kept the myometrium (muscle of the uterus) quiet, preventing it from prematurely expelling the fetus. The luteolytic prostaglandin $F_2$alpha is released from the placenta and the uterine wall as a result of stimulation from increased levels of glucocorticoid hormones from the adrenal glands of the fetus. The prostaglandin also causes a rise in the dam's estrogen level. The combined estrogen and prostaglandin levels increase the myometrium's sensitivity to oxytocin, which is released from the dam's posterior pituitary gland. Oxytocin stimulates the myometrium to contract, and this starts the labor process.

## LABOR

The three distinct stages of parturition are referred to as the **three stages of labor**.

The first stage of labor consists of **uterine contractions**. The myometrium (muscle layer of the uterus) contracts as the cervix relaxes, pressing the membrane-covered fetus down against the cervix. This causes the cervix gradually to dilate. Externally, the dam appears restless and uncomfortable as a result of these uterine contractions. She may repeatedly lie down and get up and may urinate frequently. Some species, such as dogs and pigs, may attempt to build a nest into which they will deliver their young.

The second stage of labor consists of the actual **delivery of the newborn**. This is accomplished by a combination of strong uterine and abdominal muscle contractions. The dam typically lies down and strains in a rhythmic pattern of contractions that gradually become stronger and closer together. Rupture of the "water bags," the amniotic and allantoic sacs of the placenta, usually precedes the actual delivery of the newborn.

The third stage of labor consists of **delivery of the placenta** (afterbirth). The placenta separates from the wall of the uterus and is expelled by weaker uterine contractions. The dam often eats the placenta. See Figure 20-12.

| TABLE 20-2 | Gestation Periods of Selected Species | |
|---|---|---|
| **SPECIES** | **RANGE** | **APPROXIMATE GESTATION PERIOD** |
| Alpacas | 335-345 days | 11 months |
| Camels | 360-420 days | 13 months |
| Cats | 56-69 days | 2 months |
| Cattle | 271-291 days | 9 months |
| Dogs | 59-68 days | 2 months |
| Elephants | 615-650 days | 21 months |
| Ferrets | 42 days | 6 weeks |
| Goats | 146-155 days | 5 months |
| Hamsters | 19-20 days | 3 weeks |
| Horses | 321-346 days | 11 months |
| Humans | 280 days | 9 months |
| Llamas | 330-360 days | 11.5 months |
| Pigs | 110-116 days | 3 months, 3 weeks, and 3 days |
| Porcupines | 205-217 days | 7 months |
| Rabbits | 30-32 days | 1 month |
| Sheep | 143-151 days | 5 months |

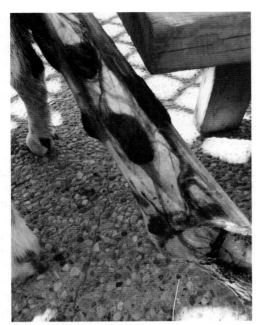

**FIGURE 20-12** Afterbirth of an African Pygmy Goat during the third stage of labor. The goat is off the figure to the left. Mild traction is being applied to the placenta to aid its passage. (Photograph by the author and used with permission from the Red River Zoo, Fargo, ND; www.redriverzoo.org)

 **CLINICAL APPLICATION**

### Dystocia

Usually parturition comes off without a hitch. After all, animals have been giving birth for millions of years without any help. However, sometimes problems develop that interfere with the birth process, causing **dystocia**, or a difficult birth. The most common causes of dystocia include a fetus that is too large for the dam to pass and a fetus that is in the wrong position for delivery, which is called an *abnormal presentation*. Abnormal presentations may involve deviations in the position of the head, one or more legs, or the overall orientation of the fetus from the normal snout-first or rear-legs-first position. Sometimes the fetus can be pushed back far enough to allow it to be repositioned for delivery; this is called *repelling* the fetus. At times this is not possible, and the fetus must be removed surgically by an operation called a *cesarean section, or C-section*. In some cases, particularly in cattle, when the fetus is dead, it may have to be cut up (called an *embryotomy*) into small enough segments to be removed through the birth canal to save the life of the dam.

In multiparous species, such as dogs, cats, and pigs, that normally give birth to multiple offspring, the second and third stages of parturition intermix with one another. Typically newborns and placentas are delivered alternately; that is, after a newborn is delivered, its placenta is usually expelled before the next newborn is delivered.

Table 20-3 lists the names for offspring of selected species.

## INVOLUTION OF THE UTERUS

After parturition is complete, the uterus immediately begins contracting down to its nonpregnant size through a process

| TABLE 20-3 | Offspring Names of Selected Species | | |
|---|---|---|---|
| **SPECIES** | **OFFSPRING** | **SPECIES** | **OFFSPRING** |
| Alpaca | Cria | Hedgehog | Pup |
| Ass/Donkey | Foal | Horse | Foal |
| Camel | Calf | Llama | Cria |
| Cat | Kitten | Monkey | Infant |
| Cattle | Calf | Mouse | Pup |
| Chicken | Chick | Mule | Foal |
| Cockroach | Nymph | Octopus | Fry |
| Deer | Fawn | Otter | Pup |
| Dog | Puppy | Parrot | Chick |
| Elk | Calf | Pig | Piglet |
| Ferret | Kit | Rabbit | Kit |
| Fly | Maggot | Rat | Pup |
| Gerbil | Pup | Sheep | Lamb |
| Goat | Kid | Snake | Hatchling |
| Goose | Gosling | Swan | Cygnet |
| Guinea Pig | Pup | Wolf | Pup |
| Hamster | Pup | Worm | Wormlet |

called **involution of the uterus**. At the placental attachment site(s), the endometrium sloughs (dies and detaches) into the lumen of the uterus, and the exposed areas heal over. The myometrium slowly continues to contract, squeezing the contents of the uterus out through the birth canal as the organ returns to its nonpregnant size. Initially the discharge contains fresh blood resulting from separation of the placenta from its attachment site(s). Pressure from the continued uterine contractions usually stops the bleeding relatively quickly. The discharge gradually turns darker as dead tissue is liquefied and sloughed from the uterine wall. It generally takes from a few weeks to a month or more for involution to be complete.

> ✓ **TEST YOURSELF 20-3**
> 1. What are the basic events of the three trimesters of pregnancy?
> 2. Describe the three stages of labor.
> 3. Why is it important that uterine contractions continue after the fetus and placenta have been delivered?

## MAMMARY GLANDS AND LACTATION

Once parturition is completed, the newborn animal must be nourished and cared for during the **neonatal period**. The mammary glands are very important now.

### CHARACTERISTICS

The mammary (milk) glands are specialized skin glands. They produce colostrum and milk, which are needed by the newly born animal during the crucial first few hours, days, and weeks of life. Although, strictly speaking, they are not part of the reproductive process, their function is vital to the survival of the newborn, therefore we discuss them along with pregnancy.

Mammary glands are present in both male and female animals, although they can be difficult or impossible to find in stallions. They normally only function in females because males do not secrete the proper blend of hormones to make them work. (It is theoretically possible to make a bull give milk with administration of the proper combination of hormones, but who would want to milk him?)

## SPECIES DIFFERENCES

Mammary glands look very different among common species of animals. Their number varies, from a low of two in horses to a high of 14 in swine, and their locations range from the inguinal (groin) region alone in cattle and horses, to locations that span the inguinal, abdominal, and thoracic regions in dogs, cats, and swine. Also, considerable variety is found in the number of openings from which milk emerges in the teats or nipples. Cattle, sheep, and goats only have one opening per teat, whereas dogs can have up to 20 openings per nipple. (Humans have up to 24 openings per nipple.) The mammary gland characteristics of some common species are listed in Table 20-4.

## UDDER OF THE COW

Because they are so large and specialized, a cow's mammary glands, commonly known as the **udder**, seem like exaggerated caricatures of other species' mammary glands. Their general makeup, however, is just a larger version of other animals' mammary glands. For this reason, we use them as our model mammary system (Figure 20-13).

The udder of the cow consists of four mammary glands that are called **quarters**. Each quarter is a completely separate unit from the other three. They each have their own milk-secreting systems and ducts leading down to their own teats. This has important clinical significance if infection of the mammary gland, a condition called **mastitis**, develops.

| TABLE 20-4 | Mammary Gland Characteristics of Some Common Species | | |
|---|---|---|---|
| **SPECIES** | **USUAL NUMBER OF GLANDS** | **LOCATION OF GLANDS** | **NUMBER OF OPENINGS IN TEATS OR NIPPLES** |
| Cats | 10 | Inguinal, abdominal, and thoracic regions | 3-7 |
| Cattle | 4 | Inguinal | 1 |
| Dogs | 10 | Inguinal, abdominal, and thoracic regions | 8-20 |
| Goats | 2 | Inguinal region | 1 |
| Horses | 2 | Inguinal region | 2-4 |
| Humans | 2 | Thoracic region | 15-24 |
| Pigs | 14 | Inguinal, abdominal, and thoracic regions | 2-3 |
| Sheep | 2 | Inguinal region | 1 |

Infection does not spread directly from one quarter to another. It has to spread down through the teat and duct system of one quarter and up another, or on rare occasions, it can spread systemically (through the bloodstream). The spread of mastitis in a herd can be prevented through good milking hygiene, which includes milking infected cows last and keeping facilities clean.

The udder of a high-producing dairy cow can weigh more than 100 lb at milking time. It needs a strong suspensory system to support the heavy weight and attach the udder to the body wall. This suspensory system consists of a slinglike arrangement of ligaments that run down the center and around the sides of the udder. The median suspensory ligament contains many elastic fibers so that it can stretch. It passes down the center (along the median plane) between the left and right halves of the udder. The lateral suspensory ligaments are composed largely of strong but relatively inelastic collagen fibers. They pass down and around the lateral sides of each half of the udder. The strong lateral ligaments provide firm support for the udder, and the elastic medial ligament acts as a shock absorber for the udder as the animal moves around. *Note:* When the udder is empty, the teats point pretty much straight down. When the udder is full of milk, however, the teats angle off to the left and right sides a bit. This is due to stretching of the elastic median ligament that runs down the center of the udder.

## ALVEOLI AND DUCT SYSTEM

The milk-secreting units of the mammary gland are small structures called **alveoli**. Each alveolus is a tiny, saclike arrangement of cells that secretes milk into an equally tiny tube called the **alveolar duct**. The alveoli are arranged like clusters of grapes around the alveolar ducts. The tiny alveolar ducts join to form larger ducts, which join to form even larger ducts, and so on. The duct system of the mammary gland is similar to the arrangement of branches in a tree. The clusters of alveoli would be similar to the leaves, and the duct system would be like the small tree branches joining to form larger branches. The largest ducts (similar to the trunks of trees) empty into a large space called the **gland sinus**, located just above (dorsal to) the teat. The gland sinus is continuous with the **teat sinus** inside the teat. The two large sinuses form a space shaped like an upside-down pear. They are the spaces where milk accumulates when **milk let-down** (described later) has occurred. The milk can be readily extracted from these large spaces by the suckling of a nursing newborn or the gentle vacuum of a milking machine.

At the tip of the teat is the **streak canal**, which is the passageway from the teat sinus to the outside. It is surrounded by elastic fibers and a ringlike sphincter muscle that keeps it closed most of the time. This helps minimize milk leakage.

## MAMMARY GLAND DEVELOPMENT

The mammary glands stay small and undeveloped until puberty (the time of sexual maturity). Up until that time,

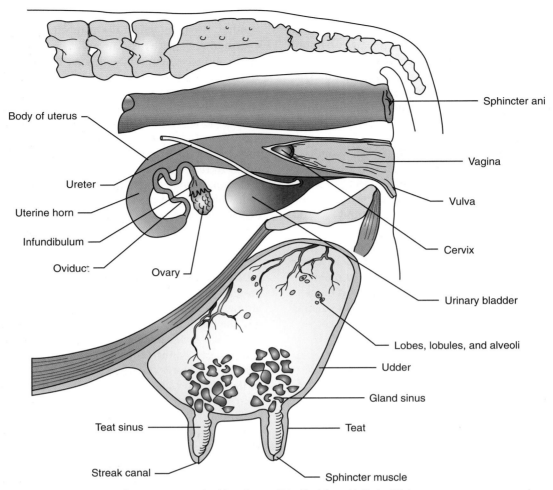

**FIGURE 20-13** Reproductive system and udder of cow. (Modified from McBride DF: Learning veterinary terminology, ed 2, St Louis, 2002, Mosby.)

the proper mix of hormones has not occurred to stimulate their growth and development. Once estrous cycles begin at puberty, however, the mammary glands respond to the new hormones flowing through the body by enlarging and gearing up to produce milk.

A complex balance of hormones stimulates the mammary glands to develop. Most of the anterior pituitary hormones are involved in the process either directly or indirectly. Prolactin and growth hormone directly encourage mammary gland development. Follicle-stimulating hormone (FSH) and luteinizing hormone (LH) stimulate the ovaries to produce estrogen and progesterone during each heat cycle. The estrogen and progesterone encourage the alveoli and duct systems of the mammary glands to develop. Thyroid-stimulating hormone and adrenocorticotropic hormone (ACTH) influence the process indirectly through their target organs (the thyroid gland and the adrenal cortex). The levels of these various hormones must be balanced precisely for complete mammary gland development to take place. Abnormally high levels of any hormones, such as might occur when thyroid hormone or corticosteroid drugs are

administered to a young animal, can actually inhibit normal mammary gland development.

## LACTATION

The physical growth and development of the mammary glands are the first steps in making them able to produce milk. The rest takes place during pregnancy.

**Lactation** is the process of milk production. It begins toward the end of pregnancy and is obvious at the time of parturition. Prolactin and growth hormone from the anterior pituitary gland and hormones from the adrenal cortex are involved in getting lactation started.

## COLOSTRUM

Before it starts to produce milk, the mammary gland produces a sort of premilk secretion called **colostrum**. Colostrum has a different appearance and a different composition than normal milk. It contains larger amounts of proteins, lipids, and amino acids than milk and also contains high levels of various essential vitamins. It supplies important nutrients to the newborn and has a laxative effect that helps clear the dark, sticky **meconium** from the newborn's intestinal tract.

Probably the most critical of colostrum's roles is the transfer of what is called **passive immunity** from the dam to the newborn. Among the proteins in colostrum are high levels of immunoglobulins, also called **antibodies**, that are an important part of the body's defense against infection. The antibodies in the colostrum are specific for disease-causing organisms that the dam has been exposed to or vaccinated against. If the newborn drinks sufficient colostrum during the first few hours after birth, the large antibody molecules will be absorbed intact into its bloodstream. This provides it with important passive immunity, in which complete, preformed antibodies help protect it against disease-causing microorganisms until its own immune system matures sufficiently to protect it. If colostrum is not consumed within the first few hours, the lining of the newborn's intestine can no longer absorb the large antibody molecules intact. They will be broken down by the digestive process, and passive immunity will not be transmitted. Youngsters that do not get sufficient colostrum in that critical early neonatal period are much more prone to diseases. Even if they do not die of early infections, they are typically weaker and do not grow as rapidly as animals that consumed colostrum at the appropriate time.

## CLINICAL APPLICATION

### Passive Immunity and Vaccinations

The passive immunity that newborns acquire from drinking **colostrum** is important to their early survival. However, it can interfere with early vaccinations, particularly in puppies and kittens. If a puppy or kitten is vaccinated while it still has a high level of antibodies from its mother in its bloodstream, the vaccine will be inactivated and will not stimulate the animal's immune system to manufacture new antibodies. So why not just wait until the passive immunity from mom wears off? The difficulty is that passive immunity lasts differing lengths of time in different animals. If you vaccinate too early, the vaccine is wasted. If you wait too long to vaccinate, the passive immunity may have worn off, leaving the animal susceptible to infection. The level of passive antibodies in the young animal's bloodstream can be tested, but this is expensive. The most practical solution is to give the young animal a series of vaccinations spread out over the period when protection from passive immunity is most likely to end. Specific vaccination protocols differ, but the first vaccination is usually given somewhere around 6 to 8 weeks of age, with subsequent vaccinations given every 2 to 3 weeks until the animal is 14 to 16 weeks old.

## MAINTENANCE OF LACTATION

Once it has begun, lactation will continue as long as the mammary gland is emptied regularly by nursing or milking. The key is continued physical stimulation of the teat or nipple, combined with regular removal of milk from the gland. These activities send sensory nerve impulses to the brain. From there nerve pathways lead to the hypothalamus, which stimulates the anterior pituitary gland to continue its production of the hormones that keep lactation going. When nursing or milking stops, the flow of essential hormones stops also. The lack of hormonal stimulation combined with increased pressure in the gland (because it is no longer being emptied) causes lactation gradually to cease. The mammary gland "dries up." This is called **involution of the mammary gland**.

## MILK LET-DOWN

**Milk let-down** is the immediate effect of nursing or milking. When milk is produced, it accumulates in the outer reaches of the mammary gland, in the alveoli and small ducts. It does not move into the larger ducts and sinuses, where it is accessible for nursing or milking, until milk let-down occurs. When nursing or milking begins, sensory nerve impulses are sent to the brain. As we've seen, this causes the hypothalamus to stimulate the anterior pituitary gland to produce the hormones necessary to maintain lactation. However, it also has another major effect. It also causes the hypothalamus to release the hormone oxytocin from the posterior pituitary gland. The oxytocin travels to the mammary gland and causes musclelike **myoepithelial cells** around the alveoli and small ducts to contract. This squeezes milk down into the large ducts and sinuses, where it can be removed by nursing or milking. The process of milk let-down takes from a few seconds to a minute or more to produce results, so there is often a slight delay from the time a newborn starts to nurse to when the milk starts to flow freely.

### ✓ TEST YOURSELF 20-4

1. Why does mastitis in one quarter of a dairy cow's udder not necessarily spread to the other three quarters?
2. Describe the suspensory apparatus of the udder.
3. Why don't the mammary glands of male animals usually develop or secrete milk?
4. Describe the importance of colostrum to the health of a newborn animal.
5. Describe how nursing or milking causes milk let-down and also helps sustain lactation.

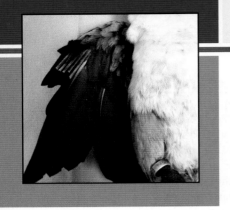

# Avian Anatomy and Physiology  21

*Lori R. Arent*

## OUTLINE

## LEARNING OBJECTIVES

*When you have completed this chapter you will be able to:*

1. Describe the anatomic structures of avian skin, beaks, and claws.
2. Describe the structure and functions of feathers.
3. List the types of feathers and the location of each type.
4. List the unique features of the avian skeleton.
5. List the unique features of avian musculature.
6. Describe the shape and general characteristics of avian eyes and explain how those characteristics affect visual acuity.
7. Describe the unique anatomic features that affect the sense of hearing in nocturnal owls.
8. List the unique anatomic features that affect the sense of taste in birds.
9. List the components of the avian digestive system and describe the functions of each.
10. List the unique features of the avian circulatory and respiratory systems.
11. Describe the composition of avian urine.
12. List and describe the unique features of the avian male and female reproductive systems.
13. List and describe the four classifications of newly hatched chicks.

*Airsac* e**ə**r-sahck

*Alula* **ahl**-yuh-luh

*Appendicular skeleton* ahp-ehn-**dihck**-ū-l**ə**r **skehl**-ih-tuhn

*Apteria* ahp-**teer**-ē-uh

*Auricular* ohr-**rihck**-yuh-l**ə**r

*Axial skeleton* **ahck**-sē-ahl **skehl**-ih-tuhn

*Barb* bahrb

*Barbule* **bahr**-būl

*Blood feather* bluhd **fehth**-**ə**r

*Brood patch* brood pahtch

*Bursa of Fabricius* **buhr**-suh of fah-**brihsh**-uhs

*Choanae* **kō**-ah-nē

*Clutch* kluhtch

*Coccygeal vertebrae* kohck-**sihj**-ē-ahl **vərt**-eh-brā

*Columella* kohl-yuh-**mehl**-ah

*Cone* kōn

*Coprodeum* kōp-rō-**dē**-uhm

*Crop* krohp

*Determinate layer* dih-t**ə**r-mih-niht **lā**-**ə**r

*Fault bar* fahlt bahr

*Feather follicle* **fehth**-**ə**r **fohl**-ih-kuhl

*Fibrous tunic* **fī**-bruhs **too**-nihck

*Fovea* **fō**-vē-uh

*Gizzard* **gihz**-**ə**rd

*Glenoid cavity* **glē**-noyd **kahv**-ih-tē

*Gular fluttering* gyoo-luhr **fluht**-**ə**r-ihng

*Hamuli* **hahm**-yuh-lī

*Heterophil* **heht**-**ə**r-ō-fihl

*Hock* hohck

*Indeterminate layer* ihn-dih-**t**ə**r**-mih-niht lā-**ə**r

*Keel* kēl

*Keratin* **ke**ə**r**-ah-tehn

*Mesobronchi* mē-sō-brohn-kī

*Molting* **mohlt**-ihng

*Mute* mūt

*Nape* nāp

*Neural tunic* n**ə**r-ahl **too**-nihck

*Nictitating membrane* **nihck**-tih-tā-tihng **mehm**-brān

*Operculum* ō-**pehr**-kyoo-luhm

*Parabronchi* pe**ə**r-ah-brohn-kī

*Patagium* puh-**tā**-jē-uhm

*Pellet* **pehl**-iht

*Pecten* **pehck**-tehn

*Pectoral crest* **pehck**-t**ə**r-ahl krehst

*Pectoralis* **pehck**-tah-rahl-ihs

*Periderm* pe**ə**r-ih-d**ə**rm

*Precocial* prē-**kō**-shuhl

*Proctodeum* prohck-tuh-**dē**-uhm

*Pterylae* **tehr**-uh-lē

*Pygostyle* **pī**-guh-stīl

*Remiges* **rehm**-ih-jēz

*Renal portal system* **rē**-nuhl **pohr**-tehl **sihs**-tehm

*Retrices* **reht**-ruh-sēz

*Rod* rohd

*Sclerotic ring* skleh-**rah**-tihck rihng

*Semialtricial* seh-mē-ahl-**trihsh**-uhl

*Semiprecocial* seh-mē-prē-**kō**-shuhl

*Shell gland* shehl glahnd

*Supracoracoideus* soo-prah-kohr-uh-**koy**-dē-uhs

*Synsacrum* sihn-**sā**-kruhm

*Syrinx* **sihr**-ihncks

*Talon* **tahl**-uhn

*Trochanter* trō-**kahn**-t**ə**r

*Tympanic membrane* tihm-**pahn**-ihck **mehm**-brān

*Uncinate process* **uhn**-suh-nāt **proh**-sehs

*Urodeum* y**ə**r-ō-**dē**-uhm

*Uropygial gland* y**ə**r-ō-**pihj**-ē-ahl glahnd

*Uterus* **ū**-t**ə**r-uhs

*Uveal tunic* **ū**-vē-ahl **too**-nihck

*Vent* vehnt

*Zygodactyl* zī-gō-**dahck**-tihl

## INTRODUCTION

A feathered marvel. There is no better way to describe the avian creature. Over 10,000 unique bird species grace our planet (Table 21-1), modeling colors from the brilliant hues of tropical species to the earthy tones of many birds of prey. They are masterpieces of beauty and function. Over the course of time, a body containing specialized structures and organ systems evolved to dominate a realm not shared by many other creatures: the sky. From the outer protective layers to the inner workings of the reproductive system, a bird is designed to fly. Let us take a look at this unique design and explore the wonders of the avian body.

| TABLE 21-1 | Bird Classification | |
|---|---|---|
| | Class: Aves; Orders: 29 with worldwide distribution (Gill, 1995) | |
| **ORDER** | **SPECIES** | **DESCRIPTION** |
| Anseriformes | Waterfowl—mallards, ducks, geese, swans | Aquatic birds with webbed feet and flattened bills with toothlike edges |
| Apodiformes | Swifts | Small aerial birds that eat insects on the wing |
| Caprimulgiformes | Nighthawks, goatsuckers, frogmouths | Nocturnal species that eat insects on the wing |
| Charadriiformes | Shorebirds, gulls, terns | Wading or swimming birds |
| Ciconiiformes | Herons, wood storks | Wading birds with long legs and bill; feed on aquatic life |
| Columbiformes | Pigeons, doves | Birds that eat grain, small seeds, and corn |
| Cuculiformes | Cuckoos | Slender birds with rounded wings, curved upper mandible; live in forests and eat caterpillars |
| Falconiformes | Hawks, eagles, falcons, vultures, osprey | Diurnal flesh eaters, with the exception of vultures; have sharp, hooked bills and strong feet for capturing live prey; some scavenge |
| Galliformes | Game birds—chickens, turkeys, quail, grouse, pheasant | Heavy-bodied land birds with short, rounded wings and curved upper bill; capable of short flights |
| Gaviiformes | Loons | Birds specialized for swimming and diving; live primarily on water |
| Gruiformes | Cranes, rails, coots | Wading birds with long legs; feed on a variety of insect, aquatic, and rodent species |
| Passeriformes | Perching birds—starlings, crows, swallows, ravens, finches, songbirds | Vary in size, have three toes in front and one behind and a well-developed syrinyx |
| Piciformes | Woodpeckers—common flickers | Strong, sharp bill for boring holes into tree trunks for insects; stiff tail used as prop |
| Procellariiformes | Albatrosses | Birds of oceans, found mostly in the Antarctic, South America, Africa, Australia; have pronounced hook at end of their bills and external nostrils modified into tubes |
| Psittaformes | Psittacines—parakeets, parrots, budgerigars, cockatiels, cockatoos | Brightly colored tropical birds with strong, heavily curved beaks and short legs |
| Sphenisciformes | Penguins | Flightless birds in southern hemisphere, adapted for living in cold water |
| Strigiformes | Owls | Mostly nocturnal, large-headed, short-necked birds of prey with large eyes and facial disc |
| Struthioniformes | Ostriches | Large, flightless birds of Africa; also bred in captivity in Australia, Europe, and United States |

Orders not described: Casuariiformes (emus, cassowaries), Coliiformes (mousebirds), Coraciiformes (kingfishers, bee-eaters, hoopoes), Dinornithiformes (kiwis), Musophagiformes (turacos and plaintain eaters), Pelecaniformes (pelicans, gannets, cormorants), Phoenicopteriformes (flamingos), Podicipediformes (grebes), Rheiformes (rheas), Tinamiformes (tinamous), Trogoniformes (trogans).

From Gill FB: Ornithology, ed 2, New York, 1995, Macmillan.

## TOPOGRAPHY

Our study of birds begins with the identification of external features (Figure 21-1). Many of these are used for identification of wild birds in the field and, in a clinical setting, for indication of illness or trauma. Familiarizing yourself with the locations of these structures will aid in your understanding of their function.

## INTEGUMENT

A bird's body is covered by skin and its derivatives: the beak, claws, and feathers. These structures cover and protect the internal organs and block the entrance of disease-causing organisms.

### SKIN

The skin of birds consists of two layers: an outer layer called the *epidermis* and an inner layer called the *dermis* (Figure 21-2). The epidermis is relatively thin and consists of flattened epithelial cells that produce **keratin**, a tough fibrous protein necessary for the production of scales, feathers, and the outer sheaths of beaks and claws. The inner layer of skin (dermis) is thicker and consists of a tough, fibrous connective tissue. It stores fat for nutrition and insulation and supplies a pathway for nerves, blood vessels, and muscles to reach the epidermis. Smooth muscles in the dermis innervate **feather follicles** to help in the regulation of heat. During hot weather, depressor muscles press the feathers against the body to promote heat loss. When a bird gets cold or does not feel well, it looks "fluffed" because erector muscles in the dermis elevate the body feathers to trap warm air near the body.

### GLANDS

Unlike mammals, birds do not possess sweat glands. Feathers cover such a large portion of a bird's body that sweat glands would not be effective. The one major skin gland that most birds do possess is called the **uropygial gland**, or *preen gland*. It is located on the dorsal surface at the upper base of the tail (Figure 21-3). The act of preening stimulates this gland to secrete an oily, fatty substance. A bird uses its beak to spread this oil throughout its feathers to clean and waterproof them. The gland varies in size and structure and is relatively large in aquatic species, such as waterfowl and ospreys. The gland is completely lacking in some parrots, ostriches, and in a few other species.

### BEAKS

One derivative of a bird's skin is its beak, or bill. It consists of an upper and lower mandible and is covered with a tough, horny keratin layer that grows continuously. Beaks vary in their hardness and flexibility, depending on their function. Some birds use their beaks to crack seeds and nuts (parrots), tear food into bite-sized pieces (hawks), capture food (herons and woodpeckers), preen their feathers or those of a mate,

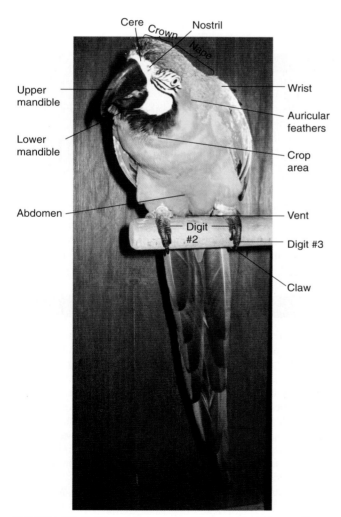

**FIGURE 21-1** External features of a Blue and Gold Macaw (*Propyrrhura maracana*). (Photo by Gail Buhl.)

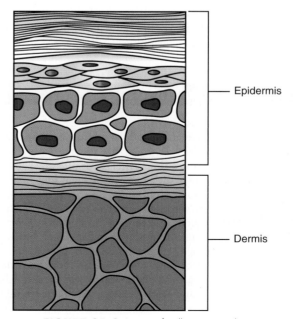

**FIGURE 21-2** Layers of cells in avian skin.

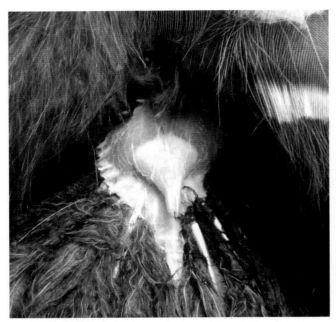

**FIGURE 21-3** Uropygial gland of a Barred Owl *(Strix varia)*.

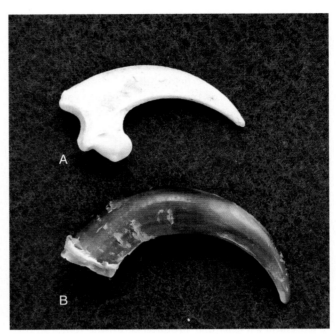

**FIGURE 21-4** Talon of an American Bald Eagle *(Haliaeetus leuco-cephalus)*. **A,** Bone; **B,** sheath.

pick up and hold things such as food and nesting material as they fly and climb, and sometimes to protect themselves.

## CLAWS

Claws possess a horny sheath derived from specialized scales at the end of each toe. Like beaks, they grow continuously. Species differ in the type of claws they possess, based on their perching habits and method of procuring food. For example, ground feeders, such as chickens and pheasants, have short, sharp claws that are used to scratch the ground for food; birds of prey have claws called **talons** that are long, sharp, and rounded to catch and kill their prey (Figure 21-4); vultures, which are scavengers, have short, blunt claws; and climbing birds, such as woodpeckers and nuthatches, have strongly curved claws for gripping.

 **TEST YOURSELF 21-1**

1. What structures are derivatives of a bird's skin and what are they made of?
2. Define the function of the uropygial gland. Do all birds possess this gland?
3. Describe the basic anatomy of a bird's beak and claws. When trimming these structures, what should you be careful to avoid?

## FEATHERS

Birds are unique in the animal kingdom in that they possess feathers. Feathers are outgrowths of skin that are made of protein; once completely developed, they are nonliving

## CLINICAL APPLICATION

### Coping Beaks and Nails

In the wild, the shape and length of a bird's beak and claws are maintained by daily activities that provide natural wear. For example, after completing a meal, birds often **feak**, or rub, their beaks on a rough surface to clean them and maintain their shape. In captivity, birds are provided with limited wearing surfaces, and some birds, such as psittacines and birds of prey, require frequent **coping**, or trimming and reshaping, of their beaks and nails. Without this maintenance, beaks can become so long that a bird has a difficult time eating, and they can develop large cracks and chips that can cause permanent damage to the beak's growth plate, located near the **cere**. Claws can become so long and sharp that they cause uneven weight bearing on the foot pads or puncture the bottom of a foot.

This can result in pad abrasions, blisters, swelling, abscess formation, and, in severe cases, degeneration of the bones in the feet (osteomyelitis). The term often used to describe these conditions of the avian foot is *bumblefoot*.

Coping beaks and claws must be done with care, because both of these structures have a blood and nerve supply that can be hit if they are trimmed too deeply. Beaks can be coped using a fingernail file or a rotary tool. Claws can be trimmed using a cat or dog nail trimmer, depending on the size of the bird. If bleeding occurs, hemostasis can be achieved by applying topical cauterizing agents, such as silver nitrate or "Quick-stop." The nails of parrots are often trimmed with a rotary tool, which cauterizes a blood vessel if it is hit.

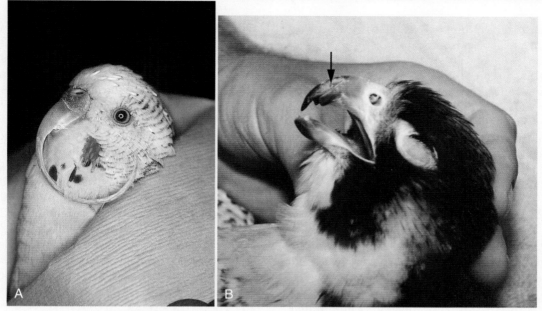

Abnormal beaks. **A**, Severely overgrown beak of a Budgerigar *(Melopsittacus undulates)*. **B**, Cracked beak of a Peregrine Falcon *(Falco peregrinus)*. (**A** from Samour J: Avian medicine, Philadelphia, 2000, Mosby.)

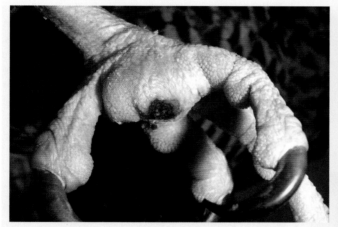

Severe bumblefoot on the metatarsal pad of a Gyrfalcon *(Falco rusticolus)*.

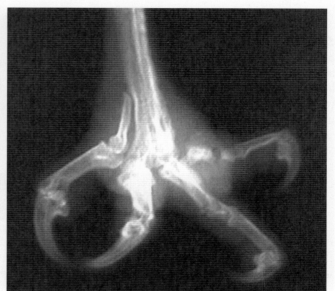

Osteomyelitis of digit number four.

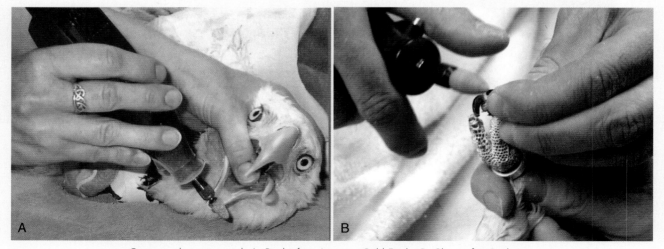

Coping with a rotary tool. **A**, Beak of an American Bald Eagle. **B**, Claws of a Cockatoo.

structures that have sensation only at the base, where they originate from a follicle under the skin.

## FUNCTIONS

Feathers serve several important functions. First, they are necessary for flight. A bird without a proper complement of flight feathers simply cannot fly. Second, feathers protect the thin skin from trauma, rain, and excessive radiation from sunlight. They also assist in thermoregulation and camouflage and are used in many communication behaviors, such as courtship, defense, and recognition.

## STRUCTURE

Six types of feather cover a bird's body. The most visible feathers, that give shape to a bird, are called *contour feathers.* Contour feathers have the most compact microstructure and consist of several components (Figure 21-5, *A*).

**INFERIOR UMBILICUS.** This structure is a tiny opening at the base of the feather, where it inserts into the skin. When a new feather is developing, it receives nourishment from blood vessels that pass through this opening.

**SUPERIOR UMBILICUS.** This structure is a tiny opening on the feather shaft, where the webbed part of the feather begins. In some birds, including several species of parrots, hawks, herons, and grouse, it gives rise to an afterfeather, which is an accessory feather thought to provide additional insulation to retain body heat.

**CALAMUS.** Also called the *quill*, the calamus is the round, hollow, semitransparent portion of a feather that extends from the inferior umbilicus to the superior umbilicus.

**RACHIS.** The rachis is the main feather shaft.

**VANE.** The vane is the flattened part of a feather that appears weblike, on each side of the rachis. It consists of numerous slender, closely spaced **barbs**. The barbs give rise to **barbules**, which have rolled edges and tiny hooklets known as **hamuli**. These hooklets interlock each barb with an adjacent one, forming a tightly linked, flexible web (see Figure 21-5, *B*). The degree of tightness varies with the species. For example, the contour feathers of owls have fewer barbules than do those of hawks. The result is a looser feather weave that feels softer and allows air to pass through, creating silent flight.

## TYPES OF FEATHER

**CONTOUR FEATHERS.** Contour feathers typically cover a bird's body and constitute the flight feathers of the wings and tail (Figure 21-6, *A*). The flight feathers in the wing are commonly called **remiges**, and the tail feathers are called **retrices**. Small contour feathers, called **auriculars**, are found around the external ear openings and improve a bird's hearing ability. They are especially numerous in some species of parrots and hawks, and in owls. Contour feathers are moved by muscles attached to the walls of the follicles.

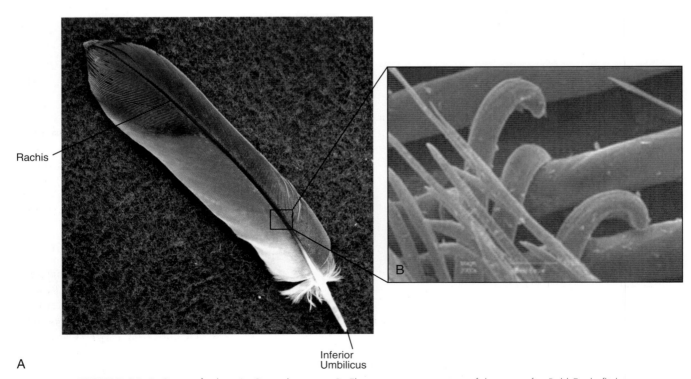

Rachis

Inferior
Umbilicus

A

**FIGURE 21-5** Contour feather. A, General structure. B, Electron microscopic view of the vane of a Bald Eagle flight feather.

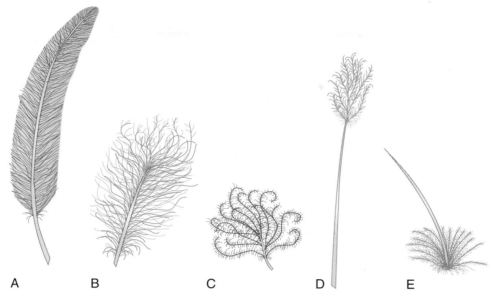

**FIGURE 21-6** Types of feather. **A**, Contour. **B**, Semiplume. **C**, Down. **D**, Filoplume. **E**, Bristle.

**SEMIPLUME FEATHERS.** Semiplume feathers possess a main rachis with barbs that lack barbules and hooklets (see Figure 21-6, *B*). They are commonly found under contour feathers, especially on the sides of the abdomen and along the neck and back. Like down feathers, semiplumes provide insulation. They also provide flexibility for the movement of the contour feathers and help with buoyancy in water birds.

**DOWN FEATHERS.** Down feathers are soft, fluffy feathers that lack a true shaft, barbules, and hooklets on their barbs (see Figure 21-6, *C*). They are located next to the skin under contour feathers, and they function primarily as insulation.

**FILOPLUME FEATHERS.** Filoplume feathers have a bare shaft that lacks barbs on the majority of its length, except at the tip (see Figure 21-6, *D*). They are located on the **nape** and upper back near contour feathers, and their follicles contain sensitive nerve endings that may play a sensory role in controlling feather movement. Slight movements of the contour feathers are transmitted to pressure and vibration receptors in the skin via the filoplume feathers.

**BRISTLES.** **Bristles** are modified contour feathers with a stiff rachis and few barbs at the base (see Figure 21-6, *E*). They are thought to serve a bird's sense of touch. Depending on the species, they may be found in various locations. Crows, ravens, and woodpeckers have bristles around their nostrils; owls have them around the mouth and sometimes around the toes, as do grouse; other birds have bristles around their eyes (Figure 21-7).

**POWDER DOWN FEATHERS.** Powder down feathers are unusual feathers that never stop growing. They grow continuously at the base and disintegrate at their tip, creating

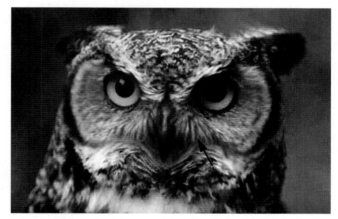

**FIGURE 21-7** Bristles on the face of a Great Horned Owl *(Bubo virginianus)*.

a waxy powder that is spread throughout the rest of the plumage to clean it and provide waterproofing. Powder down feathers are most highly developed in herons and bitterns, especially on the breast, belly, and back; they can be found more diffusely scattered in parrots and hawks. Birds without a **uropygial gland** have abundant powder down feathers.

## LOCATION

Contrary to their appearance, feathers do not originate from the entire body. They are located in specific tracts, called **pterylae**, which are separated by bare areas of skin called **apteria** (Figure 21-8). However, the feathers in these tracts overlap one another to create the fully feathered look.

## FEATHER DAMAGE

Feathers are durable structures but still can be damaged. External parasites, such as some species of feather mite, can

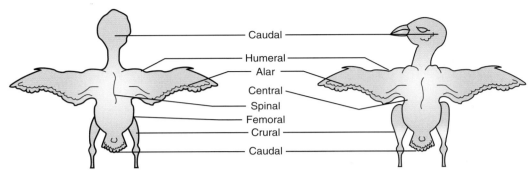

**FIGURE 21-8** Feather tracts.

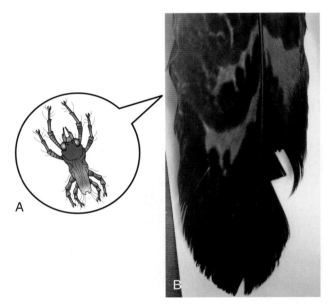

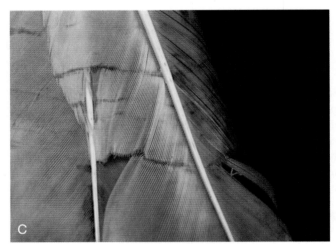

**FIGURE 21-9** Feather damage. **A**, Feather mite (not drawn to scale). **B**, Mite damage on the tail feather of a Great Gray Owl *(Strix nebulosa)*. **C**, Fault bars on the tail feather of a Red-Tailed Hawk.

chew and consume parts of the feather vanes, creating weak points (Figure 21-9, *A* and *B*). Damage also can occur from daily wear and tear. Often, the lighter tips of a bird's flight and tail feathers are worn off by the roughness of daily activities, giving the feathers a more iridescent appearance. In some species, such as Mallard ducks *(Anas platyrhynchos)* and European Starlings *(Sturnus vulgaris)*, this is most noticeable in the spring, when males of many species have lost their light feather tips and look more colorful before the breeding season.

Another cause of feather damage occurs during a feather's growth phase. If a feather is stressed during its growth, even for a few hours, there is an interruption in its blood flow. What develops is called a **fault bar**, or stress bar, which is characterized by a weakened area on the feather vane, where the barbs lack barbules (Figure 21-9, *C*). When the stressor is removed, the blood supply is returned and normal development continues. The most common stressor is a poor diet. An insufficient food supply or a food supply deficient in essential nutrients often creates fault bars on developing feathers. This can have a severe effect on the plumage of

nestling birds, because all of their flight feathers grow in at the same time. Any stressor that temporarily depletes the blood supply to these feathers creates fault bars on all of them.

## MOLTING

The process of feather replacement is called **molting**, and it occurs once to several times a year depending on the species. Molting occurs in a species-specific pattern that allows a bird to continue normal activities, such as procuring food, escaping from predators, reproducing, and finding safe roosting sites. In most species, feather replacement is symmetric; one or two pairs of flight feathers are molted at a time so that a bird still can fly adequately. One major exception is found in many species of waterfowl, which molt their flight feathers all at once after the breeding season. They are flightless during this time but can forage by grazing on land or in the water.

Between 4% and 12% of a bird's body weight is made up of feathers. Replacing them is a very energy-demanding process that requires a well-balanced diet. In many North

## CLINICAL APPLICATION

### Feather-Picking Disorder

One condition seen in many species of psittacine and some human-imprinted raptors is feather picking. Birds with this disorder preen excessively, removing most to all of their body feathers, especially on their chest and legs. Also, in severe cases, the skin surrounding the feathers is self-mutilated.

Causes of this disorder are either pathologic or psychologic. In the first category, toxins, bacteria, viruses, fungi, parasites, and malnutrition all can lead to feather picking. To determine the cause, a thorough physical examination must be conducted. Radiographs, blood samples for complete blood count and serum chemistry, cytology of feather pulp or of a local skin scraping, feather biopsy, and endoscopy are all diagnostic tools that can be used. If the problem does not appear to be physiologic, then attention must be turned to psychologic causes. These may include changes in the environment, diet, human exposure, boredom, sexual frustration, anxiety, or exposure to new pets. Many species of parrot, especially African Greys *(Psittacus erithacus)*, are very sensitive to these types of conditions.

Treatments for the disorder vary with the cause. Bacterial, viral, parasitic, and fungal infections can be treated with established protocols, and diet can be improved and varied. However, treatment for psychologic causes is more difficult, especially if the disorder cannot be attributed to a specific event or situation. Most often, changing components of the care and management of the bird is required, with no guarantee of inhibiting the feather-picking behavior.

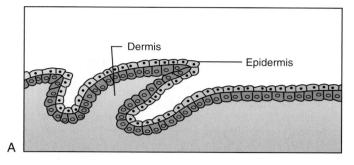

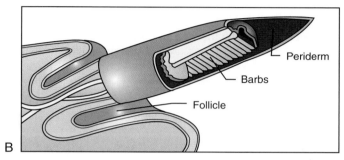

**FIGURE 21-10** Stages of feather growth. **A,** Feather papilla. **B,** Newly developing feather.

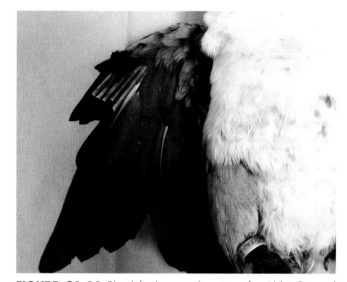

**FIGURE 21-11** Blood feathers on the wing of a White-Breasted Caique *(Pionites leucogaster).*

American species, the major annual molt is timed so that it occurs between the end of the breeding season and the beginning of migration. Food is usually abundant during this time, and a bird's energy can be directed to its growing feathers.

Feathers develop from papillae in the dermis layer of the skin (Figure 21-10, *A*). These papillae are located in the feather tracts and contain germ cells with the genetic information that dictates the type, size, and color of feathers. These cells are "activated" by physiologic and environmental factors. Increasing day length stimulates the pituitary and thyroid glands to produce hormones that stimulate molting, and sex hormones also may play a concurrent role.

Molting begins when a newly developing feather pushes an old one out (Figure 21-10, *B*). It then emerges from the skin and is covered by an epidermal covering called the **periderm**. As a bird begins to preen a growing feather, it gently removes the periderm, which can be seen as small, white flakes in the plumage. Blood vessels from the dermis reach into the new feather (through the superior umbiculus) to provide nourishment. When a feather is fully grown, the blood dries up, and the rachis is pinched closed under the skin.

During feather development, a growing feather is called a **blood feather**. Blood can be seen in the proximal part of the feather shaft during the entire growth phase

(Figure 21-11). Injury to a blood feather not only results in bleeding but can prevent a feather from developing normally until molted again.

### ✓ TEST YOURSELF 21-2

1. List three major functions of feathers.
2. What types of feather are the flight and tail feathers? Describe their microstructure.
3. Define a fault bar. What causes it?
4. What is a blood feather?
5. How do the wing and tail feathers differ between predatory and prey bird species?

## CLINICAL APPLICATION

### Clipping Wing Feathers

Many pet bird owners desire to have their bird's flight feathers clipped. The goal of clipping flight feathers is not to make a bird completely flightless, it is to prevent a bird from gaining lift while still allowing it to glide safely to the ground. This prevents a bird from injuring itself when out of its cage and prevents accidental escape. Numerous pet birds are lost every year because they fly out of open doors and windows.

Several patterns are used to clip a bird's wing feathers. The one chosen depends on the owner's wishes and the personal preference of the clinician. One technique that many practitioners prefer is to trim the outermost five to seven flight feathers under the overlying coverts, giving a smooth appearance to the wing. Another technique leaves the outer two to four primary

flight feathers intact and then trims the next five to seven flight feathers underneath the overlying covert feathers. One problem encountered with this pattern is that the long outer primaries are vulnerable to breakage. Whichever technique is used, the clipping should be done symmetrically on both wings.

Another consideration in feather clipping involves the presence of blood feathers. If blood feathers are present, it is advisable to wait until those feathers are completely developed before any are trimmed. If blood feathers are cut or damaged, a significant amount of bleeding often occurs. If waiting is not an option, completely developed feathers can be trimmed such that one feather remains intact on each side of every blood feather. Intact feathers on each side are needed to protect a growing feather from injury.

## CLINICAL APPLICATION

### Treating a Damaged Blood Feather

If a developing feather is cut, nicked, or otherwise damaged, it will often bleed profusely. To treat minor nicks or cuts, pressure can be applied to the affected area and, when dry, "Quick-stop" or a tissue glue may be applied to ensure coagulation. If more severe injury to a blood feather occurs, the most appropriate way to treat it depends on the type of bird. Many pet bird species are considered prey species and their major flight feathers are loosely seated in the follicles. Therefore, it is acceptable gently to pull out a damaged feather and pack the skin opening with "Quick-stop."

However, because developing feathers have a good nerve supply, anesthetizing the patient to prevent pain or discomfort

may be appropriate before pulling a large feather. If bleeding is persistent after a feather is pulled, the skin opening can be sutured closed for a few days to promote hemostasis, but it should be reopened to allow normal healing and new feather growth to begin.

In predatory bird species, such as birds of prey, the feathers are seated very strongly in the follicles, and pulling out a flight or tail feather can result in permanent follicle damage that results in abnormal feather growth or prevention of growth altogether. In these species, the proper approach to treating a damaged blood feather is to stop the bleeding and allow the damaged feather to be removed by the bird or to be molted during its normal cycle.

## MUSCULOSKELETAL SYSTEM

Feathers are not the only components of a bird that make it unique. A mammal or reptile with feathers still could not fly. Specially designed body systems that complement the feathers are necessary to create a structure that can support aerial locomotion. The first two systems we are going to look at are the skeleton and musculature.

### SKELETON

Although muscles do the work to create specific movements, they must be supported by a sturdy framework (Figure 21-12). In birds, this framework is highly specialized, because it must support two very different modes of locomotion: walking and flying. As we will see, the special design of the avian skeleton includes many unique features that all contribute to the creation of a remarkably lightweight but sturdy structure. The lightweight nature of the skeleton was a key component in the evolution of flight and can be explained by several general modifications:

- Reduction in the number of bones
- Fusion of bones to form plates that provide strength and simplify movements

- Reduction in the density of bones, which are relatively thin but strengthened by a network of internal bony braces
- Loss of internal bone matrix (the bones of birds are generally hollow and filled with air spaces)

Additional features of the avian skeleton that contribute to its lightness can be seen throughout its structure. To study these, we can divide the skeletal components into two major sections: the *axial skeleton* and the *appendicular skeleton*. The bones that provide the general framework of the avian body include the skull, vertebral column, and sternum and are collectively called the **axial skeleton**. The wings, shoulder bones, legs, and pelvic bones support locomotion and are collectively called the **appendicular skeleton**.

### AXIAL SKELETON

**SKULL.** The bird skull possesses several adaptations for lightness (Figure 21-13). The bones of the skull are thinner than in other animals, and instead of supporting heavy teeth, the jaws extend into a keratinized bill. The shape of the bill varies with the species, and it consists of a lower and upper component. The lower bill hinges on two small, movable bones called the *quadrates*. The upper bill has a somewhat

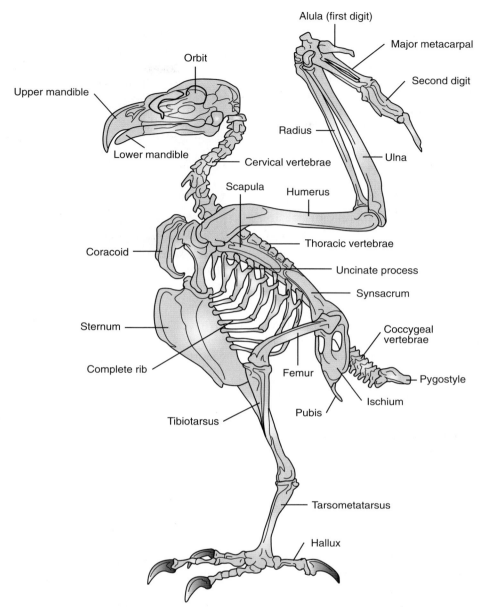

**FIGURE 21-12** Skeleton of a hawk.

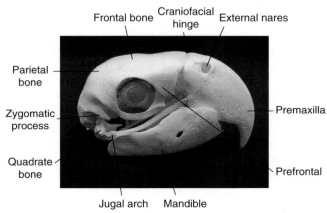

**FIGURE 21-13** Skull of a Blue and Gold Macaw.

flexible attachment to the skull and can move, although only slightly. Thus, birds actually can move their upper and lower bills independently, which gives them greater control in manipulating food and increases their gape. The gape is the size of the bird's mouth when open; the larger the gape, the larger the pieces of food that can be ingested.

Another prominent feature of the skull is the eye sockets. Good vision is important for an aerial creature, and thus a large portion of a bird's skull is devoted to supporting and protecting the eyes. The avian skull has large eye sockets that are bordered by a ring of protective bony plates called the **sclerotic ring**. In most species, a relatively small portion of the skull is devoted to the olfactory system and, as we will later see, the size of the ear canal varies with the species and its lifestyle.

**VERTEBRAL COLUMN.** The vertebral column of birds is similar to that of other animals in that it consists of five general groups of vertebrae: *cervical, thoracic, lumbar, sacral,* and *coccygeal.* Birds have fewer vertebrae than other animals in the three central regions, but they have more vertebrae in the cervical and coccygeal areas, allowing greater mobility of their neck and tail, respectively.

*CERVICAL VERTEBRAE.* The first cervical vertebra, the atlas, contains a single condyle (ball and socket type of structure) for attachment to the skull. This allows a greater range of head movements when compared with mammals, which have two condyles attaching the skull to the vertebral column. In addition, birds have more cervical vertebrae than mammals, ranging from 11 in parakeets to 25 in swans, whereas all mammals have seven. In birds, these vertebrae have special connecting surfaces that allow movement, thus contributing to the flexibility of their necks.

*THORACIC VERTEBRAE.* The thoracic vertebrae are rigid and provide a strong support for the rib cage. In birds, the first few ribs are relatively short and incomplete. The other ribs are complete, attach to the underside of the sternum, and possess a projection called the **uncinate process** that overlaps the adjoining rear rib to strengthen the rib cage (see Figure 21-12). One exception to the rigidity of these vertebrae is found in penguins; these birds swim like fish and require a high degree of flexibility in their backs.

*LUMBAR AND SACRAL VERTEBRAE.* These two groups of vertebra are also rigid. Several of the distal lumbar vertebrae fuse with the sacral vertebrae and the first few **coccygeal vertebrae** to form a light, strong, bony plate called the **synsacrum.** This plate in turn fuses with the pelvis to provide a stiff framework for support of the legs. When a bird lands, the synsacrum acts as a shock absorber to protect the legs and backbone from injury.

*COCCYGEAL VERTEBRAE.* Birds have an average of 12 coccygeal vertebrae. The first few are mobile to allow movement of the tail feathers during flight. The rest are fused into a bony structure called the **pygostyle** that supports the tail feathers.

**STERNUM.** In most species of bird, the sternum is large and concave. It not only protects the chest from traumatic injuries but also acts as the place of origin of the flight muscles (see Figure 21-18 later in the chapter). In strong fliers, the sternum has a large bony ridge, or **keel,** to which the muscles attach (Figure 21-14). In flightless birds, such as the ostrich, the sternum lacks a keel entirely.

### APPENDICULAR SKELETON
**PECTORAL GIRDLE.** The pectoral (shoulder) girdle consists of three pairs of bones: the *coracoids, scapulas,* and *clavicles* (see Figure 21-14). On each side, the coracoid and scapula are joined, forming a depression called the **glenoid**

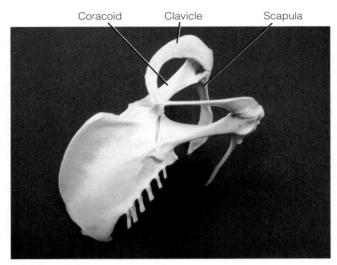

Coracoid    Clavicle    Scapula

**FIGURE 21-14** Anatomy of the pectoral girdle of a Rough-Legged Hawk *(Buteo lagopus).*

**cavity**, or *triosseal canal.* The wing attaches to the body by forming a joint in this cavity. During contraction of the powerful flight muscles, the strong, broad coracoids help to protect the sternum; the scapulas, positioned along the backbone, help protect the rib cage; and the clavicles, also known as the *wishbone,* are positioned outward and forward from the body and keep a bird's shoulders separated. Trauma to the pectoral girdle is not uncommon when birds collide with glass windows and doors (Box 21-1).

**WINGS.** The wings are connected to the body by forming a joint with the shoulder girdle. This joint is highly flexible, allowing rotation of the wing in several planes. The humerus extends from the shoulder to the elbow joint and possesses a **pectoral crest** for the attachment of wing muscles (Figure 21-15). The length of the humerus varies among species, being relatively short in birds that depend primarily on flapping flight and relatively long in birds that glide and soar.

The elbow joint is less flexible than the shoulder, and it only allows wing movement parallel to the wing. The radius and ulna extend from this joint to the wrist. In birds, the ulna has a larger diameter than the radius (it is the weight-bearing bone) and acts as an attachment point for the secondary flight feathers. These two bones create the forearm of the wing and slide past each other slightly during flight.

Extending from the shoulder to the wrist is a web of skin called the **patagium**, or *propatagium.* This skin is lightly vascularized and possesses a ligament that runs along its cranial edge. It provides elasticity to the wing and assists in the aerodynamics of flight. If a bird damages its patagium, it may be grounded permanently.

The wrist joint consists of two bones and, like the elbow, allows movement only in the plane of the wing. The first finger, called the **alula** bone, originates from the wrist and carries the alula feathers, which are important for steering. The major and minor metacarpal bones extend from the wrist and join with the second and third fingers near the

"Polly," a 7-year-old female Cockatiel, was presented to the veterinary clinic in the afternoon of 3/13. According to the owner, "Polly" had been perched on her shoulder the previous morning, was spooked by the household cat, and flew hard into the kitchen window. Subsequently, she appeared dazed, would not eat, and stood on the bottom of her cage.

Subjective: Adult female cockatiel with recent window strike. On a pelleted diet and no history of egg laying. Lethargic with eyes closed, feathers fluffed, slight left wing droop at shoulder.

Objective: Weight = 93 g, T = 106.5°F, RR = 45 per minute, HR 300 bpm. Small amount of blood present in oral cavity. Crepitation of L shoulder girdle during extension of L wing. PE otherwise WNL.

Assessment: Probable L shoulder girdle trauma, anorexia, lethargy.

Plan:
1. Whole body radiographs (VD/R lateral): closed simple midshaft fracture of L coracoids.
2. CBC/Avian Chemistry Panel: WNL except for elevated CPK (2300 IU) and low normal calcium (8.0 mg/dl).
3. LRS SQ at 50 ml/kg.
4. Meloxicam PO at 0.5 mg/kg q24h.
5. Stabilize overnight and consider release tomorrow.
6. Provide small convalescent cage with soft substrate.
7. Client education: cage rest with reduced activity for a minimum of 3 weeks, maintain Polly in small convalescent cage with a floor perch and food and water dishes on floor, administer meloxicam daily for 10 days (can be placed in favorite food), offer extra calcium (e.g., cuttle bone, egg with shell), discuss feather trimming.
8. Dispense meloxicam as per order.

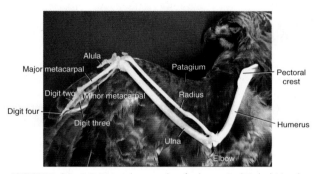

**FIGURE 21-15** Wing bones identified in a Red-Tailed Hawk.

distal end of the wing. These two fingers, along with the metacarpal bones, support the primary flight feathers.

**PELVIC GIRDLE.** The pelvic girdle provides a rigid framework for support of the legs (Figure 21-16). Each side is made up of three bones that join where the leg attaches to the body: the *ileum* is relatively broad and is fused to the synsacrum; the *ischium* and *pubis* are thin and long and are fused to the anterior ileum and directed rearward, parallel to the backbone. The distal ends of these three bones are not fused, leaving the lower part of the pelvis open. This provides room for the abdomen and facilitates egg laying in hens.

**LEGS.** The hip joint in birds is well hidden by thigh muscles and is the place where the femur attaches to the pelvis. The femur is often referred to as the *drumstick* and is relatively short but wide. It ends at the knee joint (stifle), where it is directed a little forward so that the lower part of a bird's leg is placed under its center of gravity. Similar to the pectoral crest of the humerus, the femur possesses two crests called the *greater* and *lesser* **trochanters**, where leg muscles attach. Two bones are located in the middle section of the leg, called the *tibiotarsus* and *fibula*. The fibula is relatively small in

diameter and acts as a splint. These two bones end at the ankle or **hock** joint, and the ankle itself consists of a single, elongated bone called the *tarsometatarsus*.

**FEET.** The bottom of a bird's foot is called the **metatarsal pad**. It is surrounded by two, three, or four toes, with the majority of species possessing four. Often one toe faces the rear and the other three face forward, which is called *anisodactyl*. However, in some species, such as parrots and woodpeckers, the second and third toes face forward, and the first and fourth are directed backward; this is known as **zygodactyl**. Owls, ospreys, and cuckoos also have this arrangement, but the fourth toe is opposable and can face either forward or backward.

The digits are referred to by a numbering system based on the number of joints they have. The rear toe is digit number one and has one joint, where it hinges to the metatarsal pad. Digit two is the innermost, medial digit and possesses two joints. The middle toe is digit three; it has three joints. The outer, lateral toe has four joints and is digit four.

## MUSCLES

The average bird has 175 to 200 muscles, many of which have been placed ventrally, near the center of gravity. Reptiles, the avian predecessor, have muscles on their dorsal surface. In birds, these have been replaced with strong plates of fused vertebrae, which protect the skeleton during contraction of the powerful flight muscles.

### CLASSIFICATION

As in other animals, the muscles of birds are classified as *smooth* or *striated* and *voluntary* or *involuntary*. Many of the muscles that contain smooth muscle fibers are also involuntary, stimulating the movement of the internal organs. Many muscles with striated fibers are skeletal and are associated with bone movement, so they are under voluntary control.

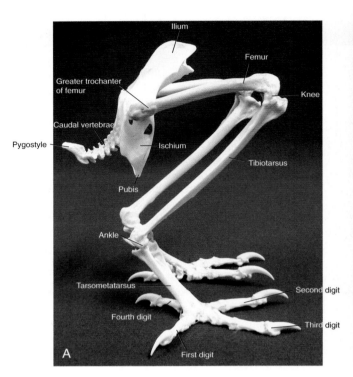
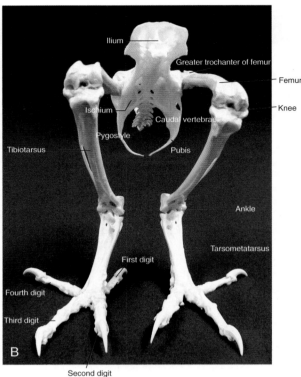

**FIGURE 21-16** Anatomy of the leg bones and pelvic girdle of a Great Horned Owl. **A**, Lateral view. **B**, Ventral view.

## CLINICAL APPLICATION

### Handling Birds

Understanding bird anatomy is critical to handling them safely and effectively. Different types of bird have different protective strategies and you must quickly restrain them and protect yourself from what can hurt you. For example, heron species will strike at your eyes with their long sharp bills and birds of prey have sharp beaks and talons, both of which they will use to defend themselves. Psittacines have extremely hard, sharp beaks and strong jaws that can inflict serious bite wounds. These birds are often grabbed/restrained by covering the body with a towel, quickly restraining the neck with one hand and gaining control of the legs/feet

with the other hand. The wings are contained with aid from the towel.

No matter which species you handle, for your safety and that of the patient, it is critical to have a firm hold. People that are afraid of hurting a bird while restraining it are often the ones who get hurt or allow a co-worker to be hurt. As you will learn later, birds have complete tracheal rings, so neck holds are safe if indicated. One action to be cautious about, however, is applying excessive pressure over the keel. Birds don't possess a diaphragm (inspiratory muscle), and air is pushed not pulled into the respiratory system. Thus, it is important not to press down on the keel too hard or this will prevent the passage of air.

---

Cardiac muscle is also striated but has its own intrinsic rhythm that does not require external innervation.

The skeletal muscles of birds can have white or red muscle fibers. Some muscles consist primarily of one type or the other, but many have a mixture of both. People celebrating the Thanksgiving holiday with a traditional turkey dinner are familiar with these fibers as they are often referred to as the "light meat" and "dark meat," respectively. White fibers are thick and have a low blood supply, have little myoglobin for carrying oxygen, and use stores of glycogen to sustain muscle contraction. They predominate in the flight muscles of short-distance fliers, such as chickens, quail, grouse, and many other gallinaceous birds that have rapid takeoffs but are capable of only short flights. If these birds are forced to fly repetitively,

they quickly become fatigued and cannot fly at all until they recover. In contrast, red fibers are thinner and have a rich supply of blood, fat, myoglobin, and mitochondria. Using these components, they can produce enough energy to sustain muscle contractions for long periods. Red fibers are found in the flight muscles of long-distance fliers, including many species of songbirds, water birds, pigeons, and birds of prey.

### WING MUSCLES

Wings possess several pairs of muscles that are each responsible for a specific action or counteraction: raising or depressing the leading edge of the wing, pulling the wing forward or backward, extending or flexing the wing, or controlling movements of the alula bone (thumb) (Figure 21-17). However, the

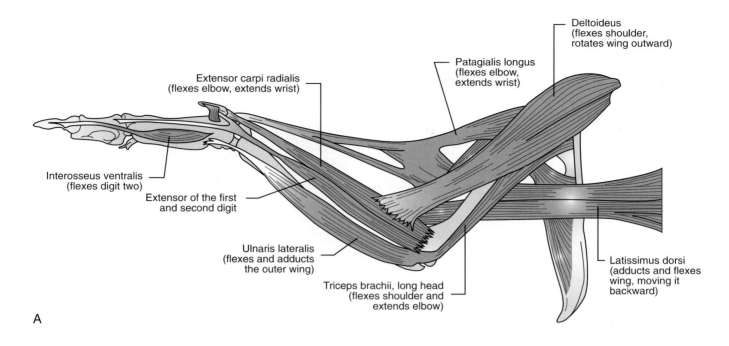

Deltoideus
(flexes shoulder,
rotates wing outward)

Patagialis longus
(flexes elbow,
extends wrist)

Extensor carpi radialis
(flexes elbow, extends wrist)

Interosseus ventralis
(flexes digit two)

Extensor of the first
and second digit

Ulnaris lateralis
(flexes and adducts
the outer wing)

Triceps brachii, long head
(flexes shoulder and
extends elbow)

Latissimus dorsi
(adducts and flexes
wing, moving it
backward)

A

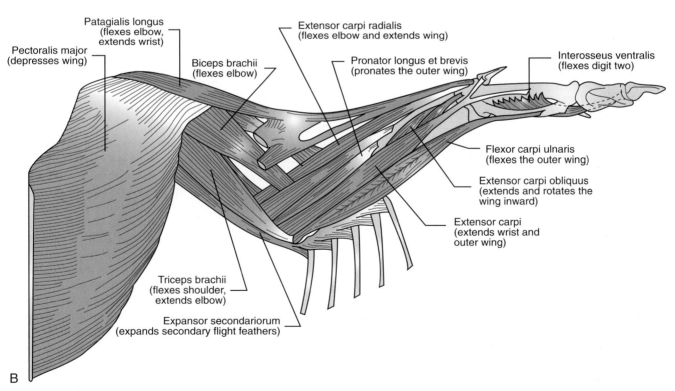

Patagialis longus
(flexes elbow,
extends wrist)

Extensor carpi radialis
(flexes elbow and extends wing)

Pectoralis major
(depresses wing)

Biceps brachii
(flexes elbow)

Pronator longus et brevis
(pronates the outer wing)

Interosseus ventralis
(flexes digit two)

Flexor carpi ulnaris
(flexes the outer wing)

Extensor carpi obliquus
(extends and rotates the
wing inward)

Extensor carpi
(extends wrist and
outer wing)

Triceps brachii
(flexes shoulder,
extends elbow)

Expansor secondariorum
(expands secondary flight feathers)

B

**FIGURE 21-17** Wing muscles and their function. **A,** Dorsal view. **B,** Ventral view.

two most prominent muscle pairs are those responsible for depressing and elevating the wing. Both pairs originate on the sternum but differ in where they insert (Figure 21-18). The larger, more superficial muscle is called the **pectoralis,** and it inserts on the underside of the humerus. When it contracts, it depresses the wing, causing the downstroke. This stroke requires a large muscle because it works against two resistant forces: gravity and a tight wing structure formed when the leading edge of each flight feather touches the adjacent feather. Because of its relatively large size and accessibility, the pectoralis is the muscle of choice for administering intramuscular injections, such as vitamins and antibiotics.

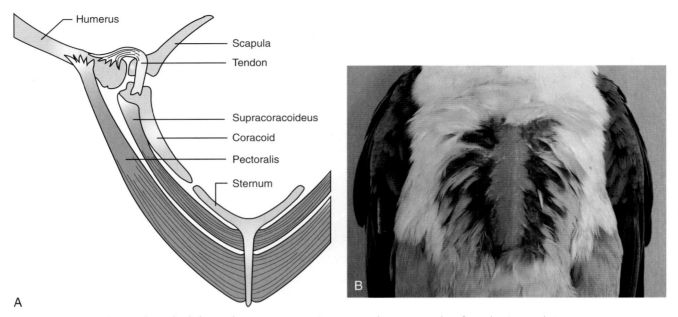

A

B

**FIGURE 21-18** Flight muscles. **A,** Cross section. **B,** Pectoralis major muscles of a White-Breasted Caique.

The smaller, deeper flight muscle is called the **supracoracoideus**; it turns into a tendon that passes through the glenoid cavity formed by the shoulder girdle and inserts on top of the humerus. When it contracts, it causes the counteraction, which is the elevation of the wing during the upstroke. During this stroke, the flight feathers separate slightly from each other, allowing air to pass through. This creates less resistance and allows the wing to move more easily. In strong, long-distance fliers, the two pairs of flight muscles constitute between 20% and 25% of a bird's weight.

### LEG MUSCLES

Like the wing muscles, the leg muscles also have been moved close to the center of gravity. The majority are located in the thigh region over the femur, a smaller number are located over the tibiotarsus, and very few are found over the tarsometatarsus (Figure 21-19). The large group of muscles over the femur can control movements in the distal leg and toes via strong tendons. For example, in perching species, tendons that control movement of the toes originate from flexor muscles in the thigh and extend over the heel joint into the digits. Extensor tendons run down the front of the tibiotarsus and metatarsus, whereas the flexor tendons run along the back. The flexor tendons sit in a groove at the top of the metatarsus. When a bird bends its legs to perch, the tendons also bend and pull the toes closed around the perch. This is called the *perching reflex* and allows a bird to grip its perch firmly while sleeping.

### MUSCLES OF THE HEAD AND NECK

The most pronounced muscles of the head are the jaw muscles, which control the beak. The extent of this musculature varies among species and is generally correlated with a bird's diet. For example, species such as parrots use their beaks to crack open large, coarse seeds, so they have relatively large and strong jaw muscles compared with species, such as doves, that consume smaller seeds, or those that consume insects.

A bird has great flexibility in its neck. It has several thin, stringy neck muscles that weave through each other and allow movement in different directions. Some muscles are attached to the connective tissue, or fascia, of adjacent neck muscles. When one muscle is stimulated, neighboring muscles contract, making a variety of movements possible. This is best demonstrated in parrot species that move their heads up and down, left and right, and many combinations thereof.

One highly specialized neck muscle in birds is referred to as a *hatching muscle*. This muscle, located on the dorsal side of a chick's head, develops during the embryonic stage and is needed to help a chick break out of its shell. It is largest a day or two before hatching, and once a chick reaches the outside world it rapidly atrophies.

From the tip of a bird's beak all the way down to the tips of its claws, a bird's bone and muscle framework is uniquely designed to support aerial locomotion. Now, let us take a peek at the organ systems that actually drive this incredible flying machine.

> ✓ **TEST YOURSELF 21-3**
> 1. Describe the attachment of the skull to the vertebral column. What does this type of attachment provide?
> 2. List the bones in the avian wing from the shoulder to the wing tip.
> 3. List the bones in the avian leg beginning at the hip and extending down to the toes.
> 4. List the two types of skeletal muscle fiber and describe their energy use.
> 5. Why can a bird perch while sleeping?

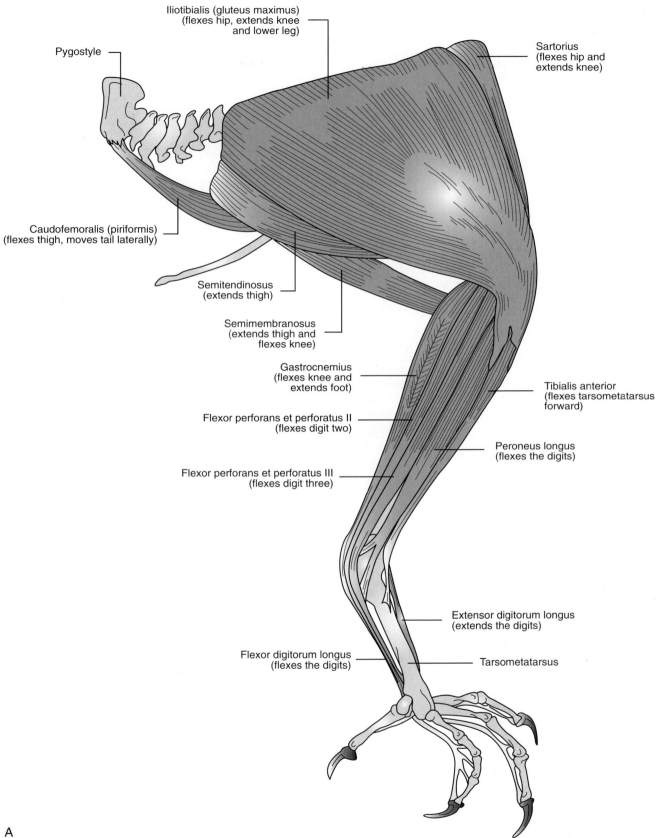

Iliotibialis (gluteus maximus)
(flexes hip, extends knee
and lower leg)

Pygostyle

Sartorius
(flexes hip and
extends knee)

Caudofemoralis (piriformis)
(flexes thigh, moves tail laterally)

Semitendinosus
(extends thigh)

Semimembranosus
(extends thigh and
flexes knee)

Gastrocnemius
(flexes knee and
extends foot)

Tibialis anterior
(flexes tarsometatarsus
forward)

Flexor perforans et perforatus II
(flexes digit two)

Peroneus longus
(flexes the digits)

Flexor perforans et perforatus III
(flexes digit three)

Extensor digitorum longus
(extends the digits)

Flexor digitorum longus
(flexes the digits)

Tarsometatarsus

**A**

**FIGURE 21-19** Leg muscles and their function. A, Lateral view.

*Continued*

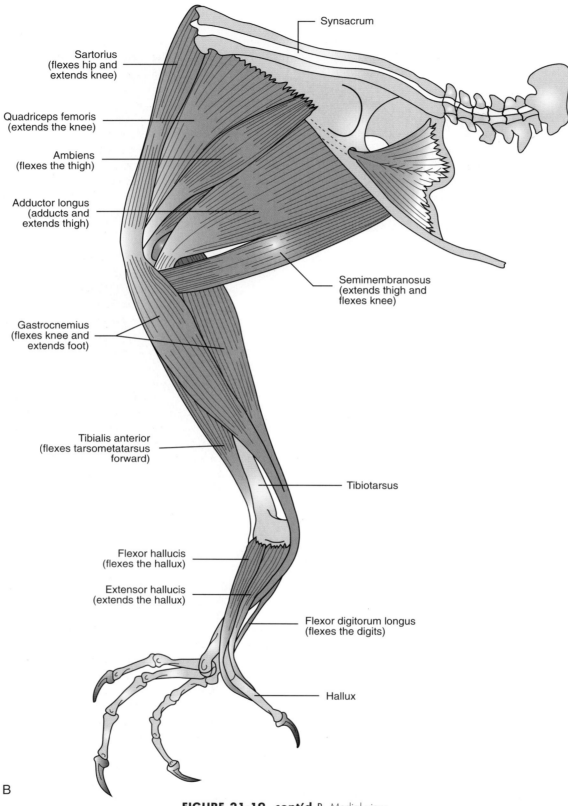

**FIGURE 21-19, cont'd** B, Medial view.

## SENSE ORGANS

The term "bird brain" has been used in reference to a small brain and therefore a lack of intelligence. This usage is misleading; in fact, the avian brain is large in proportion to its body size compared with the brains of all other vertebrates, with the exception of mammals. The location of the control centers within the brain that receive nervous stimuli from the senses is similar to that in mammals (see Chapter 10). In birds, the control centers for vision and hearing are relatively large, whereas those for taste, touch, and smell are relatively small (Figure 21-20).

## VISION

The phrase "I'm going to watch you like a hawk" alludes to the fact that the sense of vision is highly developed in birds. An aerial creature needs good vision to fly at variable speeds, find food, escape predators, identify individuals, and participate in courtship rituals. The optic lobes take up the majority of the midbrain, and a large part of the avian skull is devoted to housing and protecting the eyes. The shape of the eyes is determined by the orbits. Unlike mammals, which all have round eyes, bird eyes can be round, flat, or tubular, depending on the species. Generally, diurnal birds have round or relatively flat eyes (hawks and swans, respectively), whereas nocturnal species (owls) have tubular eyes (Figure 21-21). In tubular eyes, the diameter of the pupil is large relative to the size of the retina, and thus more light can be gathered. The eyes fill the eye sockets, leaving little room for muscles or movement.

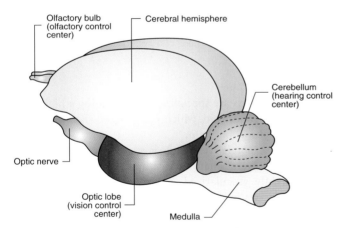

**FIGURE 21-20** Bird's brain. Side view.

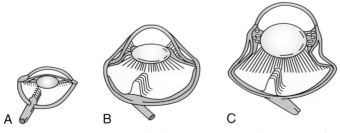

**FIGURE 21-21** Shapes of the avian eye. A, Flat. B, Round. C, Tubular.

In birds, the position of the eyes on the head differs among species and appears to depend on their feeding habits. For example, seed and grain eaters have eyes placed laterally to allow them to view potential predators from many angles. Owls have eyes that primarily face forward, thereby increasing their binocular vision but reducing their overall field of vision. Perhaps the most unusual placement occurs in bitterns, which have eyes placed low on their heads. These heronlike birds feed in shallow water and may use the low eye placement to get a better view of the water. Also, when an intruder approaches, a bittern goes into a protective posture in which it freezes in an erect position with its bill tip facing directly up. This puts its eyes in the best position to view the intruder.

### ANATOMY OF THE EYE

The general structure of the avian eye is similar to that of mammals, with a few exceptions (Figure 21-22, *A*). The avian eye consists of three layers of tissue. The outermost layer is referred to as the **fibrous tunic**. It consists of the *sclera* in the back, which functions to protect the eye, and toward the front it becomes the transparent *cornea*. At this transition point, the sclera is reinforced by a ring of small bones called the *sclerotic ring*.

The cornea is protected by three eyelids: an *upper lid*, a *lower lid*, and a third lid called the **nictitating membrane** (Figure 21-23). This membrane is thin and transparent and consists of specialized epithelial cells that brush moisture over the eye from the nasal corner laterally. It possesses striated muscles that allow a bird to control its movement voluntarily. In many species of diving birds, such as loons and some ducks, the nictitating membrane has a clear window in its center to act as a contact lens under water.

The middle layer is referred to as the **uveal tunic**. It is a vascular, pigmented layer consisting of the *choroid* in back, the *iris* in front, and *ciliary*, or *striated, muscles*. In birds, the iris contains striated muscles that allow voluntary control over the size of the pupils. Thus, a pupillary light response is not a good diagnostic indicator in birds.

The inner layer is referred to as the **neural tunic**. It consists of the *retina*, which is composed of photoreceptor cells and neural cells that transmit light images to the brain.

The lens and anterior chamber of the avian eye are similar to those of mammals, as is the posterior chamber (vitreous) with the exception of the presence of the **pecten**. The pecten is a highly vascular, ribbonlike structure attached to the retina (see Figure 21-22, *B* and *C*). It floats in the vitreous humor in the direction of the lens and is believed to distribute nutrition to the eye. More than 30% of traumatized wild birds suffer from hemorrhages arising from the pecten. These are only detected when the intraocular eye structures are examined (Korbel, 2001).

### PHOTORECEPTION

Birds possess **rods** and **cones** that are similar in function to those in mammals (see Chapter 10). Nocturnal birds, such as many species of owls, have more rods than cones in their

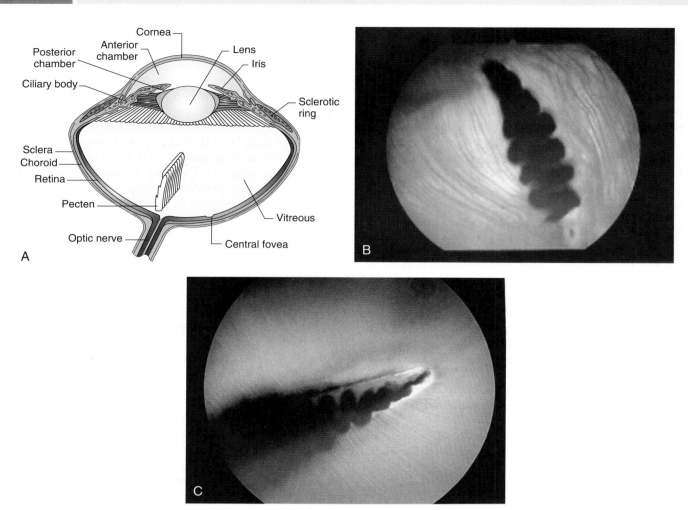

**FIGURE 21-22** The avian eye. **A**, Diagram of transverse section. **B**, Ophthalmoscopic view through the pupil of intra-ocular structures in Great Horned Owl (nocturnal bird). **C**, Ophthalmoscopic view through the pupil of a Red-Tailed Hawk (diurnal bird). (**B** and **C**, Courtesy of R. Korbel.)

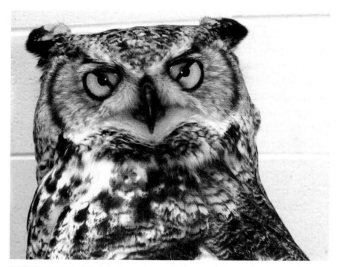

**FIGURE 21-23** Nictitating membranes of a Great Horned Owl. (Photo by Gail Buhl.)

retinas. These rods are specialized in containing a high concentration of rhodopsin, which is the night-vision pigment that aids in absorbing light.

Birds have a relatively high level of visual acuity that results from several anatomic features. First, a bird's retina is only lightly vascularized. A reduced number of blood vessels decreases interruption of an image as it reaches the back of the eye. Second, a bird's retina is packed with photoreceptor cells—sometimes twice as many as in other vertebrates. Think about the difference between a 2 and a 10 megapixel digital camera. The more megapixels a camera has, the greater the picture clarity achieved. The avian eye has more cells that receive and transmit information, thus resulting in a clearer image in the brain. A third factor that contributes to the superior visual acuity of birds is the connection between the photosensitive cells and nerve fibers. In many avian species, each cone has a single connection with a bipolar nerve cell. This means that each cone has individual representation in the brain. In mammals, multiple cones converge on a bipolar cell, and thus their information is pooled, leading to a lower level of visual acuity.

Like the eyes of other vertebrates, the avian eye possesses a central, funnel-shaped area containing a high concentration of cones. This area is called the central **fovea** and is the area of sharpest vision. However, many diurnal birds, such as parrots, hawks, and hummingbirds, also have a second fovea placed temporally. This provides another highly sensitive area and helps in binocular vision.

## COLOR VISION

Cone cells in the retina are responsible for processing color images. Each cone contains one colored oil droplet. Diurnal birds typically have yellow, red, green, and orange droplets, whereas nocturnal birds have pale or transparent droplets. How these droplets function is not completely understood, but they have a role in increasing the receptive ability of visual pigments.

## VISUAL SPECTRUM

Birds can see a wide spectrum of light wavelengths. Although they cannot see infrared light, many diurnal species can see ultraviolet (UV) light. For example, American Kestrels, which are small falcons *(Falco sparverius)*, can find a mouse by seeing the UV light reflected off its urine. The ability to detect differences in the reflection of UV light is important in other species as well. Some use this ability for distinguishing between ripe and unripe fruit, and others use it to identify males versus females in species that have similar plumages. Ostriches and nocturnal species, such as owls and kiwis, cannot detect UV light.

## HEARING AND EQUILIBRIUM

Hearing is another extremely important sense for birds. It is critical for daily activities, such as finding food, hiding from predators, defending territories, and communicating with other members of a family or flock. Although the structure

of the avian ear is simpler than that of mammals, it has exceptional acoustic ability.

## ANATOMY OF THE EAR

A bird's ears are located on the sides of its head, behind and slightly below its eyes. They consist of three ear chambers: *external, middle,* and *inner* (Figure 21-24). The external ear is an opening that funnels sound into the eardrum. It is often bordered with special auricular feathers that protect the ear during turbulent flight and yet still allow sound to pass through.

The external ear is separated from the middle ear by the **tympanic membrane**. The middle ear consists of a single bone, the **columella**, which connects to the inner ear and acts as a funnel to transmit sound; this contrasts with mammals, which possess three middle ear bones. The *cochlear window* is located adjacent to where the columella connects with the inner ear. It has a flexible membrane that protects the inner ear from pressure damage.

The inner ear is similar to that in mammals. It consists of a membranous labyrinth, which functions to maintain balance and equilibrium, and the cochlea, which converts sound waves into nerve impulses that are sent to the brain for processing.

## HEARING IN NOCTURNAL OWLS

Hearing in birds reaches its highest level of development in highly nocturnal owls, such as the Common Barn Owl *(Tyto alba)*, Long-Eared Owl *(Asio otus)*, and Northern Saw-Whet Owl *(Aegolius acadicus)*. These species can hunt mice and voles in extremely low light conditions, relying on their incredible hearing ability to capture prey. They have a fleshy flap of skin, called the **operculum**, at each external ear opening that helps to funnel the sound into the ears (Figure 21-25, *A*). In addition, their ear openings are asymmetric,

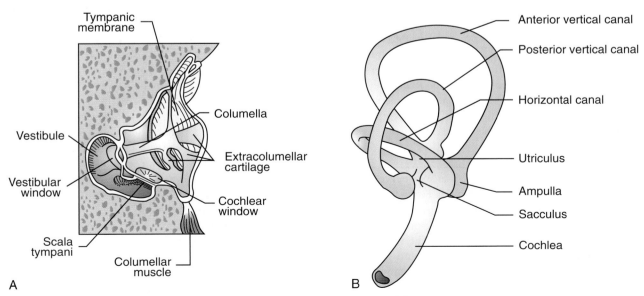

**FIGURE 21-24** Anatomy of the avian ear. **A,** Middle ear. **B,** Inner ear.

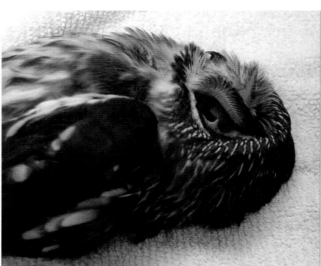
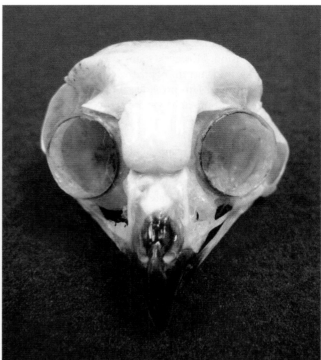

**FIGURE 21-25** Ears of an owl. A, Operculum and outer ear of a Northern Saw-Whet Owl *(Aegolius acadicus)*. B, Skull of Northern Saw-Whet Owl showing asymmetric ear placement.

with one slightly above the midpoint of the eye and the other slightly below it (Figure 21-25, *B*). This feature helps with the vertical location of sound. These nocturnal owls also have large eardrums, columellae, and cochleas, and also a well-developed acoustic center in the hindbrain. In the Common Barn Owl, the number of auditory neurons this center receives is about 95,000, compared with 27,000 in the Carrion Crow *(Corvus corone)* (Welty and Baptista, 1988).

## TASTE

Birds have a relatively poor sense of taste. They possess taste buds, but these are few in number and are scattered on the sides of their tongue and soft palate. Compared with humans, who have about 10,000 taste buds, some parrots have up to 400, and adult domestic pigeons *(Columba livia)* only have about 50 to 60 (Terres, 1980). Based on experiments with pigeons and chickens, sensitivities and thresholds for bitter, salty, and sour tastes appear to be species specific.

## TOUCH

The skin of birds contains two types of sensory nerve ending that respond to pain, heat, cold, and touch. For many species, the sense of touch is important for finding food. Therefore the nerve endings responsible for touch are often prevalent in the tongues, palates, and bills of birds. The first type of nerve ending is called a *Grandry's corpuscle*, and groups of these are located in the tongue and palate of many species that dig for food, such as woodcock and sandpipers (Figure 21-26, *A*). The second type of nerve ending is called a *Herbst*

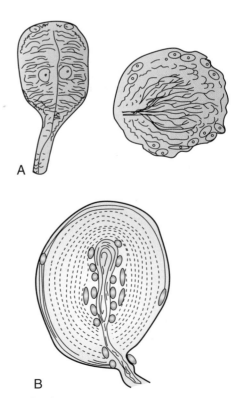

**FIGURE 21-26** Touch corpuscles. A, Grandry's. B, Herbst.

*corpuscle* (Figure 21-26, *B*). These are also often located in areas of the mouth, such as on the tongues of woodpeckers, on the palates and beaks of ducks, and on the mouth folds of young birds. In addition, Herbst corpuscles are located in the cloaca, legs, wings, uropygial gland, and the bases of many feathers, including the primary flight feathers. These corpuscles are very responsive to even the slightest feather movement. This characteristic explains why birds are sensitive when just the tips of their feathers are touched.

## SMELL

The sense of smell varies widely in birds. In a few species, such as the Turkey Vulture *(Cathartes aura)*, Northern Bobwhite Quail *(Colinus virginianus)*, and albatrosses, the sense of smell appears to be well developed and important for

locating food. Water birds have a less developed but adequate sense of smell. Goslings learn to accept or reject food by smell at an early age, and Mallard hens emit a breeding odor that stimulates drakes. The sense of smell in passerines and raptors is thought to be poor, but additional research needs to be conducted.

## ENDOCRINE SYSTEM

The function of the endocrine system in birds is similar to that in mammals (see Chapter 11). The hormones produced by the glands influence many body systems and control such things as the stress response, courtship and reproduction, body growth, and, in birds, the process of molting. There are seven major endocrine glands; and the pancreas, in addition to having a digestive function, also has an endocrine component (Figure 21-27). As we continue our study of the avian body, we will touch on the function of some of these glands and the substances they produce (Box 21-2).

## DIGESTIVE SYSTEM

Birds have a rapid metabolic rate and thus a high energy demand. To meet this need, they have a digestive system that

---

> **✓ TEST YOURSELF 21-4**
>
> 1. What are the two most important senses in birds?
> 2. Which eye structures are found in birds but not in mammals?
> 3. Where are the bird's ears located?
> 4. Name the two types of sensory nerve ending in the skin and describe where they are located.

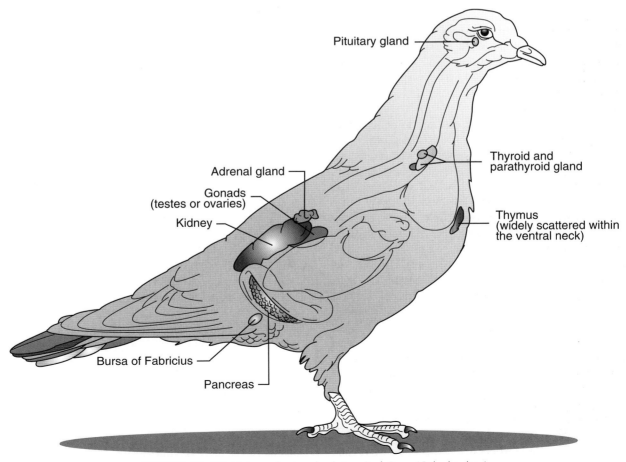

**FIGURE 21-27** Major endocrine glands in a Rock Dove *(Columbia livia)*.

**BOX 21-2** | Avian Endocrine Glands and Their Function

**Adrenal Gland**

Secretes a stress hormone (corticosterone), sex hormones (androgens in males and estrogens and progesterone in females), and hormones that control concentrations of minerals in the body.

**Bursa of Fabricius**

Stimulates production of antibodies and lymphocytes.

**Gonads**

Testes in the male produce testosterone, ovaries in the female produce estrogens and testosterone. These regulate the secondary sex characteristics and control behavioral responses to the opposite sex.

**Pancreas**

Synthesizes hormones that regulate blood sugar and sugar metabolism in the liver (insulin, glucagon, and somatostatin). Also produces pancreatic polypeptide that inhibits gastrointestinal motility and secretion and induces a sense of satiety.

**Parathyroid Gland**

Produces parathormone that regulates calcium and phosphorus levels in the body.

**Pituitary Gland**

Anterior lobe secretes hormones that regulate other glands: thyroid-stimulating hormone (thyroid), adrenocorticotropic hormone (adrenal glands), follicle-stimulating hormone, luteinizing hormone, prolactin (female reproductive system). Posterior lobe secretes antidiuretic hormone to conserve water in the kidney and oxytocin to stimulate uterine contractions for egg laying.

**Thymus Gland**

Stimulates production of antibodies and lymphocytes.

**Thyroid Gland**

Secretes thyroxin to regulate growth of the body and feathers and may stimulate the migration urge.

---

can absorb energy from foods in a rapid and efficient manner with relatively little waste. Depending on the species of bird and its diet, birds assimilate between 60% and 99% of the energy in the food they consume.

## ANATOMY

The basic anatomy of a bird's digestive system is similar to that of reptiles and mammals. However, it has been refined and adapted to meet the high and variable energy demands of different bird species (Figure 21-28).

### BEAKS AND BILLS

The beaks of birds vary with their diet and foraging strategies. Seed eaters have a thick beak that acts as a forceps and crushes their food; woodpeckers have a heavy, blunt beak that acts as a chisel to bore holes; raptors have a sharp-edged, hooked beak for tearing meat; and shorebirds have a long, delicate beak to probe for food in sandy areas. Beaks enable birds to find, grab, and sometimes kill food items and to tear food into smaller pieces to begin the digestive process.

### MOUTH

A bird's mouth consists of a hard upper palate, a soft lower palate, a distinctive tongue, salivary glands, and scattered taste buds (see Figure 21-37). In some species of finches and pelicans, the soft palate enlarges to become a pouch for temporary storage of food. The tongue aids in manipulating food and moving it to the back of the mouth for easy swallowing. In parrots it is highly muscular, but in many other species it has few muscles and is moved by muscles of the jaw apparatus. Most birds have salivary glands located in the back of the mouth (pharynx), but seed eaters also have them in the soft palate. In these birds, the saliva moistens and lubricates dry seeds, and the glands secrete a starch-digesting

enzyme. Some species, such as swifts and swallows, use dried saliva to build nests, and woodpeckers use their sticky saliva to hold on to insects.

### ESOPHAGUS

The esophagus is a somewhat muscular tube that extends from the pharynx to the stomach along the right side of the neck. The lining contains mucous glands that lubricate food to facilitate its passage into the stomach. In several species, the esophagus expands over the interclavicular space to create a **crop**, which is a storage pouch for food. This crop can be a dilation of the esophagus, as seen in some fish eaters; a single pouch, as seen in parrots, grain eaters, and hawks; or a double pouch, as seen in pigeons. Birds that have well-developed crops generally eat a few larger meals per day instead of foraging and nibbling all day long.

Little if any digestion occurs in the crop. Its main function is to store, lubricate, and regulate the passage of food. In some species, it is modified for additional purposes. For example, in pigeons and doves, the mucosal lining of the crop thickens at breeding time and is broken down to form "pigeon milk" that is fed to recently hatched chicks. Also, the crop lining in insect-eating birds consists of a heavy epithelium to give protection from insects that are swallowed alive.

### STOMACH

A bird's stomach consists of two separate components: the *glandular stomach* and the *muscular stomach*. The anterior, glandular stomach is called the **proventriculus**. This structure is unique to birds and is the organ in which chemical digestion begins. Its mucosa consists of columnar epithelial cells and mucosal glands that produce mucus to moisten food. The submucosal layer possesses digestive glands. These glands secrete pepsin, which begins the breakdown of proteins, and hydrochloric acid, which increases the acidity of

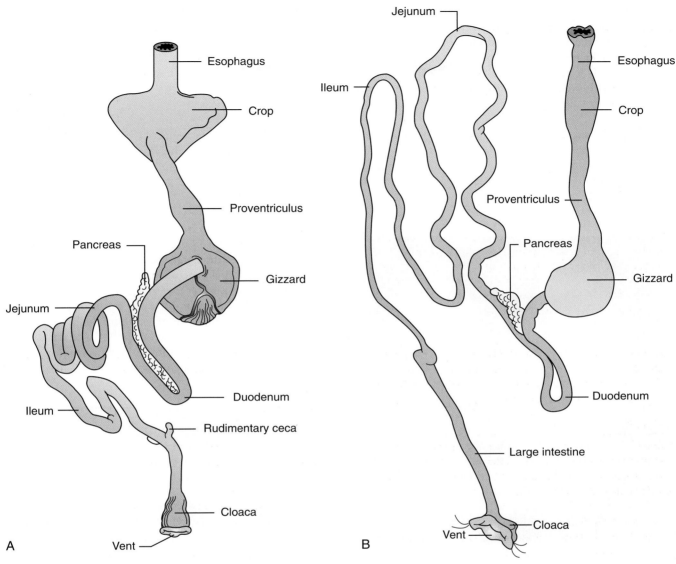

**FIGURE 21-28** General diagrams of avian digestive system. **A**, Rock Dove. **B**, Hawk.

the stomach to enhance the action of digestive enzymes. In birds, the gastric juices can have a pH between 0.7 and 2.5.

The muscular stomach is called the **ventriculus** or **gizzard**. It consists of distinct bands of striated muscles that work to grind food components, such as bones, scales, and nuts. Also, many seed eaters and grain-eating birds actively seek and ingest small pieces of grit to aid in grinding food. In chickens, this grit enhances the digestibility of grain by about 10% (Welty and Baptista, 1988).

Some characteristics of the gizzard are species specific. For example, the thickness of its walls varies with diet. Grain eaters, such as turkeys, have the thickest gizzard walls and can pulverize hard objects, such as steel needles and walnuts. The gizzard walls in carnivores are relatively thin, and those in omnivores are quite variable. In addition, the gizzards of owls, hawks, swifts, grouse, and herons grind indigestible food components into a **pellet** that is then regurgitated (Figure 21-29). Egestion of pellets in these species can

be used as a clinical indicator of normal gastrointestinal motility.

### LIVER

The liver in birds is bilobed, and the right lobe is usually larger than the left. The liver stores excess fats and sugars, makes certain proteins, produces bile to neutralize the stomach acid and emulsify fats, and excretes waste products from the blood.

### PANCREAS

The pancreas is a relatively large gland in birds and rests in the loop of the duodenum. It is larger in fish eaters and grain eaters and smaller in carnivores. It serves both an exocrine and endocrine function (see Chapter 11). In birds, the endocrine portion of the pancreas occupies more tissue mass than in mammals, and the distribution of endocrine cells within the pancreas is more random.

## DUODENUM

The duodenum, or small intestine, is the major organ responsible for the digestion and absorption of nutrients. In meat and fruit eaters, it is relatively short and thin walled. In seed eaters, it is long with several loops. In fish eaters, the duodenum is also relatively long but small in diameter.

## CECA

Ceca are paired sacs located at the junction of the small and large intestines in some species. Although their function continues to be studied, they appear to be important for water reabsorption and the bacterial fermentation of cellulose. The output from these sacs is dark brown and moist and has a distinctive odor. It is excreted a few times per week, independently of the intestinal fecal material. Ceca are present in ducks, geese, Galliformes, and owls but are absent in other species, such as parrots, hawks, passerines, and woodpeckers.

## LARGE INTESTINE

The large intestine is the segment that extends from the end of the small intestine to the cloaca. Its major role is the reabsorption of water and minerals.

## CLOACA

The cloaca is located at the end of the digestive tract and is divided into three sections. The anterior section is called the **coprodeum** and receives excrement from the intestine. The **urodeum** receives discharge from the kidneys and genital ducts. The posterior **proctodeum** is accessed by the other two sections, and it stores the excrement (see Figure 21-40). It is closed by a muscular anus that has powerful ejection muscles for the elimination of waste products through an opening called the **vent** (see Figure 21-28). The waste products are organized into a **mute**, consisting of a dark fecal center surrounded by a ring of urates (Figure 21-30).

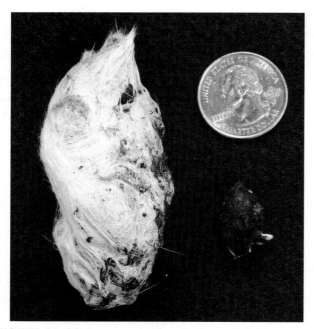

**FIGURE 21-29** Regurgitated pellets. **A**, Snowy Owl (*Nyctea scandiaca*). **B**, Northern Saw-Whet Owl.

---

### ✓ TEST YOURSELF 21-5

1. Which endocrine gland secretes hormones that regulate molting and the migratory urge?
2. List the endocrine and exocrine functions of the pancreas.
3. On which side of the neck is the esophagus located in birds? Does this differ from mammals?
4. List the two separate components of the avian stomach and their functions.
5. What is a mute? What can it tell us about the health of a bird?

---

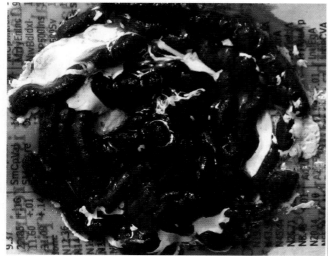
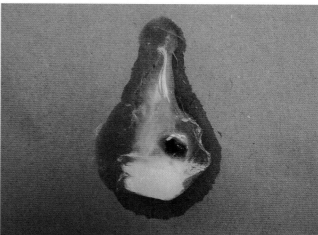

**FIGURE 21-30** Normal mutes. **A**, Blue and Gold Macaw. **B**, Red-Tailed Hawk.

## CLINICAL APPLICATION

### Mutes: A Diagnostic Tool

Evaluation of a bird's mutes is an important diagnostic tool in assessing overall health. In many species the mutes normally have a dark fecal center surrounded by a white ring of urates. However, the color and consistency of a bird's mutes can be altered by diet, parasites, or disease, and any change in an individual bird's normal excreta should be investigated to discover the cause. For example, parrots fed a fruity, pelleted diet often have a variety of colors to their mutes, and hawks fed day-old cockerels will have gold fecal centers in their mutes instead of dark ones. These are normal changes and can be explained by the diet. Birds suffering from the actions of some intestinal parasites, such as coccidia, often have a tinge of green in their output, and sometimes blood. An infection with clostridial bacteria often presents as a copious amount of light brown runny mutes. These conditions need to be diagnosed and treated.

Obtaining a complete patient history is important in evaluating these clinical observations. This is easy in the case of pet birds; however, for wild birds with unknown histories, extensive laboratory testing may be necessary to explain abnormal output from the digestive and urinary systems. Tests performed often include fecal analysis for parasites, fecal Gram stain for bacteria, a complete blood count, and a chemistry profile to assess organ function. Blood lead levels are also checked in wild species highly vulnerable to lead poisoning, such as Bald Eagles (*Haliaeetus leucocephalus*), Golden Eagles (*Aquila chrysaetos*), and vultures, as well as in pet birds.

## CIRCULATORY SYSTEM

It has been said that the way to a man's heart is through his stomach. Although this phrase does not directly refer to the physiologic functions of the two organs, it can be used to explain an important connection between them. The digestive system, as mentioned previously, functions to break down foodstuffs into nutrients that can be absorbed into the blood. From there, the circulatory system takes over to deliver nutrient-rich blood to the tissues and remove metabolic waste. The circulatory system also functions to carry oxygen, minerals, and hormones to cells; in addition, blood helps to control and prevent diseases, and to maintain body temperature.

## ANATOMY

### HEART

In birds, as in mammals, the driving force behind this delivery system is a four-chambered heart that consists of a right atrium, right ventricle, left atrium, and left ventricle (Figure 21-31, *A*). The right side of the heart is smaller and less muscular, pumping blood only to the lungs. The left side is larger, and it has well-developed muscles that pump blood to the rest of the body. The heart is located in the cranial portion of the thoracoabdominal space (Figure 21-31, *B*). It is enclosed by a thin, fibrous pericardial sac, which contains fluid that aids in the lubrication of the heart muscle. This sac adheres to several internal surfaces to keep the heart anchored in place.

### VESSELS

The heart is supported by a group of vessels that provide channels for the passage of blood. Arteries carry oxygenated blood from the heart to the tissues, and veins carry blood containing metabolic waste products away from the tissues and back to the heart (Figure 21-32, *A*). Capillaries are small vessels in which the exchange of gases and nutrients occurs. To meet the specific demands of the avian

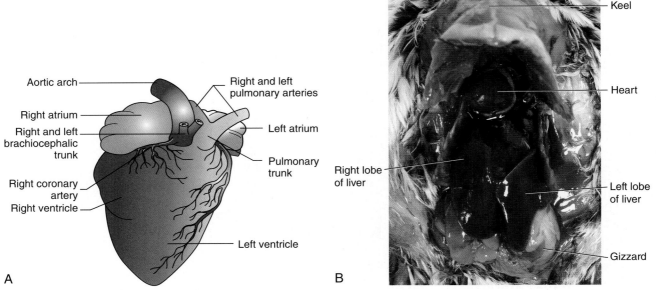

**FIGURE 21-31** The avian heart. **A**, Diagram of ventral surface. **B**, Location of the heart in a Coturnix Quail (*Coturnix japonica*).

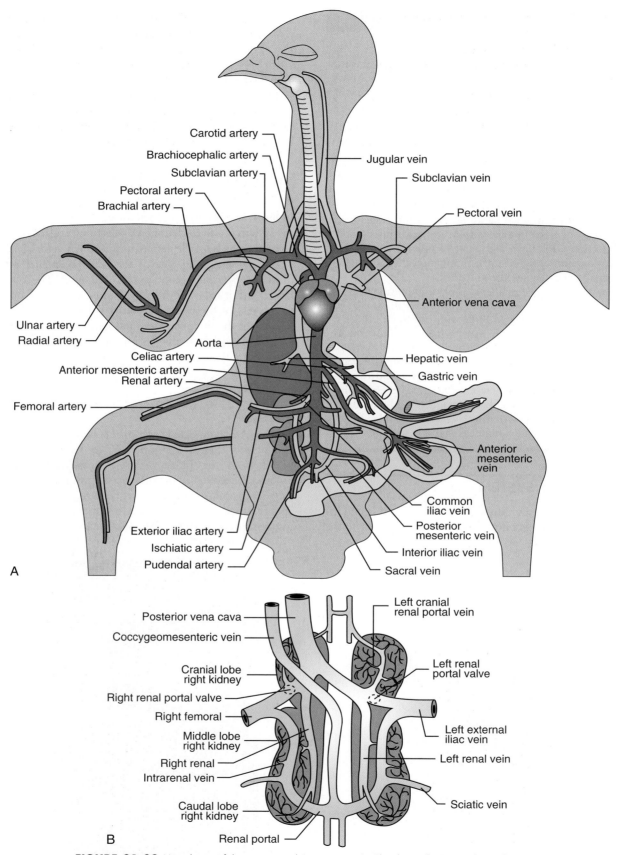

Carotid artery

Brachiocephalic artery

Subclavian artery

Pectoral artery

Brachial artery

Jugular vein

Subclavian vein

Pectoral vein

Ulnar artery

Radial artery

Aorta

Celiac artery

Anterior mesenteric artery

Renal artery

Femoral artery

Anterior vena cava

Hepatic vein

Gastric vein

Anterior mesenteric vein

Common iliac vein

Posterior mesenteric vein

Interior iliac vein

Sacral vein

Exterior iliac artery

Ischiatic artery

Pudendal artery

A

Posterior vena cava

Coccygeomesenteric vein

Cranial lobe right kidney

Right renal portal valve

Right femoral

Middle lobe right kidney

Right renal

Intrarenal vein

Caudal lobe right kidney

Renal portal

Left cranial renal portal vein

Left renal portal valve

Left external iliac vein

Left renal vein

Sciatic vein

B

**FIGURE 21-32** Vasculature of the avian circulatory system. **A**, Blood vessels. **B**, Renal portal system.

body, some of these vessels are highly specialized in the following ways:

- The pectoral and brachial arteries, which provide blood to the flight muscles and wings, respectively, are relatively large.
- Birds possess a **renal portal system** (Figure 21-32, *B*) that begins and ends in a network of capillaries. Blood returning from the extremities via the iliac veins travels to the kidneys. Valves at the junction of the iliac veins and renal (kidney) veins steer blood either to the kidneys, so metabolic waste products can be removed, or directly to the heart via the posterior vena cava.
- Many aquatic and terrestrial species possess a countercurrent system of heat exchange in their lower extremities (Figure 21-33). This system consists of a network of arteries and veins that are placed close together. Heat from arterial blood traveling to the lower extremities is transferred to the cooler, venous blood returning to the heart. Thus blood reaching the lower extremities is cooler, and less of a temperature gradient exists with the environment. This feature reduces the amount of heat loss.

## BLOOD FLOW

Birds are active creatures and have a relatively high body temperature—between 37° and 42°C (Ritchie, Harrison, and Harrison, 1994). To maintain this temperature and

generate body heat, they also have a relatively fast metabolism. This places high demands on the circulatory system to deliver oxygen and nutrients to the tissues quickly and efficiently. These demands are met with a relatively fast heart rate; smaller birds have faster heart rates than larger species (Table 21-2) and, consequently, more rapid blood flow. In unstressed chickens, it takes only 6 seconds for blood to make a complete circuit from the heart through the body and back (Welty and Baptista, 1988).

| TABLE 21-2 | Heart Rates in Clinically Normal Birds | |
|---|---|---|
| **BODY** | **RESTING HEART** | **RESTRAINED HEART** |
| **WEIGHT (g)** | **RATE (beats/min)** | **RATE (beats/min)** |
| 25 | 274 | 400-600 |
| 100 | 206 | 500-600 |
| 200 | 178 | 300-500 |
| 500 | 147 | 160-300 |
| 1000 | 127 | 150-350 |
| 1500 | 117 | 120-200 |
| 2000 | 110 | 110-175 |
| 5000 | 91 | 105-160 |
| 10,000 | 79 | 100-150 |

From Ritchie B, Harrison G, Harrison L: Avian medicine: principles and application, Lake Worth, FL, 1994, Wingers Publishing.

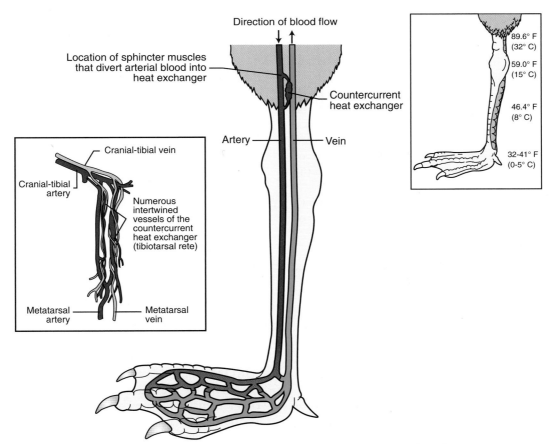

**FIGURE 21-33** Countercurrent heat exchange system in the leg of a gull.

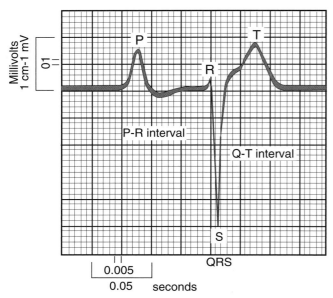

**FIGURE 21-34** Electrocardiogram of a healthy racing pigeon.

## ELECTROCARDIOGRAM

As a bird's heart chambers contract and relax, the resulting changes in electrical voltage can be detected by placing electrodes in strategic locations on the wings and legs. The voltage changes are converted into visual peaks and valleys with the help of an electrocardiograph (ECG) machine. The ECG consists of *P, QRS,* and *T* waves that correspond to the following muscular activities (Figure 21-34):

P wave—contraction and relaxation of the atria

QRS wave complex—contraction of the ventricles

T wave—relaxation of the ventricles

In birds, the existence of the *Q* wave is in question. In many species, such as chickens and turkeys, it is believed to be completely absent, but in other species, such as some ducks, it appears to be prominent. The time intervals represented in the ECG are relatively fixed, with the exception of the *T* to *P* interval, which changes based on changes in the heart rate.

The ECG is an important tool to monitor a patient's stability during anesthesia and to diagnose malfunctions of the heart and major vessels.

## BLOOD

We previously mentioned that the heart drives the circulatory system; the transport vehicle that it drives is the blood. Blood is made up of several components, and it functions to carry nutrients, oxygen, and hormones to cells; to carry metabolic wastes from cells to the lungs and kidneys; to control and prevent disease; and to regulate a bird's body temperature. Blood consists of red cells, white cells, platelets, and plasma (Figure 21-35).

### ERYTHROCYTES

Erythrocytes, or red blood cells, are oval, nucleated, and larger than those in mammals (Figure 21-35, *A*). In most species, they are formed in the bone marrow of adult birds, but in passerines (songbirds), they are formed in the spleen and liver. The red cells possess hemoglobin for carrying oxygen to the tissues. The total number of red blood cells is dependent on several factors, including age, sex, diet, and time of year. In general, the percentage of red blood cells to total blood volume in a healthy adult bird should fall between 35% and 55%.

### LEUKOCYTES

Leukocytes, or white blood cells, are important in helping fight disease. In adult birds, white blood cells are primarily produced by the spleen. In young birds, they are also formed by the liver, kidneys, pancreas, and the **bursa of Fabricius**, which is located on the dorsal wall of the proctodeum in the cloaca. There are several types of white cell, and each type has a different function.

**HETEROPHILS.** These cells are equivalent to the mammalian neutrophil. They are generally round, have a bilobed nucleus with clumped chromatin, and have rod-shaped, red–orange granules in the cytoplasm (Figure 21-35, *A*). **Heterophils** are phagocytic cells that engulf foreign matter. A rise in the number of heterophils is usually seen with the onset of acute diseases.

**EOSINOPHILS.** These cells are the same as the mammalian eosinophils. They are round cells with a lobed nucleus and large, red–orange, round granules in the cytoplasm (Figure 21-35, *B*). Their numbers increase in response to allergic reactions and heavy internal parasite loads.

**BASOPHILS.** These cells are identified by a round, centrally placed nucleus and they stain dark blue (Figure 21-35, *C*). The function of basophils is still being investigated.

**MONOCYTES.** These are phagocytic cells that act as a body's second line of cellular defense. The nucleus is often shaped like a kidney bean and can be located centrally or off to one side (Figure 21-35, *D*). An increase in monocyte production is often seen in cases of tuberculosis and aspergillosis.

**LYMPHOCYTES.** These cells are the essential components of the immune system. Their eccentrically placed nucleus is round and contains densely clumped chromatin (Figure 21-35, *E*). They are produced by the thymus and bursa of Fabricius; lymphocytes originating from the bursa of Fabricius produce humeral antibodies to help fight off infections.

### THROMBOCYTES

Thrombocytes are nucleated cells that act as platelets. They are smaller than red blood cells and have a large, round to oval nucleus (Figure 21-35, *C*). They are important in blood clotting and are produced by the bone marrow in adult birds.

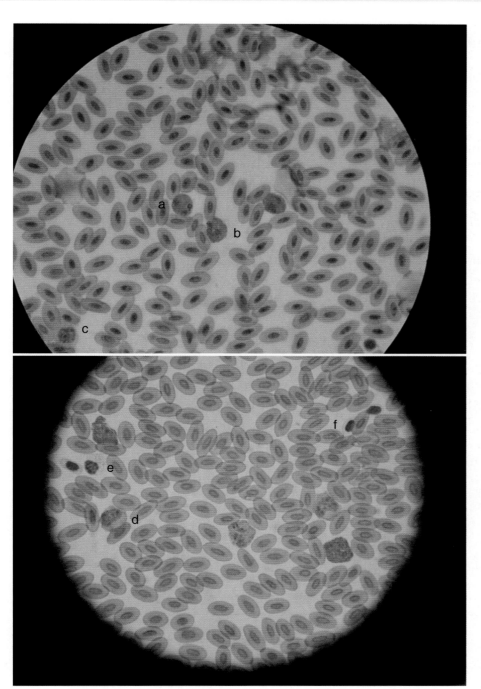

**FIGURE 21-35** Avian blood cells. *a*, Eosinphil. *b*, Heterophil. *c*, Lymphocyte. *d*, Monocyte. *e*, Basophil. *f*, Thrombocyte. (Courtesy Jamie Karlin.)

## PLASMA

The plasma is about 80% water. The remaining 20% consists of a variety of substances, including salts, glucose, fats, amino acids, hormones, antibodies, vitamins, enzymes, waste products, and special blood proteins. These proteins are important for providing the osmotic pressure to maintain normal levels of water and blood in the tissues.

### TEST YOURSELF 21-6

1. What is the renal portal system?
2. What is the body temperature range of birds?
3. Describe the components of an avian ECG.
4. How do avian red blood cells differ from those in mammals?
5. List the three veins that are commonly used for venipuncture in birds. Where are they located?

## RESPIRATORY SYSTEM

Because of the fast metabolism and high energy level of birds, the delivery of oxygen and removal of carbon dioxide from the body tissues must be quick and efficient. To accommodate this need, birds possess a respiratory system with highly specialized components (Figure 21-36).

### Sites of Venipuncture

Blood samples are taken for a variety of diagnostic purposes. In birds, blood can be drawn most easily from one of three vessels: a *jugular vein*, a *brachial vein*, or a *medial metatarsal vein*. The jugular veins are located ventrally, on each side of the trachea. The right jugular is larger than the left and is most commonly used for venipuncture in psittacines. The brachial vein is located on the ventral side of the wing, extending over the elbow and up the humerus. About halfway up the humerus, it joins the cutaneous ulnar vein and increases slightly in size. In raptors, the brachial vein is often used to take blood samples or insert temporary catheters for repeated intravenous treatments. The medial metatarsal vein is located on the ventral medial side of the leg, extending from the metatarsus dorsally over the heel joint. Blood samples are sometimes taken from this site in raptors, but it is more commonly used for waterfowl species.

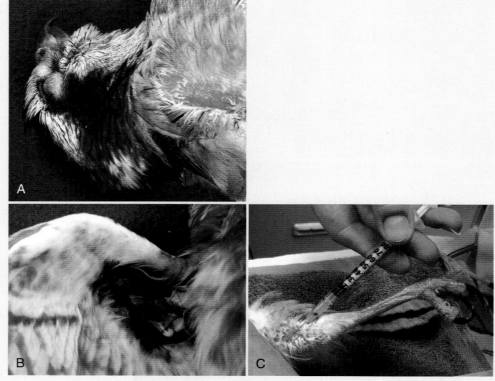

Venipuncture sites in birds. **A**, Jugular vein (Northern Goshawk, *Accipiter gentilis*). **B**, Brachial vein (Northern Saw-Whet Owl). **C**, Median metatarsal vein (Red-Shouldered Hawk).

## ANATOMY
### ORAL CAVITY

The oral cavity contains several structures involved in respiration (Figure 21-37). The glottis is the opening of the trachea, which is located at the back of the tongue. Air is directed to the glottis via the mouth and nasal chambers. These two are linked via the **choanae**, which are two internal nares that open from the nasal chambers into the roof of the mouth. The larynx, a cartilaginous structure surrounding the glottis, has ligaments and muscle attachments that enable it to act as a valve to prevent solids and liquids from entering the trachea and lungs. It does not function in the production of sound as in mammals.

### TRACHEA

The trachea consists of cartilaginous rings that are held together by bands of fibrous connective tissue. In a few species, such as swans and Whooping Cranes (*Grus americana*), the trachea is very long and coiled. For species that migrate at high altitudes, the long trachea helps provide moisture to the inhaled air and aids in the production of sound.

### SYRINX

The enlargement of the trachea above the sternum is called the **syrinx**. It is essentially the voice box of a bird and contains muscles, **air sacs**, and vibrating membranes (Figure 21-38). To create sound, air from the lungs and air sacs is forced over the membranes during expiration, causing changes in muscle tension and air pressure. These changes cause vibrations of the membranes. The complexity of a bird's vocalizations depends on the number of muscles present. Birds capable of complex vocalizations, such as many species of songbirds, have an average

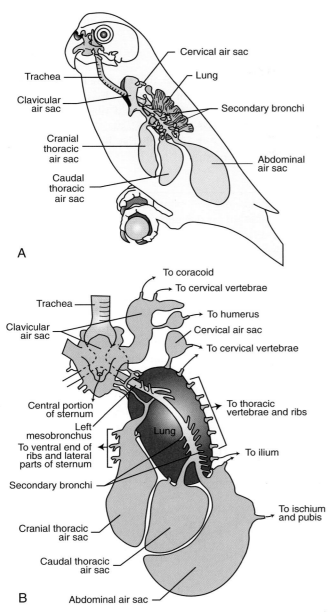

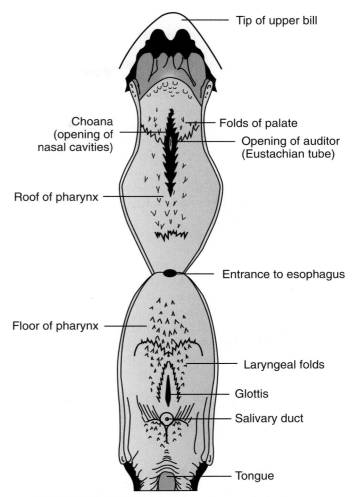

**FIGURE 21-36** Diagram of the avian respiratory system. **A,** Lateral view. **B,** Ventral view.

**FIGURE 21-37** Diagram of the oral cavity of a budgerigar.

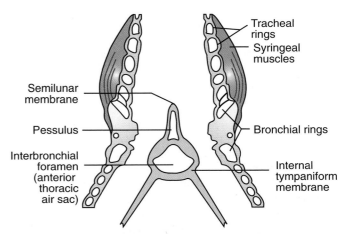

**FIGURE 21-38** Cross section of the syrinx.

of seven pairs, whereas, on the other end of the spectrum, storks, vultures, and ostriches do not have any. Parrots fall in the middle, with three pairs of muscles in their syrinx.

## BRONCHI
At the level of the sternum, the trachea bifurcates into two branches called the *bronchi*. These branches pass through the ventral side of each lung and end in the posterior air sacs. Once they enter the lung, the bronchi lose their reinforcing cartilaginous rings and are called **mesobronchi**. The mesobronchi give rise to four to six *ventrobronchi*, or secondary bronchi, which in turn divide into the **parabronchi**. The parabronchi are connected to air capillaries, where gas exchange occurs.

## PARABRONCHI
These small, parallel tubes originate from the ventrobronchi in the lungs and are connected to the tiny openings of air capillaries. The air capillaries, in turn, are surrounded by small blood capillaries. Gas exchange occurs between these two groups of capillaries.

## AIR SACS

Air sacs are thin-walled, lightly vascularized, transparent membranes that make up about 80% of the total volume of the respiratory system. There are nine air sacs, four of which are paired. The pairs include cranial thoracic, caudal thoracic, cervical, and abdominal air sacs. The unpaired sac is the interclavicular air sac, which is located in the thoracic inlet between the clavicles. Air sacs are connected to the primary bronchi (abdominal sacs) or ventrobronchi (cervical, cranial thoracic, caudal thoracic, and interclavicular sacs) and serve the following functions:

- They act as reservoirs for air, and provide warmth and moisture to facilitate the diffusion of air through the lung capillaries.
- They help in thermoregulation, cooling the body by the internal evaporation of water.
- They help provide buoyancy to water birds. Many species of penguins and diving birds have large posterior and abdominal sacs, the volume of which can be adjusted during diving and floating.

Diverticula of some of the air sacs penetrate the skeleton. In many species, the interclavicular sac extends into the humerus bones, sternum, syrinx, and pectoral girdle. The abdominal sacs often extend into the legs and pelvic girdle (see Figure 21-36, *B*).

## LUNGS

In the avian respiratory system, the lungs are relatively small, occupying only about 2% of the total body volume. They are attached to the thoracic vertebrae and ribs and are bright red, highly vascularized, and inelastic. They house the network of blood and air capillaries between which the exchange of gases occurs.

## AIRFLOW

Two inhalations and two expirations are required to transport one pocket of air through the entire respiratory system (Figure 21-39). To begin the cycle, the first inhalation involves an expansion of the thoracoabdominal space which creates a gradient that brings air into the body. Birds do not have a diaphragm, the major inspiratory muscle in mammals. Most of the air flows into the posterior air sacs (abdominal and caudal thoracic), where it is warmed and humidified. With the first expiration, this air is pushed into the lungs, where gas exchange occurs. The second inspiration results in the air moving out of the lungs and into the anterior air sacs

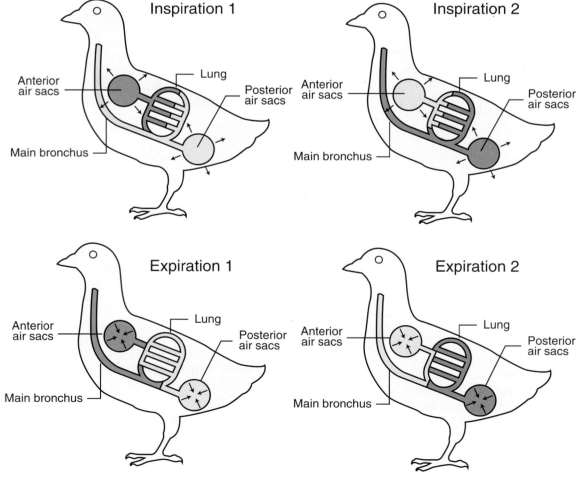

**FIGURE 21-39** Diagram of airflow through a bird's respiratory system.

(cranial thoracic, cervical, interclavicular), and the second expiration results in the air leaving the body through the trachea.

The key factor in the flow of air through a bird's respiratory system is that air is pushed, not pulled, into the lungs. More than any other group of animals, birds truly can get a "breath of fresh air." As previously mentioned, a bird's lungs are inelastic; they do not inflate and deflate as in mammals. Fresh air flows in a continuous, unidirectional path in the lungs and does not get mixed with dirty air containing waste products. This unique feature allows each breath of air to reach the lung capillaries with the maximum amount of oxygen possible—close to the 21% present in atmospheric air. In contrast, the lungs of mammals inflate and deflate, always leaving a quantity of residual air. When new air comes in, it mixes with the air remaining in the lungs, diluting the percentage of oxygen available for gas exchange.

Another unique feature of the avian respiratory system that contributes to its high efficiency is the flow between the air and blood capillaries. The air capillaries are positioned at right angles to the blood capillaries so that carbon dioxide is continually removed from the blood and oxygen is continually added.

## RESPIRATORY RATE

The breathing rate of birds varies with species, activity level, age, sex, time of day, and outdoor temperature. Smaller birds usually breathe faster than larger birds, and birds in flight have a higher respiratory rate than nonflying birds. In a thermoneutral environment, chickens at rest breathe 16 to 18 times per minute (Terres, 1980), whereas red-tailed hawks breathe about 40 times per minute (Chaplin, Mueller, and Degernes, 1989). One studyfound that, at rest, house sparrows breathe 50 times per minute; when held in the hand, 102 times per minute; and when released and flying around a room, 212 times per minute. The variability in rate under different conditions can make it difficult to use respiratory rate as a diagnostic tool.

## THERMOREGULATION

In addition to the exchange of gases, the respiratory system in birds also helps in thermoregulation. Air in the lungs picks up heat radiated by warm body tissues and blood and removes it from the body during the breathing process. The evaporation of water via the air sacs, lungs, and mouth cavity helps to cool the body to maintain a safe core temperature. This is most critical when outdoor air temperatures rise or when a bird participates in strenuous exercise, such as flight.

To increase the amount of cooling, a bird can increase the airflow over its mouth, pharynx, bronchi, and air sacs by increasing its breathing rate. This often results in panting or **gular fluttering**. The latter is often seen in doves, Great Blue Herons (*Ardea herodias*), pigeons, quail, and owls, and it involves rapid vibrations of the upper throat patch.

In addition to a bird's ability to use its respiratory system to remove excess heat, birds can control their body temperature in several other ways. To keep cool, birds bathe or reduce their activity level during the warmest parts of the day. Some species, such as Turkey Vultures and Wood Storks (*Mycteria americana*), defecate on their legs for evaporative cooling. As mentioned previously, birds also can adjust the position of their body feathers to promote both heat loss and retention. To retain heat, many land and water species possess a special artery–vein arrangement in their lower extremities that acts as a countercurrent heat exchange system to limit heat loss through their bare legs (see Figure 21-33). Birds also change their posture to conserve heat. This may involve perching on one leg to reduce exposure of bare skin to cold air or tucking thee beak behind the feathers on their back. Shivering to increase muscle heat production and moving to more protected locations also help to prevent loss of body heat during times of cold stress. In some smaller species, such as hummingbirds, short-term *nocturnal torpor*—in which body temperature is decreased by several degrees and heart rate and oxygen consumption are reduced—is another mechanism of heat conservation.

**TEST YOURSELF 21-7**
1. Where does gas exchange occur in the avian respiratory system?
2. List the nine air sacs and describe their main function in respiration.
3. Do birds have a diaphragm?
4. Describe the path of one breath of air through the respiratory system.

 **CLINICAL APPLICATION**

### Toxic Fumes

The large volume of space present in a bird's respiratory tract, the unidirectional flow of air, and the spatial relationship between the air and blood capillaries create an extremely efficient system that is highly sensitive to gaseous molecules in the air. Fumes from disinfectants, such as concentrated bleach; heated Teflon-coated pans or light bulb covers; moth balls (naphthalene); oil-based paints and varnishes; and exhaust fumes can cause illness and even death in birds. Symptoms of exposure to noxious fumes are rapid in onset and may include loss of balance, so a bird may fall off its perch and stand fluffed on the floor. Other symptoms are respiratory râles, or raspy breathing sounds; tail bobbing, in which the tail moves with each labored breath; and severe respiratory distress. Depending on the source of the fumes and extent of exposure, death can occur quickly. Diagnosing the problem relies on obtaining a detailed patient history. Treatment revolves around providing support to the respiratory system, which includes reducing stress, providing oxygen therapy and warmth, placing an air sac cannula to assist with the movement of air, and sometimes administering a mild diuretic to remove fluid from the lungs. However, because of the low rate of survival after exposure to toxic vapors, it is critical to educate all bird owners on the potential deadly effects of fumes to prevent exposure in the first place.

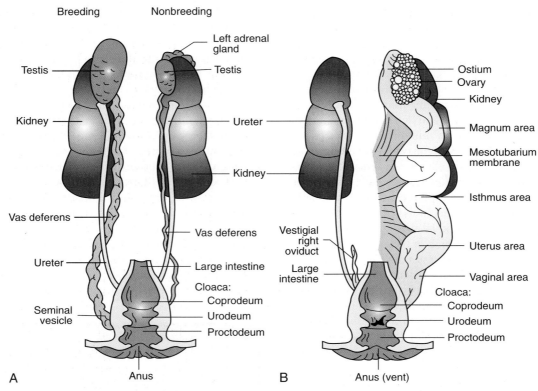

**FIGURE 21-40** Avian urogenital system. **A,** Male. **B,** Female.

## UROGENITAL SYSTEM

The urogenital system encompasses both the urinary and the reproductive systems. Although these systems have very different functions, they are often studied together because of their close anatomic relation in a bird's body (Figure 21-40).

## URINARY SYSTEM

Like that of mammals, the avian urinary system consists of two main components: *kidneys* and *ureters.* The main function of the urinary system is to remove nitrogenous waste products from the blood and eliminate them from the body; however, it also plays a role in maintaining the osmotic balance of electrolytes and salt in the blood and body tissues.

### ANATOMY
**KIDNEYS.**  The kidneys in birds are located dorsally, in the slight depression formed at the level of the synsacrum. They are elongated and consist of three divisions, each of which is layered, with an exterior cortex and an interior medulla. Within each layer, the divisions subdivide into lobules that possess nephrons, which are the "workhorses" of the urinary system. These nephrons radiate around a central vein (Figure 21-41). Unlike mammals, birds do not possess a renal pelvis, and thus the gross anatomy of the kidneys looks more homogeneous.

Each nephron consists of a glomerulus and a tubule. The glomerulus is a filter that removes wastes, salt, glucose, gases, and water from the blood and passes them on to its tubule.

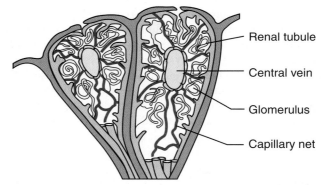

**FIGURE 21-41** Internal anatomy of the avian nephron.

The two types of tubules are *looped* and *unlooped.* The looped tubules, called the *loops of Henle,* resemble those in mammalian nephrons and are located in large nephrons in the medulla of the kidney. The unlooped tubules are located in the smaller, cortical nephrons and resemble those of reptiles. In both types of tubule, water, salt, and glucose are selectively reabsorbed into the blood through capillaries, and the waste products are concentrated and passed into collecting ducts that empty into the ureters. Between 66% and 99% of the water filtered into the kidney glomeruli is reabsorbed in the tubules.

**URETERS.**  The ureters are an extension of the main collecting ducts. They are surrounded by smooth muscle and can "milk" urates from the kidney or inhibit their flow into the cloaca. Urine passing through the ureters ends in the urodeum of the cloaca and is either moved upward to the colon and ceca for further reabsorption of water or propelled outward through a bird's vent, which is the sphincter separating the cloaca from the outside.

## URINE COMPOSITION

In chickens, the nitrogenous wastes eliminated by the kidneys consist of 75% uric acid, 10% to 15% ammonia, 2% to 10% urea, 1% to 5% creatine, and 2% amino acids (Welty and Baptista, 1988). Clearly, the predominant component is uric acid and not urea, as in mammals. This finding is significant for several reasons. First, uric acid is more efficient in eliminating nitrogen; each molecule removes twice as much nitrogen as a urea molecule. Second, uric acid conserves water because it is relatively insoluble and can be eliminated with only a small volume of water. It takes 60 ml of water to excrete 1 g of urea, whereas it only takes 1.5 to 3 ml of water to excrete the same amount of uric acid. Finally, the production of uric acid is critical to the survival of embryos within the egg. The only waste products that can be eliminated through an eggshell are gases. Other waste products must be stored in the egg throughout the embryo's development. Because urea requires a relatively large volume of water for excretion, the egg would not have enough room to house it. Also, high quantities of urea are toxic and would kill the embryo. As it is, the relatively small amount of nontoxic uric acid produced can be stored in the egg with no ill effects.

The final waste product is eliminated from the body as a paste. It is usually excreted in combination with a small quantity of fecal material from the digestive system. Collectively, the excreted product is called a *mute*, and, in a healthy bird, it is characterized by a dark fecal center—the color of which will vary with a bird's diet—surrounded by a ring of white urates (see Figure 21-30). Diet, internal parasites, toxins, and certain illnesses can all cause changes in the color of a bird's mutes.

## REPRODUCTIVE SYSTEM

Finally, we have reached the system responsible for creating the little package of genetic material that will develop into another amazing avian creature. Like most of the body systems in birds, the reproductive system is highly specialized and unique. The entire process of reproduction is periodic and under hormonal control. In temperate-zone birds, increasing daylight stimulates the hypothalamus to secrete substances that travel to the pituitary and cause the release of hormones that directly affect the reproductive process.

### ANATOMY

The major reproductive organs are called *gonads*. In males, these are the testes, and in females, the ovaries. In both sexes, the organ on the left side of the body is larger; in females, the right ovary is rudimentary and does not function at all. During the nonbreeding season, the gonads are relatively small. As the breeding season approaches, hormones stimulate enlargement of the gonads, with up to a 300-fold increase

in size of the testes in males. After the season ends, the gonads shrink. This is another adaptation that has allowed birds to reduce unnecessary weight for flight. Many species migrate long distances during the nonbreeding season and do not need to carry large, inactive gonads.

## MALE REPRODUCTIVE SYSTEM

The testes in birds are bean-shaped organs located ventral to the anterior part of the kidney (see Figure 21-40, *A*). Their anatomy and function are similar to those in mammals, because they produce the spermatozoa that are genetically ready to penetrate a developing ovum.

The spermatozoa of birds resemble tadpoles with relatively large heads and mobile tails. They swim out of the testes in seminal fluid produced by tubules in the testes, unlike mammals, whose seminal fluid is produced by accessory glands. The spermatozoa travel down a curvy, ciliated tube, called the *vas deferens*, to a storage pouch called the *seminal vesicle*. The temperature in this pouch is about 4° C cooler than the core body temperature and can safely house the heat-sensitive spermatozoa.

**COPULATION.** To pass sperm to the female, copulation must occur. This behavior is stimulated by androgens, which are male hormones produced in the testes by the cells of Leydig. The androgens travel to the hypothalamus in the brain and stimulate copulatory behavior. Copulation is achieved in one of two ways. In some species, such as ducks, geese, Galliformes, storks, and flamingos, a grooved, erectile penis is attached to the wall of the cloaca to help transfer sperm into the female's vagina. However, in most species, sperm transfer occurs when the male and female bring their cloacae into close proximity. In pigeons, 200 million sperm are transferred during a single copulatory event. In the domestic chicken, 8 billion sperm are transferred (Welty and Baptista, 1988).

## FEMALE REPRODUCTIVE SYSTEM

Eggs, or ova, are produced from follicles in the cortex of the ovary (see Figure 21-40, *B*) and are released in a manner similar to those of mammals. Several factors, including increasing day length, stimulate the anterior pituitary gland to secrete follicle-stimulating hormone (FSH), which increases the size of the follicles, and luteinizing hormone (LH), which stimulates both discharge of an egg from its follicle and development of the interstitial cells that produce sex hormones.

**OVULATION.** Ovulation is the process whereby the ovum leaves its follicle and enters the oviduct. This duct consists of three layers: an outer *connective tissue layer*, a middle *muscular layer* that moves the egg down the oviduct by peristalsis, and an inner *glandular layer* that secretes various substances that are added to the egg during its passage. Lengthwise, the avian oviduct can be divided into the following five sections:

1. Infundibulum—possesses folds that grab an ovum as it comes out of the ovary.

2. Magnum—secretes layers of albumin (egg white) around the egg.
3. Isthmus—deposits the keratin shell membrane.
4. **Uterus**—deposits watery albumin, a hard external shell, and pigmentation; large and muscular, it is also called the **shell gland**, and an egg spends the most time here.
5. Vagina—secretes mucus to assist in egg laying; stores sperm for hours to several days.

Eggs come in different colors and may have speckles, blotches, or other irregular markings, depending on how much they move when the tiny pigment glands apply color. During the egg production process, hormones alter a female's blood composition. Estrogen produced from the interstitial cells of the ovary stimulates a 3-fold to 18-fold increase in fatty substances in the blood. Hormones from the thyroid, adrenals, and pancreas are responsible for doubling the blood sugar concentration, and the ovary and parathyroid glands stimulate an increase in blood calcium.

**CLUTCH.** The group of eggs that a female lays and incubates is called a **clutch**. Clutch size varies among species but is fairly constant from year to year. Many species lay one egg per day. Others, such as ducks and geese, lay eggs every other day. Some larger species, such as eagles and condors, may lay at 4- to 5-day intervals.

The total number of eggs that a female can lay varies with the species. The two types of egg layers are *determinate* and *indeterminate*. **Determinate layers**, such as budgies, crows, and passerines, have a specific number of follicles that develop in the ovary. Once these are laid, the clutch is complete, even if the eggs are removed. **Indeterminate layers**, such as parrots, poultry, and birds of prey, can produce more eggs than their normal clutch size and will continue to lay eggs if their eggs disappear. Visual, tactile, and hormonal influences cause them to stop laying when their clutch is complete. This concept has been used to incubate eggs of endangered species artificially, because the eggs can be removed and incubated elsewhere, allowing an endangered hen to lay more eggs.

**INCUBATION.** Eggs must be kept warm and humidified during their development. An average incubation temperature for many species is 35° C. When a female bird is ready to lay her eggs, the pituitary acts again to secrete prolactin, which decreases the activity of the FSH and LH and promotes broodiness, or incubation behavior. Hormones also stimulate the development of a **brood patch**, which is an area of skin on the lower abdomen where heat is transferred to the egg. The hen plucks the feathers in this area because of the influence of prolactin, and estrogen stimulates thickening and wrinkling of the epidermis and an increase in the size and number of blood vessels.

The amount of time required for an egg to complete its development varies with the species. Generally, smaller birds have shorter incubation times than larger birds (Table 21-3).

| TABLE 21-3 | Average Clutch Size and Incubation Period for Select Avian Species | |
|---|---|---|
| **SPECIES** | **AVERAGE CLUTCH SIZE** (number of eggs) | **AVERAGE INCUBATION PERIOD** (days) |
| Budgerigar (Melopsittacus undulatus) | 4-6 | 18 |
| Blue and Gold Macaw (Propyrrhura maracana) | 2-4 | 23-27 |
| Cockatiel (Nymphicus hollandicus) | 4-8 | 21 |
| Congo African Grey (Psittacus erithacus) | 2-4 | 28-29 |
| Yellow-Naped Amazon (Amazona ochrocephala) | 3-4 | 26-28 |
| Zebra Finch (Taeniopygia guttata) | 3-8 | 14 |
| American Bald Eagle (Haliaeetus leucocephalus) | 2-3 | 35 |
| American Robin (Turdus migratorius) | 3-4 | 12-13 |
| Rock Dove (Columbia livia) | 2 | 18 |
| Royal Albatross (Diomedea epomophora) | 1 | 70-80 |

### CLINICAL APPLICATION

#### Egg Binding

Eggs passing through the oviduct sometimes get lodged. This condition is called **egg binding**, and it is seen most often in small companion birds, such as parakeets, canaries, finches, and cockatiels. Birds suffering from this condition may be sluggish and reluctant to fly or perch, or they may stand with a wide stance, droop their wings, have paralysis of the rear limbs, be anorexic, or have strained abdominal movements. Malformed eggs, excessive egg production, obesity, vitamin deficiencies, inactivity, environmental stress, or malfunction of the oviduct muscles can all result in egg binding. Removing the lodged egg may require drug therapy, such as oxytocin or prostaglandin to stimulate contraction of the uterus, or it may require manual manipulation of the patient. The latter may include massaging the abdomen, administering an enema to lubricate the urodeum, or inserting a speculum into the urodeum to facilitate egg passage. If these techniques are unsuccessful, more intricate procedures may be necessary.

### THE CHICK

From hatchlings to adults, the rate of development and life span of birds varies dramatically among its numerous species (Table 21-4). A chick hatches from the egg with the help of powerful neck muscles and a specialized egg tooth on the outside of a chick's bill (Figure 21-42). The neck muscles atrophy greatly after hatching, and the egg tooth disappears.

The sex of the chick is determined by the genetic information passed on by the female. The female chromosome, *Z*, is

| TABLE 21-4 | Life Spans of Common Pet Bird Species | |
| --- | --- | --- |
| **BIRD** | **MAXIMUM (YEARS)** | **AVERAGE (YEARS)** |
| African Grey Parrot (Psittacus erithacus) | 50 | 15 |
| Amazon Parrot | 80 | 15 |
| Budgerigar (Melopsittacus undulates) | 18 | 6 |
| Canary | 20 | 8 |
| Cockatiel (Nymphicus hollandicus) | 32 | 5 |
| Conure | 25 | 10 |
| Domestic Pigeon (Columbia livia) | 26 | 15 |
| Eclectus Parrot | 20 | 8 |
| Grey-Cheeked Parakeet (Brotogeris pyrrhopterus) | 15 | 8 |
| Guoldian Finch (Chloebia gouldiae) | Unknown | 4 |
| Macaw | 50 | 15 |
| Mynah | 8 | 3 |
| Pionus Parrot | 15 | 5 |
| Rainbow Lorikeet (Trichaglassus haematadus) | 15 | 3 |
| Rosella | 15 | 3 |
| Sulfur-Crested Cockatoo (Cacatua galerita) | 40 | 15 |
| Superb Parrot (Polytelis swainsonii) | 36 | 6 |
| Toucan | Unknown | 4 |
| Zebra Finch (Taeniopygia guttata) | 17 | 5 |

From Ritchie B, Harrison G, Harrison L: Avian medicine: principles and application, Lake Worth, FL, 1994, Wingers Publishing.

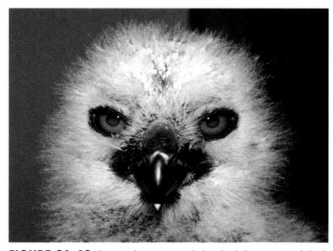

**FIGURE 21-42** Egg tooth on a recently hatched Great Horned Owl. (Photo by Gail Buhl.)

dominant in eggs; the male chromosome, *W*, is recessive. Females can lay two types of egg: those with a male chromosome *(ZW)*, and those without *(ZZ)*. Sperm all have the same sex chromosome—*WW*. Therefore only when the female contributes the *W* chromosome will a male result.

When hatched, chicks differ in the amount of feather cover they have, the status of their eyes (open or closed), and

their mobility. The four different classifications of newly hatched chicks are as follows:

- **Altricial**—Some chicks are hatched with their eyes closed and their skin bare. They require a great deal of care before they can leave the nest. Parrots and songbirds fall into this category.
- **Semialtricial**—At hatching, these chicks are covered with down and are immobile. They may have their eyes open, such as herons and hawks, or closed, like owls.
- **Precocial**—These chicks are covered with downy feathers, have their eyes open, and are quite mobile, leaving the nest quickly. Ducks and geese are good examples.
- **Semiprecocial**—Some species, such as gulls and terns, are born with a downy covering and open eyes, but move only a short distance from the nest and are fed by their parents. Chicks develop at varying rates into adult birds.

> ✓ **TEST YOURSELF 21-8**
>
> 1. What is the major component in the nitrogenous waste of birds? What are the advantages to producing this type of waste?
> 2. Explain how sperm are transferred from the male to the female in birds.
> 3. List the five sections of the avian oviduct and their functions.
> 4. What is the average incubation temperature?
> 5. What is a brood patch and how does it relate to incubation?
> 6. Describe the four classifications of newly hatched chicks.

## SUMMARY

With the general description of newly hatched chicks, we have come to the end of our brief study of the anatomy and physiology of birds. For most undomesticated species, a chick emerges from its shell and over the next few weeks to months develops physically and psychologically into a being destined to fly. Its body systems mature with all the specialized features needed to make this one act possible.

Outwardly, the bird is covered in a lightweight coat of feathers that efficiently traps air, providing insulation and enabling lift. Each of the many feather types is important in carrying out a specific function for survival. Only birds have feathers, and it is one of the most obvious features unique to them. The musculoskeletal system of birds is remarkably light, efficient, and strong. Powerful flight muscles are located ventrally along the central axis of the animal. Dorsally, fused vertebrae form a rigid plate that anchors the skeleton and protects it from the crushing forces of the flight muscles. A reduction in the number and density of bones, many of which are pneumatic (air filled), further optimizes both the skeleton's strength and its lightness. Vision and hearing are famously acute in birds because they rely on these senses for mating, defending territories, and locating prey. The digestive and urinary systems are efficient in processing food without the long-term storage of weighty excrement seen in mammals. Birds lack bladders. Feces and urates are expelled forcefully together from a single vent and, in some species, indigestible components of food are crushed in and then regurgitated from the gizzard, in the form of a pellet.

Birds are metabolically active creatures with a relatively high body temperature, and heart and respiratory rates. Respiration is designed to maximize gas exchange and enables birds to fly at high altitudes without succumbing to hypoxia. Two inhalations and two expirations are needed to circulate one pocket of air through the entire respiratory system. The air moves in only one direction through the avian respiratory system rather than in two directions as seen in mammals. Diverticulae of the respiratory system form a series of air sacs that make up the largest portion of the respiratory system (80%); the lungs make up a relatively small portion. These sacs are contiguous with pneumatic bones and add to a bird's buoyancy in water. In addition, the red blood cells are nucleated and much larger than mammalian erythrocytes, making them particularly efficient at carrying oxygen. Like air through the lungs, oxygen-rich blood moves quickly through the bird. Indeed, it takes only 6 seconds in resting chickens for blood to circulate through the entire body and return to the heart.

Even the reproductive system complies with the avian mission to be as light as possible. During the nonbreeding and migratory periods, sex organs such as the testes and ovaries are atrophied and small. However, when needed, after migration and during the breeding season, these gonads hypertrophy into much larger, functional sex organs. Like many reptiles, birds lay eggs. The number of eggs and frequency of egg laying vary among species. Once hatched, precocious chicks can feed themselves whereas altricial young may be fed by regurgitation from adults. Birds do not nurse their young and lack the heavy, milk-filled mammary glands of mammals.

In all of these ways, birds are truly remarkable. Although there are some mammals, such as bats, that fly, only birds dominate the skies. No other animal can fly as high, as far, and as continuously without rest. Every aspect of avian anatomy and physiology has evolved in some way to perform this single, miraculous feat.

## REFERENCES AND FURTHER READING

Altman R, Clubb S, Dorrestein G, et al: Avian medicine and surgery, Philadelphia, 1997, WB Saunders.

Anderson Brown AF, Robbins GES: The new incubation book, Blaine, WA, 2002, Hancock House.

Calder WA: Respiratory and heart rates of birds at rest. Condor 70(4):358–365, 1968.

Campbell T, Ellis C: Avian and exotic animal hematology and cytology, ed 3, Hoboken, NJ, 2007, Wiley.

Chaplin S, Mueller L, Degernes L: Physiological assessment of rehabilitated raptors prior to release. Wildlife J 12(1):7–8, 17–18, 1989.

Dorst J: The life of birds, vol 1, New York, 1974, Columbia University Press.

Faaborg J: Ornithology: an ecological approach, Englewood Cliffs, NJ, 1988, Prentice-Hall.

Freethy R: How birds work, Gloucester, UK, 1982, Blandford Books.

Gill F: Ornithology, ed 2, New York, 1995, WH Freeman.

Harrison G, Lightfoot T: Clinical avian medicine, vol 1, Palm Beach, FL, 2006, Spix Publishing.

Harrison G, Lightfoot T: Clinical avian medicine, vol 2, Palm Beach, FL, 2006, Spix Publishing.

King AS, McLeeland J: Form and function in birds, vol 2, London, 1981, Academic Press.

Korbel R: Klinischer untersuchungsgang. In Koenig H, Liebich HG, editors: Anatomie und propaedeutik des gefluegels, Stuttgart, New York, 2001, Schattauer Verlag.

Pettingill OS Jr, editor: Seminars in ornithology, Ithaca, NY, 1972, Cornell Laboratory of Ornithology.

Ritchie B, Harrison G, Harrison L: Avian medicine: principles and application, Lake Worth, FL, 1994, Wingers Publishing.

Samour J: Avian medicine, ed 2, Philadelphia, 2008, Elsevier Health Sciences.

Silverman S, Tell L: Radiology of birds: an atlas of normal anatomy and positioning, Philadelphia, 2009, Elsevier Health Sciences.

Stettenheim P: The integument of birds. In Farner DS, King JR, editors: Avian biology, vol 2, New York, 1972, Academic Press.

Terres JK: The Audubon Society encyclopedia of North American birds, New York, 1980, Alfred A Knopf.

Tully T, Dorrestein G, Jones A: Handbook of avian medicine, ed 2, Philadelphia, 2009, Elsevier Health Sciences.

Welty JC, Baptista L: The life of birds, ed 4, Orlando, FL, 1988, Saunders College Publishing.

Whittow GC: Sturkie's avian physiology, ed 5, San Diego, 2000, Academic Press.

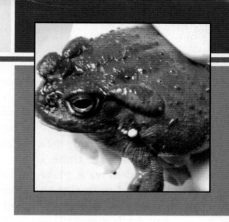

# 22 Amphibian and Reptilian Anatomy and Physiology

*Ryan DeVoe*

## OUTLINE

## LEARNING OBJECTIVES

*When you have completed this chapter you will be able to:*

1. List the taxonomic orders in the classes Reptilia and Amphibia.
2. Define *ectothermic* and explain how ectothermic animals regulate their body temperature.
3. List the unique features of the reptilian and amphibian integumentary systems.
4. Describe the process of ecdysis.
5. List the unique features of reptilian and amphibian vision and hearing.
6. List the components of the reptilian and amphibian heart and describe the flow of blood through the heart.
7. Describe the unique features of the reptilian and amphibian respiratory and gastrointestinal systems.
8. Describe the structure of the kidneys of reptiles and amphibians.
9. Describe the factors that determine the sex of the offspring of reptiles and amphibians.
10. List the unique features of the musculoskeletal systems of reptiles and amphibians.

## VOCABULARY FUNDAMENTALS

*Acrodont teeth* **ahck**-ruh-dohnt tēth
*Aglyphous* ah-**glī**-fuhs
*Anapsid skull* ah-**nahp**-sihd skuhl
*Behavioral thermoregulation* bē-**hāv**-yər-uhl thər-mō-rehg-ū-**lā**-shuhn
*Bidder's organ* **bihd**-dərz **ohr**-gahn
*Carapace* **keər**-ah-pās
*Chromatophore* **krō**-maht-uh-fōr
*Conus papillaris* **kō**-nuhs pah-puh-**leər**-ihs
*Diaphragmaticus* dī-ah-frahm-**aht**-uh-kuhs
*Diapsid skill* dī-**ahp**-sihd skihl

*Ecdysis* **ehck**-dih-sihs
*Ectothermic* ehck-tō-**thər**-mihck
*Endolymphatic sac* ehn-dō-lihm-**fah**-tihck sahck
*Faveloli* fah-vē-**ō**-lī
*Foramen of panizza* fohr-**ā**-mehn *of* pah-**nēz**-ah
*Hemipenes* hehm-ih-**pē**-nēz
*Heterophil* **heht**-ər-ō-fihl
*Lissencephalic* lihs-ehn-seh-**fahl**-ihck
*Melanomacrophage* mehl-ahn-ō-**mah**-krō-fāj
*Multicameral lung* muhl-tī-**kahm**-ər-ahl luhng
*Nuptial pad* **nuhp**-shuhl pahd

*Opisthoglyphous* ah-pihs-thuh-**glī**-fuhs
*Oviparous* ō-**vihp**-eɔr-uhs
*Oviposition* ō-vih-pō-**zihsh**-uhn
*Parietal eye* pah-**rī**-eh-tahl ī
*Paucicameral lung* paw-sē-**kahm**-ɔr-ahl luhng
*Plastron* **plahs**-truhn
*Pleurodont teeth* **ploor**-uh-dohnt tēth
*Preferred optimal temperature zone* prih-**fɔrd**
   **ohp**-tuh-muhl **tehm**-pɔr-uh-chɔr zōn
*Proteroglyphous* prō-tɔr-uh-**glī**-fuhs
*Septum* **sehp**-tuhm

*Sexual dimorphism* **sehck**-shū-ahl dī-**mawr**-fihz-uhm
*Spectacle* **spehck**-tah-kuhl
*Solenoglyphous* sohl-en-ō-**glī**-fuhs
*Splenopancreas* spleh-nō-**pahn**-krē-ahs
*Tail autonomy* tāl aw-**tohn**-uh-mē
*Thecodont teeth* **thē**-kuh-dohnt tēth
*Thrombocyte* **throhm**-bō-sīt
*Unicameral lung* ū-nih-**kahm**-ɔr-uhl luhng
*Vitellogenesis* vī-tehl-lō-**jehn**-eh-sihs
*Viviparous* vī-**vihp**-eɔr-uhs
*Vomeronasal organ* vohm-ɔr-ō-**nā**-zahl **ohr**-gahn

## INTRODUCTION

There are more than 4000 species of amphibian and 7700 species of reptile found on the earth today. Amphibians and reptiles, collectively referred to as *herptiles*, comprise an extremely varied group of animals, and it is difficult to make many generalizations regarding their form and function. This chapter covers some of the more interesting and clinically applicable features of the anatomy and physiology of amphibians and reptiles.

## TAXONOMY

The class *Reptilia* includes four orders:
1. *Crocodylia* (alligators and crocodiles).
2. *Squamata* (snakes and lizards).
3. *Chelonia* (turtles and tortoises).
4. *Rhyncocephalia* (tuataras).

Only a relatively few species within a number of different orders are commonly seen in captivity (Table 22-1).

The class Amphibia is made up of three orders:
1. *Gymnophiona* (caecilians).
2. *Anura* (frogs and toads).
3. *Caudata* (salamanders and newts).

Most people are familiar with the general body structure of anurans and salamanders, but may have never seen a caecilian. Caecilians are legless and have elongated bodies much like a snake or eel. They are found in both terrestrial and aquatic habitats. As with reptiles, only a relatively few species are commonly kept in captivity (Table 22-2).

## METABOLISM

Amphibians and reptiles are commonly referred to as **ectothermic**, or cold-blooded. Ectothermic animals are unable to generate body heat internally, therefore their body temperatures are dependent on environmental temperatures. Other ectothermic animals include fish and invertebrate species. Some reptiles are able to raise their body temperatures via metabolic processes. The two notable examples are

| TABLE 22-1 | Taxonomy of Commonly Kept Reptile Species | |
|---|---|---|
| **ORDER** | **FAMILY** | **SPECIES** |
| Squamata | Colubridae | Kingsnake (*Lampropeltis getula*) |
| | Boidae | Boa Constrictor (*Boa constrictor*) |
| Squamata | Iguanidae | Green Iguana (*Iguana iguana*) |
| | Agamidae | Bearded Dragon (*Pogona vitticeps*) |
| | Geckkonidae | Leopard Gecko (*Eublepharus macularius*) |
| Chelonia | Emydidae | Box Turtle (*Terrapene* spp.) |
| | Testunididae | African Spurred Tortoise (*Geochelone sulcata*) |
| Crocodylia | Alligatoridae | Alligator (*Alligator mississippiensis*) |
| | Crocodilydae | Nile Crocodile (*Crocodylus niloticus*) |

| TABLE 22-2 | Taxonomy of Commonly Kept Amphibian Species | |
|---|---|---|
| **ORDER** | **FAMILY** | **SPECIES** |
| Anura | Ranidae | American Bullfrog (*Rana catesbeiana*) |
| | Bufonidae | American Toad (*Bufo americanus*) |
| Caudata | Ambystomidae | Tiger Salamander (*Ambystoma tigrinum*) |
| | Salamandridae | Red-Spotted Newt (*Notopthalmus viridescens*) |
| Gymnophiona | Caecilidae | Mexican Caecilian (*Dermophis mexicanus*) |

Leatherback Sea Turtles, which are able to generate body heat internally, and pythons, which elevate their body temperature via muscular contractions when incubating eggs.

Herptiles maintain their body temperatures in an appropriate range through a process called **behavioral thermoregulation**. Through behavioral thermoregulation, amphibians and reptiles are able to regulate their body temperatures precisely according to metabolic need. Movements within the thermal gradient of their habitat, as well as postural changes, enable herptiles to adjust their body temperatures as needed. For instance, many herptiles bask in the sun to elevate body temperature, and will seek shade when they need to cool down. A snake trying to conserve body heat will coil tightly to decrease its surface area and consequently heat loss, whereas a hot snake will uncoil to accomplish the opposite. Some animals, such as chameleons, can actually adjust the color and pattern of their skin to increase or decrease the absorption of thermal energy from the sun. All of the aforementioned are examples of behavioral thermoregulation.

Ectothermy is directly related to the energy conservation strategies employed by amphibians and reptiles. Compared to mammals, herptiles are incredibly energy efficient. They are able to manipulate their body temperatures behaviorally to match changing metabolic needs. For instance, a quiescent herptile will usually choose to maintain its body temperature in the low end of its preferred range, whereas an animal digesting a meal will likely choose higher temperatures to support the metabolic demands of digestion. In some pythons, the gastrointestinal tract and associated organs, such as the liver and pancreas, actually fluctuate in size drastically depending on food intake. This allows the animal to conserve energy by not supporting a large tissue mass that is not in use.

An ectotherm's ability to thermoregulate effectively is entirely dependent on access to temperatures within the animal's **preferred optimal temperature zone (POTZ)**. The POTZ is a range of temperatures in which the animal can perform all necessary metabolic functions. This principle becomes very important when maintaining herptiles in captivity. If not provided with an appropriate thermal gradient, the herptile will not be able to thermoregulate efficiently. When provided with inappropriately low temperatures, ectothermic animals can suffer from digestive problems, immunosuppression, and other disorders. If kept at temperatures that are too high, the animal is forced to maintain a high metabolic rate and may suffer from energy deficits.

The efficiency of ectothermy allows many herptiles to survive on very small amounts of food. Some sit-and-wait predators, such as large pythons, may only consume a few large meals during the course of a year. Insectivorous herptiles can survive on minute fractions of what would be required to maintain a bird of equal size.

A disadvantage of ectothermy is that activity of herptiles is limited by the availability of appropriate environmental temperatures. For this reason, herptiles that reside in temperate areas go through periods of hibernation, or *brumation*, when temperatures drop out of the range in which the

animal can remain active. Herptiles that are hibernating do not feed and are minimally active until environmental temperatures return to the POTZ.

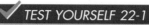

### TEST YOURSELF 22-1

1. What are the four orders of living reptiles? What are the three orders of amphibians?
2. Define *ectothermic*.
3. What is a *preferred optimal temperature zone*?
4. How does an ectothermic animal maintain an appropriate body temperature?

### CLINICAL APPLICATION

#### Drug Administration

It is important that ectothermic animals be kept within their preferred optimal temperature zones when receiving drug therapy. If a drug is administered to an ectothermic animal kept outside its POTZ, it may not be absorbed, distributed, metabolized, or eliminated as expected. This can result in ineffective treatment if the drug is not properly absorbed and distributed. Toxicity can occur when metabolism or elimination is affected. Toxicity is also possible when an animal receives a number of doses at suboptimal temperatures, and the drug pools at the injection sites or in the gastrointestinal tract instead of being absorbed systemically. When this occurs, the animal may effectively receive a toxic dose when it is warmed and therefore capable of absorbing the medication.

### INTEGUMENT

The skin of reptiles is keratinized and varies in appearance according to species. The integument has three components: the *subcutaneous space, dermis,* and *epidermis.* The subcutaneous space is typically limited in most reptiles, and the skin is relatively inelastic, making administration of subcutaneous fluids difficult in comparison to most domestic mammals. The dermis is made up of dense connective tissue and contains blood and lymph vessels, nerves, and **chromatophores**, which are pigment-containing cells. Chromatophores allow some lizards, such as chameleons, to change their skin color and pattern drastically. Some lizards and crocodilians have bony plates within the dermis called *osteoderms* that provide protection. Most reptiles have distinct scales that are formed by a folding of the epidermis. Scales can vary greatly in size and shape. The epidermis can form unique structures, such as crests, tubercles, spines, and dewlaps. Instead of eyelids, snakes have modified scales that cover the eyes; these scales are called the **spectacle**, or *brille* (Figure 22-1).

Scale and scute nomenclature is important for species identification and medical recording (Figure 22-2). Different forms of keratin are found in the scales and the interscalar skin. Alpha keratin is softer and more flexible and is found

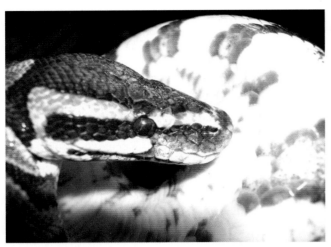

**FIGURE 22-1** The spectacle, or brille, of a Ball Python (*Python regius*).

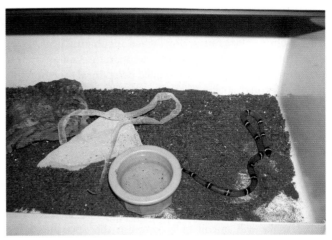

**FIGURE 22-3** Milksnake (*Lampropeltis triangulum*) with recently shed skin. Snake skin is usually shed in one piece.

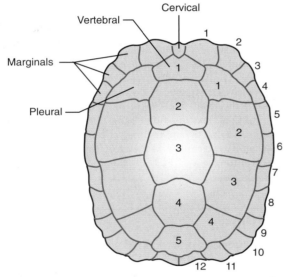

**FIGURE 22-2** Chelonian carapace illustrating nomenclature of scutes. (Redrawn from O'Malley B: Clinical anatomy and physiology of exotic species, New York, 2005, Elsevier Saunders.)

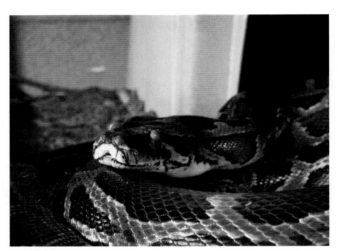

**FIGURE 22-4** Opacification of the spectacle in a Burmese Python (*Python molurus*) indicating impending ecdysis.

in the interscalar skin. Beta keratin is relatively rigid and is found in the scales.

One of the unique and most clinically important features of the reptilian integument is the process of **ecdysis**, or shedding of the skin. Ecdysis occurs as a reptile grows and in response to skin injury. The process of ecdysis is under the control of the thyroid gland. Some reptiles shed the skin completely in one large piece, such as snakes and some lizards (Figure 22-3), whereas others shed in a piecemeal fashion. Many species of lizard consume the dead skin, or exuvia. The shed cycle is initiated by cellular replication in the epidermis, followed by secretion of lymph containing enzymes between the old and new epidermal layers. This results in dulling of the skin color and opacification of the spectacle in snakes (Figure 22-4). The dullness and opacification resolve as the lymph is reabsorbed a few days prior to

actual shedding of the old skin. Actual shedding of the skin is typically accomplished by mechanical rubbing on objects in the environment.

The epidermis of amphibian skin typically has a single or very few layers of keratinized cells, which makes it extremely permeable. Aquatic amphibians have no keratinized cells in their epidermis. The dermis contains chromatophores and many glands that produce secretions that help protect the amphibian's skin. Some glands within the dermis and epidermis produce toxic secretions that are important defense mechanisms for animals that have them (Figure 22-5).

The dermis is firmly attached to the underlying musculature and bone in salamanders and caecilians, making subcutaneous space minimal to nonexistent. Anurans have more significant amounts of subcutaneous space, because the attachments of the dermis are much looser. Amphibians regularly shed the outer layers of the epidermis and usually consume the exuvia.

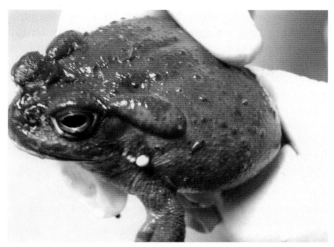

**FIGURE 22-5** Parotid gland in a Colorado River Toad (*Bufo* sp.). The gland is the raised oval structure caudal to the eye.

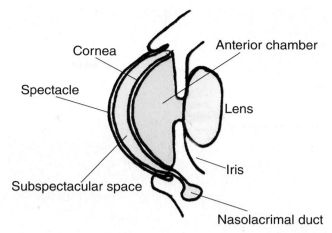

**FIGURE 22-6** Cross section of the anterior portion of a snake eye.

The extremely permeable nature of amphibian skin allows them to absorb all the water they need from the environment, thus amphibians do not drink. Areas of increased permeability, referred to as *drink patches*, are usually present on the ventral surfaces that most frequently come in contact with water.

---

**✓ TEST YOURSELF 22-2**

1. Ecdysis in reptiles is under the control of what hormone?
2. What is a *drink patch*?

---

 **CLINICAL APPLICATION**

### Dysecdysis

Dysecdysis, or abnormal shedding, can occur for a variety of reasons. Sometimes the cause is as simple as low relative humidity in the environment or a lack of appropriate cage features to rub on to begin the shed. Shedding difficulties can also be caused by dehydration due to systemic illness, dermatitis, skin wounds, and malnutrition. Dysecdysis is frequently caused by external parasites, such as the snake mite (*Ophionyssus natricis*).

Occurrence of dysecdysis should prompt a review of husbandry parameters and the correction of any problems. Most cases can be resolved simply by soaking the reptile in a container of warm water for an hour or two. Most of the adhered skin will typically fall off following the soak, or can be removed manually with ease. The removal of retained spectacles in snakes should be attempted with caution. Typically, retained spectacles can be removed with a cotton-tipped applicator or masking tape following soaking.

Failure to correct cases of dysecdysis can result in dermatitis, dyspnea caused by obstructed nares, and continued problems with future sheds. Annular rings of retained shed skin around the toes and tails of lizards can result in ischemic necrosis and sloughing of tissues.

## VISION

There are many important differences between mammalian and herptile eyes. Even among the amphibians and reptiles, there are significant anatomic differences between families.

Reptiles are similar to birds in that the iris is made up of skeletal muscle and is under voluntary control. Therefore, the mydriatic agents used to dilate the pupil for ophthalmic examinations in mammals are not effective in reptiles. A direct pupillary light response is usually noted, but consensual reflexes are often not seen.

### PERIOCULAR STRUCTURES

Some species of lizard, especially those inhabiting sandy, dry areas, have lower eyelids that are very thin. The relative transparency of these lids allows for some vision even when the eyelids are closed. In most species, the lower lid is more mobile than the upper. Crocodilians are the exception, because their upper lids are more mobile. Like birds, some reptiles have cartilaginous pads, or tarsal pads, in their eyelids.

The third eyelid, or *nictitans*, is very well developed and mobile in a variety of reptiles. Crocodilians have nictitans that they use to protect the eyes while swimming under water and procuring prey. Snakes and lizards that do not possess true eyelids do not have nictitans.

Snakes and some species of lizard do not possess true eyelids. Instead these species have a clear, fused scale called the *spectacle*, or *brille*, which covers and protects the eye. The tear film is retained between the cornea and the spectacle in the subspectacular space. The tears drain into the mouth through the nasolacrimal duct system (Figure 22-6).

Most reptiles have poorly developed extraocular muscles, therefore the globe tends to be relatively immobile. The chameleons are exceptions in that they have well-developed extraocular muscles. These extraocular muscles allow the eyes to move freely and independently of one another.

Chelonians do not possess nasolacrimal ducts. The tears spill over the lid margin, so some degree of epiphora is normal in healthy animals (Figure 22-7).

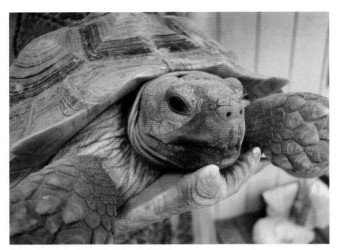

**FIGURE 22-7** African Spurred Tortoise *(Geochelone sulcata)*. A small amount of epiphora is normal in this tortoise owing to the lack of a nasolacrimal duct system.

Most reptiles possess both *lacrimal glands* and *harderian glands*. Typically the harderian gland lies medial to the eye in the rostral aspect of the orbit, whereas the lacrimal gland is typically in a caudodorsal position. Both glands produce secretions that combine to form the tear film. Only the harderian gland is found in snakes.

The eyelids develop at metamorphosis in most salamanders, frogs, and toads. Eyelids are absent in some species of completely aquatic frogs and salamanders. Caecilians' eyes are covered with skin in a manner somewhat analogous to the spectacle in snakes. The presence of periocular glands varies according to species. Only the harderian gland is present in anurans and caecilians, whereas some salamanders have both lacrimal and harderian glands.

The eyes of many amphibian species protrude ventrally into the oral cavity when the animal swallows. The movement of the eyes helps propel food from the oral cavity into the esophagus. Animals that have lost eyes may have difficulty swallowing.

## THE GLOBE AND INTRAOCULAR STRUCTURES

Most reptiles possess scleral bones, or ossicles, the exceptions being snakes and crocodilians. The ossicles help the eye maintain its shape and provide protection from trauma.

The lens is more fluid in reptiles than in mammals, especially in chelonians, in which accommodation is performed by the lens being squeezed through the pupil. The lens is more rigid in snakes, and the ciliary bodies are very closely associated with the root of the iris. Accommodation in snakes is accomplished by the lens moving back and forth as a result of changes in pressure within the aqueous and vitreous humors.

All reptiles have avascular retinas. All nutrition and waste removal within the eye is performed by choroidal vessels or modified vessels that protrude into the vitreous humor. Lizards possess a structure analogous to the avian pectin

called the **conus papillaris**. The conus extends into the vitreous humor from the optic disc and is probably involved in providing nutrition and removing waste. Crocodilians have a tapetum, whereas other reptiles do not.

Tuataras and some lizards have a well-developed **parietal eye** located dorsally on the head. This structure has a rudimentary retina and cornea but no iris, lids, or musculature. A connection exists between the parietal eye and sections of the brain, including the pineal gland. The exact function of the parietal eye is unknown, but it is thought to play a role in light-cycle–mediated hormone function.

---

✓ *TEST YOURSELF 22-3*
1. Which reptiles have a tapetum?
2. How does the reptile iris differ from that of mammals? Why is this clinically important?
3. The nasolacrimal duct system is absent in what order of reptiles?

---

🔍 **CLINICAL APPLICATION**

### Hypovitaminosis A
Diets deficient in vitamin A can result in abnormal cell growth within epithelial tissues. With hypovitaminosis A, the epithelial cells become flattened and lose their ability to perform normal functions. This change is called *squamous metaplasia*, and it frequently affects epithelial tissues associated with the lacrimal and harderian glands. The metaplastic cells can no longer produce a normal tear film and sloughed cells build up and obstruct the glandular ducts. Damage to the cornea and conjunctival tissues can occur because of decreased tear production and bacterial or fungal infection. Treatment involves addressing any secondary infections that may have occurred and correcting the vitamin A deficiency, but caution should be used, because vitamin A toxicity commonly occurs in chelonians treated with parenterally delivered vitamin A preparations. Dietary supplementation is usually a safer alternative. Also, it is important to keep in mind that the functions of other organs may be disrupted, because other epithelial tissues can be affected, including those in the kidneys and liver.

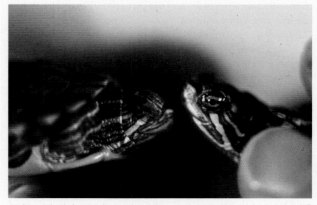

Red-Eared Slider Turtles *(Chrysemys scriptae)*. The turtle on the left suffers from hypovitaminosis A. Notice the closed, swollen eyelids as compared to the normal turtle on the right.

# CARDIOVASCULAR SYSTEM

The location of the heart within the body cavity varies according to species. In chelonians, the heart lies on the midline just caudal to the thoracic girdle and ventral to the lungs. The heart in most lizards lies within the thoracic girdle. The hearts of some lizards, such as monitors, tegus, and crocodilians, lie farther back in the coelomic cavity, and some are almost in the middle. Cardiac location varies in snakes according to species, but usually the heart is found at the junction of the first and second thirds of the animal's body length. Snakes' hearts are fairly mobile within the coelomic cavity, which facilitates the ingestion of large prey.

The cardiac structure of reptiles is significantly different from that of mammals. Most reptiles have three-chambered hearts, with two atria and one common ventricle (Figure 22-8). However, the single ventricle functions as a four-chambered heart, and therefore oxygenated and deoxygenated blood rarely mix. Three regions exist within the ventricle and are functionally separate: the *cavum venosum, cavum arteriosum*, and the *cavum pulmonale.* The cavum pulmonale receives blood from the right atrium and directs flow into the pulmonary circulation. The cavum arteriosum receives blood from the pulmonary veins and directs oxygenated blood to the cavum venosum. The paired aortic arches arise from the cavum venosum and lead to the systemic circulation.

Differential blood flow and separation of oxygenated and deoxygenated blood are maintained by pressure differences in the outflow tracts and a muscular ridge that partially separates the cavum venosum and cavum pulmonale (Figure 22-9). In times of oxygen deprivation, such as when some reptiles dive or when snakes consume large prey, reptiles can shunt blood away from the lungs. Right-to-left cardiac shunting is facilitated by an increase in pulmonary vascular

resistance. Resumption of breathing results in a decrease in pressures within the pulmonary vasculature and a restoration of pulmonary blood flow.

Crocodilians are the only reptiles that possess four-chambered hearts comparable to those of mammals and birds. Even so, crocodilian cardiac anatomy is quite different from what is seen in birds and mammals. Crocodilians possess two aortas, the right arising from the left ventricle and the left from the right ventricle. Both aortas route blood to the systemic circulation. The right and left aortas are connected near the base of the heart by the **foramen of Panizza**. The foramen allows blood from the right ventricle to bypass the pulmonary circulation when necessary. A valve exists at the opening of the pulmonary artery that has interdigitating muscular projections, hence the commonly used name *cog-wheel valve.* When the animal holds its breath, the cog-wheel valve closes, and blood that would have normally entered the pulmonary circulation is diverted into the left aorta and the systemic circulation.

The amphibian heart is three-chambered and similar in anatomy and function to that of snakes, lizards, and chelonians. The interatrial septum is fenestrated in caecilians and most salamanders; in anurans, it is not.

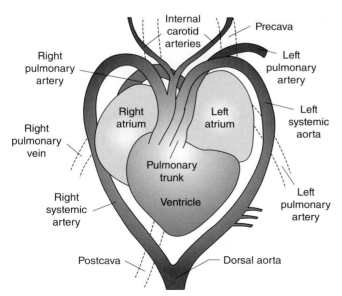

**FIGURE 22-8** Ventral view of a lizard heart. (Redrawn from Mader D: Reptile medicine and surgery, ed 2, St Louis, 2006, Saunders.)

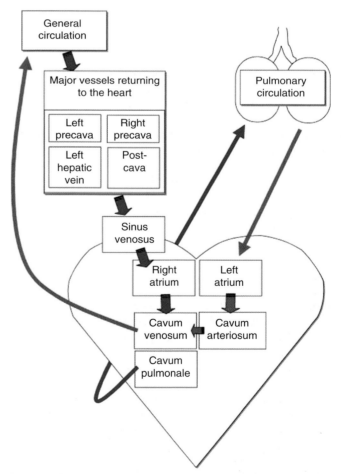

**FIGURE 22-9** Diagram of blood circulation in the noncrocodilian heart. (From Mader D: Reptile medicine and surgery, ed 2, St Louis, 2006, Saunders.)

The heart rate of reptiles depends on species, size, temperature, activity level, and metabolic function. An equation employing metabolic scaling for determination of the "appropriate" heart rate in reptiles has been proposed:

$$\text{Heart rate} = 33.4 \times (\text{weight in kilograms}^{-0.25})$$

This equation assumes that the reptile is within its preferred optimal temperature zone.

Lizards possess a vasovagal reflex that can be induced by applying gentle pressure to both eyeballs through closed lids. Pressure on the eyeballs causes a drop in heart rate and blood pressure, and induces a catatonic state from which the lizard easily recovers upon cessation of the pressure and mild stimulation.

Cardiac monitoring can be difficult in reptiles, but direct cardiac movement is easily observed in most snakes and lizards with caudally positioned hearts. When the animal is placed on its back, the motion of the ventral scutes or scales is usually visible. Auscultation is possible but difficult owing to the low-amplitude sounds produced by the reptilian heart. Placement of a thin, moist towel between the bell of the stethoscope and the animal can help cut down on incidental noise as the scales scrape against the bell. Electrocardiography and cardiac ultrasound can also be employed, but the lack of normal values and methods for standardized examination makes the interpretation of results difficult.

The vascular anatomy of herptiles is similar to that of mammals and birds. Reptiles and amphibians are unique in that they have very well developed lymphatic systems with large lymph vessels found near arteries and veins. Large dilations of the lymph vessels occur roughly where lymph nodes would be found in mammals, though reptiles have no lymph nodes. Instead, the walls of some lymph vessels contain smooth muscle that actively pumps lymph through the vasculature; these structures are known as *lymph hearts*. The presence of the large lymph vessels in association with blood vessels results in relatively frequent lymph contamination of a sample during venipuncture.

## BLOOD

Reptilian red blood cells are oval in shape, nucleated, and larger than those of mammals (Figure 22-10). Erythropoiesis takes place in the bone marrow, and the erythrocytes contain hemoglobin, which allows them to carry oxygen to tissues. The reptilian erythrocyte is relatively long lived, with a life span in some species of 600 to 800 days. Immature erythrocytes are occasionally seen in the circulation of normal animals, especially in juveniles or in animals undergoing ecdysis.

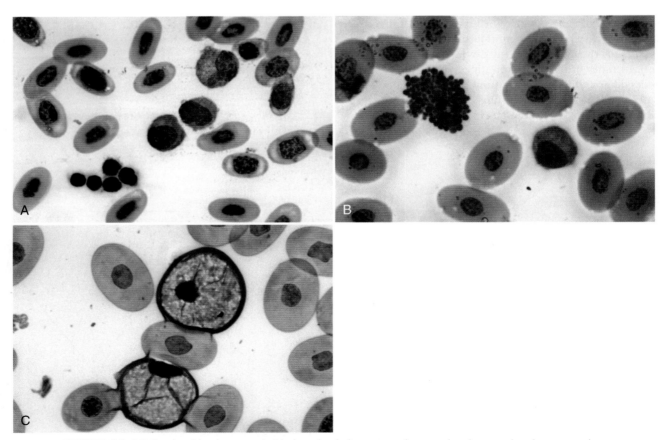

**FIGURE 22-10** Reptilian blood smears. **A,** Nucleated polychromatic erythrocytes, lymphocytes, thrombocytes, and an azurophilic monocyte. **B,** Basophil and azurophilic monocyte. **C,** Heterophils.

**Heterophils** are analogous to mammalian neutrophils. They differ from neutrophils in that they do not possess peroxidase and acid phosphatase, which are enzymes involved in breaking down necrotic material. Given that reptiles lack these enzymes, they produce caseous pus instead of liquid material. Heterophils are involved in the phagocytosis of foreign materials. Reptilian heterophils are very similar in appearance to avian heterophils; the cells are typically round with eosinophilic rod-shaped granules in the cytoplasm, and the nuclei are round to oval in shape.

*Eosinophils* are easily confused with heterophils. They are similar in appearance but differ in that the cytoplasmic granules are round instead of rod shaped. In some chelonians, eosinophils may account for over 20% of circulating white blood cells.

*Basophils* are small, round cells with deep blue cytoplasmic granules. These granules can often obscure the nucleus. Like eosinophils, basophils can normally make up a large percentage of circulating leukocytes in normal chelonians.

*Lymphocytes* can vary in size, and large and small lymphocytes are found together. Lymphocytes are usually round and have large nuclei. Lymphocytes typically have a large nucleus-to-cytoplasm ratio and no cytoplasmic granules. In most reptiles, the lymphocyte is the predominant leukocyte in circulation.

Monocytes are the largest leukocytes in the reptile circulation. The nuclei may be oval or lobed. The cytoplasm in monocytes is typically blue–gray and may contain small vacuoles or fine granules. The monocytes of some reptiles, namely snakes, may have small azurophilic granules in the cytoplasm and therefore are sometimes referred to as *azurophils*. Because these cells are simply a monocyte variant, they are more appropriately labeled *azurophilic monocytes*.

**Thrombocytes** perform the same function as mammalian platelets. Thrombocytes are small oval nucleated cells with clear cytoplasm. The cytoplasm is usually colorless, but may contain small granules.

---

### ✓ TEST YOURSELF 22-4

1. How many cardiac chambers do noncrocodilian reptiles and amphibians have?
2. Right-to-left cardiac shunting serves what function in reptiles?
3. What is the main difference between a *heterophil* and a *neutrophil*?
4. What is the function of a lymph heart?

---

## RESPIRATORY SYSTEM

The anatomy and physiology of the reptilian respiratory system differ significantly from those of mammals. Reptiles are capable of functioning with very low oxygen levels, accounting for many unique features. Owing to their relatively large pulmonary volume, efficient anaerobic metabolism, and cardiac shunting capabilities, reptiles are capable of surviving for long periods of time without breathing.

### CLINICAL APPLICATION

### Blood Collection

Blood collection can be very difficult in amphibians and reptiles, because there are usually no externally visible vessels, therefore it is important to know vascular anatomy to be successful in obtaining usable samples. The vessel most commonly used for blood collection in reptiles is the ventral coccygeal vein, which courses on the midline just ventral to the vertebrae of the tail. This vessel is accessible in snakes, lizards, crocodilians, and salamanders.

Obtaining a blood sample from chelonians presents additional challenges because of the presence of the shell. A variety of options exist, and which one to use depends on the size and species of the turtle or tortoise. The jugular vein, dorsal coccygeal vein, and brachial vein are all used with success, as is the subcarapacial sinus formed by the confluence of the common intercostal veins and the caudal branch of the external jugular vein.

Cardiac puncture can be performed safely on most reptiles and amphibians as long as they are securely restrained or anesthetized. Other options for blood collection include the ventral abdominal vein in amphibians and lizards and the postoccipital sinus in crocodilians and chelonians.

---

Respiration in reptiles is driven by oxygen levels ($PO_2$) in the blood. This is in contrast to mammals, in which $CO_2$ levels are the primary determinants of respiratory rate and tidal volume.

The *glottis* of most amphibians and reptiles is easily located in the rostral portion of the oral cavity (Figure 22-11); it is found behind the tongue in all species, and in snakes it is very mobile. The mobility of the snake glottis makes it capable of protruding from the mouth, allowing respiration during ingestion of prey. The glottal opening, which is only open during respiration, is bordered by paired arytenoid cartilages. Amphibians and reptiles do not have vocal cords and are therefore only capable of limited

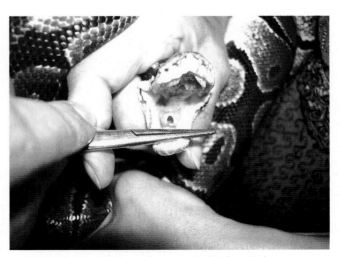

**FIGURE 22-11** Open glottis in a Ball Python *(Python regius).*

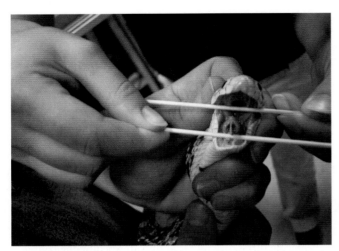

**FIGURE 22-12** Bullsnake *(Pituophis melanoleuca)* glottis showing the preglottal keel.

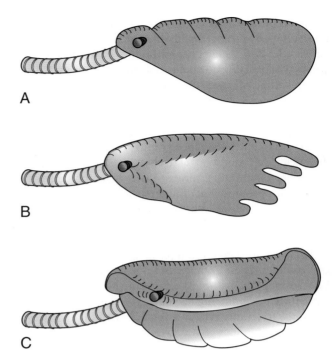

**FIGURE 22-13** Different lung structures found in reptiles. **A**, Unicameral. **B**, Paucicameral. **C**, Multicameral. (Redrawn from O'Malley B: Clinical anatomy and physiology of exotic species, New York, 2005, Saunders.)

vocalization: all species hiss; some grunt, such as chelonians and crocodilians; and some, like crocodilians, bellow. The calling sounds produced by frogs and toads are produced by vocal sacs that arise from the trachea. Movement of air in and out of the vocal sacs produces the sound. Some species of snake possess a *glottal keel* (Figure 22-12), which increases the volume of vocalizations.

Chelonians posses complete cartilaginous tracheal rings, whereas the rings of all other reptiles are incomplete. The tracheal bifurcation occurs in the cervical area of chelonians, but it is lower in other reptiles and is usually found around the base of the heart.

Three distinct lung structures are found in reptiles (Figure 22-13). The most primitive is the **unicameral lung**, which is found in snakes and some lizards. The unicameral lung is a simple, saclike structure. The cranial portion of the unicameral lung typically contains the tissues involved in gas exchange, and the relatively avascular caudal portion is comparable to the avian air sac. The **multicameral lung** is found in chelonians, some lizards, and crocodilians. The multicameral lung is divided into many compartments and possesses intrapulmonary bronchi. An intermediate lung structure, the **paucicameral lung**, shares characteristics of both the unicameral and multicameral lungs. Paucicameral lungs are found most notably in iguanas and chameleons.

The lungs of amphibians are typically simple, saclike structures with little if any partitioning. Some species of salamander do not have lungs at all and rely entirely on cutaneous respiration.

The pulmonary tissue of amphibians and reptiles grossly has a honeycomb appearance (Figure 22-14). The openings of the honeycomb terminate in gas-exchange structures called **faveoli**. Unlike mammalian alveoli, the faveoli are fixed structures that do not expand or contract. The faveoli are surrounded by capillary beds, where the blood takes up oxygen and releases carbon dioxide.

Reptiles do not have true diaphragms, therefore they must rely on different methods of respiration. Most

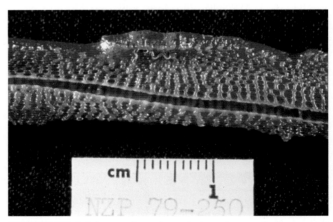

**FIGURE 22-14** Inner surface of a snake lung showing the honeycomb structure. The intrapulmonary trachea is seen running the length of the section. A lungworm is also present.

chelonians and some lizards possess membranous separations between the lungs and the other coelomic viscera that are somewhat analogous to the mammalian diaphragm, although these membranes are not directly involved in the respiratory cycle. Reptiles rely on the action of the intercostal muscles and other parts of the axial musculature to perform the active phases of respiration.

A unique variation in respiration is utilized by crocodilians, which respire through the function of a *hepatic piston*. Crocodilians have a muscular **septum** caudal to the lungs that is somewhat analogous to the mammalian diaphragm, and the cranial aspect of the liver is attached to this septum. The **diaphragmaticus** muscle attaches the caudal aspect of the liver to the pubis. Contraction of the diaphragmaticus moves the postpulmonary septum caudally through the liver, resulting in inflation of the lungs.

Pumping of the buccal cavity and pharynx provides the primary means of pulmonary ventilation in amphibians. Gas exchange can also occur across the mucous membranes of the buccal cavity and pharynx. Many aquatic chelonians are also capable of exchanging gases across the mucous membranes of the pharynx and cloaca.

Old World chameleons have an air sac that arises from the ventral aspect of the trachea in the cervical region. This structure is probably involved in behavioral displays and does not have gas-exchange capabilities. Snakes are unique in that most only have a single right lung. The left lung is present in some species, such as boas and pythons, but is reduced in size. A tracheal lung is present in some snake species and is presumed to allow for some degree of gas exchange during ingestion of prey.

> **TEST YOURSELF 22-5**
> 1. Which reptiles have complete tracheal rings?
> 2. Where does gas exchange take place in the reptilian lung?
> 3. Describe the three different lung structures found in reptiles.

## EARS AND HEARING

The ears are found on both sides of the head and caudal to the eyes in most amphibians and reptiles. The tympanum is easily observed in most species, but lies in a depression and may be covered by folds of skin in some lizards and crocodilians. Like birds, reptiles have a single bone in the middle ear called the *columella*. The columella connects to the tympanum and the quadrate bone, and it transmits vibrations to the oval window of the cochlea, which is part of the inner ear. Vibrations transmitted from the columella to the inner ear are converted to nerve impulses that travel to the brain via the vestibulocochlear nerve.

Reptiles possess semicircular canals comparable to those found in mammals and birds; these fluid-filled canals control balance and equilibrium.

Snakes do not have external ears; their columella articulates distally with the quadrate bone. Articulation of the columella with the quadrate bone allows snakes to be sensitive to ground vibrations that are transmitted through the mandibles. Snakes are also able to hear aerial sounds, especially those of lower frequency. Salamanders and caecilians are somewhat like snakes in that they do not have tympanic membranes and their columella is sometimes degenerate.

Snakes, frogs, toads, and some lizards possess **endolymphatic sacs** associated with their middle ears; these sacs function as calcium-secreting glands. Some, for example those of geckos in the genus *Phelsuma*, are so large they pass

through the skull and bilaterally into the cervical region. These glands are involved in maintaining calcium homeostasis, particularly during egg formation and metamorphosis, in amphibians.

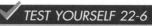

> **TEST YOURSELF 22-6**
> 1. What is the name of the single bone found within the middle ear of a reptile?
> 2. Which reptiles do not have external ear openings?

### CLINICAL APPLICATION

#### Aural Abscesses

Middle ear infections are frequently encountered in both wild and captive chelonians. These infections result in the accumulation of caseous purulent material within the middle ear that results in outward bulging of the tympanum (see figure). The abscess can be unilateral or bilateral and is sometimes larger than the animal's head.

Aural abscesses are likely to result from the ascension of bacteria from the oral cavity into the middle ear through the auditory tube. A variety of bacteria are commonly cultured from these abscesses. Predisposing factors include unsanitary captive conditions and nutritional deficiencies, namely hypovitaminosis A. Hypovitaminosis A results in squamous metaplasia of epithelial surfaces and can affect the middle ear, making it more susceptible to infection.

Treatment requires incising the tympanum and removing the caseous material, followed by thorough flushing. After surgery has been performed, antibiotic therapy, continued flushing, and elimination of predisposing factors complete the therapy.

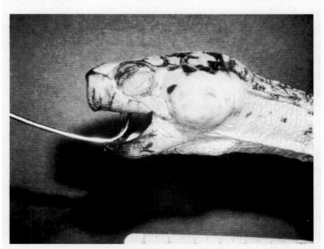

Aural abscess in a Box Turtle (*Terrapene* sp.).

## GASTROINTESTINAL TRACT

Reptiles are remarkable in the wide variety of feeding strategies employed across the class. Carnivorous, omnivorous, and herbivorous reptiles all exist. Snakes and crocodilians are strict carnivores, whereas all three feeding strategies are

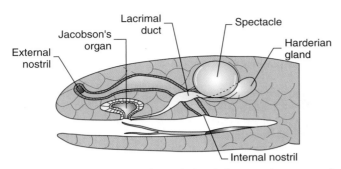

**FIGURE 22-15** Diagram of a snake head illustrating the structure of the vomeronasal organ. (Redrawn from O'Malley B: Clinical anatomy and physiology of exotic species, New York, 2005, Saunders.)

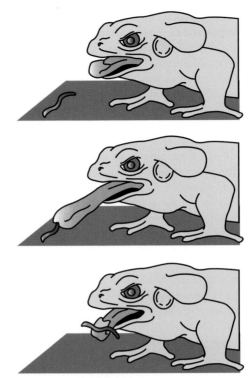

**FIGURE 22-16** Lingual flipping mechanism for prey capture in an anuran. The sequence shows how the tongue unfolds and the rostroventral surface adheres to the prey.

represented among the lizards and chelonians. All adult amphibians are carnivores as well. Some animals have highly specialized diets and only consume specific foods or prey. Examples include snakes such as the King Cobra *(Ophiophagus hannah)*, which preys exclusively on other snakes; the Caiman Lizard *(Dracaena paraguinesis)* feeds only on snails. It is important to know these specialized dietary requirements when attempting to maintain a species in captivity. If incorrect food is offered, acceptance may be poor and nutritional deficiencies can occur.

Snakes and lizards, such as monitors and tegus, have tongues that are deeply forked and function as a particle delivery system for the **vomeronasal organ**. The vomeronasal organ is an accessory olfactory organ (Figure 22-15). The forking of the tongue allows detection of particle gradients across the sampled area, enabling animals to follow scent trails efficiently. Most lizards have fairly mobile tongues, which they use frequently to taste items they encounter. Chameleons have highly specialized projectile tongues designed for capturing prey at long distances. The tongue is long and has a sticky end that sticks to the prey. Muscular connections between the tongue, a specialized hyoid apparatus, and the sternum allow the tongue to be extended to lengths longer than the body in most chameleons. Turtles and tortoises typically have thick, fleshy tongues that are relatively immobile. The Alligator Snapping Turtle has a uniquely adapted tongue, which resembles a small pink worm. The turtle wiggles this tongue with the mouth open to attract prey. Crocodilians have immobile tongues that are attached along their entire length to the intermandibular space. Crocodilians also have muscular flaps arising from the base of the tongue and dorsal pharynx that allow them to open their mouths while submerged without ingesting or inhaling water.

Tongue structure varies according to species in amphibians. All species, except aquatic anurans, salamanders, and caecilians, use the tongue for capturing prey. Anurans and most terrestrial salamanders grasp food through a process called *lingual flipping*, in which the caudodorsal aspect of the fleshy tongue is flipped forward into a cranioventral position (Figure 22-16). Sticky secretions on the surface of the tongue cause the prey to adhere, allowing it to be pulled into the mouth. Lungless salamanders are able to project their tongues much like chameleons when feeding.

There are numerous salivary glands in the oral cavities of most reptiles. The salivary secretions facilitate the ingestion of large prey by providing lubrication. As in mammals, the saliva also has enzymatic properties that aid digestion. The venom glands of some snakes are modified salivary glands and are found in the upper jaw below the eyes. In venomous lizards, members of the genus *Heloderma*, the venom glands are found along the lateral aspects of the lower jaws.

The dentition of reptiles varies significantly according to family. Turtles and tortoises have no teeth but possess keratinized beaks similar to those of birds, called *tomia*. Among the other reptiles, three types of dentition exist: *thecodont*, *pleurodont*, and *acrodont* (Figure 22-17). **Thecodont teeth**, in which the teeth arise from sockets in the skull bones, are found only in crocodilians. **Acrodont teeth**, in which the teeth are fused to the biting edges of the mandible and maxillae, are found in some species of lizards, such as those in the family Agamidae. **Pleurodont teeth** are attached to the periosteum on the medial aspects of both the mandibles and maxillae. Snakes and iguanid lizards have pleurodont dentition. Thecodont and pleurodont teeth are replaced periodically during the life of the animal, whereas acrodont teeth do not grow back if lost or broken.

Snakes are unique in that they possess six rows of teeth: two on the mandibles, two on the maxillae, and two on the palatine/pterygoid bones (Figure 22-18). Venomous snakes

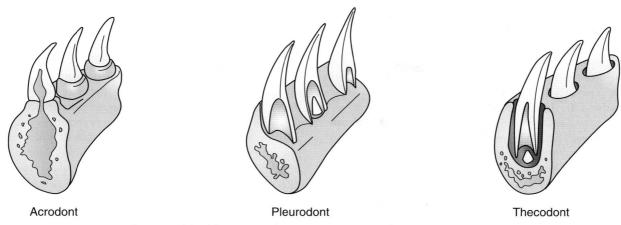

Acrodont          Pleurodont          Thecodont

**FIGURE 22-17** Illustration of the different types of reptile dentition. (From O'Malley B: Clinical anatomy and physiology of exotic species, New York, 2005, Saunders.)

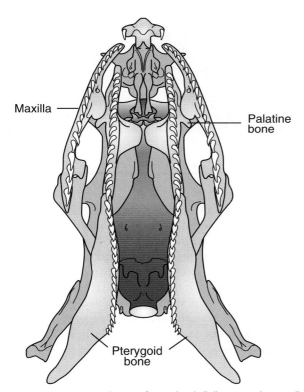

Maxilla

Palatine bone

Pterygoid bone

**FIGURE 22-18** Ventral view of a snake skull illustrating the maxillary and palatine/pterygoid teeth. (From O'Malley B: Clinical anatomy and physiology of exotic species, New York, 2005, Saunders.)

have specialized dentition for venom delivery and are divided into three categories: *solenoglyphous snakes*, or *vipers*; *proteroglyphous snakes*, or *elapids*; and *opisthoglyphous snakes*, or rear-fanged *colubrids*. **Proteroglyphous** and **opisthoglyphous** snakes have fangs that are fixed in an upright position. The fangs of **solenoglyphous** snakes fold against the roof of the mouth when the mouth is closed and are moved into an erect position when the snake bites. Nonvenomous snakes are referred to as **aglyphous**, meaning they are without fangs. The venom-delivering teeth are comparable to

hypodermic needles in that they are hollow with an opening near the end through which the venom is expelled. The fang receives venom through a duct from the venom gland at its base. When delivering a bite, muscles surrounding the venom gland contract to force venom out through the fang. Venomous snakes are capable of controlling the amount of venom delivered with each bite. The primary function of snake venom is for procurement of food; its use for defense is secondary. It should also be noted that enzymes found in snake venom perform an important role in the digestion of prey.

With the notable exception of bufonid toads, most amphibians have teeth. Caecilians and salamanders have both maxillary and mandibular teeth, and some species have palatal teeth. Maxillary dentition occurs sporadically in anuran species, and only one species is known to have mandibular teeth. Some species of frog have well-developed cutting plates on their rostral mandibles called the *odontoid process*.

The reptilian esophagus is relatively thin and distensible in most species, especially in those adapted for consuming large prey. Some reptiles have unique esophageal structures that reflect the type of prey they consume. Sea turtles have conical projections that line the esophagus, and these aid in swallowing slippery food items.

The stomach varies in size and shape according to species and is involved in both chemical and mechanical digestion of food. Snakes have stomachs that are very distensible but often not grossly distinct from the esophagus and duodenum. In crocodilians, the body of the stomach is made up of thick muscle comparable to that of the avian gizzard. Like that of mammals, the pH of the reptilian stomach is usually quite acidic, ranging between 2 and 3 in healthy animals. Hydrochloric acid, pepsinogen, and other enzymes are involved in the chemical digestion of food held in the stomach.

The amphibian gastrointestinal tract is relatively short and simple. The esophagus is very short and wide, especially in anurans. Anurans are capable of prolapsing their stomach through the mouth and cleaning it off after they have ingested an undesirable item. Gastric prolapse can also be seen with some methods of anesthesia or as a terminal event in dying animals. Unlike the intestinal tract in mammals, the amphibian intestinal tract is not easily divided into distinct regions. The liver and gallbladder are usually found close together, and the livers of amphibians often contain aggregations of melanin-containing macrophages called **melano-macrophages**. These cells are involved in immune function and can give the liver a mottled black appearance. The amphibian liver performs the same functions as in other vertebrates. The pancreas is usually found between the stomach and the proximal segments of intestine.

The structure of the reptilian intestinal tract is extremely variable, according to species and, consequently, diet. Herbivores tend to have longer intestinal tracts than carnivores, and omnivores fall somewhere between the two. Snakes have relatively straight intestinal tracts with only minor winding found in the small intestine. The colon can be large and complex in herbivorous species that rely heavily on hindgut fermentation for digestion. In some species, such as the Green Iguana, the colon is partitioned as an adaptation for more efficient hindgut fermentation. Cecae are found in herbivorous lizards and chelonians and also serve as a site for hindgut fermentation. The cecum is absent or rudimentary in carnivorous chelonians, lizards, snakes, and crocodilians.

The liver in reptiles is usually quite large and consists of at least two lobes in most species. The exceptions are snakes, which have a large, elongated, single-lobed liver. Typically the liver makes up approximately 3% to 4% of the body weight in lizards and snakes, although the size can vary with season, nutritional status, and other factors. Most reptiles have a gallbladder, which is variable in size and position; the gallbladder in snakes is found caudal to the liver, near the spleen and pancreas. Blood is supplied to the liver by the hepatic artery and portal vein.

The reptilian liver performs the same functions as the mammalian liver; it excretes bile for digestion, performs metabolic degradation, and produces various substances. Normally, the liver can be dark brown to black in color. Certain metabolic states, such as **vitellogenesis**, can cause a normal change in color of the liver. For example, during vitellogenesis the liver can take on a yellow color due to fat accumulation. This should not be misinterpreted as pathologic hepatic lipidosis. As in amphibians, reptilian livers also often contain large numbers of melanomacrophage centers, which can result in a mottled appearance.

The pancreas is typically found within the mesentery in close proximity to the stomach or duodenum. In snakes, the pancreas is found near the pylorus of the stomach near the gallbladder and spleen. In some snake species and in chelonians, the spleen and pancreas are combined to form a single organ, called the **splenopancreas**. The pancreatic ducts enter the duodenum in most species. In chelonians, the pancreatic ducts and the bile ducts enter the pyloric region of the stomach.

The reptilian pancreas performs both exocrine and endocrine functions. As in mammals, the pancreas produces a variety of digestive enzymes, including but not limited to amylase, chymotrypsin, trypsin, and chitinase. The exact makeup of pancreatic secretions is dependent on species and diet, and the function of enzymes depends on appropriate temperature. Pancreatic islets are found throughout the pancreas in reptiles and contain glucagon-secreting alpha cells, insulin-secreting beta cells, and other cells capable of secreting somatostatin and pancreatic polypeptide. Glucagon and insulin are involved in the maintenance of blood glucose levels in mammals, but it is important to note that blood glucose levels in reptiles are much more variable because of the fluctuations in metabolic rate related to ectothermy.

Figures 22-19 through 22-22 illustrate the gastrointestinal tract and other aspects of internal anatomy of a chelonian, lizard, snake, and frog, respectively.

---

✓ **TEST YOURSELF 22-7**
1. What is the function of the vomeronasal organ?
2. Name the different types of dentition found in reptiles.
3. Which amphibians do not have teeth?
4. What herptiles are capable of gastric prolapse as a method of emptying their stomachs?

---

## CLOACA

All amphibians and reptiles possess a common outflow tract for the gastrointestinal and urogenital tracts called the *cloaca*. The cloaca is made up of three chambers: the *coprodeum*, *urodeum*, and *proctodeum* (Figure 22-23). In some species, the cloacal chambers are distinctly separated by muscular sphincters; in other species, they are less discrete. The coprodeum is the most cranial chamber and receives the rectum. The urodeum is the middle chamber, where the urogenital openings, urethra, and male reproductive organs

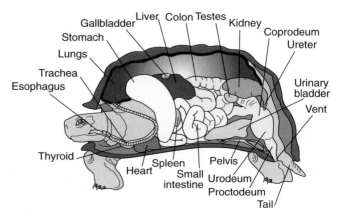

**FIGURE 22-19** Cross section showing the internal anatomy of a chelonian. (Redrawn from O'Malley B: Clinical anatomy and physiology of exotic species, New York, 2005, Saunders.)

bladder. The urinary bladder, if present, is connected to the urodeum by a short, broad urethra. The urine enters the bladder for storage through the urodeum. It is important to note that crocodilians, snakes, and some species of lizard do not possess urinary bladders. When the bladder is absent, any storage of urine occurs in the cloacal chambers or the rectum.

Reptile kidneys do not have a distinct renal pelvis. Instead, the distal tubules of the nephrons join into collecting ducts, which eventually come together and form the ureter. Unlike those of mammals, the reptile nephron does not have a loop of Henle, so reptiles are incapable of producing urine more concentrated than their blood. When water conservation is necessary, reptiles are able to absorb additional water from the urine through the wall of the urinary bladder, rectum, or cloaca, which results in voided urine that is somewhat concentrated.

Following the distal tubule of the nephron, a sexual segment is found, the cells of which enlarge when high levels of reproductive hormones are in circulation. These sexual segments are believed to add secretions to the seminal fluid in male reptiles, but their exact function is unknown.

Other unique physiologic characteristics allow reptiles to conserve water very efficiently, even though they are unable to produce concentrated urine. The first is the production of uric acid as a protein waste product in terrestrial reptiles. Uric acid is relatively insoluble in blood and is voided via secretion from the renal tubules. Because uric acid is secreted rather than filtered, very little urine is needed to excrete it from the body. (Production of uric acid is also functionally important for embryos in the egg, because it is relatively insoluble and nontoxic, therefore relatively large amounts can be stored in the egg without adverse effects.) Aquatic or semiaquatic reptiles produce ammonia, urea, or both as a waste product; these are much more soluble but also more toxic than uric acid. The aquatic environment allows these reptiles to pass large amounts of urine to eliminate waste products without risk of dehydration.

The second characteristic that allows water conservation is the presence of a renal portal system (see Chapter 18). The renal portal veins arise from the veins of the tail and hindlimbs, if such are present. The renal portal vessels lead to capillary beds; these perfuse the renal tubules but bypass the glomeruli. This anatomic configuration allows the reptile to discontinue blood flow to the glomeruli and decrease urine production during times of dehydration, while maintaining blood flow to the renal tubules. By maintaining blood flow to the tubules, ischemic necrosis is avoided and uric acid secretion continues.

Following excretion by the kidneys, uric acid combines with minerals to form potassium or calcium salts. These uric acid salts, or urates, are passed with the feces and urine and appear as a white, chalky substance (Figure 22-25).

Amphibian kidneys are somewhat more primitive than reptilian kidneys. In addition to filtering the blood, amphibian kidneys also filter coelomic fluid via openings called *nephrostomes* that connect the coelomic cavity to the renal

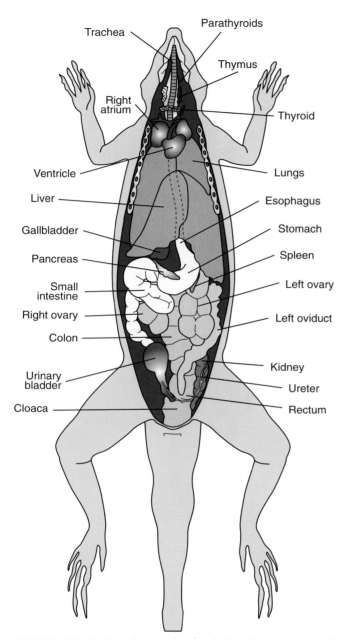

**FIGURE 22-20** Ventral view of a female lizard showing internal anatomy. (Redrawn from O'Malley B: Clinical anatomy and physiology of exotic species, New York, 2005, Saunders.)

of crocodilians and chelonians are found. The proctodeum is the last chamber before the vent and often contains glandular tissue.

## KIDNEYS

The kidneys of reptiles differ significantly in structure and function from those of mammals. In crocodilians, turtles, and most lizards, the kidneys are oblong, smooth-surfaced structures found in the caudal coelomic cavity. Snakes possess kidneys that are lobulated and grossly resemble a stack of melted coins (Figure 22-24). The ureters empty into the dorsolateral aspect of the urodeum instead of the urinary

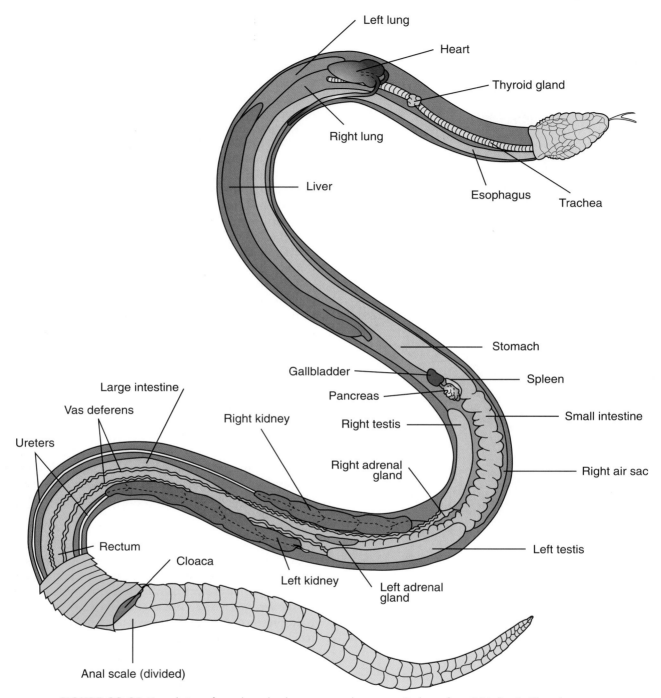

**FIGURE 22-21** Ventral view of a male snake showing internal anatomy. (Redrawn from O'Malley B: Clinical anatomy and physiology of exotic species, New York, 2005, Saunders.)

tubules. The kidneys of amphibians are usually lobulated and are found in the caudodorsal coelomic cavity. Larval and aquatic amphibians typically produce and excrete ammonia as a nitrogenous waste product. Amphibians that lead more terrestrial life-styles excrete considerable amounts of urea, and some specialized species of tree frogs (*Phyllomedusa* spp.) that inhabit relatively arid areas have even evolved to produce uric acid. As in reptiles, the amphibian kidney is incapable of producing urine more concentrated than the blood. Thus, species with less access to water need to produce

less toxic, more soluble nitrogenous waste products to conserve water. All amphibians have urinary bladders and a cloacal anatomy similar to those of reptiles.

## REPRODUCTIVE SYSTEM

### MALE ANATOMY

All male reptiles have internal testes. They are located in the dorsal coelomic cavity in close proximity to the caudal vena

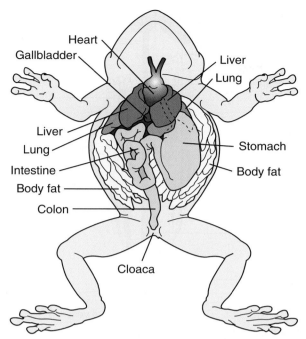

**FIGURE 22-22** Ventral view of a frog showing internal anatomy. (Redrawn from O'Malley B: Clinical anatomy and physiology of exotic species, New York, 2005, Saunders.)

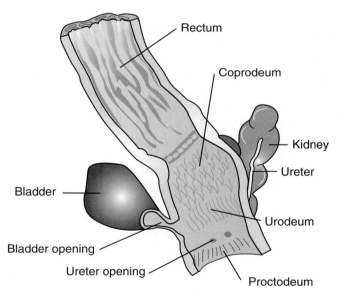

**FIGURE 22-23** Illustration of the distal colon, cloaca, bladder, and kidney of a lizard. (From O'Malley B: Clinical anatomy and physiology of exotic species, New York, 2005, Saunders.)

---

✔ *TEST YOURSELF 22-8*

1. Given that reptiles are unable to produce concentrated urine, how do they conserve water?
2. What nitrogenous waste products are produced most frequently by aquatic amphibians? What nitrogenous waste products are produced by terrestrial amphibians?
3. What is the purpose of the renal portal system?
4. Where do the ureters terminate in reptiles and amphibians?

---

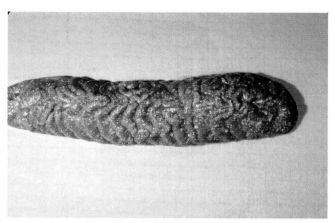

**FIGURE 22-24** Snake kidney. The white mottling is due to uric acid deposits; this snake suffered from gout.

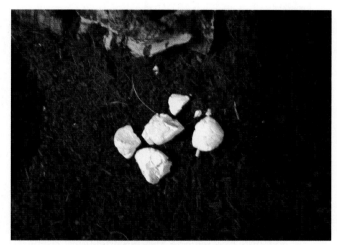

**FIGURE 22-25** Urates from a snake.

cava, aorta, and adrenal glands. The *ductus deferens* leads from the testes to the dorsal wall of the urodeum. Most male reptiles also have a sexual portion to the kidney tubules, which develops in response to high levels of circulating sex hormones. These areas of the renal tubules probably provide secretions that contribute to the seminal fluid.

Male reptiles all possess copulatory organs, and fertilization is internal. The copulatory organs of reptiles vary in structure according to family. Crocodilians and chelonians have a phallus that originates in the floor of the cloaca. This phallus is composed of erectile tissue and forms a trough, through which semen is transmitted to the female's cloaca. The phallus has no function in urination. Male snakes and lizards possess paired structures, called **hemipenes**, that can be everted from the tail base through the vent (Figure 22-26). These hemipenes also form a trough through which semen is carried and serve no purpose in urination.

## FEMALE ANATOMY

All female reptiles have paired ovaries, which are found in the dorsal coelomic cavity in close proximity to the caudal vena cava, aorta, and adrenal glands. The paired oviducts

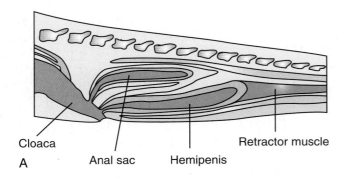

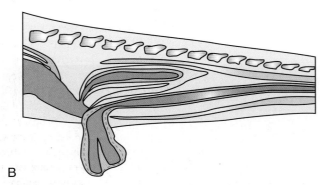

**B**

**FIGURE 22-26** Cross section of a snake tail showing the hemipenes in both the resting **(A)** and everted **(B)** positions. (From O'Malley B: Clinical anatomy and physiology of exotic species, New York, 2005, Saunders.)

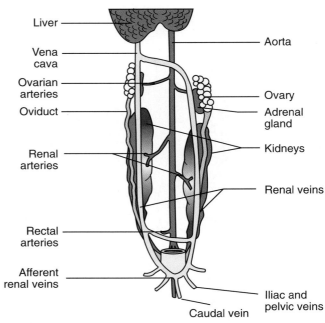

**FIGURE 22-27** Diagram illustrating the reproductive anatomy of a female lizard. (From O'Malley B: Clinical anatomy and physiology of exotic species, New York, 2005, Saunders.)

lead to the cloaca and terminate at the genital papillae in the dorsal wall of the urodeum (Figure 22-27). The oviducts are divided into five regions: the *infundibulum, magnum, isthmus, uterus,* and *vagina*. Ova from the ovaries are released to the oviducts during ovulation. The albumen and shell are added in the oviduct in **oviparous** species prior to egg laying. The fetuses are retained in the uterine portion of the oviduct for development in **viviparous** species.

## REPRODUCTIVE CYCLE

The quiescent ovary is covered with small, inactive follicles. When certain environmental cues are encountered, estrogen and follicle-stimulating hormone (FSH) are released; this causes development and maturation of the follicles via a process called *vitellogenesis*, which is the process of adding vitellogenin, a lipid substance, to the yolk within the developing follicle. Vitellogenin is formed by the liver from mobilized fat, and during vitellogenesis the liver often takes on a yellow color. Large amounts of calcium are also added to the yolk during this process. Circulating calcium levels tend to be very high in reptiles during vitellogenesis, because calcium is mobilized by bone to supply the developing follicles.

Following maturation of the follicles, a surge of luteinizing hormone (LH) causes ovulation, and the ova are released from the follicles and taken up into the oviducts. In the oviducts, the albumen, shell membranes, and shell are laid down prior to the egg being laid. In all viviparous

reptiles, some degree of support of the fetus is continued by the female, and some lizards possess true placentas.

## OVIPOSITION

Many reptiles dig nests and therefore need suitable substrate to lay eggs. If not provided with suitable nesting material, some female reptiles will be reluctant to lay and may experience dystocia. Most snakes readily make use of enclosed egg-laying chambers lined with moist substrate. Chelonians and lizard species, such as iguanas and chameleons, will often excavate deep holes to deposit their eggs in; they should be provided with suitable nesting material when **oviposition** is imminent.

Few reptiles show any interest in their eggs or offspring after oviposition or parturition. Exceptions include crocodilians, which protect their nests and provide protection for the young for a period of time following hatching. Pythons and cobras protect their nests until hatching.

## EGG INCUBATION

The anatomy of the reptilian egg is comparable to that of the avian egg. Refer to Chapter 21 for a description of the avian egg.

Successful hatching of eggs requires appropriate environmental conditions in the nest. Temperature, humidity, and gas composition of the environment must be within acceptable ranges for healthy embryos to develop. The substrate on which eggs are incubated must retain an appropriate amount of moisture without encouraging growth of bacteria and fungi (Figure 22-28). Incubation time and temperature vary according to species; incubation time can range from a few weeks to well over a year. Typically, eggs will hatch faster if

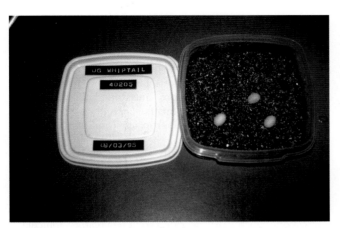

**FIGURE 22-28** Incubating lizard eggs in vermiculite substrate.

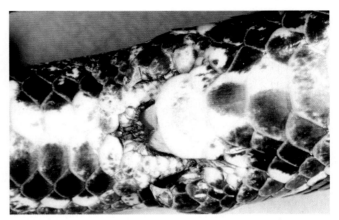

**FIGURE 22-29** Pelvic spurs of a male African Rock Python (*Python sebae*).

incubated at temperatures at the high end of the acceptable range. Some species of chelonian require a diapause during incubation for the embryos to develop normally and proceed to hatching. A diapause occurs when incubation temperatures drop and development stops for a period of time; development resumes when temperatures rise again.

Reptile eggs do not need to be rotated during incubation, unlike bird eggs. The embryonic membranes and shell membranes form attachments within a few days of oviposition that solidly anchor the developing embryo within the shell. Repositioning eggs following development of these attachments can destroy the embryo.

## SEX DETERMINATION

Sex in reptiles is determined by either the genotype or the temperature at which the eggs are incubated. Sex chromosomes are not present in species such as crocodilians, chelonians, tuataras, and some lizards, therefore egg incubation temperature determines the sex of the hatchling. In general, higher incubation temperatures produce males and lower temperatures produce females in crocodilians and lizards, but the opposite is true for chelonians. In nature, there is typically a temperature range within the nest that allows the production of a mixed clutch of male and female hatchlings. Reptiles that possess sex chromosomes differ from mammals in that the females are the heterozygous sex *(ZW)* and males are homozygous *(ZZ).*

## SECONDARY SEXUAL CHARACTERISTICS

Snakes do not tend to show significant **sexual dimorphism**. Many times, the tail is longer and thicker in males owing to the presence of the hemipenes. In boids, pelvic spurs can be larger in males; pelvic spurs are remnants of the pelvic limbs, and these are used by males to provide tactile stimulation to females during courtship (Figure 22-29).

Male chelonians often have a concave **plastron**, which allows closer apposition of the cloacas when the male mounts the female. The vent is also located in a more distal position in males for the same reason. Other, less reliable, keys to sexing chelonians are eye color, **carapace** shape, and the length of claws on the forelimbs.

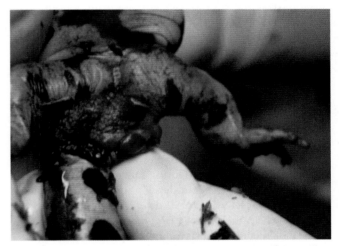

**FIGURE 22-30** Cloacal glands in a male Tiger Salamander (*Ambystoma tigrinum*). The glands are the bulging tissue behind the legs at the base of the tail.

Some lizards show significant dimorphism that is readily apparent, even to the untrained eye. A good example is the Jackson's Chameleon (*Chameleo jacksonii*); the males have three well-developed horns on their faces, and the females have none. In Green Iguanas, the males are larger with more pronounced dewlaps and crests. Hemipenal bulges can also be detected in the tail base of some male lizards. Iguanids and geckonids have femoral or precloacal pores that are frequently more developed in males.

Crocodilians sometimes display significant differences in size as adults, and the males are clearly larger than the females.

## AMPHIBIAN REPRODUCTION

Sexual dimorphism is present in many amphibians. In some species of poison dart frogs, the males have enlarged toe pads. The tympanic membranes are larger in some male anurans. Male salamanders possess prominent cloacal glands (Figure 22-30) that are visible around the vent. Some male anurans and newts develop rough **nuptial pads** on their limbs in response to testicular hormones. These nuptial pads help the male grasp the female during fertilization. Male anurans will also call when conditions are appropriate.

Amphibians have paired gonads, which are found in the dorsocaudal coelomic cavity. Male toads possess ovarian remnants associated with the testes called the **Bidder's organs**.

The majority of caecilians are viviparous and most anurans and salamanders are oviparous. Internal fertilization occurs in caecilians and most salamanders. Caecilians evert a portion of their cloaca, the *phallodeum*, to deposit semen into the female's cloaca. Male salamanders deposit packets of sperm called *spermatophores* onto substrate; these are subsequently picked up by the female salamander's cloaca. Female salamanders can store sperm for extended periods of time in pockets within the cloaca called *spermatotheca*. In anurans, fertilization is external; male frogs and toads fertilize the eggs as they are laid, while grasping the female in an embrace called *amplexus*.

Amphibian eggs are usually deposited in or near water, because *larvae*, amphibian young, are typically water dependent. Some anurans and most salamanders display some form of parental care of eggs or young. Many amphibians that display parental care will carry the eggs or young on their backs, on their legs, or in pouches found on the dorsal or ventral surfaces.

Larval anurans, or tadpoles, lead completely aquatic lives prior to metamorphosis. Tadpoles have round bodies and laterally compressed tails. During metamorphosis, tadpoles lose their gills and tails and develop limbs. Metamorphosis is usually complete within 90 days in most species. Some species, such as the Bullfrog (*Rana catesbiana*), are capable of delaying metamorphosis for up to 2 years. Metamorphosis is stimulated by thyroid hormones.

Some larval salamanders have forms similar to those of tadpoles, but they do not lose their tails when they change to their adult form. Many species of salamander bypass the larval stage and hatch in their adult form. Some species of salamander, such as the Axolotl (*Ambystoma mexicanum*) are *neotenic*, which means they retain their larval form into adulthood.

---

 **CLINICAL APPLICATION**

### Preovulatory Follicular Stasis and Egg Binding

Many factors are involved in stimulating and maintaining normal reproductive function in reptiles. These factors include nutrition, temperature, humidity, light cycle, and suitable egg-laying environments. Disruption of normal function can occur when inappropriate conditions occur in captive settings.

Preovulatory follicular stasis occurs when large, mature follicles develop on the ovaries but ovulation fails to occur. These mature follicles take up space within the coelomic cavity and can cause decreased feed intake owing to impingement on the stomach. Also, retained follicles are prone to infection, which can lead to sepsis. Preovulatory follicular stasis is usually corrected by surgical removal of the ovaries (ovariectomy).

Egg binding can be caused by all of the aforementioned factors, but most frequently it seems to be the result of inadequate calcium balance due to poor nutrition or conditions that result in mechanical obstruction of the oviducts. If no obstructions are present, oviposition can be encouraged by providing appropriate environmental conditions and nesting substrate, as well as correction of any nutritional deficits. If all conditions are considered normal, and the animal is healthy, oxytocin can be used effectively to stimulate oviduct contractions and oviposition in most chelonians. The effectiveness of oxytocin is variable, but is generally poor, in other reptile species. Surgical removal of the eggs or the reproductive tract should be pursued when oviduct or cloacal obstruction occurs, or in animals unresponsive to conservative therapy.

---

species, and the gland can be seen as diffuse tissue in the cervical region. The size of the thyroid gland varies according to season and metabolic state. Thyroid hormone is involved in the process of ecdysis and growth.

Also found in the cervical region are the parathyroid glands and ultimobrachial bodies. These glands are separate from the thyroid and can be difficult to find grossly. The parathyroid glands secrete parathormone and the ultimobrachial bodies produce calcitonin. Both hormones are involved in calcium and phosphorus homeostasis (see Chapter 11).

The adrenal glands are usually found in the ligaments that suspend the gonads (mesorchium or mesovarium) and are therefore in close proximity to the gonads. The exceptions are chelonians and crocodilians, in which the adrenals lie against the kidneys. The adrenal glands are usually red or yellow and can become enlarged with stress. Reptilian adrenal glands produce the same hormones as avian glands: *epinephrine*, *norepinephrine*, *aldosterone*, and *corticosterone*. There is no distinct separation between the adrenal cortex and the medulla in reptilian adrenal glands.

The exact location of the various endocrine organs in amphibians varies greatly according to species. In general, the form and function of these organs are comparable to what is observed in reptiles. Thyroid hormone is responsible for stimulating metamorphosis and ecdysis in amphibians.

---

### ✔ TEST YOURSELF 22-9

1. How is sex determined in reptiles that do not possess sex chromosomes?
2. What are the names of the male copulatory organs in snakes and lizards?
3. Describe the process of fertilization in salamanders.
4. What is vitellogenesis?

---

## ENDOCRINE SYSTEM

With the exception of lizards, all reptiles have a single thyroid gland. It is tan in color and found ventral to the trachea and cranial to the great vessels of the heart. In crocodilians, the thyroid is bilobed with a thin isthmus in between. Lizards have variable thyroid gland structure among the various

### Nutritional Secondary Hyperparathyroidism

Nutritional secondary hyperparathyroidism occurs frequently in herbivorous or omnivorous reptiles that receive diets deficient in calcium or vitamin D, or in animals not provided with access to adequate ultraviolet radiation. In response to low calcium availability, the parathyroid glands secrete high levels of parathormone, which results in resorption of calcium from the skeletal system, retention of calcium by the kidneys, and increased intestinal absorption of calcium. These effects maintain normal blood calcium levels, which are necessary for life. If the nutritional or environmental deficits are not corrected, bones become depleted of minerals, are weakened, and are prone to pathologic fractures. In an effort to provide support to the limbs, fibrous connective tissue develops in place of bone, in a condition called *fibrous osteodystrophy.*

Hypocalcemia can develop if the bones become completely depleted of calcium. Clinical signs associated with hypocalcemia include constipation, anorexia, muscle weakness, muscle tremors, and seizures. Many animals can recover if provided with supportive care, appropriate environmental conditions, and an appropriate diet.

## NERVOUS SYSTEM

The neuroanatomy of reptiles follows the basic vertebrate design with a central nervous system consisting of a brain and a spinal cord. There are three major divisions within the reptilian brain: the *forebrain*, which comprises the olfactory lobes, cerebral hemispheres, and a diencephalon; the *midbrain*, made up of the optic lobes, cerebral peduncles, and nerve fibers connecting the hindbrain to the forebrain; and the *hindbrain*, which is the cerebellum and medulla oblongata. Peripheral nerves provide motor and sensory innervation.

The reptilian brain is **lissencephalic**, meaning there are no gyri or sulci present on the surface. In terms of evolution, reptiles were the first group to have a cerebral cortex separated into hemispheres and to have a brain offset from the spinal cord and extending back over the diencephalon.

The two meninges in reptiles are the *pia–arachnoid layer* and the *dura mater.* The pia–arachnoid layer is vascular and lies directly on the surface of the brain and spinal cord. The dura mater lies over the pia–arachnoid layer and is relatively avascular.

Unlike mammals, reptiles do not have a *cauda equina*, and the spinal cord extends to the tip of the spine.

Reptiles are the lowest vertebrates to have 12 cranial nerves; fish and amphibians have only 10. The spinal nerves of reptiles are also advanced beyond those of fishes and amphibians, and only sensory fibers are found in the dorsal roots and motor fibers in the ventral roots.

Reptiles depend more on spinal segmental reflexes and locomotion centers for the control of movement than they do cerebral stimulation. As a result, body movements are more autonomous in reptiles than in mammals and birds. Because of their spinal autonomy, reptiles with spinal cord injuries usually have a much better prognosis than do mammals with comparable lesions.

The amphibian nervous system is more primitive than that of reptiles. Amphibian brains are well adapted to support basic functions such as sight, olfaction, and movement, but they have very limited integrative capabilities. The spinal cord extends to the tip of the tail in amphibians and caecilians. In frogs and toads, the spinal cord ends in the lumbar region and a cauda equina is present. Much like reptiles, amphibians are heavily dependent on spinal segmental reflexes to control movement.

## MUSCULOSKELETAL SYSTEM

### SKULL

There is extreme variation in the skulls of the different reptile orders. The different types are divided into two general categories: *anapsid* and *diapsid* (Figure 22-31). Chelonians possess **anapsid skulls**, which do not have temporal openings. All other reptiles possess **diapsid skulls**, which means they *do* have temporal openings in the skull. Unique skulls are found in the lizards and snakes, which have skulls that are designed to have significant flexibility. This flexibility allows for ingestion of large prey. Snake skulls in particular are extremely mobile, because the mandibular symphysis is not fused in snakes, rather it is connected by ligaments. This flexible connection of the rostral mandibles allows the

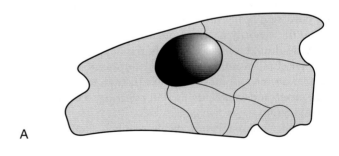

A

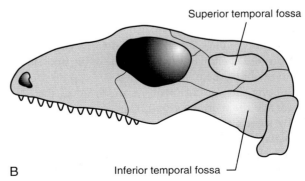

Superior temporal fossa

Inferior temporal fossa

B

**FIGURE 22-31** Illustration of anapsid and diapsid skull types. **A**, Anapsid skulls are found in chelonians. **B**, Diapsid skulls are found in crocodilians, tuataras, snakes, and lizards.

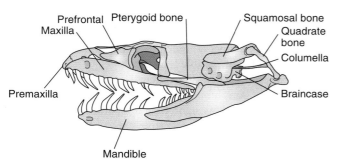

**FIGURE 22-32** Skull of a nonvenomous snake. (Redrawn from O'Malley B: Clinical anatomy and physiology of exotic species, New York, 2005, Saunders.)

jaws to move independently of one another and literally "walk" forward when prey is ingested. Other adaptations include the presence of quadrate bones, which allow the mouth to open very wide, and movable bones that make up the maxillae and palate (Figure 22-32).

The skulls of anurans are typically broad and fenestrated, with fewer bones than those of other amphibians. The parts of the skull involved with olfaction and hearing are better developed than they are in salamanders and caecilians, but the palate is poorly developed, and the dentition is reduced.

Caecilians have compact, well-ossified skulls, and the dentition is well developed. Salamander skulls generally represent an intermediate between caecilian and anuran skulls.

## AXIAL SKELETON

With the exception of chelonians, the spines of reptiles are extremely flexible in comparison to those of mammals. This is possible because reptilian spines are not required to support significant amounts of weight, as most reptiles spend the majority of their time with their bellies in contact with the ground. Unlike mammals, it is not possible to divide the vertebral regions of reptiles into cervical, thoracic, lumbar, sacral, and caudal regions. Instead, the terms *presacral*, *sacral*, and *caudal* are used in referring to reptilian vertebral regions.

Another unique feature of the reptilian axial skeleton is the presence of a single occipital condyle that forms the articulation between the skull and spine. This allows for increased mobility of the head on the spine but also makes this connection relatively fragile, necessitating care when restraining reptiles. Most reptiles have well-developed ribs that help support the body wall and assist in respiration. The exceptions are chelonians, in which the spine and ribs are fused to the bony shell.

The bony shell of chelonians is made up of the *dorsal carapace* and the *ventral plastron*. The bone is covered externally by keratinized scutes. Some chelonians, such as Box Turtles, have hinged plastrons that allow them to withdraw into their shells and close up completely for protection.

Many lizard and salamander species are capable of losing their tails via a defensive mechanism called **tail autonomy**. Tail autonomy allows lizards to drop their tails when being pursued or attacked by a predator. The discarded tail usually continues to wiggle about, which is intended to draw the attention of the attacker while the lizard makes its escape. The tails of lizards capable of autonomy have fracture planes along which they break. When tails are lost this way, there is usually little or no blood loss, because the muscles of the tail contract strongly, and the blood vessels are occluded. The lost tail can regenerate with a stiff, cartilaginous rod that replaces the spine in the tail. In lizards, the regenerated tail is usually smaller and stiffer than the original. The regenerated tails of salamanders usually closely resemble the original.

The number of vertebrae found in amphibians varies greatly. Caecilians can have up to 250, salamanders from 30 to 100, and anurans from six to nine. With the exception of the first cervical vertebra, the atlas, the vertebrae of caecilians are indistinguishable. In salamanders and anurans, the vertebrae are somewhat more differentiated, because these animals also possess sacral vertebrae. In anurans, the vertebrae are fused, and the last caudal vertebra is called the *urostyle*. Ribs are well developed in caecilians, poorly developed in salamanders, and absent in anurans. Caecilians lack a sternum, whereas it exists as a small cartilaginous plate in salamanders. Anurans have a well-developed, ossified sternum.

## APPENDICULAR SKELETON

The skeletal structures of reptilian limbs are comparable to those of mammals, with a few exceptions. In reptiles, the pectoral girdle consists basically of a scapula and coracoid bone, which have muscular attachments to the body. The bones of the pectoral limbs articulate with the scapula and coracoid bones and consist of a humerus, radius, ulna, carpal bones, metacarpal bones, and phalanges. The pelvis of a reptile articulates with the sacral vertebrae and forms the connection between the spine and pelvic limb. The pelvic limb consists of the femur, tibia, tarsal bones, metatarsal bones, and phalanges. Reptiles typically have five digits on both front and rear feet. Exceptions occur, such as in crocodilians, which have only four digits on the hind feet. In most reptiles, the hindlimbs are longer than the forelimbs.

Snakes, obviously, are devoid of limbs, though some species, such as pythons and boas, have vestigial pelvic limbs. These vestigial limbs are referred to as *spurs* and are found on either side of the vent. The spurs are used in courtship behavior and can be larger in males. Some species of lizards also have rudimentary limbs that move in a manner similar to those of snakes. These legless species of lizards all retain vestigial thoracic and pelvic limb structures.

The pectoral girdle of salamanders consists of the *precoracoid*, *coracoid*, and *scapula*. All of these structures are cartilaginous, and they are ossified only at the point where they articulate with the humerus. The pectoral girdle of anurans is more complex and completely ossified. It is made up of the *scapula, clavicle,* and *coracoid*. The skeletal structure of the pectoral limb is comparable to that of reptiles, with the exception of the fused radius and ulna, called the *radioulna*, which is found in anurans. Anurans and salamanders typically have four toes on the pectoral limbs.

Concertina

Lateral undulation

Sidewinding

Rectilinear

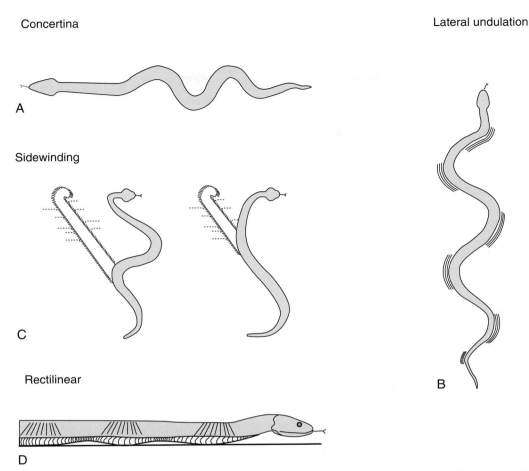

A

C

D

B

**FIGURE 22-33** Different methods of locomotion employed by snakes. **A,** Concertina—the back half anchors while the front half moves forward, and vice versa. **B,** Lateral undulation—when the body comes in contact with an object or rough surface, it thrusts itself forward. **C,** Sidewinding—this is used by desert species on loose sand and involves moving laterally by throwing the body in loops sideways. **D,** Rectilinear—this is used by large snakes, such as boas and pythons, which use the ventral skin and attached muscle to pull themselves forward in a straight line, similar to a caterpillar. (Redrawn from O'Malley B: Clinical anatomy and physiology of exotic species, New York, 2005, Saunders.)

The pelvic girdle of amphibians consists of the *ilium, ischium,* and *pubis.* The pelvic limb of anurans is elongated in comparison to the forelimb and is well adapted to swimming and jumping. The skeletal structure of the amphibian hindlimb is comparable to that of other vertebrates, the exception being the elongated metatarsal bones in anurans, which are known as the *astragalus* and *calcaneum.* Five toes are typically present on the hindlimbs of anurans and salamanders.

## MUSCLES

The muscular structure of four-limbed amphibians and reptiles varies according to species, but is somewhat analogous to the muscular structure in mammals.

Snakes have well-developed epaxial muscles, as well as segmental muscles that attach the ventral scutes to the ends of the ribs. This muscular arrangement allows a number of effective methods of locomotion (Figure 22-33).

Amphibian and reptilian muscles are incapable of sustained aerobic metabolism and switch quickly to anaerobic metabolism with prolonged physical exertion. Anaerobic metabolism is less efficient than aerobic metabolism and results in rapid buildup of lactate. Lactate decreases the pH of the blood and tissues and is metabolized slowly by reptiles. For this reason, reptiles are unable to sustain physical activity and are capable of only short bursts of motion.

> ✓ *TEST YOURSELF 22-10*
> 1. What adaptations are found in the snake skull that allow the ingestion of large prey?
> 2. What is tail autonomy?
> 3. What is unique about the attachment between the skull and cervical spine of a reptile?
> 4. Why are reptiles unable to sustain physical activity for long periods of time?

## SUMMARY

Amphibians and reptiles are remarkable creatures. Collectively known as herptiles, they differ from mammals in extraordinary ways. For example, unlike mammals, herptiles are ectothermic, and regulate their body temperature by adjusting their posture and by moving to areas that are cooler or hotter as needed. Herptiles consist of four orders of reptiles and three orders of amphibians.

Like that of mammals, the skin of reptiles includes an epidermis, dermis, and subcutaneous space. The epidermis of most reptiles has distinct scales and can form unique structures such as crests, tubercles, and spines. The dermis is composed of dense connective tissue, which may contain bony plates for protection. Reptiles shed their skin as they grow, in a process called echysis. The epidermis of amphibians, in contrast, is very thin and permeable, which allows them to absorb all the water they need percutaneously. They do not, therefore, need to drink. Like reptiles, amphibians shed the outer layer of the epidermis and often consume the exuvia.

The cardiovascular system of herptiles is quite different from that of mammals. Remarkably, most reptiles and all amphibians have a three-chambered heart, not four as mammals do, consisting of two atria and one large ventricle. Heart rate depends on species, size, temperature, activity level, and metabolic function. Therefore, it can be challenging to determine whether or not a herptilian patient has an abnormal heart rate. The lymphatic system in herptiles is very well developed with large lymph vessels. Herptiles have no lymph nodes but instead possess sections of special lymph vessels that include smooth muscles in the vessel wall. These specialized lymph vessels (known as lymph hearts) actively pump lymph through the vasculature. Unlike that of mammals, reptilian blood contains oval, nucleated red blood cells and phagocytic heterophils. The enzyme-rich neutrophil of mammals liquefies necrotic debris and produces fluid, white pus. In contrast, heterophils in reptiles lack these enzymes and therefore produce solid, cheeselike pus.

Reptiles have a remarkably large pulmonary volume, efficient anaerobic metabolism, and cardiac shunting capabilities that enable them to survive for long periods of time without breathing. They can function with very low oxygen levels and may possess one of three different types of lung (unicameral, paucicameral, or multicameral) depending on species. In contrast, the lungs of amphibians are typically simple saclike structures, and some species, such as salamanders, lack lungs entirely and exchange gases through their skin instead. The pulmonary tissue in herptiles has a honeycomb appearance and terminates in gas-exchange structures called faveoli (rather than alveoli, which are found in mammals).

Interestingly, all adult amphibians are carnivorous, whereas reptiles may be herbivorous, omnivorous, or carnivorous depending on species. Snakes and crocodilians are strict carnivores, whereas various species of lizards and chelonians may utilize any one of the three feeding strategies. Snakes and lizards use their flickering tongues to detect their prey by capturing ambient particles in the air. The tongue is subsequently inserted into the vomeronasal organ located in the roof of the mouth. There, the molecules stimulate sensory input, enabling the animal to track its prey or find water, for example. The rest of the gastrointestinal tract in reptiles is

quite variable among species, but most herptiles have the usual parts: teeth, salivary glands, esophagus, stomach, liver, gallbladder, intestinal tract, pancreas, spleen, and cloaca. The size and structure of these organs are highly variable among species. Similarly, great variability exists in the structure of the urogenital system and the location, size, shape, and number of the kidneys, ureters, urodeum, bladder, and adrenal glands. With respect to the reproductive system, all male reptiles have internal testes and most possess a sexual portion to the kidney tubules that develops in response to high levels of sex hormones. Male snakes and lizards possess paired structures called hemipenes, which are everted through the vent for mating. The hemipenes form a trough through which semen is carried. However, the phallus has no role in urination. Once fertilized, females can either lay eggs (oviparous) or deliver live offspring (viviparous). Gender in reptiles is determined by either the genotype or the temperature at which the eggs are incubated. Sex chromosomes are not present in some species such as crocodilians, therefore sex is determined during incubation. In crocodilians and lizards, higher temperatures produce males and lower temperatures produce females. In other species, the reverse may be true.

Reptiles have a cerebral cortex separated into two hemispheres. However, the reptilian brain contains no sulci or gyri on its surface and is therefore called lissencephalic. Reptiles do not possess a cauda equine, so the spinal cord extends to the tip of the tail. They are also the lowest vertebrates to have 12 cranial nerves, whereas amphibians have 10. Both reptiles and amphibians depend more on segmental reflexes and locomotion centers for the control of movement than they do on cerebral stimulation. The amphibian brain is well adapted to support basic functions such as sight, olfaction, and movement, but they have very limited integrative capabilities.

The axial and appendicular skeletons of reptiles and amphibians differ from those of mammals in many ways. With the exception of chelonians, the reptilian spine is extremely flexible and is divided into the presacral, sacral, and caudal vertebral regions, rather than cervical, thoracic, sacral, and caudal as seen in mammals. A single occipital condyle forms the articulation between the skull and spine. The number of vertebrae and the presence of ribs vary from species to species. The skeletal structures of reptilian limbs are comparable to those of mammals, with a few exceptions. Unlike mammals, the pectoral girdle of a reptile consists of a scapula and coracoid bone. In most reptiles the hindlimbs are longer than the forelimbs. Snakes are devoid of limbs entirely, though a few species have vestigial hindlimbs.

Lastly, the muscular systems of amphibians and reptiles are incapable of sustaining aerobic metabolism for a long time. Consequently, they are capable of only quick bursts of motion. So, if you can avoid getting caught after the startling thrust forward and powerful chomp of an alligator, you stand a good chance of getting away … a helpful titbit to take with you on your next trip to the bayou. Carnivorous herptiles tend to lie in wait for their prey, but when they move … they move VERY fast!

## FURTHER READING

Duellman W, Trueb L: Biology of amphibians, Baltimore, 1994, Johns Hopkins University Press.

Mader D: Reptile medicine and surgery, ed 2, St Louis, 2006, Saunders.

McArthur S, Wilkinson R, Meyer J: Medicine and surgery of tortoises and turtles, Ames, IA, 2004, Blackwell Publishing.

O'Malley B: Clinical anatomy and physiology of exotic species, New York, 2005, WB Saunders.

Pough FH, Andrews RM, Cadle JE, et al: Herpetology, ed 3, Upper Saddle River, NJ, 2004, Prentice-Hall.

Wright K, Whitaker B: Amphibian medicine and captive husbandry, Malabar, FL, 2001, Krieger Publishing.

# Glossary

## A

**A bands**  Large, dark bands in a skeletal muscle fiber that alternate with lighter I bands to give a striped appearance to skeletal muscle fibers under a microscope. The A bands are composed of thick filaments of the contractile protein myosin.

**abduction**  The joint movement whereby an extremity is moved away from the median plane.

**abomasum**  The "true stomach" of the ruminant; secretes acids, mixes and contracts ingesta, and moves liquid chyme into the small intestine.

**absorptive cell**  A cell commonly found in the small intestine that can absorb nutrients from the luminal surface via phagocytosis and pinocytosis. Absorptive cells have large surface areas as a result of the presence of microvilli. The expanded surface area increases the absorptive capability of the cell.

**accommodation**  The focusing of the lens of the eye to allow close-up and distant vision. It is accomplished by the muscles of the ciliary body that apply or relieve tension on the suspensory ligaments that attach it to the lens.

**acetabulum**  The socket portion of the ball-and-socket hip joint. It is formed at the junction of the ilium, ischium, and pubic bones of the pelvis.

**acetylcholine**  A neurotransmitter associated with somatic nerves and with parasympathetic nervous system effects even though it is used in the preganglionic neuron in both the sympathetic and parasympathetic nervous systems; has a stimulatory effect on the gastrointestinal tract, it increases secretions and muscle contractions in the esophagus, stomach, ruminant forestomachs, intestine, and colon.

**acetylcholinesterase**  The enzyme that breaks down acetylcholine.

**acids**  Substances that dissolve in water to yield hydrogen ions and produce a solution with a pH less than 7.

**acinar gland**  The secretory units of exocrine glands that contain one or more saclike structures.

**acrodont teeth**  Dentition in which the teeth are fused to the biting edge of the mandible and maxillae, found in some species of lizards.

**acromegaly**  A form of gigantism that results from an excess of growth hormone (GH).

**acrosome**  The caplike structure that partially covers the head of a spermatozoon. It contains digestive enzymes that are activated when the sperm enter the female reproductive tract. These help the cell penetrate through the layers around the ovum to fertilize it.

**ACTH**  See *adrenocorticotropic hormone.*

**actin**  A protein that forms microfilaments. It is found in the cytoskeleton, in myofibrils of muscle fibers, and in spindle fibers during cell division.

**actin filaments**  Formed of one of the two contractile proteins of muscle (the other is myosin), these slide over each other to produce the shortening of the muscle cell that we refer to as *muscle contraction.*

**activation energy**  The minimum energy required for a chemical reaction to occur.

**active immunity**  Activation of the immune system by either administration of a vaccine that contains a modified antigen or exposure to the antigen (e.g., by disease).

**active site**  The specific area on an enzyme that connects with a substrate to cause a chemical reaction.

**active transport**  The process that moves ions or molecules across the cell membrane and against the concentration gradient; requires energy.

**adaptive immunity**  Portion of the immune system that is able to target specific antigens.

**adduction**  The joint movement whereby an extremity is moved toward the median plane.

**adenine (A)**  One of the nucleotides present in both DNA and RNA. It is a purine base that pairs with RNA's uracil and DNA's thymine.

**adenosine diphosphate (adp)**  Adenosine diphosphate is the "discharged" form of adenosine triphosphate (ATP). It is a nucleotide that contains two phosphoric acid groups. When a phosphate group is split off of an ATP molecule to produce ADP, energy is released that powers the sliding of the actin and myosin filaments in muscle over each other. When the phosphate group is reattached, which requires another energy source, ADP is converted back to ATP, and the molecule is ready to provide energy again.

**adenosine monophosphate (amp)**  A nucleotide that contains one phosphoric acid group. AMP is produced by the hydrolysis of one high-energy phosphate bond of ADP. This releases energy that can be used by cells or phosphorylated back into ADP.

**adenosine triphosphate (atp)**  A high-energy molecule produced in the mitochondria of cells. It is a nucleotide that contains three phosphoric acid groups. When a phosphate group is split from an ATP molecule to produce ADP, energy is released that powers the sliding of the actin and myosin filaments in muscle over each other. When the phosphate group is reattached, which requires another energy source, ADP is converted back to ATP and the molecule is ready to provide energy again. The more active a cell or body part is, the more ATP it will have produced and stored. For instance, muscles have a great deal of stored ATP, whereas fat has relatively little.

**ADH**  See *antidiuretic hormone.*

**adipocyte**  A type of fixed cell in the connective tissue that stores fat (lipids) in its cytoplasm. The nucleus and other organelles are pushed to the periphery of the cell.

**adipose**   Fat.

**adipose cells**   See *adipocyte*.

**adipose connective tissue**   A subclass of connective tissue proper, adipose connective tissue is a vascularized type of connective tissue whose general functions are to protect, insulate, and provide a major source of energy to the body. Adipose connective tissue can occur as either brown or white adipose tissue. White adipose tissue, found commonly throughout the body, is a storage area for lipids. These lipids may be used for the production of energy, or ATP. Brown adipose tissue, found in neonates and hibernating species, has its lipids converted to heat.

**ADP**   See *adenosine diphosphate*.

**adrenal cortex**   The outer portion of the adrenal gland that produces glucocorticoid, mineralocorticoid, and sex hormones.

**adrenal glands**   Two endocrine glands located near the cranial poles of the kidneys. Each consists of an outer cortex and an inner medulla.

**adrenal medulla**   The inner portion of the adrenal gland that produces the hormones epinephrine and norepinephrine.

**adrenergic neurons**   Neurons that secrete catecholamines (e.g., norepinephrine) as their neurotransmitter.

**adrenocorticotropic hormone (ACTH)**   A hormone secreted by the anterior portion of the pituitary gland, which in turn activates the cortex of the adrenal gland. The adrenal cortex then releases its own hormones. ACTH is vital to the normal function and development of the adrenal cortex.

**adult hemoglobin**   The primary type of hemoglobin found in the red blood cells of animals from a couple of weeks to a couple of months after birth.

**aerobic metabolism**   Oxygen-consuming metabolism. The type of metabolism in muscle in which the supply of available oxygen is sufficient to keep up with the energy needs of the muscle fibers. Aerobic metabolism extracts the maximum amount of energy from glucose molecules.

**aerobic respiration**   The cell function that produces chemical energy with the use of oxygen.

**afferent**   A directional term meaning *toward* some reference point.

**afferent glomerular arterioles**   The smallest arteriole branches that carry blood into the renal glomerulus for filtration.

**afferent nerve**   Nerve that carries impulses toward the central nervous system.

**afterbirth**   The name given to the placenta at parturition because it is delivered *after* the newborn.

**agglutination**   Precipitation or clumping of antigen–antibody complexes; one of the methods by which the immune system neutralizes antigens.

**aglyphous**   Referring to having solid teeth, without a groove for venom (used to classify snake groups).

**agranulocytes**   White blood cells without cytoplasmic granules. The agranulocytes are the monocytes and the lymphocytes, also known as *nongranulocytes*.

**air sacs**   Nine thin, transparent membranes found in birds that are connected to the primary and secondary bronchi and act as reservoirs for air entering and leaving the lungs.

**albumin**   Protein manufactured by the liver that plays an important role in maintaining the osmotic fluid balance between capillaries (blood) and tissues; a lack of albumin results in movement of fluid from the capillaries into the tissues, producing edema and fluid accumulation in body cavities.

**aldosterone**   A mineralocorticoid hormone secreted by the cortex of the adrenal gland. It stimulates the kidney to conserve sodium ions and water and to eliminate potassium and hydrogen ions.

**alimentary canal**   Also called the *digestive tract,* this encompasses all of the parts of the digestive system that transport food from the mouth to the anus: the mouth, esophagus, stomach, small and large intestines, and anus.

**alkaline**   The adjective that describes substances with a pH above 7 (basic). Basic, or alkaline, solutions have fewer hydrogen ions (or more hydroxide ions) than pure water.

**allantoic sac**   Part of the placenta. It is a fluid-filled sac formed by the allantois that surrounds the amniotic sac.

**allantois**   Part of the placenta. It is the membrane that forms the allantoic sac.

**all-or-nothing principle**   The principle that an individual muscle fiber either contracts completely or does not contract at all.

**alopecia**   Loss of hair.

**alpha cells**   Cells in the pancreas that produce glucagon.

**alpha helix**   The coiled structure in a complex protein composed of hydrogen bonds and amino acids.

**alpha$_1$-adrenergic receptors**   Receptors associated with the sympathetic nervous system response; these receptors, when stimulated by catecholamines, cause vasoconstriction.

**altricial**   Chicks that are hatched with their eyes closed and their skins bare and that are immobile.

**alula**   Bone in birds that originates from the wrist and is comparable to the first digit; carries feathers that aid in steering.

**alveolar ducts**   The smallest air passageways in the lungs. The alveolar ducts carry air to the alveolar sacs.

**alveolar glands**   Secretory units of exocrine glands that are saclike in form; also called *acinar glands.*

**alveolar sacs**   Clusters of alveoli at the ends of the alveolar ducts. The alveoli are arranged like bunches of grapes.

**alveoli (singular, alveolus)**   Microscopic, thin-walled sacs surrounded by networks of capillaries. The interface between the wall of the alveoli and the wall of the capillary is where the actual exchange of gases takes place in the lungs.

**amino acids**   The basic building blocks of peptides and proteins; those organic compounds, numbering around 80, that are have both an amino group ($NH_2$) and a carboxyl group (COOH). Amino acids make up proteins when joined together in peptide bonds. They occur naturally in all plants and animals.

**aminopeptidase**   Protease secreted in an inactive form from the pancreas and activated by trypsin.

**amnion**   Part of the placenta. It is the membrane that forms the fluid-filled amniotic sac.

**amniotic sac**   Part of the placenta. It is the fluid-filled sac that immediately surrounds the developing fetus.

**amoeboid motion**   Amoeba-like movement accomplished by the extension of pseudopodia to create a streaming movement of cytoplasm.

**amorphous**   Having no defined shape.

**AMP**   See *adenosine monophosphate*.

**amphiarthrosis**   A slightly movable cartilaginous joint, such as the pelvic symphysis.

**ampulla**   An enlargement in each semicircular canal that contains the receptor structure (the crista).

**ampulla of the vas deferens**　An enlargement of the vas deferens just before it enters the urethra. It is present in some species and absent in others.

**amylase**　Enzyme produced by the pancreas and, in some species, the saliva; attacks starch and breaks it into disaccharides (which contain two simple sugar molecules).

**amyloid**　An excessive amount of a waxlike, proteinaceous substance in the body's tissue.

**anabolism**　The form of metabolism by which cells build complex compounds from simpler ones; the opposite of catabolism. The process by which the cell uses energy to manufacture large molecules from smaller ones; these molecules are used to maintain the cell and carry out metabolic processes.

**anaerobic**　A biochemical pathway that can function without oxygen. The term also may be used to describe microbes that can live in the absence of oxygen.

**anaerobic glycolysis**　An alternative expression for glycolysis, referring to the fact that the reaction does not require oxygen.

**anaerobic metabolism**　Non–oxygen-dependent metabolism. The type of metabolism in muscle that occurs when the need for energy to produce muscular activity exceeds the available oxygen supply. Anaerobic metabolism is not as efficient as aerobic metabolism and results in the formation of lactic acid as a by-product. Lactic acid can cause discomfort in muscle tissue and requires oxygen for conversion back to glucose.

**anaerobic respiration**　The cell function that produces energy chemically without the use of free oxygen.

**anagen phase**　The active phase of hair growth.

**anal sacs**　Perianal sacs, containing apocrine and sebaceous glands, that are located at the 5 o'clock and 7 o'clock positions relative to the anus. The sacs reside between the internal and external sphincters of carnivores and produce a strong-smelling fluid when expressed; they are important for fecal territorial marking and are expressed during fearful episodes.

**analgesia**　Decreased perception of pain.

**anaphase**　The phase of mitosis when the daughter chromosomes begin to migrate to their respective centrioles, away from the center of the dividing cell.

**anaphylaxis**　A severe, potentially life-threatening, allergic response.

**anapsid skulls**　Skulls of primitive reptiles (all extinct except turtles) that have no openings in the temporal region.

**anatomy**　The study of the form and structure of an animal body and its parts. Through anatomy we can describe where things are located in or on the animal body and what they look like.

**anconeal process**　A beak-shaped process at the proximal end of the trochlear notch of the ulna. When it fails to unite with the ulna, an ununited anconeal process can cause the elbow joint to become unstable, leading to lameness.

**androgens**　Hormones that promote the development of male characteristics; male sex hormones. The principal androgen is testosterone.

**anemia**　Decreased oxygen-carrying capacity of the blood caused by insufficient numbers of red blood cells, decreased hemoglobin concentration, or a combination of both of these conditions.

**anesthesia**　Complete loss of sensation.

**anestrus**　The period when the ovary "shuts down" between the estrous cycles or breeding seasons of some animal species.

**angle**　The angle of the hoof wall as viewed from a lateral aspect when the foot is flat on the ground.

**anions**　A negatively charged atom or molecule; a negatively charged ion.

**anisodactyly**　Toe position in which three toes face forward and once faces the rear.

**antagonist**　Something that opposes the action of something else. An antagonist muscle or muscle group directly opposes the action of a "prime mover" muscle or muscle group that is directly producing a desired movement.

**antebrachium**　The "forearm" region of the thoracic limb.

**anterior**　A directional term meaning *toward the front* (of a human body).

**anterior chamber**　The portion of the aqueous compartment of the eye in front of (rostral to) the iris.

**anterior pituitary gland**　The adenohypophysis; the rostral portion of the pituitary gland that produces seven hormones, many of which influence other endocrine glands.

**antibodies**　Proteins produced by plasma cells (transformed B lymphocytes) in response to the presence of an antigen. A specific serum antibody is generated for a specific antigen.

**anticlinal vertebra**　The thoracic vertebra whose spinous process projects straight up dorsally in contrast to the caudally inclined spinous processes cranial to it and the cranially inclined spinous processes caudal to it. It acts as a landmark on radiographs of the thoracolumbar region, particularly in dogs, in which it is the 11th thoracic vertebra.

**anticoagulant**　A substance that prevents blood from clotting when it is added to the blood.

**anticodon**　The triplet pair of nucleotides in transfer RNA (tRNA) that corresponds to the triplet bases or codons of messenger RNA (mRNA).

**antidiuretic hormone (ADH)**　A hormone released by the posterior pituitary. It facilitates water conservation in the body by promoting water reabsorption from urine in the collecting ducts. Low levels of ADH cause diabetes insipidus, a condition that results in excessive water loss from the body through increased urine volume.

**antigens**　Cells or organisms that are "not self." An antigen also can be a structure on a cell membrane that the body recognizes as foreign. The presence of an antigen initiates an immune response in a healthy animal.

**antiparasitic drug**　A drug that kills parasites.

**antiport system**　When two separate materials are moved across the plasma membrane in opposite directions at the same time.

**antitussive drug**　A drug that suppresses the cough reflex.

**antrum**　(1) The fluid-filled space within an ovarian follicle. (2) The muscular part of the stomach that is responsible for grinding of food; located between the body of the stomach and the pylorus.

**anucleated**　Having no nuclei.

**anuria**　Condition in which no urine is being passed from the body.

**aorta**　Major artery of the systemic circulation that receives blood from the left ventricle.

**aortic valve**　A semilunar valve; it separates the left ventricle and the aorta.

**apex (of a tooth)**　The tip of the tooth root where the blood and nerve supply enter the tooth; the uppermost point of a structure.

**apical surface**   The side of an epithelial cell that faces in toward the body cavity.

**apocrine gland**   A gland whose secretions contain some of its cellular material. Part of the secretory cell is destroyed and must regenerate before the cell can secrete again. Examples of these glands are mammary glands and some sweat glands.

**apocrine sweat glands**   Exocrine glands that secrete substances into the hair follicle, rather than directly to the skin surface.

**aponeurosis**   A broad sheet of fibrous connective tissue that attaches certain muscles to bones or to other muscles.

**apoptosis**   Programmed cell death.

**appendicular skeleton**   The bones of the limbs (appendages).

**apteryia**   Bare areas of the skin of birds where feathers do not originate.

**aqueous compartment**   The compartment of the eye in front of (rostral to) the lens and ciliary body. It contains a watery fluid, called *aqueous humor,* and is subdivided by the iris into the anterior chamber and the posterior chamber.

**aqueous humor**   The watery fluid that fills the aqueous compartment of the eye. It is produced in the posterior chamber and drained from the anterior chamber by the canal of Schlemm.

**arachnoid**   The delicate, weblike layer of the meninges between the dura mater and the pia mater.

**areolar connective tissue**   A soft, spongy connective tissue, also known as *loose connective tissue.* It is located throughout the body and is composed of a soft ground substance, numerous cell types (white blood cells, fibroblasts, macrophages), and all three types of fiber (elastic, reticular, and collagenous).

**arrector pili muscle**   Smooth muscle that is attached to the base of the hair follicle. It is responsible for the involuntary "hair raising" response to cold, fear, or aggression.

**arthrodial joint**   A gliding joint in which two flat, articular surfaces rock on each other. This type of joint usually allows only the movements of flexion and extension.

**articular cartilage**   The thin layer of hyaline cartilage that covers the articular surfaces of long bones in synovial joints. It forms a smooth layer over the joint surfaces of the bones, which decreases friction and allows free joint movement.

**articular process**   The process of a vertebra that forms a synovial joint with an adjacent vertebra.

**articular surface**   The smooth joint surface of a bone that contacts another bone in a synovial joint.

**arytenoid cartilages**   Two of the cartilages of the larynx. The vocal cords attach to the arytenoid cartilages. The arytenoid cartilages and the vocal cords form the boundaries of the opening into the larynx (glottis).

**ascites**   An abnormal condition in which an excessive amount of fluid accumulation is present in the abdominal cavity. Abdominal distention or a potbellied appearance can be clinically evident.

**asternal rib**   A rib whose costal cartilage joins the costal cartilage of the rib ahead of it instead of directly joining the sternum.

**ataxia**   Incoordination. An ataxic animal makes jerky, spastic movements.

**atlas**   The first cervical vertebra. It forms the atlantooccipital joint with the occipital bone of the skull and the atlantoaxial joint with the axis (the second cervical vertebra).

**atom**   The smallest unit of an element having all the characteristics of that element. It consists of a positively charged nucleus surrounded by a system of negatively charged electrons.

**atomic nucleus**   A dense region at the center of an atom consisting of positively charged protons and uncharged neutrons.

**atomic number**   The number of protons found in the nucleus of an atom. In a neutrally charged atom, the atomic number is also the number of electrons.

**atomic weight**   The average mass of an atom of an element. Generally equal to the atomic mass of the protons and neutrons in the atom, because the electrons are so tiny they are almost irrelevant to the mass.

**atony**   Lack of normal muscle tone.

**ATP**   See *adenosine triphosphate.*

**ATP synthase**   The enzyme in the mitochondria of body cells that functions as a tiny "molecular machine" to regenerate ATP from ADP and detached phosphate groups. It is powered by the proton gradient present across interior mitochondrial membranes.

**atrophy**   Shrinkage.

**auricle**   Ear-shaped appendage of either atrium of the heart.

**auriculars**   Small contour feathers located around the external ear openings in birds.

**auscultation**   Listening, with the ear or with a stethoscope, to sounds produced within the body.

**autoimmune disease**   An abnormal condition in which the body starts recognizing some of its own cells as "not self" and initiates an immune response to destroy them.

**autolysis**   The self-digestion of tissues or cells by enzymes that are released by their own lysosomes.

**autonomic nervous system**   The part of the nervous system that controls smooth muscle, cardiac muscle, and endocrine glands automatically without conscious control; has motor and sensory branches.

**autonomic reflex**   A reflex that results in stimulation or inhibition of smooth or cardiac muscle or endocrine gland function; mechanisms of homeostasis are autonomic reflexes.

**avascular**   Without a blood supply.

**axial skeleton**   The bones along the central axis of the body; made up of the skull, the hyoid bone, the spinal column, the ribs, and the sternum.

**axis**   The second cervical vertebra. It forms the atlantoaxial joint with the first cervical vertebra, the atlas.

**axon**   Extension of the neuron that conducts the nerve impulse away from the cell body to the terminal bouton (synaptic bulb) at the end of the neuron.

**azotemia**   A buildup of waste materials, particularly creatinine and BUN, in the blood because of insufficient removal of these substances by the kidneys.

## B

**B lymphocyte**   The type of lymphocyte that is responsible for humoral immunity through its transformation into a plasma cell and production of antibodies.

**ball-and-socket joint**   Also called a *spheroidal joint,* it consists of a spherical joint surface (the ball) that fits into a closely matching, concave joint surface (the socket). The shoulder and hip joints are ball-and-socket joints. Ball-and-socket joints allow the greatest range of joint movement.

**barbs**   Slender projections off the main feather shaft. Barbs make up the vanes on each side of the shaft.

**barbules**   Microscopic projections of feather barbs that help maintain a contour feather's structure.

**barrel**   Trunk of the body—formed by the rib cage and the abdomen.

**basal bodies**   A pair of tubular structures. Each is composed of nine microtubules surrounding another pair of microtubules. Basal bodies act as the base of cilia and flagella.

**basal surface**   The side of an epithelial cell that faces a lower level of connective tissue.

**basement membrane**   A noncellular, collagen-based structure that supports epithelial tissue.

**bases**   Substances that dissolve in water to yield hydroxyl ions and give the solution a pH greater than 7.

**basopenia**   Theoretically, a decrease in the total number of basophils in peripheral blood. This condition is difficult to describe because basophils normally are rarely found in peripheral blood.

**basophilia**   An increase in the total number of basophils in peripheral blood.

**basophil**   One of the granulocytic white blood cells, characterized by the presence of numerous, dark blue-staining granules in its cytoplasm.

**behavioral thermoregulation**   Carried out by cold-blooded animals that move into and out of relatively warm locations to regulate body temperature.

**belly**   The thick, central portion of a muscle.

**beta cells**   Cells in the pancreas that produce insulin.

**beta$_1$-adrenergic receptors**   Receptors associated with the sympathetic nervous system response; these receptors, when stimulated by catecholamines, tend to cause an increase in the rate and force of contraction of the heart.

**beta$_2$-adrenergic receptors**   Receptors associated with the sympathetic nervous system response; these receptors, when stimulated by catecholamines, tend to cause dilation of the bronchioles and vasodilation of some blood vessels.

**beta oxidation**   The breakdown of fatty acid chains into two carbon fragments in the mitochondria. These two carbon fragments can be broken down further into ketone bodies and acetyl CoA.

**bicarbonate**   Often referred to as *sodium bicarbonate,* it acts as a buffer in the secretions (e.g., pancreatic juice, saliva) to reduce the acidity of the stomach or rumen; also helps to buffer the pH of the blood.

**Bidder's organs**   Undeveloped ovaries located anterior to the testes in male toads. Environmental and physiologic influences enable the male to become female.

**bifurcation of the trachea**   The division of the trachea at its caudal end into the left and right main bronchi, which enter the lungs.

**bilateral symmetry**   The concept that the left and right halves of an animal's body are mirror images of each other. Paired structures, such as the kidneys, are located one on each side of the body, and single structures, such as the heart, are located near the median plane.

**bile acids**   Hydrophilic (water-loving) molecules with a hydrophobic (water-hating) end that are secreted by the liver into the duodenum; these combine with fat droplets to make them more water soluble.

**bilirubin**   The yellow breakdown product of hemoglobin.

**biologic value**   The percentage of absorbed protein that is retained by the body. Biologic value is a measure of the body's ability to convert absorbed protein into body tissue.

**biopsy**   The removal of a small sample of tissue for microscopic examination. This procedure is often but not exclusively used to determine whether a tumor is benign or malignant.

**blast**   A cell in the production stage of a particular substance.

**blastic transformation**   Through this process, B lymphocytes become plasma cells that produce antibodies.

**blastocyst**   The stage of development of a zygote that is ready for implantation in the uterus. It is shaped like a tiny, hollow ball of cells with a "bump" on one side that eventually develops into the embryo.

**bloat**   The accumulation of gas within the rumen or monogastric stomach that causes severe distention.

**blood–brain barrier**   The functional barrier between the capillaries in the brain and the nervous tissue; composed of capillary walls, without the openings found in other capillaries, and glial cells.

**blood feather**   A developing feather that contains blood in its shaft for growth and nourishment.

**body condition scoring (BCS)**   Use of a numerical scale to indicate the amount of fat in an animal's body.

**body of the penis**   The largest portion of the penis. It contains the majority of the erectile tissue of the organ.

**body of the stomach**   The central part of the stomach, between the fundus and the antrum.

**bolus (of food)**   Amount of food swallowed at one time.

**bone cortex**   The outer layer of a bone that is composed of compact bone.

**bone marrow**   The soft material that fills the spaces inside bones. Two types of bone marrow are *red bone marrow,* which forms blood cells, and *yellow bone marrow,* which consists primarily of adipose connective tissue (fat).

**bones of the cranium**   The bones of the skull that surround the brain. The externally visible bones of the cranium are the occipital bone, the interparietal bones, the parietal bones, the temporal bones, and the frontal bones. The internal (hidden) bones of the cranium are the sphenoid bone and the ethmoid bone.

**bones of the face**   The skull bones that do not surround the brain. The externally visible bones of the face are the incisive bones, the nasal bones, the maxillary bones, the lacrimal bones, the zygomatic bones, and the mandible. The internal (hidden) bones of the face are the palatine bones, the pterygoid bones, the vomer bone, and the turbinates.

**bovine spongiform encephalopathy (BSE)**   Also known as *mad cow disease.* This disease was first contracted by cows in Great Britain that had consumed the flesh of sheep thought to carry infectious prions.

**Bowman's capsule**   Part of the renal corpuscle. It consists of two layers: an inner, *visceral layer* that lies directly on the glomerular capillaries and an outer, *parietal layer*. It functions as a plasma filter in the process of urine formation.

**brachium**   The upper arm. The area of the thoracic limb between the elbow and the shoulder.

**brachycephalic**   Short-faced. Brachycephalic breeds of dogs include Boston Terriers, Pugs, English Bulldogs, and Pekingese.

**brainstem**   The connection between the rest of the brain and the spinal cord, composed of the medulla oblongata, the pons, and the midbrain; heavily involved in autonomic control functions related to the heart, respiration, blood vessel diameter, swallowing, and vomiting.

**breathing**   The movement of air into and out of the lungs. Also known as ventilation.

**brisket**   Area at the base of the neck between the front legs that covers the cranial end of the sternum.

**bristle**   Modified contour feather with a stiff rachis and few barbs at the base; found around the eyes, mouth, nostrils, and toes of some bird species, these serve a tactile function.

**broad ligaments**   Paired sheets of connective tissue that suspend the uterus from the dorsal part of the abdominal cavity and attach it to the abdominal wall. They are often subdivided into the mesovarium, which supports the ovary; the mesosalpinx, which supports the oviduct; and the mesometrium, which supports the uterus.

**bronchi**   The largest air passageways in the lungs. The left and right main bronchi are formed by the bifurcation of the trachea. The main bronchi divide into smaller and smaller branches within the lungs.

**bronchial tree**   The air passageways in the lungs between the main bronchi and the alveoli. The branching nature of the bronchi as they form smaller and smaller air passageways resembles the branching of a tree.

**bronchioles**   Some of the smallest branches of the bronchial tree. The bronchioles subdivide down to the alveolar ducts, which are the smallest air passageways that lead directly to the alveolar sacs.

**bronchitis**   A lower respiratory tract infection affecting the lining of the larger air passageways in the lungs. Bronchitis can be a serious disease because the inflammatory fluids and excess mucus resulting from the irritation are difficult for the animal to cough up from down deep in the lungs.

**bronchoconstriction**   Contraction of the smooth muscle that surrounds the air passageways in the lungs. Bronchoconstriction narrows the air passageways. It can be physiologic, as when a mild degree of bronchoconstriction reduces the work of moving air in and out of the lungs at rest. Bronchoconstriction also can be pathologic, for example when inhaled irritants cause severe bronchoconstriction that makes breathing very difficult.

**bronchodilation**   Relaxation of the smooth muscle that surrounds the air passageways in the lungs. Full bronchodilation causes the air passageways to dilate to their full diameters. Physiologic bronchodilation occurs during intense physical activity, when maximum air must be moved into and out of the lungs. A class of drugs called *bronchodilators* can be used to help relax severe bronchoconstriction, such as might occur in an asthmalike condition.

**brood patch**   Area of thickened skin on the lower abdomen of birds, from which feathers are plucked to allow transfer of heat to eggs during incubation.

**brown adipose tissue**   *Brown fat;* commonly found throughout the body of hibernating species and neonates. It is a specialized form of adipose tissue that releases its stored lipid reserves in the form of heat. This is accomplished because of the high degree of vascularization and concentration of mitochondria found in brown adipose tissue.

**brush border**   Microvilli on the free surfaces of intestinal epithelial cells and kidney tubule cells that resemble the bristles of a brush.

**buccal cavity**   Although this translates literally to *cheek cavity,* the buccal cavity usually refers to the mouth or oral cavity; pronounced "BHU-kal."

**buccal surface**   The surface of the caudal part of the upper and lower arcade teeth that face the cheeks; *bucco* is Latin for *cheeks.*

**buffer**   A substance that minimizes the change of the acidity of a solution when an acid or base is added to the solution.

**bulb of the glans**   An enlargement in the penis of the dog and related species. It is made up of erectile tissue that slowly engorges with blood during copulation. When muscles surrounding the vagina and vulva of the female clamp down on the enlarged bulb, the male cannot withdraw the penis. He typically dismounts and turns so that the two animals are tail to tail. This position is known as the *tie* and usually lasts 15 to 20 minutes, after which the animals can separate.

**bulbar conjunctiva**   The transparent membrane that covers the front (rostral) portion of the eyeball.

**bulbourethral glands**   Male accessory reproductive glands that secrete a mucus-containing fluid just before ejaculation that lubricates the urethra for the passage of semen and clears it of urine. Bulbourethral glands are present in all common domestic animals except dogs.

**bumblefoot**   General term for pathology of the avian foot. Includes cuts, abrasions, blisters, ulcers, punctures, and infections.

**bursa of Fabricius**   Specialized organ in birds that is necessary for B-lymphocyte development. Mammals do not have this organ, but B (bursa-derived) lymphocytes were so named before their development in mammalian lymphatic tissue was determined.

## C

**calcaneal tuberosity**   Large process of the fibular tarsal bone that projects upward and backward; commonly referred to as the *point* of the hock; site of attachment of the gastrocnemius (calf) muscle; equivalent to the human heel.

**calcified**   Hardening of organic tissue by the deposit of lime and calcium salts.

**calciotropic**   Involved in the regulation of calcium levels in body.

**calcitonin**   The hormone secreted by the thyroid gland that prevents the level of calcium in the blood from getting too high.

**callus**   The healing tissue between the ends of a fractured bone that is eventually replaced by true bone as the fracture heals.

**calorigenic**   Heat producing.

**CAMs**   See *cell adhesion molecules.*

**canal of Schlemm**   The structure that drains aqueous humor from the anterior chamber of the eye. It is located at the edge of the anterior chamber, where the iris and the cornea meet.

**canaliculi**   Tiny channels through the matrix of bone. Threadlike projections from osteocytes communicate with each other and with blood vessels through the canaliculi.

**cancellous bone**   Spongy bone. A form of bone composed of a seemingly random arrangement of *spicules* of bone separated by spaces filled with bone marrow. Appears spongelike to the naked eye. Found in the ends (epiphyses) of long bones and the interiors of short bones, flat bones, and irregular bones.

**canine parvoviral enteritis** Caused by the canine parvovirus, this infectious disease has an extremely high mortality rate in puppies. Infections occurring in utero are known to cause acute myocarditis and overall poor health in the litter. Because it tends to attack cells in the mitotic phase, rapidly dividing epithelial tissue is particularly affected by parvoviral infections. Vomiting, diarrhea, bloody stool, and dehydration are clinical signs of disease. An immunization is available.

**canine teeth** Sharp, pointed teeth between the most caudal incisors and the most rostral premolars.

**cannon bones** The large metacarpal and metatarsal bones of the horse.

**canthus** The corner of the eyelids where they come together. Each eye has a medial and a lateral canthus.

**capacitation** The process spermatozoa undergo in the female reproductive tract that increases their fertility before contact with the ovum. Part of the process exposes the digestive enzymes in the acrosome. This helps the cell penetrate through the layers surrounding the ovum.

**capillary refill time (CRT)** The time it takes for mucous membranes to return to their normal, pink color after being pressed to a white color. If the return to normal color is too slow, it can indicate poor peripheral blood perfusion.

**capsular space** The space between the visceral and parietal layers of Bowman's capsule.

**carapace** The dorsal shell of turtles and tortoises.

**carbohydrate metabolism** Metabolic processes that store and release energy contained within carbohydrates for the purposes of growth, repair, and normal function of the body.

**carbohydrates** One of the essential nutrients necessary for all life functions; sugars. They are a quick source of energy and may be stored in the body as glycogen.

**carboxypeptidase** Protease secreted in an inactive form from the pancreas and activated by trypsin.

**cardia** The part of the stomach where the esophagus enters.

**cardiac muscle** Striated, involuntary muscle that is found exclusively in the heart. Cardiac muscle is influenced by the autonomic nervous system. It has one centrally located nucleus and intercalated discs that form special connections between the muscle branches.

**cardiac output** The amount of blood that leaves the heart.

**cardiac sphincter** The smooth muscle sphincter around the entrance of the esophagus into the stomach.

**cardiac tamponade** A condition in which the heart becomes unable to expand normally between contractions because of pressure from fluid in the pericardial space.

**carnassial teeth** In the dog, the large, first lower molar tooth and fourth upper premolar tooth. The carnassial teeth have deep roots.

**carnivore** An animal whose diet is primarily meat.

**carpal bones** The bones of the carpus. Consist of two parallel rows of short bones located between the distal ends of the radius and ulna and the proximal ends of the metacarpal bones.

**carpus** The joint composed of the carpal bones. Referred to as the "knee" of the horse and the "wrist" of humans.

**carrier proteins** Any protein that facilitates diffusion of a specific molecule through the cell membrane.

**cartilage** An opaque, dense connective tissue composed of a relatively small number of cells that are contained within a nonliving matrix. Cartilage absorbs shock and protects the epiphysial ends of bones. Cartilage is not innervated or vascularized, which makes it resistant to pain but also to healing. It is found in joints, body structures such as the ears and nose, the costal cartilage of the rib cage, and the fetal skeleton.

**cartilaginous joint** A joint in which the bones are united by cartilage; also called an *amphiarthrosis*. Only a slight rocking motion is permitted between the bones.

**caruncle** Numerous mushroomlike structures in the lining of the uterus of ruminant animals. They join with the cotyledons of the placenta to form placental attachment sites called *placentomes*.

**catabolism** The breaking down of nutrients into smaller and simpler materials for use by the cell to release energy; the opposite of anabolism.

**catagen phase** The transitional phase between anagen and telogen phases of the hair growth cycle.

**catalase** An enzyme found in almost all cells that breaks down hydrogen peroxide into water and oxygen.

**catalyst** Substance that induces chemical reactions by lowering the activation energy needed.

**catecholamines** The group of neurotransmitters that includes norepinephrine, epinephrine, dopamine, and others with similar chemical properties.

**cations** Positively charged ions.

**caudal** A directional term meaning toward the tail end of an animal.

**caveolae** Tiny invaginations of the plasma membrane of vertebrate cells, particularly endothelial and fat cells, which are believed to initiate endocytosis, oncogenesis, and the formation of plaque in blood vessels. The invaginations are approximately 50–100 nm in size and are composed of protein, cholesterol, and other lipids. Caveolae may also play a role in the uptake of pathogenic bacteria and certain viruses.

**cecocolic orifice** The opening between the cecum and the colon; most developed in the horse and other nonruminant herbivores.

**cecum** The blind pouch leading off from where the ileum meets the colon; in nonruminant herbivores, the cecum can be well developed, with a base, body, and apex (tip).

**cell** The most basic structural unit of all animals and plants. Cells make up all tissues of an organism and perform all of the functions by which life is defined, including growth, reproduction, and metabolism.

**cell adhesion molecules (CAMs)** Glycoproteins that aid not only in the bonding of cells but also in lubricating the movement of one cell past another. They also help to transport specialized cells to areas of need.

**cell membrane** The selectively permeable outer membrane of the cell that is composed of a phospholipid bilayer, protein, and cholesterol; also called the *plasma membrane* or *plasmalemma*.

**cell metabolism** Functions that break down nutrients, produce ATP, use ATP, and create complex molecules from simple ones.

**cell-mediated immune response** Response of the body's cells that regulates the destruction of infectious bacteria and viruses during specific immune responses.

**cell-mediated immunity**    The portion of the immune system that produces "killer" cells that directly attack foreign invaders.

**cellular respiration**    The oxidation of organic material to yield energy, carbon dioxide, and water.

**cellulase**    An enzyme that breaks down the sugar cellulose.

**cellulose**    A complex carbohydrate that makes up the cell walls and fibers of plant tissue. Herbivores digest cellulose through microbial fermentation. Cellulose is not digested by carnivores and most omnivores.

**cementum**    The hard connective tissue that covers the root of a tooth and helps secure it in its bony socket.

**central canal**    Small diameter canal, filled with cerebrospinal fluid, in the center of the spinal cord that is continuous with the ventricles of the brain.

**central nervous system (CNS)**    The brain and spinal cord.

**central sulcus**    The central depression of the frog in the equine hoof.

**centriole**    A tubular organelle composed of nine triplets of microtubules that aids in the process of cell division. Centrioles split in two and migrate to opposite poles of a dividing cell to organize the spindle fibers, enabling the cell to divide in two.

**centromere**    Also called a *kinetochore;* the protein disc that holds a pair of chromatids together as a chromosome and then holds that chromosome to a spindle fiber during cell division.

**centrosome**    An area of condensed cytoplasm located near the nucleus that contains the centrioles of the cell.

**cere**    Fleshy colored skin located at the base of the upper beak in many bird species; supplied with touch corpuscles.

**cerebellar dysfunction**    Caused by inflammation, underdevelopment, or degeneration of the cerebellum, the condition is characterized by an exaggerated and awkward gait, usually resulting from hyperextension of the legs. Cerebellar dysfunction does not cause any degree of paralysis, partial or complete.

**cerebellum**    Second largest component of the brain; allows the body to have coordinated movement, balance, posture, and complex reflexes.

**cerebral cortex**    Gray matter that makes up the outer layer of the cerebrum.

**cerebral hemispheres**    The two halves of the cerebrum.

**cerebrospinal fluid (CSF)**    Fluid that bathes and protects the brain and spinal cord from the hard inner surface of the skull and spinal vertebrae.

**cerebrum**    That portion of the brain responsible for functions most commonly associated with "higher-order" behaviors (learning, intelligence, awareness); receives and interprets sensory information, initiates conscious (voluntary) nerve impulses to skeletal muscles, and integrates neuron activity that is normally associated with communication, expression of emotional responses, learning, memory and recall, and other behaviors associated with conscious activity.

**cervical vertebrae**    The bones of the neck portion of the spinal column.

**cervix**    The sphincter muscle "valve" between the uterus and the vagina; controls access to the lumen of the uterus from the vagina. It is normally closed except during breeding and parturition.

**chemical bond**    A force by which atoms are bound in a molecule. The types of chemical bond are covalent bonds, ionic bonds, and hydrogen bonds.

**chemical control system**    The respiratory control system that monitors the pH of the blood and its content of $O_2$ and $CO_2$. If any of the measured values varies outside preset limits, the chemical control system initiates changes in the breathing pattern to bring them back into balance.

**chemical digestion**    The breakdown of food by the action of chemicals or enzymes.

**chemical element**    Any of 116 known substances that cannot be separated into smaller substances. The smallest unit of an element is an atom.

**chemical equation**    A symbolic representation of a chemical reaction. Arrows are used to denote in which direction the reaction is occurring. Chemical symbols are used to denote the reactants and products of the reaction.

**chemical reaction**    A process that results in the creation of new chemicals, involving changes in the movement of electrons in forming and breaking chemical bonds.

**chemical signaling**    The specific interaction of hormones and neurotransmitters with cell surfaces for the purpose of changing cell activity.

**chemical symbol**    The abbreviation of the name of a chemical element. Used to identify the element in the Periodic Table of the Elements.

**chemotaxis**    The movement of white blood cells into an area of inflammation in response to chemical mediators released at the site by injured tissue or other white blood cells.

**chestnut**    Believed to be the vestigial remnants of carpal and tarsal bones or extra toes possessed by ancestors of the modern horse; they are horny, keratinized growths located on the medial forearms and hocks of horses.

**chief cells**    Cells in the stomach that produce the enzyme precursor pepsinogen.

**choanae**    Two internal nares that open from the nasal chambers into the roof of the mouth of birds.

**cholecystokinin (CCK)**    A hormone released by the duodenum when chyme enters from the stomach. It slows gastric emptying and motility while increasing intestinal motility. It also stimulates the pancreas to release digestive enzymes into the duodenum.

**cholesterol**    A steroid alcohol that is found in many fat-based tissues throughout the body. Cholesterol can be synthesized in the body or obtained from the diet.

**cholinergic neurons**    Neurons that secrete acetylcholine as their neurotransmitter.

**cholinergic receptors**    Receptors for acetylcholine; may be muscarinic or nicotinic receptors.

**chondroblasts**    Fixed cells that form cartilage.

**chondrocyte**    Mature cartilage cell.

**chondroitin sulfate**    A glycosaminoglycan found in cartilage.

**chondronectin**    An adhesive glycosaminoglycan found in cartilage.

**chordae tendineae**    Fine, threadlike cords that connect the two atrioventricular valves to the appropriate papillary muscles in the ventricles.

**chorion**    Part of the placenta; the outermost layer that attaches to the uterine lining. The chorion is linked to the fetus by the umbilical cord.

**chorionic gonadotropin**    A hormone produced by the placenta of a pregnant animal.

**choroid**   A portion of the uvea, or middle vascular layer, of the eye. The choroid consists mainly of pigment and blood vessels and is located between the sclera and the retina.

**chromatids**   Strands of genetic material that, when joined together with another chromatid by a centromere, form a chromosome.

**chromatin**   A material that is composed of DNA and proteins and makes up chromosomes.

**chromatophore**   Any pigment cell or color-producing plastid.

**chromosomes**   Threadlike accumulations of DNA in the nuclei of cells that are particularly visible during mitosis. The DNA of the chromosomes contains the genetic material of the cell. The number of chromosomes is constant within a given species.

**chyle**   The milky lymph from the intestines consisting primarily of small molecules of absorbed fats.

**chylomicrons**   Microscopic particles of fat found in chyle and blood. Their numbers are highest after a meal.

**chyme**   The semifluid, partially digested food that leaves the stomach and enters the duodenum.

**chymotrypsin**   Protease secreted in an inactive form from the pancreas and activated by trypsin.

**cilia**   Hairlike processes of the luminal surfaces of cells that assist in the movement of mucus, fluid, and solid material across the cell surface.

**ciliary body**   A portion of the uvea, or middle vascular layer, of the eye. The ciliary body is a ring-shaped structure located immediately behind the iris. It contains the ciliary muscles that adjust the shape of the lens and the cells that produce aqueous humor.

**ciliary muscles**   Multiunit smooth muscles of the ciliary body that adjust the shape of the eye's lens.

**circular muscle**   The smooth muscle in the muscle layer of the gastrointestinal tract that encircles the organ and causes mixing or segmental contractions; plays a role in peristalsis; sphincters are made of concentrated circular muscle.

**circulating pool of neutrophils**   Neutrophils found in the peripheral blood flowing through the center of blood vessels.

**circumduction**   A joint motion whereby the distal end of an extremity moves in a circle.

**cisterna**   A reservoir that stores fluid.

**citric acid cycle**   A complicated metabolic pathway that is included in the metabolism of fats, proteins, and carbohydrates and that involves the oxidation of pyruvic acid and the release of energy. Also called the *Krebs cycle* and the *tricarboxylic acid cycle.*

**claws**   Accessory appendages of the integumentary system, present mainly in carnivores, used for grasping prey and self-defense.

**cleavage**   The process of very rapid cell division after an ovum has been fertilized. The cells divide so rapidly that they do not have time to grow appreciably between divisions. The number of cells increases rapidly, but the overall size of the cell mass does not increase much.

**clitoris**   One of the structures of the vulva of the female. Homologous to the penis of the male, the clitoris contains erectile tissue and is richly supplied with sensory nerve endings.

**clutch**   The total number of eggs laid in a single nesting period.

**CNS**   See *central nervous system.*

**coated pit**   Parts of the cell membrane that have a hairlike coating necessary for endocytic functions. These portions of the cell membrane pinch off to form vesicles that aid in the intracellular transport of materials.

**coccygeal vertebrae**   The bones of the tail portion of the spinal column.

**coccyx**   The human "tailbone." It consists of four to five coccygeal vertebrae fused into a solid structure.

**cochlea**   The snail shell-shaped cavity in the temporal bone of the skull that contains the hearing portion of the inner ear.

**cochlear duct**   A long, fluid-filled tube that runs the length of the cochlea. It contains the receptor organ of hearing (the organ of Corti).

**codon**   The genetic code of an amino acid expressed in DNA or messenger RNA as three bases.

**coenzyme**   An organic molecule that is required by an enzyme to carry out a metabolic reaction. Coenzymes, such as nicotinamide adenine dinucleotide (NAD), are often derived from vitamins.

**cofactors**   Elements, such as coenzymes, that act concurrently with another element to carry out a chemical reaction.

**coffin bone**   The distal phalanx bone of the horse.

**collagenous fiber**   A structural protein that is commonly located in tendons and ligaments.

**collateral sulcus**   Deep ridge on either side of the frog that separates it from the bars in the equine hoof.

**collateral**   Located on both sides.

**collecting ducts**   The system of tubules that collects tubular filtrate from the distal convoluted tubules and carries it to the renal pelvis. They are not considered part of the nephron.

**colloidal**   Referring to a gelatinous and viscous fluid.

**colloids**   Emulsions; heterogeneous mixtures that contain much larger sized solutes than those found in solutions.

**colon**   The last large component of the intestinal tract; responsible for absorption of water and electrolytes; extensively developed in nonruminant herbivores, such as horses.

**colostrum**   The initial secretion of the mammary gland before milk is produced. Colostrum is rich in nutrients, has a laxative effect on the newborn, and contains antibodies to the diseases the dam has been exposed to or vaccinated against. If the newborn drinks the colostrum within the first few hours of birth, the large antibody molecules will be absorbed intact by the intestine and impart passive immunity to the young animal.

**columella**   The middle ear bone in birds.

**columnar epithelial cells**   Tall, thin epithelial cells with nuclei located at the basal end; often ciliated.

**columnar epithelium**   Epithelium composed of columnar cells.

**common bile duct**   The duct leading from the gallbladder to the duodenum; may be formed by the merging of the cystic duct from the gallbladder and the hepatic duct from the liver.

**common vaginal tunic**   The outer connective tissue sac that surrounds the testis. It is derived from the layer of parietal peritoneum that was pushed ahead of the testis as it descended through the inguinal ring. Also called the *parietal vaginal tunic.*

**compact bone**   Heavy, dense bone made up of tiny, tightly compacted, laminated cylinders of bone called *Haversian systems;* makes up the shafts (diaphyses) of long bones and the outer surfaces of all bones.

**complement**   A group of inactive enzymes (proteins) in plasma that can be activated to rupture the cell membrane of a foreign cell. Complement can also act as an opsonin.

**compound**   A substance made up of two or more elements.

**compound follicles**   Follicles through which more than one hair emerges.

**compound gland**   An exocrine gland with branched ducts.

**concentration gradient**   The spectrum between the area of highest concentration and the area of lowest concentration.

**conduction of the action potential**   Another name for a nerve impulse.

**condyle**   A large, rounded articular (joint) surface. Examples are found on the distal ends of the humerus and femur.

**cones**   Photoreceptors in the retina of the eye that perceive color and detail.

**congenital**   Present at birth.

**congestive heart failure**   Failure of the heart to maintain circulatory equilibrium with resulting congestion of the venous system. It is characterized by edema of the lungs, enlargement of the heart, increase in heart rate, and dilation of peripheral blood vessels.

**conjunctiva**   The thin, transparent membrane that covers the front portion of the eyeball and lines the interior surfaces of the eyelids.

**conjunctival sac**   The space between the bulbar and palpebral portions of the conjunctiva; the space between the eyelid and the eyeball.

**connective tissue**   Tissue made up of cells and extracellular substances that connect and support cells and other tissues.

**connective tissue papilla**   The base of the hair follicle that ultimately provides the material necessary to create hair.

**connective tissue proper**   Includes all types of connective tissue except for bone, blood, and cartilage. Connective tissue proper is divided into two subclasses: *loose connective tissue* and *dense connective tissue*.

**connexon**   Proteinaceous channel that aids in the intercellular transport of nutrients.

**contact inhibition**   That property that inhibits cells from dividing when in proximity to other cells.

**contact signaling**   Cell-to-cell recognition, which is important in immune responses to infection.

**contractile proteins**   Proteins that are essential to muscle contractions, such as myosin and actin.

**contractility**   The inherent ability of the heart to develop a force by contracting, which increases chamber pressures.

**contralateral reflex**   Reflexes that are initiated on one side of the body and travel to the opposite side to produce their effect.

**contrast radiography**   Radiographs (x-rays) taken after a contrast medium has been introduced into the patient's body to make organs or structures more visible on the finished image.

**conus papillaris**   A structure histologically similar to the pectin (a vascular structure in avian eyes). Found in the eyes of lizards and closely related reptiles.

**coping**   The process of trimming and shaping a bird's beak.

**coprodeum**   Anterior section of the avian cloaca that receives excrement from the intestine.

**copulation**   The act of breeding; consists of intromission of the penis into the vagina, thrusting, and ejaculation.

**corium**   The dermis of the skin.

**cornea**   The clear "window" on the front of the eye that admits light to the interior of the eye; part of the outer, fibrous layer of the eyeball.

**cornification**   Formation of a layer of tough keratin on an epithelial surface.

**cornual process**   The "horn core" of horned animals; a process of the frontal bone. The hollow cavity within the cornual process is continuous with the frontal sinus (the paranasal sinus of the frontal bone).

**corona glandis**   The widest portion of the glans penis of the horse.

**corona radiata**   A thin layer of granulosa cells that surrounds the ovum as it develops in the ovarian follicle and after it is released by ovulation.

**coronary band**   The part of the hoof that articulates with the skin.

**coronary corium**   The part of the corium that has differentiated to provide nourishment to the hoof at the site of the coronary band.

**corpus callosum**   White fibers that connect and provide communication pathways between the two cerebral hemispheres.

**corpus cavernosum penis**   The larger of the two erectile tissue structures in the body of the penis. It is located dorsal to the smaller corpus cavernosum urethrae.

**corpus cavernosum urethrae**   The smaller of the two erectile tissue structures in the body of the penis. It forms a "sleeve" around the urethra and is located ventral to the larger corpus cavernosum penis.

**corpus hemorrhagicum**   The blood-filled remnant of the ovarian follicle immediately after ovulation.

**corpus luteum**   Literally "yellow body." The solid endocrine structure that forms from the empty ovarian follicle after ovulation. Under stimulation from luteinizing hormone from the anterior pituitary gland, the granulosa cells left in the empty follicle multiply to form the solid corpus luteum. It produces progestin hormones, principally progesterone, that are necessary for the maintenance of pregnancy.

**cortex**   (1) The outer, superficial layer of an organ or structure. (2) The outer portion of the kidney. It contains the renal corpuscles, proximal convoluted tubules, distal convoluted tubules, collecting ducts, and peritubular capillaries. (3) In hair, it is the layer surrounding the medulla, composed of hard keratin.

**costal cartilage**   The cartilaginous, ventral portion of a rib.

**cotyledon**   Numerous areas on the surface of the placenta of ruminant animals that join with the caruncles in the lining of the uterus to form placental attachment sites called *placentomes*.

**cotyledonary placental attachment**   The type of placental attachment found in common ruminant animals. It consists of numerous cotyledons on the surface of the placenta joining with caruncles in the lining of the uterus to form attachment sites called placentomes.

**cough**   A protective response to irritation or foreign material in the trachea or bronchi. The sudden, forceful expiration of air is intended to force the irritant or foreign material up and out of the respiratory tract. Productive coughs are moist and generally help an animal to clear mucus and other matter from the airways. Nonproductive coughs are dry and generally not beneficial to the animal.

**covalent bond**   Chemical bonds in which electrons are shared.

**cranial nerves**   Set of 12 pairs of nerves originating directly from the brain; may be sensory or motor or may contain both sensory and motor nerves.

**cranial–sacral system** Another term that defines the parasympathetic nervous system, based on the fact that the parasympathetic nerves emerge from the cranial nerves and from the sacral spinal cord segments.

**cranial** A directional term meaning *toward the head* of an animal.

**cranium** The cranial portion of the dorsal body cavity, formed from several skull bones. It houses and protects the brain. It is the reference point for the directional term *cranial*.

**creatine phosphate (CP)** The molecule in muscle cells that splits to release the energy necessary to reattach the detached phosphate group to an adenosine diphosphate (ADP) molecule to convert it back to the high-energy molecule adenosine triphosphate (ATP).

**cremaster muscle** The bandlike muscle that raises and lowers the testes in the scrotum to help control their temperature. The testes must be maintained at a temperature slightly cooler than body temperature to produce spermatozoa.

**Creutzfeldt–Jakob disease** A disease in humans that was discovered by Hans Gerhard Creutzfeldt and Alfons Maria Jakob. The disease has no known cure and causes a fatal spongiform encephalopathy. Prions are known to be the infectious agent.

**cribriform plate** The sievelike area of the ethmoid bone through which the many branches of the olfactory nerve pass from the upper portion of the nasal cavity to the olfactory bulbs of the brain.

**cricoid cartilage** One of the cartilages of the larynx. The cricoid cartilage is ring-shaped. It helps form and support the caudal portion of the larynx.

**crista** The short name for the receptor structure of the semicircular canals.

**crista ampullaris** The full name of the receptor structure of the semicircular canals.

**cristae** The folds within the mitochondria that increase ATP output by increasing the surface area and thus the number of reaction sites.

**crop** Dilated portion of the esophagus in some species of bird that acts as a storage pouch for food.

**cross-bridges** Tiny "levers" on the myosin filaments of muscle. A muscle cell contracts by ratcheting the cross-bridges back and forth to pull the thinner actin filaments toward the center of the myosin filaments.

**crossed extensor reflex** Reflex initiated by a stimulation of a limb that results in extension of the limb on the other side of the body.

**crown** (1) Top part of the head. (2) The enamel-covered, exposed part of a tooth.

**CRT** See *capillary refill time*.

**crude protein** The total nitrogen content of a feed multiplied by 6.25. The crude protein gives a close approximation of the protein content in a particular feed.

**crura** A portion of the roots of the penis. The connective tissue bands that attach the penis to the brim of the pelvis.

**cryptorchidism** The condition of one or both testes failing to descend into the scrotum. Cryptorchidism in animals may be unilateral (one side only) or bilateral (both sides).

**crypts** Invaginations in the intestinal mucosa that produce the cells that form the villi.

**cuboidal cells** Cube-shaped cells with centrally located nuclei.

**cuboidal epithelium** Epithelium composed of cuboidal cells.

**cumulus oophorus** The small mound of granulosa cells on which the oocyte sits as it develops in the ovarian follicle.

**cupula** The gelatinous structure that sits on top of the receptor hairs in the crista ampullaris of the semicircular canals.

**cutaneous membrane** Also known as the *integument*. The outer layer (epidermis) is composed of keratinized stratified squamous epithelium. This helps to waterproof and prevent dehydration of the body. The inner layer or *dermis* is composed of dense irregular connective tissue, as well as collagenous and elastic fibers. This also helps the cutaneous membrane by giving it reinforcement and flexibility.

**cutaneous muscles** "Skin muscles"; thin muscles in the connective tissue beneath the skin. When a cutaneous muscle contracts, it causes the skin to twitch.

**cuticle** The single layer of cells that make up the outermost layer of the hair shaft.

**-cyte** Suffix meaning cell.

**cytochromes** Essential to the final stage of the electron transport system, this copper-containing complex of enzymes transfers electrons to oxygen. The oxygen in turn can bond with hydrogen, thus producing water.

**cytokines** Signaling molecules responsible for cell movement/signaling.

**cytokinesis** The separation of the cytoplasm into two separate daughter cells during the mitotic stage of cell division called *telophase*.

**cytologist** One who studies cells.

**cytoplasm** The part of the cell's protoplasm that is located outside the nuclear envelope.

**cytosine (C)** One of the nucleotides present in both RNA and DNA. It is a pyrimidine base that pairs with RNA and DNA's guanine.

**cytosis** The active transport of materials into or out of the cell. The transported material is bound by a membrane.

**cytoskeleton** The internal structure of the cell that maintains the cell's shape and aids in some functions. The cytoskeleton is composed of three types of filament: *microfilaments, microtubules,* and *intermediate filaments*.

**cytosol** The fluid component of protoplasm that acts as its base.

**cytotoxic T cells** Also known as *killer cells* or *killer T lymphocytes*. They attach to antigenic cells and destroy them, but they are not themselves damaged.

**D**

**DCT** See *distal convoluted tubule*.

**deamination** The process during catabolism in which the amino group $NH_2$ is removed.

**decomposition reaction** A chemical reaction in which a complex reactant is divided into simpler molecules or elements. The opposite of a synthesis reaction.

**deep** A directional term meaning toward the center of the body or a body part; see *internal*.

**defecation** The expelling of feces.

**defibrillation** The process of sending an electrical current through the heart to restart coordinated pumping activity and restore regular rhythm.

**dehydration synthesis** The combination of two or more simple materials to form one or more complex materials by removing water. For example, two monosaccharides can combine to form a disaccharide:

**delivery of the newborn** Passage of the newborn animal through the vagina from the uterus to the outside world. Accomplished by a combination of uterine and abdominal muscle contractions.

**delivery of the placenta** Passage of the placenta through the vagina from the uterus to the outside world after delivery of the newborn. Accomplished by a combination of uterine and abdominal muscle contractions.

**deltoid crest** See *pectoral crest.*

**dendrites** The receptive sites of the nerve cell; they extend from the cell body, giving the cell a starlike shape; they receive stimuli and convey them as nerve impulses to the cell body.

**dens** Process on the cranial end of the second cervical vertebra (axis) that fits into the caudal end of the first cervical vertebra (atlas).

**dense bodies** Structures in smooth muscle cells to which the small contractile units of actin and myosin attach. The dense bodies of smooth muscle correspond to the *Z* lines of skeletal muscle to which the actin filaments attach.

**dense connective tissue** A highly fibrous connective tissue with little vascularization. It functions to reinforce and bind body structures. Dense connective tissue is of two types: *dense regular* and *dense irregular.*

**dense irregular connective tissue** A collagen-based fibrous connective tissue that is found in the dermis, spleen, and liver. It has thicker bundles of fiber than dense regular connective tissue and is designed to withstand tension from multiple directions.

**dense regular connective tissue** Tightly bound, minimally vascularized fibrous connective tissue found in ligaments, tendons, and fascia. In ligaments it binds joints, whereas in tendons it binds muscle to bone. In fascia, it helps support surrounding tissues.

**dental formula** The shorthand abbreviation that shows the number of incisors (I), canines (C), premolars (P), and molars (M) that a species has; the first number of the pair indicates the number of teeth in half of the upper arcade; the second number indicates the number of teeth in half of the lower arcade; lowercase letters indicate deciduous teeth; for example: I3/3 C1/1 P2/2 M3/3.

**dental pad** The hard, thick connective tissue pad that ruminants have in the space occupied by upper incisor teeth in other species.

**dental prophylaxis** The cleaning of teeth; slang is *dental prophy.*

**dentin** The layer surrounding the tooth pulp; more dense than bone but not as dense as the overlying enamel.

**deoxyhemoglobin** Hemoglobin that is not carrying any oxygen; also known as *empty hemoglobin.*

**deoxyribonucleic acid** Referred to as *DNA.* The genetic material of a living thing, found in strands called *chromatin* within the nucleus of the cell.

**depolarization** A reduction in the voltage across a neuron or muscle cell membrane from its normal polarized state (resting membrane potential). This results in an action potential (nerve impulse) in the case of a neuron or the initiation of contraction in the case of a muscle cell.

**dermis** The deep, connective tissue portion of the skin that contains blood vessels, glands, and hair follicles.

**desmosome** A type of intercellular attachment found in epithelial tissue. The bond is formed from the interlocking of filaments that connect the plasma membranes of adjacent cells.

**determinate layer** Species that can lay only the number of eggs in a normal clutch size.

**development** The growth of an organism to full size or maturity.

**dewclaw** A toe that does not reach the ground, such as the first digit of dogs and cats and the rudimentary medial and lateral toes of cattle.

**diabetes insipidus** A disease resulting from a deficiency of antidiuretic hormone from the posterior pituitary gland. It results in polyuria and polydipsia.

**diabetes mellitus** A disease resulting from a deficiency of the hormone insulin from the pancreatic islets. The lack of insulin prevents glucose from entering cells and being used as an energy source. This results in signs that include hyperglycemia, glycosuria, polyuria, polydipsia, polyphagia, weight loss, and weakness.

**diapedesis** The process by which white blood cells leave capillaries and enter tissue by squeezing through the tiny spaces between the capillary cells.

**diaphragm** The thin, dome-shaped sheet of muscle that forms the boundary between the thoracic and abdominal cavities. A muscle that helps produce inspiration when it contracts. The diaphragm is dome-shaped at rest, with its convex surface directed cranially. When it contracts, the dome of the diaphragm flattens out, which increases the volume of the thoracic cavity and causes air to be drawn into the lungs.

**diaphragmatic flexure** Where the left dorsal colon of the horse bends back on itself to form the right dorsal colon.

**diaphragmaticus** Diaphragm.

**diaphysis** The shaft portion of a long bone.

**diapsid skulls** Skulls of various reptiles (lizards, snakes, crocodiles) with two pairs of temporal openings behind each eye.

**diarthrosis** A freely movable synovial joint.

**diastole** The part of the cardiac cycle associated with relaxation of the atria and ventricles and the filling of the chambers with blood.

**diencephalon** Serves as a nervous system passageway between the primitive brainstem and the cerebrum; three major structures of the diencephalon are the *thalamus,* the *hypothalamus,* and the *pituitary.*

**diestrous** Animals that have two estrous cycles per year.

**diestrus** The active luteal stage of the estrous cycle. During this period, the corpus luteum has reached maximum size and is producing maximum amounts of progestin hormones.

**differentiation** The progressive acquisition of individual characteristics by cells to enable them to perform different functions.

**diffuse placental attachment** A loose form of placental attachment to the uterine wall; attachment sites are spread diffusively over the whole surface of the placenta and the whole lining of the uterus; found in horses, swine and camelids.

**diffusion** The tendency for molecules to move from an area of high concentration to an area of low concentration.

**digestive enzyme** An enzyme in the digestive tract that aids the breakdown of complex food substances into simpler molecules that can be absorbed into the bloodstream.

**digestive system** The collection of organs that take in, digest and absorb food for use by the body to maintain health and normal function. This system includes all structures of the mouth, esophagus, stomach, and the small and large intestines. Although not part of the digestive tract, accessory digestive organs such as the gallbladder and pancreas provide secretions that aid in the chemical part of the process.

**digestive tract** Also called the *alimentary canal,* this encompasses all of the parts of the digestive system that transport food from the mouth to the anus: mouth, esophagus, stomach, small and large intestines, and anus.

**digit** A toe made up of two or three bones called *phalanges.*

**dilated cardiomyopathy** Enlargement of the heart resulting from dilation of the heart's chambers and thinning of the ventricular walls. If left untreated, the condition will ultimately lead to heart failure.

**dipeptide** A molecule that consists of two amino acids joined by a single peptide bond.

**diploid chromosome number** The chromosome number in all of an animal's cells except for the gametes (reproductive cells). It is always an even number.

**disaccharide** "Two sugars"; includes sucrose, maltose, isomaltose, and lactose.

**discoid placental attachment** Attachment of the placenta to the uterus in a single, disc-shaped area; found in primates, rabbits, and many rodents.

**distal convoluted tubule (DCT)** The last tubular part of the nephron before it enters the collecting duct. DCTs are found in the kidney's cortex.

**distal phalanx bone** The phalanx that is located most distally from the body; the tip of the digit.

**distal sesamoid bone** The *navicular bone* of horses. It is located in the digital flexor tendon deep in the hoof behind the joint between the middle and distal phalanges.

**distal** A directional term used only for extremities of the body. It implies a position or direction *away from* the body proper.

**disulfide bonds** Strong covalent bonds that unite amino acids in globular protein formations.

**diuresis** Producing and passing large amounts of urine.

**DNA polymerase** An enzyme that reestablishes the double helix of DNA by uniting the nucleotide bases with their corresponding base pairs. This creates a new strand for each original DNA strand.

**dolichocephalic** Long-faced. The Rough Collie is a dolichocephalic dog breed.

**dopamine** A catecholamine neurotransmitter.

**dorsal** A directional term meaning *toward the top* of an animal when it is standing on all four legs; toward the backbone.

**dorsal body cavity** The space in the skull and spinal column that contains the brain and spinal cord. The portion in the skull is called the *cranium,* and the portion in the spinal column is called the *spinal canal.*

**dorsal horn** The area of the spinal cord's gray matter "butterfly" where the neurons that forward sensory (afferent) nerve impulses to the brain or other parts of the spinal cord are located.

**dorsal nerve root** The branch off each side of the spinal cord between each set of adjacent vertebrae that conducts sensory impulses into the spinal cord from the periphery of the body.

**dorsal plane** An anatomic reference plane that divides the body into dorsal (upper) and ventral (lower) parts that are not necessarily equal.

**double helix** Also called the *Watson–Crick helix;* the double coils seen in DNA that contain specific nucleotides whereby one set determines the corresponding set.

**dressing forceps** A tweezerlike surgical instrument with serrated tips used to grasp gauze sponges and other surgical materials. It is not intended for use on tissue.

**duct** A tubelike channel that provides an exit route for secretory or excretory products.

**duodenum** The first segment of the small intestine after the stomach. Chyme enters the duodenum from the stomach.

**dura mater** The thick outermost layer of the meninges that covers the brain and spinal cord; it is considered to be the toughest of the meninges.

**dysfunction** Abnormal functioning of an organ or body part.

**dystocia** A difficult birth. Dystocias usually result from a fetus that is too large for the birth canal or one that is oriented inappropriately for delivery.

**E**

**eardrum** Common name for the tympanic membrane. The paper-thin, connective tissue membrane that is tightly stretched across the opening of the external ear canal into the middle ear.

**eccrine glands** Exocrine glands that secrete substances directly onto the skin without the loss of cellular material. They contain simple, coiled, tube structures for excretory purposes.

**eccrine sweat glands** Sweat glands that cover the entire surface of the body of some animal species for the purpose of thermoregulation.

**ecdysis** Shedding of the skin of reptiles.

**eclampsia** A condition seen in lactating dogs and cats that results from hypocalcemia. Early signs of eclampsia include muscle tremors and spasms.

**ectothermic** "Cold-blooded," not internally regulated. Body temperature varies with the environment. Includes all animals except mammals and birds.

**edema** An abnormal accumulation of fluid, either localized or generalized, within the tissues or cavities of the body.

**effector cell** A cell such as a muscle or gland cell that carries out some action when stimulated by a nerve impulse.

**efferent** A directional term meaning *away from* some reference point.

**efferent ducts of the testes** The passageways that allow spermatozoa to move from the rete testis to the head of the epididymis.

**efferent glomerular arterioles** Arterioles that leave the glomeruli of the kidney. They are carrying blood that has been filtered by the glomeruli, so it contains less water. Blood in the efferent glomerular arterioles has a higher concentration of blood cells and plasma proteins than blood in the afferent glomerular arterioles.

**efferent nerve** Nerve that carries impulses away from the central nervous system.

**effusion** Excess fluid that has escaped into a body cavity to the detriment of normal body function.

**egg binding** The condition resulting when an egg gets stuck in the oviduct of a bird.

**eicosanoids** Any of a group of substances derived from 20-carbon unsaturated fatty acids, such as arachidonic acid. Includes prostaglandins, leukotrienes, and thromboxanes. They are the principal mediators of inflammation.

**ejaculation** The reflex expulsion of semen from the penis.

**elastase** Protease secreted in an inactive form from the pancreas and activated by trypsin.

**elastic cartilage** Also called *yellow cartilage;* similar to hyaline cartilage, except that it is more opaque and contains many elastic fibers. It is found in the external ear and in the epiglottis.

**elastic connective tissue** Connective tissue composed of large numbers of elastic fibers; found in tissues that expand and contract, such as the lungs and vocal cords.

**elastic fibers** Fibers composed of elastin. Elastic fibers form a delicate mesh in tissues.

**electrocardiogram** A recording of the electrical activity of the heart.

**electrolyte** A substance that conducts an electric current in solution.

**electron** A lightweight subatomic particle that carries a negative charge. Together with the nuclei, they make up the atom; they are the particles responsible for chemical bonding.

**electron microscope** A powerful microscope that magnifies a sample by using an electron beam for illumination.

**electron shell** The grouping of electrons around the nucleus of an atom. The electron shell is determined by the energy level of the electron. The electrons in the outer electron shell are the ones responsible for chemical reactions.

**electron transport system** The final and most productive stage of cellular respiration, which takes place inside the mitochondria.

**electrostatic attraction** The attractive force between two particles of opposite electric charge. The force is proportional to the magnitude of the charge and inversely proportional to the distance between the particles.

**element** Any of 116 known substances that cannot be separated into smaller substances. The smallest unit of an element is an atom.

**embryo** The name generally given to the developing offspring during the first trimester of pregnancy. During this period, the newly implanted zygote and its placenta are getting themselves organized and the body tissues, organs, and systems begin to form.

**embryonic hemoglobin** Hemoglobin found in red blood cells during early fetal life.

**emulsification** The mixing of fat or oil and water by agitation or shaking.

**enamel** Outer coating layer of the crown of a tooth; toughest substance in the body.

**endocardium** The innermost layer of the heart.

**endochondral bone formation** The type of bone formation whereby bone grows into and replaces a cartilage model. This is the method by which most bones form in a developing fetus, starting with cartilage "prototypes" that are gradually replaced by bone. It is also the means by which long bones increase in length at the epiphyseal (growth) plates. New cartilage is created on the outside surfaces of the plates, and bone replaces old cartilage on the inside surfaces. This allows the bones to increase in length as the animal grows.

**endocrine glands** Glands or cells that release their regulatory products (hormones) directly into the bloodstream. Endocrine glands control most metabolic functions. Examples of endocrine glands include the pituitary, parathyroid, and pancreas.

**endocrine system** The system of glands that controls and regulates body functions through the internal secretion of hormones. The hormones are released directly into the bloodstream, which allows them to exert their actions on target cells throughout the body.

**endocrinology** The study of the endocrine system.

**endocytosis** The taking in of a material from the outside of the cell by creating a "mouth" with the plasma membrane. The membrane engulfs the material and pinches off at the ends to form a vesicle. Endocytosis includes the processes of pinocytosis and phagocytosis.

**endolymph** The fluid in the receptor structures of the inner ear.

**endolymphatic sacs** Sacs that are located in the inner ear and contain endolymph.

**endomysium** The thin, delicate layer of connective tissue that surrounds each individual skeletal muscle fiber.

**endoplasmic reticulum (ER)** A system of channels within the cell that run from the nucleus to the exterior cell membrane. The two forms of ER have their own functions. *Rough ER* is the site for protein synthesis, and *smooth ER* is the site for lipid synthesis.

**endosteum** The fibrous membrane that lines the hollow interiors of bones.

**endothelium** Derived from mesothelium, the endothelium is composed of simple squamous epithelium. It lines the heart, blood vessels, and serous cavities of the body.

**endotracheal (ET) intubation** The placement of a soft rubber or plastic ET tube through the larynx and into the trachea to establish an open airway.

**endotracheal (ET) tube** A soft rubber or plastic tube that is passed through the larynx and into the trachea to establish an open airway; often used to administer inhalation anesthetics.

**energy of activation** The amount of energy necessary to initiate a reaction.

**enteric** Referring to the intestine.

**enteritis** Inflammation of the intestines.

**enterogastric reflex** The reflex in which the presence of food in the stomach stimulates motility and digestive secretions in the intestine.

**enzyme** A specialized globular protein that carries out and/or speeds up chemical reactions in the body by acting as a catalyst and lowering the temperature necessary for the reaction to take place. Specific enzymes are exclusive to specific reactions, and although they may change the rate of reaction, they are never changed or used up themselves in the process.

**eosinopenia** A decrease in the total number of eosinophils in peripheral blood.

**eosinophil** The granulocytic white blood cell characterized by the presence of numerous red-staining granules in its cytoplasm.

**eosinophilia** An increase in the total number of eosinophils in peripheral blood.

**epicardium** Outermost layer of the heart.

**epidermal** Referring to the epidermis.

**epidermal orifice** The opening of the hair follicle through which the hair emerges.

**epidermis** Composed of keratinized stratified squamous epithelium, it is the outermost layer of the skin.

**epididymis** The ribbonlike structure that lies along the surface of the testis. It is actually one long, convoluted tube that links the efferent ducts with the vas deferens. Spermatozoa are stored in the epididymis as they await ejaculation.

**epidural anesthesia** The administration of anesthetic agents into the space between the dura mater and the surrounding bone of the vertebrae.

**epiglottis** The most rostral of the laryngeal cartilages. It projects forward from the ventral portion of the larynx, and its bluntly pointed tip usually tucks up behind the caudal rim of the soft palate when the animal is breathing. When the animal swallows, the epiglottis is pulled back to cover the opening of the larynx, like a trapdoor.

**epimysium** The tough, connective tissue layer that covers and delineates individual muscles. It surrounds groups of skeletal muscle fascicles.

**epinephrine** Commonly called *adrenaline.* A hormone secreted by the medulla of the adrenal gland under stimulation by the sympathetic portion of the autonomic nervous system. It produces part of the fight-or-flight response that results when an animal feels threatened.

**epiphyseal plate** The growth plate of a long bone. Epiphyseal plates are located at the junction of the proximal and distal epiphyses with the diaphysis. They are areas where long bones increase in length by the process of endochondral bone formation. When an animal reaches its full size, the epiphyseal plates of its bones completely ossify and the bones cease their growth.

**epiphysis** The end of a long bone. Each long bone has a proximal and a distal epiphysis.

**epithelial tissues** A collection of tissues that are made up of layers of cells that line and cover body surfaces. These cells may be in single layers or multilayered and can regenerate quickly.

**epithelialization** The rapid division of epithelial cells around a wound edge. Epithelialization attempts to cover the opening of a wound. This process is assisted by the contraction of collagen fibers, which bring the edges of the epithelial layer into close opposition.

**equator** The center of the spindle apparatus where the chromosomes line up during metaphase in cell division; also known as the equatorial plate.

**equilibrium** (1) The balance of solutes and solution between the inside and outside of the cell. For example, in the case of salts and water, the concentrations on either side of the cell membrane will be in a state of equilibrium. (2) The sense that helps an animal maintain its balance by keeping track of the position and movements of its head.

**erectile tissue** A spongy network of fibrous connective tissue and blood sinuses. When more blood flows into erectile tissue than leaves it, the sinuses engorge with blood and create hydraulic pressure that enlarges and stiffens the organ in which the erectile tissue is located.

**erection** Enlargement and stiffening of an organ that contains erectile tissue, such as the penis, clitoris, or nipple.

**ergots** Believed to be the vestigial remnants of metacarpal and metatarsal pads, these are the horny, keratinized growths located behind the fetlocks of all equids.

**eructation** The expulsion of gases orally; burping or belching.

**erythrocytes** Also called *red blood cells* or *red corpuscles,* these cells are anucleated and biconcave in shape. They are responsible for carrying oxygen from the lungs to tissues. Erythrocytes are formed in the red bone marrow of adults and in the liver, spleen, and marrow of a fetus. They are also manufactured in the spleens of anemic and ill adults.

**erythropoiesis** Production of erythrocytes.

**erythropoietin** The hormone produced by the kidney that stimulates the red bone marrow to increase its production of red blood cells.

**esophageal groove** See *reticular groove.*

**essential amino acid** An amino acid that cannot be produced in sufficient amounts in the body; therefore, it must be obtained in the diet. Different species have different essential amino acid needs.

**essential fatty acids** Unsaturated fatty acids such as linolenic, arachidonic, and linoleic fatty acids that are necessary for normal body functions yet are not synthesized by the body in sufficient amounts; therefore, they must be supplemented in the diet.

**essential nutrients** A select group of nutrients that cannot be manufactured in the body from the "building-block" molecules amino acids, monosaccharides, glycerol, and fatty acids. Animals must obtain essential nutrients from their diet.

**estrogens** Hormones that promote the development of female characteristics; female sex hormones.

**estrous** An adjective used with the noun "cycle" to refer to the entire reproductive cycle in females.

**estrous cycle** The period from the beginning of one heat period to the beginning of the next. It includes the stages of proestrus, estrus, metestrus, and diestrus.

**estrus** The heat period; the stage of the estrous cycle when the female is sexually receptive to the male and will allow breeding to take place.

**ethmoid bone** A skull bone; an internal bone of the cranium. The single ethmoid bone is located just rostral (ahead of) the sphenoid bone. It contains the cribriform plate, which transmits the many branches of the olfactory nerve to the olfactory bulb of the brain.

**ethmoidal sinus** The paranasal sinus in the ethmoid bone of a horse or human.

**eukaryotes** This classification of cells is found in all living things, such as plants and mammals, except for prokaryotes. Eukaryotes have a true nucleus that contains chromosomes and has a nuclear envelope. They also have membrane-bound organelles.

**Eustachian tube** The tube that connects the middle ear cavity with the pharynx. It allows equalization of the air pressure on the two sides of the tympanic membrane.

**euthanize** To end an animal's life humanely.

**exchange reaction** A chemical reaction in which chemical substances exchange molecules or elements to form different chemical substances. A combination of decomposition and synthesis reactions.

**excising** Removing all or part of a tissue or organ by cutting it out surgically.

**excitatory neurotransmitters** Chemicals released by neurons at the synapse that tend to cause excitation or depolarization of other neurons or target tissues.

**excretion** The elimination of waste materials from the cell or body.

**excretory ducts** Ducts that transport waste products or secretions out of an organ or gland.

**exocrine glands** Glands that release their secretions through ducts that lead directly to the location intended to be controlled. Some examples include sweat glands and salivary glands.

**exocytosis** The passage of materials too large to diffuse though the cell membrane by packaging them in vesicles, transporting them to the cell membrane, and then pressing them out of the cell.

**exons** Parts of a gene's DNA sequence that are coded. Exons are separated by noncoding portions, called *introns,* which are spliced out to join the exons together to form messenger RNA.

**expiration** Exhalation; the process of pushing air out of the lungs.

**expiratory muscle** A muscle whose action is to decrease the size of the thoracic cavity; this squeezes air out of the lungs, thereby producing expiration (exhalation).

**extension** The joint movement that increases the angle between two bones.

**external** An alternative directional term for *superficial.* External also means toward the surface of the body or a body part.

**external acoustic meatus** The bony canal in the temporal bone that leads into the middle and inner ear cavities of the bone. In the living animal, it contains the external ear canal.

**external auditory canal** The tube that begins at the base of the pinna and carries sound waves to the tympanic membrane. In most domestic animal species, it is L shaped, with a vertical portion leading down to a horizontal portion.

**external ear** The outer portion of the ear. It consists of the structures that collect and transmit sound waves to the middle ear: the *pinna,* the *external auditory canal,* and the *tympanic membrane.*

**external respiration** The process of respiration that occurs in the lungs. Oxygen and carbon dioxide are exchanged between the air inhaled into the alveoli of the lungs and the blood in the capillaries that surround them.

**extracellular fibers** The fibers of connective tissue located outside cells that perform a variety of functions depending on the degree of their elasticity or concentration.

**extracellular fluid** The fluid located outside the cell.

**extracellular matrix** The nonliving substance found between cells that provides support and nourishment.

**extraocular muscles** The small skeletal muscles that move and position the eyeballs.

**extravascular hemolysis** Destruction of red blood cells outside a blood vessel.

**exudate** The accumulation of fluid, pus, or serum in a cavity or tissue. Fluid or serum has often leaked through vessel walls or capillaries into the adjoining space.

**eyelids** The conjunctiva-lined folds of skin that protect and cover the eyeball.

**F**

**fabella** One of two small sesamoid bones located in the proximal gastrocnemius (calf) muscle tendon just above and behind the femoral condyles of dogs and cats.

**facet** A flat articular surface, for example those between carpal bones and between the radius and ulna.

**facilitated diffusion** The diffusion of molecules across the cell membrane with the aid of carrier proteins. This reaction is unable to be performed as simple diffusion, and it requires no energy or ATP.

**false vocal cords** The vestibular folds; connective tissue bands in the larynx of nonruminant animals in addition to the vocal cords. The false vocal cords are not involved in voice production.

**fascia** An arrangement of dense regular connective tissue that lies over muscle. This layer helps to support, separate, and connect muscles to other structures.

**fascicle** A group of skeletal muscle fibers bound together by a layer of fibrous connective tissue called the *perimysium.*

**fat soluble** A molecule, such as a vitamin, that can dissolve in fat.

**fatty acids** The organic compounds of hydrogen, oxygen, and carbon that, when mixed with glycerol, form fat. There are several types of fatty acid. *Saturated fatty acids* are solid at room temperature and have no double bonds in their carbon chain. *Unsaturated fatty acids,* such as those in olive oil, are liquid at room temperature and have one or more double bonds. *Polyunsaturated fatty acids* contain two or more double bonds. *Volatile fatty acids* are created in the rumen and reticulum of ruminant animals, such as cows, through the process of cellulose fermentation and are essential for energy production. All fatty acids are insoluble in water.

**fault bar** Area on a feather vane that lacks barbules, also called a *stress bar;* caused by an interruption of the feather's blood supply during development.

**faveoli** Minute pits or depressions.

**feak** The act of rubbing the beak on a rough surface to clean it and maintain its shape.

**feather follicle** Depression in the skin that gives rise to and stabilizes a new feather.

**feedback system** A system by which the level of a hormone in the blood affects the gland that produced it. Negative feedback decreases further hormone production and positive feedback increases further hormone production.

**feline panleukopenia** Caused by the feline parvovirus, this infectious disease has an extremely high mortality rate in kittens. Infections in intrauterine cases are known to cause miscarriages, as well as fetal and newborn deaths. Because the virus tends to attack cells in the mitotic phase, epithelial tissue is at high risk of attack as a result of its constant cell division. Therefore characteristics of feline panleukopenia include vomiting, diarrhea, and dehydration. Vaccines are available.

**female pronucleus** The name for the nucleus of an ovum after the head of a spermatozoon has penetrated into the cell (fertilization of the ovum) but before the nuclei of the sperm (the male pronucleus) and ovum have come together. When the female and male pronuclei combine, the diploid chromosome number is restored and the genetic makeup of the offspring is determined.

**femur**   The long bone of the thigh region. It forms the hip joint with the pelvis at its proximal end and the stifle joint with the tibia at its distal end.

**fenestrations**   Small openings or holes (literally, *windows*); in the walls of the glomerular capillaries, fenestrations allow certain molecules to leave that would normally be too large to escape.

**fermentation**   Anaerobic oxidative decomposition of cellulose into simpler compounds, such as volatile fatty acids. The enzymes that break down the cellulose are produced by microorganisms, which are contained in the rumen or cecum of herbivores.

**fermentative digestion**   Digestive process in which food is broken down by enzymes produced by microbes.

**fertilization**   The physical entry of the head of a spermatozoon into an ovum, which is then called a zygote. The nuclei of the ovum and sperm merge, establishing the genetic makeup of the future offspring.

**fetal development**   The second stage (trimester) of pregnancy during which all the cells, tissues, organs, and systems of the fetus develop from primitive, undifferentiated stem cells.

**fetal growth**   The third stage (trimester) of pregnancy during which all parts of the fetus grow in size and complexity to prepare for the transition to a free-living, independent existence after parturition (the birth process).

**fetal hemoglobin**   The predominant hemoglobin in red blood cells during the later part of gestation. It is gradually replaced by adult hemoglobin during the first few weeks to months after birth.

**fetlock joint**   The lay term for the most proximal joint of the equine digit, which is the joint between the large metacarpal or metatarsal and the proximal phalanx. The proximal sesamoid bones are located on the palmar (front leg) or plantar (rear leg) surface of this joint.

**fetus**   The name given to the developing offspring, beginning about the second trimester of pregnancy. The body tissues, organs, and systems develop in the early fetal period, and then the offspring grows to its full birth size.

**fibrin**   A protein created when thrombin acts on fibrinogen. Fibrin is essential to the coagulation of blood. It forms a lattice of interwoven fibers around blood cells and platelets that solidify to form a blood clot.

**fibrinogen**   A protein formed in the liver and released into the bloodstream, especially in the presence of inflammatory processes. Fibrinogen, when acted on by thrombin, forms fibrin, which creates the meshwork of a blood clot.

**fibrinolysis**   Destruction of the fibrin strands that make up the matrix of a clot; part of the process of the breakdown of a clot.

**fibroblast**   Fixed cell involved in the development of connective tissue. Fibroblasts can differentiate into chondroblasts and osteoblasts to create substances specific to their cell type.

**fibrocartilage**   Found between the vertebrae of the spine, fibrocartilage is different from other types of cartilage in that it has no perichondrium. In addition, it possesses dense bundles of collagenous fibers but few chondrocytes. It is usually found intermingled with hyaline cartilage and has an excellent ability to resist compression.

**fibrocyte**   Mature, fiber-forming cell.

**fibrous adhesions**   Fibrous connections that are generated during the healing process; often seen in the abdominal and thoracic cavities after surgical procedures.

**fibrous joint**   An immovable joint; also known as a *synarthrosis*. The bones of a fibrous joint are firmly united by fibrous tissue. The sutures that unite most of the skull bones are fibrous joints.

**fibrous tunic**   Outer layer of tissue of the eye, composed of the sclera at the back and the cornea in front.

**fibula**   A thin bone located beside the tibia in the lower region of the pelvic limb. It is a complete bone in the dog and cat, but only the proximal and distal ends are present in horses and cattle. The fibula does not support any appreciable weight. It mainly acts as a muscle attachment site.

**fight-or-flight response**   A whole-body response resulting from an animal feeling threatened that prepares the body for intense physical activity. It results from a combination of direct sympathetic nerve stimulation and the release of epinephrine and norepinephrine into the bloodstream from the medulla of the adrenal gland. Effects in the body include increased heart rate and output, increased blood pressure, dilated air passageways in the lungs, and decreased gastrointestinal function.

**filtration**   The passage of a fluid, in response to pressure, through a semipermeable membrane that allows the liquid portion to pass through but not cells and large molecules such as proteins.

**fimbriae**   The muscular, fingerlike projections that form the fringe of the infundibulum of the oviduct. The fimbriae feel their way across the surface of the ovary to where follicles are developing. They help position the infundibulum so that the ovum or ova will be guided into the oviduct when ovulation occurs.

**first-intention healing**   Healing that occurs in tissues in which the wound edges are held in close apposition to one another, as in the case of a sutured wound. Little to no granulation tissue is formed. There is generally minimal scarring.

**fission**   The asexual division of an organism or cell into two individual "daughter" cells.

**fissures**   Deep grooves found in the cerebral cortex.

**fixator**   A muscle that stabilizes a joint so that other muscles can produce effective movements of other joints.

**fixed cells**   One of the two subdivisions of connective tissue cells. Fixed cells are stationary within the connective tissue and perform functions such as matrix production and regulation.

**flagellum (plural, flagella)**   The primary means of motility for spermatozoa and unicellular organisms. This threadlike tail propels the organism by means of a whiplike movement.

**flank**   Lateral surface of the abdomen between the last rib and the hind legs.

**flat bone**   Bones that are relatively thin and flat. They consist of two thin plates of compact bone separated by a thin layer of cancellous bone. Many of the skull bones are flat bones.

**flexion**   The joint movement that decreases the angle between two bones.

**floating rib**   The most caudal one or two ribs in the rib cage. A rib whose costal cartilage does not unite with anything but ends in the muscle of the thoracic wall.

**fluid mosaic**   The constantly changing pattern of proteins and fluid between the two sides of the liquid bilayer.

**follicle**   A fluid-filled structure or cavity. An ovarian follicle consists of an oocyte surrounded by fluid and the follicular cells that produced it. Thyroid follicles are microscopic and consist of small globules of thyroid hormone precursor surrounded by simple cuboidal cells.

**follicle-stimulating hormone (FSH)** The anterior pituitary hormone that stimulates the growth and development of follicles in the ovaries of the female. In the male, it stimulates spermatogenesis in the seminiferous tubules of the testes.

**follicular atresia** The shrinkage of ovarian follicles that began developing but stopped.

**follicular cells** The cells that surround oocytes in ovarian follicles. Also known as *granulosa cells*. They produce estrogenic hormones in developing follicles.

**foramen (plural, foramina)** A hole in a bone.

**foramen magnum** The large hole in the occipital bone through which the spinal cord exits the skull.

**foramen of Panizza** A shunt connecting the left and right aorta in the crocodile heart; important in switching from terrestrial to aquatic circulatory patterns.

**forestomachs** Prestomach chambers in a ruminant animal. Includes the reticulum, rumen, and omasum.

**fossa** A depressed or sunken area on the surface of a bone. Fossae are usually occupied by muscles or tendons.

**fossa glandis** A shallow depression at the tip of horse's penis from which the urethral process protrudes.

**fovea** Depression in the retina of the eye containing a high concentration of cone photoreceptor cells.

**free radicals** Molecules that contain an odd number of electrons, making them highly reactive with other molecules. They bond to other molecules in the body, creating a new free radical that often causes a chain reaction of free radical formation.

**freely permeable** Those structures that allow the passage of fluids.

**frog** The thick triangular pad located on the plantar and palmar surfaces of the horse's hooves. It is one of the important structures of the "circulatory pump" in the equine foot.

**frontal bones** Skull bones; external bones of the cranium. The two frontal bones make up the "forehead" region of the skull. They contain the large frontal sinuses. The cornual process (horn core) in horned animals is an extension of the frontal bone.

**frontal plane** A human anatomic reference plane that divides the body into anterior and posterior parts. Equivalent to the dorsal plane of four-legged animals.

**frontal sinus** The large paranasal sinus in the frontal bone of the skull.

**functional group** Unique, specific groups of atoms within molecules that are responsible for the characteristic chemical reactions of those molecules.

**functional proteins** Complex proteins bearing a spherical shape. They are highly biochemically active. Also called *globular proteins*.

**fundus of eye** The caudal interior surface of the eye. It includes the retina and the optic disc.

**fundus of stomach** The blind pouch of the stomach that relaxes and distends with food.

# G

**G cells** Cells in the antrum of the stomach that produce gastrin.

**GABA** Gamma-aminobutyric acid; inhibitory neurotransmitter.

**GAGs** See *glycosaminoglycans*.

**gallbladder** The muscular, blind sac underneath the liver that stores bile until it is needed; cholecystokinin stimulates the gallbladder to contract, forcing the bile into the cystic duct and common bile duct and then into the duodenum.

**gamete** A reproductive cell—spermatozoon in the male or ovum in the female. Gametes have half the number of chromosomes (the haploid chromosome number) present in all other body cells (the diploid chromosome number).

**ganglion (plural, ganglia)** Cluster of neuron cell bodies outside the CNS.

**gap junctions** Proteinaceous pores that exist in the intestinal epithelial cells of most animals. These pores allow the passage of nutrients, as well as providing a channel for intercellular communication.

**gastric** Referring to or pertaining to the stomach.

**gastric atony** The state in which the stomach is very relaxed or has little or no muscle tone.

**gastrin** A hormone produced in the lining of the stomach when food arrives. It stimulates the gastric glands to secrete hydrochloric acid and digestive enzymes to start the digestive process and causes the fundus to relax.

**gastritis** Inflammation of the stomach.

**gastrointestinal tract** The part of the digestive tube composed of the stomach, small intestine, and large intestine.

**general anesthesia** Complete loss of sensory perception accompanied by loss of consciousness.

**general senses** The senses that are distributed throughout the body. Their receptors are fairly simple, and they keep the central nervous system informed about general conditions inside and outside the body.

**genes** Specific sites on chromosomes that dictate heredity. Some genes may control one specific phenotypic trait, whereas other traits require many genes for proper expression. Pairs of genes that control the same trait and are located on the same part of paired chromosomes are called *alleles*.

**genetic code** The unique order of pyrimidine- and purine-based nucleotides that govern the arrangement and transmission of genetic information in all living things, with the exception of RNA-based viruses.

**genetic material** Materials, such as DNA, that perpetuate the genetic code through the function of reproduction.

**gestation** The period of pregnancy.

**GFR** See *glomerular filtration rate*.

**GI tract** Abbreviation for *gastrointestinal tract*.

**gingiva** The epithelial tissue that composes the "gums."

**ginglymus joint** A hinge joint in which one articular surface swivels around another. The only movements possible are flexion and extension.

**gizzard** Muscular stomach in birds that grinds food into a digestible form.

**gland sinus** The large space in the mammary gland into which the large milk ducts empty. It is located just dorsal to the teat.

**glandular epithelium** Epithelial tissue composed of one cell (goblet cell) or groups of cells that produce and secrete substances into the lumen.

**glans of the penis** The distal, free end of the penis. It is richly supplied with sensory nerve endings.

**glenoid cavity** The concave articular surface of the scapula; the socket portion of the ball-and-socket shoulder joint. In birds, the wing is attached to the body by forming a joint in the depression.

**glial cells**   Cells in the nervous system that support and protect neurons.

**gliding joint**   An arthrodial joint in which two flat articular surfaces rock on each other. The carpus is an example of a gliding joint.

**globular proteins**   Complex proteins bearing a spherical shape.

**glomerular capillaries**   Part of the renal corpuscle. Urine production begins here when plasma is filtered out of the glomerular capillaries and into the capsular space of Bowman's capsule.

**glomerular filtrate**   The fluid that has been filtered out of the glomerular capillaries and into the capsular space.

**glomerular filtration rate (GFR)**   The rate at which plasma is filtered into the capsular space. It is expressed in milliliters per minute.

**glomerulus**   The tuft of capillaries found in the renal corpuscle; also called *glomerular capillaries.*

**glottis**   The opening into the larynx. The arytenoid cartilages and the vocal cords form the boundaries of the glottis.

**glucagon**   A hormone produced by the pancreas that raises blood glucose.

**glucocorticoid hormones**   A group of hormones with similar actions, secreted by the cortex of the adrenal glands. The most prominent effect of these hormones is to raise the level of glucose in the bloodstream.

**gluconeogenesis**   The production of glucose from amino acids that occurs in the liver.

Glucose + Galactose = Lactose + Water

**glucose**   Monosaccharide (simple sugar) that is used by the body for energy.

**glucosuria**   See *glycosuria.*

**glycerol**   The main component of triglycerides present in all fats. Triglycerides are soluble in water and alcohol.

**glycine**   Inhibitory neurotransmitter.

**glycocalyx**   Composed of glycoproteins, the outer covering of the cell that not only aids in cell adhesion but also allows the cell to be identified by other cells.

**glycogenesis**   The creation of glycogen from glucose in the liver.

**glycogenolysis**   The breaking apart of glycogen into glucose molecules.

**glycolipid**   A compound composed of a carbohydrate, usually in the form of sugar, and a fatty acid together in a compound.

**glycolysis**   The first step of cellular respiration that converts glucose into lactate or pyruvate and releases a small amount of ATP.

**glycoprotein**   A compound composed of a carbohydrate, usually in the form of sugar, and a protein.

**glycosaminoglycans (GAGs)**   Carbohydrates composed of amino sugars, which are found in proteoglycans.

**glycosuria**   The presence of glucose in the urine.

**goblet cell**   A type of cell, located in the respiratory and intestinal tracts, that secretes mucus.

**Golgi apparatus**   An organelle located near the nucleus that looks like sacs that are stacked and flattened at the ends. It is believed to be involved in the synthesis of glycoproteins, lipoproteins, and enzymes.

**gonad**   The organ that produces the reproductive cells; the testis in the male and the ovary in the female.

**gonadotropin**   A hormone that stimulates the growth and development of the gonads (ovaries and testes). Usually refers to follicle-stimulating hormone (FSH) or luteinizing hormone (LH).

**granulation tissue**   The new vascular and cellular tissue formed during the restoration of wounded tissue. It mostly consists of connective tissue and new blood vessels.

**granulocytes**   White blood cells that are characterized by the presence of granules in their cytoplasm. The granulocytes are neutrophils, eosinophils, and basophils.

**granulopoiesis**   A general term for the production of any or all of the granulocytes.

**granulosa cells**   The follicular cells of the developing follicle. They produce estrogenic hormones.

**gray matter**   That part of the CNS made up of neuron cell bodies.

**greater curvature of the stomach**   The larger, outer curve of the stomach.

**gristle**   Lay term for *cartilage.*

**gross anatomy**   The study of body structures that are visible without additional aid to the naked eye.

**ground substance**   The shapeless, viscous matrix present in connective tissue in which cells receive nutrients and void waste products. It also helps to protect the body from infectious agents by acting as a barrier.

**growth hormone (GH)**   The anterior pituitary hormone that promotes body growth in young animals and helps regulate the metabolism of proteins, carbohydrates, and lipids in all of the body's cells.

**growth one phase (G1)**   Part of interphase, during cell division. The cell enlarges and organelles replicate over time, which varies between cell types.

**growth plate**   The epiphyseal plate of a long bone. Located at the junction of the proximal and distal epiphyses with the diaphysis. Growth plates are areas where long bones increase in length by the process of endochondral bone formation. When an animal reaches its full size, the growth plates of its bones completely ossify and the bones cease their growth.

**growth two phase (G2)**   Part of interphase, during cell division. During this phase, enzymes and proteins are synthesized and the centrioles complete their replication.

**guanine (G)**   One of the nucleotides present in both RNA and DNA. It is a purine base that pairs with DNA and RNA's cytosine.

**gubernaculum**   The short, inelastic band of connective tissue that attaches the testes to the scrotum. Growth of the embryo, while the gubernaculum stays the same length, results in movement of the testes caudally and ventrally. Eventually, they descend through the inguinal rings into the scrotum.

**gular fluttering**   Rapid vibrations of the upper throat patch in many species of owls, herons, quail, pigeons, and doves. Used to increase cooling by the evaporative loss of heat from air passed over the oral cavity.

**gustatory sense**   The sense of taste.

**gut**   Also called the *gastrointestinal tract.* Includes the stomach, small intestine, and large intestine.

**gut-associated lymph tissue (GALT)**   Lymphoid tissue scattered throughout the lining of the intestine. It is often compared with the bursa of Fabricius in birds, where B lymphocytes are processed.

**gyrus (plural, gyri)**   The folds that provide the wrinkled appearance of the surface of the cerebral hemispheres.

## H

**hair bulb**    The bulbous portion of the hair follicle, located within the dermis, that provides the material for hair production.

**hair follicle**    Tubelike invaginations of the epidermis that traverse the dermis and pass into the connective tissue, where the hair is rooted. The arrector pili and sebaceous glands are located in close proximity to the hair follicle.

**hamuli**    Microscopic hooks that link the barbules of feathers together.

**haploid chromosome number**    The chromosome number in the gametes (reproductive cells). It is half the diploid chromosome number that is present in all other body cells.

**haptoglobin**    A transport plasma protein that carries free hemoglobin from intravascular hemolysis to the macrophages of the mononuclear phagocyte system in the liver for further breakdown.

**hard palate**    The bony roof of the mouth; the division between the mouth and the nasal cavity. The soft palate is immediately caudal to the hard palate. The hard palate is made up of portions of the maxillary and palatine bones.

**hardware disease**    A disease in ruminant animals caused by irritation of the lining of the reticulum by swallowed metal objects.

**haustra**    Sacculations of the colon and cecum.

**Haversian canal**    The central canal that runs the length of a Haversian system. The Haversian canal contains the blood vessels, lymph vessels, and nerves that supply and nourish the osteocytes.

**Haversian system**    The microscopic, laminated cylinders of bone that make up compact bone. Oriented lengthwise in a long bone, Haversian systems consist of a central Haversian canal surrounded by concentric layers of bone. Osteocytes in their lacunae are present at the junctions of the bony layers of the Haversian system.

**head**    A spheroidal articular surface on the proximal end of a long bone; present on the proximal ends of the humerus, femur, and ribs. The head of a bone is joined to the shaft by an area that is often narrowed, called the *neck*.

**health**    A state of normal anatomy and physiology that allows the body to function normally.

**hearing**    The auditory sense; the mechanical sense that converts the sound wave vibrations of air molecules to nerve impulses that are interpreted by the brain as sounds.

**heart rate**    How often the heart contracts, usually stated in beats per minute.

**heatstroke**    A dangerous body reaction to prolonged heat exposure. As the animal's core temperature rapidly rises, the animal becomes weak and confused and may lapse into unconsciousness, which can lead to convulsions and death. Heatstroke often occurs in animals that are locked in automobiles in the hot summer sun or confined in sunny areas without water or access to shade. Heatstroke victims must be cooled rapidly to prevent brain damage and death.

**heel**    The most posterior region of the hoof.

**helper T cells**    The most numerous of the T lymphocytes. They help the immune response by secreting substances known as *lymphokines* into the surrounding tissue, which increases activation of B lymphocytes and cytotoxic T cells.

**hematocrit**    The percentage of a total blood sample volume made up of red blood cells; the laboratory test performed to determine the percentage of red blood cells in a blood sample; also known as the *packed cell volume (PCV)*.

**hematopoiesis**    Blood cell production.

**hematopoietic tissue**    Tissue that produces blood cells. Red bone marrow is hematopoietic tissue.

**hemidesmosomes**    The half-units of desmosomes.

**hemipenes**    Saclike projections from the posterior cloaca of male snakes and lizards, which together act as a penis and are inserted into the cloaca of the female.

**hemoconcentration**    A condition resulting from a loss of plasma from blood into tissue. The cells become more concentrated in the plasma. This condition is commonly seen in a dehydrated animal.

**hemodilution**    A condition resulting from excess fluid entering blood from tissue or from intravenous injection of fluids. The cells become more diluted in the plasma. This condition can result from overhydration of an animal with intravenous or subcutaneous fluids.

**hemoglobin**    The protein molecules found inside red blood cells that are responsible for carrying oxygen molecules.

**hemoglobinemia**    Hemoglobin in plasma. The red blood cell membrane has ruptured, resulting in the release of hemoglobin. Hemoglobinemia is the result of intravascular hemolysis.

**hemoglobinuria**    Free hemoglobin found in urine. The degree of intravascular hemolysis was great enough to release large amounts of hemoglobin. The excess hemoglobin, over what could be bound to haptoglobin and carried to the liver, is eliminated in urine.

**hemolytic anemia**    An anemia caused by the hemolysis (rupture) of red blood cells; may be caused by an autoimmune disorder or the toxic effects of certain chemicals, or may be congenital.

**hemorrhaging**    The abnormal loss of blood from damaged blood vessels. It can be severe and may occur from arteries, veins, and capillaries.

**hemostasis**    Controlling bleeding; stopping the flow of blood out of a damaged blood vessel.

**hemothorax**    Blood present in the pleural cavity as a result of a condition such as pneumonia, cancerous tumors, or trauma.

**heparin**    A polysaccharide manufactured by mast cells that acts as an anticoagulant to help continue the increased blood flow during the inflammatory response.

**hepatic**    Referring to the liver.

**hepatic duct**    The duct that carries bile from the liver to the gallbladder in those species that have a gallbladder.

**hepatic lobes**    The large divisions of the liver seen grossly during surgery or dissection.

**hepatic lobules**    The microscopic divisions of the liver.

**hepatic portal system**    The blood vessels that carry blood from the capillaries of the intestine directly to the sinusoids of the liver.

**herbivore**    An animal whose diet is primarily plants.

**heterophil**    Phagocytic avian white blood cell equivalent to the mammalian neutrophil; generally round, containing a bilobed nucleus with clumped chromatin and rod shaped, red–orange granules in the cytoplasm.

**hexose sugar**   A simple sugar, such as glucose or fructose, that has six carbon atoms per molecule.

**hibernate**   To arrive at a deep state of sleep, nearly to the degree of a comatose state. During hibernation, an organism's metabolism and body temperature are in a significantly lowered state.

**hibernating gland**   An alternate nomenclature for brown adipose tissue, owing to its glandular appearance and its vital role in providing body heat to an animal during hibernation.

**hiccups**   Spasmodic contractions of the diaphragm accompanied by sudden closure of the glottis causing the characteristic "hiccup" sound. They are usually harmless and temporary.

**high-energy bonds**   Phosphate bonds in ADP and ATP containing large amounts of energy. The ATP molecule is used to move the energy to the cell. When the phosphate bond is broken, the energy contained in the bond is available to do cellular work.

**hilus**   The isolated area of some organs where blood vessels and other structures, such as nerves, enter and leave. For example, the hilus of the kidney is the indented area on the medial side where blood or lymph vessels and nerves enter and leave and where the ureters leave the organ. The hilus of the lung is where air passageways, blood, lymph vessels, and nerves enter and leave.

**hindgut**   The location of the microbial fermentation chambers in simple-stomached herbivore species, such as the horse and the rabbit; the cecum and colon.

**hinge joint**   A joint where one surface swivels around another like a door hinge; also called a *ginglymus joint.* The only movements possible in a hinge joint are flexion and extension. The elbow joint is an example of a hinge joint.

**hip dysplasia**   A disorder of the hip joint in which the normally tight-fitting ball-and-socket hip joint is abnormally loose. The looseness (laxity) of the dysplastic joint allows the head of the femur to "rattle around" in the acetabulum, resulting in damage to the joint surfaces and osteoarthritis development. Movement of the damaged hip causes pain.

**histamine**   Produced by mast cells from histidine during tissue injury, this biochemical increases blood flow and heart rate during the inflammatory response.

**histiocytes**   Macrophages located in loose connective tissue.

**histology**   The microscopic study of the structure of tissues and organs; microanatomy.

**histone**   A globular protein found in the cell nucleus that connects with nucleic acid to form nucleoproteins. Histones form a complex with DNA in chromatin and act as regulators of gene activity.

**hock**   Ankle joint, or tarsus; joins the tibiotarsus and the tarsometatarsus of birds.

**holocrine gland**   A gland whose granular secretions contain not only the secretory product but also the cells themselves. Holocrine gland cells are destroyed in the process of secretion. The sebaceous gland is an example of a holocrine gland.

**homeostasis**   A state of equilibrium maintained in the body by feedback and regulatory processes in response to internal and external changes; the maintenance of balance in the body. The concept of homeostasis includes the many mechanisms that monitor critical levels and functions in the body and stimulate corrective actions when things stray from normal. By keeping important activities within relatively narrow ranges, the process of homeostasis helps maintain normal body structure, function, and therefore health.

**homogeneous**   Having a uniform composition.

**homologous**   Similar in basic structure and from the same embryological origin. The penis of the male and the clitoris of the female are homologous structures.

**hoof wall**   The external, cornified portion of the hoof. It grows constantly downward from the coronary band to the sole. The deepest layer articulates with the corium by way of the laminae.

**Hooke, Robert**   Robert Hooke, in 1665, was the first person to identify the structure of the cell under a microscope.

**hormones**   Chemical messengers of the body that are produced and excreted by endocrine glands for the purpose of regulating specific organs or cells.

**horn tubes**   Minute lines that traverse the hoof wall vertically from the germinating layer of the coronary band to the sole.

**horn**   A horny, keratinized extension of the frontal bone in ruminate ungulates. At its root, it arises from the corium. Epidermal in origin, horns vary in shape and size depending on age, sex, and species.

**humerus**   The long bone of the brachium or upper arm.

**humoral immunity**   A type of defensive immune response regulated by B lymphocytes. When B lymphocytes are activated by the presence of an antigen, they transform into plasma cells that produce antibodies against the antigen.

**hyaline cartilage**   A bluish, translucent cartilage present in the costal cartilage, trachea, and embryonic skeleton. Hyaline cartilage is composed of densely packed collagen fibers and is covered by the perichondrium, except when present as articular cartilage in joints.

**hyaluronic acid**   A small protein containing no sulfate that acts as an intercellular material present in the *zonula adherens.* It is important in the formation of tight junctions.

**hyaluronidase**   An enzyme contained within white blood cells or infectious bacteria that hydrolyzes hyaluronic acid.

**hydraulic pressure**   Pressure exerted by confined fluids. During erection of the penis, more blood enters the erectile tissue of the penis than leaves it. The resulting hydraulic pressure produces enlargement and stiffening of the penis.

**hydrogen bonds**   Weak bonds that unite hydrogen with nitrogen or oxygen.

**hydrolysis**   One of the most basic and prevalent life processes. Hydrolysis breaks down more complex materials into simpler ones by adding water. Water breaks down or dissociates into a hydrogen atom (H) and a hydroxyl group (OH), which cling to individual parts of the material, thus separating it into two simpler materials.

**hydrophilic**   The tendency of a tissue to absorb or be attracted to water.

**hydrophobic**   The tendency of a tissue to be repelled by water or to be insoluble.

**hydrostatic pressure**   The force that propels a liquid.

**hyoid apparatus**   The hyoid bone.

**hyoid bone**   The bone in the neck region that supports the base of the tongue, the pharynx, and the larynx and aids the process of swallowing. It is usually referred to as a single bone, but it is composed of several portions. The hyoid bone is attached to the temporal bone by two small rods of cartilage.

**hyperadrenocorticism**   Excessive secretion of hormones from the cortex of the adrenal gland; also called *Cushing's syndrome.*

**hyperbilirubinemia**    An excess amount of bilirubin in plasma.

**hypercalcemia**    An excess level of calcium in the blood.

**hyperemia**    The reddish tinge of mucous membranes caused by an excessive flow of blood to the extremities.

**hyperglycemia**    Too high a level of glucose in the blood.

**hypermetria**    A condition in which voluntary movements become jerky and exaggerated.

**hyperplasia**    Excessive development of a body part as a result of an abnormal proliferation of cells.

**hyperreflexive**    Reflex response that is more pronounced than normal.

**hypersegmented neutrophil**    A neutrophil that has more than five nuclear lobes when seen in peripheral blood.

**hyperthermia**    An abnormally high body temperature.

**hypertonic**    When the concentration of particles in solution is higher outside the cell. This may cause water to move from the inside to the outside of the cell to attain equilibrium. In this way, the cell shrivels and becomes crenated.

**hypoadrenocorticism**    Deficient secretion of hormones from the cortex of the adrenal gland; also called *Addison's syndrome*.

**hypocalcemia**    Too low a level of calcium in the blood.

**hypoglycemia**    Too low a level of glucose in the blood.

**hypophysis**    Pituitary gland.

**hyporeflexive**    Reflex response is less than normal.

**hypothalamus**    A portion of the diencephalon that has extensive links to the brain and to the pituitary gland. It functions as an important bridge between the nervous and the endocrine systems.

**hypothermia**    An abnormally low body temperature that slows down all metabolic processes. Hypothermia can result from prolonged exposure to cold environmental temperatures, or it may be drug induced, such as with many general anesthetic drugs. Efforts should always be made to keep anesthetized animals and animals recovering from general anesthesia warm.

**hypotonic**    When the concentration of a solution outside the cell is lower than it is on the inside of the cell, water will tend to flow into the cell toward the higher concentration. This causes swelling and possible rupture of the cell.

**hypoxia**    Oxygen deficiency; causes bluish tinge of mucous membranes. There are many causes of hypoxia, ranging from anemia to respiratory blockage.

## I

**I bands**    Large, light bands in a skeletal muscle fiber that alternate with the darker A bands to give a striped appearance to skeletal muscle fibers under a microscope. The I bands are composed of thin filaments of the contractile protein actin.

**iatrogenic**    A condition caused by medical treatment given to an animal.

**icterus**    The yellowish color given to tissues, membranes, and secretions by the presence of bile pigments; may indicate elevated levels of bilirubin, possibly resulting from liver failure; also known as *jaundice*.

**IgA**    Immunoglobulin A; it can leave blood and enter tissue, where it plays an important role in preventing diseases caused by antigens that enter the body through mucosal surfaces.

**IgD**    Immunoglobulin D; its function is unknown.

**IgE**    Immunoglobulin E; it is associated with allergies.

**IgG**    Immunoglobulin G; it is produced during the first exposure to an antigen; it is also made by newborn animals.

**IgM**    Immunoglobulin M; it is produced after an animal has been exposed to an antigen for an extended time or when an animal is exposed to an antigen for the second time.

**ileocecal sphincter**    The circular smooth muscle that regulates the movement of intestinal contents from the ileum to the cecum.

**ileum**    The last of three segments of the small intestine; it empties into the colon or cecum.

**ileus**    Lack of movement of the bowel.

**ilium**    The most cranial of the three pairs of bones that make up the pelvis. It forms the sacroiliac joint with the sacrum.

**immunization**    The process of creating immunity within an animal, usually by introducing a killed or modified culture of the infectious agent to the body to allow it to create antibodies; also called *vaccination*.

**immunoglobulins**    Created by B lymphocytes; also called *antibodies;* these protein-based molecules are produced by exposure to an infectious agent's antigen. In future encounters with the same antigen, the antibodies will identify and fight it.

**immunosuppressed**    Refers to an immune system that cannot elicit a normal immune response.

**impermeable**    Refers to structures that do not allow the passage of fluid.

**implantation**    Embedding of a developing blastocyst in the lining of the uterus.

**implantation angle**    The degree of angulation of a shaft of hair.

**incisive bones**    Skull bones that are part of the external bones of the face. The two incisive bones are the most rostral of the skull bones. In all common domestic animals, except ruminants, the incisive bones house the upper incisor teeth.

**incisors**    The most rostral teeth of the mouth that are narrowed into a sharp ridge at their tip.

**inclusion**    A temporary component of a cell that is lifeless, having been brought into the cell via phagocytosis.

**incus**    One of the three ossicles, the tiny bones that transmit sound wave vibrations across the middle ear. The incus, or anvil, is the middle of the three ossicles.

**indeterminate layer**    Species that can produce more eggs than their normal clutch size.

**infection**    Invasion and replication of microorganisms causing detrimental effects on the body.

**inferior**    A directional term meaning *toward the lower portion* of a human body.

**inflammation**    The first step in the healing process when the body is injured. Its purpose is to "clean up" the damaged area through various inflammatory processes so healing can begin.

**inflammatory process**    The series of cellular and metabolic events that take place primarily in connective tissue as the result of injury or loss of tissue. The inflammatory process acts to isolate and destroy infectious agents, as well as to prepare the tissue for healing.

**infraorbital pouch**    A pouch of cutaneous tissue found rostral to the medial canthus of the eye in sheep and other ungulates; also called the *lacrimal pouch*.

**infundibulum**    The funnel-shaped ovarian end of the oviduct. Cilia lining the infundibulum beat rhythmically to ensure passage of the ovum into the oviduct.

**inguinal pouch**   Also known as the *mammary pouch;* a pouch of cutaneous tissue found within the inguinal area of sheep.

**inguinal rings**   Slitlike openings in the abdominal muscles located in the groin (inguinal) region. The spermatic cords of the male pass through the inguinal rings from the scrotum to the interior of the abdominal cavity.

**inhibitory neurotransmitters**   Chemicals released by neurons at the synapse that tend to depress or decrease depolarization of other neurons or target tissues.

**innate immunity**   Portion of the immune system that is present at birth, and which is nonspecific.

**inner ear**   The most internal portion of the ear. It is contained in the temporal bone and contains both hearing and equilibrium structures.

**innervated**   Having a nerve supply.

**inorganic compound**   A chemical that does not contain hydrocarbon groups.

**insertion of a muscle**   The more movable of the attachment sites of a muscle. When a muscle contracts, it exerts traction on its insertion site, usually producing movement of a bone or other structure.

**inspiration**   The process of drawing air into the lungs; inhalation.

**inspiratory muscle**   A muscle whose action is to increase the size of the thoracic cavity; this causes air to be drawn into the lungs, thereby producing inspiration (inhalation).

**insulin**   A hormone produced by the beta cells of the pancreatic islets. Its main action is to allow glucose to be absorbed into body cells and used for energy; this decreases the level of glucose in the blood.

**integral proteins**   The proteins located within the lipid bilayer that create channels that aid the selective permeability of the cell membrane.

**integument**   The outer covering of the body, consisting of the skin and all of its related components, such as nails, hair, hooves, and horns.

**integumentary system**   The skin and all of its related components, such as nails, hair, hooves, and horns.

**intercalated discs**   End-to-end attachment sites between adjacent cardiac muscle cells. The intercalated discs securely fasten the cells together and also transmit impulses from cell to cell. This allows large groups of cardiac muscle cells to function as a single unit.

**intercostal space**   The space between two ribs.

**interdigital pouch**   A pouch of cutaneous tissue that exudes a waxy substance; found between the toes of sheep and other cloven-hoofed animals.

**interferon**   A substance produced by a cell after a virus has invaded it. Interferon prevents further development or spread of the virus.

**intermediate fibers**   Fibers that are specialized to the cell in which they are contained. They are composed of tough protein fibers that help to reinforce the cell.

**intermediate filaments**   See *tonofilaments.*

**internal respiration**   The exchange of oxygen and carbon dioxide between the blood in the capillaries all over the body and the cells and tissues of the body.

**internal**   An alternative directional term for *deep.* Internal also means toward the center of the body or a body part.

**interneuron**   Typically a short neuron that connects two other neurons; usually mentioned in the context of the reflex arc.

**interparietal bones**   Skull bones that are part of the external bones of the cranium. The two interparietal bones are located on the dorsal midline just rostral to the occipital bone. The interparietal bones are usually distinct in young animals, but in older animals they may fuse into one bone and may even fuse to the parietal bones and become indistinguishable.

**interphase**   The period between cell divisions during which all normal growth and functions occur.

**interpleural space**   The space between the pleural covering of the right lung and the pleural covering of the left lung. The mediastinum.

**interstitial cell**   Endocrine cells located between the seminiferous tubules of the testes. They produce androgens, the male sex hormones.

**interstitial cell-stimulating hormone (ICSH)**   The anterior pituitary hormone that stimulates the interstitial cells of the testes to produce androgens, the male sex hormones; also known as *luteinizing hormone (LH).*

**interstitial fluid**   Tissue fluid; fluid contained within the tissues, except for the fluid found within lymph and blood vessels.

**intervertebral disc**   The cartilaginous disc located between the bodies of adjacent vertebrae. It acts as a shock absorber for the vertebrae.

**intracellular fluid**   The fluid that is contained within cells.

**intramembranous bone formation**   *Membrane* bone formation. The type of bone formation that only occurs in certain skull bones when bone forms in the fibrous tissue membranes that cover the brain in a developing fetus.

**intramuscular injection**   A route of drug administration that involves injecting a drug through a hypodermic needle that has been inserted into the belly of a muscle. The large blood supply of the muscle leads to rapid absorption of the drug into the bloodstream for distribution to the rest of the body.

**intravascular hemolysis**   Destruction of red blood cells within blood vessels.

**intrinsic factor**   A protein produced by the stomach and required for absorption of vitamin B12.

**intromission**   Insertion of the penis into the vagina.

**introns**   Spaces between coded exons of a gene's DNA sequence that do not contain codes.

**involuntary muscle**   An old name for smooth muscle.

**involuntary striated muscle**   An old name for cardiac muscle.

**involution of the mammary gland**   "Drying up" of the mammary gland when the stimuli for lactation cease; the cessation of milk production with shrinkage of the mammary gland back to near its prelactation size.

**involution of the uterus**   Shrinkage of the uterus after parturition back to near its prepregnant size.

**ion**   An electrically charged atom or molecule. Cations are positively charged ions, and anions are negatively charged ions.

**ionic bond**   A type of chemical bond formed by the electrostatic attraction between two oppositely charged atoms or molecules (ions).

**ipsilateral reflex**   The reflex stimulus and response are on the same side of the body.

**iris**   A portion of the uvea, or middle vascular layer, of the eye. The iris is a pigmented, muscular diaphragm that controls the amount of light that enters the posterior part of the eyeball.

**irregular bone**   A bone whose shape does not fit into the long bone, short bone, or flat bone categories. Irregular bones either have characteristics of more than one of the other three shape categories or have a truly irregular shape. Examples include vertebrae, some strangely shaped skull bones (such as the sphenoid bone), and sesamoid bones.

**ischium**   The most caudal of the three pairs of bones that make up the pelvis.

**islets of Langerhans**   Clusters of cells in the pancreas that produce insulin, glucagon, and other endocrine products of the pancreas. Also called the *pancreatic islets.*

**isotonic**   Equal osmotic pressure present on either side of the cell membrane.

**isotope**   One of two or more atoms having the same atomic number (same number of protons) but different atomic masses (different number of neutrons).

**ivermectin**   A commonly used antiparasitic drug that works by interfering with parasites' nervous and muscular system functions, which paralyzes and kills them.

## J

**jaundice**   An abnormal condition characterized by the yellowing of the mucous membranes, skin, and sclerae as a result of excess bilirubin moving from the blood into tissues. This may be caused by liver failure, excessive destruction of red blood cells, or blockage of the bile ducts. Also known as *icterus.*

**jejunum**   The second of the three segments of the small intestine, usually the longest segment.

**joint**   The junction between two bones. Joints can be completely immovable (fibrous joints), slightly movable (cartilaginous joints), or freely movable (synovial joints).

**joint capsule**   The membrane that encloses the ends of the bones in a synovial joint; consists of an outer fibrous membrane and an inner synovial membrane that produces viscous synovial fluid which lubricates the joint surfaces.

**joint cavity**   The fluid-filled potential space between the joint surfaces of a synovial joint; the joint cavity is normally filled by the viscous, lubricating fluid (synovial fluid) produced by the synovial membrane lining of the joint capsule; also known as the *joint space.*

**joint space**   Alternate name for the *joint cavity.*

**junctional complex**   The point at which epithelial cells join to one another in very close proximity.

## K

**keel**   Bony ridge on the sternum of a bird to which the flight muscles attach.

**keratin**   A tough, waterproof protein that makes up scales, the outer sheaths of beaks and claws, and feathers; a major component of the epidermis, nails, hair, horns, and hooves.

**keratin fibers**   The strong strands of the fibrous protein keratin that are insoluble in water.

**keratinization**   The normal formation of keratin (a tough, waterproof protein) inside epithelial cells of the skin. As the epithelial cells mature, they fill with granules containing keratin.

**keratinized stratified squamous epithelium**   The epithelial classification of the epidermis. It is highly regenerative and waterproof, thereby helping the body to retain moisture and thermoregulate.

**keratinocytes**   Cells that synthesize keratin. They have three distinct stages visible in the epidermis: the *basal, prickle,* and *granular* cell stages. As keratinocytes travel progressively away from the basement membrane toward the superficial epithelium, they lose their organelles to make way for more keratin. As a result of this process, the cells die by the time they reach the surface.

**ketone bodies**   Products of lipid metabolism (lipolysis), including beta-hydroxybutyric acid, acetoacetic acid, and acetone. They are usually produced from acetyl CoA from fatty acids within the liver.

**knee**   The carpus of hoofed animals.

**Krebs cycle**   The metabolism of sugars, fatty acids, and amino acids through oxidation to produce carbon dioxide, water, and energy.

**Kupffer cells**   Macrophages present in the liver. Fifty percent of macrophages are Kupffer cells.

## L

**labia**   Literally means *lips.* The external boundary of the vulva of the female.

**labial**   Liplike or pertaining to the lips.

**labial surface**   The surface of the rostral part of the upper and lower arcade of teeth that face the lips.

**lacrimal apparatus**   The tear-producing and draining structures of the eyes.

**lacrimal bones**   Skull bones; external bones of the face. The two small lacrimal bones form part of the medial portion of the orbit of the eye and house the lacrimal sacs, which are part of the tear-drainage system of the eye.

**lacrimal gland**   The main tear-producing gland. It is located dorsal and lateral to the eyeball inside the bony orbit.

**lacrimal puncta**   Openings in the upper and lower eyelid margins located near the medial canthus of each eye. They drain tears away from the surface of the eyes.

**lacrimal sac**   A small sac that receives tears from the lacrimal puncta and sends them down into the nasolacrimal duct.

**lactation**   Milk production by the mammary gland.

**lactic acid**   A waste product of anaerobic metabolism in skeletal muscle; an end product of the metabolism of carbohydrates. It is created by the conversion of pyruvate into lactic acid after the fermentation of cellulose. The buildup of lactic acid in a muscle that has been forced into anaerobic mode by overstrenuous activity can cause discomfort.

**lactic acidosis**   In the ruminant, this is the same as *grain overload* and *rumen acidosis;* a condition in which too much carbohydrate is available to the rumen microbes, resulting in production of large amounts of lactic acid and subsequently causing severe changes in the rumen microflora and systemic acidosis.

**lacunae**   Small cavities within the matrix of some connective tissues, such as cartilage and bone, within which cells (chondrocytes and osteocytes) are contained.

**lamina propria**   The areolar connective tissue located in the mucous membranes.

**laminae**   The interdigitations between the corium and hoof that serve as the attachment sites between the hoof and coffin bone.

**laminitis**   Manifests itself as extreme pain and heat in the equine hoof because of swelling and inflammation of the sensitive laminae. It most often affects equids in their front feet, but in severe cases, it may involve all four feet. There are many causes, such as ingesting large quantities of grains and carbohydrates, drug reactions, retained placenta, and trauma. In severe cases, the coffin bone may penetrate the sole of the hoof; also called *founder.*

**Langerhans cells**   The macrophages of the epidermis that phagocytize invading microorganisms and serve as antigen-presenting cells.

**lanolin**   Fat-based secretion of the sheep's sebaceous glands; a by-product of the wool industry, it is used for lotions and ointments.

**laryngeal hemiplegia**   The medical name for what is commonly called *roaring,* a condition often seen in horses. It is produced by paralysis of the muscles that tighten the arytenoid cartilages and vocal cord on one side, usually the left, of the larynx. The result is that the paralyzed vocal cord partially obstructs the glottis and causes difficulty breathing, particularly when the animal tries to breathe heavily when exercising. Vibrations of the paralyzed vocal cord produce a characteristic roaring sound as the animal breathes.

**laryngoscope**   An instrument used to aid the passage of an endotracheal tube through the glottis and down into the trachea. The laryngoscope consists of a handle that contains batteries and a long, narrow blade with a small light source near the end of it. The blade is used gently to press the tip of the epiglottis ventrally, exposing the opening of the glottis.

**laryngospasm**   A spasmodic closure of the opening of the glottis; often occurs in cats during endotracheal intubation because of the sensitivity of a cat's larynx.

**larynx**   The "voice box"; a short, irregular tube of cartilage and muscle that connects the pharynx with the trachea. Its functions are voice production, preventing foreign material from being inhaled, and controlling airflow to and from the lungs.

**lateral cartilages**   Two large bands of cartilage contained within the equid hoof that, in conjunction with the frog and digital cushion, aid in venous return.

**lateral ventricles**   Blind pouches that project laterally between the vocal cords and the vestibular folds in the larynx of a non-ruminant animal.

**lateral**   A directional term meaning *away from the median plane* (center line) of the body.

**lesser curvature of the stomach**   The smaller, inner curve of the stomach.

**leukemia**   "White blood"; a cancer or malignancy of one type of white blood cells. Production of that type of cell is abnormal and uncontrolled.

**leukocytes**   Also called *white blood cells,* leukocytes come in many different varieties, including basophils, eosinophils, neutrophils, lymphocytes, and monocytes. They may be granulated or non-granulated and are capable of amoeboid motion. The main function of leukocytes is body defense.

**leukocytosis**   An increase in the total number of white blood cells in peripheral blood.

**leukopenia**   A decrease in the total number of white blood cells in peripheral blood; also called *leukocytopenia.*

**leukopoiesis**   A general term for production of white blood cells.

**leukotrienes**   Eicosanoids formed from the activation of white blood cells. They act to sustain inflammation in asthmatic and allergic reactions.

**ligaments**   Bands of fibrous connective tissue that are present in and around many synovial joints. When present, ligaments connect the bones of the joint to each other.

**ligands**   Small molecules that bond to larger chemical groups or molecules.

**ligated**   Surgically tied off, as with blood vessels; usually done with suture material.

**limbus**   The junction of the cornea and sclera of the eye.

**linea alba**   The sheet of fibrous connective tissue (aponeurosis) that connects the abdominal muscles from each side on the ventral midline.

**lingual surface**   The surface of the lower arcade of teeth that faces the tongue; *lingua* is Latin for *tongue.*

**lipase**   Enzyme produced by the pancreas and, in some species, the saliva; breaks apart fats into their components.

**lipid bilayer**   A double-layered membrane made of phospholipids, such as the cell membrane and nuclear envelope.

**lipids**   The group of fatty or fatlike substances that are insoluble in water. Alcohol, ether, chloroform, and other nonpolar substances can, however, dissolve them.

**lipolysis**   The breakdown of fats.

**lipoprotein**   A molecule that contains both a lipid and a protein. They often function as transmembrane proteins to transport molecules across cell membranes or transport proteins for the movement of fat molecules in the blood.

**lissencephalic**   Associated with a malformation of the gyri in the cerebral cortex. In dogs, it is associated with behavioral abnormalities, visual deficits, ataxia, and seizures.

**lobe**   Each cerebral hemisphere is divided by sulci into lobes; different lobes of the cerebral hemispheres specialize in certain functions.

**lobes (of the lung)**   Subdivisions of the lungs. Lung lobes are defined by major branches of bronchi entering them, rather than by grossly visible grooves and clefts.

**local anesthesia**   Loss of sensation from a localized area of the body.

**long bone**   Bones that are longer than they are wide. Most of the limb bones, such as the humerus, femur, and radius, are long bones.

**longitudinal fissure**   Prominent groove that divides the cerebrum into right and left cerebral hemispheres.

**longitudinal muscle**   The muscle in the intestinal tract layer that is responsible for shortening segments of the intestine when it contracts; is involved with peristaltic movement.

**loop of Henle**   The middle part of the tubular portion of a nephron. It has a descending part that travels from the cortex to the medulla and an ascending part that travels back to the cortex. The loop of Henle is located between the proximal convoluted tubule and the distal convoluted tubule.

**loose connective tissue**   A subclass of connective tissue proper, loose connective tissue is a vascularized type of connective tissue whose general function is to support the structures it surrounds. Types of loose connective tissue include areolar, adipose, and reticular connective tissues.

**lower arcade**   In reference to teeth, it means the teeth in the mandible, or the lower set of teeth in the mouth.

**lower respiratory tract**   All of the respiratory structures within the lungs; includes all the respiratory passages from the bronchi down to the alveoli.

**lumbar vertebrae**   The group of vertebrae located dorsal to the abdominal region.

**lumen**   The opening in the middle of the intestinal tract or any hollow organ.

**luteinizing hormone (LH)**   The anterior pituitary hormone that stimulates ovulation in most species and then causes the empty follicle to develop into the corpus luteum.

**luteolysis**   Destruction of the corpus luteum.

**lymph**   Excess tissue fluid that is picked up by lymph vessels and returned to peripheral blood.

**lymphocytes**   Nongranulocytic white blood cells that are involved in the immune response. The two types of lymphocyte are *T lymphocytes,* which are involved with cell-mediated immunity, and *B lymphocytes,* which are involved with humoral immunity.

**lymphocytosis**   An increase in the number of lymphocytes in peripheral blood.

**lymphokines**   Proteins that develop on the surface of helper T lymphocytes. The lymphokines activate killer T lymphocytes, which are responsible for cell-mediated immunity.

**lymphopenia**   A decrease in the number of lymphocytes in peripheral blood.

**lysosome**   An organelle that fights pathogens, repairs damaged tissues, and aids in intracellular digestion by engulfing materials within its membrane-bound vesicle bodies. It contains the digestive enzymes that help destroy microorganisms that have been phagocytized by the neutrophil.

## M

**macrominerals**   Minerals, such as calcium, phosphorus, magnesium, sodium, potassium, chlorine, and sulfur, that are required in larger quantities than other minerals.

**macromolecule**   A large molecule consisting of smaller units linked together, such as a polysaccharide or polypeptide.

**macrophages**   Phagocytic cells that can engulf relatively large cells or bits of debris. They may be fixed in place, or they may travel around in the tissues. Mature macrophages may become more mobile during times of infection and inflammation.

**macroscopic anatomy**   Also called gross anatomy; the study of body parts large enough to be seen without magnification, such as a lung, leg, or brain.

**macula**   A patch of sensory epithelium in the vestibule of the inner ear. It consists of hair cells covered by a gelatinous mass containing otoliths. The macula senses the position of the head.

**male pronucleus**   The name for the nucleus of a spermatozoon after its head has penetrated into the ovum (fertilization of the ovum) but before the nuclei of the ovum (the female pronucleus) and the sperm have come together. When the female and male pronuclei combine, the diploid chromosome number is restored and the genetic makeup of the offspring is determined.

**malleus**   One of the three ossicles, which are the tiny bones that transmit sound wave vibrations across the middle ear. The malleus, or hammer, is the outermost of the three ossicles and is attached to the tympanic membrane.

**mandible**   A skull bone; one of the external bones of the face. The mandible is the lower jaw, the only movable skull bone. The mandible houses all of the lower teeth. It is usually referred to as a single bone, but in dogs, cats, and cattle, the two halves of the mandible are separate bones joined by a cartilaginous mandibular symphysis at the rostral end.

**mandibular symphysis**   The cartilaginous joint (amphiarthrosis) that unites the two sides of the mandible at the rostral (front) end.

**manubrium**   The first, most cranial sternebra. Its full name is *manubrium sterni.*

**marbling**   The common name for fat deposits in the connective tissue layers of meat (skeletal muscle).

**marginal pool of neutrophils**   Neutrophils found lining the walls of small blood vessels, mainly in the spleen, lungs, and abdominal organs. These neutrophils are not circulating but are moving slowly along the walls of the vessels.

**mast cell**   A transient cell of connective tissue containing heparin and histamine used in the inflammatory response. Mast cells recognize foreign invaders and release granules of histamine and heparin to increase blood flow. They resemble basophils, but they do not circulate in blood.

**mastication**   Chewing.

**mastitis**   Infection of a mammary gland.

**matrix**   The intercellular material of connective tissue.

**matter**   Anything that has mass and exists as a solid, liquid, or gas.

**mature follicle**   An ovarian follicle that is fully developed and ready for ovulation; also known as a *vesicular follicle* or a *Graafian follicle.*

**maxilla**   The bone of the upper jaw.

**maxillary bones**   Skull bones; external bones of the face. The two maxillary bones make up most of the upper jaw and house the upper canine teeth, if present, and all of the upper cheek teeth (premolars and molars).

**maxillary sinus**   The paranasal sinus in the maxillary bones.

**mechanical control system**   The respiratory control system that sets inspiration and expiration limits for normal resting breathing; operates on the basis of stretch receptors in the lungs that communicate with the respiratory center in the brainstem.

**mechanical digestion**   The physical breakdown of food into small particles.

**meconium**   Dark, tarry material in the intestine of a newborn animal. The first feces passed by the newborn.

**medial**   A directional term meaning *toward the median plane* (center line) of the body.

**median plane**   An anatomic reference plane. A median plane is a sagittal plane that runs down the center of the body and divides it into equal left and right halves. It is also called a *midsagittal plane.*

**mediastinum**   The area of the thorax between the lungs. It contains the heart and most of the other thoracic structures, such as the trachea, esophagus, blood vessels, nerves, and lymphatic structures.

**medulla**   (1) The inner, deep layer of an organ or structure. (2) The inner part of the kidney. It contains the loop of Henle, peritubular capillaries, and collecting ducts. (3) The innermost layer of a hair strand, made of two or three layers of flexible, soft keratin.

**medulla oblongata**   The part of the brainstem just above (cranial to) the spinal cord.

**megaesophagus**   A condition in which the esophagus loses muscle tone and dilates into a flaccid, saclike structure.

**megakaryocytes**   Large, multinucleated cells in red bone marrow that are the parent cells of platelets. Platelets are formed when chunks of cytoplasm break off a megakaryocyte and enter the circulation.

**meibomian glands**   The tarsal glands of the eyelid margins. They produce a waxy substance that helps prevent tears from overflowing onto an animal's face.

**meiosis**   The *reduction division* that reproductive cells undergo during their development. It results in a reduction of the chromosome number from the normal diploid number to the haploid number (half of the diploid number).

**Meissner's corpuscles**   The oval, tactile nerve endings, both myelinated and unmyelinated, found within the dermal papillae of the epidermis. Sensitive to light touch, they are especially common in body parts with no hair follicles, such as the soles of the feet.

**melanomacrophage**   A histocyte laden with phagocytosed melanin. Also called *melanophages.*

**melanin**   That sulfurous pigment produced by melanocytes, especially when stimulated by sunlight. Melanin is present in the skin, hair, choroid of the eye, and abnormally in melanomas.

**melanocyte**   A cell located within the lower epidermis that processes tyrosinase and melanin. Melanin, contained within melanosomes, is transferred to keratinocytes by way of the melanocyte's long projections.

**melanocyte-stimulating hormone (MSH)**   The anterior pituitary hormone that apparently influences the pigment cells of the skin (the melanocytes). Its precise role in the body of mammals is not well understood.

**melanosomes**   Granules filled with melanin that are transferred from the melanocytes to the keratinocytes.

**melatonin**   A hormonelike substance produced by the pineal body. It apparently affects moods and wake–sleep cycles and may affect the timing of seasonal estrous cycles in some species.

**membrane potential**   The difference in voltage that exists on either side of a cell membrane caused by the different concentrations of positive and negative charges.

**membrane proteins**   Proteins imbedded in the cell's membrane that function as cell receptors and membrane transport molecules.

**membrane receptors**   The integral proteins and glycoproteins that form binding sites; may aid in contact signaling.

**memory cells**   After an initial immune response, lymphocytes that are programmed to remember the antigen that caused the immune response and to produce a more rapid immune response to that antigen the second time the body is exposed to it.

**meninges**   Set of connective tissues that surround the brain and spinal cord; the three layers of the meninges, from outside to innermost layer, are the dura mater, the arachnoid, and the pia mater.

**meniscus**   One of two concave, half moon-shaped, cartilaginous structures on the proximal surface of the tibia that help support the condyles of the femur.

**Merkel's cells**   Thought to aid in tactile sensory function, these cells are located in small numbers within the epidermal–dermal junction.

**Merkel's disc**   The junction formed by Merkel's cells and sensory nerves.

**merocrine gland**   A gland whose secretions contain none of its cells, thus leaving the gland cells intact. Examples include salivary and sweat glands.

**mesobronchi**   In the avian respiratory system, bronchi that have entered the lung and lost their reinforcing cartilaginous rings.

**mesoderm**   The middle layer of fetal body tissues. Located between the outer layer (ectoderm) and the inner layer (endoderm), the mesoderm gives rise to all connective and muscle tissues.

**mesothelium**   A layer of cells that lines the body cavities of the fetus and that covers the serous membranes in adult animals.

**messenger RNA (mRNA)**   One of the main components of protein synthesis; mRNA transfers the specific amino acid sequence of the genetic code of DNA to the cytoplasm, where protein is synthesized.

**metabolic turnover**   The continuous breakdown of old cells and body matter to be replaced with new cells and body matter.

**metabolism**   All of the complex, interrelated chemical processes that make life possible. Its two fundamental components are *anabolism* and *catabolism.*

**metabolites**   Substances that are produced during metabolism.

**metacarpal bones**   Bones of the forelimb that lie between the carpal bones and phalanges.

**metaphase**   The phase of mitosis when the newly formed chromosomes align on a medial plane or "equator" between the two centrioles located at each end of the dividing cell.

**metaphase plate**   During metaphase, the site where chromosomes line up and are evenly distributed.

**metatarsal bones**   The bones of the pelvic limbs located between the tarsus and the phalanges.

**metatarsal pad**   The bottom of a bird's foot; the large rear footpad of animals such as cats and dogs located over the ventral surface of the junction between the metatarsal bones and the proximal end of the phalanges.

**metestrus**   The stage of the estrous cycle after ovulation, when the corpus luteum develops. It occurs between estrus and diestrus.

**micelle**   A very small droplet of fat surrounded by hydrophilic (water-loving) molecules that allow it to move readily in the liquid environment of the small intestine.

**microbe**   A microscopic organism that may or may not cause disease.

**microfilament**   Closely associated with microtubules, these submicroscopic structures are found in most cells and are composed mostly of actin.

**microglial cells**   Macrophages located in brain tissue.

**microminerals**   A group of minerals called the *trace elements,* such as copper, iron, boron, molybdenum, and cobalt, which are required by the body in minute amounts.

**microscopic anatomy**   The study of anatomic parts too small to be seen with the unaided eye, such as cells and tissues.

**microtome**   A cutting instrument used to make extremely thin slices of tissue for microscopic study.

**microtrabeculae**   A component of the cytoskeleton thought to add form, support, and substance to the cell's inner anatomy.

**microtubules** Tiny, hollow, tubelike structures that aid certain cells with rigidity and transportation. They also form the spindle fibers in the process of mitosis.

**microvilli** Fingerlike protrusions of the luminal surfaces of some epithelial cell membranes that increase a cell's exposed surface area.

**micturition** The process of expelling urine from the body; also called *urination* or *uresis*.

**midbrain** The mesencephalon.

**middle ear** The middle portion of the ear; an air-filled cavity in the temporal bone of the skull. It contains the ossicles and the opening of the Eustachian tube. The middle ear amplifies and transmits sound wave vibrations from the tympanic membrane to the cochlea of the inner ear.

**milk fever** A disease seen in lactating cattle that results from hypocalcemia. The signs of milk fever include muscle weakness and an inability to stand.

**milk let-down** The immediate effect of nursing or milking. The movement of milk from the alveoli and small ducts down into the larger ducts and sinuses, where it is accessible for nursing or milking. It results from the release of oxytocin from the posterior pituitary gland. The oxytocin causes myoepithelial cells surrounding the alveoli and small ducts of the mammary gland to contract, squeezing the milk into the lower parts of the gland.

**mineralocorticoid hormones** A group of hormones secreted by the cortex of the adrenal glands that regulate the levels of some important electrolytes in the body. The principal mineralocorticoid hormone is aldosterone.

**minute volume** The volume of air that an animal breathes in and out during 1 minute. It is calculated by multiplying the animal's tidal volume by its respiratory rate, which is the number of breaths taken per minute.

**mitochondria** Intracellular organelles, which are the primary sources of ATP formation for aerobic cell respiration. Contain DNA and RNA, making the mitochondria capable of their own protein synthesis and replication.

**mitochondrial matrix** The enzyme-rich liquid in the mitochondria that surrounds the cristae and provides them with the enzymes necessary for the proper function of the Krebs cycle.

**mitosis** Cell division of somatic cells for growth and to replace old or dead cells; the type of cell division that occurs in all body cells except the reproductive cells. When cells divide by mitosis, the chromosomes first duplicate themselves and then pull apart into two daughter cells. This preserves the diploid chromosome number.

**mitotic phase** The period during which cell division occurs. It is divided into the main phases of interphase, metaphase, anaphase, and telophase.

**mitral valve** Also called the *left atrioventricular valve;* separates the left atrium and ventricle and protects the pulmonary venous system from the high pressures in the left ventricle during systole.

**mixed exocrine glands** Exocrine glands, such as salivary glands, that can produce both mucous and serous secretions.

**mixed nerve** A nerve made up of both sensory nerve fibers and motor nerve fibers.

**mixture** A mixture is a combination of two or more substances. There are three types of mixture: solutions, colloids, and suspensions.

**modulation** Regulating or changing something. In the process of nociception, dorsal horn neurons in the spinal cord can modulate pain impulses before they reach the brain. This can take the form of amplification or suppression of the pain impulses. See *wind-up.*

**molars** The grinding teeth located at the back of the mouth.

**molecule** The smallest particle of a substance, composed of two or more atoms, that retains the properties of the substance.

**molting** Process of feather or hair replacement; occurs one to several times a year, depending on the species.

**monoamine hormones** Hormones derived from amino acids such as tyrosine and tryptophan. Their name comes from the fact that they retain one amino group.

**monocyte** A large, phagocytic white blood cell. It is the largest white blood cell normally found in peripheral blood; it is an agranulocyte.

**monocytopenia** A decrease in the number of monocytes in peripheral blood.

**monocytosis** An increase in the number of monocytes in peripheral blood.

**monoestrous** An animal that has only one estrous cycle each year.

**monogastric** Having one stomach; usually refers to nonruminant animals that do not rely on gastric fermentative processes to any great extent.

**monoglyceride** A product of triglyceride breakdown; made from one fatty acid plus a glycerol molecule.

**mononuclear phagocyte system** A collective term for monocytes and tissue macrophages found throughout the body.

**monosaccharides** Simple sugars; single sugar molecules, including glucose, galactose, and fructose.

**morphologic** The unique structures and forms of each individual organ, tissue, cell, or the organism as a whole.

**morula** The solid mass of cells into which the zygote has developed a few days after fertilization of the ovum. It resembles a tiny raspberry.

**motor nerve** Nerve that carries efferent impulses to muscles, although motor function may be used to describe any nerve that carries an efferent impulse, including those that supply endocrine glands and tissues that are not muscle.

**motor neuron** A neuron carrying impulses from the CNS to a peripheral effector organ such as a muscle or gland.

**motor unit** One nerve fiber and all the skeletal muscle fibers it innervates. Motor units with small numbers of muscle fibers per nerve fiber are capable of fine, delicate movements. Motor units with large numbers of muscle fibers per nerve fiber are capable of large, powerful movements.

**mRNA** See *messenger RNA.*

**mucin** The main constituent of mucus, produced by goblet cells in the respiratory and intestinal tracts. It is composed of proteoglycans.

**mucosa** The inner layer of the intestinal tract; this layer usually contains glands that secrete into the lumen of the gastrointestinal tract.

**mucous** An adjective to describe something pertaining to mucus or structures that either secrete or are covered by mucus.

**mucous cells** Cells in the lining of the stomach that produce mucus, which helps prevent autodigestion of the stomach.

**mucous membrane** The mucus-producing layer of stratified squamous or columnar epithelium found over the lamina propria. It is present in organs that have contact with the outside of the body. Mucus production in mucous membranes is commonly found in the digestive, respiratory, and reproductive tracts, with the exception only of the urinary tract. The mucus secreted in them helps to fight infection because it is loaded with antibodies. Mucus also helps to absorb nutrients and lubricate surfaces.

**mucous secretions** Viscous secretions composed mostly of glycoproteins.

**mucus** Complex, gel-like substance that is secreted by goblet cells or other mucous glands; acts as a lubricant and protective barrier.

**multicameral lung** A multichambered lung.

**multicellular** Composed of many cells.

**multinucleated** Having more than one nucleus.

**multiparous** An animal that normally gives birth to more than one offspring at parturition.

**multiunit smooth muscle** The type of smooth muscle composed of individual smooth muscle cells or small groups of cells. Found where small, delicate involuntary contractions are needed. Multiunit smooth muscle requires nerve impulses to stimulate its contractions.

**muscarinic receptor** A type of cholinergic receptor that binds with acetylcholine.

**muscle spindle** A sensory organ located within muscle that detects stretch of the muscle.

**muscle tissue** A collection of tissues that support the body and enable it to move, thermoregulate, and transport materials. Some muscles may be controlled voluntarily, whereas others act involuntarily. Examples of involuntary muscle include cardiac and smooth muscle; voluntary muscle includes all of the skeletal muscles.

**mutagen** An agent that can create a transmissible genetic change in an organism's DNA.

**mutation** A sudden and irreversible genetic change that causes a difference between offspring and their parents.

**mute** Organized waste product of birds that is ejected from the cloaca by the muscular anus; normally consists of a dark fecal center surrounded by a ring of white urates.

**myelin** Fatty substance that covers some axons. When fixed for microscopic examination, it appears white, hence myelinated neurons make up the "white matter" of the brain and spinal cord.

**myelin sheath** Cell membrane of glial cells (e.g., oligodendrocytes, Schwann cells) wrapped around an axon; increases speed of impulse conduction along the axon.

**myelography** The radiographic (x-ray) procedure of injecting contrast media into the subarachnoid space to visualize better the outline of the spinal cord.

**myocardium** The middle layer of the heart and the main muscle layer responsible for contraction during systole.

**myoepithelial cells** Cells in the mammary glands that have characteristics of both muscle cells and epithelial cells. They surround the alveoli and small ducts of the glands. When stimulated by the hormone oxytocin, they contract, squeezing milk down into the large ducts and sinuses; see *milk let-down*.

**myofibrils** Microscopic, fiberlike structures that occupy most of the cytoplasm (sarcoplasm) in skeletal muscle cells. Myofibrils are composed of filaments of the contractile proteins actin and myosin and are packed together longitudinally in the muscle cells.

**myoglobin** A protein in muscle cells that has properties similar to hemoglobin. It can store and release large quantities of oxygen to fuel aerobic metabolic processes in the muscle cells.

**myometrium** The muscle layer of the uterus.

**myosin filaments** One of the two contractile proteins of muscle (actin is the other one) that slide over each other to produce the shortening of the muscle cell that we refer to as *muscle contraction*.

**myosin** A protein present in muscle fibers that aids in contraction and makes up the majority of muscle protein.

**myosphitis** Inflammation of a voluntary muscle that causes pain and stiffness.

## N

**NAD+** See *nicotinamide adenine dinucleotide.*

**NADH** See *nicotinamide adenine dinucleotide.*

**nape** Back of the neck.

**nares** The nostrils.

**nasal bones** Skull bones that are part of the external bones of the face. The nasal bones form the bridge of the nose, or the dorsal part of the nasal cavity.

**nasal conchae** Skull bones that are part of the internal bones of the face; also known as the *turbinates*. The nasal conchae are four thin, scroll-like bones that fill most of the space in the nasal cavity. The turbinates are covered by the moist, vascular lining of the nasal passages. Their scroll-like shape helps the nasal lining warm and humidify the inhaled air and trap tiny particles of inhaled foreign material.

**nasal meatus** Any of the main passageways in the nasal cavity. The nasal cavity is subdivided by the dorsal and ventral nasal turbinates into three main passageways: the *dorsal, middle,* and *ventral* nasal meatuses. A small fourth passageway, the *common nasal meatus,* is continuous with the three main passageways.

**nasal passages** The convoluted air passageways in the nose that conduct air between the nostrils and the pharynx.

**nasal septum** The midline barrier that separates the left and right nasal passages.

**nasolacrimal duct** The tube that carries tears from the lacrimal sac to the nasal cavity.

**natural killer (NK) lymphocytes** Lymphocytes that are neither T lymphocytes nor B lymphocytes but have the ability to kill some types of tumor cell and cells infected with various viruses.

**navicular bone** The distal sesamoid bone of the horse. The navicular bone is located deep in the hoof behind the joint between the middle and distal phalanges.

**neck** The area of a bone that joins the head with the main portion of the bone.

**necrotic** Refers to the death of a particular portion of tissue.

**negative (nitrogen) balance** When the rate of protein loss in feces and urine exceeds the amount of protein ingested.

**neonatal period** The first few weeks and months after birth.

**nephron** The basic functional unit of the kidney. It is composed of the renal corpuscle and the tubule system, which is made up of the proximal convoluted tubule, loop of Henle, and distal convoluted tubule.

**nephrosis** An abnormal condition of the kidney involving degenerative changes, particularly in the renal tubules; may be associated with protein loss in the urine, which leads to a systemic hypoproteinemia.

**nerve** A bundle of myelinated nerve fibers in the peripheral nervous system that conduct sensory and/or motor impulses to and from the central nervous system and the periphery of the body.

**nerve fiber** An axon.

**nerve impulse** A wave of cell membrane depolarization that travels from the point of stimulus down the length of a nerve cell process.

**nervous tissue** A collection of tissues that collect, process, and convey information. Nervous tissue includes the brain, spinal cord, and nerves. Sensory (afferent) nerves convey information about the body's surroundings to the brain, whereas motor (efferent) nerves send instructions from the brain to the body. Some nervous tissues, called *mixed nerves,* can perform both functions.

**neural tunic** Inner layer of the eye, consisting of the retina.

**neuroglia** Auxiliary cells in the nervous system that support and protect the neurons. Examples include oligodendrocytes, microglia, and astrocytes.

**neurology** The study of the nervous system.

**neuromuscular junction** The "connection" between the end bulb of a motor nerve fiber and a skeletal muscle cell. There is actually a tiny space, called *the synaptic space,* between the end of the nerve fiber and the sarcolemma of the muscle fiber.

**neurons** Cells of the nervous system that are structurally composed of a cell body (perikaryon), dendrites, and an axon. They not only initiate nerve impulses but also conduct them.

**neurotransmitter** A chemical released by the presynaptic neuron that diffuses across the synaptic cleft, binds with the receptor on the postsynaptic membrane, and stimulates (excitatory neurotransmitter) or inhibits (inhibitory neurotransmitter) the postsynaptic neuron. Neurotransmitters also stimulate effector cells such as muscle or gland cells.

**neutral fats** A lipid composed of three fatty acids and a glycerol. Also known as *triglycerides.*

**neutralize** To cause the pH of a solution to approach 7 (neutral).

**neutron** A subatomic particle with no electrical charge that joins with the protons to make up the entire mass of the nucleus.

**neutropenia** A decrease in the number of neutrophils in peripheral blood.

**neutrophil** A granulocytic white blood cell. Neutrophils are phagocytes and are known as the first line of defense against invading microorganisms because of their fast response time.

**neutrophilia** An increase in the number of neutrophils in peripheral blood.

**nicotinamide adenine dinucleotide (NAD⁺ or NADH)** The coenzyme used in many oxidation–reduction functions. When oxidized, it is written as *NAD⁺.* In its reduced form, having given up an electron, it is written as *NADH.*

**nicotinic receptor** A type of cholinergic receptor that binds with acetylcholine.

**nictitating membrane** Thin, translucent third eyelid that moves across the eye from the medial canthus laterally to moisten and protect the eye. A T-shaped plate of cartilage covered by conjunctiva. It has lymph nodules and a gland that contributes to the tear film on its ocular surface. No muscles attach to the third eyelid. Its movements are entirely passive.

**nitrogen balance** When the rate of protein synthesis equals the rate of protein breakdown in the healthy animal. In other words, the amount of nitrogen ingested in the form of protein equals the amount excreted in urine and feces.

**nociception** Pain perception.

**nociceptors** Pain receptors.

**nodes of Ranvier** Myelin gaps in the covering of the axon between adjacent Schwann cells that are involved in rapid conduction of nerve impulses along the axon.

**nonessential amino acid** An amino acid that is produced in the body in sufficient amounts; it does not have to be supplemented by diet. Different species produce different nonessential amino acids; therefore, what may be nonessential in one species may be essential in another.

**nonspecific immunity** Protects an animal against anything the body recognizes as foreign. It involves inflammation, phagocytosis, and the protective barrier of the skin and mucous membranes, which prevent antigens from entering the body. The immune system is not activated during nonspecific immunity.

**nonsteroidal anti-inflammatory drug** A drug that relieves pain (analgesia) and reduces inflammation but that is not related to the glucocorticoid hormones from the adrenal cortex. Glucocorticoid-like drugs are commonly referred to clinically as *corticosteroids.* Carprofen and meloxicam are examples of nonsteroidal anti-inflammatory drugs used in veterinary medicine.

**nonstriated involuntary muscle** An old name for *smooth* muscle.

**norepinephrine** A hormone secreted by the medulla of the adrenal gland under stimulation by the sympathetic portion of the autonomic nervous system. It produces part of the fight-or-flight response that results when an animal feels threatened.

**nuclear envelope** A double-layered membrane made of lipids that surrounds the nucleus and separates the inner nucleoplasm from the outer cytoplasm; also called *nuclear membrane.*

**nuclear membrane** See *nuclear envelope.*

**nuclear pores** Pores that traverse both layers of the nuclear envelope, allowing the inflow of protein molecules and the outflow of RNA molecules.

**nuclei** Clusters of neuron cell bodies within the CNS.

**nucleic acids** The class of substances that include RNA and DNA, located within the cells of all living things. They are extremely dense and are composed of complex patterns of pentose sugars, phosphoric acids, and the nitrogen bases (purines and pyrimidines).

**nucleolus (plural, nucleoli)** The dark, spherical object contained within the nucleus that is the site of ribosomal RNA synthesis. Nucleoli are composed of DNA, RNA, and protein. Each cell's nucleus may have more than one nucleolus.

**nucleoplasm** The gelatinous substance that is the protoplasm of the nucleus.

**nucleotides** The combinations of phosphoric acid, pentose sugars, and pyrimidine or purine bases that make up nucleic acids.

**nucleus**   The part of the cell that contains DNA and aids in several body functions, including reproduction, metabolism, and growth.

**nuptial pads**   Dark, rough calluses on the undersides of the fore-limbs of male frogs that give males a better grip on the female during amplexus (external fertilization of eggs by the male).

**nutrient foramen**   A large channel through the cortex of a large bone through which large blood vessels pass carrying blood to and from the bone marrow.

## O

**obturator foramina**   A pair of large holes in the pelvis located on either side of the pelvic symphysis. The role of the obturator foramina seems to be to lighten the pelvis because no large nerves or vessels pass through them.

**occipital bone**   A skull bone that is one of the external bones of the cranium. The occipital bone is the caudal-most bone of the skull. It forms the atlantooccipital joint with the first cervical vertebra via the occipital condyles. The large foramen magnum in the occipital bone is where the spinal cord exits the skull.

**occipital condyle**   One of two articular surfaces on the occipital bone. The occipital condyles are located on either side of the foramen magnum and form the atlantooccipital joint with the first cervical vertebra (the atlas).

**occlusal surface**   The surface of the tooth that meets the surface of another tooth in the opposite arcade (e.g., the surfaces between the upper and lower premolars).

**olecranon process**   The large process on the proximal end of the ulna that forms the point of the elbow. The olecranon process is the site where the tendon of the powerful triceps brachii muscle attaches.

**olfactory sense**   The sense of smell. The receptors for smell are located in the nasal passages.

**oligodendrocytes**   Glial cells in the brain and spinal cord whose cellular membrane forms the myelin sheath for axons in the CNS.

**oligopeptides**   Chains of 2-20 amino acids; also called *polypeptides*.

**oliguria**   Passing small amounts of urine.

**omasum**   A chamber of the ruminant forestomach that absorbs nutrients and water.

**omentum**   The supportive mesenteries which arise from the greater and lesser curvatures of the stomach.

**omnivore**   An animal whose diet is a mixture of plants and meat.

**oncogene**   A gene, often carried by tumor viruses, that causes malignancy in cells.

**oncotic pressure**   The difference between the osmotic pressure of blood and the osmotic pressure of interstitial fluid or lymph.

**oocyte**   The immature form of the female reproductive cell.

**oogenesis**   The production of female reproductive cells (ova) in ovarian follicles.

**operculum**   Fleshy flap of skin at the external ear openings of some species that aids in funneling sound into the ear; flap of skin covering the ear of many owl species.

**opisthoglyphous**   Referring to snakes with grooved rear fangs for venom delivery.

**opsonin**   Plasma protein, usually an immunoglobulin, that coats an antigen, usually a microorganism, making it more attractive to phagocytes.

**opsonization**   The process by which opsonins coat an antigen to make it more susceptible to phagocytosis.

**optic disc**   The area of the retina where nerve fibers on its surface converge to form the beginning of the optic nerve. It contains no photoreceptors and is the blind spot of the eye.

**orchiectomy**   A surgical procedure by which the testes are removed from a male animal; castration.

**organ of Corti**   The receptor organ of hearing located in the cochlea. It consists of hair cells with a gelatinous structure (the tectorial membrane) resting on the hairs surrounded by fluid. Vibrations of the fluid cause distortion of the hairs, which generates nerve impulses that are interpreted by the brain as sound.

**organ**   A group of tissues that work together for common purposes.

**organelles**   Specialized structures within a cell that carry out specific functions for that cell. Examples of organelles include mitochondria, Golgi apparatus, lysosomes, and ribosomes.

**organic compounds**   A compound containing hydrocarbon groups.

**organism**   A living individual, animal, or plant, unicellular or multicellular, that is capable of independent existence.

**origin of a muscle**   The more stable of the attachment sites of a muscle. When a muscle contracts, its origin attachment sites do not move much. This provides stability so that the insertion of the muscle can move bones or other structures.

**oropharynx**   The portion of the pharynx caudal to the mouth through which food and air both pass.

**os cordis**   The visceral bone in the heart of cattle that helps support the valves of the heart.

**os penis**   The visceral bone in the penis of dogs that partially surrounds the penile portion of the urethra.

**os rostri**   The visceral bone in the snout of swine that strengthens it for the rooting behavior of pigs.

**osmoregulators**   Proteins that regulate and adjust the osmotic pressure between the cell and extracellular fluids. Examples include albumin and enzymes.

**osmosis**   The passive movement of water through a semipermeable membrane into a solution where the water concentration is lower.

**osmotic diuresis**   Diuresis produced by excess dissolved substances in the fluid circulating through the tubules of the nephrons. The excess glucose in the tubular fluid of animals with diabetes mellitus produces an osmotic diuresis that results in polyuria.

**osmotic pressure**   The force of fluid moving from one side of a semipermeable membrane to the other side because of differences in solute (dissolved substance) concentrations on the two sides of the membrane. Under osmotic pressure, fluid moves from the side of the membrane with lower solute concentration to the side with higher solute concentration in an attempt to equalize the concentrations on both sides of the membrane.

**ossicles**   Skull bones that are the bones of the ear. The ossicles are six tiny bones, three on each side, in the middle ear that transmit sound wave vibrations from the tympanic membrane to the inner ear. From the outside in, they are the malleus, the incus, and the stapes.

**ossification**   The mineralization or hardening of bone.

**osteoarthritis**   Inflammation of a joint characterized by progressive deterioration of the articular cartilage.

**osteoblasts** The cells that produce bone.

**osteoclasts** Large, multinuclear cells of the bone that absorb bone and reshape and remodel damaged bones.

**osteocyte** Mature bone cell. The osteocytes are located in spaces in the ossified matrix called *lacunae.*

**osteomyelitis** A inflammatory bacterial infection of bone, often resulting in local bone death.

**otoliths** The literal meaning of otolith is *ear stone.* Otoliths are tiny crystals of calcium carbonate that lie in the gelatinous matrix that covers the hair cells of the macula (the sensory epithelium of the vestibule). The otoliths help the macula keep track of the position of the head.

**oval window** The membrane-covered opening into the cochlea that the stapes lies against. Vibrations of the oval window membrane set the fluid in the cochlea in motion; this stimulates the sensory structures in the organ of Corti and produces the nerve impulses that are interpreted by the brain as sound.

**ovarian follicle** The fluid-filled structure in the ovary in which immature oocytes develop into mature ova. The lining cells of the follicle, the granulosa cells, produce estrogen hormones.

**ovaries** The female gonads; they produce the female reproductive cell, the ovum, as well as estrogen and progestin hormones; homologous to the testes of the male.

**oviduct** Also called the *Fallopian tubes* or *uterine tubes;* the oviduct, by way of ciliary movement, transports ova from the ovary via the infundibulum to the uterus; the site of fertilization in many species; tubular extension of the uterine horn.

**oviparous** Producing eggs in which the embryo develops outside the female's body, as in birds.

**oviposition** The act of laying eggs.

**ovulation** The traumatic rupture of a mature ovarian follicle that releases the ovum.

**ovum (plural, ova)** The mature female reproductive cell. The ovum is released from the mature follicle into the oviduct for fertilization by spermatozoa. The female gamete.

**oxidation** When a substance is combined with oxygen, or when an atom loses electrons and thereby becomes more positively charged.

**oxidative phosphorylation** A process that allows free energy within the mitochondria to be used in the form of ATP.

**oxyhemoglobin** Hemoglobin that is carrying oxygen attached to iron molecules.

**oxyntic cells** Slightly older term for *parietal cells;* gastric gland cells that produce hydrochloric acid.

**oxytocin** One of the posterior pituitary hormones. It is produced in the hypothalamus and then stored and released from the posterior pituitary gland. It stimulates contraction of the myometrium of the uterus at breeding and parturition and contraction of the myoepithelial cells of the lactating mammary gland.

## P

**Pacinian corpuscle** Tactile nerve endings located within the subcutaneous tissue of the skin. These nerves can sense deep and heavy pressure, as well as stretch.

**packed cell volume (PCV)** The percentage of red blood cells in a blood sample; also known as the *hematocrit.*

**pain** An unpleasant sensory response caused by the stimulation of pain receptors in the body.

**palatal surface** The surface of the upper arcade of teeth that faces the inside of the mouth; *palatal* means the teeth are facing the hard or soft palate.

**palatine bones** Skull bones that are part of the internal bones of the face. The two palatine bones make up the caudal portion of the hard palate.

**palmar** The caudal surface of the forelimb from the carpus distally.

**palpate** To examine parts of the body by touching and feeling them.

**palpebral conjunctiva** The transparent membrane that lines the inner portion of the eyelid.

**palpebral reflex** Reflex closure of the eyelids when the medial canthus of the eyelids is touched; used in anesthesia monitoring to assess depth of anesthesia.

**pampiniform plexus** The network of veins in the spermatic cord of the male. It is derived from the testicular vein and surrounds the testicular artery. It functions as a heat-exchange mechanism that helps keep the testes slightly cooler than the rest of the body without cooling the body as a whole. Warm blood coming down the testicular artery is cooled by the blood in the pampiniform plexus; at the same time, the blood in the plexus, which is returning to the systemic blood supply, is warmed by the blood in the artery.

**pancreas** Endocrine and exocrine gland that produces and secretes digestive enzymes into the intestine and produces hormones, including insulin and glucagon.

**pancreatic islets** The endocrine portion of the pancreas; composed of thousands of microscopic clumps of cells scattered throughout the organ; also called the *islets of Langerhans.*

**papilla** (1) A nipplelike protuberance. (2) In birds, depressions in the feather tracts that give rise to new feathers.

**papillary layer** Layer of loose connective tissue that is intimately adjoined to the epidermis.

**papillary muscles** Muscular, nipplelike projections in the heart that anchor the chordae tendineae. When contracted, papillary muscles act to open the atrioventricular heart valves.

**parabronchi** Subdivisions of the secondary bronchi in birds; connected to air capillaries with which gas exchange occurs.

**paraffin** A fine, purified hydrocarbon wax that is used to preserve tissue samples and support them so that they can be sliced into thin sections for microscopic examination.

**paralyzed** Referring to the condition of temporary or permanent loss of muscle power or sensation.

**paramecium** A single-celled, ciliated protozoan.

**paranasal sinus** A space within a skull bone that is an outpouching of the nasal cavity. Depending on the species, paranasal sinuses are found within the frontal bones, maxillary bones, sphenoid bones, and ethmoid bones; commonly referred to by the term sinus.

**parasympathetic nervous system** Part of the autonomic nervous system that is responsible for the "rest-and-restore response"; also called the *craniosacral system* because of the location of the parasympathetic nerves emerging from the brainstem and sacral vertebral segments.

**parathyroid glands** Endocrine glands consisting of several small nodules located in, on, or near the thyroid gland. They produce parathyroid hormone.

**parathyroid hormone (PTH)** The hormone secreted by the parathyroid gland that prevents the level of calcium in the blood from getting too low; also called *parathormone*.

**paresis** Partial or incomplete paralysis.

**paretic** Referring to a part of the body that suffers from paresis.

**parietal** Pertaining to the wall of an organ or cavity.

**parietal bones** Skull bones that are among the external bones of the cranium. The two parietal bones form the dorsolateral walls of the cranium. They are large and well developed in the dog and cat but relatively small in horses and cattle.

**parietal cells** Cells in the gastric glands that secrete hydrogen and chloride ions to form the hydrochloric acid in the stomach.

**parietal eye** Part of the epithalamus; usually associated with the pineal gland; may be photoreceptive in some species and is associated with the endocrine system. Found in lizards and snakes. Also referred to the *parietal organ* or *third eye*.

**parietal layer** The layer of pleura or peritoneum that lines the thorax or abdomen, respectively.

**parietal vaginal tunic** The thick outer connective tissue layer around the testis and spermatic cord. Derived from parietal peritoneum. Also called the *common vaginal tunic*.

**partial pressure** In a mixture of gases, the partial pressure is the portion of the overall pressure each gas exerts. It can be calculated for a particular gas by multiplying the total pressure of the gas mixture by the percentage content of that particular gas.

**parturition** The birth process.

**parvovirus** A virus of the family Parvoviridae that is highly contagious and often deadly.

**passive immunity** The transmission of intact, preformed antibodies from one animal to another. The antibody molecules can help protect the recipient animal from disease-causing agents. An important source of passive immunity is colostrum, the first secretion of the mammary gland after parturition. If it is drunk by the newborn within the first few hours after birth, the antibody molecules will be absorbed into the bloodstream intact and help protect the newborn; however, after that time, the antibody molecules will be broken down by digestion and not absorbed intact.

**pastern** Area of the proximal phalanx of hoofed animals.

**patagial ligament** Ligament that runs along the leading edge of the patagium of birds, allowing extension and flexion of the wing.

**patagium** Lightly vascularized web of skin in birds extending from the shoulder to the wrist; provides elasticity to the wing during flight.

**patella** The kneecap; the largest sesamoid bone in the body. The patella is located on the front surface of the stifle joint in the tendon of the large quadriceps femoris muscle. It rides in the trochlea of the femur.

**patellar ligament** The name given to the quadriceps femoris tendon distal to the patella. It helps provide stability to the stifle joint.

**patent ductus arteriosus** Persistent fetal connection between the aorta and the pulmonary artery that can result in congestive heart failure if not corrected.

**pathogen** A microorganism that can cause a disease.

**pathogenicity** Disease-causing potential of a microorganism. Virulence.

**paucicamerial lung** A lung with four chambers.

**PCT** See *proximal convoluted tubule*.

**PCV** See *packed cell volume*.

**pecten** (1) Dark, ribbonlike structure attached to the retina and extending into the vitreous humor in the eye of birds; thought to provide nourishment to the eye.

**pectin** Sugar polymer commonly found in fruits.

**pectoral crest** Thin, widened area on the proximal humerus where the wing muscles of a bird attach. Also called the *deltoid crest*.

**pectoralis** Large flight muscle originating from the keel and inserting on the humerus of birds; contraction results in the downstroke.

**pellet** Tight bundle of indigestible food components (small bones, fur, feathers) that is eliminated by regurgitation by some species of birds.

**pelvic flexure** Where the left ventral colon of the horse bends back on itself to begin the left dorsal colon.

**pelvic limb** The hindlimb.

**pelvic symphysis** The cartilaginous joint (amphiarthrosis) that unites the two halves of the pelvis ventrally; the pubic symphysis.

**pelvis** The most proximal bony structure of the pelvic limb. Also known as the *os coxae*. The pelvis attaches to the sacrum dorsally at the sacroiliac joints and forms the hip joints with the heads of the femurs.

**penis** The male copulatory organ; homologous to the clitoris of the female.

**pentose sugar** A simple sugar that has five carbon atoms per molecule. An important component of riboflavin and ribonucleic acid (RNA).

**pepsin** A protease activated from pepsinogen in the stomach.

**pepsinogen** The enzyme precursor secreted by the chief cells in the stomach; pepsinogen is activated to pepsin.

**peptidase** Enzyme that breaks peptides into amino acids, dipeptides, and tripeptides.

**peptide** A molecule containing two or more amino acids joined together. Peptides combine to form proteins.

**peptide bond** Covalent joining of one amino acid to another to form a peptide.

**peptide hormone** Hormone consisting of chains of amino acids.

**perception** The conscious recognition of something; for example, in the process of nociception, pain nerve impulses are perceived in the brain.

**pericardial fluid** The transudate fluid secreted into the pericardial sac around the heart. It helps to lubricate the surface of the heart as it beats.

**pericardium** Tissue that forms a sac around the heart to protect it and to control the movement of the heart within the thorax.

**perichondrium** The fibrous connective tissue surrounding the external surface of cartilage. The perichondrium is vascularized and provides a limited amount of nutrition to the cartilage.

**periderm** Epidermal covering of a new feather as it emerges from the skin.

**perikaryon** The cell body of the neuron; soma.

**perilymph** The fluid that surrounds the membranous portion of the inner ear, where the sensory receptors of the inner ear are found.

**perimysium**    The fibrous connective tissue layer in skeletal muscle that surrounds groups of muscle fibers and binds them into groups called fascicles.

**perinuclear cisterna**    The space between the internal and external layers of the nuclear envelope.

**periosteum**    The fibrous membrane that covers the outsides of bones except for their articular (joint) surfaces.

**peripheral blood**    Blood outside bone marrow that is flowing around the body in blood vessels.

**peripheral nervous system (PNS)**    Nerves outside the central nervous system (i.e., outside the brain and spinal cord).

**peripheral proteins**    Proteins located on the inside of the cell's lipid bilayer that have enzymatic capabilities. These proteins are less mobile than integral proteins because they are attached directly to the cytoskeleton.

**peristalsis**    A rhythmic, wavelike motion that progressively moves through a tubular organ, such as the small intestine. Peristalsis assists in the movement of food through the alimentary canal. It is an involuntary movement that is stimulated when the tube is distended.

**peritoneal fluid**    A fluid secreted by the peritoneum in the abdomen. It lubricates the internal organs as they move over one another.

**peritoneum**    The thin membrane in the abdominal cavity that covers the abdominal organs (the visceral layer of peritoneum) and lines the abdominal cavity (the parietal layer of peritoneum). A potential space between the two layers contains a small amount of lubricating fluid that allows abdominal structures to slide smoothly over each other.

**peritonitis**    Inflammation of the peritoneum.

**peritubular capillaries**    Capillaries that branch off from the efferent glomerular arterioles. They flow through the kidney closely associated with the tubules of the nephron and eventually converge and leave the kidney as the renal vein. Tubular secretion and reabsorption are associated with the peritubular capillaries.

**peroxidase**    A catalyst (enzyme) that converts free radicals into hydrogen peroxide, a function that is essential for cellular respiration.

**peroxisome**    Found in high numbers in the kidney and liver cells of most vertebrate animals, this single-membraned vesicle detoxifies the body by releasing catalase and other enzymes.

**petechiae**    Small hemorrhages found on the skin, mucous membranes, and serosal surfaces anywhere in the body.

**pH**    A chemical concept defined as the negative logarithm of the hydrogen ion concentration. It is a number that indicates relative acidity or alkalinity. The pH ranges from 0 to 14. The lower the pH, the more acidic the environment, and the higher the pH, the more alkaline the environment. A pH of 7 is neutral (neither acidic nor alkaline).

**phagocytize**    The verb describing ingestion of solid material by a cell.

**phagocytosis**    Ingestion of microorganisms or other substances by phagocytic cells (neutrophils, monocytes, and macrophages).

**phagosome**    The vesicle formed by phagocytosis, which contains material to be digested.

**phalangeal bones**    The bones that compose the digits.

**phalanx (plural, phalanges)**    A bone of a digit (toe or finger).

**pharynx**    The throat; a common passageway for the respiratory and digestive systems.

**pheomelanin**    A sulfur-based, yellow–brown pigment that produces a reddish color in hair.

**phonation**    Voice production.

**phospholipid**    A molecule composed of three parts: *phosphorus, fatty acids,* and a *nitrogenous base.* Any lipid that contains phosphorus. Phospholipids are the main components of the cell membrane.

**phosphorylation**    The addition of phosphorus to an organic compound.

**photoreceptors**    The sensory receptors that convert photons of light energy to nerve impulses that are interpreted by the brain as vision; the rods and cones.

**physiology**    The study of the functions of the animal body and its parts. Through physiology, we can describe how parts of the body work and what their functions are.

**pia mater**    The innermost layer of the meninges.

**pigmentation**    The degree of coloration, dependent on the concentration of melanin. Higher concentrations of melanin (pigment) will create a darker color.

**pillars**    Muscular folds that divide the sacs of the rumen.

**pineal body**    A structure in the brain located at the caudal end of the deep cleft that separates the two hemispheres of the cerebrum, just rostral to the cerebellum. It produces the hormone-like substance melatonin that appears to influence the body's biological clock.

**pinna**    The externally visible part of the ear that collects sound waves and funnels them down into the external ear canal; the ear flap.

**pinocytosis**    The ingestion by a cell of liquid material through endocytosis ("cell drinking").

**pitting edema**    The condition in which dents are left behind in moist, edematous tissue when pressed firmly.

**pituitary fossa**    A depression in the dorsal surface of the sphenoid bone that houses the pituitary gland in the living animal.

**pituitary gland**    The master endocrine gland. A pea-sized endocrine gland located at the base of the brain; made up of the anterior pituitary gland, which produces seven known hormones, and the posterior pituitary gland, which stores and releases two hormones from the hypothalamus; also called the *hypophysis.*

**pivot joint**    A joint that allows only a rotary motion. The only true pivot joint in most animal bodies is the atlantoaxial joint between the first and second cervical vertebrae; also called a *trochoid joint.*

**placenta**    A life-support system for a developing fetus; a multilayered, fluid-filled, membranous sac that surrounds the fetus and links it to the blood supply of the uterus. There is normally no direct mixing of fetal and maternal blood, but the blood vessels are close enough to each other that nutrients, wastes, and respiratory gases are easily exchanged between the fetal and maternal bloodstreams. It is also an important endocrine organ. At parturition, it is delivered last; so it is sometimes referred to as the *afterbirth.*

**placentome**    The attachment site with the uterine lining for cotyledonary placentas. It is formed from the tight connection of a cotyledon on the surface of the placenta with a caruncle in the lining of the uterus. Normally, large numbers of placentomes link the placenta with the uterus.

**plane of reference** Any of four basic imaginary slices through an animal body oriented at right angles to each other. They provide points or areas of reference for descriptions of direction or location. The four anatomic planes of reference are the *sagittal plane, median plane, transverse plane,* and *dorsal plane.*

**plantar** The caudal surface of the hindlimb from the tarsus distally.

**planum nasale** The topmost plane of the muzzle in such species as cats, dogs, pigs, and sheep.

**planum nasolabiale** The topmost plane of the muzzle including the upper lip in such species as horses and cows.

**plaque** A flat, thickened site present in the desmosomes of the epithelial tissue.

**plasma** The liquid matrix of blood, which contains proteins and suspended cells. Plasma also contains diffused gasses, electrolytes, and a variety of biochemicals.

**plasma membrane** See *cell membrane.*

**plasmalemma** See *cell membrane.*

**plastron** The ventral shell of turtles and tortoises.

**platelets** Also known as *thrombocytes.* Platelets are small pieces of cytoplasm that break off cells in the bone marrow (megakaryocytes) and enter peripheral blood. They are involved in hemostasis by helping plug leaks in blood vessels and initiating the blood-clotting process. The majority (two-thirds) of the body's platelets are found in the spleen; the rest are circulating through the blood.

**pleomorphic** Varying shapes; used to describe a monocyte nucleus that can take on many shapes without dividing into distinct segments.

**pleura** The thin membrane in the thoracic cavity that covers the thoracic organs (the visceral layer of pleura) and lines the thoracic cavity (the parietal layer of pleura). A potential space between the two layers contains a small amount of lubricating fluid that allows the thoracic structures to slide smoothly over each other as they and the thorax itself move.

**pleural fluid** The transudate fluid secreted by the serous membranes of the pleural cavity. It helps to lubricate the lungs during respiration.

**pleurodont teeth** Teeth fused with the inner surface of the jaw (alveolar ridge), not in sockets.

**pluripotent stem cell** Primitive cell type found in red bone marrow. It is the cell type from which all blood cells are formed.

**pneumonia** A lower respiratory tract infection affecting the tiny bronchioles and alveoli in the lungs. Pneumonia can be a serious disease because the inflammatory fluids and excess mucus that are produced by the irritation are difficult for the animal to cough up from deep in the lungs.

**pneumothorax** Air in the chest; an abnormal condition resulting from air leaking into the thoracic cavity from the lung or the outside world. It can result in collapse of the lung in that area because of loss of the normal partial vacuum in the thorax.

**PNS** See *peripheral nervous system.*

**podocytes** Meaning "foot cells." Podocytes make up the visceral layer of Bowman's capsule in the kidney. Podocytes form a permeable covering on the outside of the glomerular capillaries.

**point** The portion of the frog that points towards the toe of the horse's hoof.

**polar** Having the quality of defined direction.

**polar body** A "garbage can" for excess chromosomes. The polar body is a by-product of ovum development in the ovarian follicle; it will not develop into a mature ovum.

**polar molecule** A molecule with oppositely charged ends.

**poll** Top of the head between the bases of the ears.

**polled breeds** Hornless animals from species that normally produce horns. The breeder achieves this by consistently selecting polled offspring in their breeding lines. An example of a common polled beef breed is the Hereford.

**polychromasia** "Many colors"; this term is used to describe immature red blood cell cytoplasm when it is still metabolically active and has started producing hemoglobin. This condition results in both acidic (red) and alkaline (blue) stain being taken up by the cytoplasm, giving it a lavender color.

**polycythemia** An abnormal increase in the number of red blood cells in the circulation.

**polydipsia** Excessive thirst.

**polyestrous** An animal that has continual estrous cycles if she is not pregnant. As soon as one cycle ends, another begins.

**polymorphonuclear** A term that describes a nucleus that can have many shapes.

**polypeptide** Chains of more than 10 amino acids; also called *oligopeptides.*

**polyphagia** Excessive appetite.

**polysaccharide** "Many sugars"; a carbohydrate containing many monosaccharides that may be released in the process of hydrolysis. Polysaccharides are divided into two groups: *cellulose* and *starch.*

**polyunsaturated** Describes a fatty acid in which more than one double bond is present in the carbon chain.

**polyuria** Production of an excessive volume of urine.

**pons** A part of the brainstem located just rostral to the medulla oblongata.

**pore** A minute opening or space.

**portal system** An arrangement of blood vessels that carries blood from one organ or tissue directly to another organ or tissue before returning it to the heart.

**positive nitrogen balance** When the amount of protein ingested is greater than the amount excreted.

**posterior chamber** The portion of the aqueous compartment of the eye behind (caudal to) the iris.

**posterior pituitary gland** The neurohypophysis; the caudal portion of the pituitary gland that stores and releases two hormones (antidiuretic hormone and oxytocin) that are produced in the hypothalamus.

**posterior** A directional term meaning toward the back of a human body.

**postganglionic neuron** In reference to the autonomic nervous system, it is the second of two neurons that typically make up the nerves of the autonomic nervous system; so called because this neuron originates from a ganglion and carries the impulse from it to the target organ or tissue.

**postprandial lipemia** A condition of cloudy plasma that results from small fat particles found in blood soon after eating.

**postsynaptic neuron** The neuron that contains the receptors to which a released neurotransmitter binds, causing depolarization or inhibition of depolarization of the neuron.

**precocial**    Chicks that are hatched with downy feathers and their eyes open and that are mobile.

**precursor**    Something that precedes or develops into something else.

**preganglionic neuron**    In reference to the autonomic nervous system, it is the first of two neurons that typically make up the nerves of the autonomic nervous system; so called because the first neuron is located "before" the ganglion.

**prehend**    To grasp.

**prehensile**    Capable of grasping.

**prehension**    Grasping.

**premolars**    The teeth rostral to the molars.

**prepuce**    The skin-covered sheath around the free end of the penis.

**pressure**    The sense of something pressing on the body surface; often combined with the tactile sense, which is the sense of touch.

**pressure gradient**    The spectrum between an area of highest pressure and an area of lowest pressure.

**presynaptic neuron**    The neuron that is stimulated by the depolarization wave to release a neurotransmitter into the synapse.

**primary growth center**    The main growth area of a bone developing by the endochondral (cartilage) method. Primary growth centers are the areas of bone development that are located in the main portions of the cartilage rod bone templates in a developing fetus.

**primary hairs**    The large, straight hairs predominant in complex hair follicles.

**primary structure**    A long chain of amino acids held together with peptide bonds.

**prime mover**    A muscle or muscle group that directly produces a desired movement.

**prion**    A small, protein-based particle that is both infectious and resilient yet not a living pathogen.

**process**    A general name for a lump, bump, or other projection on a bone. Processes can be either articular processes, which contribute to joint formation, or nonarticular processes, which are usually sites where tendons attach.

**proctodeum**    Posterior section of the cloaca of birds that is accessed by the coprodeum and urodeum and stores the excrement until it is eliminated.

**product**    The new substance created by the interaction of two or more chemical substances.

**product molecules**    The product of an enzyme reaction caused by the enzyme's ability to weaken the bonds of the substrate molecule.

**proestrus**    The stage of the estrous cycle when follicles are actively developing and growing in the ovary. As they grow, the follicles produce rising levels of estrogens, which gradually induce the physical and behavioral changes that prepare the animal for breeding.

**progesterone**    The principal progestin hormone produced by the corpus luteum of the ovary. It helps prepare the uterus for implantation of the fertilized ovum and helps maintain pregnancy once it begins.

**progestins**    Hormones produced by the corpus luteum of the ovary. They are necessary for the maintenance of pregnancy, particularly during the early gestational period. The principal progestin hormone is progesterone.

**prohormone**    A hormone precursor that has minimal hormonal effect by itself.

**prokaryotes**    Included in the kingdom Monera, these unicellular organisms have no true nucleus, nuclear envelope, or membrane-bound organelles. Bacteria and cyanobacteria are included in this classification.

**prolactin**    The anterior pituitary hormone that helps trigger and maintain lactation.

**promoters**    Codes within the DNA sequence that indicate where RNA synthesis should begin.

**proper vaginal tunic**    The inner connective tissue sac that surrounds the testis. It is derived from the visceral peritoneum that covered the testis during its early development in the abdominal cavity. Also known as the *visceral vaginal tunic.*

**prophase**    The phase during mitotic division when chromatin becomes visible and organizes into chromosomes by joining two strands via a centromere. The nuclear envelope and the nucleoli also disappear, and the centrioles divide and replicate, traveling to either "pole" of the cell.

**propionic acid**    One of the key volatile fatty acids produced by anaerobic, fermentative metabolism in the rumen.

**proprioception**    The sense of body position and movement. Stretch receptors in skeletal muscles, tendons, ligaments, and joint capsules send impulses to the nervous system to keep it informed of the positions and movements of the various body parts.

**prostaglandins (PGs)**    Hormonelike substances that are produced and exert many effects locally in a variety of body tissues. Sometimes called *tissue hormones* because they regulate biochemical activities in the tissues where they are formed.

**prostate gland**    The male accessory reproductive gland that generally surrounds the urethra; it lies just distal to the urinary bladder. The prostate gland is the only accessory reproductive gland in the dog, so it is quite large in that species.

**proteases**    Enzymes that break down the basic structure of a protein by hydrolyzing the peptide bonds between the amino acids.

**proteasome**    A tiny organelle found in both the nucleus and the cytoplasm that breaks down individual proteins no longer needed by the cell. The proteasome is a complex of proteins with a hollow core containing proteases. Individual proteins, tagged for destruction by the protein ubiquitin, are drawn into the core and degraded. Short chains of amino acids are expelled from the proteasome.

**protective proteins**    Proteins that are a component of the immune response, such as antibodies.

**protein**    Large organic compounds that are composed of amino acids held in peptide bonds to form polypeptides. They are synthesized by all living things and are essential for the basic maintenance of animal tissue.

**proteoglycan**    The viscous intercellular material located in the gaps between the adjacent cells in the zonula adherens. It is composed of polysaccharide chains and small proteins.

**proteroglypous**    Associated with the Proteroglyphae group of snakes with hollow fangs that are venomous but not aggressive.

**proton**    A subatomic particle with a positive charge that, along with the neutrons, makes up the entire mass of the nucleus. The number of protons defines the atom as a specific element.

**protoplasm**    The viscous fluid found within the cell.

**proud flesh**  The condition occurring when excess amounts of new tissue, known as *granulation tissue,* develop in an otherwise nonhealing wound; also known as exuberant granulation tissue.

**proventriculus**  Anterior glandular stomach of birds in which chemical digestion of proteins begins.

**provitamin**  A molecule, such as beta carotene, from which an animal can manufacture a vitamin.

**proximal**  A directional term used only for extremities of the body. It implies a position or direction *toward* the body proper.

**proximal convoluted tubule (PCT)**  The first part of the tubular portion of a nephron. Its lumen is a continuation of the capsular space of Bowman's capsule in the renal corpuscle. The majority of tubular reabsorption takes place from the PCT.

**proximal sesamoid bones**  Paired sesamoid bones in the legs of horses. They are located in the large digital flexor tendons behind the fetlock joints (the joints between the large metacarpal and metatarsal bones and the proximal phalanges).

**pruritus**  Itching; often caused by parasitic infestations or allergic reactions.

**pseudocyesis**  Pseudopregnancy; an abnormally prolonged and exaggerated diestrus period that results in an animal acting and looking pregnant when it is not. Most cases resolve spontaneously.

**pseudopod (plural, pseudopodia)**  "False foot"; the temporary extension of the cell's membrane and cytoplasm either for locomotion or to engulf nourishment.

**pseudopregnancy**  See *pseudocyesis.*

**pseudostratified columnar epithelium**  Single-layered columnar cells that appear to be stratified because of the positioning of their nuclei. These epithelia are often ciliated and are good at moving material across their surfaces.

**pterygoid bones**  Skull bones that are part of the internal bones of the face. The two pterygoid bones support part of the lateral walls of the pharynx (throat).

**pterylae**  Seven tracts of skin where feathers originate.

**pubis**  The smallest and most medial of the three pairs of bones that make up the pelvis. The pubis forms the cranial portion of the floor of the pelvis.

**pulmonary**  An adjective referring to the lungs.

**pulmonary artery**  Artery arising from the right ventricle that delivers blood into the pulmonary circulation.

**pulmonary circulation**  The part of the circulatory system that delivers unoxygenated blood to the lungs and oxygenated blood to the left side of the heart.

**pulmonary valve**  A semilunar valve; it separates the right ventricle and the pulmonary artery during ventricular diastole.

**pulp**  The latticelike material in the center of the tooth, which contains the nerve and blood supply.

**pupil**  The opening in the center of the iris.

**pupillary light reflex (PLR)**  Reflex in which light is shone into one eye, and the pupil constricts in both eyes.

**pustules**  Small, pus-filled elevations of the skin that are easily expressed.

**pygostyle**  Bony plate in birds formed by the fusion of several coccygeal vertebrae; supports the tail feathers.

**pyknotic**  The term used to describe a nucleus that has died. The chromatin has become densely compacted, so no pattern is visible.

**pyloric antrum**  The portion of the stomach between the body and the pylorus. The pyloric antrum grinds up swallowed food and helps regulate hydrochloric acid production.

**pyloric sphincter**  Ring of circular smooth muscle between the duodenum (small intestine) and the stomach; regulates the movement of the liquid chyme from the stomach to the intestine.

**Pylorus**  The portion of the stomach that connects with the duodenum (small intestine).

**Q**

**quarters**  (1) The common name for the mammary glands that make up the udder of the cow. (2) The medial and lateral regions of the hoof.

**queen**  A sexually mature, intact female cat.

**R**

**radioactive isotope**  An unstable isotope of an element that decomposes spontaneously by emission of subatomic particles and radiation.

**radius**  One of the two bones (the ulna is the other) that form the antebrachium, or forearm. The radius is usually the main weight-bearing bone.

**rafts**  Free-floating, specialized regions in the plasmalemma, and also in the membranes of the Golgi and lysosomes. Called *lipid rafts,* they serve as a construction site for signalling molecules. They regulate protein trafficking, the fluidity of the membrane and neurotransmission.

**ramus of the mandible**  The vertical portion of the mandible located at its caudal end. The ramus is where the powerful jaw muscles attach to the mandible.

**reabsorption**  The process by which some constituents of plasma that were filtered out of the plasma by the glomerulus are returned to the bloodstream. Water, glucose, amino acids, and sodium are some of the substances that are reabsorbed.

**reactants**  Substances initially involved in a chemical reaction.

**receptor**  In the context of the nervous system, a specialized protein to which neurotransmitters bind.

**receptor-mediated endocytosis**  A very specialized form of endocytosis that only allows the cell to incorporate those materials that have protein receptor sites specifically for that material on the cell.

**rectum**  The last portion of the large intestine, located between the colon and the anus. The rectum stores feces until defecation.

**red bone marrow**  The hematopoietic (blood cell-forming) type of bone marrow.

**red pulp**  The area of the spleen that is filled with blood sinusoids and macrophages.

**reflex**  A rapid, automatic response to a stimulus, intended to protect the body and maintain homeostasis.

**reflex arc**  The reflex arc is composed of the sensory receptor, sensory neuron, interneuron(s), motor neuron, and target tissue or organ involved with a stimulus and reflex response.

**refractory period**  The period in the depolarization–repolarization cycle when the neuron cannot be stimulated to depolarize (absolute refractory period) or can only be depolarized with a greater than normal stimulation (relative refractory period).

**regional anatomy**   A method of studying anatomy that examines all the component structures that make up each region of the body. For example, the regional approach to abdominal anatomy would examine all the cells, tissues, organs, muscles, blood vessels, and nerves that are present in the abdomen.

**regulatory proteins**   Those proteins essential to maintaining normal body function, including insulin and many other hormones.

**regurgitation**   The movement of food back up the esophagus toward the mouth; in contrast to vomiting, regurgitation usually involves undigested food and occurs without the violent abdominal contractions associated with vomiting. Regurgitated material usually does not contain stomach acid.

**relaxin**   A hormone produced late in pregnancy that helps relax ligaments between the bones around the birth canal in preparation for parturition. Depending on the species it may be produced by the corpus luteum of the ovary, the uterus, or the placenta.

**remiges**   The primary and secondary flight feathers in the wing.

**renal artery**   The major arterial blood supply to the kidney. It is a branch of the aorta and enters the kidney at the hilus. After entering the kidney, it begins branching into progressively smaller vessels that eventually become the glomerular vessels.

**renal corpuscle**   The first part of the nephron. It is composed of the glomerular capillaries and Bowman's capsule. The capsular space of the renal corpuscle continues as the proximal convoluted tubule.

**renal pelvis**   The collection point for tubular filtrate as it leaves the collecting ducts. When the fluid enters the renal pelvis, it is in the form of urine that must be eliminated from the body. The renal pelvis continues as the ureter that carries urine to the urinary bladder.

**renal portal system**   In birds, the network of veins that transport blood from the extremities to the capillaries of the kidneys before returning it to the heart.

**renal vein**   The major vein that drains the kidney. It is formed from venules that are formed by convergence of the peritubular capillaries. It leaves the kidney at the hilus.

**renin**   A hormone released in the kidney (by the juxtaglomerular cells of the afferent glomerular arterioles) in response to low blood pressure.

**renin–angiotensin–aldosterone system**   A sequence of hormonal reactions, initiated by the kidneys in response to low blood pressure, which result in vasoconstriction and increased blood volume.

**repolarization**   The process following depolarization wherein potassium ions diffuse rapidly out of the neuron.

**reproductive cells**   Cells found in the ovary and testis that carry the genetic code. Each cell (called an ovum and sperm for female and male, respectively) contains one half of the genetic code, which is expressed as a haploid number of chromosomes. The gametes.

**reproductive system**   The group of organs that function to produce offspring. The organs of the reproductive system include not only those of the genital tract, such as the ovaries and testes, but also all the organs of the endocrine system that regulate reproductive hormones.

**residual volume**   The volume of air remaining in the lungs after the maximum amount of air has been forced out by expiration.

**respiration**   The movement of oxygen from the outside air to the cells in an animal's body, and the movement of carbon dioxide in the opposite direction.

**respiratory center**   The area in the brainstem that controls the breathing process.

**respiratory system**   The group of organs that function to fortify blood with oxygen and remove carbon dioxide. The respiratory system includes the lungs, the trachea, and the respiratory center in the medulla oblongata. Supportive thoracic muscles and the diaphragm also play important roles in respiration.

**resting membrane potential**   The electric charge of some cells at rest, caused by differing concentrations of ions inside and outside the cell membrane.

**resting state**   In reference to neurons, more sodium ions are outside the cell membrane than inside, and more potassium ions are inside the cell; it is the state of the neuron before stimulation.

**rete testis**   A complex of ducts in the testis that conduct spermatozoa from the seminiferous tubules to the efferent ducts.

**reticular cell**   Phagocytic cells of reticular connective tissue. Reticular cells are particularly important in lymphatic and hematopoietic tissue.

**reticular connective tissue**   Connective tissue composed of networks of reticular fibers and cells; found principally in bone marrow, lymph nodes, blood vessels, liver, and kidney.

**reticular fibers**   Extremely fine fibers in reticular connective tissue.

**reticular groove**   A muscular groove found in young ruminants that conveys milk and liquids from the cardia directly to the omasum; also called the *esophageal groove.*

**reticular layer**   Layer of irregular connective tissue that composes the majority of the dermis. It is intimately associated with the papillary layer by collagen fibers.

**reticuloperitonitis**   Also called *hardware disease;* inflammation and infection of the reticulum and abdominal cavity that can occur in ruminants due to irritation from sharp objects that have been swallowed.

**reticulorumen**   Pertaining to both the reticulum and rumen; often describes the contractions of the rumen and reticulum together.

**reticulum**   The most cranial part of the forestomach; it has a honeycomb appearance inside.

**retina**   The inner nervous layer of the eye where the photoreceptors are located. The refractive structures of the eye form an image on the retina that is converted to nerve impulses by the photoreceptors (the rods and cones). The nerve impulses from the retina are transmitted by the optic nerve to the brain, where they are converted to visual images.

**retinal degeneration**   The progressive degeneration of the rods and cones, eventually leading to blindness. It occurs as an inherited disease in dogs and as a result of taurine deficiency in cats.

**retractor penis muscle**   An elastic, bandlike muscle that pulls the nonerect penis of animals with a sigmoid flexure back into its S-shaped configuration.

**retrices**   Tail feathers.

**retroperitoneal**   Behind the parietal layer of peritoneum that lines the abdominal cavity, outside the abdominal cavity proper.

**ribonucleic acid**   See *RNA.*

**ribosomal RNA (rRNA)**   One of the main components of ribosomes; aids in protein synthesis and the combination of amino acids to create protein molecules.

**ribosome** An organelle composed of ribonucleic acid, located on the rough endoplasmic reticulum or suspended in the cytoplasm, where protein synthesis takes place.

**ribs** Long bones of the axial skeleton that form the lateral walls of the thorax. Their dorsal portions are made of bone and form synovial joints with the thoracic vertebrae. Their ventral portions are made of cartilage (the costal cartilages).

**rigor mortis** Literally, *stiffness of death.* The stiffness of skeletal muscles that usually occurs shortly after death. It results from insufficient sources of energy in muscle fibers to allow them to relax.

**RNA (ribonucleic acid)** The nucleic acid used in protein synthesis. It differs from DNA, because it uses ribose instead of deoxyribose and also because RNA's pyrimidine, uracil, replaces DNA's thymidine. The three types of RNA are *transfer RNA (tRNA), messenger RNA (mRNA),* and *ribosomal RNA (rRNA).*

**RNA polymerase** An enzyme that aids in transcription by converting DNA base sequences into RNA base sequences.

**roaring** See *laryngeal hemiplegia.*

**rods** Photoreceptors in the retina of the eye that perceive dim light images in shades of gray.

**root** The anchor of the hair that attaches it to the connective tissue layer.

**root hair plexus** The arrangement of sensory nerves located at the root of the hair follicle that enable it to sense touch.

**roots of the penis** The structures that attach the penis to the brim of the pelvis. They consist primarily of the two connective tissue crura covered by the ischiocavernosus muscles.

**rostral** A directional term meaning *toward the tip of the nose.* Rostral is generally used to describe positions and directions only on the head, where the term *cranial* loses its meaning.

**rotation** A joint movement that consists of a twisting motion of a part on its own axis.

**rough endoplasmic reticulum (rough ER)** The portion of the ER that is studded with ribosomes and is involved in protein synthesis.

**round ligament of the uterus** A cord of fibrous tissue and smooth muscle contained in the free edge of a lateral fold of the broad ligament in the female. Extends from the tip of the uterine horn caudally and ventrally to the area of the inguinal ring.

**round window** The membrane-covered opening into the cochlea that functions as a pressure-relief device. When the stapes pushes on the membrane covering the oval window, the fluid in the cochlea pushes on the membrane covering the round window, making it bulge outward. When the stapes pulls on the oval window membrane, the round window membrane bulges inward. This allows the fluid in the cochlea to vibrate freely with the movements of the ossicles and stimulate the hearing receptors in the cochlea.

**rRNA** See *ribosomal RNA.*

**rugae** Folds of the inner lining of the stomach.

**rumen** A large, fermentative section of the forestomachs of ruminants; the rumen is responsible for production of volatile fatty acids, microbial protein, and other essential nutrients needed by the ruminant.

**ruminant** An herbivore that has a large fermentative section of forestomach called a *rumen;* cattle, sheep, and goats are examples of ruminants.

**rumination** The process of regurgitating coarse food from the reticulorumen, rechewing the food, and swallowing it again; also called "chewing the cud."

## S

**SA node** See *sinoatrial node.*

**saccule** One of two saclike spaces (the utricle is the other one) in the vestibule that contain sensory structures that monitor the position of the head.

**sacral vertebrae** The vertebrae of the pelvic region. The sacral vertebrae fuse into a solid structure called the *sacrum,* which forms a joint with the ilium of the pelvis on each side called the *sacroiliac joint.*

**sacroiliac joint** The joint between the pelvis and the sacrum that joins the pelvic limb to the axial skeleton.

**sacrum** The solid structure formed by the fusion of the sacral vertebrae.

**sacs** Blind pouches.

**sagittal plane** An anatomic reference plane; the sagittal plane runs lengthwise, dividing the body into left and right parts that are not necessarily equal halves; see *median plane.*

**saliva** The liquid secretion of the salivary glands. Saliva is secreted into the mouth in response to food, stimulation of the mouth, or thinking about eating; in most species, it contains enzymes and buffers.

**salivary glands** Glands located in and around the mouth that produce saliva; include the parotid, mandibular, and lingual salivary glands.

**salt** Any ionic compound composed of positively charged cations and negatively charged anions so that the product is electrically neutral.

**saltatory conduction** The skipping of the depolarization wave (action potential) in a myelinated axon from one node of Ranvier to the next node of Ranvier; means "leaping" conduction.

**sarcolemma** The cell membrane of a muscle cell.

**sarcomere** The basic contracting unit of skeletal muscle. It consists of the actin and myosin filaments between Z lines in a muscle cell. Myofibrils are composed of many sarcomeres stacked end to end.

**sarcoplasm** The cytoplasm of a muscle cell.

**sarcoplasmic reticulum** The organelle in a muscle cell that is equivalent to the endoplasmic reticulum of other cells. It stores calcium ions ($Ca^{2+}$) necessary to initiate the muscle contraction process. Release of $Ca^{2+}$ from the sarcoplasmic reticulum is stimulated by a nerve impulse.

**saturated fatty acids** Such as those found in animal fats; have no double bonds in their carbon chains and can therefore accommodate the maximum number of hydrogen atoms; are solid at room temperature.

**scapula** The shoulder blade; the most proximal bone of the thoracic limb. In domestic animals, no bony connection exists between the scapula and the axial skeleton.

**Schleiden, Mathias** Mathias Schleiden's work with plant tissue helped him to develop the cell theory, which states that all living things are composed of cells.

**Schwann cells** Glial cells associated with peripheral nerves whose cellular membrane forms the myelin sheath for axons in the PNS.

**Schwann, Theodor**   German anatomist whose work with animal tissue helped to develop the cell theory, which states that all living things are composed of cells.

**sclera**   The white portion of the eye; part of the outer, fibrous layer of the eyeball.

**sclerotic ring**   Bony plates that act as a protective border of the eye sockets.

**scrapie**   A contagious and fatal disease caused by prions, occurring in both sheep and goats; the incubation period is around 2 years before symptoms, such as a disabled gait, appear. This eventually leads to prolonged illness, resulting in death.

**scrotum**   The sac of skin that houses the testes and, by raising or lowering them, helps control their temperature.

**seasonally polyestrous**   An animal that has continuous estrous cycles during a certain portion, or portions, of the year and no estrous cycles at other times.

**sebaceous glands**   Simple holocrine glands that secrete an oily substance called *sebum* through the hair follicle.

**sebum**   Secretion of the sebaceous gland containing oils and epithelial cells. It is released into the hair follicle to lubricate the hair and skin.

**secondary growth center**   Secondary areas of growth in bones developing by the endochondral (cartilage) method. Secondary growth centers are areas of bone development located outside the main portions of the cartilaginous bone templates in a developing fetus.

**secondary hair**   The smaller, yet most numerous hairs in an animal's undercoat.

**second-intention healing**   Healing of wounds that are not sutured and that form granulation tissue. Epithelialization, fibrosis, and contraction of the wound are part of the healing process.

**secretin**   A hormone produced in the lining of the duodenum, when chyme enters from the stomach. It stimulates the pancreas to release a fluid rich in sodium bicarbonate to help neutralize the acidic chyme. It inhibits gastric motility and delays gastric emptying.

**secretion**   The process by which a cell or gland produces and expels some useful product; also used to refer to the product itself.

**secretory granules**   Materials that have been brought into the cell and are separated from the cytoplasm by a single membranous boundary.

**secretory unit**   The portion of a multicellular exocrine gland that is composed of secretory cells and produces a secretion.

**segmental contractions**   Alternating contractions of the circular muscles in the intestine; they mix the intestinal contents and slow their transit time.

**selectively permeable**   Structures that allow some things to pass through but not others.

**semialtricial**   Chicks that are hatched with downy feathers, are immobile, and may or may not have their eyes open.

**semicircular canals**   Three semicircular canals in each inner ear that are part of the vestibular system. They sense rotary motion of the head.

**seminal vesicles**   Accessory reproductive glands that contribute various materials to semen. Seminal vesicles are present in all common domestic animals except the dog and cat.

**seminiferous tubule**   The site where spermatogenesis (spermatozoa production) takes place in the testis.

**semiprecocial**   Chicks that are hatched with downy feathers and open eyes but that are not mobile.

**senescence**   The process of aging.

**sensory nerves**   Nerves that carry afferent impulses from sensory receptors toward the central nervous system.

**sensory neuron**   Neuron carrying impulses toward the CNS.

**sensory receptor**   A modified nerve ending that converts mechanical, thermal, chemical, or electromagnetic stimuli into nerve impulses that travel to the CNS and are interpreted as the appropriate sensation.

**septic pericarditis**   Infection, and resulting inflammation, of the pericardium of the heart. In ruminant animals often caused by the penetration of sharp foreign objects that have been swallowed through the wall of the reticulum and diaphragm, and into the pericardium. See *hardware disease*.

**septum (plural, septa)**   A partition or dividing structure in an organ or area.

**serosa**   The outermost layer of the intestinal tract.

**serous membrane**   A membrane that lines a serous cavity, such as the thorax or abdomen. Serous fluid produced by serous membranes helps lubricate organs.

**serous secretions**   Thin, watery secretions; transudates.

**Sertoli cells**   Large "nurse" cells to which spermatozoa are attached during their development. Sertoli cells normally produce small amounts of estrogen hormones. If they grow abnormally and form a Sertoli cell tumor, the unusually high amount of estrogens produced by the tumor can cause feminization of the affected male animal.

**serum**   The fluid portion of blood that has had the clotting factors removed. Serum is produced by letting a blood sample clot before the fluid is removed.

**sesamoid bones**   Bones present in some tendons where they change direction markedly over joints. Sesamoid bones act as bearings over the joint surfaces, allowing powerful muscles to move the joints without the tendons wearing out as they move over the joints.

**sex chromosomes**   Two of the normal diploid chromosome complement. The sex chromosomes determine the genetic sex of the individual. If there are two $X$ sex chromosomes, the individual is genetically female. If there is an $X$ and a $Y$ sex chromosome, the individual is genetically male.

**sex hormones**   Hormones that target the reproductive tissues. The male sex hormones are the androgens, and the female sex hormones are the estrogens.

**sexual dimorphism**   The male and female of the species look distinctly different from one another. Sexual dimorphism occurs in many avian species.

**shaft of the mandible**   The horizontal portion of the mandible that houses all the lower teeth.

**shaft**   The keratinized, visible portion of hair that extends above the surface of the epithelium.

**shell gland**   Muscular section of the oviduct in birds where the egg shell is applied; also called the *uterus*.

**short bone**   A small bone shaped like a small cube or marshmallow. The bones of the carpus are examples of short bones.

**short-chain fatty acids**   See *volatile fatty acids*.

**sigh** A deeper than normal breath. A sigh may correct a minor oxygen or carbon dioxide imbalance in the blood, or it may expand the lungs a little more than the normal breaths do. Sighs can have an emotional basis also.

**sigmoid flexure** The S-shaped bend in the nonerect penis of the bull, ram, and boar.

**simple ciliated columnar epithelium** Single-layered, columnar-shaped epithelium containing cilia; found in the oviduct.

**simple columnar epithelium** Single-layered columnar epithelium found in the stomach and intestines because of its ability to absorb and secrete.

**simple cuboidal epithelium** Single-layered, cube-shaped epithelium found in the ovaries and in many of the ducts of the body because of its ability to aid in secretion.

**simple diffusion** The ability of some molecules, such as oxygen, water, and carbon dioxide, to pass through the cell membrane without the aid of carrier proteins.

**simple epithelium** Epithelium composed of a single layer of cells.

**simple gland** An exocrine gland with unbranched ducts.

**simple squamous epithelium** Delicate, single-layered, flat-celled epithelium found in the alveoli of the lungs and lining blood vessels.

**simple sugars** Monosaccharides, such as glucose and fructose.

**sinoatrial (SA) node** A group of specialized cardiac muscle cells in the wall of the right atrium of the heart that act as the heart's pacemaker. The impulse that starts each heartbeat is initiated in the SA node.

**sinus hairs** See *tactile hairs.*

**sinuses** Also known as the *paranasal sinuses;* outpouchings of the nasal passages that are housed within spaces in areas of the skull bones.

**sinusitis** Inflammation and swelling of the lining of a paranasal sinus.

**skeletal muscle** Multinucleated, striated, voluntary muscle that enables conscious movement of an animal; the type of muscle that moves the bones of the skeleton and is under conscious control.

**skeletal muscle fiber** A skeletal muscle cell. Because of their long, thin fiberlike appearance, skeletal muscle cells are often called skeletal muscle fibers.

**skull** The collective name of the 37 or 38 bones of the head. The skull is the most complex part of the skeleton. It houses the brain and all the special sense organs.

**small ribonucleoproteins** RNA–protein complexes that remove noncoded introns from messenger RNA and splice together the coded exons to create a complete and identical copy of the DNA gene.

**smell** The olfactory sense; a chemical sense that detects odor molecules in the inhaled air. The olfactory epithelium is located high in the nasal passages.

**smooth endoplasmic reticulum (smooth ER)** The portion of the ER that is without ribosomes and is involved in the synthesis of lipids.

**smooth muscle** Nonstriated, involuntary muscle having only one nucleus per cell; the type of muscle found in soft internal organs and structures. Smooth muscle gets its name because its cells do not have a striped appearance under the microscope, in contrast to skeletal and cardiac muscle cells. Smooth muscle is not under conscious control. Smooth muscle is found in the digestive tract, where it assists with the movement of food through the gut (peristalsis).

**sneeze** A protective reflex stimulated by irritation or foreign matter in the nasal passages. Consists of a sudden, forceful expiration of air that is directed through the nose and mouth in an effort to eliminate the irritant.

**sodium cotransport** The process by which glucose and amino acids are passively reabsorbed back into the circulation in the proximal convoluted tubule. These two substances bind to the transport protein to which sodium is also attached. When the sodium is actively transported into the tubular epithelial cells, the glucose and amino acids follow.

**sodium–potassium pump** Active transport molecule that moves sodium molecules out of the neuron and potassium molecules into the neuron to maintain the resting state.

**soft palate** The soft mucosal flap that extends caudally from the hard palate on the roof of the mouth.

**sole of hoof** The concave plantar or palmar portion of the hoof. The sole is avascular and lacks innervation.

**solenoglyphous** Having hinged, hollow fangs that fold back when the mouth is closed. Refers to snakes with mobile fangs that can be moved to give the best position for envenomation of the prey. Includes vipers, puff adders, and rattlesnakes.

**solute** Substance that is dissolved in another substance. The component of a solution that is present in the lesser amount.

**solutions** Homogeneous mixtures of two or more substances. The components can be gases, liquids, and/or solids.

**solvent** A substance in which another substance is dissolved.

**soma** The cell body of a neuron; perikaryon.

**somatic cells** Nonreproductive cells found throughout the body, containing a diploid number of chromosomes and replicating themselves through the cell division process of mitosis.

**somatic nervous system** Conscious or voluntary nervous system controlling skeletal muscles; somatic motor function is the efferent branch, and somatic sensory function is the afferent branch.

**somatic reflex** A reflex resulting in the stimulation or inhibition of skeletal muscle contraction.

**special senses** Taste, smell, hearing, equilibrium, and vision. The organs of special sense are organized into complex structures that are all located in the head.

**specialization** The ability of an organism to differentiate to acquire new characteristics.

**specialized connective tissue** Tissue including bone, blood, and cartilage. Specialized connective tissue may be subdivided into *supportive connective tissue,* which includes bone and cartilage, and *vascular connective tissue,* including blood.

**specific immunity** Reactions of the immune system aimed at destroying specific antigens.

**spermatic cords** Cordlike connective tissue structures that enclose blood vessels, nerves, lymphatic vessels, and the vas deferens as they pass between the testes and the abdominal cavity through the inguinal rings.

**spermatogenesis** The production of spermatozoa in the testis.

**spermatozoon (plural, spermatozoa)** The male reproductive cell. The male gamete.

**sphenoid bone** A skull bone that is one of the internal bones of the cranium. The sphenoid bone forms the floor of the cranium and contains a depression, the pituitary fossa, that houses the pituitary gland.

**sphenoidal sinus** The paranasal sinus in the sphenoid bone.

**spheroidal joint**   A ball-and-socket joint, such as the shoulder or hip joint.

**sphincter muscle**   A circular muscle that surrounds and controls flow through an orifice.

**spinal canal**   The long, flexible, caudal portion of the dorsal body cavity formed by the adjacent arches of the vertebrae of the spine. It houses and protects the spinal cord.

**spinal column**   Also known as the *vertebral column;* the collective name for the cervical, thoracic, lumbar, sacral, and coccygeal vertebrae.

**spinal nerves**   Nerves of the peripheral nervous system that originate from the spinal cord.

**spindle apparatus**   The structure that during mitosis connects to the centromeres of the chromosomes for the purpose of division.

**spindle fibers**   Visible during the metaphase stage of cell division, the fusiform structure is made up from the microtubules that extend from the centrosomes. These fibers aid in mitosis by connecting to the cell's chromosomes at their centromeres, creating the pull necessary to divide them.

**spinous process**   The single, dorsally projecting process of a vertebra.

**splenopancreas**   Pertaining to the spleen and pancreas.

**spliceosomes**   Specialized areas in the nucleus created by small ribonucleic proteins that remove noncoded introns from messenger RNA.

**splint bones**   The vestigial metacarpal and metatarsal bones of a horse's leg. There are two splint bones in each leg: one on each side of the cannon bone (the large metacarpal or metatarsal bone).

**squamous cell carcinoma**   Composed of squamous epithelium, these cancerous masses are locally invasive and also may metastasize. They occur in a variety of species, most commonly on the conjunctiva, skin surface, urogenital tissue, mouth, and stomach.

**squamous cells**   Flat cells that make up squamous epithelia.

**squamous epithelium**   Epithelium composed of squamous cells.

**stages of labor**   The three main parts of the parturition (birth) process. Stage 1 consists of uterine contractions that force the membrane-covered fetus against the cervix, causing it to dilate. Stage 2 is the delivery of the newborn animal by a combination of uterine and abdominal muscle contraction. Stage 3 is delivery of the placenta by a combination of uterine and abdominal contractions.

**stapes**   One of the three ossicles, which are the tiny bones that transmit sound wave vibrations across the middle ear. The stapes, or stirrup, is attached to the membrane that covers the oval window of the cochlea. It is the innermost of the three ossicles.

**steatorrhea**   Fatty, greasy stools.

**sternal flexure**   Where the right ventral colon of the horse bends to form the left ventral colon on the ventral floor of the peritoneal cavity.

**sternal rib**   Rib whose costal cartilage directly joins the sternum.

**sternebra**   A bone of the sternum.

**sternum**   The breastbone; the series of rodlike bones called *sternebrae* that form the floor of the thorax.

**steroid hormone**   Hormone whose structure is derived from cholesterol.

**steroids**   Lipids characterized by a carbon skeleton that contains four fused rings. Cholesterol and the steroid hormones are examples of steroids in the animal body.

**stifle joint**   The joint between the femur and the tibia. In humans, it is called the *knee joint.*

**storage proteins**   Proteins that are stored for later use, such as those found in egg whites.

**stratified cuboidal epithelium**   Multilayered, cube-shaped epithelium found in excretory tracts of the body.

**stratified epithelium**   Epithelium composed of layers of cells.

**stratified squamous epithelium**   Epithelial tissue composed of multiple layers of flat squamous cells; found in the epidermis of the skin, vagina, mouth, and anus; possesses the ability to regenerate rapidly.

**stratum basale**   See *stratum germinativum.*

**stratum corneum**   The horny layer of the epidermis lying most superficially on the skin's surface. The cells of this layer are anucleated and keratinized, being the dead remnants of keratinocytes. This is the predominant layer of the epidermis.

**stratum germinativum**   The base layer of the epidermis, composed of a single layer of cuboidal cells that divide to replenish the constantly eroding superficial layer of the epidermis.

**stratum granulosum**   The granular layer of epidermis containing keratohyaline and lamellated granules, located between the stratum germinativum and the stratum lucidum. This layer of the epidermis aids in waterproofing the skin.

**stratum lucidum**   The clear layer of epidermis present only in very thick skin, such as that of the paw pads; located beneath the stratum corneum.

**stratum spinosum**   The prickle cell layer; the weblike layer of epidermis dense with intercellular attachments; located between the stratum granulosum and the stratum basale.

**streak canal**   The passageway at the tip of the teat of the cow that carries milk from the teat sinus outside the body.

**stretch reflex**   Reflex initiated by stretch receptors within a muscle that results in contraction of the muscle to compensate for the stretching.

**striated**   Striped.

**striated muscle**   Muscle that looks striped because of alternating light and dark bands. Examples of striated muscle are skeletal and cardiac muscle.

**stroke volume**   The amount of blood ejected with each cardiac contraction.

**stroma**   The foundation-supporting tissues of organs.

**structural proteins**   Proteins that form body structures, such as hair and collagen.

**subcutaneous layer**   The layer of adipose tissue located beneath the epidermis and dermis that insulates and protects the body.

**submucosa**   The second innermost layer of the intestinal tract; lies between the mucosa and the muscle layer.

**substrate**   Substance acted on by an enzyme. May also be used to describe nesting material.

**sulcus (plural, sulci)**   Groove, especially shallow grooves in the cerebral cortex.

**superficial**   A directional term meaning *toward the surface* of the body or a body part; see *external.*

**superior**   A directional term meaning *toward the head* of a human.

**superovulation**  Production of an abnormally high number of ova in the ovaries induced by the administration of drugs with follicle-stimulating hormone activity. Usually done as the first step in transfer of embryos to other animals.

**suppressor T cells**  Lymphocytes that inhibit helper T cells and cytotoxic T cells by negative feedback. They also prevent B lymphocytes from transforming into plasma cells. These cells provide the means by which the immune response can be shut down.

**supracoracoideus**  Small, deep flight muscle originating on the keel and inserting on the top of the humerus; contraction results in the upstroke.

**surfactant**  A component of the fluid that lines the alveoli in the lungs. Surfactant helps reduce the surface tension of the fluid, which helps prevent the alveoli from collapsing shut as air moves in and out during breathing.

**suspensions**  Heterogeneous mixtures containing large solutes that readily separate from the solution when there is no movement of the suspension.

**suspensory ligament of the ovary**  The cranial edge of the broad ligament in the female that extends cranially and dorsally from the ovary and attaches to the body wall in the area of the last rib.

**suspensory ligaments**  The tiny ligaments that attach to the periphery of the lens of the eye and connect it to the ciliary body. They are the means by which the ciliary muscles exert and relieve tension on the lens to adjust its shape for near and far vision.

**sutures**  The immovable fibrous joints that unite most of the skull bones; also known as *synarthroses.*

**sweat glands**  Coiled glands, either *merocrine* or *apocrine,* located in the corium of all or some of the body's subcutaneous flesh depending on the species. Where present, the ducts of these glands pass through the dermis to the surface of the epidermis, where the sweat evaporates, aiding in thermoregulation.

**sympathetic ganglion chain**  Series of ganglia located outside the thoracolumbar area of the spinal column and associated with the sympathetic nervous system.

**sympathetic nervous system**  Part of the autonomic nervous system that is responsible for the "fight or flight" response; also called the *thoracolumbar system* because of the location of the sympathetic nerves emerging from the thoracic and lumbar vertebral segments.

**symport system**  A system in which all of the substances are moved in the same direction.

**synapse**  The junction between two neurons or between a neuron and another target cell.

**synaptic cleft**  Physical gap between two communicating neurons or between a neuron and its target cell.

**synaptic end bulb**  Button at the end of the axon that releases the neurotransmitter; also called *synaptic knob* or *terminal bouton.*

**synaptic knob**  See *synaptic end bulb.*

**synaptic transmission**  The continuation of the nerve impulse across the synapse from one neuron to another or from one neuron to its target cell.

**synarthrosis**  An immovable fibrous joint; for example, the sutures that unite most of the skull bones.

**synergist**  Something that aids the action of something else. A synergistic muscle contracts at the same time as a prime mover and assists it in carrying out its action.

**synovial fluid**  Viscous fluid formed by the lining layer of the joint capsule of a synovial joint; lubricates the joint surfaces.

**synovial joint**  A freely movable joint; also known as a *diarthrosis.*

**synovial membrane**  The membrane that lines joint capsules. It is composed of connective tissue and produces synovial fluid, which helps reduce friction in the joint.

**synsacrum**  Strong bony plate created by fusion of the distal lumbar vertebrae, the sacral vertebrae, and the first few coccygeal vertebrae of birds. It fuses with the pelvis and provides a stiff framework to support the legs.

**synthesis reaction**  A chemical reaction in which elements or simple molecular reactants are combined into a more complex product. The opposite of a decomposition reaction.

**synthetic phase (S phase)**  The period spent by the cell in preparation for cell division, in which the cell begins to replicate and synthesize DNA.

**syrinx**  Enlargement of the trachea above the sternum of birds. Contains muscles, air sacs, and vibrating membranes that collectively form the voice box.

**system**  Groups of organs that are involved in a common set of activities.

**systematic anatomy**  A method of studying anatomy that examines each system of the body (e.g., skeletal system, reproductive system) as a separate topic.

**systemic circulation**  The part of the circulatory system that provides blood flow to and away from all of the body tissues except the lungs.

**systole**  The part of the cardiac cycle associated with contraction of the ventricles and atria and ejection of blood into the arterial systems.

**T**

**T lymphocyte**  The type of lymphocyte that is responsible for cell-mediated immunity.

**T tubules**  Transverse tubules; a system of tubules in a skeletal muscle cell that extend from the sarcolemma (cell membrane) into the depths of the cell. They help carry an impulse caused by nerve stimulation of the muscle cell into its interior.

**tachycardia**  A rapid heart rate.

**tactile elevations**  Small elevations located throughout the surface of the epidermis, usually containing a tactile hair; important in the perception of touch.

**tactile hairs**  Hairs sensitive to touch.

**tactile sense**  The sense of touch.

**tail glands**  An oval region filled with many sebaceous and apocrine glands, located on the dorsal surface of the tail. It aids in scent marking and in personal identification in certain mammals including the domestic dog and cat.

**tailhead**  Dorsal part of the base of the tail.

**talons**  The claws of birds of prey.

**tapetum**  A shortened name for the tapetum lucidum.

**tapetum lucidum**  A highly reflective area of the choroid in the back of the eye of most domestic animals (except swine). It acts as a light amplifier to aid low-light vision by reflecting light back through the photoreceptors after it has passed through them once.

**target**  An organ or tissue that responds to a particular hormone.

**tarsal bones**   The bones of the tarsus, consisting of two rows of short bones located between the distal ends of the tibia and fibula and the proximal ends of the metatarsal bones.

**tarsal glands**   The meibomian glands of the eyelid margins. They produce a waxy substance that helps prevent tears from overflowing onto an animal's face.

**tarsus**   The joint composed of the tarsal bones; referred to as the *hock* in most animals and the *ankle* in humans.

**taste**   The gustatory sense; a chemical sense that detects taste molecules dissolved in the saliva in the mouth.

**teat sinus**   The large space within the teat of the cow that fills with milk when milk let-down occurs.

**tectorial membrane**   The gelatinous sheet that lies on the hair cells of the organ of Corti in the cochlea. Movements of the cochlear fluid produced by sound wave vibrations cause the tectorial membrane to distort the sensory hairs, producing nerve impulses that the brain interprets as sound.

**telodendron**   The branched end of an axon; each branch terminates in a neurotransmitter-filled synaptic end bulb.

**telogen effluvium**   "Blowing the coat"; the overall hair loss that occurs from the hair follicles being in a synchronized telogenic phase. It may be brought on by many factors, such as stress, medication, malnutrition, and postpartum hormonal changes in dogs.

**telogen phase**   The resting phase of hair growth.

**telophase**   The phase of mitosis when the daughter chromosomes return to being long-fiber chromatids, the nuclear envelope and nucleoli reappear, and the cell has completed its formation of two completely independent daughter cells.

**temperature sense**   The sense of hot and cold.

**temporal bones**   Skull bones that are part of the external bones of the cranium. The two temporal bones form the lateral walls of the cranium, contain the middle and inner ear structures, and are the skull bones that form the temporomandibular joints with the mandible (lower jaw).

**temporomandibular joint (TMJ)**   The hinge joint on each side of the lower jaw (mandible) that connects it with the rest of the skull. Each joint is formed by the convex condyle of the mandible articulating with the concave articular surface on the ventral portion of each temporal bone.

**tendons**   Fibrous connective tissue bands that connect skeletal muscles to bones.

**terminal bouton**   Button at the end of the axon that releases the neurotransmitter; also called the *synaptic end bulb* or *synaptic knob*.

**terminators**   Codes within the DNA sequence that indicate where RNA synthesis should end.

**testes**   The male gonads. They produce the male reproductive cells, spermatozoa, as well as androgen hormones.

**testosterone**   The principal male sex hormone.

**tetraiodothyronine (T₄)**   Thyroxine; thyroid hormone that is largely converted to $T_3$ before exerting an effect on target cells.

**thalamus**   Part of the diencephalon that acts as a relay station for regulating sensory impulses to the cerebrum.

**thecodont teeth**   Teeth held in sockets.

**thermolabile enzymes**   Enzymes that are affected by changes in temperature and are therefore changed in structure themselves.

**third eyelid**   The nictitating membrane. A T-shaped plate of cartilage covered by conjunctiva. It has lymph nodules and a gland that contributes to the tear film on its ocular surface. No muscles attach to the third eyelid. Its movements are entirely passive.

**thoracic cavity**   The chest cavity. It is separated from the abdominal cavity by the thin, sheetlike diaphragm.

**thoracic duct**   A large lymph vessel found in the thorax. It empties its contents of lymph into large blood vessels in the thorax.

**thoracic limb**   The front limb.

**thoracic vertebrae**   The group of vertebrae located dorsal to the thoracic region.

**thoracolumbar system**   Sympathetic nervous system; so named because most of the nerves of the sympathetic nervous system emerge from the thoracic and lumbar segments of the spinal cord.

**thorax**   Another name for the thoracic, or chest, cavity.

**threshold**   The required level of stimulation, or degree of change in a cell's electrical potential, necessary to initiate an action potential.

**threshold stimulus**   The minimum stimulus that will generate a nerve impulse.

**thrombocytes**   Also known as *platelets*. Platelets are small pieces of cytoplasm that break off megakaryocytes in the bone marrow and enter peripheral blood. They are involved in hemostasis and the blood-clotting process.

**thrombopoiesis**   The production of platelets.

**thromboxane**   An eicosanoid produced by platelets that causes vasoconstriction and promotes the clumping of platelets.

**thymine (T)**   Part of one of the nucleotides present only in DNA. It is a pyrimidine base that pairs only with adenine.

**thymopoietin**   A hormonelike substance produced by the thymus. It influences the development of T cells, important components of an animal's cell-mediated immunity.

**thymosin**   A hormonelike substance produced by the thymus. It influences the development of T cells, important components of an animal's cell-mediated immunity.

**thymus**   An organ that is important in the development of a young animal's immune system. It produces hormonelike substances, such as thymopoietin and thymosin.

**thyroid cartilage**   One of the cartilages of the larynx. It is shaped as a V that forms and supports the ventral portion of the larynx. The human thyroid cartilage is commonly referred to as the "Adam's apple."

**thyroid gland**   An endocrine gland made up of two parts, located on either side of the larynx, in the neck region. It produces thyroid hormone and calcitonin.

**thyroid hormones**   The collective name given to two hormones produced by the thyroid gland—$T_3$ and $T_4$. They help an animal generate body heat; influence the metabolism of proteins, carbohydrates, and lipids; and encourage the growth and development of young animals.

**thyroid-stimulating hormone (TSH)**   The anterior pituitary hormone that stimulates the growth and development of the thyroid gland and causes it to produce its hormones.

**thyroxine**   See *tetraiodothyronine*.

**tibia**   The main weight-bearing bone of the lower leg. It forms the stifle joint with the femur proximal to it and the hock with the tarsus distal to it.

**tibial crest**  A longitudinal ridge on the front of the proximal end of the tibia.

**tidal volume**  The volume of air breathed in and out in one breath. It varies according to the body's needs. The tidal volume is lowest at rest and higher during physical activity.

**tie**  The process by which male and female dogs become temporarily "attached" to each other as a part of the breeding process. Muscles in the female clamp down around the enlarged bulb of the glans of the penis, making it impossible for the male to withdraw the penis for a time. The male dismounts and turns so that the two animals stand tail to tail. The tie lasts about 15 to 20 minutes and does not seem uncomfortable to either animal.

**tight junction**  A type of intercellular connection that is impermeable to leaks. Passage of extracellular substances can occur only through the cell itself. Tight junctions are formed by the fusion of one cell's plasma membrane to another cell's plasma membrane.

**tissue forceps**  A tweezerlike surgical instrument with delicate tips; used for grasping and moving tissue. The delicate tip is designed to be gentle on the tissues it grasps.

**tissue**  A group of cells that are similar in structure and perform the same function. The four basic tissues in the animal body are *epithelial tissue, connective tissue, nervous tissue,* and *muscle tissue.*

**toe**  The most anterior region of the hoof.

**tonofilaments**  Thin filaments that provide the structural support for certain membrane junctions. Tonofilaments are especially important in tissue that needs to flex.

**touch**  The tactile sense; the sensation of something being in contact with the surface of the body.

**trace elements**  Microminerals; minerals required in minute amounts relative to the macrominerals.

**trachea**  The windpipe; the tube that extends from the larynx down into the thorax, where it divides into the left and right main bronchi that enter the lungs. The trachea is held open by incomplete hyaline cartilage rings that are spaced along its length.

**transamination**  The process of amino group transfer to other amino acids or within the same compound.

**transcription**  The process of transcribing the genetic code from DNA and RNA through protein synthesis using messenger RNA.

**transduction**  Conversion of a sensory stimulus to a nerve impulse.

**transfer RNA (tRNA)**  The type of RNA that transfers amino acids to the ribosome for protein synthesis. Each of the 20 amino acids has its own specific type of tRNA, which places it in the appropriate order for the specific type of protein being synthesized. The nucleotides or anticodons of tRNA base-pair with the codon triplets of mRNA to accomplish the process.

**transient cells**  One of the two subdivisions of connective tissue cells, transient cells have a mobile existence, traveling in and out of the connective tissue as needed.

**transitional epithelium**  Epithelium that can stretch and contract without damage. Transitional epithelium is found lining the urinary bladder and ureters. The appearance of the epithelial cells varies depending on the level of tension on the tissue.

Transitional epithelium therefore may appear columnar, cuboidal, or squamous.

**translation**  Referring to the process of protein synthesis using messenger RNA to transfer genetic information in the form of nucleotides into amino acid form. This process occurs in the cytoplasm on ribosomes.

**transmission**  Conduction of a nerve impulse along a nerve fiber.

**transport proteins**  Proteins that transport substances, such as hormones, from their origin to where they are needed.

**transudate**  A thin fluid containing small amounts of protein or no protein that has been passed through a membrane. Normal serous fluid is a transudate.

**transverse plane**  An anatomic reference plane across the body that divides it into cranial (head-end) and caudal (tail-end) parts that are not necessarily equal.

**transverse process**  A lateral-projecting process of a vertebra.

**transverse tubules**  See *T tubules.*

**triacylglycerols**  Neutral fats; triglycerides.

**tricuspid valve**  Also called the *right atrioventricular valve;* separates the right atrium and ventricle.

**triglyceride**  A glycerol composed of three fatty acids; the main storage form of water-insoluble lipids.

**trigone**  The triangular body of the urinary bladder located between the openings of the ureters and the urethra.

**triiodothyronine (T$_3$)**  The main active thyroid hormone.

**trimesters**  The three main divisions of pregnancy. They are not equal thirds, but they give a convenient way to describe the events occurring during pregnancy.

**tripeptide**  A peptide that consists of three amino acids.

**tRNA**  See *transfer RNA.*

**trochanter**  Greater and lesser; areas on the femur where leg muscles attach.

**trochoid joint**  Also known as a *pivot joint;* one bone pivots on another in a rotary motion. The only true pivot joint in the bodies of most domestic animals is the joint between the first and second cervical vertebrae.

**trypsin**  A protolytic enzyme formed in the intestines by the cleavage of trypsinogen by enterokinase.

**trypsinlike immunoreactivity (TLI) test**  Test that identifies the presence of pancreatic trypsin in the blood; a positive test result is suggestive of pancreatic disease.

**trypsinogen**  Precursor for trypsin secreted from the pancreas.

**tubular filtrate**  The glomerular filtrate after it has passed into the proximal convoluted tubule. It will be called the *tubular filtrate* throughout its entire journey through the nephron tubules even though its chemical composition will change many times before it enters the collecting duct.

**tubular gland**  Secretory unit of exocrine glands either containing or composed of tubules.

**tubulin**  A protein present in the microtubules that gives support to the microtubule and also aids in the motility of the cell.

**tubuloacinar**  Referring to secretory units of exocrine glands that possess both tubular and acinar (or alveolar) parts.

**tunica albuginea**  The tough, fibrous connective tissue capsule of the testis.

**turbinates**   Skull bones that are part of the internal bones of the face; also known as the *nasal conchae*. The turbinates are four thin, scroll-like bones that fill most of the space in the nasal cavity. The turbinates are covered by the moist, vascular lining of the nasal passages. Their scroll-like shape helps the nasal lining warm and humidify the inhaled air and trap tiny particles of inhaled foreign material.

**twitch contraction**   A single skeletal muscle fiber contraction. It can be divided into three phases: a brief, latent phase; a longer, contracting phase; and an even longer relaxation phase.

**tylotrich hairs**   Tactile hairs used to aid in the perception of touch. They are located in close association with tactile elevation, or tylotrich, pads.

**tympanic membrane**   The eardrum. The paper-thin, connective tissue membrane that is tightly stretched across the opening of the external ear canal into the middle ear.

**tyrosine melanin**   The pigment that produces brown–black colors in hair.

**U**

**udder**   The collected inguinal mammary glands. As of cattle, horses, sheep, goats and camelids.

**ulna**   One of the two bones (the radius is the other) that form the antebrachium, or forearm. The ulna forms a major portion of the elbow joint with the distal end of the humerus.

**umbilical arteries**   Arteries that carry carbon dioxide-rich, waste-filled blood from the fetus to the placenta through the umbilical cord.

**umbilical cord**   The link between the fetus and the placenta. It is a cordlike structure that contains blood vessels and a drainage tube from the urinary bladder of the fetus (the urachus).

**umbilical vein**   The vein in the umbilical cord that carries oxygen and nutrient-rich blood from the placenta to the fetus.

**uncinate process**   Projection on a complete rib of birds that overlaps the adjoining rear rib to strengthen the rib cage.

**ungual process**   The process on the distal end of the distal phalanx of dogs and cats that is surrounded by the claw in the living animal.

**ungula**   An alternate name for the *hoof*.

**ungulate**   The taxonomic classification of animals that includes all hoofed animals, both wild and domestic.

**unicameral lung**   A one-chambered lung.

**unicellular exocrine gland**   The only known example is the goblet cell. It is a ductless exocrine gland that secretes mucus. Goblet cells are located in the respiratory and intestinal tracts.

**uniparous**   An animal that normally gives birth to only one offspring at parturition.

**unsaturated fatty acids**   Breakdown products of fat metabolism. Unsaturated refers to the fact that not all the chemical binding sites of the molecules are filled. They have one or more double bonds in their carbon chains and are liquid at room temperature. If one double bond is present, the fatty acid is monounsaturated. If more than one double bond is present, the fatty acid is polyunsaturated. Examples are found in plant oils and include arachidonic, linolenic, and oleic acids.

**upper arcade**   In reference to teeth, it means the teeth in the maxillary and incisive bones; the upper set of teeth in the mouth.

**upper respiratory tract**   The respiratory structures outside the lungs. Includes the nose, pharynx, larynx, and trachea.

**urachus**   A tube in the umbilical cord that drains urine from the fetus's urinary bladder into the allantoic sac of the placenta.

**uracil (U)**   Part of one of the nucleotides present only in RNA. It is a pyrimidine base that pairs only with RNA's adenine.

**urea**   A nonprotein source of nitrogen produced in the liver that is used by rumen microbes. One of the final products of protein metabolism.

**uremia**   Urine in the blood. Refers to a buildup of waste materials, especially urea, in the blood because of insufficient removal by the kidneys.

**uresis**   Expelling urine from the body; also called *micturition* or *urination.*

**ureters**   The muscular tubes that leave the kidney at the hilus and connect to the urinary bladder. They move urine to the bladder by peristaltic smooth muscle contractions.

**urethra**   The tube that connects the urinary bladder with the outside world. In the female, it only conducts urine. In the male, it conducts urine and semen.

**urethral process**   The distal end of the urethra of the male horse that extends from a shallow depression, the fossa glandis, at the tip of the penis.

**urinary calculi (singular, calculus)**   Uroliths or urinary tract stones.

**urinary stones**   See *uroliths.*

**urination**   See *uresis.*

**urodeum**   Section of the cloaca of a bird that receives waste products from the kidneys and genital ducts.

**urolithiasis**   An abnormal condition characterized by the presence of urinary tract stones.

**uroliths**   Urinary tract stones; precipitated aggregates of mineral crystals that form macroscopic stones or sand anywhere in the urinary tract.

**uropygial gland**   Also called the *preen gland;* secretes an oily substance that cleans and waterproofs feathers.

**uterine contractions**   Contractions of the myometrium, the smooth muscle layer of the uterine wall.

**uterus**   The womb; where the fertilized ovum implants and lives while it grows and develops into a new animal.

**utricle**   One of two saclike spaces (the saccule is the other one) in the vestibule of the inner ear that contain sensory structures that monitor the position of the head.

**uvea**   The middle, vascular layer of the eye. It includes the choroid, the ciliary body, and the iris.

**uveal tunic**   Vascular, pigmented, middle tissue layer of the eye, consisting of the choroid, iris, and ciliary muscles.

**V**

**vacuole**   A clear space in the cytoplasm of a cell; it is surrounded by cell membrane. Phagocytized microorganisms are found in vacuoles.

**vagina**   The tube that connects the cervix with the vulva. It receives the erect penis at breeding and serves as the birth canal at parturition.

**vaginal tunics**   Two connective tissue layers that surround the testes in the scrotum. They are derived from layers of peritoneum that were pushed ahead of the testes when they descended through the inguinal rings into the scrotum.

**vagus nerve**   The nerve of the parasympathetic nervous system that is involved in regulating gastrointestinal motility and secretion; acetylcholine is the neurotransmitter of the vagus nerve. The 10th cranial nerve.

**vas deferens**   The muscular tube that carries spermatozoa and the fluid they are suspended in from the epididymis to the urethra for emission as a component of semen.

**vascularized**   Region of the body supplied with a blood source via blood vessels.

**vaults**   Small transport structures that shuttle molecules to and from the nucleus in the cell.

**velvet skin**   The soft skin on the antlers of deer that provides a vascular source necessary during the early seasonal growth of the antler. Later in the season, the buck will scrape the velvet off, allowing the antler to harden. These hardened antlers are used for sparring with competing males during the breeding season. The velvet is often eaten by the buck because of its high nutritive value.

**vent**   Opening of the cloaca to the outside in birds.

**ventilation**   The movement of air into and out of the lungs. Also known as breathing.

**ventral**   A directional term meaning *toward the bottom surface* of an animal when it is standing on all four legs; toward the belly.

**ventral body cavity**   The large space in the body that is divided by the thin, sheetlike diaphragm muscle into the cranial thoracic cavity (chest) and caudal abdominal cavity (belly).

**ventral horn**   The area of the spinal cord's gray matter "butterfly" where the neurons that transmit motor (efferent) nerve impulses to the spinal nerves are located.

**ventral nerve root**   The branch off each side of the spinal cord between each pair of adjacent vertebrae that conducts motor impulses from the spinal cord to effectors in the periphery of the body.

**vertebra**   One of the bones of the spinal column.

**vertebral column**   Also known as the *spinal column;* the collective name for the cervical, thoracic, lumbar, sacral, and coccygeal vertebrae.

**vesicle**   A small sac that contains fluid.

**vestibular folds**   The false vocal cords; connective tissue bands in the larynx of a nonruminant animal, in addition to the vocal cords. The vestibular folds are not involved in voice production.

**vestibule of the ear**   The portion of the inner ear that senses the position of the head. Its sensory epithelium is contained in two saclike spaces: the *utricle* and the *saccule.*

**vestibule of the vulva**   The entrance into the vulva; the short space between the labia and the entrance into the vagina. The urethra of the female opens into the vestibule.

**VFAs**   See *volatile fatty acids.*

**villi**   Fingerlike projections on the surface of the small intestine that increase the surface area for absorption; contain the microvilli brush border that digests nutrients.

**virulence**   A specific pathogen's ability to invade a host's tissues. Determined by virulence factors. Pathogenicity.

**virulent**   Capable of causing disease.

**virus**   The simplest organism, composed of DNA or RNA, surrounded by a protein sheath and sometimes an additional envelope. Viruses cannot live or reproduce independently; therefore, they must establish a parasitic relationship with another cell to perform these functions. Individual viruses are identifiable by their antigens.

**viscera (singular, viscus)**   Refers to the soft, internal organs enclosed within a body cavity, such as the lungs, kidneys, and intestines. The term is used to describe the organs of the abdominal and thoracic cavities.

**visceral**   Pertaining to the soft internal organs.

**visceral layer**   The layer of pleura or peritoneum that lies directly on the surface of organs in the thorax or abdomen.

**visceral sensations**   Miscellaneous interior body sensations. They include hunger and thirst and stretching sensations from hollow internal organs.

**visceral skeleton**   Bones formed in soft organs (viscera). Examples include the os penis in the penis of a dog, the os cordis in the hearts of cattle, and the os rostri in the snouts of swine.

**visceral smooth muscle**   The type of smooth muscle found in the walls of many soft internal organs, such as the intestine, urinary bladder, and uterus. Its cells are linked to form large sheets that show rhythmic waves of contraction without external nerve stimulation.

**visceral vaginal tunic**   The thin, inner connective tissue layer that is tightly adherent to the surface of the testis and the structures of the spermatic cord. Derived from visceral peritoneum.

**vitamin D**   A fat-soluble vitamin essential for life in most organisms. Vitamin D enables the body to use calcium and phosphorus and is necessary for the formation of healthy teeth and bones. Vitamin D may be found in many common food sources, as well as being produced in the skin when it is exposed to ultraviolet rays in sunlight. An insufficient amount of vitamin D can cause rickets or osteomalacia.

**vitellogenesis**   The formation of yolk in the vitellarium (gland) in egg-laying species.

**vitreous compartment**   The compartment of the eye behind (caudal to) the lens and ciliary body. It contains a soft, gelatinous fluid called *vitreous humor.*

**vitreous humor**   The soft, gelatinous fluid that fills the vitreous compartment of the eye.

**viviparous**   Giving birth to living young that develop within the maternal body. Occurs in placental mammals but also in some reptiles and amphibians.

**vocal cords**   Two fibrous connective tissue bands attached to the arytenoid cartilages that stretch across the lumen of the larynx and vibrate as air passes over them; also known as the *vocal folds.*

**vocal folds**   See *vocal cords.*

**volatile fatty acids (VFAs)**   Also called *short-chain fatty acids,* these are the main energy source of ruminants. They are created by the microbial fermentation of cellulose in the rumen and in the colon of nonruminant herbivores. Common VFAs include acetic acid and propionate.

**Volkmann's canal**   One of countless tiny channels through the matrix of bone that bring blood in from the periosteum to the Haversian canals in the centers of the Haversian systems. The Haversian systems run lengthwise in long bones. Volkmann's canals come in at right angles to the Haversian systems and join with the Haversian canals.

**voltage**　The potential electrical energy created by separation of opposite electric charges on either side of the cell membrane.

**voluntary muscle**　Also known as *skeletal muscle;* muscle involved in the conscious movements of the body.

**voluntary striated muscle**　An old name for *skeletal* muscle.

**vomer bone**　A skull bone that is one of the internal bones of the face. The vomer bone forms part of the nasal septum.

**vomeronasal organ**　Also called *Jacobson's organ.* It consists of two long, thin sacs situated on either side of the nasal septum, which is accessible via a pit in the roof of the mouth. It is part of the animal's olfactory system.

**vulva**　The external portion of the female reproductive system. It consists of the vestibule, the clitoris, and the labia.

## W

**water soluble**　Refers to a molecule that is hydrophilic and soluble in water.

**wave of depolarization**　The opening of sodium channels, starting at the point of stimulus and continuing down the length of the neuron to the end of the axon; also called the *nerve impulse* and the *propagation of the action potential* along the neuron.

**white adipose tissue**　*White fat;* found commonly throughout the body. It is used for thermoregulation, protection, and support of the body and its organs. It is also a storage compartment for lipids. White adipose tissue is highly vascularized so that the lipids contained within can be readily converted to energy via triglyceride metabolism.

**white line**　The white or light-colored region that marks where the wall and sole of the hoof adjoin.

**white matter**　Myelinated axons in the CNS.

**white pulp**　The area of the spleen that contains lymphocytes.

**whole blood**　Blood that contains plasma and all the formed elements (cells and platelets).

**wind-up**　An exaggerated pain response that can be produced when the spinal cord is bombarded with severe or chronic pain impulses. It can result in severely painful responses to stimuli that would normally not be distressful.

**withdrawal reflex**　Reflex arc in which a painful stimulus on the skin causes contraction of the affected limb; also called the *flexor reflex.*

**withers**　Area dorsal to the scapulas.

**wool-type hairs**　Hair coat composed primarily of secondary hairs, as seen in sheep.

## X

**xiphoid, xiphoid process**　The last, most caudal sternebra.

## Y

**yawn**　A slow, deep breath taken through a wide-open mouth. It may be stimulated by a slight decrease in the blood oxygen level, or it may just be due to boredom, drowsiness, or fatigue.

**yellow bone marrow**　The most common type of bone marrow in adult animals. Yellow bone marrow consists mainly of adipose connective tissue (fat). It does not produce blood cells, but it can revert to red bone marrow if the body needs greater than normal blood cell production.

## Z

**Z line**　The dark line in the center of the light band (I band) of skeletal muscle. Z lines are actually discs to which the actin filaments are attached. They look like lines because of the angle at which they are usually viewed.

**zona pellucida**　Thick, gel-like glycoprotein layer that surrounds the cell membrane of a developing oocyte in an ovarian follicle, and an ovum after ovulation.

**zonary placental attachment**　The type of placental attachment to the uterus that is in a belt-shaped area that encircles the placenta; found in dogs and cats.

**zygodactyly**　Toe position in some birds in which the fourth digit is opposable and can be positioned forward or to the rear.

**zygomatic arches**　Bony arches below and behind the eyes of common domestic animals. In dogs and cats, they form the widest part of the skull. The zygomatic arches are made up of the rostral-facing zygomatic process of the temporal bone joined with the caudal-facing temporal process of the zygomatic bone.

**zygomatic bones**　Skull bones that are part of the external bones of the face. The zygomatic bones form a portion of the orbit of the eye and the rostral portion of the zygomatic arch.

**zygote**　The fertilized ovum.

# Index

Note: Page numbers followed by "*f*" refer to illustrations; page numbers followed by "*t*" refer to tables; page numbers followed by "*b*" refer to boxes.